Textbook of Microbiology

Textbook of Microbiology

Vasant Baradkar

Associate Professor
Department of Microbiology
Topiwala National Medical College
and BYL Nair Charitable Hospital
Mumbai

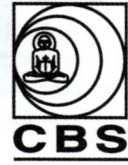

CBS

CBS Publishers & Distributors Pvt Ltd

New Delhi • Bengaluru • Chennai • Kochi • Kolkata • Mumbai
Hyderabad • Nagpur • Patna • Pune

Textbook of Microbiology

ISBN: 978-93-86478-14-6

First Edition: 2017

Published by Satish Kumar Jain and produced by Varun Jain for

CBS Publishers & Distributors Pvt Ltd

4819/XI Prahlad Street, 24 Ansari Road, Daryaganj, New Delhi 110 002, India.
Ph: 23289259, 23266861, 23266867   Fax: 011-23243014   Website: www.cbspd.com
                                                                                   e-mail: delhi@cbspd.com; cbspubs@airtelmail.in.
Corporate Office: 204 FIE, Industrial Area, Patparganj, Delhi 110 092
Ph: 4934 4934   Fax: 4934 4935   e-mail: publishing@cbspd.com; publicity@cbspd.com

Branches

• **Bengaluru:** Seema House 2975, 17th Cross, K.R. Road, Banasankari 2nd Stage, Bengaluru 560 070, Karnataka
  Ph: +91-80-26771678/79   Fax: +91-80-26771680   e-mail: bangalore@cbspd.com
• **Chennai:** No. 7, Subbaraya Street, Shenoy Nagar, Chennai 600 030, Tamil Nadu
  Ph: +91-44-26680620, 26681266   Fax: +91-44-42032115   e-mail: chennai@cbspd.com
• **Kochi:** Ashana House, 39/1904, AM Thomas Road, Valanjambalam, Ernakulam 682 016, Kochi, Kerala
  Ph: +91-484-4059061-65,67   Fax: +91-484-4059065   e-mail: kochi@cbspd.com
• **Kolkata:** No. 6/B, Ground Floor, Rameswar Shaw Road, Kolkata-700014 (West Bengal), India
  Ph: +91-33-2289-1126, 2289-1127, 2289-1128   e-mail: kolkata@cbspd.com
• **Mumbai:** 83-C, Dr E Moses Road, Worli, Mumbai-400018, Maharashtra
  Ph: +91-22-24902340/41   Fax: +91-22-24902342   e-mail: mumbai@cbspd.com

Representatives

• **Hyderabad** 0-9885175004   • **Nagpur** 0-9021734563   • **Patna** 0-9334159340
• **Pune**   0-9623451994

Printed at International Print - O - Pac Limited, Noida, UP, India

to

My father Sh Purushottamrao
My mother Smt Sumitra
My wife Swati
and
My sons Pushkaraj & Shubhankar

for their love which made
everything possible

Preface

This book is written in a manner to cover the syllabi of medical and paramedical students as well as it is useful for laboratory persons. Special efforts have been made to increase clinical judgment of the students. Use of real diagrams, as many as possible, is helpful so that students can understand and assimilate the knowledge without giving too much stress to their imagination. Students can reproduce information in examination. All the topics are covered precisely which act as a base for the students to prepare for higher examinations. Recent advances in diagnosis, treatment and vaccination is included in each topic. Various flowcharts are given under pathogenesis to make it easy to understand. Epidemiological features of infectious diseases are given with special reference to the Indian context.

I welcome all the suggestions and hope that students and teachers will extend their support by giving me their valuable suggestions and comments.

Vasant Baradkar

Acknowledgments

I would like to thank my teachers who are my role models, and who set examples in teaching. I am indebted Mr Rajesh Bhalani of Bhalani Publishers and Mr Satish Kumar Jain of CBS Publishers & Distributors Pvt Ltd who helped to make my dream come true by publishing my work. I am thankful to Dr Prachi Jawale for helping in correction of the manuscript. I would like to thank my family for patiently enduring the writing of the book. I thank Manoj Rajbhar for doing DTP work.

Vasant Baradkar

Contents

Contents

Contents

Introduction

Medical microbiology is the study of organisms that cause human infections, diseases they produce, their diagnosis, their prevention by vaccines, chemo-prophylaxis and treatment.

History

Antony van Leeuwenhoek who had the habit of grinding lenses, first observed bacteria under microscope.

Major development in the field was brought by Louis Pasteur.

LOUIS PASTEUR (Fig. 1.1)

He was a French chemist. His discovery of fermentation built up his interest in further research into microbiology.

He is known as the **father of modern microbiology**. His important contributions are as follows:
- He coined the term 'microbiology'.
- He identified silkworm disease. He established that fermentation was the result of microbial activity. He also showed that different types of fermentation are associated with different organisms.

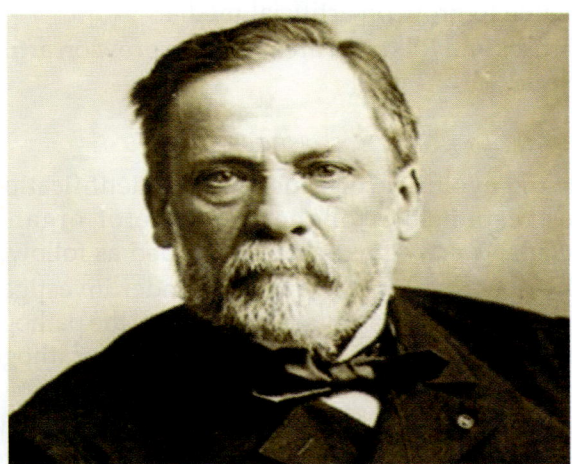

Fig. 1.1: Louis Pasteur

- He developed the techniques of bacteriology.
- He introduced the techniques of sterilization, e.g. steam sterilizer, autoclave, hot air oven, flaming, and pasteurization.
- He also proved that microbes arose from their like and not *de novo*. He along with Robert Koch showed that living organisms were the cause of disease.
- He established the importance of cotton plugs for protection of culture media from aerial contamination.
- He suggested method of pasteurization of milk.
- He introduced concept of liquid media and used nutrient broth for culture of bacteria.
- He introduced the use of complex media.
- He accidentally observed that culture of *Chicken cholera* bacillus left on the bench for several weeks lost its pathogenic property but retained its ability to protect the birds against subsequent infection. This led to the process of attenuation and development of live vaccines (1880).
- He prepared anthrax vaccine by attenuating anthrax bacilli at high temperature (42–43°C) in 1881. In 1881, he took part in a public trial of his vaccine against anthrax in domestic animals. He coined the term 'vaccine' for such prophylactic preparations. He also proved that inoculation of vaccine in animals induces specific protection against anthrax.
- He developed a vaccine for rabies in 1881. He obtained fixed virus of rabies by serial intracerebral passage in rabbits. The vaccine was prepared by dried pieces of spinal cord from rabies infected with fixed virus. This was proven effective in humans when he inoculated Joseph Mister, 9-year-old boy who had been bitten badly with dog having rabies.

JOSEPH LISTER

- Joseph Lister is known as the **father of antiseptic surgery**.

- He realized that microorganisms prevalent in the atmosphere might be responsible for postoperative wound infections.
- He was interested in the prevention of postoperative sepsis.
- He introduced **antiseptic techniques** in surgery using carbolic acid as a spray during operation or on the wound in postoperative stage. It was a revolution and an important milestone in surgical practice.

ROBERT KOCH (Fig. 1.2)

- Robert Koch is known as the **father of bacteriology**.
- He invented hot air oven and steam sterilizer.
- He introduced solid media for bacterial culture. Method of isolation of bacteria in pure culture is also introduced by him.
- While in general practice in Berlin, he isolated anthrax bacillus and showed a specific organism as a cause of disease.
- He was the founder of germ theory of disease. He brought clarity in medicine—until then diseases were attributed to miasmas or mists, to punishments from Gods or devils or to unfortunate conjunctions of stars and planets.
- He became first to grow bacteria in colonies, initially on potato slices and later on, with his pupil Petri, on gelatin media.
- He perfected bacteriological techniques.
- He introduced methods for isolation of bacteria in pure cultures using solid media.

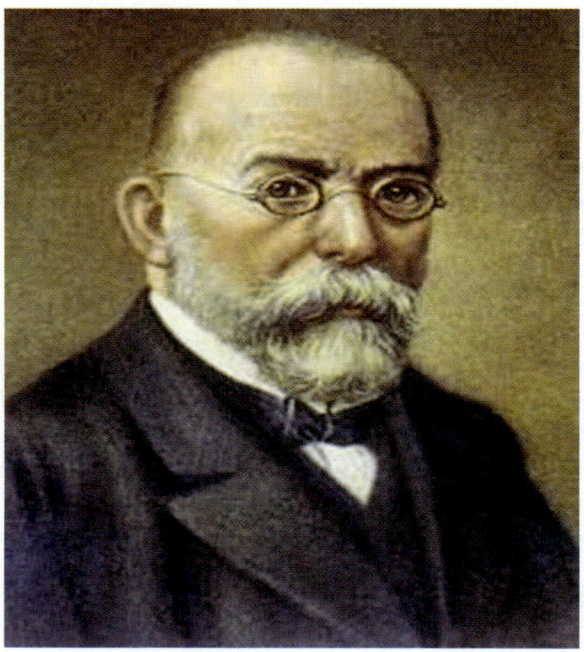

Fig. 1.2: Robert Koch

- Method of study of motility by hanging drop method is invented by him.
- He was the first to isolate anthrax bacilli in pure culture and to show spores in anthrax bacilli.
- He introduced staining techniques.
- He discovered tubercle bacilli and *Vibrio cholerae*.
- He was the first person to see motility of bacteria by hanging drop method.
- He discovered old tuberculin.

Koch's Postulates and Molecular Koch's Postulates

Robert Koch postulated the criteria for proving that a microorganism isolated from a disease was indeed caused due to it.

According to these postulates, a microorganism can be accepted as the causative agent of the disease only if the following conditions are satisfied.

- The microorganism should be constantly associated with the lesions of the disease.
- It should be possible to isolate the organism in pure culture from the lesions of the disease.
- Inoculation of such pure culture in suitable laboratory animals should produce a similar disease in animals.
- It should be possible to reisolate the organism in pure culture from lesions produced in the experimental animals.
- An additional criterion introduced subsequently states that specific antibodies to that organism should be demonstrated in the serum of patients.

These postulates have proved to be useful in confirming doubtful claims made regarding the causative agents of infectious diseases.

Exceptions to Koch's Postulates

- *Treponema pallidum* and *Mycobacterium leprae* are unable to grow on artificial media.
- Viruses and *Rickettsia* are unable to grow on artificial media.

Molecular Koch's Postulates

With the evolution of genetics and identification of genes responsible for the virulence of organism, **molecular Koch's postulates** are added as follows:

- The phenotype or the property under investigation should be significantly associated with the pathogenic strains of the species and not with nonpathogenic strains of the disease.
- Specific inactivation of gene or genes associated with virulence trait should lead to measurable decrease in pathogenicity or virulence.

- Reversion or replacement of mutated gene with wild type gene should lead to restoration of pathogenicity or virulence.

Koch's Phenomenon

Robert Koch observed that guinea pig sensitized by infection with tubercle bacilli responded with an exaggerated manner following injection of TB bacilli or its protein.

PAUL EHRLICH (Fig. 1.3)

- He is known as **father of chemotherapy**. He initialized the search for chemotherapeutic agent for killing of bacteria.
- He discovered arsenic compound for treatment of syphilis.
- He reported acid-fast nature of tubercle bacilli.
- He proposed side chain theory for antibody production.
- He introduced methods of standardizing toxin and antitoxins.

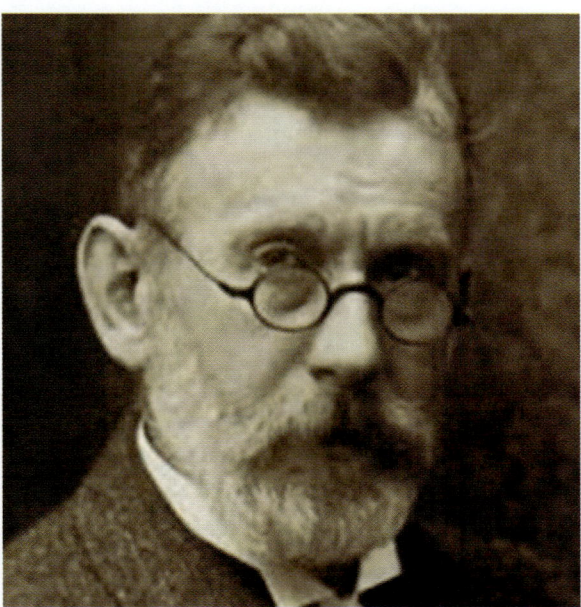

Fig. 1.3: Paul Ehrlich

Important discoveries by other scientists

Lepra bacillus	Hansen 1874
Gonococcus	Neisser 1881
Diphtheria bacillus	Klebs 1883-Loffler1884
Pneumococcus	Frankel 1886
Tetanus bacillus	Kitasato 1889
Meningococcus	Weichselbum 1887

IMPORTANT LANDMARKS IN VIROLOGY

- Pasteur while working with rabies postulated that the causative agent is ultramicroscopic.
- Yellow fever was first human disease proved to be of viral origin and it was discovered by Walter Reid 1902.
- Landsteiner demonstrated that poliomyelitis is due to filterable virus.
- Goodpasture developed techniques of viral cultivation in chick embryo.
- Bacteriophage was discovered by Twort in 1915.

SOME IMPORTANT DISCOVERIES IN IMMUNOLOGY

- Pfeiffer and Bordet contributed in understanding of complement.
- Metchnikoff discovered phenomenon of phagocytosis while Wright discovered opsonization.
- Richet for the first time observed the phenomenon of anaphylaxis.
- Jerne proposed natural selection theory of antibody formation.
- Burnet postulated clonal selection theory.
- Burnet also developed concept of immunological surveillance.
- Medawar and Burnet made first transplant successful by using immunosuppression.

OTHER DEVELOPMENTS

- Ruska developed electron microscope.
- Alexander Fleming discovered first antibiotic penicillin.

NOBEL LAUREATES IN PHYSIOLOGY AND MEDICINE

Year	Name	Work
1901	Emil A von Behring	Serum therapy
1902	Ronald Ross	Malaria life cycle
1905	Robert Koch	Tuberculosis
1907	C LA Laveran	Role of protozoa in causing disease
1908	P Ehrlich and E Metchnikof	Immunity
1913	Charles Robert Ricket	Anaphylaxis
1919	Jules Bordet	Immunity
1926	Johannes Fibiger	*Spiroptera carcinoma*
1928	Charles Nicolle	Typhus
1930	Karl Landsteiner	Discovery of human blood groups
1939	Gerhard Domagk	Prontosil
1945	A Fleming Boris Chain and Howard Walter Florey	Penicillin
1951	Max Theiler	Yellow fever
1952	Selman A Waksman	Streptomycin
1954	Franklin Enders H Weller and F C Robbins	Poliomyelitis culture in tissue
1958	George Beadle and E LTatun and Lederberg	Gene action and genetic recombination
1960	F M Burnet and P B Medawar	Acquired immunological tolerance
1965	Francois Jacob, Andre Lwoff and Jacques Monod	Genetic control of enzymes
1966	Peyton Rous	Tumor inducing viruses
1969	M Delbruck, A D Hershey and S E Luria	Replication mechanism and genetic structure of viruses
1972	Gerald M Edelman and Rodney R Porter	Chemical structure of antibodies
1975	D Baltimore, R Dulbecco and H Martin Temin	Interaction between tumor viruses and genetic material of cell
1976	Baruch S Blumberg and D Carleton Gajdusek	New mechanisms of infectious diseases dissemination
1978	Werner Arber, Daniel Nathans and Hamilton O Smith	Restriction enzymes
1980	Baruj Benacerraf, Jean Dausset and George D Snell	Immunological regulation by cell surface
1984	Niels K Jerne, Georges J F Kohler and Cesar Milstein	Control of immune system and monoclonal antibodies
1987	Susumu Tonegawa	Generation of antibody diversity
1989	J Michael Bishop and Harold Varmus	Origin of retroviral oncogenes
1996	Peter C Doherty and Rolf M Zinkernagel	Specificity in cell-mediated defense
1997	Stanley B Prusiner	Prions
2005	Barry J Marshall and J Robin Warren	*Helicobacter pylori*
2008	Herald Hausen and Francoise Barre-S and L Montagnier	Human papillomaviruses, human immunodeficiency virus
2011	Bruce A Beutler, Jules A Hoffman, Ralph M Steinman	Activation of innate immunity, and dendritic cells and their role in adaptive immunity
2012	Sir John B Gurdon, Shinya Yamanaka	Mature cells can be programmed to become pluripotent

2

Microscopy and Staining Reactions

Bacteria are unicellular prokaryotic organisms without chlorophyll and do not show true branching, except in *Actinomyces*.

Microorganisms belong to the kingdom Protista which is further divided into prokaryotes and *eukaryotes*. Bacteria (and blue green algae) are prokaryotess while fungi, algae and protozoa are eukaryotes (Table 2.1).

TABLE 2.1: Differences between prokaryotes and eukaryotes

Character	Prokaryotes	Eukaryotes
Nucleus		
Nuclear membrane	Absent	Present
Nucleolus	Absent	Present
DNA		
Chromosome	One, circular	More than one, linear
Mitotic division	Absent	Present
Cytoplasm		
Streaming	Absent	Present
Pinocytosis	Absent	Present
Mitochondria	Absent	Present
Lysosomes	Absent	Present
Golgi apparatus	Absent	Present
Endoplasmic reticulum	Absent	Present
Chemical composition		
Sterols	Absent	Present
Muramic acid	Present	Absent
Diaminopimelic acid	Present in some	Absent
Other	Always unicellular	Unicellular or multicellular
	Reproduction by binary fission	Reproduction sexual or asexual
	Ribosomes are small	Ribosomes are large

Size of Bacteria

The unit used to measure the size of bacterium is micron, which is one-thousandth of a milimeter. One nanometer is one-thousandth of a micron, while one Angstrom unit is one-tenth of a nanometer. The size of medically important bacteria falls in the range of 2–5 μ in length and 0.2–1.5 μ in diameter.

MICROSCOPY

Light (Optical) Microscope (Fig. 2.1)

Purpose of Microscope

- Increases the size of organisms. This is called **magnification**.
- Another purpose of using microscope is that it increases the **resolution** or resolving power of microscope.

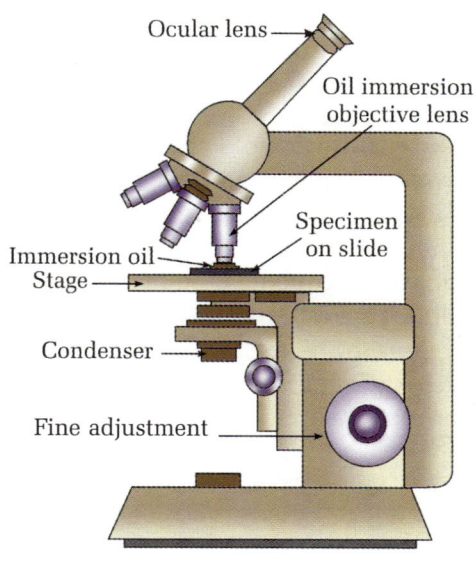

Fig. 2.1: Light microscope

Parts of Microscope

The **mechanical system** consists of base, handle, mechanical stage on which slide is placed, screws are used for fine adjustment and coarse adjustments. Microscope has a light source and the optical system of lenses made up of eyepiece (which is near to eye) and objectives (near object, i.e. organisms present on slide). As it has more than one lens, it is also called compound microscope. Condenser passes light into slide.

Objective lenses: They are three of types:
1. Low power objective (×10)
2. High power objective (×40)
3. *Oil immersion (×100)*: The oil having same refractive index as that of glass is used, hence oil placed between slide and objective avoids refraction of light and which passes directly into eyepiece, so that maximum illumination is achieved.

Eyepiece: It is usually ×10; it magnifies further the real image of object formed by objective.

Condenser: It focuses light on object.

Iris diaphragm: It is used to control the rays of light entering.

Mirror: It collects and reflects light on object, the flat surface is used when light source is normal, concave surface is used with artificial source of light.

Total magnification: An object (e.g. bacterium) is first magnified by objective and again by eyepiece, hence total magnification is magnification of eyepiece × magnification of objective. Thus, total magnification at ×10 eyepiece with ×10 objective is ×100; similarly, magnification of high power is ×400 while that of oil immersion is ×1000.

Resolution: It is defined as the distance that must separate two points, if they are to be seen as two distinct images. The resolution power of human eye is 0.2 mm, while resolution of light microscope is 0.2 μ. The electron microscope has the highest resolution of 0.1 nanometre. The resolution is inversely proportional to the wavelength, hence as electrons have shortest wavelength (wavelength is 0.005 nm as compared to 5000 nm of wavelength of light ray), it has highest resolution.

Adjustment of Contrast and Positions of Condenser

The different preparations observed under microscope in clinical microbiology laboratory are wet mounts (e.g.

urine mount, fluid mount, stool mount) and stained slides (Gram stained, Z-N stained slide, peripheral blood smear stained for malarial parasites).

As a stained slide has contrast given by different dyes used in different stages of staining, it requires maximum illumination under oil immersion. For this, condenser should be at highest position and iris diaphragm is fully opened. In case of unstained wet mounts, there is not much difference between refractive index of object and surrounding medium, hence contrast is achieved by partially closing iris diaphragm and lowering condenser. Thus in low power, the position of condenser is lowest, for high power, the position is midway and for oil immersion it is at highest position.

Care of microscope: When it is not in use, cover it. When carrying it from one place to another, hold it with handle and base. Clean the lenses with soft lens paper and xylol.

Wet Mount

It is used to see organisms in specimens directly, e.g. bacteria in urine wet mount or stool mount. A drop of specimen or suspension of bacteria in suitable solvent is taken on a clean grease-free slide and a cover slip is placed over it. The preparation is observed under high power (×400) by properly adjusting contrast.

Hanging Drop Method

A drop of specimen or bacterial suspension is taken on a coverslip. Cavity slide is taken; on the corners of the cavity, wax is applied. Coverslip is touched with glass slide (facing cavity downside towards coverslip) (wax helps for adhesion), and then it is inverted, so that the drop will be hanging from coverslip in the cavity. This preparation is first observed under low power to focus the edge of the drop. Then switch on to high power to obverse the motility of organisms. The edge is focused because it gives good contrast and at edge it is easy to differentiate true motility, from Brownian movement. If bacteria are motile, they move across the field and change their relative positions. During motility, there is altered cell behavior due to sensory transduction which is responsible for aerotaxis and phototaxis (Figs 2.2 to 2.4).

Uses of hanging drop method
- To observe darting motility of *Vibrio cholerae* in stool sample.
- To study of motility of bacteria in liquid cultures.

Other microscopes used in microbiology are as follows.

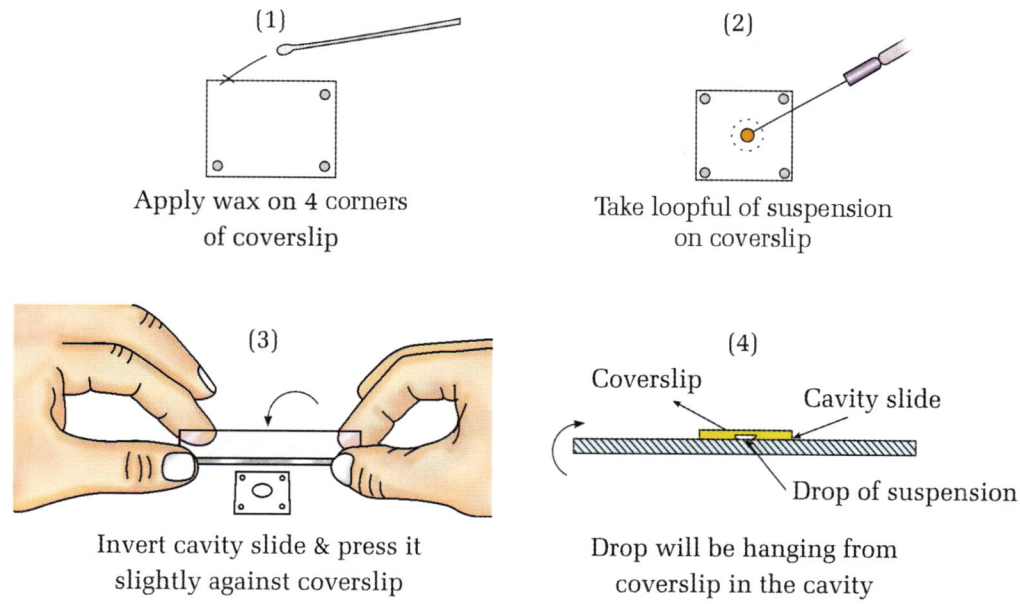

(1)

Apply wax on 4 corners
of coverslip

(2)

Take loopful of suspension
on coverslip

(3)

Invert cavity slide & press it
slightly against coverslip

(4)

Coverslip

Cavity slide

Drop of suspension

Drop will be hanging from
coverslip in the cavity

Fig. 2.2: Hanging drop method

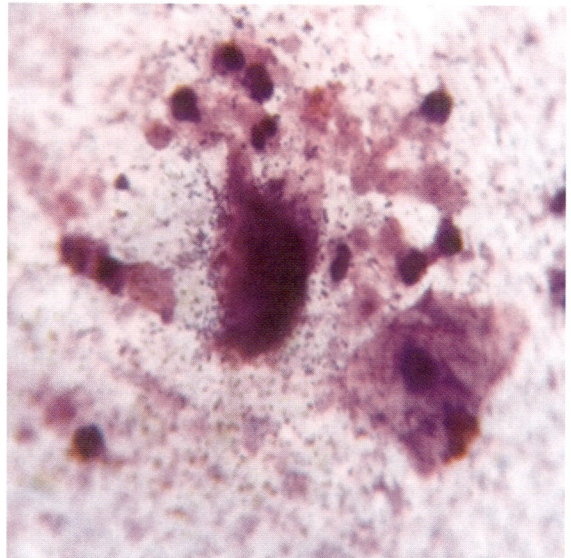

Fig. 2.3: Appearance of epithelial cell in Gram smear

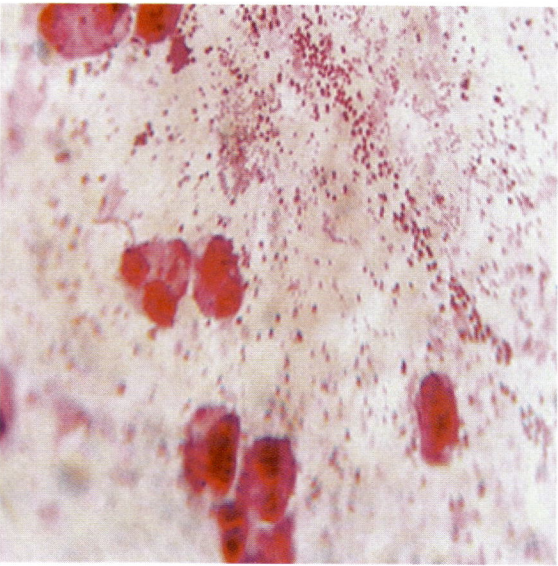

Fig. 2.4: Appearance of pus cells in Gram stain

Phase Contrast Microscope (Fig. 2.5)

It is used to improve the contrast between cells and surrounding medium. The phase contrast microscope takes the advantage that the wavelengths of light passing through the cells and surrounding medium are in different phases due to differences in their refractive indices. These phase differences are again further magnified by using the phase plate or special ring in the objective of the phase contrast microscope, leading to formation of dark image on light background or light and dark bands of different objects.

Uses

- Phase contrast microscope is used for demonstration of motility of bacteria like darting motility of *Vibrio.*
- This microscope is also used to detect delicate or fine bacteria, as *Treponema pallidum.*
- This microscope is used in detection of *Leptospira* in urine.
- It is to find out microfilariae in wet blood mounts.
- It is for demonstration of *Trichomonas vaginalis* in urethral discharge.
- It is used for demonstration of *Campylobacter* in watery stool.

Phase Contrast Microscope Optical Train

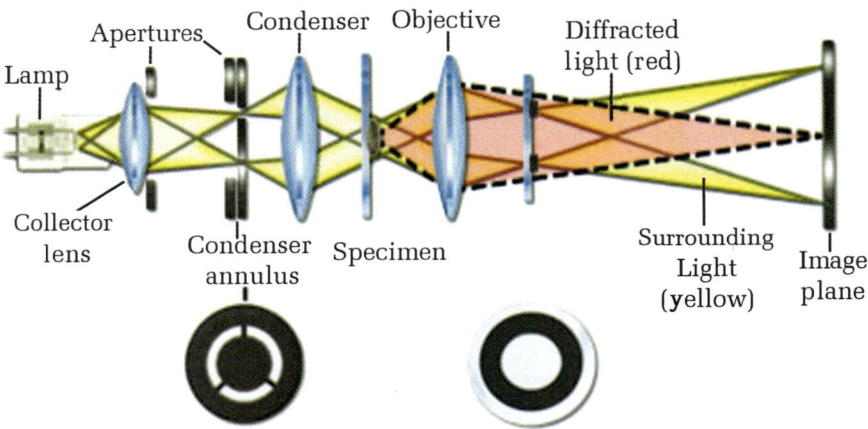

Fig. 2.5: Principle of phase contrast microscope

Dark Field or Dark Ground Microscope

The objects are illuminated with oblique rays of light instead of straight light. This is possible by using a special dark ground condenser in which cental part is blackened and it deflects light off a mirror an oblique angle. This creates a 'dark field' that contrasts against the highlightened edge of specimens and results when oblique rays are reflected from the edge of specimen into objective of the microscope (Fig. 2.6).

Uses

• Demonstration of *Treponema pallidum* in exudate from the ulcer.
• *Leptospira* can be demonstrated in urine sample.
• Demonstration of motility of bacteria like darting motility of *Vibrio*.
• It is used to find out microfilariae in wet blood mounts.

Fluorescent Microscope

Light has visible spectrum and invisible spectrum. UV rays are used in this microscope instead of light rays and fluorescent dye is used as a stain which stains organisms (Fig. 2.7).

The microscope converts invisible spectrum into visible spectrum, hence organisms are seen as bright objects against dark background as if they are self-illuminating.

Mercury vapor lamp is used as source of light. The light beam which is generated is reflected by concave mirror. It is then projected through collecting lenses to excitation filters, which emits a fluorescent light beam. A reflecting mirror directs the beam from underneath the stage, through the condenser into specimen, and the fluorescence pattern is viewed through ocular lenses.

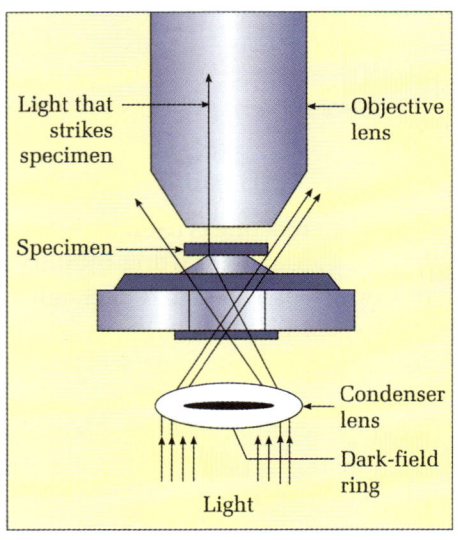

Fig. 2.6: Dark ground condenser

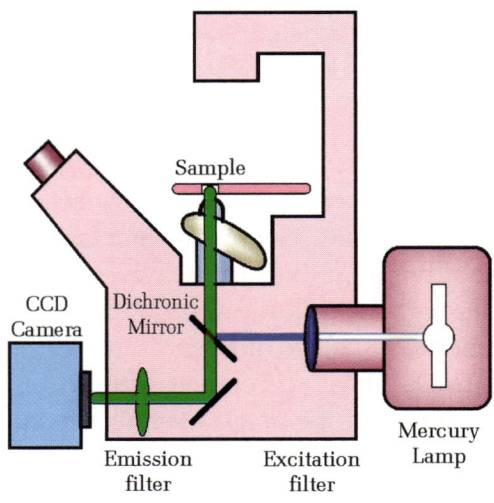

Fig. 2.7: Fluorescent microscope

Uses

- Phenolic auramine is used for screening *Mycobacterium tuberculosis* in sputum.
- Acridine orange causes DNA to fluoresce green and RNA, orange red. Fluorescent staining is recommended for rapid identification of *Trichomonas vaginalis* and clue cells in vaginal discharge.
- Calcofluor white is used for staining fungi in specimens.
- It is also used for *meningococci* and *gonococci*.
- *Direct immunofluorescence*: In this, antibody against the organism to be seen is tagged with fluorescent stain and that fluorescent is used for staining the smears.
- It is used for *Streptococcus pyogenes* in nasopharyngeal secretions.
- Demonstration of *Chlamydia* in genital specimens and corneal scraping from a case of Trachoma.
- Demonstration of *HSV* in different samples. Biopsy may be used for diagnosis of encephalitis.
- Detection of rabies viral antigens in corneal scrapings for the antemortem diagnosis of rabies.

Electron Microscope

Electron microscope uses electromagnetic fields as lenses and beams of electrons are used as light source. The microscope has the highest **resolving power,** i.e. **0.2 nanometer** because resolving power is reciprocal of wavelength and electrons have shortest wavelength. The high resolving power enabled scientists to observe very minute structures of prokaryotes and eukaryotes.

There are mainly two types of electron microscopes mostly used, i.e. scanning electron microscope **(SEM)** and transmission electron microscope **(TEM).**

Transmission electron microscope (Fig. 2.8) was first to be developed and uses a beam of electrons projected from an electron gun and directed or focused by electromagnetic condenser lenses on to a thin film. As electrons strike the specimen, they are differentially scattered by number and mass of atoms in the specimens, some electrons pass through the specimen and are condensed and focussed by electromagnetic objective lenses which represent an image of the specimen to the projector lens system for further magnification. The image is visualized by allowing it to impinge on a screen that fluoresces when struck with electrons. The image is recorded on a photographic film.

SEM has comparatively low resolution. It is used to provide three-dimensional images of the surface of objects. Electrons are focused by means of lenses into a very fine point. The interaction of electrons with specimens results in release of different forms of radiations (secondary electrons) from the surface of material which can be captured by appropriate detector, amplified, and imaged on a television.

An important technique in electron microscope **is shadowing.** This involves deposition of a thin layer of heavy material, e.g. platinum on specimen, by placing it in the path of a beam of metal ions in a vacuum. The beam is directed at a low angle to the specimen so that it acquires a shadowing in the form of an uncoated area on the other side. When a beam of electrons is passed through the coated preparation in electron microscope, a positive print is made from negative image, a three-dimensional effect is achieved (Table 2.2).

Epifluorescence Microscope

It is the simplest form of fluorescent microscope.

The examples are:

1. *Autofluorescence*: A few organisms, as **cyclospora,** fluoresce when kept under UV lamp.
2. *Phenolic auramine* is used to stain smear from sputum for demonstration of *Mycobacterium tuberculosis*.

Confocal Scanning Laser Microscope

It couples a laser light source to a light microscope. In this microscope, a laser beam is bounced off a mirror that directs the beam through a scanning device. The laser beam is directed through a pinhole that precisely adjusts the plane of focus of beam to a given vertical layer within the specimen.

By precisely illuminating only a single plane of the specimen, illumination intensity drops off rapidly below and above the plane of focus and stray light rays from other planes of focus are minimized. Thus in a relatively thick specimen, various layers can be observed by adjusting the plane of focus of laser beam. Cells are often stained with fluorescent dye to make

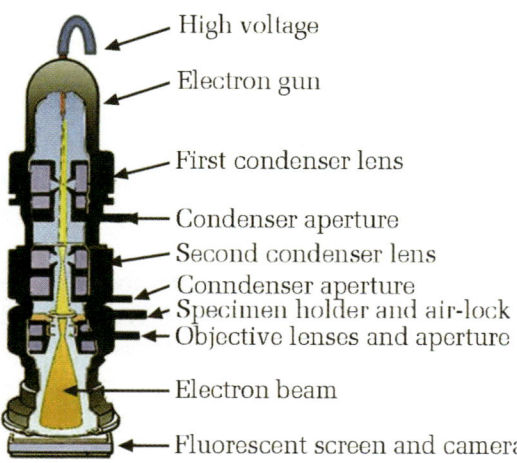

High voltage
Electron gun
First condenser lens
Condenser aperture
Second condenser lens
Conndenser aperture
Specimen holder and air-lock
Objective lenses and aperture
Electron beam
Fluorescent screen and camera

Fig. 2.8: Transmission electron microscope

TABLE 2.2: Comparison between light microscope and electron microscope

Property	Light microscope	Electron microscope
Source	Visible light	Electrons
Lenses used	Glass	Electromagnetic lenses
Focusing	Mechanically	Current to magnetic lenses adjusted
Source of contrast	Differential light refraction based on refractive indices. In colored preparations, stains give contrast	Scattering of electrons
Resolution	0.2 μm	0.1–0.5 nm
Magnification	1000 on oil immersion	1 Lakh

them more visible. Alternately, false color images can be generated by adjusting the microscope in such a way as to make different layers take on different colors.

STAINING METHODS OF BACTERIA

In wet mount, e.g. urine mount, it becomes difficult to obverse bacteria as there is no major difference between refractive index of bacteria and refractive index of the surrounding medium.

To increase the contrast, we use coloring agent called stain. The **stain** is a coloring agent used to stain tissues while dye is used for nonliving agent.

Classification of Stains

Stains are salts and can be classified as **acidic,** if the coloring component is present in acidic part, while in **basic** dyes, the coloring agent is present in basic component of the salt. As bacteria have acidic protoplasm, basic dyes are used to stain bacteria while acidic stain is used to stain background, for the demonstration of capsule, e.g. Nigrosin or India ink preparation.

Another way to classify stains is one which stains the organisms and kills it called as **supravital,** while vital stains retain the viability. During the staining, the heat fixation and the stains kill bacteria. But 100% killing is ensured only by using potassium permanganate. This method is specially used for staining the smear containing the anthrax bacilli.

Vital stain is able to differentiate between living cells and dead cells. Living cells exclude the dye hence stain negatively while dead cells take the stain positively. The examples include eosin, trypan blue and neutral red.

Intravital staining is done by injecting stain in body (*in vivo*).

Different Types of Stains

- *Simple stain*: Staining agent stains the organisms as well as background. Methylene blue is the example of simple stain.

- *Negative staining*: It is used to demonstrate the capsule of organisms and stains the background. As mentioned above, Nigrosin or India ink is used to demonstrate capsule. To prepare this, one drop of the stain is taken on a glass slide, to this added small portion of colony of organism or specimen, coverslip is placed and the preparation is observed under ×10 and ×400.

Differential Staining Methods

By these methods bacteria can be differentiated into two different groups. For example, by Gram staining, bacteria are classified into two groups, i.e. Gram-positive which appear violet while Gram-negative bacteria appear red. By ZN staining, we can differentiate into acid-fast (red) from nonacid-fast (blue).

Special Staining Methods

- **Albert's staining** is used for *Corynebacterium diphtheriae*. The metachromatic granules appear dark green to black as compared to bacterium which appears green in color.
- **Giemsa staining** is useful for **staining plague bacillus** which shows **bipolar staining**.
- **Gimenez** is used for *Chlamydia*.
- **Fluorescent staining** (phenolic auramine).
  I. It is used for staining TB bacilli in sputum sample. The method has the advantage that it screens bacilli under ×400, hence rapid screening is possible in a set up where large number of sputum samples have to be screened daily. The Z-N staining requires observation under ×100 which takes more time.
  II. Acridine orange causes DNA to fluoresce green, and RNA orange red. This method is recommended for rapid identification of *Trichomonas vaginalis*, Clue cells in vaginal discharge. It can also be used for *meningococci* and *gonococci*.
  III. Calcofluor white is used for staining fungi in specimens.

- **Wayson's stain** is used for *Yersinia pestis,* it shows bipolar staining due to condensation of protoplast at the ends giving safety pin appearance. By this method, *Yersinia pestis* bacillus is stained blue and ends are pink.
- **Polychrome methylene blue staining** demonstrates capsule of *Bacillus anthracis* by McFadyean method.
- **Silver impregnation method:** Because of deposition of silver salts, which apparently increase the thickness of the structures and make fine structures visible.

Silver impregnation methods used are:
a. **Fontana's staining** is used for the demonstration of *Treponema pallidum* in secretion taken from the base of genital ulcer.
b. **Levaditi** staining is used for demonstration of Spirichaetes in tissue, i.e. demonstration of *Treponema pallidum* in liver biopsy of a child suffering from congenital syphilis.

GRAM'S STAINING

How to Prepare a Smear?

Smears should be evenly spread over an area of 15–20 mm.
- *Purulent specimen:* Use sterile wire loop, pick up specimen and make a thin preparation.
- *Sputum:* Use a clean stick to pick up purulent part of sputum. Soak the stick in Na⁻ hypochlorite solution before discarding.
- *Non-purulent fluids:* Centrifuge, mix the sediment and use for smear preparation.
- *Swabs:* Roll the swab over the slide.
- *Feces:* Use a clean stick to transfer mucus and purulent part on a slide.
- *Culture:* Smear prepared from a colony is called **secondary smear**. Emulsify colony in sterile distilled water or saline and make a thin preparation. If there is growth in broth culture, transfer it on slide with sterile loop.
- *Urine:* Take one loopful on slide and allow it to air dry, without spreading. This is important because by this method, if after staining, we observe average one bacterium per field, it corresponds to 10^5 bacteria per ml of urine. This test is used as **screening method for** urine (for significant count).
- *Skin slit smears for lepra bacilli:* The material is collected with scalpel blade and tissue juices transferred on slide.

Drying and Fixing the Smear

Smear is allowed to air dry and fixed with heat. The purpose of fixation is that the smear should not be washed away during the staining procedure and to preserve the microorganisms.

Heat fixation: For the fixation of smears, pass the slides; smear facing upwards, three times through the frame.

Note: Passing through the flame three times, it should be possible to touch the slide on back of hand without feeling uncomfortable, if felt uncomfortable, means too much heat has been applied.

Other Fixation Methods

- *Alcohol fixation:* This type causes less damage to bacteria and pus cells, hence useful especially for intracellular bacteria as meningococci and gonococci which are inside the pus cells. For fixing these, 2–3 drops of absolute methanol or ethanol are used.
- For the detection of *Mycobacterium tuberculosis,* smears are fixed with 2 drops of 70% v/v methanol or ethanol (absolute methanol can also be used but 70% is sufficient for MTB). Leave alcohol for at least 2 minutes. Alcohol ensures the killing of MTB but heat is not sufficient.
- **4% solution of K-permanganate** solution is useful for fixation of dangerous organisms as anthrax bacilli.
- **Formaldehyde solution** is sometimes recommended for MTB.

Procedure of Gram's Staining (Fig. 2.9)

I. To a heat fixed smear, crystal violet or gentian violet is added.

II. The smear is washed with tap water.

III. Gram's iodine is added to the slide, which acts as **mordant** (which brings the staining reaction).

IV. After washing with tap water, smear is decolorized by acetone or alcohol. This is continued till last drop from the slide is colorless.

V. After washing with tap water, counterstain saffranin is added. Wash with tap water, air dry and focus under oil immersion.

The **Standiforts** modification used for **gonococci** which uses **malachite green** as counterstain. Diluted carbol fuschin (1 in 10 dilution) is used for staining *Campylobacter, Vibrios, Vincent's bacilli, Haemophilus and Yersinia.*

Gram-positive bacteria take primary stain and do not get decolorized and appear violet color while Gram-negative bacteria take primary stain but after decolorization, loose primary stain and take the counterstain, hence appear red.

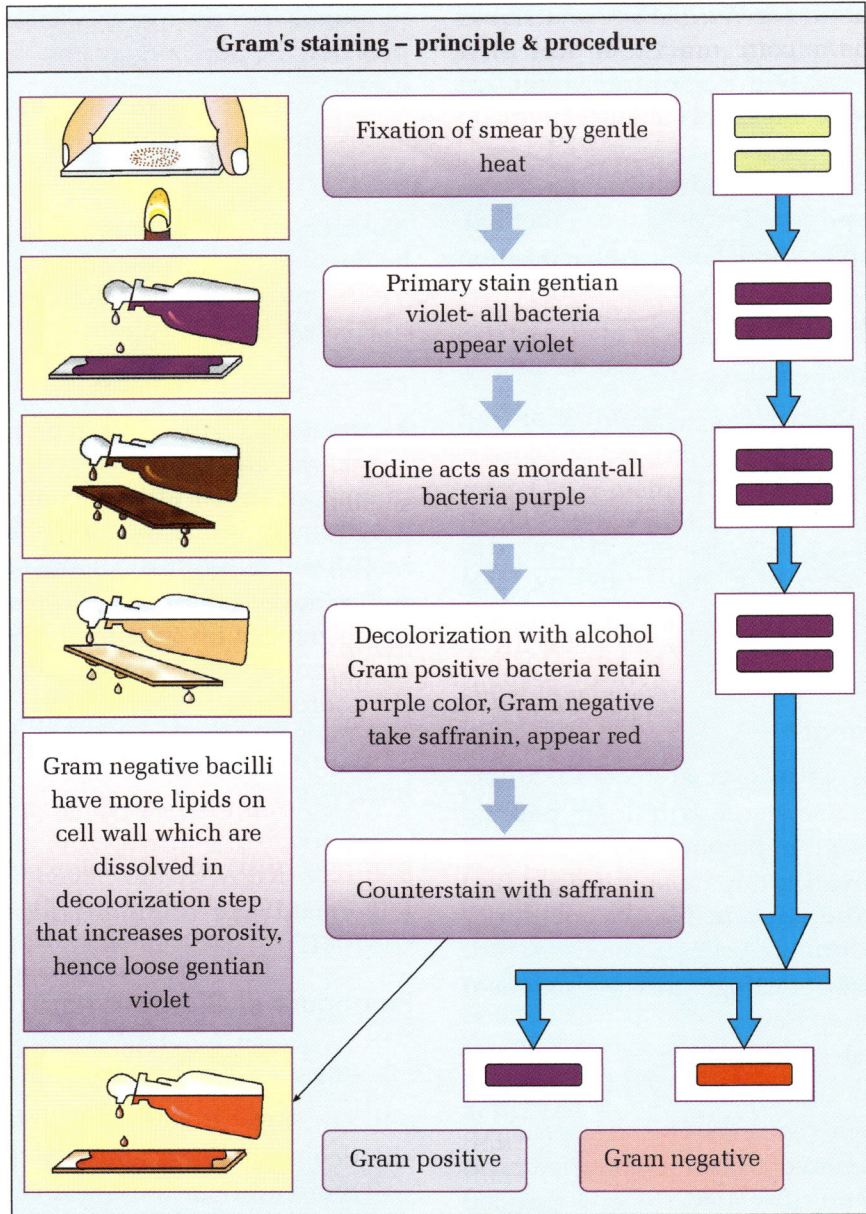

Fig. 2.9: Gram's staining

Principles of Gram Staining

1. Gram-positive bacteria have more acidic protoplasm and the primary stain, stains more intensely.

2. During decolorization, after addition of acetone or alcohol, the lipids present on the cell wall of Gram-negative bacteria (Gram-positive bacteria have more protein on cell wall) get dissolved increasing the porosity of cell wall, hence Gram-negative bacteria loose primary stain and take counterstain.

3. Cell wall of Gram-positive bacteria has potassium ribonucleotide which forms complex with primary stain and iodine complex, which helps to maintain the complex.

4. Cell wall of Gram-positive bacteria are composed of many layers of murein. The layer is so thick that it impedes passage of hydrophobic compounds. Hence, Gram-positive bacteria have the capacity to retain primary dye-iodine complex.

Conditions in which actual Gram reaction of bacteria may be altered:

- If the slide is over decolorized, Gram-positive bacteria may appear Gram-negative. This mistake can be overcome by using control smears.

- If damage to cell wall occurs, Gram reaction may be changed.

- If Gram staining is performed from very old cultures, Gram variable reaction may occur.
- Some bacteria have the inherent property that they may occur Gram variable, e.g. *Clostridium welchii*.
- Staining also depends upon the stage of bacilli during their growth cycle.

The examples **of Gram-positive cocci** (cocci are spherical):

A. Staphylococci, *Streptococcus pyogenes, Streptococcus pneumoniae, Enterococcus* species, *Peptostreptococcus* species.

B. The examples of Gram-negative cocci are meningococci, gonococci.

C. Examples **of Gram-positive bacilli**: *Bacillus antracis, Bacillus cereus, Corneybactrium diphtheriae,* all *Clostridium* species as *Clostridium tetani, Clostridium welchii, Clostridium botulinum, Mycobacterium tuberculosis.* (**Note:** For this bacterium, Z-N staining is preferred.)

D. Examples of Gram-negative bacilli are *E.coli, Klebsiella,* and *Salmonella.*

Importance of Gram's Staining (Application)

- Gram reaction gives knowledge of **growth requirements** of bacteria and thus selection of media. Depending on Gram reaction, proper culture media are chosen for isolation of bacteria from specimens. For example, if Gram-positive cocci are seen in primary stain from specimens, blood agar is selected for isolation, if Gram-negative bacilli as *E. coli* are suspected in urine, we choose MacConkey's medium, in addition to blood agar, for differentiation of lactose fermenters from nonlactose fermenters.
- Similarly biochemical reactions are selected on the basis of Gram reaction.
- Selection of antibiotics may be done based on Gram reaction.

IMPORTANCE OF PRIMARY SMEAR (SMEARS PREPARED FROM SPECIMENS)

- If a case of diphtheria is suspected and if findings of Gram reaction on smear prepared from nasopharyngeal secretions showing Gram-positive bacilli with Chienese letter pattern, provisional report that organisms resembling *Corynebacterium* seen, can be given so that treating clinicians can immediately start anti-diphtheric serum to give immediate protection.
- Similarly if the smear is prepared from muscle piece or wound swab from a suspected case of gas gangrene, the report of box car Gram-positive bacteria with minimum pus cells gives presumptive

diagnosis of gas gangrene in which immediately antigas gangrene serum is given to the patient as lifesaving therapy, followed by surgical treatment.

ZIEHL-NEELSEN STAINING (ACID-FAST STAIN) (Fig. 2.10)

Acid-fast staining is discovered by Ehrlich and subsequently modified by Ziehl and Neelsen.

Principle

Acid-fast bacilli have high contents of lipids, fatty acids, alcohols and mycolic acids present on cell wall. The integrity of cell wall is also important for acid fastness of bacteria. During primary staining with heating, temporary, small pores are opened and the primary stain, i.e. carbol fuschin penetrates the cell. Acid-fast organisms thus are difficult to stain but once stained, they retain primary stain (they hold acids fast), hence appear red colored. Nonacid-fast bacteria take the counterstain, i.e. methylene blue and appear blue.

Other effects of presence of lipids, fatty acid on cell wall of *Mycobacterium*: Because of these nutrients also reach slowly; the bacteria have high generation time, take longer period to form colonies on medium. Other effect is presence of caseation necrosis in tubercle formation.

The primary stain, carbol fuschin, contains basic fuschin and phenol. Basic fuschin is coloring agent while phenol itself acts as mordant. (As mordant is present in primary stain, this staining method has only three steps as compared to Gram staining in which addition of Gram's iodine is separate step.)

How to Judge whether the Sputum Sample is Proper for Processing?

If we perform the gross examination of the sample and if the sample contains thick purulent material, it means a suitable sample and if sample collected by patient is salivary, it is not proper for processing. In revised national tuberculosis control programme (RNTCP), at least two samples are processed.

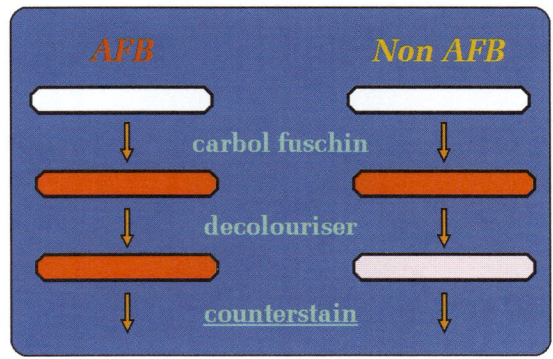

Fig. 2.10: Z-N (acid-fast) staining

Procedure

Smear is prepared from the thick purulent part of sputum and spread evenly on a glass slide (diameter of smear should be 15–20 mm) and fixed by gentle heat.

- Carbol fuschin is poured on slide covering the smear completely. The slide is gently heated from the underneath until steam just start coming. (Vigorous heating is avoided.) During heating, temporary pores are opened up causing entry of carbol fuschin. These pores are again closed. This step is done for 5 minutes.
- Decolorization is done with 25% sulphuric acid until the smear is pinkish on washing (2–4 minutes). Counter-staining is done for half minute by Loeffler's methylene blue. The smear is washed with tap water, air dried and observed under oil immersion.

Number of samples recommended for examination for AFB, under **RNTCP:** Currently **two samples** are recommended, of which first is early morning sample (produced by coughing in open space).

For urine sample, centrifuge whole early morning sample of each day for three days. Take the sediment for preparing smear.

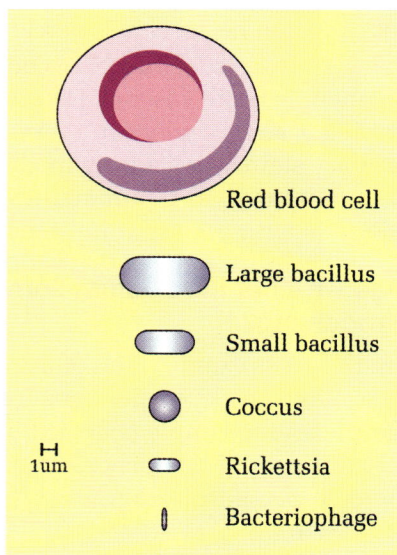

Red blood cell

Large bacillus

Small bacillus

Coccus

⊢ 1um

Rickettsia

Bacteriophage

Fig. 2.11: Comparison of size of different organisms with size of RBC

Result: Acid-fast bacteria take the primary stain and resist decolorization, hence appear pink or red, while nonacid-fast bacteria appear blue and pus cells appear blue in color.

Typical *Mycobacterium tuberculosis* bacillus appears straight or slight curved red or pink rods with **"beaded appearance"**.

Other acid-fast structures are:

Bacteria
- Atypical mycobacteria
- *Mycobacterium leprae* (5% H_2SO_4)
- *Nocardia* (1% H_2SO_4)
- *Rhodococcu equi*
- *Brucella abortus* (special modified staining is used)
- *Legionella micdadei*
- Spores of bacteria

Parasites
- *Cryptosporidium*
- *Isospora belli*
- *Cyclospora*
- Egg of *Taenia saginata*

Other acid-fast structures: Sperms, bacterial spores.

MODIFICATIONS OF Z-N STAINING

- Instead of 20% H_2SO_4, 3% acid alcohol can be used as decoloring agent.
- As lepra bacilli are less acid-fast, 5% H_2SO_4 is used as decoloring solution.
- 1% H_2SO_4 solution is used for Nocardia.
- Modifications of Z-N methods are also used to stain other acid-fast structures as cysts of *Cryptosporidium* and *Isospora* (0.5% H_2SO_4).
- **Brucella differential stains** are used for demonstration of *Brucella abortus* in stained smear. Dilute carbol fuschin is allowed to act without heating for 15 minutes. The slide is decolorized by 0.5 acetic acid for 15 seconds, washed with tap water, stained with Loffler's methylene blue for one minute.

3

Morphology of Bacteria

DIFFERENT SHAPES OF BACTERIA

- Cocci are spherical or oval-shaped (kokos means berry), e.g. staphylococci.
- Some cocci are not perfectly spherical, they may be lanceolate or flame-shaped as pneumococci.
- Bacilli (bacillus means rod) are rod-shaped, e.g. *E. coli* (Fig. 3.1).
- Coccobacilli are ovoid bacteria, e.g. *Acinetobacter*.
- **Vibrios** are coma-shaped curved rods.
- **Spirilia** are rigid spiral forms.
- **Spirochaetes** are thin, fine spiral forms.
- **Actinomyces** are branching filamentous forms like fungal elements but they are thin (this appearance is similar to sun rays; actis meaning ray, mykes meaning fungus).
- **Mycoplasmas** are cell wall deficient, hence show no stable morphology. They may show disc shape, oval or filamentous structures.
- When cell synthesis becomes defective, bacteria are converted into protoplasts, spheroplasts or L forms.

DIFFERENT ARRANGEMENTS OF BACTERIA

- Gram-positive cocci arranged in grape-like clusters are *staphylococci* (Fig. 3.2).
- Gram-positive cocci arranged in chains are strepto-cocci, e.g. *Streptococcus pyogenes* (Fig. 3.3).
- Gram-positive cocci arranged in pairs are called diplococci as *pneumococci* (Fig. 3.4).
- Oval cocci in pairs showing 'spects-like appearance' are *enterococci*.
- Gram-negative cocci may be arranged in pairs, e.g. *Gonococcus* or *Meningococcus* (Fig. 3.5).
- Gram-positive cocci arranged in group of fours (tetrads) are *micrococci* while groups of eight are *Sarcina*.
- Bacilli arranged single (Fig. 3.6) or arranged in pairs are called diplobacilli.

- Bacilli may be arranged in chains as in *Bacillus anthracis* (chain of bacilli is surrounded by capsule giving bamboo stick appearance).
- Some bacilli are arranged at angles to each other giving cuneiform or Chinese letter appearance as seen in *Corynebacterium diphtheriae*.

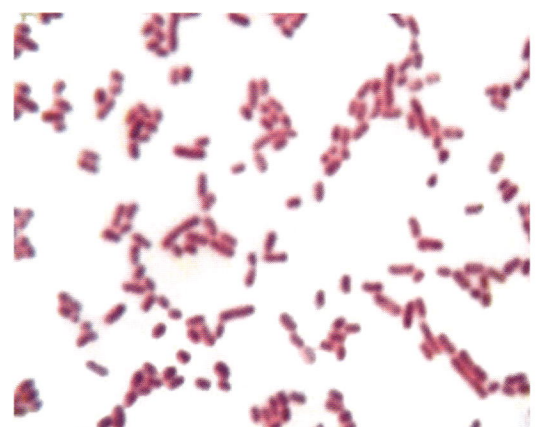

Fig. 3.1: Gram-negative bacilli—*E. coli*

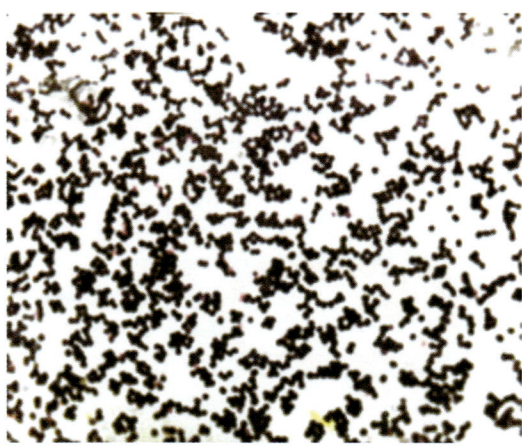

Fig. 3.2: Gram-positive cocci in clusters—*Staphylococcus aureus*

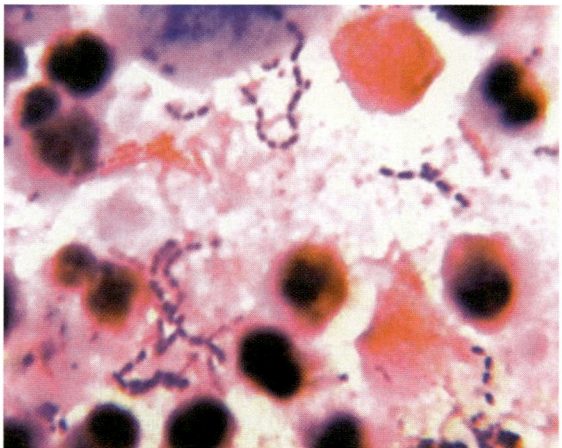

Fig. 3.3: Gram-positive cocci in chain—*Streptococcus pyogenes*

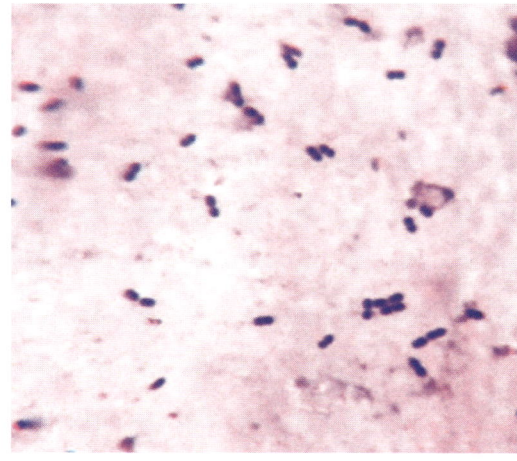

Fig. 3.4: Gram-positive cocci in pairs—pneumococci

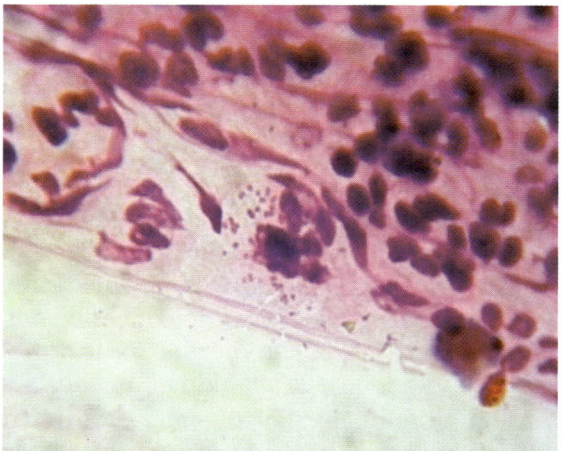

Fig. 3.5: Gram-negative cocci in pairs—*Gonococci*

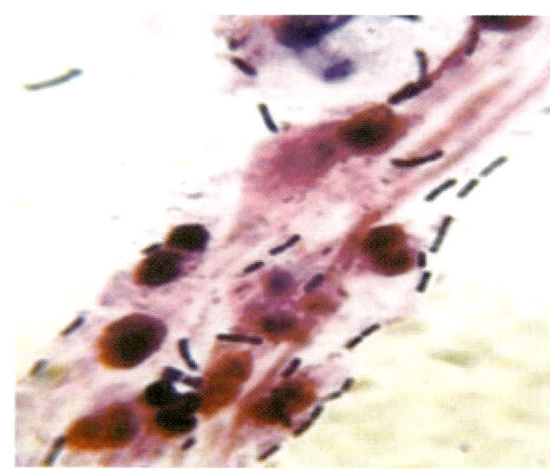

Fig. 3.6: Gram-positive bacilli

STRUCTURE OF BACTERIAL CELL

The **cell envelope,** i.e. outer layer, is divided into cell wall and cytoplasmic membrane or plasma membrane which encloses protoplasm made up of cytoplasm, cytoplasmic inclusions and nuclear body. *Cytoplasm* contains nucleoid, ribosomes, mesosomes, inclusions and sometimes plasmids. Some bacteria may have capsule. Flagellum is the organ of locomotion while fimbria are meant for attachment or adhesion (Fig. 3.7).

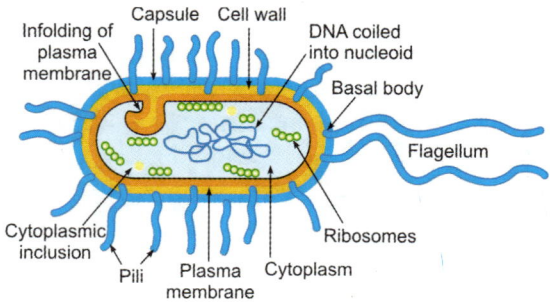

Fig. 3.7: Structure of bacterial cell

Cell Wall

It is a covering of a bacterium which performs many functions as follows:

- It gives shape and rigidity to the bacterium.
- It has role in division of bacteria as well as serving as primer for its own biosynthesis.
- Structure of cell wall is such that various parts of it act as antigens.
- It has receptors for bacteriophages which help in phage typing, similarly it has role in colicin typing.
- Cell wall of Gram-negative bacteria has lipo-polysaccharides which act as endotoxin and responsible for the toxemia.
- Cell wall has invasive property, for example, outer membrane proteins of Gram-negative bacteria, as *Shigella*, have invasive property.
- It acts as gateway for nutrients.
- It is selectively permeable, one layer of Gram-negative cell wall—outer membrane proteins—prevents passage of larger molecules.

• Certain drugs act on cell wall and inhibit bacteria, e.g. penicillin acts on cell wall of staphylococci.

Composition of Cell Wall (Fig. 3.8)

It is 10–25 nm in thickness and shares 20–30% of dry weight of bacteria.

Bacterial cell wall has strength because of presence of a layer composed of a substance called peptidoglycan or mucopeptide or murein.

In **Gram-positive** bacteria, peptidoglycan forms as many as **40 sheets**, while in Gram-negative bacteria one or two such sheets are present.

The composition of cell wall varies from Gram-negative bacteria to Gram-positive bacteria. The peptidoglycan in both acts as backbone and is made up of N-acetylmuramic acid and N-acetylglucosamine linked (Fig. 3.9) by beta 1–4 linkages.

Cell wall of Gram positive is thick. Teichoic acids and tecouronic acids are present on cell wall. These acids form 50% dry weight of cell wall. In addition, Gram-positive walls may have polysaccharide molecules.

The teichoic acids are of two types, wall teichoic acid (WTA) and membrane teichoic acids which are covalently linked to membrane glycoproteins.

Functions of teichoic acids: They form antigens of Gram-positive cocci, e.g. *Streptococcus pneumoniae*. Teichoic acids bear Forssman antigen. In case of *Streptococcus pyogenes*, teichoic acids in association with 'M' protein form microfibrils which help in attachment. They act as antigens and also act as substrate for many reactions.

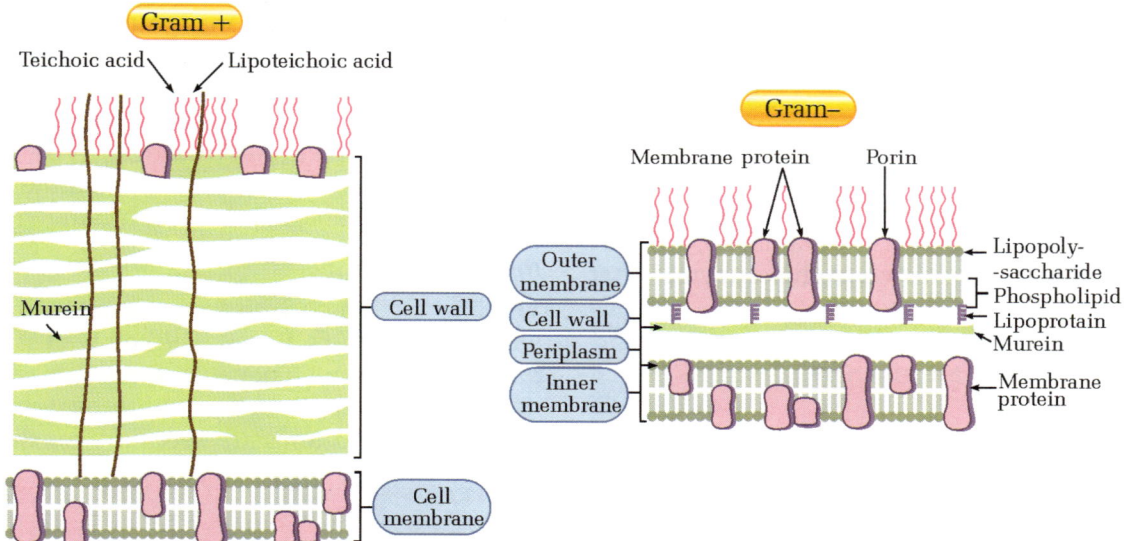

Fig. 3.8: Cell wall of Gram-positive and Gram-negative bacteria

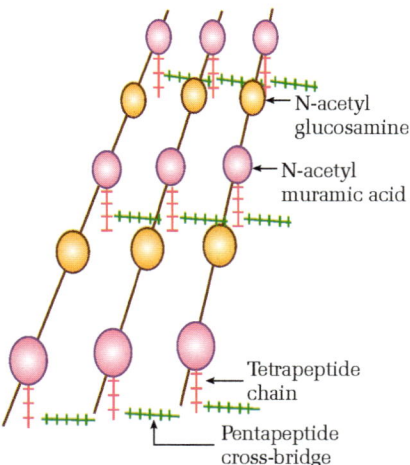

Fig. 3.9: Basic unit of cell wall

Teichuronic acids are synthesized when phosphate supply is limited.

Cell Wall of Gram-negative Bacilli

Gram-negative bacteria have thin cell wall without teichoic acids and have many layers.

Inner layer is made up of peptidoglycan. Outside the peptidoglycan, cell wall contains lipoprotein layer, outer membrane and lipopolysaccharides.

Lipoprotein layer has Braun's lipoprotein which is joined to peptidoglycan and it stabilizes the outer membrane.

Outer membrane: It is bilayered structure, it has special channels called **porins**. Porins permit passive diffusion of sugars, amino acids; they exclude hydrophobic molecules. The proteins called outer membrane proteins (OMP). OMP C, D, F cause diffusion of maltose along with Pho E, LamB. The Tsx is bacteriophage receptor, Omp A acts as sex pilus receptor. Porin acts as gateway for nutrients and antibiotics, it has invasive property also.

Apart from this, outer membrane proteins contain proteins involved in transport of specific molecules as vitamin B_{12}, iron siderophore complex. Some proteins of outer membrane act as phospholipases, proteases.

Lipopolysaccharide (LPS)

- **It has lipid 'A'** having endotoxic activity.
- *Core oligosaccharide*: It includes sugars and it is genus-specific. Lipooligosaccharides are small glycoproteins, they are antigenic. Epitopes on it mimic host structures and evade immune responses (*H. ducrei*, meningococci, gonococci, *H. influenzae*).
- *Polysaccharide or 'O' antigen*: Presence of peculiar sugars on it gives species-specific antigens.

Periplasmic Space

The space between outer and inner membrane is called periplasmic space. It contains proteins specific for substrates, hydrolytic enzymes (β-lactamases), proteins that help in taking nutrients and other enzymes that inactivate antibiotics.

Differences between cell wall of Gram-positive and Gram-negative bacteria are given in Table 3.1.

Methods of Demonstration of Cell Wall

- Differential staining methods as Gram's staining, Z-N staining
- Electron microscope
- *Plasmolysis*: When intact bacteria are inoculated in solution of very high solute concentration, protoplast shrinks; the cytoplasmic membrane is retracted. This process is called **plasmolysis**
- Staining method is **Chain's** method

- Reaction with antibody
- Microdissection

Cell Wall Defective Bacteria

L Forms

These are the abnormal forms of bacteria without cell wall. Due to absence of cell wall, the shape is irregular. The name 'L' forms are given, because they are first isolated from Pasteur Institute by Kleinberg-Nobel. L forms may be produced spontaneously or they may be formed by inhibition of the cell wall synthesis in presence of substrates as penicillin. They are difficult to culture; culture is possible in a medium with high osmotic pressure. They are unstable and may revert back, if the inducing agent is removed. Colonies of an organism having 'L' form on solid medium are small 'fried egg' like. They are nonpathogenic to experimental animals, but if there is infection of the organism which has produced L forms, it may cause relapse or difficult to treat with antibiotic which act on cell wall. L forms are the stable forms as compared to protoplasts and spheroplasts. L forms resemble with *Mycoplasma* in many aspects like morphology, type of growth, filterability, it was also postulated that the *Mycoplasma* represents the stable L forms of an unknown bacterium.

Protoplast

These forms are derived from Gram-positive bacteria which are unstable forms. The cell wall is lost due to action of lysozyme. They may grow in size, but do not multiply in a medium with high osmotic pressure. Hypertonic conditions are necessary for their growth.

Spheroplasts

These forms retain at least some part of cell wall. They are produced in presence of penicillin. They are osmotically less fragile forms. They are derived from Gram-negative bacteria. These forms are produced in the presence of toxic agents and penicillin, but can revert back, if the toxic agent is removed.

TABLE 3.1: Differences between cell wall of Gram-positive and Gram-negative bacteria

	Gram-positive	*Gram-negative*
Thickness	Thick (approx. 80 nm)	Thin (2–8 nm)
Variety of amino acids	Few	Many
Lipids	Absent or few (2–5% only)	Present (15–20%)
Teichoic acids	Present	Absent
Aromatic sulfur containing amino acids	Absent	Present
	More sensitive to cell wall attacking antibiotics	Less sensitive
	No toxic property of cell wall	Cell wall has toxic property due to LPS
Rigidity	More rigid	Less rigid

Cytoplasmic Membrane (Plasma Membrane)

It is a unit membrane composed of phospholipids and 200 different kinds of proteins. Sterols are absent except in *Mycoplasma*.

Functions

- Selective permeability and transfer of solutes. The enzyme permease which plays role in passage through membrane.
- Presence of polymerizing enzymes which manufacture substance of cell wall.
- It also bears enzymes and carrier molecules that function in biosynthesis of DNA, cell wall polymers, membrane lipids.
- Transport of electrons and oxidative phosphorylation in aerobic bacteria.
- It has receptors and proteins of chemotactic system and sensory transduction system.
- Excretion of enzymes.

Cytoplasm

It contains organic and inorganic substances forming colloidal system. Ribosomes, mesosomes, inclusions and vacuoles are present in cytoplasm. Endoplasmic reticulum and mitochondria are absent. It does not have internal mobility, i.e. **protoplasmic streaming.**

Ribosome and Mesosomes

Ribosomes are the sites of protein synthesis while mesosomes are the sites of respiration. Mesosomes are formed from plasma membrane by invagination of plasma membrane into cytoplasm.

Functions of Mesosomes

I. They are the sites of respiratory enzymes for bacteria.
II. They coordinate nuclear and cytoplasmic division.
III. They are responsible for compartmentation of DNA during sporulation.

Intracytoplasmic Inclusions

Cytoplasm of bacteria may contain various **inclusions** depending upon the organism.

Examples of inclusion are volutin granules (present in *Corynebacterium diphtheriae*), which are source of polymetaphosphate.

Nucleoid

No true nucleus is present, instead of that DNA is present in structure called **nucleoid.** There is no nuclear membrane. The nucleoid is a single continuous circular molecule (double-stranded), the chromosomal DNA is haploid and replicates by simple fission.

DNA can be made visible under light micro-scope by Feulgen staining.

Inclusion Granule

Cytoplasmic inclusions	Found in	Function
Glycogen	E. coli	Reserve of carbon and energy
Parasporal crystals	Bacillus	Unknown

Plasmids

Some bacteria may contain extrachrosomal DNA called plasmid which replicates of its own and may carry genes of drug resistance.

Flagella

Flagella are the organs of locomotion in bacteria. They are semi-rigid structure that give movement to bacteria. The flagella are 3–20 μ in length and 0.01–0.03 μ in diameter.

Energy required: The rotation is due to flow of protons. In the absence of metabolic energy, it can be driven by proton motive force generated by ionophores. Bacteria living in alkaline conditions use energy of sodium ion gradient to drive flagellar motor.

Structure

Flagellum has three distinct regions, basal body or basal structure, hook and filament (Fig. 3.10).

- *Basal body:* It has a circular structure, with central rod and it has ring-like structures (one pair in Gram-positive and two pairs in Gram-negative bacteria. (Rings L and P are absent in Gram-positive bacteria).
- *Hook:* It is the portion of flagella which connects basal body to filament, which is present within cell envelope.
- *Filament:* It is connected to hook and projects as free flagellum. Flagella are made up of flagellin.

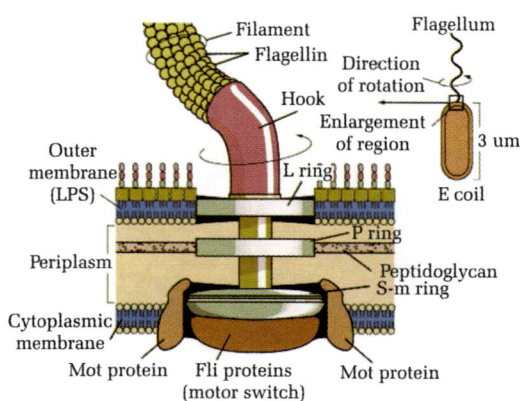

Fig. 3.10: Structure of flagella

Functions of Flagella

- They are the organs of locomotion of bacteria.
- They are antigenic in nature and antibody against them is used for diagnosis, e.g. in widal test, antibodies against flagellar antigens are used for diagnosis of enteric fever.
- Darting motility of vibrios, they act as virulence factor as they help the bacilli to penetrate through the mucus secretions.
- They also help the bacteria to move through the tissues.

Methods of Demonstration of Flagella

- Silver impregnation method
- Electron microscope
- Indirect methods as demonstration of motility by dark ground microscope, hanging drop preparation, demonstration of spreading growth in semisolid media (other indirect methods are swarming of *Proteus*, Cragies tube method)
- Leifsen method
- Ryu's method

Arrangements of Flagella (Fig. 3.11)

- **Monotrichous:** Single flagellum at one end, as present in *Vibrio cholerae.*
- **Amphitrichous:** Single flagellum at both the ends of bacteria (*Spirillium minus*).
- **Peritrichous:** Flagella all around the bacillus, e.g. *Salmonella.*
- **Lophotrichous:** Tufts of flagella at one or both ends as seen in *Spirillium.*

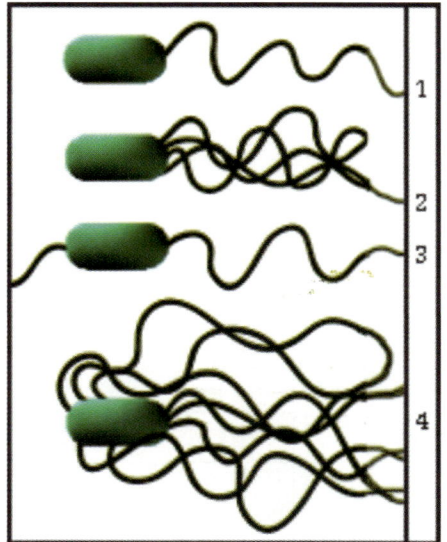

Fig. 3.11: Arrangements of flagella—(1) Monotrichous, (2) Lophotrichous, (3) Amphitrichous, (4) Peritrichous

Different Types of Motility of Bacteria

- **Darting motility:** *Vibrio cholerae (Campylobacter, Aeromonas, Plesiomonas)*
- **Active motility:** *Salmonella, Proteus*
- **Sluggishly motile:** *E. coli*
- **Nonmotile bacteria:** *Shigella, Acinetobacter*
- **Corkscrew motility:** *Spirochaetes*
- **Gliding motility:** *Mycoplasma*
- **Tumbling motility:** *Listeria monocytogenes*
- **Twiching motility:** *Kingella kingae.*

Other motile organisms without flagella are **Legionella** which is motile with apical knob, **Spirochaetes** are motile with endoflagella. (Amoeba forms pseudopodia, cilli are present on *Balentidium coli*, and flagella are present in parasites as *Leishmania donovani, Trypanosoma, Giardia,* and *Trichomonas*).

During motility, there is altered cell behavior which is brought in response to change in environment called sensory transduction. (Sensory transduction is also responsible for aerotaxis and phototaxis.)

Pili or Fimbriae

These are hair-like appendages present on a surface of bacterium rising from cytoplasmic membrane of some Gram-negative bacteria. They are short in comparison to flagella. Fimbriae, if present, are present all over the surface of bacterium. Their length (0.1μ–1μ) and breadth (10 nm) is shorter than flagella. Chemically they contain protein called **pilin.**

Types of Pili

There are two types of pili. With the help of adhesive pili, bacteria adhere to epithelial surfaces of host. Sex pili are special type as they cause attachment of two bacteria during conjugation , which is transfer of genetic material from one bacterium to other. They are longer than normal pili but they are present less in number.

They cause hemagglutination of guinea pig RBCs and may be inhibited by mannose on the basis of which they are classified as follows:

Type 1: They are mannose sensitive, they occur in *E.coli, Klebsiella, Shigella,* and *Salmonella.*

Type 2: They are devoid of adhesion and hemagglutinating property.

Type 3: They are mannose resistant, agglutinate RBCs only after heating. They are seen in some strains of *Serratia, Klebsiella.*

Type 4: They are mannose resistant and occur in *Proteus.*

Functions

1. **Sex pili** help in transfer of genetic material from one bacterium to another (male to female) by formation of conjugation tube.
2. The bacteria having pili form surface pellicle. This property is useful in identification of some bacteria.
3. **Ordinary pili** act as virulence factor by helping the bacteria to attach to epithelial surfaces causing infection. *E. coli* requires pili for adhesion to intestinal cells and then it produces enterotoxin. Similarly pathogens of genitourinary tract attach by pili.
4. Some bacteria are able to make pili as *Neisseria gonorrheae*, are able to make pili of other types and thus can still adhere to cells in presence of antibodies to their original type of pili.
5. Similar to capsule, pili inhibit phagocytosis by polymorphs.

Demonstration of Pili

- Electron microscope
- Hemagglutination with RBCs
- Surface pellicle formation in liquid medium
  Differences between flagella and fimbriae are given in Table 3.2.

Bacterial Spore (Endospore)

Spores are highly resistant stages of bacteria which are formed to survive in adverse conditions. As they are produced within the bacteria, they are called endospores. Each bacterium forms a single endospore that is released when mother cell undergoes autolysis. Single endospore on germination forms a single bacterium. Sporulation is not the method of reproduction.

List of bacteria which produce spores:
- Bacteria with bulging spores are anaerobic bacilli—*Clostridium* species.
- Aerobic bacillus produces nonbulging spores which are called *Bacillus anthracis*.
- Cocci producing spores are *Sporosarcina*.
- **Other bacteria** known to produce spores are *Sporolactobacillus, Sporotomaculum, Thermoactinomyces,* and *Sporomausa.*

TABLE 3.2: Differences between flagella and fimbriae	
Flagella	*Fimbriae*
Larger and thicker	Smaller and thinner
Organ of motility	Organ of adhesion
They are not straight	They are straight
Arise from cytoplasm or cytoplasmic membrane but not attached to cell wall	Attached to cell wall

Properties of Bacterial Spores (Fig. 3.12)

Core: It is spore's protoplast which contains nucleic acid and all components of the protein synthesizing apparatus and energy generating system which is based on glycolysis. Cytochromes are absent and short electron pathway involving **flavoproteins** is utilized.

Heat resistance of spores is due to their dehydrated stage and presence in large amounts of **calcium dipocolinate.**

Spore wall: Innermost layer surrounding the core of spore which contains peptidoglycans. On germination, it becomes vegetative cell wall.

Cortex: A thickest layer surrounding the inner spore membrane. It contains abnormal peptidoglycan which has a few cross linkages as compared to vegetative cell. Its autolysis is important in germination.

Coat: This layer makes spore resistant to chemical. It is made up of keratin-like protein.

Exosporium: It is made up of proteins, lipids, and carbohydrates. The function is unknown and this layer may be present or may not be present.

Sporulation: Role of Sigma Factor (Fig. 3.13)

Sporulation takes place under unfavorable conditions for bacteria. Initially a clear area occurs in protoplasm of bacteria. This area becomes opaque. Condensation of nuclear material occurs, forming fore spore. The cell membrane grows to form spore wall around it. Cortex surrounds it and multilayered spore coat is formed. The changes which occur represent a true process of differentiation. Products of some genes produce different parts of spores. The changes involve alternation of transcriptional specificity of RNA polymerase core protein and one or other promoter specific proteins called **sigma factor.**

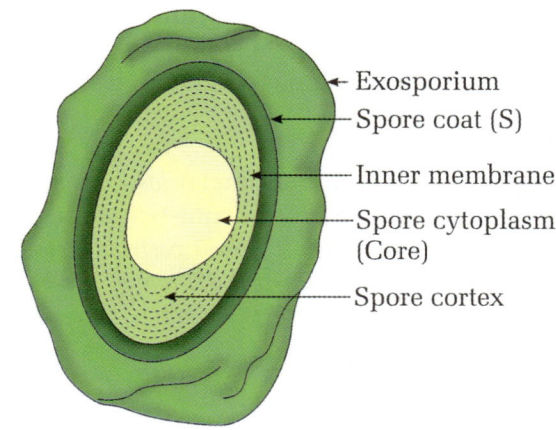

Exosporium
Spore coat (S)
Inner membrane
Spore cytoplasm (Core)
Spore cortex

Fig. 3.12: Structure of bacterial spore

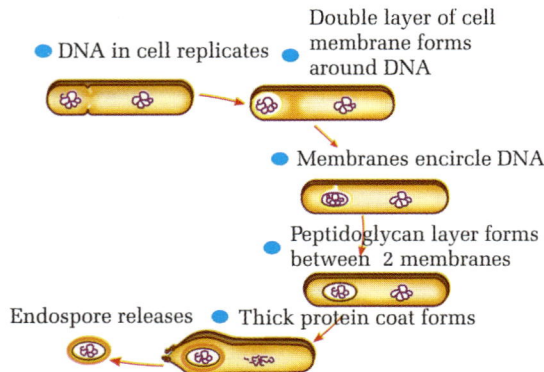

Fig. 3.13: Formation of endospores by sporulation

During vegetative growth, a sigma factor called **sigma prime** predominates, during sporulation other sigma factors are formed that cause spore genes to be expressed at various times in specific locations (differentiation of vegetative cell to spore **takes 7 hours** under standard laboratory conditions).

Germination of Spores

This occurs when condition becomes favorable. One spore on germination produces a single bacterial cell. Different stages of germination are as follows:

Activation: Once spores are produced from a vegetative form of bacterium, they are not converted into vegetative form, they take some time unless favorable conditions are available. Damage to spore coat is produced by heat, abrasion, acidity, free sulfhydryl compounds.

Initiation: Different bacteria different receptors which identify different signals in favorable conditions in the medium. The binding of receptor molecules of spore to different signals initiate germination of spores by breaking it peptidoglycan of spore cortex. Water is taken up; calcium dipocolinate is released, and a variety of substances are degraded.

Outgrowth: A new bacterial cell with spore protoplast comes out. A period of active synthesis occurs which terminates the cell division is called outgrowth.

Positions, Shapes of Spores

Location of spores may be terminal (*Clostridium tetani*—bulging terminal spore gives drumstick appearance), subterminal as seen in *Clostridium perfringens,* central bulging spore is seen in *Clostridium novyi* non-bulging central spore is seen in *Bacillus anthracis.*

Methods of Demonstration of Spores

Modified acid-fast stain: On a heat-fixed smear, pour carbol fuschin and with intermittent heating keep for 8–10 minutes. Decolorize with 0.5% H_2SO_4 or 2% nitric acid in absolute alcohol. Wash and counterstain with methylene blue for 1 minute.

Moller method: Heat-fixed smear is placed over a beaker with boiling water. As steam starts condensing, the undersurface of slide, add malachite green. Keep it for 2 minutes. Counterstain with dilute carbol fuschin.

Capsule

Many bacteria produce large amounts of polymers which is mostly polysaccharide in nature called glycocalyx. A condensed well-defined layer surrounding cell that excludes particles as Nigrosin is called capsule. If the polymers are loose and not organized, it is called **slime layer**.

Types

Based upon the chemical nature of capsule, the different types of capsule are as follows:
- Polysaccharide capsule is present in *Streptococcus pneumoniae, Klebsiella pneumoniae,* and *Cryptococcus neoformans.*
- Polypeptide capsule is seen in *Bacillus anthracis;* while *Yersinia pestis* capsule contains proteins.
- Teichoic acid is seen some capsulated types of *Streptococcus pyogenes.*

Functions of Capsule

- Capsule acts as a virulence factor for the bacteria. Capsule inhibits phagocytosis, thus escapes phagocytic killing. Being the outermost layer, it protects bacterium from external environment.
- As capsule is antigenic, its identification helps in diagnosis of infection, e.g. rapid diagnosis of meningitis caused by capsulated organisms as *Pneumococcus* is possible by detection of capsular antigen in CSF by latex agglutination test.
- Antibody to capsular antigen is protective hence capsule acts as a vaccine candidate, for example, 'Hib' vaccine of *Haemophilus influenzae.* Similarly capsular vaccine against most prevalent strains of bacteria, Pneumococci is used to produce pneumococcal vaccine.
- It plays role in formation of biofilms.
- Glycocalyx protects from desiccation.

Methods of Demonstration of Capsule

Negative staining with India ink or with Nigrosin (Fig. 3.14).

Special capsular staining methods
- *Anthony or Hiss method:* Treat freshly prepared smear with hot crystal violet for one minute. Wash with 20% solution of copper sulfate and blot. Capsule is blue and bacillary body is deep purple.

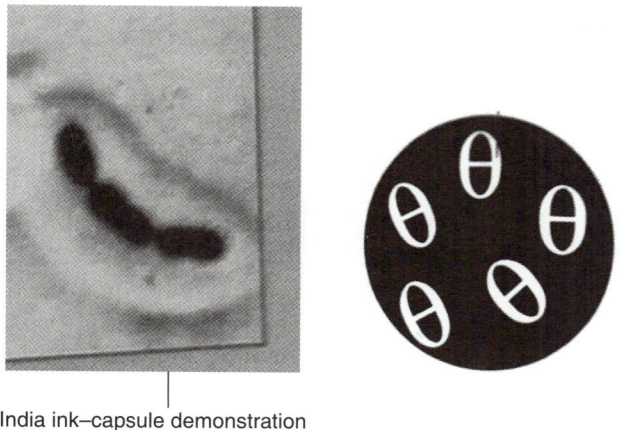

India ink–capsule demonstration

Fig. 3.14: Capsulated diplococci

- Muir's staining.
- Mayer mucicarmine.

Microcapsule and Macrocapsule

Microcapsule which cannot be detected by light microscope having small width less than 0.2µ, while macrocapsule has width more than 0.2µ, and detected by light microscope.

List of Capsulated Organisms

Bacteria

Polysaccharide capsule is seen in:
1. *Streptococcus pneumoniae*
2. *Klebsiella pneumoniae*
3. *Haemophilus influenzae*
4. *Meningococci*
5. *Bordetella*
6. *Yersinia pestis*
7. *Vibrio parahemolyticus*
8. *Clostridium perfringens*
9. Rare strains of *E. coli* which cause neonatal meningitis
10. Some isolates of *Staphylococcus aureus*.

Polypeptide capsule: *Bacillus anthracis*

Hyaluronic acid: *Streptococcus pyogenes*

Fungi
- *Cryptococcus neoformans*
- *Rhodotorulla*

Bipolar staining is seen in
1. *Yersinia pestis*
2. *Calmatobacterium granulomatous*
3. *Pseudomonas mallei*
4. *Pseudomonas pseudomallei*
5. *Vibrio parahemolyticus*
6. *Haemophilus ducreyi*

Volutin granules (metachromatic granules) (polar bodies) are common in *Corynebacterium diphtheriae, Gardenella vaginalis, Spirillium* sp., mycobacteria, and *Argobacterium tumefaciens.*

Volutin granules are basophilic bodies consisting of polymetaphosphate. Granules appear reddish with polychrome methylene blue or toludine blue **(metachromasia)**. Special stains used to stain granules are Albert's stain and Nasser's stain.

List of Organisms with Polar Flagella
- *Vibrio cholerae*
- *Campylobacter* species
- *Helicobacter pylori*
- *Aeromonas, Plesiomonas, Pseudomonas*
- *Legionella*

Pleomorphism: Some bacterial species show variation in size and shape of individual cells, e.g *Proteus* sp.

Involution form: Some species of bacteria show swollen, aberrant forms on ageing especially in the presence of high salt concentration.

The diagrammatic presentation of different bacteria is given in Fig. 3.15.

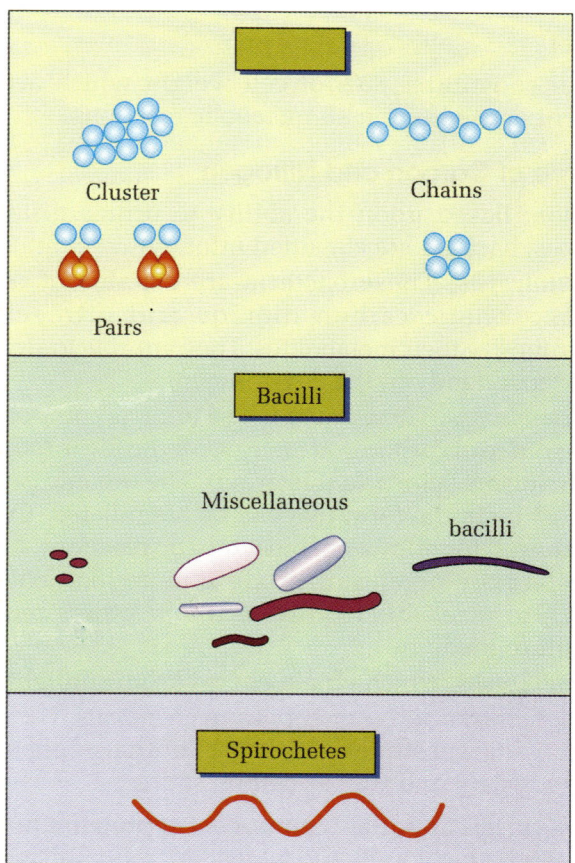

Fig. 3.15: Morphological forms of various bacteria

4

Physiology of Bacteria

BACTERIAL NUTRITION

For the growth of bacteria, following are the growth requirements:

- Water
- Source of carbon and nitrogen
- Inorganic salts
- Growth factors
- Conditions of incubation which include pH, temperature, O_2, CO_2, moisture and light.
- Source of energy

Water

Water constitutes 80% of cell weight which acts as solvent or medium in all metabolic reactions.

Source of Carbon and Nitrogen

Carbon: Based upon the ability to utilize different sources, bacteria are classified into:

a. *Autotrophs*: These bacteria are capable of using atmospheric carbon dioxide and nitrogen to synthesize their metabolites. They are able to survive independently in the environment.

b. *Heterotrophs*: These bacteria use organic compounds as source of carbon and energy. Medically important organisms belong to this group. The organic carbon must be in the form that can be assimilated. CO_2 is required for number of biosynthetic reactions. Many respiratory organisms produce more than enough CO_2 to meet this requirement, but others require culture medium.

c. *Phototrophs*, which obtain energy from sunlight.

d. *Chemotrophs* derive energy from chemicals. They use inorganic substrate as hydrogen or thiosulphates as a reductant and CO_2 as carbon source.

Nitrogen: It is important component of proteins, nucleic acids and other compounds. Most microorganisms can use ammonia as a source of nitrogen. Production of ammonia (NH_3) from deamination of amino acids is called ammonification.

Inorganic Salts

Trace sodium, potassium, manganese, calcium, phosphates, sulfates are known as growth factors or bacterial vitamins.

These are required for enzyme function. Mg and Fe are found in porphyrin derivatives. Mg and K are essential for function of ribosomes. Ca^{++} is required for constitution of cell wall of Gram-negative bacilli. In formulating medium, it is necessary to provide all these nutrients in the medium.

Sulfur source: Similar to nitrogen, sulfur acts as component of organic cell substrates. Most microorganisms can use sulfate as a source of sulfur, reducing sulfate to the level of H_2S. Some organisms can assimilate H_2S directly from the growth medium.

Phosphorus source: It is required as a component of ATP, nucleic acids and coenzymes.

Growth Factors

Some bacteria require particular substances as growth factors like vitamins, amino acids, purines and pyrimidines.

Some organic compounds which are required for cell growth and which are not produced by bacterium but present in the culture medium are known as growth factors. If suitable nutrients are provided in the medium, bacterial cell produces building blocks required for themselves. Each of these essential compounds is synthesized by enzymatic reactions and the enzyme is coded by a gene. If mutation is produced in bacterium, bacterium may loose capacity to form growth factors. If bacterium cannot synthesize the essential compounds, they should be provided in culture medium. The compound becomes growth factor for that organism.

Thus, in general, for growth of micro-organisms, the following nutrients must be provided:

Hydrogen donors and acceptors about 2 g/L, carbon source about 1 g/L, nitrogen source about 1 g/L, minerals: Sulfur and phosphorus about 50 mg/L each, trace elements: 0.1–1 mg/L, growth factors: amino acids—50 mg/L, and vitamins: 0.1–1 mg/L each.

Conditions of Incubation

Conditions of growth or the factors affecting growth of bacteria:

1. Temperature

Most of the human pathogens grow best at the 37°C. On the basis of temperature requirements, bacteria are classified as follows:

Psychrophilic: These bacteria grow optimally below 15°C and capable of growing at 0°C. They grow best at low temperatures (–5 to –15°C) and found in Arctic and Antarctic regions. These are soil saphrophytes.

Mesophilic: Bacteria which grow best at temperature 25–40°C are called mesophilic. They cause infections of warm-blooded animals. Human pathogens are mesophilic.

Thermophilic: These bacteria grow optimally at temperature greater than 45°C (55–80°C), most of them are spore bearers, e.g. *Clostridium* species, *Bacillus* sp. The lowest temperature which kills a bacterium under standard conditions in a given time is known as **thermal death point.**

2. pH

The optimum pH of most of the pathogens is 7.2–7.6 **(neutralophiles)**, growth is poor at pH 6 and above pH 9, and exceptions are *Lactobacilli*, which grow at acidic pH and *Vibrio* at pH 9. Some bacteria which require low pH 3 are **acidophiles**, those bacteria which require high pH 10.5 are **alkaliphiles**.

The upper end of temperature range tolerated by any given species correlates with thermal stability of that species. Microorganisms share with plants and animals the heat shock proteins response, a transient synthesis of a set of heat shock proteins.

3. Effect of Light

Some bacteria grow in dark. Photochromic atypical mycobacteria produce pigment in dark also.

4. Moisture

Fastidious bacteria require 60–70% humidity for their growth. They are called 'humidophilic'. To provide this condition, water-filled pans is placed at the bottom of incubator.

5. Gaseous Requirements

Carbon dioxide: Capnophilic bacteria are those require additional carbon dioxide **(5–10%)** for their growth, e.g *Brucella, pneumococci, Neisseria* species.

Such conditions can be produced by two ways:
- Special CO_2 incubator
- Candle extinction jar in which inoculated plate is kept. A candle is light up, a lid is placed cover jar—before candle flames out, it uses same O_2 producing CO_2.

6. Oxygen Requirements (Table 4.1)

- *Aerobic bacteria* require oxygen for their growth. Obligatory aerobes are strict aerobes which will grow only in presence of oxygen. Examples are *Vibrio cholerae, Mycobacterium tuberculosis.*
- *Anaerobic bacteria* grow in absence of oxygen. Strictly anaerobes die on exposure to oxygen. Example of obligate anaerobe is *Clostridium novyi.*
- Most of the bacteria of medical importance are *facultative anaerobes* which are ordinarily aerobic but also grow in absence of oxygen, e.g. *E. coli, Proteus* sp., *Salmonella* sp.
- *Microaerophilic organisms*: Those grow best in presence of low oxygen tension, e.g. *Leptospira, Campylobacter* sp., *Actinomyces israelii*. An oxygen 5–7% is used. This can be done by evacuation replacement method with N_2 as the major replacement gas and 5–10% CO_2. Some commercial systems used are Campy–Pak system (BBL) or Campylobacter Gas Generating kit (Unipath) (described in detail in the Campylobacter chapter).

TABLE 4.1: Different terms used based on different growth conditions		
Terms used	*Property*	*Example of organisms*
Growth atmosphere Strict (obligate) aerobe	Requires aerobic atmosphere for their growth	*Pseudomonas aeruginosa*
Strict (obligate) anaerobe	Will not tolerate oxygen	*Bacteroides fragilis*
Facultative anaerobe	It grows best aerobically	*E. coli, S. aureus*
Aerotolerant anaerobe	Anaerobic but tolerates exposure to air	*Clostridium perfringens*
Microaerophilic	Requires/prefers low oxygen	*Helicobacter* sp., *Campylobacter jejuni*
Capnophilic	Requires increased CO_2 levels	*Neisseria* spp.

Source of Energy in Aerobic and Anaerobic Bacteria

- **Aerobic bacteria** obtain energy through oxidation involving oxygen as terminal electron acceptor. In aerobes, the carbon and energy source may be oxidized to CO_2 and water. Energy is obtained by production of energy rich phosphate bonds and conversion of adenosine diphosphate (ADP) to adenosine triphosphate (ATP). The process is called **oxidative phosphorylation.**
- **Anaerobic bacteria** use other organic compounds as terminal electron acceptor. They obtain energy by fermentation. They use nitrates or sulfates as electron acceptors. In their metabolism, the series of oxidation and reduction reactions takes place, in which carbon and energy sources act as electron donor and acceptors. This process is called fermentation during which various energy rich phosphate bonds are formed by introduction of organic phosphate into intermediate metabolites. This is called **substrate level phosphorylation.** The energy rich phosphate groups are used for conversion of ADP to ATP.

The reasons why some bacteria are anaerobic are:
- The anaerobes do not have catalase, which breaks down H_2O_2 into H_2 and O_2.
- They contain enzyme superoxide dismutase.
- They may contain enzymes which are active only in anaerobic conditions (oxidation reduction).

Oxidation reduction (Redox) potential: In the production of suitable conditions for anaerobes, the important thing is the state of oxidation reduction of environment. The oxidizing or reducing condition is determined by the readiness of the system to accept or donate electrons. This is called redox potential.

Methods of detection of redox potential:
1. The electric potential difference between the medium and unattackable electrode kept within it is the redox potential.
2. Use of oxidation reduction indicators, which show different colors at different conditions and have pH range.

METHODS OF ANAEROBIASIS (GROWTH CONDITIONS OF ANAEROBIC BACTERIA)

1. *Displacement of oxygen with other gases (Fig. 4.1)*: For this method, McIntosh and Filde's jar is used. The jar has two openings, one is outlet which is connected to a vacuum pump and inlet which is connected with external gaseous cylinder containing CO_2, N_2, H_2. Palladised asbestos is the catalyst used, which is placed underside of the lid and it catalyses the reaction between remaining O_2 and H_2 to produce some amount of water.

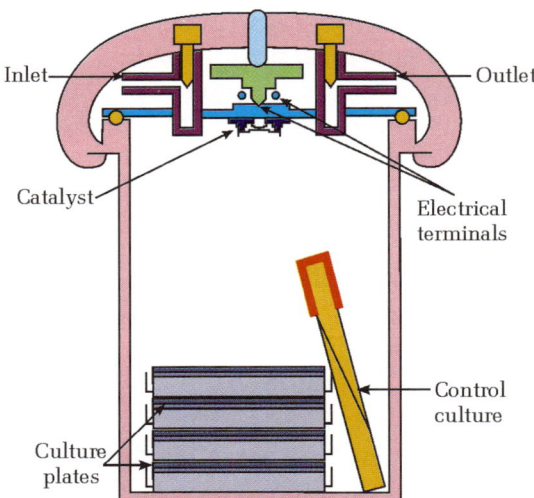

Fig. 4.1: McIntosh and Filde's anaerobic jar

Procedure: Culture media on which specimen is inoculated are placed at the bottom of jar. The catalyst is kept on underside of lid, and lid is closed. It is tightened with the help of screws. Inlet is closed. The outlet is connected to a vacuum pump so that the whole air and oxygen is removed; this is indicated by drop in pressure. Then the outlet is closed and inlet is opened, which is connected to a gas cylinder of mixture of gases so that pressure inside also increase. When remaining O_2 reacts with H_2 again, there is fall in pressure. The inflow of gases is repeated so that pressure becomes normal (90% H_2 + 10% CO_2 or 10% H_2 + 10% CO_2 + 80% N_2).

Quality control of working of jar: When culture plates are placed inside, outer tube of jar is connected to a test tube containing methylene blue as anaerobic indicator which is colorless at reduced conditions and becomes blue on oxidation, i.e. exposure to oxygen. This tube is heated while attaching so that initially the indicator is colorless and it should remain colorless at the end of anaerobic cycle. In some jars, the control tube is placed inside the jar itself.

2. *Gas pak system*: The gas pak contains mixture of chemicals in disposable envelope. A chemical reaction generates CO_2 and H_2. The gas pak after addition of the proper solvent is kept inside of the jar and lid is closed. Catalyst in the envelope permits combination of H_2 and O_2. These systems are commercially available and effective but they are costly.

The method is simple. There is no need of vacuum gas (cylinder or other source) and catalyst, but it is expensive.

3. *Anaerobic media*:
Robertson's cooked meat medium: This medium consists of meat particles of ox heart in nutrient broth. The unsaturated fatty acids in the medium provides the

anaerobic conditions. Also other reducing substances such as glutathione, cysteine utilizes oxygen and helps in anaerobiasis. The heating of medium before use removes the dissolved oxygen. The one more advantage of this medium is that if *Clostridia* are suspected, proteolytic and the saccharolytic conditions produced by *Clostridium tetani* and *Clostridium perfringens* respectively are observed in the medium.

Thioglycollate broth: This is another anaerobic medium. Haemin and vitamins are added to make it more enriched for the growth of nonsporing anaerobes.

Liquid media: The addition of reducing substances makes the medium anaerobic. Reducing substances are 1% glucose, 0.1% ascorbic acid and 0.1% cysteine. Liquid media are pre-reduced by holding in boiling water bath for 10 minutes to remove the dissolved oxygen, and then cooled quickly to 37°C just before use; sterile preparations of heat labile substances should be added after this heat treatment.

The effectiveness of reducing substances can be increased by making a liquid medium semisolid with addition agar (0.05–0.1%).

4. *Hungate procedure*: It is more meticulous procedure to prevent entry of air during preparation, inoculation and incubation, first developed by Hungate. All the manipulations are done under oxygen free conditions. Surface colonies are grown in roll tubes in which a thin layer of agar coats the inside of the tube. The medium must be transparent for surface colonies to be visible. This procedure uses blood agar.

5. *Anaerobic cabinets or chambers*: These are commercially produced for processing of specimens and subsequent incubation of cultures and subcultures in an oxygen free atmosphere enriched with 5–10% CO_2.

6. *Anoxmat*: This is an automated system. It evacuates the air from jar and replaces hydrogen from an external cylinder as McIntosh jar. The advantage is it is easier to handle, disadvantage is its cost.

BACTERIAL GROWTH AND MULTIPLICATION (Fig. 4.2)

It occurs by simple binary fission by which each bacterium will form two equal daughter cells. When maximum growth occurs and a critical mass is achieved, cell starts division. Double-stranded DNA separates into two single strands which form their complementary strands, thus two new double-stranded DNA molecules are formed which are equally distributed in two cells. A transverse septum grows across the cell from cell membrane, cell material is deposited and two cells get separated.

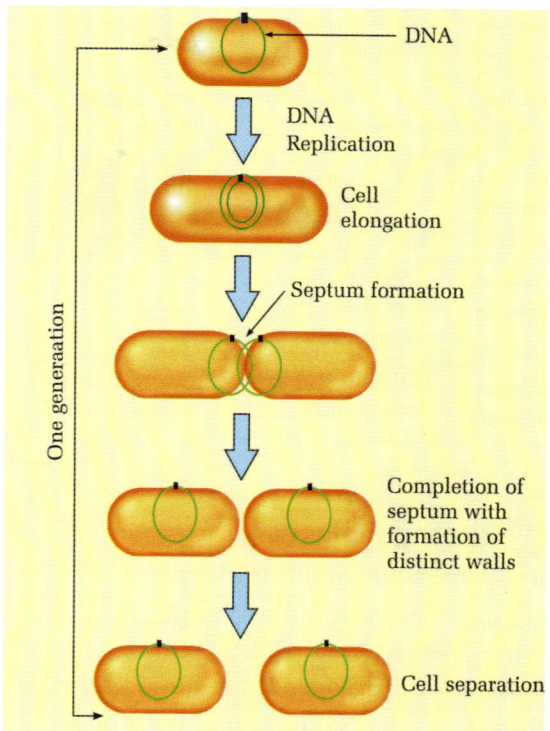

Fig. 4.2: Bacterial cell division

Bacteria divide by binary fission.

Generation or **population doubling time**: It is interval of time between two cell divisions. It is time required for parent cell to produce daughter cells. Generation time for coliform bacilli is 20 minutes, while for TB bacilli, it is 20 hours and for lepra bacilli, it is 20 days (Table 4.2).

During the bacterial growth, there is increase in size and increase in number. When maximum size is achieved multiplication starts. In the pool of multiplying bacilli, total count increases and it is the combination of live bacilli and dead bacilli.

Total counts of bacteria are the total of living and dead cells.

TABLE 4.2: Generation time of different organisms

Organism	Situation	Generation time
Viruses	In cell	<1 hour
Staphylococci		20–30 minutes
Salmonella	*In vitro*	24 hours
typhimurium	*In vivo*	5–12 hours
M. tuberculosis	*In vitro*	20 hours
	In vivo	Many days
Lepra bacillus	*In vivo*	2 weeks
Treponema pallidum	*In vivo*	30 hours

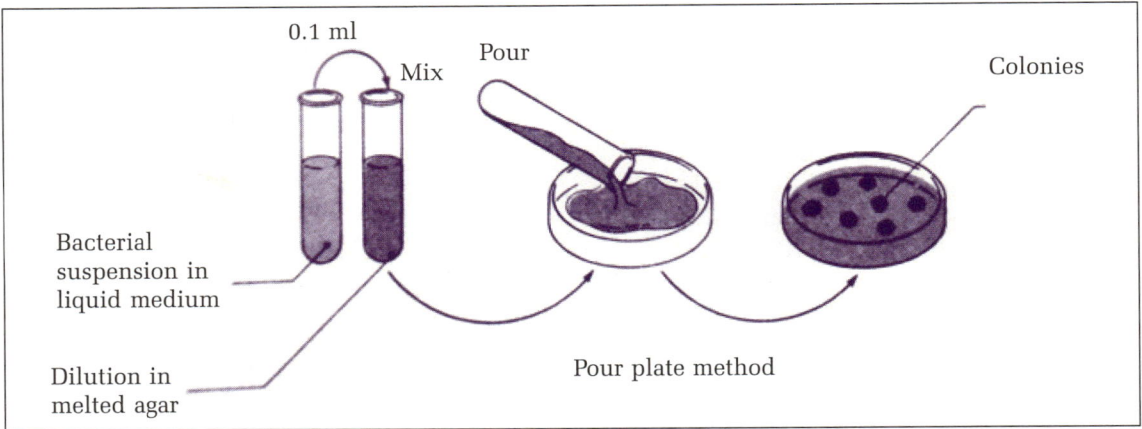

Fig. 4.3: Pour plate method

Direct Counting Methods

- Microscope with counting chamber.
- Electronic device (Coulter counter).
- Stained smear prepared by spreading a known volume of culture over a measured area of slide.
- Comparing relative numbers in smears of mixed culture with known number of other cells.
- Opacity measurements (absorptiometer, nephelo-meter).
- Separating cells by centrifugation/filtration and measuring their wet or dry weight.
- Chemical assays of cell components.
- Measuring nitrogen content.

   Viable counts are number of living cells, i.e. cells capable of multiplication.

Bacterial Counting by Pour Plate Method

Dilution method: In this method, most probable number (MPN) is calculated as it is done for counting *E. coli* in water samples to check drinking water.

Pour plate method (Fig. 4.3): This can be done for finding out bacterial counts in urine to access the significant counts. The original sample is diluted many times to decrease the population density. The most diluted samples are mixed with warm agar and poured into petridishes. Considering that each bacterium will form one colony (1 CFU= colony-forming unit), bacterial colonies on the medium are counted.

Continuous Culture

In liquid medium after many divisions, due to depletion of nutrients and accumulation of toxins, multiplication is halted and the total counts are different from viable counts. Cells can be maintained in the log phase by transferring them repeatedly into fresh medium of identical composition when they are still in log phase. The most common culture device is chemostat.

Bacterial Growth Curve (Fig. 4.4)

A bacterium is inoculated in a liquid medium at suitable temperature and pH. If we plot the graph of number of cells in relation to time, the culture passes through different phases of growth. This curve having different phases of growth is called bacterial growth curve.

Lag Phase

Immediately after the liquid medium is inoculated with the bacterium, for some time there is no increase in number of bacilli. They take some time to adapt to new environment of the medium. This phase is called as lag phase. After adaptation, bacteria take nutrients from the medium for their growth. When maximum size is achieved at the end of lag phase, bacteria start multiplying and enter in log phase. Thus in lag phase there is increase in size of bacteria but there is no increase in number.

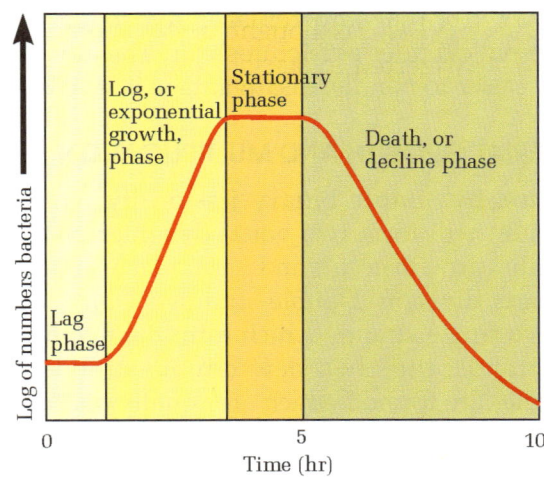

Fig. 4.4: Bacterial growth curve

Log Phase

In this phase, bacteria divide maximally hence there is exponential increase in number of bacilli. New cell material is being synthesized at a constant rate, but the new material is itself catalytic and mass increases. This continues until one of two things happen: Either one or more nutrients in the medium exhaust, or toxic metabolic products accumulate. When the cell concentration exceeds about 1×10^7/ml (in case of aerobic bacteria), the growth rate decreases until oxygen is forced into medium by agitation or by bubbling in air. When the bacterial concentration reaches $4–5 \times 10^9$/ml, the rate of oxygen diffusion cannot meet the demand even in an aerated medium, and growth is progressively slowed.

Stationary Phase

Bacteria die due to lack of nutrient or accumulation of toxic substances. An equilibrium is achieved between dying cells and new cells. Bacteria become Gram variable and show irregular staining (intracellular storage granules). Bacteria produce exotoxins and antibiotics in this phase.

Phase of Decline

In this phase, the number decrease due to cell death. Involution forms are common in this phase, cells become smaller and stain irregularly.

Important changes or characteristics of bacteria in different stages:

- *Lag phase*: Maximum size at the end
- *Log phase*: Bacterial cell stain uniformly
- *Stationary phase*: Production of toxins, antibiotics, production of spores, intracellular granules, staining irregular
- *Phase of decline*: Involution forms

A phenomenon which is called viable but not culturable (VBNC) is thought to be the result of a genetic response trigerred in starving, stationary phase cells.

Just as some bacteria form spores as a survival mechanism, others are able to become dormant without changes in morphology. When the appropriate conditions are available, VNBC resumes growth.

Maintenance of cells in the exponential phase: Cells can be maintained in exponential phase by transferring them repeatedly into fresh medium of identical composition while they are still growing exponentially. This is called continuous culture; the commonest type of continuous culture device used is chemostat. Continuous culture is more similar to conditions the bacteria get in human body.

Continuous systems can be operated as turbidostat or chemostat: In a turbidostat, the system includes an optical sensing device that measures the turbidity of cultures in the growth vessels and generates an electrical current that is used to regulate flow of fresh medium into the vessel and flow of spent medium and cells out of it. Thus the number of cells in the culture controls the flow rate and the rate of growth of culture adjusts to this flow rate.

In chemostat, the flow rate is set at a particular value and the rate of growth of culture adjusts to this flow rate.

Turbidometric methods: As bacterium may contain different particles which reduce scattering of light depending upon concentration, hence if a beam of light is passed through bacterial suspension, the amount of light transmitted through suspension may be reduced depending upon turbidity of medium. Measuring the amount of light that passes through the suspension of organisms with a spectrophotometer or optical measuring device can be used for estimating the amount of light absorbed or scattered by microorganisms proportional to the cell density.

When calibrated against bacterial suspensions of known concentration, **spectrophotometers** provide an accurate and rapid way to estimate the dry weight of bacteria by per unit volume of culture.

5

Classification, Nomenclature, Taxonomy

Taxonomy consists of classification in proper order unit-wise (group of unit called taxa); taxonomy also involves identification of unknown organism and naming it.

BACTERIAL CLASSIFICATION

The kingdom is divided into divisions, class, order, family, tribe, genus, and species (Fig. 5.1).

Phylogenetic Classification (Fig. 5.1)

Evolutionary arrangement of organisms in branching tree-like pattern is the phylogenic classification. It shows the pattern which is arranged based on evolution. It groups together the types which are related evolutionary and several groups are used as divisions, classes, orders, families, tribes, genera, and species.

Example of bacterium arranged in this classification:
Division: Protophyta
Class: Schizomycetes
Order: Eubacteriales
Family: Enterobacteriaceae
Genus: Eshcherichia
Species: coli

Adansonian Classification

It takes into consideration all the characteristics at the time of study and may not be based on phylogenetic relationship.

Molecular or Genetic Classification

The genetic relatedness is assessed by DNA hybridization or recombination. It is based on homology of DNA

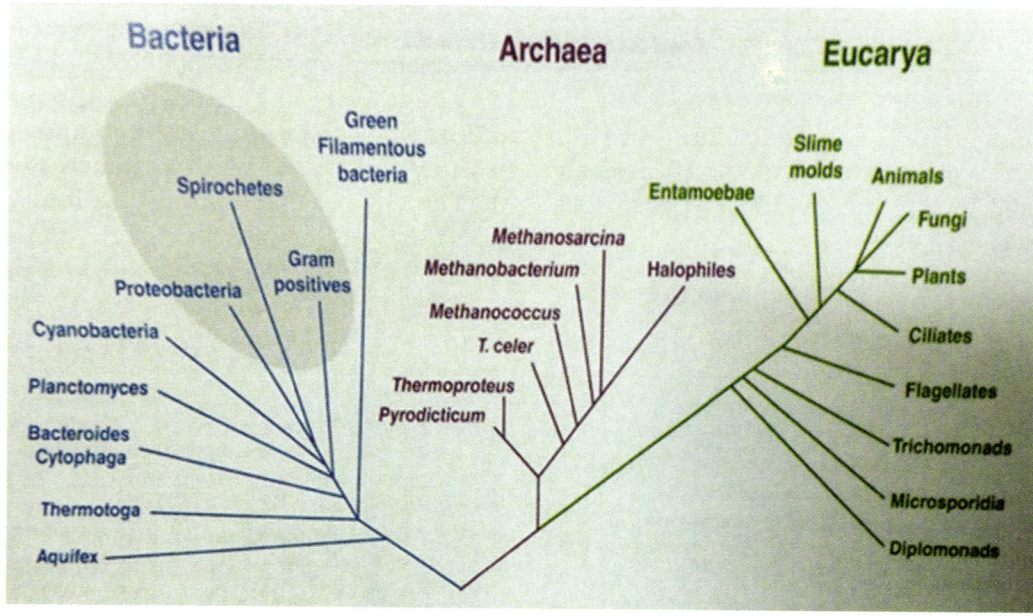

Fig. 5.1: Phylogenetic classification

sequences of the organisms. The DNA of the organism is first extracted, nucleotide sequence of DNA is studied by DNA hybridization or recombination methods.

DNA Composition

The hydrogen bonding between guanine and cytosine (G–C) base pairs in DNA is stronger than bond between adenine and thymine (A–T). Thus the melting or denaturation temperature of DNA (at which two strands of DNA separate) is primarily determined by the G+C content. At the melting temperature, the separation of the strand brings out about a marked change in the light absorption characteristics at wavelength of 260 nm and this is radially detected by spectrophotometrically.

By measuring the G+C content of a bacterium, it can be shown that there is a very wide range in the G+C component of DNA varying from about 25–80 moles% in different genera. However, for one species, the G+C content is relatively fixed or falls within a very narrow range, thus providing a basis for classification.

DNA Homology

It arranges individual organisms in groups on the basis of the homology of their DNA base sequences. Tests of DNA homology use the fact that double strand re-forms from separated strands during controlled cooling of a heated preparation of DNA. This annealing process can be readily demonstrated with suitably heated homologous DNA extracted from a single species, but it can also occur when a mixture of DNA from two related species is used; in later case, hybrid pairs of DNA strands are produced. These hybrid pairings occur with high frequency between complementary regions of DNA and the degree of hybridization can be assessed, if labeled DNA preparations are used. Binding studies with mRNA can also give information to complement these observations, which provide genetic evidence of relatedness among bacteria.

Organisms with different G+C ratios are very unlikely to show DNA homology. However, organisms with same or close G+C ratios do not necessarily show homology.

NOMENCLATURE

Organisms are given name with two components, the generic name starts with capital letter and name of species starts with small letter.

It is necessary to classify bacteria below a species level for epidemiological purpose. It is done by various typing methods. The typing methods may be based on phenotypic classification or genetic characteristics.

The name of the genus is in Latin. Name of the species is based on property of bacterium, e.g. *Staphylococcus*

albus (white colonies). The name of the species may be derived from animal origin, or name of the disease (*Vibrio cholerae* causes cholera), or the species name goes to the name of discoverer or place from which organism is isolated.

Intraspecific Classification

Typing methods for bacteria:

Phenotypic methods
- Bacteriocin typing
- Phage typing
- Biotyping based on biochemical reactions
- Serotyping by identifying the antigen by using antiserum
- Antibiogram

Genotypic methods
- Restriction fragment length polymorphism (RFLP)
- Ribotyping
- Plasmid profile

Colicin typing
- Bacteriocins are antibiotic-like substances which act on different strain of bacterium. Colins are bacteriocins produced by member of the family enterobacteriaceae. They may act on different genera of the family or different strains of the same species.
- Colicin typing uses the ability of test strain to inhibit indicator or passive strains maintained in laboratory. The pattern of inhibition is colicin type of the test strain.
- The test strain to be typed is diametrically streaked on peptone soya blood agar. The plate is then incubated at 35°C for 24 hours.
- After this incubation, the growth which is appeared on medium is removed with sterile glass slide. The plate is exposed to chloroform so that all organisms on inoculation are killed. Thereafter the plate is exposed to air for some time to remove remaining chloroform.
- Total 15 indicator strains are streaked on the plate at right angles to original growth lines of producer strains, 8 strains are inoculated on right side and 7 strains on left side.

Interpretation

After further overnight incubation at 37°C which will allow diffusion of colicins into medium during growth of producer strain to exert their antibiotic activity on particular indicator strains. The pattern of inhibition of the strains by test strain is the colicin type of the test strain.

6

Culture Media

TYPES OF CULTURE MEDIUM: LIQUID AND SOLID

When a specimen is inoculated on solid medium, if pathogens are present, they will multiply overnight and produce individual colonies. One bacterium produces one colony, i.e. colony-forming unit (CFU). The colony morphology of each bacterium varies which helps to identify the pathogen. Once the pathogen is isolated in pure form, we proceed for antibiotic sensitivity testing on Mueller Hinton agar which is a solid medium. Even if there is more than one type of colony on solid medium, with the help of colony morphology one can make out colony of pathogen from mixed population for further identification and antibiotic susceptibility testing.

When the specimen is inoculated in liquid medium the growth is seen in the form of turbidity. There is one disadvantage with the liquid medium. If mixed flora is present in specimen, we cannot differentiate the pathogen, as growth is seen as turbidity. But still there are some indications when we use liquid media.

Uses of Liquid Medium

When organisms are diluted in the specimen, we need to inoculate first large volume of specimen in liquid medium. Once turbidity appears, sub-culturing is done on solid medium.

1. Blood culture (Fig. 6.6) is first done in liquid medium.
2. Many biochemical tests media are liquid media.
3. Culturing in liquid medium is done for preparation of antigens or vaccines.
4. MIC (minimum inhibitory concentration) and MBC (minimum bactericidal concentration) is calculated in liquid media by broth dilution methods.

Solid Media

Uses

- When specimen is inoculated on solid medium, we can isolate the pathogen in pure form.

- Solid medium, i.e. Mueller Hinton agar, is used for antibiotic sensitivity testing by disc diffusion method.
- Some biochemical media are solid media.

Substances used to solidify the media are: 1. Gelatin, 2. Potato, 3. Serum or egg, 4. Agar.

Most of the solid media use agar (agar-agar) for solidification which is obtained from sea weeds.

Characteristics of agar as solidifying agent are:

- At incubation temperature, it remains as firm gel in watery solution.
- It is bacteriologically inert; it does not add any nutrition or does not contain any inhibitory substance. The melting points and solidifying points are different which are 95°C and 42°C, respectively. Also the low solidifying point of agar makes it useful because we can add heat sensitive nutrients to be mixed with it in the molten state at 45°C.

Common Contents of Media

- *Water:* Tap water is suitable for media but if supply is not proper distilled water is used.
- *Agar:* It is used in the concentration of 2–3%. It is obtained from seaweeds. New Zealand agar has twice the jellifying capacity of Japanese agar.
- *Peptone:* It contains peptones, proteases, amino acids, inorganic salt such as phosphates, potassium, and magnesium. Peptone is derived from water-soluble products obtained from heart muscle, casein, and fibrin by digestion with proteolytic enzymes.
- *Casein hydrolysate:* It contains amino acids obtained by hydrolysis of milk protein, casein.
- *Meat extract:* It is obtained by hot water extraction of lean beef which is concentrated by evaporation. Commercially prepared meat extract is known as **Lab-Lemco.**

- *Yeast extract*: It is prepared from baker's yeast, contains amino acids as growth factors (vitamin B_{12} group).
- *Blood or serum*: Oxalated sheep blood is used (5–10%).

Classification

Media are classified as solid, liquid and semisolid, simple and complex media, differential media, enriched media, enrichment media, selective media, biochemical tests media or ordinary.

a. Example of Simple (Basal) Medium

Example of **simple (basal)** solid medium is nutrient agar. The example of simple liquid medium is peptone water (Fig. 6.1).

b. Enriched Medium

If blood, serum or egg is added to basic medium to support the growth of fastidious organisms, it becomes enriched medium. The examples are blood agar (contains blood) and chocolate agar (RBCs are lysed, some substances present in RBCs are released which support the growth of specific bacteria such as *Haemophilus influenzae*, meningococci, gonococci, and *Streptococcus pneumoniae*).

Brain heart infusion broth (BHIB): It supports the growth of anaerobes as well as fungi apart from other bacteria.

Loffler's serum slope used for growth of *Corynebacterium diphtheriae* (Table 6.1).

c. Enrichment Medium (Table 6.1)

When we are trying to isolate the pathogen from a site which contains commensal flora, we add certain substances to basal liquid medium to inhibit the growth of commensals or which supports the growth of pathogen, it becomes enrichment medium. Take the

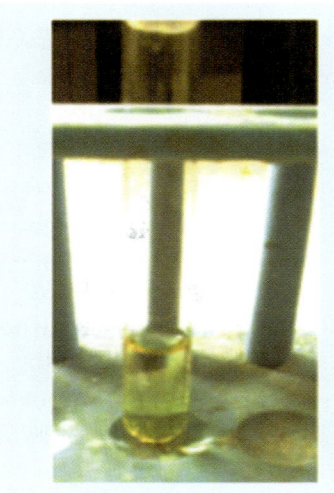

Fig. 6.1: Peptone water

example of culturing Salmonella from fecal sample. Fecal sample normally contains commensals as *E.coli*, *Proteus* and other bacteria. They will try to inhibit the growth of pathogen, i.e. *Salmonella*, we add some substances to prepare enrichment media as selenite F, tetrathionate broth. Other example of enrichment medium is alkaline peptone water for *vibrios*.

d. Selective Medium

It works on the same principle as that of enrichment medium, the difference is inhibitory substances are added to solid media to prepare selective medium. Blood potassium tellurite agar for *Corynebacterium diphtheriae*, deoxycholate citrate agar for *Salmonella* and *Shigella* and thiosulfate citrate bile salts sucrose agar for *Vibrio cholerae* are the examples of selective media.

e. Differential Media

Growth pattern of bacteria makes it possible to differentiate two groups of organisms. MacConkey's agar is able to differentiate between lactose fermenting organisms as *E.coli*, *Klebsiella* (pink colonies) from nonlactose fermenting bacteria as *Salmonella*, *Shigella*, *Proteus* which produce colorless colonies on this medium.

MacConkey's agar also acts as indicator medium which contains neutral red and sugar lactose. Due to lactose fermentation, acid pH is produced which changes color of indicator to pink.

f. Transport Media

These media maintain the viability of bacteria during transport of specimen. Commonsals may try to overgrow; this is avoided in transport media.

Stuarts transport medium is non-nutrient soft agar gel with reducing agent to prevent oxidation. Charcol neutralizes bacterial inhibitors. This medium may be used for gonococci. **Sach's buffered glycerol saline** is transport medium for enteric pathogen as *Shigella*, also Cary Blair's medium is used for *Salmonella*, *Shigella*, *Vibrio*, *Campylobacter*.

g. Complex Media

All media apart from simple media are complex media. They have added nutrients for the growth of bacteria.

h. Synthetic Media (Defined Media)

These are prepared from pure chemicals and their exact composition is known. Dubo's medium with tween 80 is example of synthetic medium.

i. Indicator Media

These media contain an indicator which changes color due to bacterial growth. MacConkey's medium, Wilson

Blair medium are examples. *Salmonella typhi* produces black colonies on Wilson Blair medium. Most of the selective media are indicator media, e.g. thiosulphate citrate bile salts agar (*Vibrio* ferments sucrose present in medium and produce yellow colonies).

Composition, uses and methods of sterilization of commonly used media are given in Table 6.1.

Nutrient Agar (NA)

It is identified by its straw color. This medium is prepared from ready to use dehydrated powder, supplied by different companies. It contains peptone, yeast extract, sodium chloride and agar (Fig. 6.2).

Method of preparation: Dissolve 2.8 gm of powder in 100 ml of distilled water by boiling.

Method of sterilization: Autoclaving at 121°C for 15 minutes. The pH should be in the range of 7.2–7.6.

Uses

- It is a simple solid medium. It can be used for antibiotic susceptibility testing.
- Oxidase positive bacteria are first subcultured from selective media on NA to perform the oxidase test.
- Similarly agglutination test with colonies is performed from NA plate.
- Bacteria grown on an agar slant can be used for the preservation of the isolates.

It is nutrient broth solidified by agar (sterilized by autoclave).

Blood Agar

It is prepared by adding blood (5%) to sterile nutrient agar that has been melted and cooled to 50°C. It is enriched medium. Some bacteria produce zone of complete lysis (clearing of medium around colonies)

TABLE 6.1: Composition, uses and methods of sterilization of commonly used media

Name of medium	Type	Main constituents	Method of sterilization	Uses
Glucose broth	Basal liquid	Nutrient broth, 0.5% glucose	Autoclave	Cultivation of fastidious organisms, some laboratories use it and along with taurocholate broth for blood culture
Tetrathionate broth	Enrichment, Liquid	Na-thiosulfate, Nutrient broth, CaCO$_3$	Autoclave	Enrichment medium for stool sample for *Salmonella* and *Shigella*
Selenite F	Enrichment, Liquid	Peptone water, Na-selenite	Autoclave	Enrichment medium for stool sample for *Salmonella* and *Shigella*
Alkaline peptone water	Enrichment, Liquid	Peptone water at pH 9	Autoclave	Enrichment medium for stool sample for *Vibrio cholerae*
Loffler's serum slope	Enriched solid slope	Glucose, Nutrient broth, horse serum	Inspissation	For *Corynebacterium* Advantage—growth appears within 6–8 hours and metachromatic granule formation enhanced
Lowenstein-Jensen medium (Fig. 6.5)	Enriched solid slope	Whole egg, malachite green, glycerol, mineral salt solution	Inspissation	Culture of *Mycobacterium tuberculosis*, atypical mycobacteria and *Nocardia*
Dorset egg medium	Enriched solid slope	Egg, nutrient broth	Inspissation	Culture of *Mycobacterium tuberculosis*
Stuart's transport medium	Transport medium		Autoclave	Swab from a case of gonococci, anaerobic transport medium
Glycerol saline	Transport medium		Autoclave	Enrichment medium for stool sample for *Shigella*
TCBS medium	Selective	Thiosulfate, citrate, bile salts, sucrose, agar	Steam at atmospheric pressure	Selective medium for stool sample for *Vibrio cholerae*
Blood potassium tellurite medium	Selective	Blood agar, Potassium tellurite	Autoclave	Selective for *Corynebacterium*

Concentration of malachite green is 0.025% which is between Petragnani medium (0.52%) and American Thoracic Society (ATS) medium which has 0.02% malachite green and it is less inhibitory and recommended for culture of sterile body fluids.

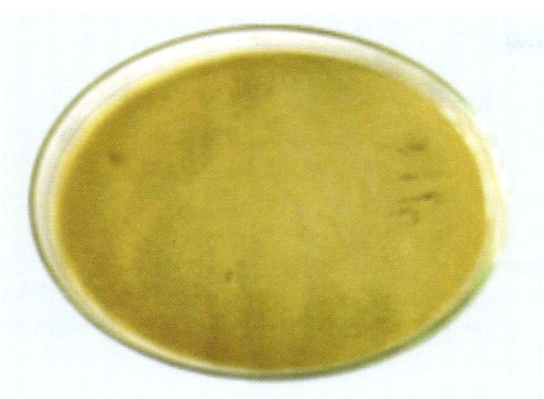

Fig. 6.2: Nutrient agar (NA)

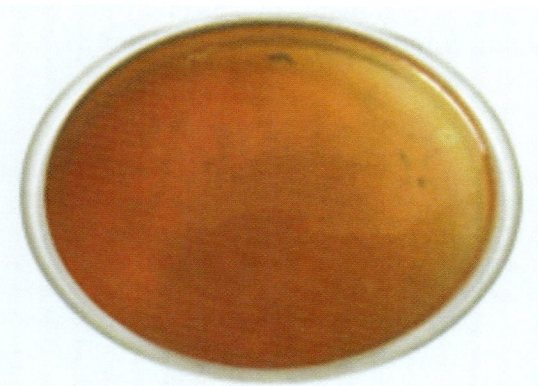

Fig. 6.3: Blood agar

MacConkey's Agar

It is differential medium used for members of family Enterobacteriaceae. It contains taurocholate as bile acid which inhibits nonintestinal bacteria and lactose with neutral red as an indicator. If NaCl is removed from the medium, swarming of *Proteus* is inhibited (Fig. 6.4).

Preparation of medium: Peptone and bile acid is dissolved by heating in water. Add agar, dissolve it in steamer or autoclave. Adjust pH to 7.5. Add lactose and neutral red—shake it, mix it and add to the medium.

Method of sterilization: Heat in autoclave with free steam (100°C) for 1 hour. The medium should be reddish brown in color. Nowadays, ready to use dehydrated power is available. The medium is used at concentration of 5.2 g in every 100 mL of water.

Storage of culture media: Prepared sterilized media in separate bottles or tube can be stored at room temperature for weeks. Keep media plates in refrigerator.

called betahemolysis. Zone of partial hemolysis is called alpha hemolysis. *Vibrio cholerae* produces hemo-digestion on blood agar which is very larger clearing of medium (Fig. 6.3).

Method of sterilization: Nutrient agar is first sterilized by autoclaving and while it is cooling, blood is added under aseptic precautions.
• BA is enriched, differential and indicator medium.

Chocolate Agar (Heated Blood Agar)

Due to its chocolate color, it is called chocolate agar. It is obtained by heating 10% sterile blood in sterile nutrient agar. Melt the agar, cool it to 75°C, add blood and mix properly. Chocolate agar has added advantage over blood agar as factor X and factor V present inside the RBCs are released which are required for the growth of *Haemophilus influenzae*.

Mueller Hinton Agar

It contains beef infusion 300 mL, casein hydrolysate 17.5 g, starch 1.5 g, distilled water 1 liter (sterilized by autoclave). This medium is used for antibiotic sensitivity by Kirby-Bauer disk diffusion method.

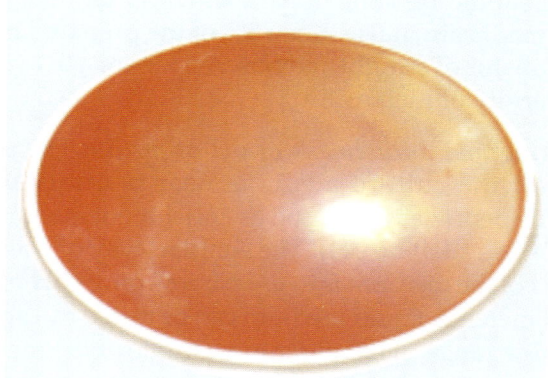

Fig. 6.4: MacConkey agar

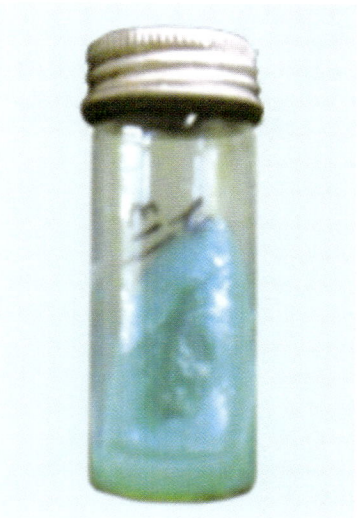

Fig. 6.5: L-J medium

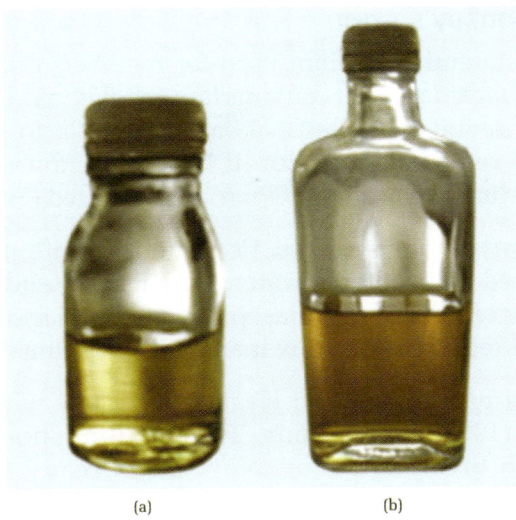

(a)   (b)

Fig. 6.6: Pediatric (a) and adult (b) blood culture bottles Hartley's broth

QUALITY CONTROL OF MEDIA

It is advised before each batch of medium is issued for use or should be done in parallel with first time when fresh media are in use. Keep 5% of the prepared media in incubator overnight and observe for growth to check the sterility of media.

Checking and adjustment of pH of media: The pH of most of the culture media is near neutral (except alkaline peptone water used as enrichment medium for vibrios has alkaline pH). The simplest way of checking the pH of the medium is to use narrow range pH papers or pH meter. A liquid medium can be tested by dipping a narrow range pH paper into a sample of the medium when it is at room temperature, comparing with color chart. An agar medium is tested by pouring a sample medium into a small beaker or petridish and when it

has solidified, laying a narrow range pH paper on its surface.

The pH of the medium is as directed in the method of preparation of medium. Minor adjustments are done using 0.1 mol/L (N/10) sodium hydroxide when the medium is too acidic and 0.1 mol/L (N/10) hydrochloric acid, if it is too alkaline.

When adjusting the pH of a large volume of the medium, it is best to do adjustments for 10 ml of medium first, then calculate the amount required for remaining volume.

Composite media are useful for identification of bacterial isolate. It becomes economical and convenient as a single composite medium indicates different properties of organism. In TSI medium, we detect fermentation and/or gas with or without H_2S.

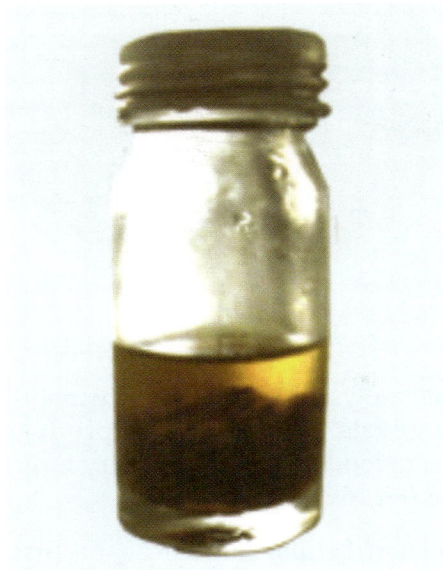

Fig. 6.7: Robertson's cooked meat medium

7

Culture Methods

Instruments used to seed culture media depend upon the nature of the medium and inoculum. Nichrome wire no. 24 SWG is generally used. One end of it is inserted into a special aluminum holder. The wire is sterilized by holding in Bunsen flame till it becomes red hot.

- *Wire loop* (Fig. 7.1): The free end is converted in the form of a loop of 2–4 mm diameter. It holds a large drop of liquid (*Note*: Presterilized loops—disposables are available in market). It is sterilized by flaming till it becomes red hot. For counting the bacterial colonies by semi-quantitative method, a standard loop is used which holds a drop of 0.001 mL. Nichrome wire is cheap. Wire loop is used to inoculate culture media, for preparation of smears, and for collection of urethral discharge directly from urethral meatus from a case of gonorrhea.
- *Straight wire*: It is used to stab cultures and for picking single colony for biochemical tests. Thick wire is used to handle tenacious growth as fungus.
- *Scalpel*: Sterile scalpel is used for making inoculations with scrapping from tissues and ulcers.
- *Pasteur pipettes*: It is capillary pipette with rubber teat.

Methods of Inoculations (Aerobic Culture Methods)

Streak method (surface plating) (Fig. 7.2): It is the most routine method for inoculation of specimens on solid media with the help of loop.

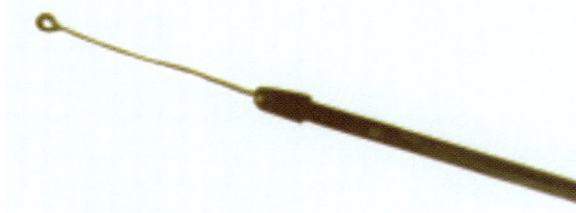

Fig. 7.1: Inoculation nichrome loop (sterilized by flamed till it becomes red hot)

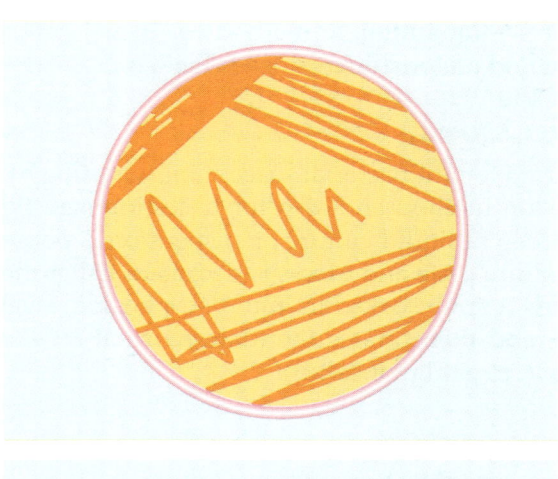

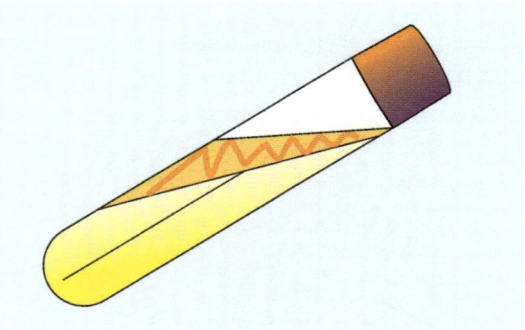

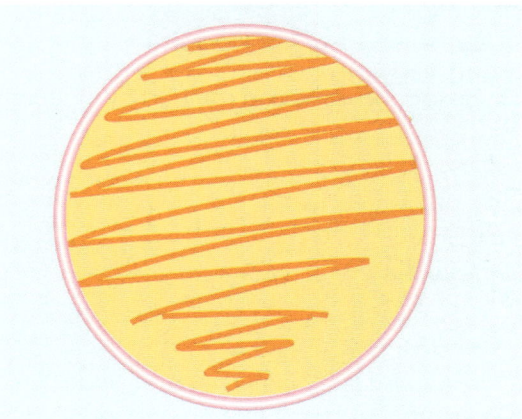

Fig. 7.2: Surface streaking methods

Hexagonal Streaking (Fig. 7.3)

- Primary inoculation can also be done from swab or other devise. The material is spread on to surface of agar making a well.
- The inoculum is spread by drawing parallel lines in different segments of the medium taking precaution of intermittent heating, to get isolated colonies (hexagonal method), confluent growth occurs at well, while individual colonies appear on the streaks away from well.
- This solves the purpose of isolation in pure form. (*Note*: While inoculating urine on primary plates for counting organisms by semiquantitative method, loop is not heated intermittently.)
- For semiquantitative method for urine, "T" shape method of spreading is used (Fig. 7.4).

Lawn Culture or Carpet Culture

It is used for antibacterial susceptibility testing by disk diffusion method and also for bacteriophage typing. Specimen of liquid culture or suspension is poured on the culture plate and excess is decanted. Other method is using a swab soaked in liquid suspension, swab the plate, and then rotates the plate twice at 60°C again swab it, to get lawn culture.

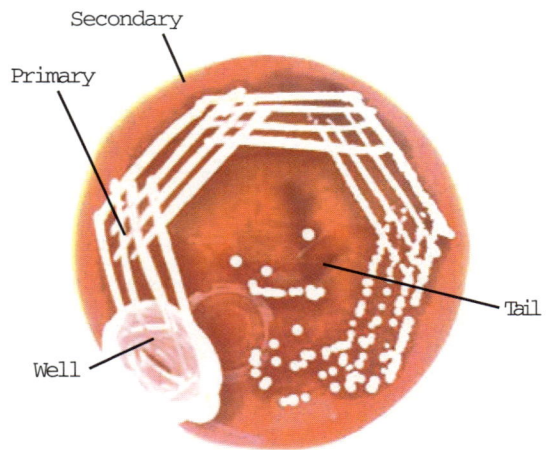

Fig. 7.3: Hexagonal streaking method by inoculation loop

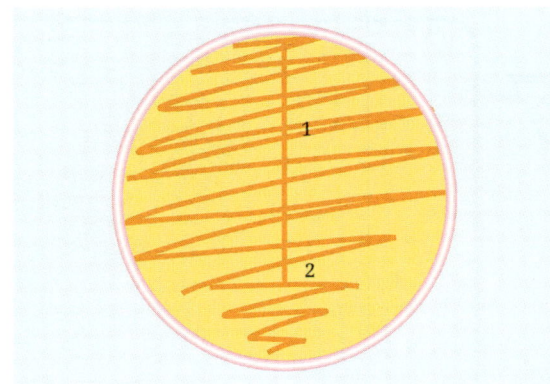

Fig. 7.4: T-shaped streaking method of inoculation used for urine sample for semiquantitative method

Stroke Culture

It is done on agar slant for pure growth of bacteria for agglutination test from colonies; as done in *Salmonella, Shigella*, and *Vibrio*.

Stab Culture

It is done by stabbing the slant with straight wire for demonstration of gelatin liquefaction test. This method of inoculation is also used for maintenance of stock cultures of bacteria in semisolid media.

Pour Plate Method

This method is used to find out quantity of bacteria in urine, for bacteriological analysis of water and to find out viable count.

The inoculum to be tested is serially diluted, e.g. urine is diluted in saline to produced dilutions as 1:2, 1:4. 1:8, etc. Known amount (1 ml) of diluted inoculum is mixed with 15 ml of melted agar at 45–50°C and mixed well in separate tubes. The contents of each tube poured on sterile agar plate, allowed to set and incubated at 37°C. The bacterial colonies which appear throughout the depth of medium are counted. The number give bacterial count per 1 ml of inoculum.

Sweep Plate Method

Culture media are rubbed over the cloths; it is useful in studying bacteria on fabrics.

8

Identification of Bacteria

Identification of bacteria is done on the basis of the following characteristics

1. Morphology
2. Colony (cultural) characteristics
3. Biochemical tests
4. Serological identification
5. *Phenotypic methods of identification of isolate*: It can be done by conventional ways by Gram's reaction, biochemical characteristics and in some bacteria by serotyping
6. Animal pathogenicity testing
7. Serological tests for detection of antigens in tissues by direct fluorescence, ELISA
8. Detection of antibodies (it is used for retrospective diagnosis of infections)
9. Various semiautomated or automated methods are available commercially as API system, Vitek systems which cause early and easy identification of bacteria
10. *Molecular methods include*: PCR, LCR, NASABA, DNA probes, hybridization, DNA chips, microarray
11. Mass spectrometry (MALDI)
12. Identification of anaerobe by analysis of fatty acids produced by gas–liquid chromatography
13. Nanotechnology

Important Cultural Characteristics (Growth) in Identification

Growth on solid media: Following colony characteristics should be noted (Figs 8.1 and 8.2):
- *Size of colony*: It may vary, it is few millimeters.
- *Shape of colony*, e.g. circular
- *Surface*: It may be smooth or rough; fresh isolates give smooth surface. Granular, rough surface usually given by *Bacillus subtilis* which is laboratory contaminant. Rarely *Pseudomonas stutzeri* produces rough surface. Smooth to rough variation of colony is seen in *Salmonella typhi*, rough variants occur in *Neisseria gonorrhoeae*.

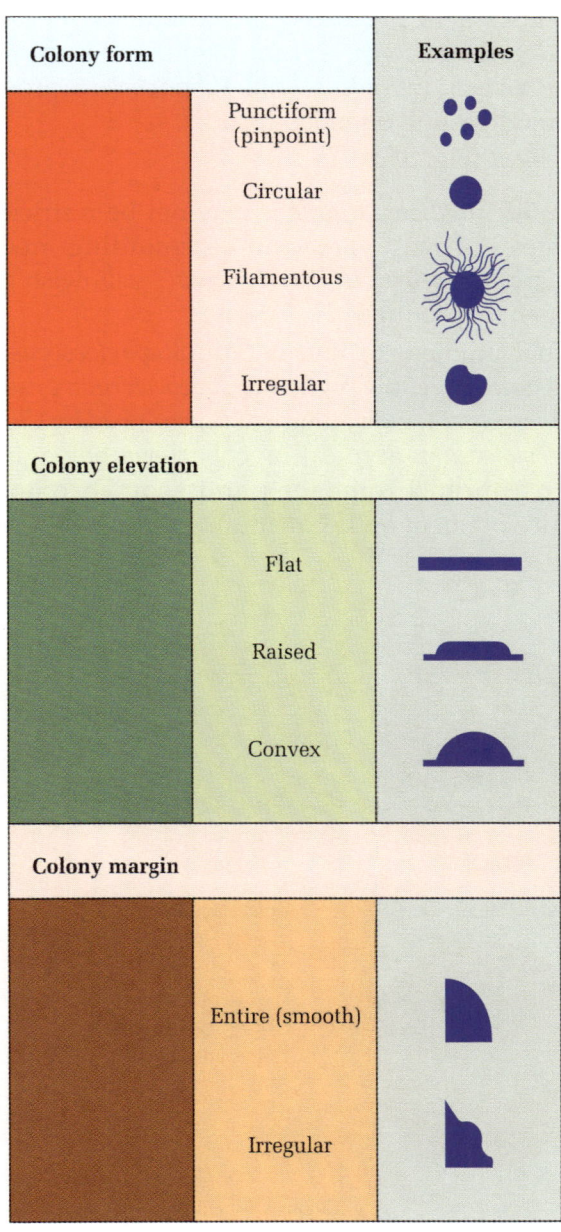

Fig. 8.1: Colony characteristics

- *Elevation*: *E. coli* produces flat colonies, *Klebsiella* produces raised dome-shaped colonies, and *Pneumococcus* forms draughtsman colonies with central umbonation, most of the members of Enterobacteriaceae form low convex colonies. *Pseudomonas* produces colonies which are slightly flat called as "effuse".
- *Edge*: Different types are entire edge or crenated or lobate or fimbriate or ciliate. Irregular edge is characteristic of *Pseudomonas aeruginosa.*
- *Consistency*: Mucoid type of colonies are seen in *Klebsiella* sp. Other types are butryous firm, friable.
- *Hemolysis on blood agar (Fig. 8.2)*: It is produced by *Staphyococcus aureus, Streptococcus pyogenes*; alpha hemolysis is produced by viridans streptococci and pneumococci. Target hemolysis is given by *Clostridium perfringens* while *Vibrio cholerae* produces hemodigestion on blood agar.
- *Pigment* (Fig. 8.3).

Diffusible pigment: Pigment may not be restricted to colonies but may spread in surrounding medium (diffusable), as seen in *Pseudomonas*—yellowish green pigment is produced.

Other pigment producers are: *Staphylococcus* produces golden-yellow pigment, *Flavobacterium* produces yellow pigment, violet pigment is produced by *Chromobacter violaceum*; atypical mycobacteria belonging to groups photochromogens and scotochromogens produce pigment on L-J medium.

Swarming: It is produced by *Proteus* on nutrient agar or on blood agar. *Clostridium tetani* may produce swarming on blood agar which is anaerobically incubated. Growth is produced in wave-like pattern.

Description of growth in liquid media
1. *The degree of growth*: Scanty, moderate, abundant
2. *Presence of turbidity and type of turbidity*: Uniform or not
3. Presence of deposit, surface pellicle (it is due to fimbria).

Gram-stained smear should be described in following heads which gives clue in identification
1. *Staining reaction*: Gram reaction may be positive or negative. Irregular staining is seen in *Mycobacterium tuberculosis* (Z-N staining). Staining may be variable as seen in *Clostridium perfringens.*
2. *Shape*: Spherical bacteria are cocci; bacilli are rod shaped, coccobacillary, or filamentous. If cocci are flame-shaped/lanceolate, they are *Streptococcus pneumoniae*. Bean-shaped cocci are seen in gonococci. Clusters are seen staphylococci while chains are seen *Streptococcus pyogenes.*

Characteristics of bacilli to be noted
1. Straight or slightly curved (*Mycobacterium tuberculosis*).
2. *Sides*: Sides are parallel in *E. coli, Klebsiella, Enterobacter* and *Citrobacter*. Convex sides are seen in plague bacillus (*Yersinia pestis*).

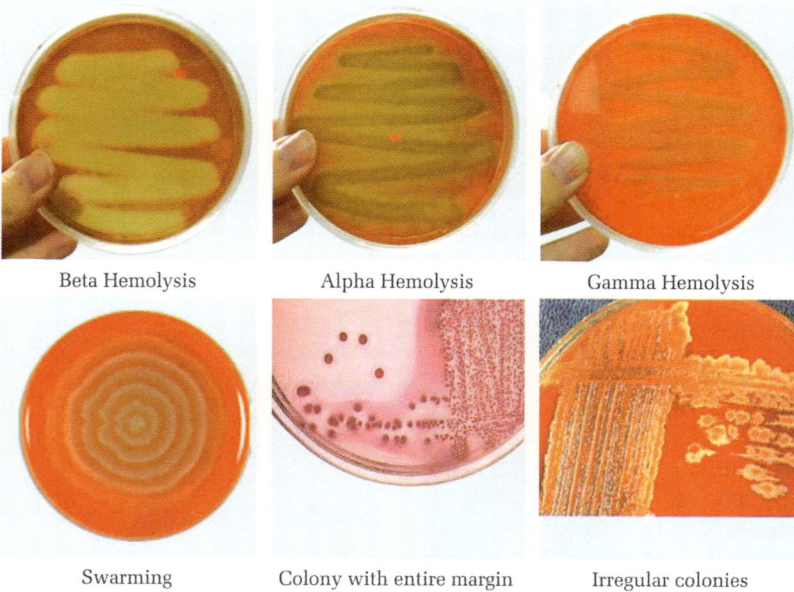

Fig. 8.2: Colony characteristic on different media

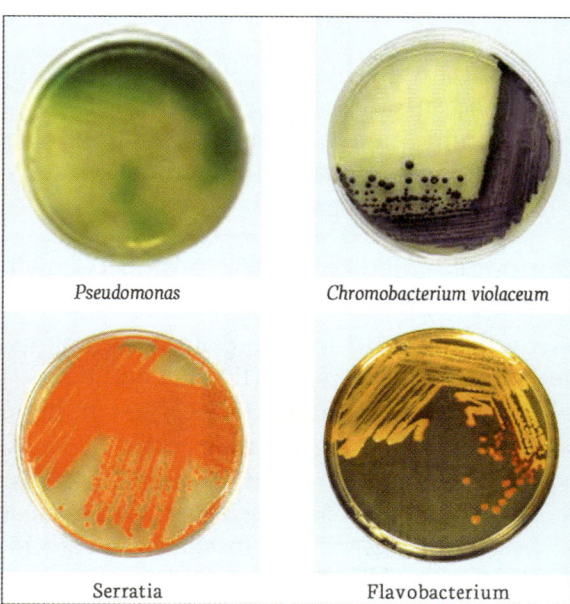

Fig. 8.3: Pigment produced by bacteria

3. *Ends*:
- Convex in *E. coli, Klebsiella pneumoniae.*
- Truncated ends are seen in *Clostridium perfringens.*

4. *Arrangement*: Bacilli in pairs are streptobacilli. Bacilli in chains and the chain surrounded by capsule seen in *Bacillus anthracis.*

5. *Uniform staining or irregular staining*: Irregular staining is seen in *M. tuberculosis.* Nonviable cells of lepra bacilli also stain irregular.

6. *Bipolar staining*: Ends are darkly stained as compared to rest bacillary body—seen in *Yersinia pestis, Vibrio parahemolyticus, Calymatobacterium granulomatis, Pseudomonas pseudomallei, Haemophilus ducreyi,* and *Pseudomonas mallei.*

7. *Arrangement*: Chinese letter pattern is seen in *Corynebacterium diphtheriae.*

Demonstration of Motility

1. Hanging drop method is used for demonstration of (darting) motility.

2. *Growth in semisolid medium* (Fig. 8.4): Semisolid medium is dispensed in sterile tubes. Inoculate with sterile wire, making a single stab down the center of tube to about half the depth of the medium. The tube is incubated at 37°C, examine after 6 hours and then after overnight incubation. If the bacterium is nonmotile, the growth is restricted along the line of inoculation of medium by stabbing and has sharply defined margins. Motile bacteria give diffuse, hazy growth that spreads from line of inoculation to surrounding medium.

   The advantages of semisolid medium:
   - As large inoculum is used, it is more sensitive for detection of motility of bacteria.
   - It is also used for the preservation of bacteria.

   Disadvantage: Different types of motility cannot be differentiated.

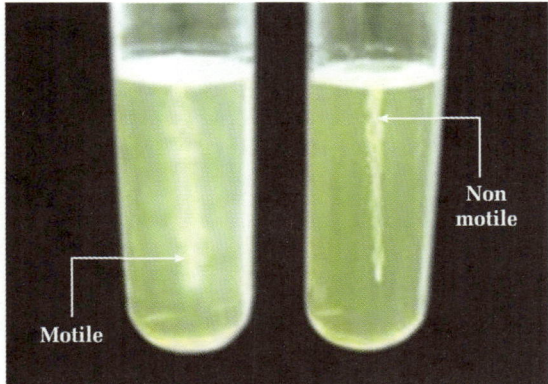

Fig. 8.4: Demonstration of motility by using semisolid medium

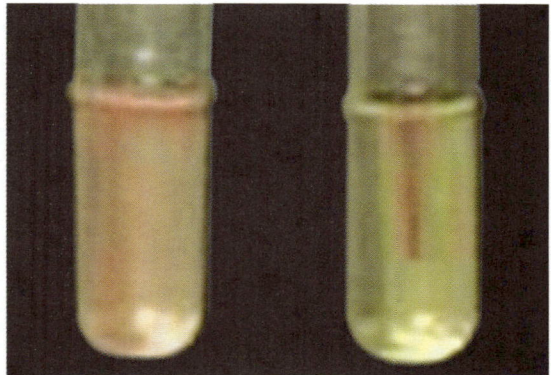

Fig. 8.5: Demonstration of motility in semisolid medium containing tetrazolium chloride

3. *Motility medium with 0.0005% tetrazolium chloride is helpful which is colorless in oxidized form; reduced state is red, indicating bacterial growth. Diffuse growth fan out from the end of inoculation (Fig. 8.5).*

BIOCHEMICAL REACTIONS

Sugar Fermentation Tests

The ability of the bacterium to ferment a specific sugar with acid or acid with gas is tested.

Rapid Carbon Utilization Test

It checks for preformed enzymes. A buffered solution of high concentration of sugar is inoculated with test organism. After 1–4 hours of incubation, the test will be positive.

Procedure: In peptone water, different sugars, as glucose, lactose, sucrose, mannitol, are taken with concentration of 1%. If sugar is fermented, acids are produced, which change the color of Andrade's indicator from yellow to pinkish red due to change of pH to acidic side and if gas is produced, it accumulates in Durham's tube placed in the medium.

IMViC Tests

These are used to distinguish different enteric Gram-negative bacteria.

Indole Test (Fig. 8.6)

Principle: Indole positive bacteria convert the amino acid tryptophan into indole which shows pink color ring at the top of tube.

Medium used: Peptone water is rich in tryptophan.

Procedure: The part of colony of bacterium is picked up with nicrome wire and emulsified in peptone water tube. The tube is incubated at 37°C for 24–48 hours. Production of Indole is tested by adding Kovac's

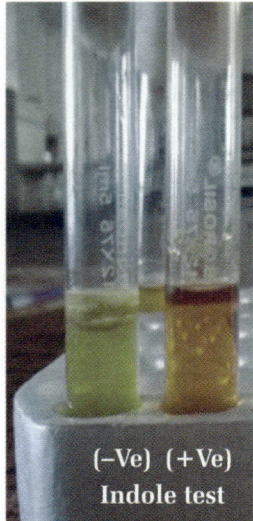

Fig. 8.6: Indole test

reagent. Xylene is added (1 mL) before the reagent. Indole is extracted by xylene. The positive test is development of pink color.

Examples of Indole positive bacteria: *E. coli, Proteus vulgaris.*

Methyl Red Test (Fig. 8.7)

The bacteria which use mixed acid fermentation pathway, produce many acids which constantly keep the pH of the medium to acidic side (below 4.4). Hence after addition of methyl red reagent to the overnight growth of bacterium in glucose phosphate broth, it shows red color.

Examples of MR positive bacteria: *E. coli, Salmonella* sp, *Proteus* species, *Shigella* species.

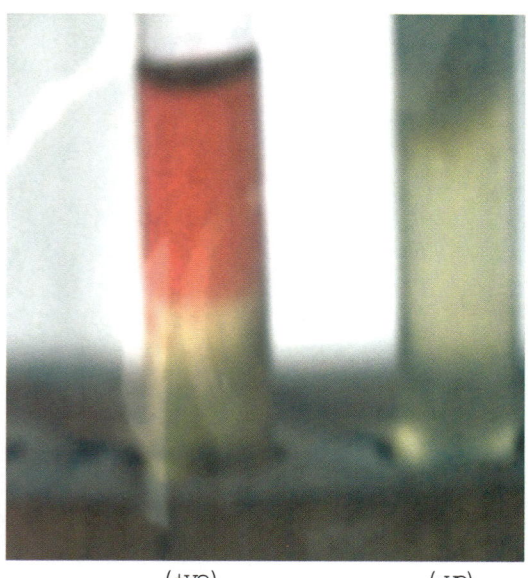

(+ve)   (–ve)

Fig. 8.7: MR test

Voges-Proskauer (VP) Test

Principle: The bacteria which utilize butelene glycol pathway produce acetyl methyl carbinol (acetoin) from pyruvic acid. In presence of alkaline atmospheric oxygen, acetoin is oxidized to diacetyl that gives pink color.

Procedure: Inoculate part of colony in glucose phosphate broth. Incuabte at 37°C for minimum 48 hours. After incubation, add 1 mL of 40% KOH and 3 mL of 5% alpha-naphthol.

Examples of VP positive bacteria: *Klebsiella* species, *Enterobacter* species, El Tor *Vibrio cholerae.*

Citrate Utilization Test (Fig. 8.8)

It detects ability of the bacteria to utilize citrate as a sole source of carbon. Bacterium will grow and give test positive.

Procedure: The part of colony of bacterium from medium is picked up to inoculate Simmon's citrate medium, the test is incubated for 18–24 hours at 37°C.

Result: Positive-change of color from green to blue or growth of bacterium on slant. The bacterium when utilizes citrate, the alkaline pH is produced which changes the color of bromothymol blue from green to blue.

If **Kosers citrate medium** is used for citrate test, it is inoculated by just touching upper part of medium which is liquid, positive result is indicated by turbidity. If bacterium is citrate negative, it will not grow, hence no turbidity will be seen.

Examples of citrate positive bacteria: *Klebsiella* species, *Enterobacter* species, *Citrobacter* species, *Pseudomonas aeruginosa.*

Examples of citrate negative bacteria: *E. coli, Shigella* species.

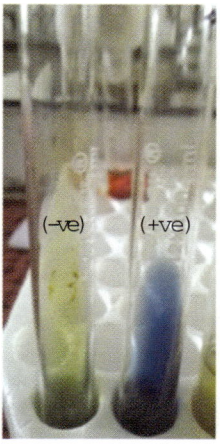

Fig. 8.8: Simon's citrate test

Oxidase Test (Cytochrome 'c' Test)

Principle of test: The bacterium which has cytochrome oxidase which catalyses transfer of electrons between electron donor in bacteria and redox dye which gets reduced to deep purple color.

Procedure

Filter paper method: A freshly prepared 1% oxidase reagent (tetramethyl paraphenylene diamine dihydro-chloride) is soaked on a filter paper. The colony of the organism is taken with sterile glass rod and touched to paper, if test is positive, color changes to deep purple within 20 seconds.

Plate method: Freshly prepared reagent is poured on suspected colony; the development of purple color occurs. This method is specially used to identify bacteria in mixed growth as *Neisseria gonorrhoeae* from urethal discharge. Positive control used for the test is a known strain of *Pseudomonas aeruginosa*. Negative control used for the test is *E. coli*.

Oxidase positive organisms: *Pseudomonas* species, *Vibrio cholerae*, meningococci, gonococci, *Aeromonas, Plesiomonas, Helicobacter pylori*.

Note: Oxidase test is used to identify all members of family Enterobacteriaceae as all of them are negative.

Oxidase test must not be performed from growth of bacteria on media containing sugars as MacConkey's; thiosulfate citrate bile salts sucrose agar (TCBS). The acidic pH produced due to fermentation of sugars in the media inhibits oxidase enzyme activity.

Nitrate Reduction Test

It determines the ability of bacteria to produce an enzyme nitrate reductase. The bacteria which reduce nitrates to nitrites or free nitrogen gas develop red color when nitrate reagent is added.

Procedure: The test bacterium is inoculated into broth containing $KMNO_4$ and incubated at 37°C. After incubation 0.1 mL nitrate reagent (Nessler's reagent) is added.

Result: Development of red color indicates positive reaction.

Examples of nitrate positive bacteria: This test is used to identify from growth whether or not the bacterium belongs to the family Enterobacteriaceae, e.g. *E. coli, Proteus* (all are positive).

Test for Production of Ammonia

Nessler's reagent is added to culture of organism in peptone water. Brown color is positive, faint yellow color is negative.

Triple Sugar Iron Test (TSI) (Fig. 8.9)

This medium is available in tube with slant and butt portions. The medium contains three sugars—glucose, sucrose, lactose. (1:10:10 proportion). Ferric salts present in the medium help to detect production of H_2S. Phenol red indicator changes color from red to yellow, if acids are fermented. Method of inoculation is important. First stab the butt portion and while coming out streak the slant. If the organism is fermenting only glucose, a slight amount of acid is produced within 6–8 hours of incubation, but as the amount of glucose is low for the growth of bacterium, bacterium attacks peptone at slant area. Also some acids produced at slant get oxidized as it is exposed to air, hence the slant will appear as alkaline again and butt remains yellow. This reaction is indicated as K (alkaline)/A (acidic). If the bacterium is fermenting lactose and/or sucrose, the amounts of acids produced are large enough so that the slant also remains yellow, A/A reaction. If H_2S is produced, blackening in the medium occurs. If acids are fermented with gas formation, it is seen in butt.

Examples of different organisms: If the organism is not fermenting even glucose reaction will remain as K/K. This type of reaction is given by nonfermenters as *Pseudomonas*.

If the bacterium is fermenting only glucose, the reaction is K/A, if along with that H_2S is produced, reaction is K/A with H_2S.

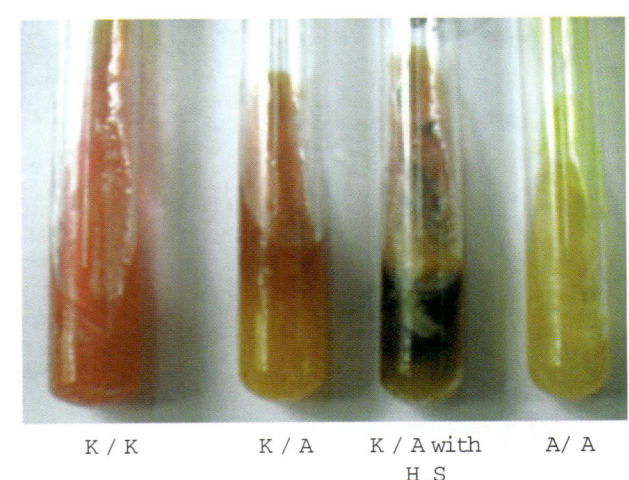

| K / K | K / A | K / A with H_2S | A/ A |

Fig. 8.9: Various reactions seen on TSI medium

E. coli	A/A with gas
Klebsiella sp.	A/A with gas
Proteus	K/A with H_2S
Pseudomonas	K/K no change
Vibrio cholerae	A/A without gas
S. typhi	K/A with H_2S
S. paratyphi A	K/A with gas no H_2S
S. paratyphi B	K/A with gas and H_2S
Morganella	K/A with gas

Urease Test: (Christensen's Urease Agar)

Principle of test: The bacterium is grown on Christensen's urease agar slant. Urease positive organisms have ability to split urea into ammonia as they have urease enzyme. Once ammonia is produced, the pH of urease medium becomes alkaline due to which urease slant turns pink. The indicator in this medium is phenol red which changes from yellow to red (Fig. 8.10).

Method of inoculation of slant: The test organism is inoculated over the whole slant and incubated at 37°C. The test is observed after 4 hours, then after overnight incubation.

Urease positive organisms: *Proteus* (gives positive results within 4 hours) and *Helicobacter pylori* give rapid urease positive. Other urease positive organisms include *Klebsiella* and yeast, i.e. *Cryptococcus*.

Phenylalanine Deaminase Test

The bacteria which give this test positive deaminate phenylalanine to phenylpyruvic acid (PPA).

Procedure: A medium containing PPA is inoculated with test bacterium, incubated at 37°C overnight. Following incubation 10% ferric acid is added. The positive result is the development of green color.

Examples of PPA positive bacteria: *Proteus, Providencia, Morganella.*

Catalase Test

Catalase positive bacteria due to presence of enzyme catalase, help to release oxygen from H_2O_2 (Fig. 8.11).

Procedure: A drop of 3% H_2O_2 is taken on slide. The test organism is picked up with sterile glass rod and touched to the drop, when test is positive, bubbles are seen. Other method is tube catalase test which is done for *M. tuberculosis*.

Uses of test: It differentiates staphylococci from streptococci which are catalase negative.

All members of the family Enterobacteriaceae are catalase positive.

Note: Catalase test is not performed from growth on blood agar which may give false positive test.

Coagulase Test

The coagulase enzyme produced by the bacteria converts fibrinogen to fibrin. Free coagulase is detected by tube method (clotting is seen). Free coagulase converts fibrinogen to fibrin by activating a coagulase reacting factor present in plasma. The bound coagulase is detected by slide method in which clumping of bacteria is seen. It converts fibrinogen directly to fibrin. This bound coagulase is also called clumping factor.

Requirements: Ideally rabbit plasma should be used otherwise EDTA anticoagulated human plasma (preferably pooled and *HIV, hepatitis* B tested) is used.

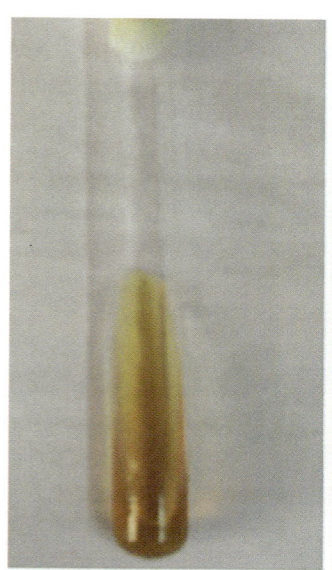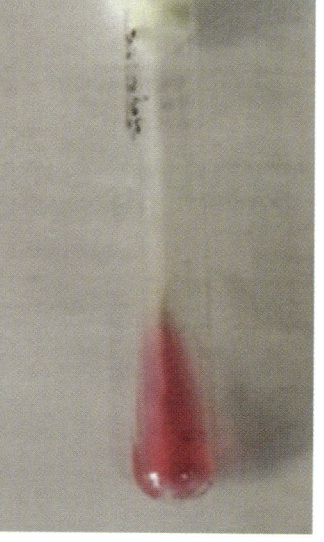

Fig. 8.10: *Urease test*: Negative (yellow) and positive (pink)

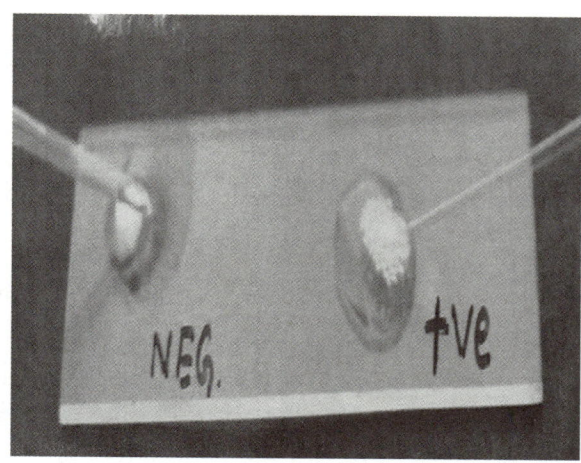

Fig. 8.11: Catalase test

Citrated plasma must not be used because citrate utilizing bacteria as *Klebsiella, Pseudomonas* may cause clotting of plasma.

Slide Coagulase Test

For detection of bound coagulase: On a grease-free slide, place two separate drops of distilled water. Pick up colonies from nutrient agar and emulsify in both the drops. Add one loopful of plasma to one of the drops, mix gently, and second drop is used to differentiate any granular appearance of organism from true clumping.

On a separate slide positive control, i.e. ATCC *Staphylococcus aureus* is tested.

Result: If test is positive, clumping appears within 10 seconds.

Tube Coagulase Test (Fig. 8.12)

- Add 0.2 mL of plasma to 0.8 mL of test broth (containing growth of organism).
- Incubate the tubes at 37°C, and examine for clotting after 1 hour, if negative, examine after 3 hours. If the test is still negative, take out tubes from incubator, keep them at room temperature overnight and observe next day.
- If clot is seen in the tube, consider it as positive, which means test organism is *S. aureus*.

Use of the test: It is used to differentiate coagulase positive *S. aureus* from coagulase negative staphylococci as *S. epidermidis* and *S. saphrophyticus*.

Bile Solubility Test

Principle of the test: A heavy inoculum of organism is emulsified in saline and sodium deoxycholate as bile salt is added which will cause clearing of turbidity within 10–15 minutes. The autolytic enzymes produced by *Pneumococcus* solubilize the peptidoglycan of cell wall, the reaction is augmented by addition of surface reducing agent as bile salts used in this test.

When ox bile (10%) or Na-deoxycolate (2%) is added to a broth culture or suspension of bacterium at neutral pH, lysis occurs, evident by clearing of the medium.

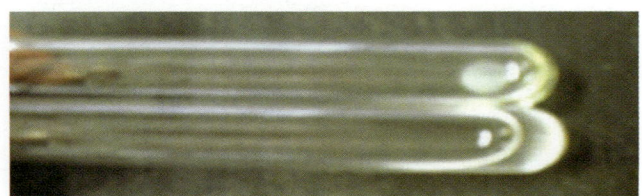

Fig. 8.12: Tube coagulase test: clot formation (coagulase positive organism upper tube, i.e. *Staphylococcus aureus*)

(Alternative test is directly performed on colonies grown on chocolate agar on which bile salt is added, showing clearing of colonies.)

Use of the test: It is used to differentiate *Streptococcus pneumoniae* which gives test positive from other alpha hemolytic streptococci as *S. viridans*.

CAMP Test (Cristie, Atkin, Munch, Peterson)

When *S. agalactie* is inoculated perpendicular to a steak of known beta hemolytic *Staph. aureus* on blood agar, after overnight incubation there is accentued zone of hemolysis of *Strep. agalactiae* near *Staph. aureus*.

Reverse CAMP Test

The alpha (α) toxin produced by *Cl. perfringens* acts synergistically with β hemolytic group B streptococci.

The test organism, *Clostridium perfringens*, is streaked in the center of the plate. *Streptococcus agalactiae* (group B) is streaked perpendicular to the *Clostridium perfringens*.

A positive reverse CAMP result for *Clostridium perfringens* is shown by the arrow-shaped zone of enhanced hemolysis pointing towards *Clostridium perfringens*.

Important

- *Clostridium perfringens* **reverse CAMP test** differs from the test used for *Arcanobacterium haemolyticum*.
- Hemolysis is **enhanced** when **Cl. perfringens** and group B streptococci grow closer.
- *Arcanobacterium* inhibits the hemolysis of *Staphylococcus aureus*.

Oxidation–Fermentation(O-F) Test (Hugh and Lefson Test)

This test differentiates between fermenters and non-fermenters that utilize glucose oxidatively.

O-F medium contains

- Agar (0.3%) is added to make medium semisolid, diffusion of acids from surface to throughout the medium is allowed, that changes the color of indicator bromothymol blue to yellow.
- Sugar (0.5–1%).
- Peptone concentration is decreased from 1–0.2%.
- Two tubes of O-F medium are inoculated with the organism. One of the tubes is covered with liquid paraffin (1 cm layer) to create anaerobic conditions. Acid production changes the color of the medium from green to yellow.
- Nonfermenters utilize sugar oxidatively, hence the tube without liquid paraffin changes from green to yellow. If the organism is fermenter, acid production takes place in both tubes.

Decarboxylase–Dihydrolase Tests

This test detects the ability of test organisms to degrade lysine, ornithine and arginine.

The enzymes remove decarboxl group in the amino acids making the environment alkaline.

Medium: Moeller's decarboxylase instead of decarboxyl medium (broth) is commonly used. Its important characteristics are:

Glucose: A small amount is present in the medium to support the growth.

Amino acid: Each medium contains one specific amino acid (i.e. ornithine, lysine, arginine).

Procedure: One each tube with broth medium is used for separate amino acids. The control tube has only the medium and it is lacking amino acid. After inoculation of tubes, mineral oil is covered over the broth which generates anaerobic conditions necessary for deamination.

The enzyme decarboxylase degrades amino acids to produce these alkaline/basic products. However, the enzyme does not do this unless the growth medium is acidified by other metabolic activities, so the test involves two distinct stages: First the microbe must acidify the medium; then the decarboxylase enzyme (if present) can metabolize the amino acid. The medium is a nutrient broth to which 0.5% amino acid is added. An important component of the medium is a modest amount of glucose, necessary for the initial acidification of the medium. The pH indicator bromocresol purple is purple at neutral or alkaline/basic pH but turns yellow at pH <5.2.

In a positive test, the microbe must first ferment the glucose present to cause the pH to drop. This is indicated by a change from purple to yellow during the first 24 hours of incubation. Once the medium has been acidified, the enzyme decarboxylase is activated. The culture is incubated an additional 24 hours at 35–37°C to allow the microbe to use the amino acid. The final results are then observed. Change back to purple from yellow indicates a positive test. Failure to turn yellow at 24 hours or failure to revert back to purple at 48 hours indicates a negative result.

NEW APPROACHES FOR THE DIAGNOSIS

Commercial systems for idenfication are available from various systems. Some are miniaturized classical biochemical tests. The incorporation of antibiotic susceptibility testing in these systems provides additional information. Dehydrated plastic cups are reconstituted when a fluid culture suspension of bacterium under investigation is injected. A biochemical profile is obtained after 18–24 hours of incubation at 37°C. The profile is translated in a neumerical code which can be read from the key (profile index). Computerized based identification systems are also available.

Sensititre Systems

It detects biochemical reactions of bacteria along with antibiotic susceptibility of microtitre plate contains dry media. Fluorescent technology detects bacterial enzyme activity and measurement of that allows determination of growth. This system can run manually or semiautomated or automated. Antibiotic susceptibility testing is also available using microtitre plate or MIC can be obtained by strips (Fig. 8.13).

API System

It is useful for final identification of bacteria. Different sets of test are used for identification of different organisms. For example, API20E is used for identification of enterobacteria along with API NE. For Staphylococcus API Staph is used and API20STREP is used for Streptococci. Similarly separate sets are used for yeasts and anaerobic bacteria.

Proper identification of member of family Enterobacteriaceae is done by API20. Suspension of bacteria is taken in stripes which detect various enzyme activity. The results are ready in four hours. There are 20 small capsules detection chambers in which bacterial suspension is taken. The result of the API20-E system can be used for identification of some nonfermentative bacilli, Gram-negative bacilli, and for anaerobic bacteria. For identification of nonfermenters, 6 additional tests are run to generate a 9-digit biotype identification number. Over 100 taxa of GNB are identified using this system.

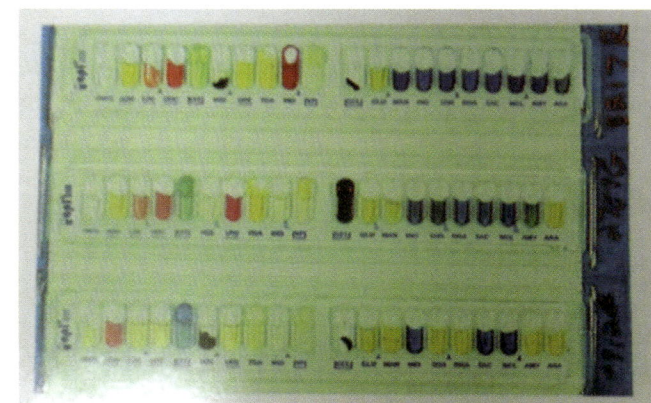

Fig. 8.13: Biochemical identification system

Monotek System

Reagent for identification are available in the paper discs to which bacterial suspension is added. Number of discs may vary, generally 17 such identification discs are used at a time. The profile of tests used obtained with this system is useful in identification of obligatory anaerobes as well as facultative enteric bacteria.

Micro ID System

Identification of member of family enterobacteriaceae is possible by using biochemical reactions. Tests for biotyping for *H. influenzae* is possible with a set of tests. There are 15 reaction chambers, and the test results can be used to generate a 5-digit identification code number. This system lists possible identification and probabilities based on the results of 15 biochemical test reactions.

Other systems

- Paper disks impregnated with biochemical substrates (Minitek, from Becton and Dickinson) are used.
- *Mastascan color system (mast group)*: It is computerized automated system. Identification of organism and pattern of distribution of specific organism in community, with details of antibiotic susceptibility testing is reported.

Automated Blood Culture Systems

These systems use equipment that automatically detects an early sign of bacterial growth in a special blood culture medium (Fig. 8.14).

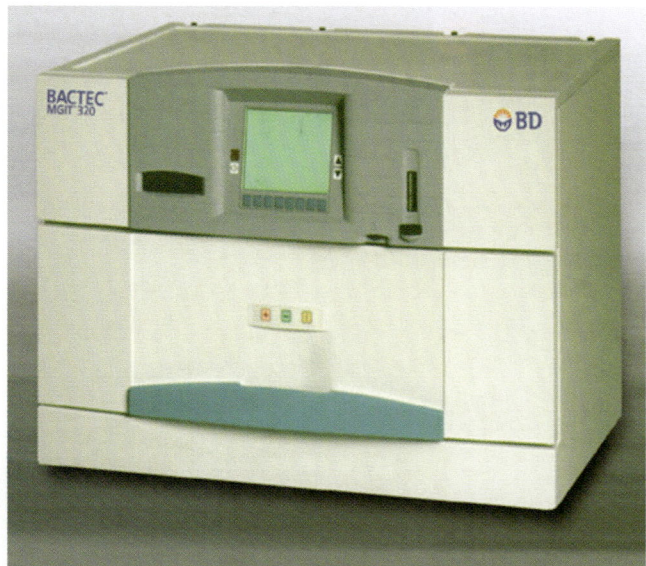

Fig. 8.14: Automated blood system—Bactec (Becton and Dickinson)

1. ***Bactec (Becton and Dickinson)***: This system was initially simple manually operated device, now it is modified to fully automated computerized assembly which detects positive blood cultures, identifies the organism. The original system used a substrate containing radiolabeled carbon, C14. If the organism is present and growing , it will use the substrate and release radiolabeled CO_2, which is detected by radio-metric method. **The new models use fluorochemical sensor and measures CO_2 induced increase in fluorescence.**

2. ***Organon Teknika BacT/alert***: It also moniters CO_2 released from substrate and reads colorimetric signals generated by exciter wavelength.

3. ***Vitek (bioMerieux)***: It measures exitor-induced fluorescence.

Molecular Methods

Samples: Blood, respiratory secretions, urine, tissue, etc.

Microbe detection procedures are classified into

a. *Direct target nucleic acid detection*: *In situ* nucleic acid detection method, e.g. FISH—fluorescent *in situ* hybridization directly in tissue.

b. *Nucleic acid purification and then detection*: It used for DNA or RNA (e.g. r-RNA, viral RNA): Target detection is done by:
   1. Dot or slot-blot hybridization
   2. Restriction fragment length polymorphism (RFLP) analysis
   3. Pulse field gel electrophoresis.

c. *Target nucleic acid amplification and detection techiniques*:
   i. *Polymerase chain reaction (PCR)*: Various modification are now available as nested PCR, multiplex PCR, real-time PCR, reverse transcriptase PCR.
   Other amplication techniques
   ii. Ligase chain assay (LCR)
   iii. Strand displacement assay (SDA)
   iv. Nucleic acid sequence based assay (NASBA)
   v. *Signal amplification assay*: Branched DNA assay.
   Of these methods, PCR is most commonly used with real-time PCR format. Latest one is loop-mediated isothermal amplication (LAMP).

LAMP

It gets the name from the fact that the final amplification product consists of a structure that contains multiple loops (repeats) of target sequence. The reaction is isothermal and consists of autocycling strand displacement DNA sysnthesis using Bst DNA polymerase and four to six primers. Amplication products can be detected in real time by precipitating DNA by adding magnesium pyrophosphate to the reaction creating turbidity that can be read visually or by using a spectrophotometer. The method is highly sensitive, detecting as few as 10 target copies per reaction.

Molecular methods are discussed in chapter of genetics
Other newer techniques used at reference center are:

a. *Gas liquid chromatography*: It is used for identification of nonsporing anaerobes and a few other organisms as *Corynebacterium diphtheriae.*

b. *Thin paper chromatography* is used for *M. tuberculosis.*

c. *MALDI-TOF*: It can be used for identification of many organisms.

Mass Spectrometry

It is used to analyse proteins or DNA. It uses method such as ionization radiation to distrupt material forming charged particles that are identified in various ways on the basis of mass or mass to charge ratio.

Nanotechnology

The nanometer refers to a unit which is one billionth of a meter (10^{-9}). The molecular and submolecular technology is evolving in the diagnosis of infectious diseases. The technology includes nanoarrays, protein arrays, nanopore technology, nanoparticles (NP) as a contrivance in immunoassays and nanosensors in others. Gold nanoparticles and quantum dots (semiconductors) are widely used. Other materials used are gallinium, phosphate, quartz, ceramic, nanobiosensors, in which antibodies based nanobiosensors are used.

Magnetic NP on antibody serves as a label for antigen, in magnetic immunoassay techniques. Here, the magnetic field generated by reaction between an antigen and magnetic labeled particles is measured.

Gold nanoparticles tagged on short segment of DNA have been used for detection of DNA sequence in sample.

Recently developed functionalized NP covalently linked to biological substances as antibodies, antigen, peptides, nucleic acids are developed.

9

Sterilization and Disinfection

Sterilization is a method by which an article or surface or medium is made free from all organisms including spores.

Disinfection is a process by which an article or surface or medium is made free of pathogenic organisms or organisms capable of producing disease. It may not ensure killing spores.

PHYSICAL METHODS OF STERILIZATION (*see* Fig. 9.6)

These include sunlight, drying, dry heat (flamming, incinerator, hot air oven), moist heat (boiling, steam under normal pressure, steam under pressure), radiation and filtration.

Sunlight: Due to presence of UV rays, it has some killing action on some organisms. It is not completely reliable.

Drying: Drying removes the water present in the organism, hence it has some effect on organisms.

HEAT (DRY HEAT STERILIZATION)

Dry heat: It is preferred for the sterilization of glassware such as petridishes, test tubes, and other materials as oils, pharmaceutical powders.

Principle of dry heat: It kills microorganisms by denaturation of proteins, toxic effects of raised electrolytes and oxidative damage (oxidizing chemical constituents).

Sterilization methods in which dry heat is used are incinerator, hot air oven, flaming and red heat.

I. Incineration (Fig. 9.1)

It uses very high temperature so that everything is converted into ash. Incinerator is used for disposal of soiled dressing, anatomical products, microbiological and pathological waste. The word incinerator comes from Greek word meaning—turn to ash. It signifies combustion process.

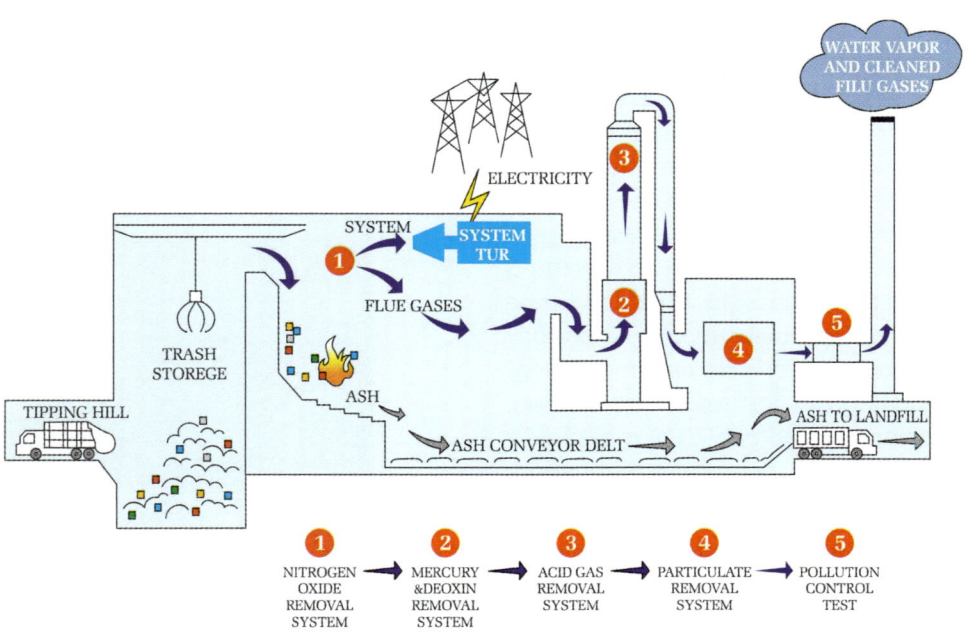

Fig. 9.1: Incinerator

Advantages
- It reduces the waste volume and weight.
- It renders the waste unrecognizable.
- It is suitable for all types of waste.
- It has heat recovery potential.
- It can treat chemotherapeutic waste.

Disadvantages
- High capital loss
- High maintenance and repair cost
- Stacks emissions
- Permission difficulties
- Public opposition

Design concept and principles of working: It is a high thermal process employing combustion of waste under controlled conditions for converting them into inert material and gases. It can be electrically operated. (Oil fired or a combination type.) The types of incinerators are:
1. Multiple chamber type
2. Controlled air and rotary kiln types
3. Rotary kiln

All have primary and secondary chamber to ensure proper combustion. Overall, the primary chamber has temperature that has pyrolytic conditions with temperature range 800+/− 50°C. The secondary chamber operates **at 1050°C +/−50°C**. The volatile fumes are released in the first chamber, whereas they are destroyed in second chamber.

1. *Multiple chamber incinerator*: Solid phase combustion takes place in primary chamber; secondary chamber is for gas phase combustion. The tertiary chamber when present condenses the gases and air particulates. They are also called excess air incinerators as excess air is present in the both chambers.
2. *Controlled air incinerator*: First chamber is operated at low air level followed by excess chamber air. Due to low oxygen in primary chamber; there is better control of particulate matter in the flue gas.
3. *Rotary kiln*: This is a cylindrical refractory lined shelled that is mounted at a slight tilt to facilitate mixing. It signifies dressings, instruments, laboratory ware and pharmaceutical products and movement of waste inside. It has provision for air circulation. The kiln acts as a primary solid phase chamber followed by secondary chamber for gaseous combustion.

Regulations and standards for biomedical waste rules: The incinerator should be two-chambered incinerator with a combustion efficiency of 99%, the temperature in the primary chamber 1050°C (+/− 50°C) with 3% O_2 in stock gas.

II. Red Heat

Red heat (flaming till article becomes red hot) is used for sterilization of inoculation loops, tips of forceps, scissors, and spatulas.

III. Flaming

It is direct exposure to flame without making it red hot. This method is used for the sterilization of glass slides, coverslips, mouth of culture tubes.

IV. Hot Air Oven (Fig. 9.2a)

It has two-walled chamber with heating elements present inside two walls and the fan ensures even distribution of heat and removes air pockets. The chamber is divided into small compartments on which different articles to be sterilized are kept.

Procedure: The articles as glassware to be sterilized are made dry before keeping into the chamber (the process of keeping articles inside is called loading). The glassware after drying is wrapped in a paper before loading so that after cycle is over, the paper maintains the sterility of the article till it is carried at the site of use. The articles are loaded in such manner that there is even distribution of heat and there is no over-crowding also. The temperature is adjusted to a required level and heating is started. The temperature is kept constant at 160°C for one hour which is called as **holding period.** The temperature is measured by thermometer. After the holding period of 60 minutes at 160°C, hot air oven is switched off and after some time (after cooling) the articles are taken out. For sharp instruments like those required for ophthalmic surgery, low temperature (150°C) for two hours (holding time) is required for sterilization. However, alternative temperatures and holding time include 170°C for one hour and 180°C for 30 minutes.

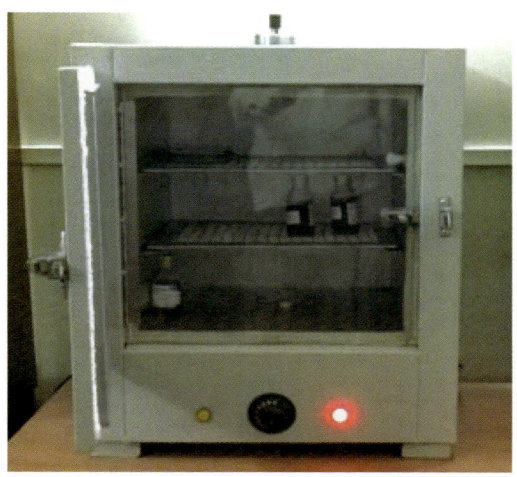

Fig. 9.2a: Hot air oven

Uses of hot air oven: Following items are sterilized by it:
- Glassware like glass syringes, petridishes, etc.
- Surgical instruments like scalpels, scissors, etc.
- Chemicals such as liquid paraffin, grease
- Cotton swabs
- Pharmaceutical products
- A lower temperature at 150°C for 2 hours is used for sharp instruments like those required for ophthalmic surgery. By exposure to lower temperature but prolonged cycle, the sharpness is maintained.

Sterilization Controls

- **Biological control:** The spore stripes of *Bacillus subtilis* subsp. *niger* (NCTC 10075 or ATCC 9372) are kept inside the oven. These spores should be destroyed, if sterilization is proper which is tested by growing the spores in Robertson's cooked meat (RCM) medium.
- Thermocouples may also be used.
- Browne's tube which shows green color after the desired temperature is reached.

STERILIZATION USING MOIST HEAT (STEAM) AT TEMPERATURE BELOW 100°C (<100°C)

a. Inspissation

Use: This method is used for sterilization and solidification of the L-J medium and Loffler's serum slope (Fig. 9.2b).

Procedure: Heating is done at 80–85°C for three consecutive days in an inspissator. In the first cycle, the vegetative organisms are killed. Spores germinate, killed in the subsequent cycles. Also bacteria which are germinated in and after 1st cycle are killed in next cycles.

b. Water Bath

It is used for the sterilization of serum or body fluids which is achieved in 1 hour at 56°C on several occasions.

c. Pasteurization of Milk

Two methods used are holder method (63°C for 30 minutes) and flash method (72°C for 20 seconds followed by cooling quickly at 13°C or lower). *Coxiella burnetii* survives holders method and killed by flash

method while *Mycobacterium, Brucella,* Salmonellae are killed by holders method.

d. Vaccine Bath

Heating for 1 hour at 60°C in vaccine bath is used for the inactivation of bacteria in the vaccine preparation.

Moist heat temperature at 100°C
  i. *Boiling:* Boiling at 100°C for 15–30 minutes is used for sterilization of scalpels, forceps, pipette, but total sterilization is not achieved.
  ii. Steam at atmospheric pressure.

Steam Sterilizer

Koch/Arnold Steamer: Media containing certain substances as sugar or gelatin are sterilized by steaming at 100°C at atmospheric pressure (Fig. 9.2c). This is done for three successive days. After each cycle of 100°C for 30 minutes, the media are incubated. If spores are present, they will germinate. Again the medium is sterilized. Thus with the three cycles, killing of bacteria and spores is achieved. This method is called **tyndalization** or **intermittent sterilization.** This method is used only for the media which contain nutritive substances which favor germination of spores. Container and medium is simultaneously sterilized. Evaporation from the medium is prevented. It requires no or a little attention and less expensive. Steamer is tinned copper cabinet with conical lid enabling drainage of steam. Perforated tray placed above the water level ensures

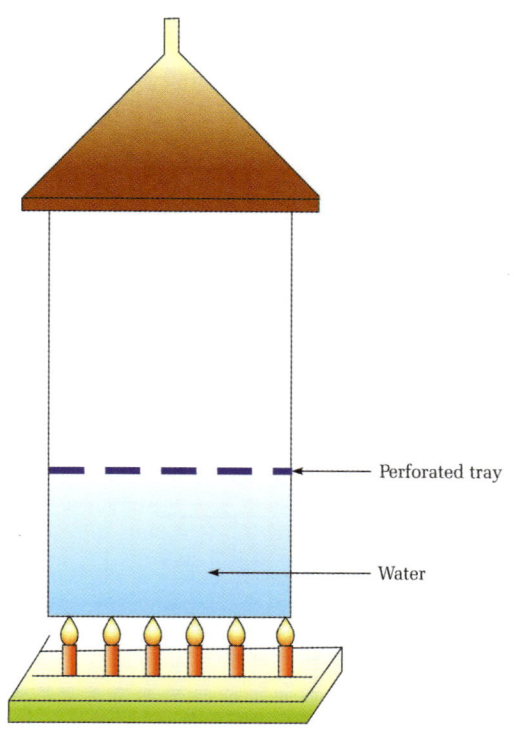

— Perforated tray

— Water

Fig. 9.2c: Koch's steamer

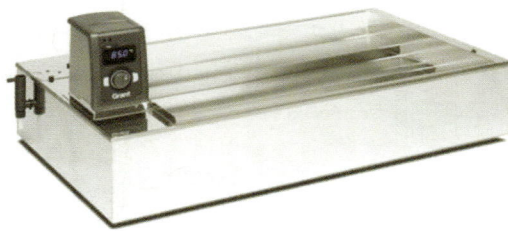

Fig. 9.2b: Inspissator

that the article to be sterilized is always surrounded by steam. Single exposure of 90 minutes is used.

Autoclave

Principle of Working

- When water boils in a closed vessel, temperature at which it boils increases according to the Boyle's law. When steam comes into contact with a cooler surface, it condenses and liberates its latent heat to the surface, e.g. 1600 mL of steam at 100°C and at atmospheric pressure, condenses into one mL of water at 100°C and releases 518 calories of heat.
- Steam above 100°C which is saturated steam, has a better killing power than dry heat.
- Saturated steam can penetrate porous material easily.
- The large reduction in volume sucks in more steam to the same site and the process continues till the temperature of the article is raised to that of steam.
- The condensed water produces moist conditions for killing the microbes.
- In the presence of moisture, spores are easily killed.

Structure of Autoclave (Figs 9.3 a,b, and 9.4)

There is vertical (or horizontal) cylinder made up of stainless steel which has lid or door which is provided with screws and washer as pressure cooker. The autoclave is heated by electricity. On the lid, there are steam outlet, safety valve and pressure gauge.

Other types of autoclaves are:
- Gravity displacement type
- Rapid cooling sterilizer

- Vacuum displacement type
- Flash autoclaving

Sterilization conditions

Temperature: 121°C

Chamber pressure: 15 lb per square inch

Holding time: 15–20 minutes

These conditions are generally used; however, sterilization can also be done at higher temperatures, at 126°C (20 lb/square inch) for 10 minutes or at 133°C (30 lb/square inch) for 3 minutes.

Working: Water is placed at the base of autoclave. There is perforated tray above the water level. Items to be sterilized are packed and placed on the tray. With the help of screws, lid is closed. Safety valve is adjusted to desired pressure. Heating is started. Steam tap is kept open, hence air present inside will come out and there will be saturated steam inside the autoclave. Tap is closed when all air is displayed. Pressure is recorded and when it becomes to the desired level, i.e. 15 pounds per square inch **holding time** is calculated (20 minutes). After the cycle is over, the instrument is switched off, autoclave is allowed to cool down, lid is opened and the articles are removed.

Precautions

- If some air remains inside, it is expelled out, otherwise it will hamper the process. To check presence of air, some water is taken in a small bowl which is hold near trap. If air is present in autoclave, bubbles will come out. If all air is expelled, bubbles will stop.

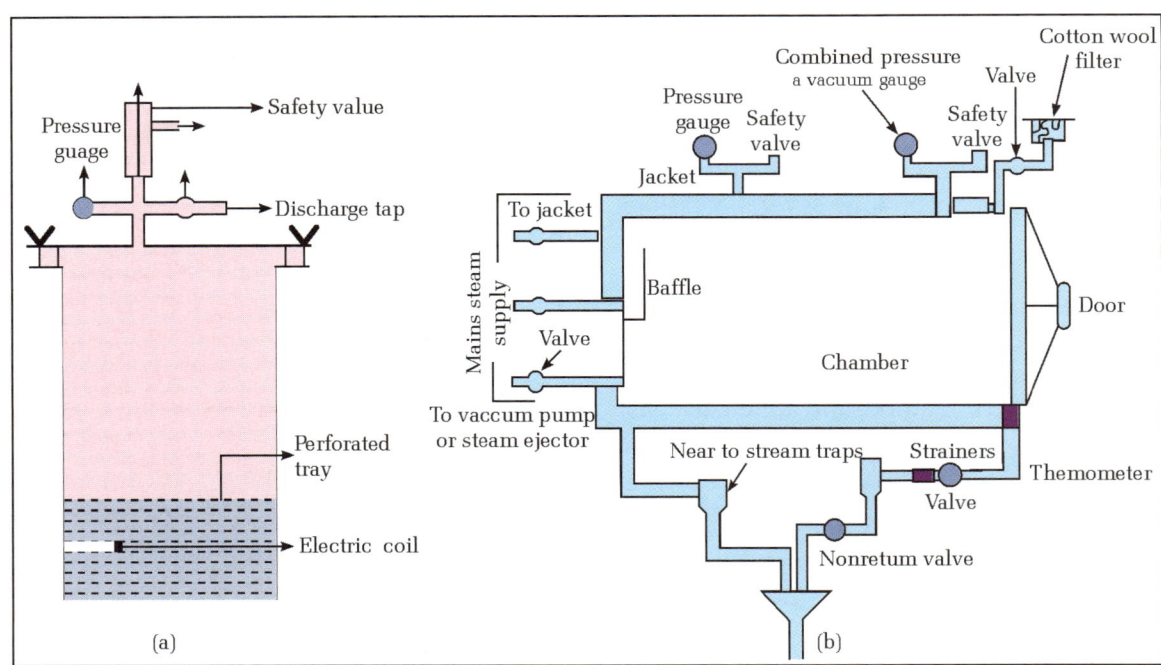

Fig. 9.3a and b: (a) Vertical autoclave, (b) Horizontal autoclave

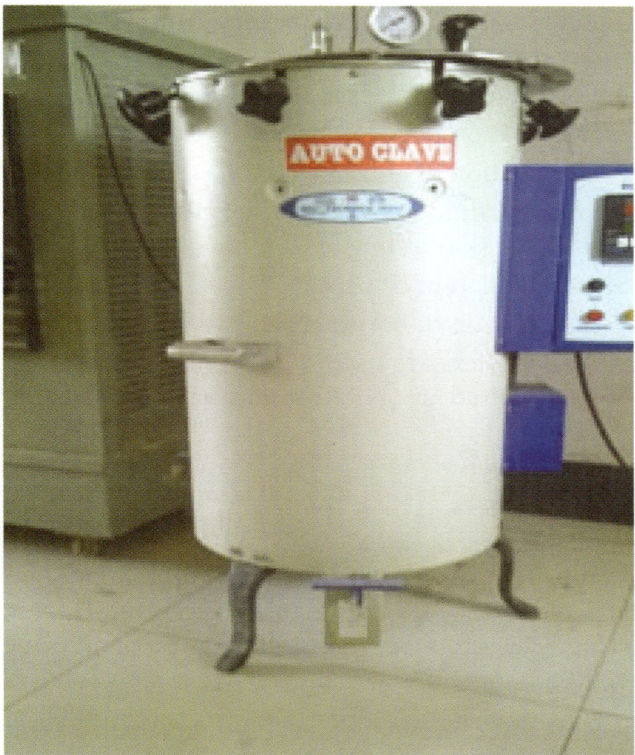

Fig. 9.4: Vertical autoclave

- The lid is to be opened when pressure inside equals to atmospheric pressure. If pressure inside is higher than the atmospheric pressure, it will cause violent boiling of the medium or liquid which may some-times come out forcefully.
- On the other hand, if we open the lid when pressure inside is low, evaporation of water occurs and quality of media is hampered.

Uses: Sterilization of culture media, rubber material, gowns, dressings, gloves, surgical instruments, distilled water, saline solution, swabs, laboratory coats, needle and syringes.

Sterilization Control

1. *Thermocouple:* It is to record the temperature directly by a potentiometer.
2. *Bacterial spores (biological control):* Spores of *Bacillus stearothermophilus* are on a strip. This control strip is placed within autoclave with each cycle. When the cycle is over, the strips are taken out and inoculated in an anaerobic medium which is incubated to look for presence of turbidity (growth). If the proper temperature is achieved, the spores on the strips will be killed, hence no growth and no turbidity will occur. It means the cycle was run properly with desired temperature, pressure, and holding time.

3. *Chemical indicators:* **Browne's tube** contains red solution which turns green, when exposed to temperature of 121°C for 15 minutes in autoclave. The disadvantage of the indicator is that it shows a color change when a desired temperature is reached but it will not indicate whether the same temperature was maintained during the holding period of 20 minutes. Chemical indicators in the form of **strips** are also available.

Gravity displacement autoclave: In this autoclave, the induced steam, which is less dense than air, forces air down and out through autoclave drain. Unfortunately, if steam does not reach the surface, this is equivalent to dry heat a process that is gently held to require 2 hours of exposure.

Vacuum displacement autoclaves: These are evacuated before induction of steam. Pulsed vacuum autoclaves are even more efficient since they go through various cycles of vacuum and steam replacement, more reliably air removal.

Hydroclave

It is classified as steam sterilizer technology. It is an innovative form of autoclave. It is a double-walled container, in which steam is injected into outer jacket to heat inner chamber containing waste. Moisture in the waste evaporates. There are paddles inside the chambers which tumble the waste continuously against the hot wall mixing it as well as fragmenting waste. In absence of enough moisture, additional steam is injected. The system operates at 132°C for 15 minutes or 121°C for 30 minutes. The waste material is dehydrated and reduced in volume. The space required to install and operate the hydroclave is size of average room.

The hydroclave is horizontally mounted and has one or more top side loading doors and a smaller unloading door at its bottom. The vessel is fitted motor driven shaft to which are attached powerful fragmenting or mixing arms, that slowly rotate inside the vessel.

When steam is introduced in the vessel jacket, it transmits heat rapidly to the wet fragmented waste, which in turn produces steam of its own.

The resultant dynamic reactions
- It sterilizes waste by high temperature and pressure steam similar to autoclave but with high temperature and pressure.
- Hydrolyses the organic components of waste.
- Fragments and totally dehydrates the waste.
- Reduces the volume by 85% and weight by 60%.
- Allows self-unloading after the treatment cycle.

Advantages
- No pretreatment of waste is required.
- Complete waste dehydration.
- Disposal costs are reduced.
- Pathological waste treatment—sterilizes, dehydrates and renders waste unrecognizable.
- Environment friendly.
- Treatment of cost is ₹ 1–2/kg, so economical.
- Simple, easy to operate and maintain.
- Operation is push button automatic.

The treatment cycle
- Loading, heating and fragmentation
- *Sterilization*: 15 minutes at 132°C
- Depressurization

Radiation

Two types of radiations are used for the sterilization—ionizing radiations and nonionizing radiations.

a. *Ionizing radiations*: X-rays, gamma rays and beta rays are used for sterilization. The advantages are that they have high penetrating power; they inactivate DNA and other components of organisms. When these rays are passed through article or medium or surface, they do not increase the temperature of the article or medium or surface, hence they are called **cold sterilization methods**.

   Uses: Disposable items as plastic syringes, swabs, catheters, fabrics, various types of rubber materials are sterilized by this method. Apart from these pharma products, oils, food products are sterilized by gamma and beta rays.

   X-rays are not recommended for sterilization as they have poor penetrating power and produce radiations.

b. *Nonionizing radiations*: Ultraviolet rays

   Uses: It is used in control of air-borne infections in operation theatres, hospital wards.

   UV rays of wavelength of 240 nm and 254 nm have high penetrating power which produces photochemical changes in cellular enzymes and other parts of cells of microorganisms as DNA, cellular proteins of organisms including spores (require double exposure) are killed by UV rays. UV rays are obtained from special UV lamps.

   Though ultrasonic and sonic vibration waves are bactericidal, they give variable results with variable bacteria.

Filtration

Uses
1. For heat labile liquids
2. To obtain bacteria free filtrates for virus isolation
3. Filter disks concentrate bacteria from samples like water for testing cholera
4. For obtaining bacterial toxins free of bacteria
5. Sterilization of sugar solutions
6. Sterilization of antisera
7. Hydatid fluid is sterilized by Seitz filter and then used for skin testing
8. Sterilization of trypsin
9. Sterilization of hormones
10. HEPA filters are used to purify large volumes of air required in operation theatre and in laminar flow.

Types of Filters

Candle filters: Berkfeld and Chamber lands filters which use unglazed ceramic filters and diatomaceous filters respectively. The filters are sterilized by autoclaving. The sample to be sterilized is passed through filters.

Asbestos filter: A metal disc is used on which asbestos disc is placed,It is assembled in the form fennel. Sterile flask is used to collect the filtered material by allowing fluid to pass through the filter. When the disk is placed inside the funnel the whole assembly is sterilized by autoclaving. Asbestos filters of various grades of porosity can be used. Example of asbestos filter is **Seitz filter** (Fig. 9.5).

Sintered glass filter: It is made up of powdered glass, the particle size of which controls the pore size of the filter. Filters can be cleaned easily; the disadvantage is the cost.

Membrane filters: Membranes made up of cellulose acetate, cellulose diacetate, polycarbonates are used. Porosity varies from 0.015–12; the filter with pore size 0.22 is mostly used. This pore size is smaller than bacteria.

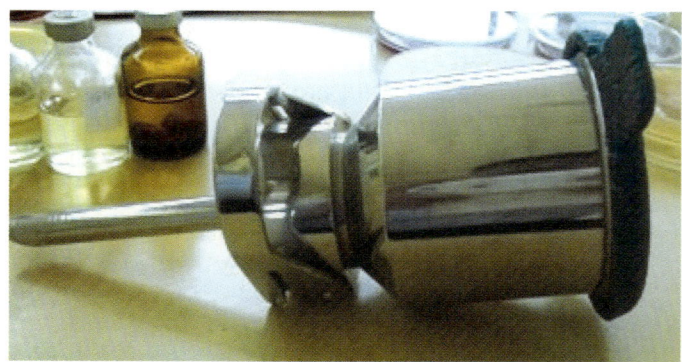

Fig. 9.5: Seitz filter

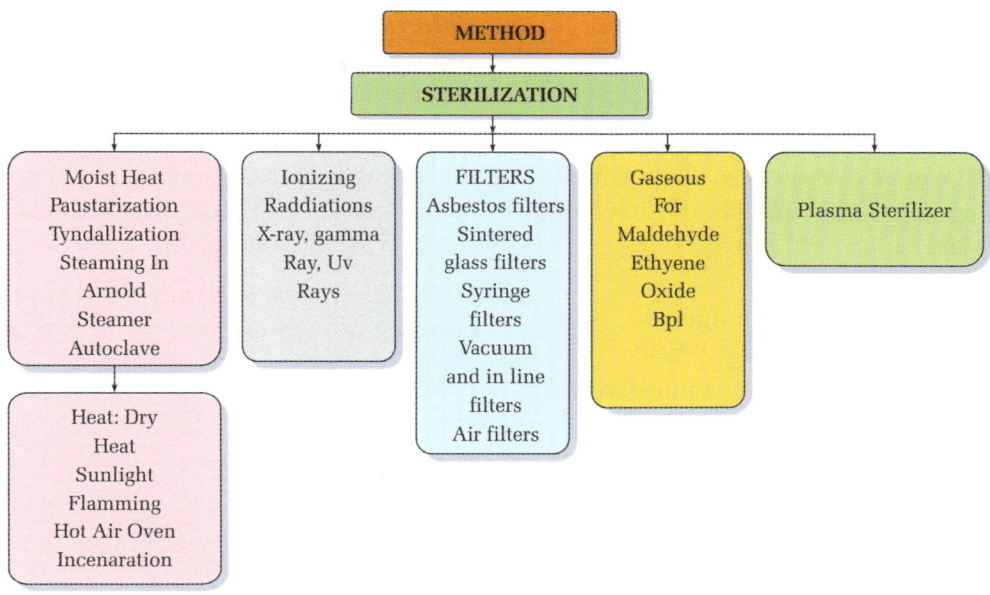

Fig. 9.6: Different methods of sterilization

Uses
- Checking of water samples
- Preparation of sterile parental fluids

Syringe filters: Membranes of 13 μm and 25 μm diameters are fitted in a holder of steel or polycarbonate. For the sterilization, the fluid is pushed with pressure by syringe.

Vacuum and in-line filters: Membranes of 25 μ and 45 μ are used and fitted with in-line filter holders or vacuum holders of borosilicate glass. Pressure filters of large membranes, 100–293 μm diameter, are held by Teflon filter or filter cartridges fitted on pressure filter holders. This is used to get **ultrapure water** for work in laboratory.

Air filters: Air is sterilized by air filters and then passed **in operation theatres or special wards**. High efficiency particulate air filters (HEPA) are used to purify large volume of air by using filters which remove particles above 0.3 micron or larger. These filters are used in **laminar flow.**

Various disinfectants and their efficiency against different organisms (Fig. 9.7):

Disinfectant	Effective			
	Bacteria	Spores	Viruses	Organic matter
Formaldehyde	+++	+++	+++	–
Gluteraldehyde	+++	+++	+++	–
Chlorine	+++	+/–	+++	+++
Phenols	++(+)	–––	+	+/–

TABLE 9.1: Summary of biological controls used in different sterilization methods (Fig. 9.6)

Autoclave	*Bacillus stearothermophilus*
Hot air oven	*Bacillus subtilis*
Ionizing radiations	*Bacillus pumilus*
Gas sterilization	*Bacillus subtilis*
Plasma sterilization	*Bacillus stearothermophilus*

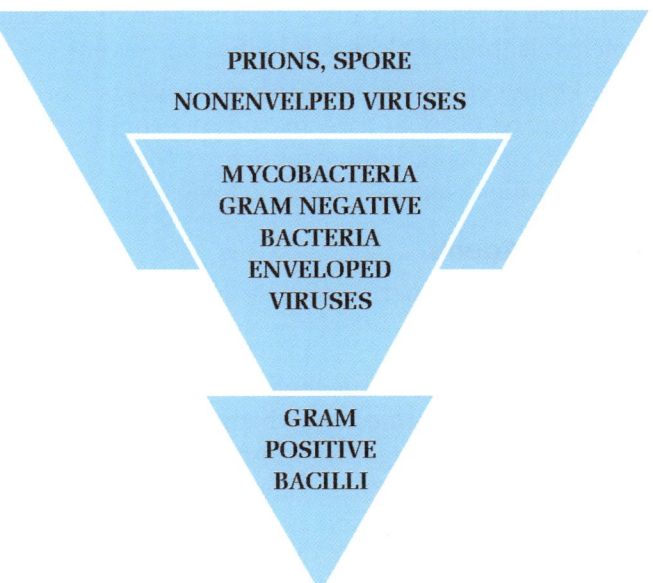

Fig. 9.7: Microorganisms arranged in decreasing order in respect to susceptibility to disinfectants

DISINFECTION

Characteristics of an ideal antiseptic or disinfectant:
- It should have a wide spectrum of activity.
- It should be active in presence of organic matter.
- It should be active in acid as well as alkaline media.
- It should have speedy action and should have high penetrating power.
- It should be stable.
- It should be compatible with other agents.
- It should not corrode metals.
- It should not cause local irritation or interfere with healing.
- It should be not be toxic, but safe and easy to use.
- It should be cheap and easily available.

Different modes of action of disinfectants
- Damage to cell wall and disruption of cell of microorganisms
- Oxidative damage
- Coagulation of proteins
- Change of proteins of microorganisms
- Inhibition of metabolism by inhibition of enzymes of microorganisms
- Inhibition of nucleic acid synthesis or change in nucleic acids
- Removal of sulfhydryl groups essential for functioning of enzymes
- Substrate competition.

Alcohol

Ethyl or isopropyl alcohol (60–70%)

Mechanism of action: It causes denaturation of bacterial proteins. Isopropyl alcohol is better, fat solvent.

Uses: Disinfection of clinical thermometers, for disinfection of skin before invasive procedures as collection of blood, lumbar puncture. Methyl alcohol used for fungal spores, vapour is toxic.

Oxidizing Agents

Halogens, H_2O_2, K-permanganate are oxidizing agents.

Halogens

- **Iodine**: Aqueous or alcoholic solution of iodine is used as a skin disinfectant which is bactericidal with moderate action against spores but active against *Mycobacterium tuberculosis* and many viruses.
- Tincture iodine which is an alcoholic solution containing 2.5% I and 2.5% KI in 90% alcohol.
- **Iodophore**: Iodine combined with surface active agents are called iodophores which are more active than tincture iodine.

Chlorine and related compounds: Chlorine releasing compounds used for purification of water (bleach), food and surface.

Treatment of spillage of blood: Place gauge piece over the blood spillage, pour 2% Na-hypochlorite solution over, keep it for 30 minutes and discard as infectious waste with gloved hands.

H_2O_2 (hydrogen peroxide): 3% solution is used for cleaning of wounds, for mouthwash and for gargles.

K-permanganate: This oxidizing agent is bactericidal and virucidal used in treatment of urethritis.

Alkylating Agents

This includes formaldehyde, gluteraldehyde and ethylene oxide gas.

Aldehydes

1. Formaldehyde: Its aqueous solution is bactericidal, sporocidal, and also effective against viruses.

Mechanism of action: It is active against amino groups.

Uses:
- For the preservation of anatomical specimen.
- Destroying spores of anthrax bacillus on wool or hairs of animals.
- Fumigation of wards and operation theaters, laboratories.
- Sterilization of bedding, clothing, instruments.

Fumigation procedure: If the area of room is 1000 cu.ft, 150 g of potassium permanganate is added to 280 mL of formalin. Before vapors start appearing, close the windows and door. Door and windows sealed for 48 hours and after that all traces of formaldehyde gas is nullified by ammonia vapors to avoid toxic effects and irritation.

Disadvantage: Formaldehyde gas coming out is irritant, which is nullified by ammonia vapors.

2. Glutaraldehyde: Percentage used is 1–2%. It is very effective against tubercle bacilli, fungi and viruses. (Less toxic and less irritant as compared to formaldehyde dye).

Uses: Sterilization of cystoscopes, bronchoscopes, corrugated rubber tubes, anesthetic tubes, face mask.

Formaldehyde gas, ethylene oxide gas and BPL are gaseous methods of sterilization.

Ethylene Oxide Gas

- This is one of the effective gaseous methods of sterilization. The processing of sterilizing items with ethylene oxide gas begins by addition of nitrogen gas to remove air or evacuating the chamber. Items sterilized must be aerated for 12 hours to remove traces of gas. Thus the entire process takes >16 hours but modified sterilizers can have short cycles.

- Toxic residues may be trapped in the wrapper or in the item.
- Polyvinylchloride and polyurethane absorb the gas fast and require long periods. The wrapper should be made up of materials which allow penetration of ethylene oxide gas. Items are then sterilized at 55°C.
- **Six variable** but independent **parameters** must be checked—gas concentration, vacuum, pressure, temperature, relative humidity and time of exposure.
- Ethylene oxide is a colorless liquid with low boiling point (10.7°C). It has high penetrating power.

Mechanism of action

- It is an alkylating agent, which inhibits amino, carboxyl, hydroxyl and sulfhydryl groups in proteins.
- It also reacts with DNA and nucleic RNA.
- N_2 and CO_2 decrease its explosive property while vapor increases its efficiency.

Uses: Temperature and/or pressure sensitive items are sterilized by ethylene oxide gas. It inactivates all microorganisms including fungal spores. It kills spores, bacteria, and viruses. It is used by manufacturer for sterilization of disposable items such as disposable needles, syringes, dental equipment, heart lung machine, respirators, sutures, clothing, books, food and tobacco.

In ethylene oxide sterilization, cold cycle operates at 37 ±5°C and hot cycle operates at 54 ±5°C.

Humidity is maintained at 40–50%.

Disadvantages: It has explosive activity, also mutagenic and carcinogenic. As it is difficult to handle being explosive, it is not suitable for sterilization of rooms and operation theatre.

Formaldehyde Gas

It is used for fumigation of operation theatres and special rooms.

Betapropoinolactone

Active against all forms of organisms, especially against viruses and used for biological products. It is used **in preparation of killed vaccines.**

Surface Active Agents

These act by reducing surface tension. They are classified as:

a. *Cationic agents*: This group includes benzalkonium chloride, cetrimide or cetavlon and quaternary ammonium compounds. These substances are efficient in killing Gram-positive bacteria than Gram-negative and no activity against MTB, bacterial spores, and viruses.

b. *Anionic agents*: They include soaps; soaps prepared from saturated fatty acids as coconut oil are effective against Gram-negative bacteria while soaps made from unsaturated fatty acids are effective against Gram-positive bacilli.

Amphoteric compounds known as tego agents which are effective against bacteria but they are not used routinely.

Phenols

Different phenolic compounds are used commonly as disinfectants. Phenol or carbolic acid (1%) is bactericidal, effective against vegetative bacteria, MTB and some fungi. It is toxic and corrosive also.

Cresol

It is used for cleaning floors and disinfection of table surfaces. If they are made in soaps, their bactericidal activity is increased, e.g. lysol is cresol in soaps.

Aniline Dyes

Aniline dyes, as crystal violet, malachite green, are active against Gram-positive organisms. **Acridine dyes** are active against Gram-negative bacilli.

Heavy metals, as silver, copper, have limited activity against bacteria.

Plasma Sterilizer (New Method of Sterilization)

Low temperature plasma is produced in a closed chamber with deep vacuum, an electromagnetic field and chemical precursor (H_2O_2 or mixture of H_2O_2 and per acetic acid). The resulting **free radicals, the chemicals and UV radiations destroy organisms and spores.**

Medical instruments are placed in the chamber, a strong vacuum is created and solution of H_2O_2 and water is automatically injected from a cassette. The solution vaporizes and diffuses in the chamber. Radiofrequency energy is applied to create an electric field, which in turn generates low temperature plasma, including free radicals. The combination of diffusion, pretreatment and plasma sterilizes the item. At the end of cycle, the radiofrequency energy is turned off, vacuum released and the chamber is filled with filtered air returning to normal pressure.

Disadvantages: Materials that absorb too much H_2O_2 (nylons), materials as some nylons that catalytically breakdown H_2O_2 and materials that react with H_2O_2 as organic dyes cannot be sterilized.

Disinfectants are divided into three groups:
a. High level disinfectants
b. Intermediate level disinfectants
c. Low level disinfectants

a. *High level disinfectants*: These methods are equivalent to that of sterilization except killing of large number of spores. These disinfectants are gluteraldehyde, hydrogen peroxide, peracetic acid and chlorine compounds. These disinfectants are used for cystoscopes and certain types of endoscopes.

b. *Intermediate level disinfectants*: These are not effective against spores. Mycobacteria and non-enveloped viruses are killed. They are useful for instruments as fiberoptic endoscopes where contamination with spores and highly resistant organisms is unlikely. These disinfectants include alcohols, phenolic compounds, and iodophores.

c. *Low level disinfectants*: These disinfectants are used for items which come in contact with patients but do not penetrate inside, e.g. stethoscopes, ECG electrodes.

The uses of different levels of disinfectants in relation to different items are given in Table 9.2.

Methods to Determine the Quality of Disinfectants

1. *Rideal-Walker tests*: Small quantities of organisms are added to varies tubes containing varying concentration of phenol as well as to tubes containing the disinfectant to be tested. The dilution of the disinfectant which sterilizes the suspension in a given time is divided by the dilution of phenol which sterilizes the same suspension at the same time is called **phenol coefficient.**

The test is easy to perform but has some disadvantage that it does not give the idea that how the disinfectant will perform in presence of organic matter.

2. *Inuse test*: The efficiency of the actual disinfectant routinely used in hospital is tested. Here, the ability of the disinfectant is determined by ability of it to inactive a particular number of a pathogenic *Staph. aureus* on a given surface within certain time.

3. *Chick-Martin test*: It is modified test, disinfectant acts in presence of organic matter. This makes natural conditions. Organic matter in the form of feces is added.

TABLE 9.2: Spaulding system of sterilization		
Class	*Definition and example*	*Level of sterilization*
Critical instruments	Equipment or devices that enter sterile body surfaces or tissues—surgical instruments, laparoscope, arthroscope, cardiac catheters	Sterilization
Semicritical instruments	Equipment or devices that come in contact with non-intact skin or mucous membranes but do not penetrate them—laryngoscope, vaginal speculum, gastroscope, colonoscope, bronchoscope, USG probe	High levels of disinfection destroys bacteria, fungi, viruses but not spores. 2% gluteraldehyde, 6% H_2O_2, pasteurization
Noncritical devices	Devices touches only skin and not mucosa—stethoscope, ECG machine, thermometer	Low or intermediate levels of sterilization kill bacteria, some fungi and enveloped viruses and mycobacteria. 3% H_2O_2, 60–90% alcohol, hypochlorite

TABLE 9.3: Summarizing different methods of sterilization used for different items	
Material	*Method*
Inoculating loop or wire	Flaming till it becomes red hot
Glassware—syringes, petridishes	Hot air oven
Disposable syringes and other disposable items	Gamma radiation, ethelene oxide
Culture media	Autoclave
L-J medium	Inspissation
Culture media containing egg, serum, glucose	Tyndallization
Toxins, sugar solutions, antibiotic solutions, hydatid fluid	Filtration
Cystoscopies and endoscopes	Gluteraldehyde
Milk	Pasteurization
Skin	Tincture iodine, 70% ethanol
Sterilization of operation theatre	Formaldehyde gas
Rubber, plastic tubes	Gluteraldehyde
Infective material as soiled dressing, beddings	Incineration

TABLE 9.4: Summary of mechanism of action of commonly used disinfectants

Material	Method
Alcohols	Denaturation of proteins
Aldehydes	Combined with nucleic acids, proteins by cross-linking and alkylating the molecules
Phenolic compounds	Denaturation of proteins
Na-hypochlorite	Oxidation of cellular materials
H_2O_2	Liberation of toxic free radicals which attack membrane, DNA
Heavy metals	Combine with bacterial proteins especially sulfhydryl groups

4. *Kelsey-Sykes test*: It takes into account, the capacity of disinfectant to retain its action on bacterium, though it is repeatedly exposed to standard bacterium (*Staphylococcus aureus, Pseudomonas, E. coli*). To a disinfectant solution, bacterium is added at 0, 10, 20 minutes. The disinfectants are incubated and transferred at 8, 18, 28 minutes, respectively. Presence or absence of growth is noted.

***Sterilization of prions*:** They are infectious proteins which are highly resistant to physical and chemical agents. Steam at 134–138°C for 18 minutes is effective in killing prions. They are sensitive to household bleach, 90% phenol and iodine.

10

Genetics

GENETICS

It is study of heredity and variation. It helps to understand the causes of the similarities and differences between parents and their progeny. All hereditary characteristics (except some RNA viruses) such as virulence, pathogenicity, and antibiotic resistance, are due to genes present in DNA. Chromosomal DNA maintains the stability within organism.

Nucleic Acids

They are of two types, DNA and RNA, which are almost similar except in RNA, the sugar is ribose and the base uracil is present instead of thymine.

Bacterial chromosome: It is haploid, with one copy of gene. In bacteria, circular chromosome is present, which is single long DNA molecule (1 mm long). There are two strands of complementary polynucleotide chains held together in a double helix. Each strand has backbone of deoxyribose and phosphate and one of the nitrogen bases are attached to deoxyribose (Fig. 10.1a). The nitrogen bases are two purines, i.e. adenine (A) and guanine (G) and two pyrimidines: Thymine (T) and cytocine (C). Two strands are held together by hydrogen bonding between bases on opposite strands such a way that hydrogen bonds are present between A–T and G–C. Adenine and thymine form one complementary base pair, while another pair is formed by guanine and cytocine. In a DNA molecule, there are equal numbers of adenine and thymine and equal numbers of guanine, cytocine.

G+C ratio: The ratio of each pair of bases is called G+C ratio. It is A+T/G+C. This ratio for a particular species is constant; hence it is used as one of genetic characteristics which determines the percentage of similarity between species, and helps in genetic classification of bacteria.

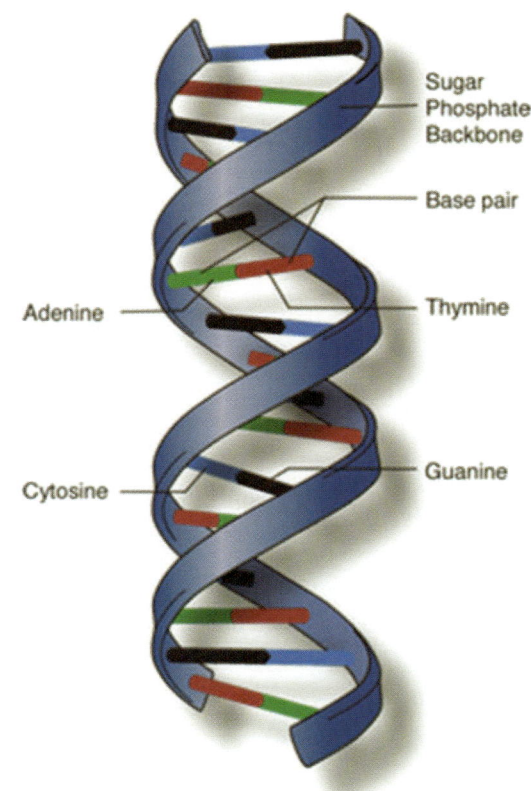

Sugar
Phosphate
Backbone

Base pair

Adenine

Thymine

Cytosine

Guanine

Fig. 10.1a: Structure of DNA

What are genes?

A segment of DNA carrying codons specifying for a particular polypeptide is called a **gene** and the total compoment of genes in a cell is genome. Genetic information is stored in DNA as a **code** which is a sequence of 3 bases, i.e. **triplet code (codon)**. A DNA molecule consists of large number of genes, each triplet codon transcribed on mRNA codes for a single amino acid. A molecule of DNA consists of a large number of genes, each gene contains hundreds of thousands of nucleotides. Bacterial chromosome consists of double-stranded DNA arranged in circular form, about 1000 µm in length. Length of DNA is usually expressed as kilobases. (1 kb = 1000 base pairs). Bacterial DNA is about 4000 kb and human genome is about 3 million kb long.

There are total 64 codons, 61 of which code for specific amino acids and 3 codons do not code for amino acid, called **nonsense codons**. Their function is to terminate polypeptide chains, hence called **stopcodons (UAA, UGA, and UAG).**

DNA replication: Two strands of DNA separate, each acts as template for producing complementary strand, thus newly formed DNA has one strand of parent DNA preserved and one strand of daughter DNA. Hence, this type of replication is called semiconservative replication. DNA-dependent DNA polymerase is important enzyme in replication, others are polymerases; polymerase III is responsible for replication while polymerase I is required for repair.

Transcription: The gene represents a code which is transcribed on mRNA and translated as a polypeptide. There are three types of RNA: rRNA, mRNA, and tRNA. RNA polymerase attaches itself to beginning of gene on DNA and synthesizes a single complementary polyribonucleotide strand, using one of the strand in DNA double helix. This is called transcription.

Genotype: It is the genetic constitution of the cell that is transmitted to its progeny.

Phenotype: It is physical expression of the genotype in the given environment. The cell may exhibit different phenotypic appearances in different situations.

Two types of variations seen in bacteria are phenotypic variation and genotypic variation. Genetic variation is mostly because of mutation.

Phenotypic variation: A bacterial cell shows different phenotypic characteristics in different conditions.

S. typhi becomes nonmotile when grown on phenol agar due to loss of flagella. This is a reversible change. If subcultured in broth, it develops flagella.

Environmental influence on synthesis of enzymes: Some of the enzymes produced by bacteria are **inducible,** they are produced in presence of inducible substance. *E. coli* has genes required for the synthesis of enzyme beta-galactosidase which is necessary for lactose fermentation. This enzyme is produced in presence of lactose (medium containing lactose such as MacConkey agar).

Enzymes which are produced irrespective of presence or absence of substrate are called **constitutive enzymes.**

MUTATION (Flowchart 10.1)

Random undirected heritable variation caused by an alteration in the nucleotide sequence at some point of the DNA of the cell is called mutation. This may occur irrespective of phenotypic change in the cell. As there is permanent alteration or change in bases of DNA, these changes may or may not lead to detectable change phenotypically, hence they are called **silent mutations**. The form in which a gene exists when a bacterium is first isolated from nature is called **wild type alleles**. The genes produced by mutations are called **mutant alleles.** Mutation rate of individual gene in bacteria ranges from 10^{-6} to 10^{-10} per bacterium per division (Fig. 10.1b).

Mutation may be **spontaneous** or **induced by some agents mutagenes** as UV rays, acridine dyes, alkalating agents, 5-bromouracil.

Mutational changes include nucleotide replacements, deletions and insertions.

A. Point Mutation

It is a mutation in which there is a change in sequence of a single nucleotide. It may be reversible. It is of two classes.

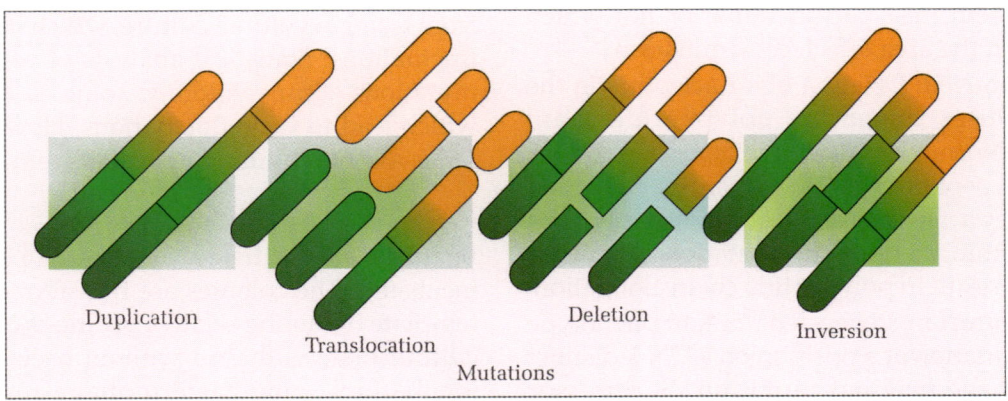

Duplication

Translocation

Deletion

Inversion

Mutations

Fig. 10.1b: Mutations

1. Base Pair Substitution

Mutants in which a single base pair (nucleotide) has been substituted by another pair. It occurs by following ways:

a. *Transposition*: Replacement of purine by purine or pyrimidine by pyrimidine (substitution of one base pair but purine to pyrimidine orientation is retained).

b. *Transversion*: Replacement of purine with pyrimidine or vice versa.

c. *Silent mutation*: It is change in DNA level that does not result in any change in amino acid in the encoded protein. This is due to more than one codon may code for an amino acid.

2. Frame Shift Mutations

One or more base pairs (nucleotides) may be inserted or deleted from DNA. This results in shifting of normal translation reading frame of coded message from the point of forming an entirely new set of codons. During translation, the coded message is read correctly up to the point of loss or addition. The subsequently codons will specify for a wrong amino acids.

B. Multisite Mutations

There is alteration of DNA involving large number of base pairs. The changes in DNA involves multisite deletions or duplications or addition.

C. Deletions and Insertions

During DNA replication, there may be insertion of base pairs or deletions of base pairs. This shifts normal reading frame of coded message, forming new triplet of codons which specify for nonspecific amino acid. These mutations are **frame shift mutations.**

Other Mutations

- *Missense mutation*: The triplet code is altered so as to specify an amino acid different from that normally located at the particular position in the protein. The resultant protein may be functional or not which depends upon the area affected by mutation.

- *Nonsense mutation*: Deletion of a nucleotide in the gene that causes premature polypeptide chain termination. Normally, any of the nonsense codons terminate polypeptide chain elongation, in production of protein, they act as stop codons. If nonsense codon is formed within the gene by mutation of a sense codon, it will result in polypeptide chain elongation.

- *Suppressor mutation*: Reversal of mutant phenotype by another mutation at a position on a DNA distinct from that of the original mutation. Suppressor mutations are classed as intragenic when second mutation occurs at site different from first in the same gene. Intergenic mutations are those when second mutation is occurring in different genes.

- *Lethal mutation*: Mutations involving vital functions and such mutants are nonviable.

- *Conditional lethal mutant*: Mutants produced may be able to live under certain conditions (permissive conditions), e.g. **temperature** sensitive mutant.

Spontaneous mutations: These are mutations taking place in absence of known mutagenic stimuli. Its frequency is one per 10^{-6}–10^{-10}.

Induced mutations: These are induced by a stimulus which may be physical as UV rays, ionizing raditions, heat or chemicals, or substances acting directly on the structure of DNA as alkylating agents.

Demonstration of mutation

- Microarrays and DNA chips
- Gene sequencing
- *Detection of phenotypic character*: It involves screening a property that is unique to mutant strain, e.g. organism's ability to grow in presence of antibiotic.

Tests for Demonstration of Mutations

Mutations can be demonstrated by gene sequencing and demonstrating phenotypic changes.

Fluctuation Test

A small portion of sensitive bacterial colonies are cultured in 100 tubes containing media and a single large volume culture. Sample from each tube is plated on medium containing bacteriophages.

Plates are incubated. After incubation, the numbers of colonies of mutant bacteria (phage resistant) are determined.

When results are observed, wide fluctuations in the number of resistant variants in small cultures are seen as compared to control with multiple samples plated from a single volume culture, which has much smaller fluctuations. Statistical analysis of results shows that mutations occur randomly, some early and some late which lead to wide fluctuations. However, in a single large volume culture, fluctuations remain within limits.

Replica Plating Method

Bacteria are cultured on master plate. Plates are incubated. The colonies are transferred using a velvet template (retaining relative positions of all colonies) on culture plate with and without bacteriophages. After incubation, some bacteriophage resistant mutants appear on plate containing bacteriophage (Fig. 10.1c).

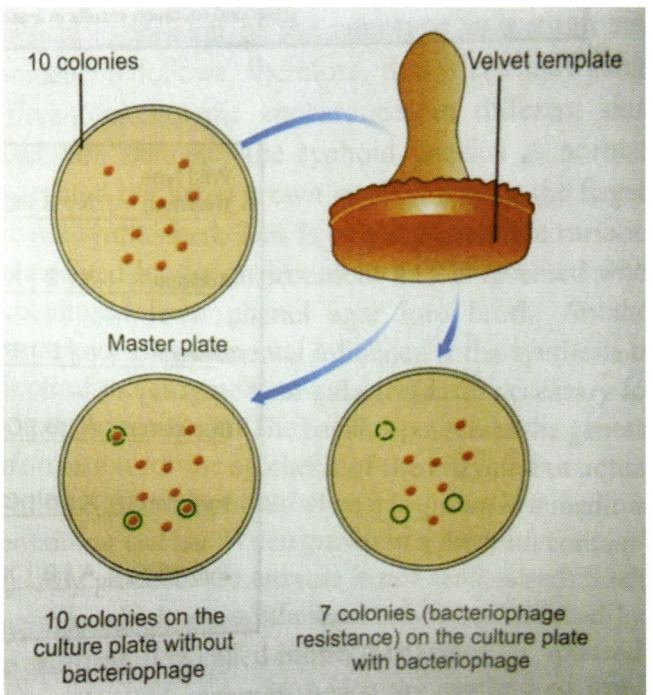

Fig. 10.1c: Replica plate method

Flowchart 10.1: Mutations

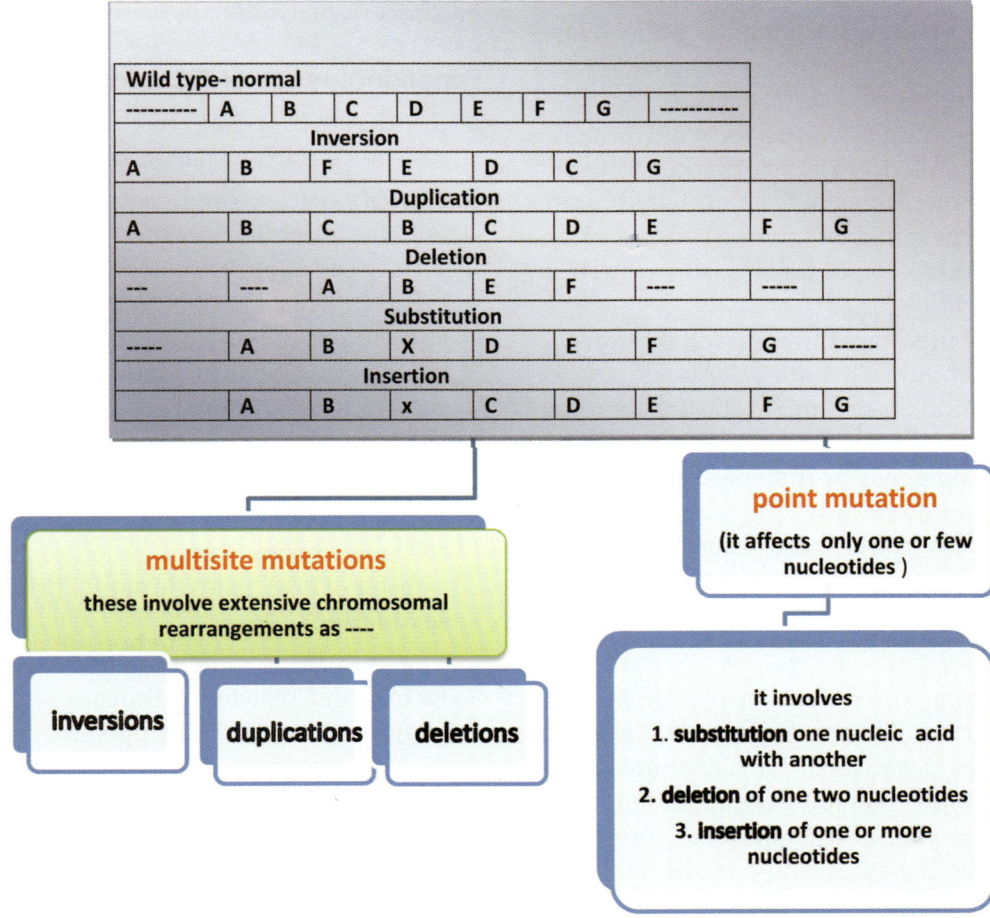

Wild type- normal								
----------	A	B	C	D	E	F	G	-----------
Inversion								
A	B	F	E	D	C	G		
Duplication								
A	B	C	B	C	D	E	F	G
Deletion								
---	----	A	B	E	F	----	-----	
Substitution								
-----	A	B	X	D	E	F	G	-------
Insertion								
	A	B	x	C	D	E	F	G

multisite mutations

these involve extensive chromosomal rearrangements as ----

inversions **duplications** **deletions**

point mutation

(it affects only one or few nucleotides)

it involves

1. **substitution** one nucleic acid with another
2. **deletion** of one two nucleotides
3. **insertion** of one or more nucleotides

The appearance of bacteriophage resistant mutants without prior contact with selective agent indicates that mutation occurred.

PLASMIDS

Plasmids are extrachromosomal genetic material (DNA) which replicate of their own, independent of chromosomal DNA (autonomous replication without dependence on chromosomes). It is double-stranded circular DNA present in cytoplasm away from chromosome in a free state and carry different genes. The larger plasmids which are **self-transferable** are called **conjugative plasmids,** which carry genes necessary for their transfer from one bacterium to another. Apart from these genes, the plasmid may carry genes of drug resistance, e.g. 'R' plasmids which carry genes for multidrug résistance.

The non-conjugative plasmids are small, non-transferable of their own as they do not have genes which take part in transfer, but can be transferred with the help of conjugative plasmids. For example, resistance determinants, bacteriocin plasmids.

Plasmids may express a phenotypic character in progeny. These are enterotoxin production, hemolysin production.

Plasmids act as **virulence factors** in many ways, which are:

- They may carry genes of drug resistance.
- Some bacteria have invasive property attributed to cell wall proteins called "virulence marker antigens" which are coded by plasmids. Such proteins are present in *Shigella* which invade mucosa causing ulcers.
- Plasmids may code for enterotoxin production, exotoxin production.
- They have the ability to get transferred by transfection (transfer without cell contact).
- Some of the plasmids may jump to chromosome and vice versa by a process called transposition hence known as jumping genes or transposons.
- They can be lost automatically. They can be extracted from a cell by chemicals and characterized. Plasmid profile is one of the genotypic typing methods of bacteria which has role in identification of source of outbreaks.

'R' plasmids: The groups of conjugative plasmids—large plasmids with **R factors**. There are two functional parts:

a. *Resistance transfer factor (RTF):* This contains, genes of autonomous replication and conjugation.
b. *Resistance determinant (r-det)* smaller component transfers drug resistance. A single factor may carry genes of resistance to many antibiotics.

General Properties of Plasmid

1. *Physical properties:* It is double-stranded circular DNA existing autonomously. The molecular weight is 10^6–10^8, they encode for 40–50 genes. They are about 1–3% of the weight of bacterial chromosome.
2. *Replication:* Plasmids carry genes for their self-replication.
3. *Curing:* They can be lost naturally or by curing agent.
4. *Incompatibility:* Two members of the same group cannot coexist.
5. *Transferability:* Some plasmids are self-transferable others are not (non-conjugative plasmids).

Types of Plasmids

Conjugative plasmids: These types of plasmids are common in Gram-negative bacilli. They are relatively large, 25–150 million daltons. Large plasmids are usually present in 1–2 copies per bacterium, their replication may be closely related to the replication of bacterial chromosome.

Nonconjugative plasmids: They are common in Gram-positive bacteria, they are small, 1–10 daltons. Some of functional types of plasmid, i.e. 'r' plasmids or bacteriocin plasmids are nonconjugative plasmids.

Functional Types of Plasmids

a. *R plasmid:* It has two component—RTF, i.e. resistance transfer factor and r-determinants.
b. *Fertility factor:* The F factor in donor cell integrate with bacterial chromosome form one large molecule. This produces high frequency recombination cells(Hfr cells, i.e. cells transfer chromosomal DNA to recipient cells with high frequency.

   The conversion of F+ cell into Hfr state is reversible, hence when 'F' factor reverts back from integrated state to free stage, it may carry some chromosal genes. Such 'F' factor with some chromosomal genes is called **Fprime**. Matting with Fprime cell, recipient cell gets chromosomal genes of host cell and this transfer of host genes through Fprime factor is called **sexduction.**
c. The two important plasmids colicinogenic (**col factor**) and resistance transfer factor (**RTF**) which give properties as colicin production and resistance to drugs are transferred by conjugation.
   COL factor: This is a plasmid responsible for the production of colicins by *E. coli*. Colicin is an antibiotic-like substance which acts on other bacteria. The plasmid or col factor is transmitted by conjugation.

Episomes

These are also extra chromosomal genetic materials which are either integrated with chromosomal DNA or exist autonomously in the cytoplasm. They are similar to plasmids (even it may not be possible to differentiate between these two hence two terms are used many times synonymously).

Transposomes (Fig. 10.2)

These are DNA sequences which have the property of moving from chromosome to plasmid or vice versa or from one plasmid to another plasmid. Hence they are also called **jumping genes** (transposons).

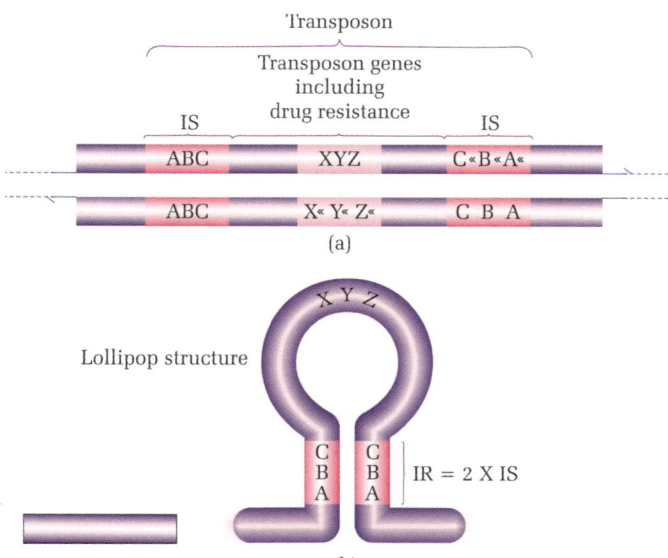

Fig. 10.2: Transposon

Transposomes do not have separate existence as plasmids. The transfer from one DNA to other is called **transposition.**

Apart from other genes, transposomes also carry genes that are required for their transfer. When they migrate they produce insertion mutants. The involvements of short transposome known as insertion elements produce many insertion mutations. Insertion elements carry genes for enzymes for their jumping character from one site to another site. As genes required for their own replication are absent on transposomes are not able to replicate autonomously. Transposomes integrate with bacterial DNA for their transmission. Transposomes are larger than 2 kb and contain resistant gene (often encoding resistance to one or more antibacterials) in addition to those required for transposition. Two ends have inserted repeat sequences which are complementary to each other but in reverse order. Each strand of transposome can form a single-stranded loop and double-stranded stem formed by terminal inverted repeat sequences with hydrogen bonds. Small transposons are called insertion sequences. There are two classes of transposomes:

1. **Composite transposomes** where two copies of an identical IS elements flank drug resistance genes.

2. **Simple transposome** is Tn3 (encoding resistance to beta lactamase).

MECHANISMS OF TRANSFER OF GENETIC MATERIAL OR GENE TRANSFER

A. Transformation (Fig. 10.3)

The genetic information transferred through free or naked DNA is called **transformation.** The soluble DNA

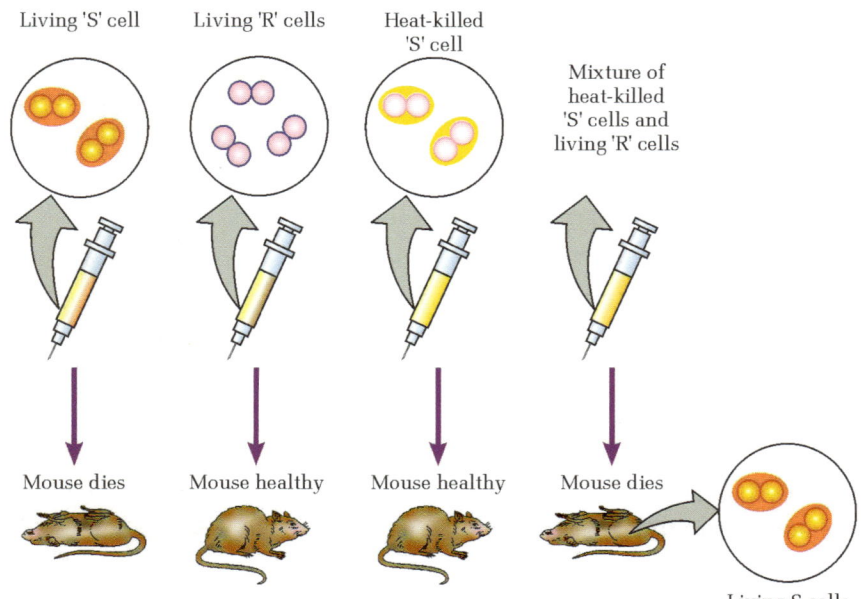

Fig. 10.3: Transformation

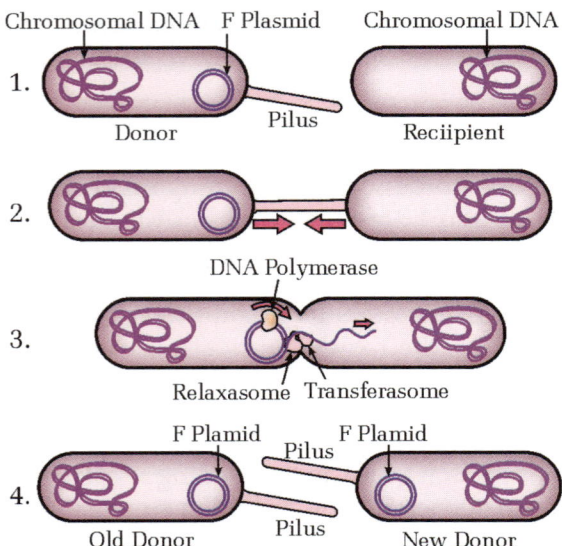

Fig. 10.4: Transfer of 'F' plasmid

is transferred from one bacterium to another, thus properties of one bacterium is transferred to another.

Transfer of genetic characteristic of one bacterium to another was first studied by Griffith, he performed experiment on pneumococcus. He injected non-capsulated strain of bacterium in mouse. He also injected killed suspension of capsulated strains of penumococcus in the same animal. The moused died and living smooth strain of pneumococcus was isolated for that mouse. He concluded that the heat killed smooth strains might have liberated some substance which converted rough strains into smooth strains and virulence of those strains increased causing death of animal.

Later on transformation was identified as mechanism responsible for the change and DNA of smooth strain which was transformed directly to non-virulent rough strains.

Mechanism of transformation: During transformation, the bacterium becomes competent and during this period of competence, the double-stranded DNA binds to sites (present during the stage of competence only). The DNA is fragmented by some enzymes. Fragmented pieces of parent bacterium are taken by recipient cells. These fragments are well placed in recipient cell.

Natural competence is not common in bacteria and some of these bacteria get transformed in presence of competence factors. Competence factors are produced at only specific point in growth cycle.

Naturally competent bacteria are the pneumococci, gonococci, meningococci, *Haemophilus influenzae* and *Bacillus subtilis*. For *Neisseria* and *Haemophilus* spp, specific DNA sequences are required for the uptake of

DNA. This uptake sequences are species specific, thus restricting the transfer to single species.

Forced transformation: Other bacteria can be forced by treatment with calcium chloride and temperature shock.

Once taken into cell, the chromosomal DNA must combine with host cell genome to maintain stability and to inherited. But if DNA is completely unrelated, the absence of homology prevents recombination and the DNA is degraded. However, plasmid DNA may be transformed into cell and expressed without recombination. Thus transformation is a strong tool for molecular genetic analyis of bacteria.

B. Transduction (Fig. 10.5)

Transfer of genetic information from one bacterium toanother through the agency of bacteriophages is calledtransduction. Bacteriophages are the viruses that infectand live on bacteria. They transfer chromosomal DNAas well as plasmid DNA.

During multiplication, maturation, and assembly bacteriophages occurs in bacterium, the progeny viruses carry some genes of host bacterium. When such progeny bacteriophages infect other bacterium, they give genes of first bacterium to second bacterium. There are two types of transduction mechanisms:

1. *Generalized transduction*: Any segment of host DNA has equal chance of being incorporated into the bacteriophage coat.

2. *Specialized transduction* in which a particular segment of host DNA is transduced, hence a particular genetic trait is transferred.

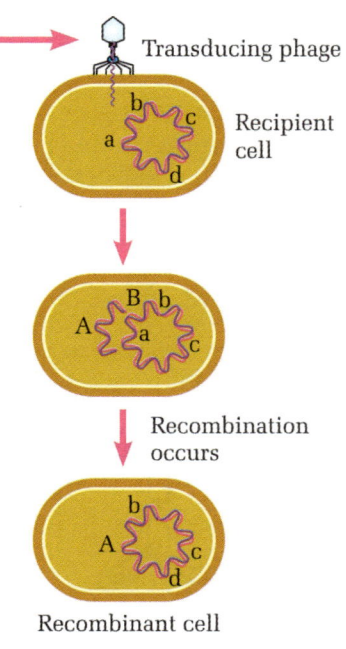

Fig. 10.5: Transduction

Bacteriophage infects bacterial cell. This is followed by release of phage nucleic acid in bacterium which starts replicating. During maturation of phage , few phage heads may enclose any fragments of bacterial DNA(generalized transduction) or particular part of bacterial DNA(specialized transduction) along with phage DNA. When such phage enters other bacterial cell, it introduces bacterial DNA which may be incorporated into bacterial chromosome.

Since the specialized transduction is based on specific chromosome—prophage interaction, only genomic DNA and not plasmid DNA is transferred by this process.

Significance

Transduction can be observed in any bacterium for which bacteriophage exists. Transduction may carry not only nuclear DNA but may also plasmid or episomes. It is an excellent tool for genetic mapping and it can be used in genetic engineering to control inborn errors of metabolisms.

Lysogenic Conversion

In transduction, adsorption of phage is followed by injection of phage DNA into bacterium. If the phage is virulent type, new phage particles formed within bacterium are released by lytic cycle. If bacteriophage is temperate phage, instead of release, its DNA gets incorporated with bacterial DNA as prophage. It multiplies synchronously with bacterial DNA, acts as additional chromosomal DNA and bacterium acquires new characteristics which are transferred to progeny bacterium. This process by which a bacterium acquires new property because of infection by bacteriophage is called lysogenic conversion. For example, diphtheria bacilli are toxigenic because of presence of TOX phage. It produces its toxin, the genes of which are coded by infecting bacteriophage. If the strain is made free from the TOX phage, the resultant bacterium will not be able to produce the toxin.

C. Conjugation (Fig. 10.6)

Transfer of genetic material in which male or donor bacterium makes contact with recipient bacterium which is female bacterium is called conjugation. The male bacterium which has genes to code for conjugation tube act as donor F+ cell. The genes for formation of conjugation tube is present on plasmid. 'F' factor is transmitted by only conjugation, when male and female cells make cell to cell contact. After F factor is transmitted, every bacterium F– gets converted in male F+.

The genetic information required for formation of conjugation tube is on 'tra' genes.

In other cases, the self-transmissible plasmid integrates with DNA of another replicon and as an extension of itself, carries a strand of DNA into recipient cell.

'F' is self-replicating plasmid and may carry genes for other properties. The plasmids control the process of conjugation, hence called transfer factor or conjugative genes. Thus 'F' factor is one of the plasmids which determines 'maleness' as well as other characteristic. For example, 'R' factor and Col factor. R determines drug resistance while Col factor causes production of colicin.

Mechanism of Conjugation

- The donor cell has genes for production of pilus; it makes contact with recipient bacterium.
- Retraction of pilus present on first bacterium mediates contact between two bacteria. There is pore formation in adjoining cell membranes of two bacteria.
- Single strand of first bacterial DNA is broken down. The broken strand enters recipient bacterium. Formation of mating signals the plasmid to begin the transfer of one strand.

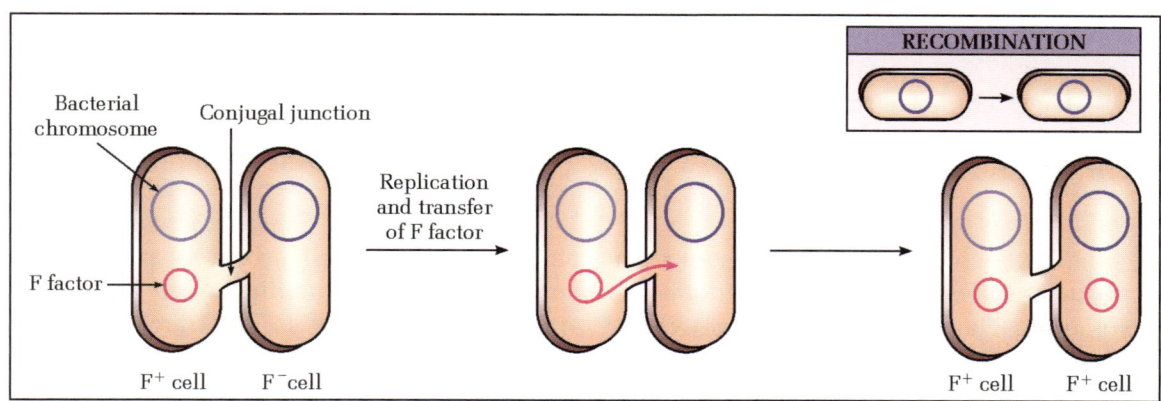

Fig. 10.6: Conjugation

- The complementary strands are produced in both, donor and recipient bacteria.
- Both cells now contain double-stranded plasmids and the mating pair separates.

The F factor in donor cell integrate with bacterial chromosome form one large molecule. This produces high frequency recombination cells (Hfr cells, i. e. cells transfer chromosomal DNA to recipient cells with high frequency.

'F' factor may revert back from recombinant state to free cells and may detach from from chromosomal DNA. It may carry some chromosomal DNA with it. Such 'F' factors with some chromosomal genes are known as F' (F prime). This F' cell may conjugate with F cell and transfer chromosomal DNA inserted in it. This is known as sexduction.

Transfer of drug resistance was first observed in Japan (1959), there were many strains of *Shigella* which were multiple drug resistant and drug resistance in *Shigella* was transferred from multiple drug resistant *E. coli*. This mechanism of drug resistance is called **transferable drug resistance or infectious drug resistance.**

Genetic Mechanisms of Acquired Drug Resistance

The drug resistance is acquired when change in DNA occurs. The change may occur by alteration of structure of chromosome called mutation or by acquisition of plasmid which is the result of exchange of genetic material in which sensitive bacterium gets extra chromosomal DNA (part of DNA) which carry genes of resistance to one or more drugs.

Mutational Drug Resistance

Mutation is a random and undirected heritable change caused by change in nucleotide sequence of the DNA of the cell. A spontaneous change in chromosomal gene which regulates susceptibility to a particular drug may occur. Such change takes place due to mutation of genes. This makes bacterium resistant to that drug. The presence of drug serves as selective mechanism to suppress susceptibility and promotes the growth of drug resistance strains. Mutational drug resistance is nontransferable. The presence of the drug itself serves as a selective mechanism to suppress susceptibility and promotes the drug resistance.

Mutational resistance is of two types:
- *Stepwise mutation*: A high level of resistance to penicillin is due to series of stepwise mutations.
- *One step mutation*: The mutants differ widely in degree of resistance which is seen in streptomycin.

In medicine, drug resistance is important as *Mycobacterium tuberculosis* may show resistance to various drugs as INH, rifampicin, streptomycin. If a single drug is given to the patient, bacilli may die initially but soon develop resistance as some mutants with change in genes occur. The consequence of this may be serious as emergence of multiple drug resistant strains. To avoid this in tuberculosis, multiple drug therapy is given. By using four drugs together, a mutant resistant to one drug is taken care by other drugs as mutational drug resistance involves one drug at one time.

Transferable Drug Resistance

As the genes are responsible for expression of drug resistance, the change in DNA may lead to resistance to antibiotic substances. As there are different mechanisms of transfer of genetic material from one bacterial cell to another, the genes of resistance will also be transferred from one bacterium to another, hence this type of resistance is called transferable drug resistance. Examples of transferable resistance include R plasmids.

Transferable drug resistance is seen in bacteria belonging to family Enterobacteriaceae, e.g. *E. coli*, *Salmonella*, *Shigella*.

Drug resistance is transferred *in vivo*, in GIT. If the person has plasmids for multiple drug resistance present in normal commensal as *E. coli* and if that person gets infection with *Salmonella*, the drug resistance may be transferred from *E. coli* to *Salmonella* in the intestine, and the organisms will be shed in feces and will be responsible for spread of multiple drug resistant *Salmonella* among many patients.

Factors which help in spread of drug resistance: In normal gastrointestinal tract, there are many factors which will prevent transfer of 'R' plasmids.

These factors include anaerobic conditions, alkaline pH, normal flora preventing the contact between sensitive bacteria and resistant bacteria. **Indiscriminate use of oral** antibiotics will kill the normal flora of GUT and hence increase conditions for transfer of drug resistance.

How R plasmid spread occurred in Salmonella?
Oral antibiotics were given along with animal feeds to animals. The transfer of 'R' factor occurred in animal intestine and animals shed multiple drug resistant *Salmonella*.

Other species or genera in which spread of R plasmids occur are *Vibrio, Pseudomonas, Providentia, Klebsiella, and Pasteurella*.

The resistance of *Staphylococcus* to penicillin is due to a plasmid which produces penicillinase which inactivates the penicillin group of antibiotics. This plasmid is lacking RTF. **The transfer occurs by transduction rather than conjugation.**

Differences between mutational and transferable drug resistance are given in Table 10.1.

TABLE 10.1: Differences between mutational and transferable drug resistance

Mutational	Transferable drug resistance
Resistance is due to mutation of gene	Resistance is due to transfer of genes of resistance
Resistance is nontransferable	Resistance is transferable from one bacterium to another bacterium from another taxa
Low degree resistance	High degree resistance
Resistance to one drug at a time	Resistance to many drugs at a time may occur
Resistance can be overcome by combination of antibiotics	Combination of antibiotics is ineffective
Virulence of mutants may low	Virulence is not decreased, or it may be enhanced
Mutants may be defective	Nondefective

Some Points to Remember

- First example of transformation in bacteria—*Pneumococcus*.
- First example of lysogenic conversion—*Corneybacterium*.
- First example of transferable drug resistance was seen in *Shigella*.

Genetic Engineering

Genetic engineering is also called recombinant DNA technology. In this method, a specific protein which is coded by a particular gene, i.e. the gene of interest is inserted in another organism which will express that gene, thus leads to large-scale production of the desired protein.

Steps

- The desired gene, for example, the gene for cytokine production, is cut by enzyme **restriction endonuclease** and isolated.
- This gene is inserted into a carrier or vector as a plasmid or bacteriophage to which it binds covalently. The inserted gene is sealed by enzyme ligase. The plasmid now becomes recombinant plasmid.
- The recombinant plasmid is inserted into bacteria as *E. coli* or yeast as *Saccharomyces* by transformation (direct transfer of plasmid from one cell to another).
- The *E.coli* is then inoculated on suitable medium; it will produce colonies thus large quantities of proteins as cytokines are produced.

Uses

- Production of vaccines as recombinant *Hepatitis B* vaccine, rabies vaccine.
- Genetic diseases may be treated by producing many copies of normal genes and injecting them in the patient.
- Production of hormones as insulin, growth hormone, production of cytokines as IL1, IL-2, TNF, enzymes as streptokinase.

DIAGNOSTIC TECHNIQUES—RECENT ADVANCES

DNA Probes

DNA probes are pieces of single stranded DNA which are either radio-labeled or chromatographically labeled so that they can be used to detect homologous DNA present in clinical specimen. As genetic sequence of organism is known, if we attach such DNA (sequence similar to the organism) to radiolabeled dye, it can be used to detect that specific organism in the clinical specimen. The nucleic acid of the organism is extracted and denatured. The DNA probe will attach to the single-stranded DNA of the organism present in the specimen and will form a double-stranded DNA, a process called genetic recombination. After recombination, radioactivity is detected. If there is no organism present, no radioactivity is detected.

Uses of DNA probes: Detection of organism especially noncultivable organisms in clinical specimens.

- List of infections which can be diagnosed includes *Chlamydia trachomatis, Mycoplasma pneumoniae, H. pylori, Mycobacterium tuberculosis, Mycobacterium avium intercellulare complex*, Herpes simplex viruses, Hepatitis B virus, Hepatitis C virus, Rotavirus, HIV, HPV, CMV, Malarial parasite, *Leishmania donovani*, enterotoxins of Enterotoxigenic *E. coli*.
- Identification of genes of bacterial resistance.
- Identification of virulence factor as outer membrane protein (OMP) of *Shigella*.
- Identification of organism from culture.
- Identification of a strain of organism which is important epidemiologically to find out the source of outbreak.

PCR (Polymerase Chain Reaction) (Karry Mullis 1983)

PCR causes amplification of specific DNA sequence or gene of interest which is then detected by any of the detection system. If small number of organisms present, their DNA is first separated and amplified so that detection is possible with increased sensitivity. Specific designed primer with specific sequences make use of ribonucleotides provided in the reaction mixture to produce multiple copies of target DNA. The reaction is carried in three steps.

- *Denaturation*: The DNA of organism is first extracted; denaturation is carried out at high temperature (94°C) so that two strands of DNA get separated.
- Annealing of primers to target DNA at 50–70°C.
- Synthesis of nucleic acids by addition of ribonucleotides and the DNA polymerase which causes extension of primers and synthesis of nucleic acids. Thus, from a single DNA, two copies of similar DNA produced (amplification).
- The denaturation of newly formed DNA occurs and such cycles are repeated so that there is exponential increase in the amount target DNA. The last step is detection of the amplified products.

Applications of PCR

Diagnosis of infectious diseases

1. **Bacterial infection:** Tuberculosis, legionellosis, *H. pylori, Chlamydia trachomatis, Mycoplasma pneumoniae.*
2. **Viruses:** HPV, HIV, hepatitis B virus, hepatitis C virus, herpes simplex viruses, CMV, measles, adenovirus.
3. **Parasites:** *Plasmodium* species, *Toxoplasma gondii.*
4. **Fungi:** *C. albicans, Pneumocystis jirovecii.*

Immunoblotting Techniques

1. *Southern blotting (EM Southern)*: Specific DNA sequences generated by restriction fragment length polymorphism are separated by gel electrophoresis. Detection is done by southern blotting, a method that uses hybridization of DNA to DNA. Restriction endonuclease breaks DNA at some specific locations producing some DNA fragments. These are separated by gel electrophoresis. They are converted into single-stranded DNA and treated with single-

stranded DNA tagged with radiolabeled dye. The DNA–DNA hybridization forms radioactive double-stranded DNA which is detected by X-ray. (Blotting is the absorption of fragment on cellulose membrane) (Fig. 10.7).

2. *Northern blotting*: It is used for analysis of RNA. The method is similar to Southern blotting (Fig. 10.8).

3. *Western blotting (WB)*: It is used for the identification and analysis of proteins. In clinical microbiology, it is a specific test for diagnosis of HIV. The antibodies are detected in patient's serum. Similarly WB is also used for diagnosis of Lyme disease (Fig. 10.9).

The test for HIV is specific as it detects antibodies against different components of HIV.

Steps

- Suspension of organisms against which antibodies are to be detected, is mechanically or chemically distrupted.
- The solubilized antigen suspension is placed on polyacrylamide gel, and proteins are separated by electrophoresis.
- The protein bands which are produced by electrophoresis are transferred from gel to nitrocellulose or other type of thin membrane.
- The nitrocellulose (or membrane) is cut into many thin strips, each carrying the pattern of protein band.
- Patient's serum is layered over the strips, antibodies will bind to each protein component represented by a band on strip.
- The pattern of band is used to detect whether the patient is infected with the organism or not.

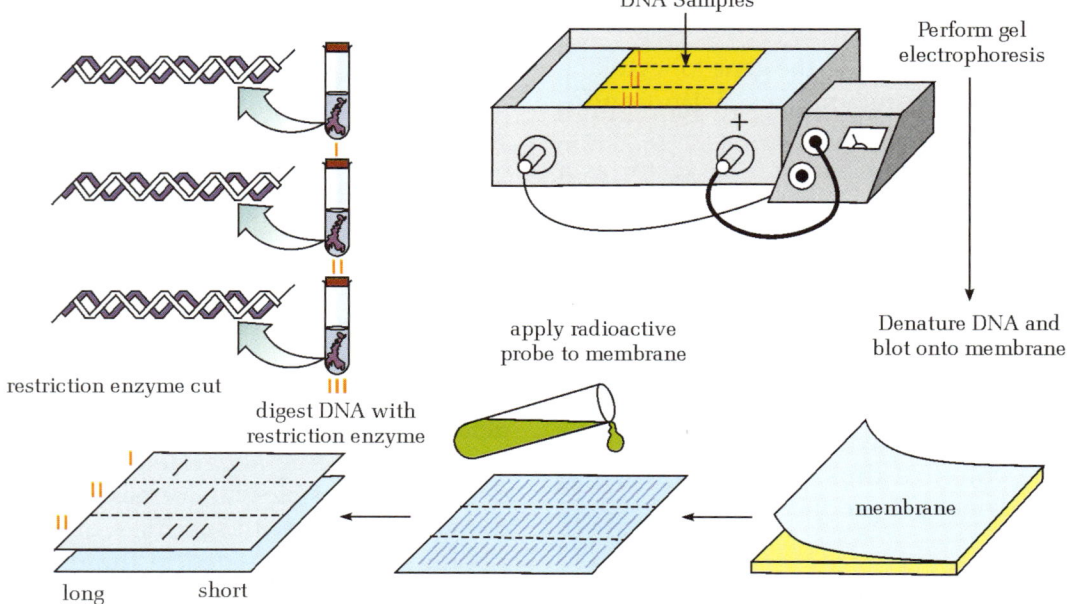

Fig. 10.7: Restriction fragment length polymorphism and Southern blotting

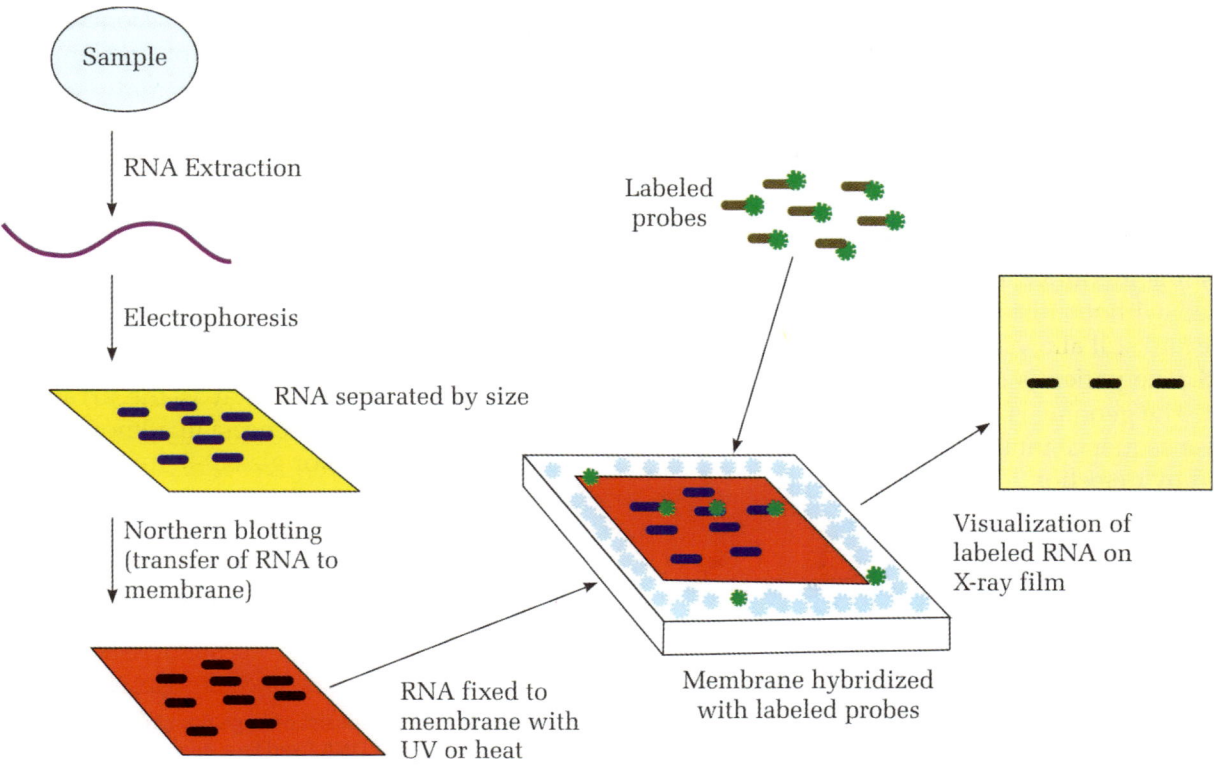

Fig. 10.8: Northern blotting

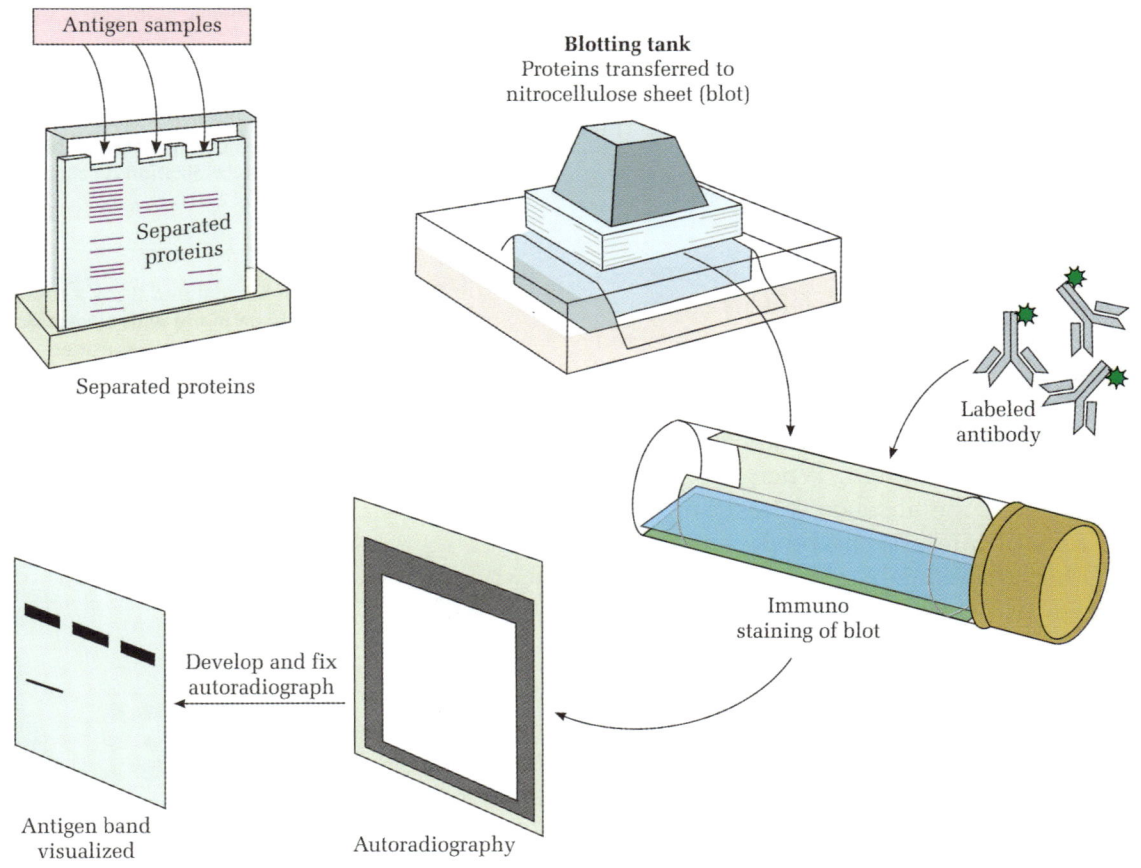

Fig. 10.9: Western blotting

Uses: Detection of antibodies against:

1. *HIV*
2. *Treponema pallidum*
3. *Herpes simplex virus-2*
4. Lyme disease

In Situ Hybridization

Organism is identified in the lesion. Tissue section is processed without disturbing the structural integrity of tissue and still allows nucleic acid present in it to be released. The patient's cells or tissue is used as solid support. The genome is denatured into a single strand with base sequence intact. Then hybridization is done followed by detection.

PNA Probes

These are synthetic pieces of DNA. They have special chemical characteristic. Negatively charged sugar phosphate of DNA is changed by using neutral polyamide. Individual nucleotide bases can be attached to this backbone of polyamide allowing probe to hybridize with it's complimentary nucleic acid targets. These probes have improved hybridization because of synthetic nature.

PNA FISH is a fluorescence *in situ* hybridization, which uses PNA probes targeting species specific rRNA sequences within organisms. After penetration of microbial cell wall, the fluorescent labeled PNA probes hybridize to multicopy rRNA sequences within the organisms, resulting in fluorescent cells.

Multiplex PCR

More than one primer pair can be used. One primer set is directed against sequences present in clinically significant bacteria. The second primer is directed against a sequence which is specific for the gene of interest. The control amplification should be always detectable after PCR and its absence indicates proper PCR conditions not maintained. When the control amplicon is detected, the absence of test amplicon (amplicon of gene of interest) can be detected more confidently. Other advantage is ability to search for different targets using one reaction. Primer pairs directed at sequences specific for organisms can be put together so that use of multiple reaction vessels can be minimised, e.g. multiplexed PCR assays containing primers to detect viral agents that cause meningitis.

Nested PCR

It involves sequential use of two primers. First set is used to amplify the target and amplicons obtained is then used as target sequence for second amplification using primers internal to those of first amplicons.

Advantage is that it is extremely sensitive and specific.

Disadvantage is that procedure requires open manipulations of amplified DNA that is readily aerosolized, causing contamination of other reaction vessels.

DNA Microarray (Fig. 10.10a; Flowchart 10.2)

DNA microarrays are based on principles of nucleic acid hybridization. The test is available in various formats; the general format is the arrangement of samples (e.g. gene sequences) in a known matrix on a solid support (nylon or glass).

Flowchart 10.2: DNA chip

> DNA chip or DNA microarray

> DNA chips consist of large no. of evenly spaced spots of DNA fixed to a microscopic slide

> Each spot is unique DNA fragment transferred by a robot from multiwell plates on a slide

> The DNA chip can be hybridised with DNA extracts from unknown isolate to produce patterns of hybridization on slide

> The patterns can be analysed using a computer & comparism can be made with electronic data and organisms can be identified

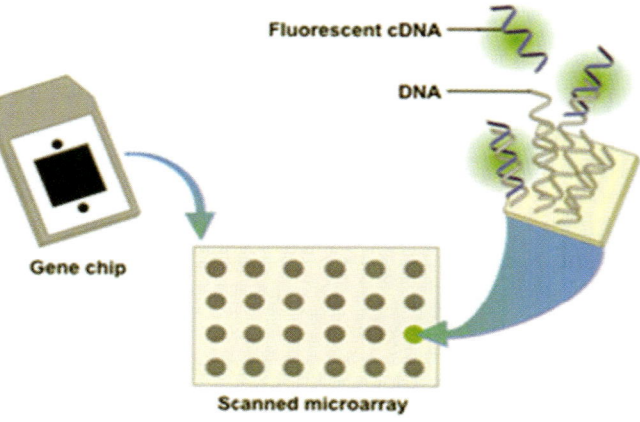

Fluorescent cDNA

DNA

Gene chip

Scanned microarray

Fig. 10.10a: DNA microarray

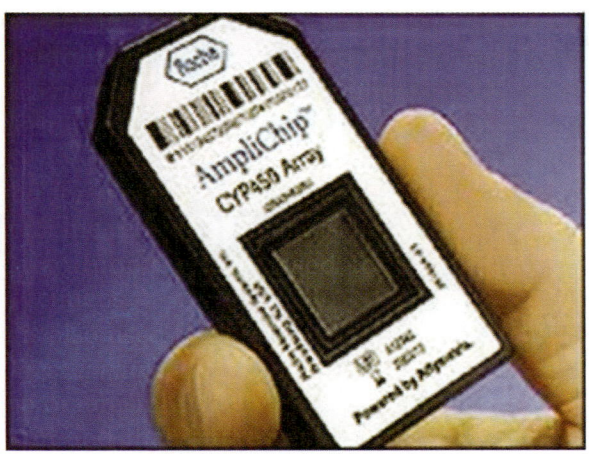

Fig. 10.10b: DNA chip

One DNA chip may have thousand spots; each spot may be less than 200 nm. Such large number of spots are applied by specialized robotics (Fig. 10.10b). Different fluorescent labeled probes of known sequences may then be simultaneously applied followed by monitoring to detect whether complimentary binding has occurred.

Flow Cytometry

- Cells in the sample are stained with fluorescent reagents to detect surface molecules and then stream on at a time past the laser.
- Each cell is measured by size (forward light scatter) and granularity (90° light scanner) as well as for red and green fluorescence, to detect two different surface markers.
- Three-dimensional plates show a whole lymphocyte population and CD8 population obtained by cell sorting stained with anti-CD 8.

It is used for counting CD4 cell; CD8 cells, CD4/CD8 ratio and these values decide when to start antiretroviral therapy for *HIV* and also used to assess the prognosis. This method is also used for the diagnosis of leukemia.

Real-time PCR

It uses automated instrument. It combines target nucleic acid amplification with qualitative and quantitative measurement of amplified products. This instrument combines thermo-cycling or target DNA amplification with ability to detect the amplified products by fluorescently labeled probes as hybrids are formed (detection in real time). As all the steps are carried in a single vessel, manipulations are avoided. It is also possible to quantitate amount products and number of copies in original specimen. The amount of time required is 20–30 minutes as compared to 4–6 hours required for conventional PCR (Fig. 10.11).

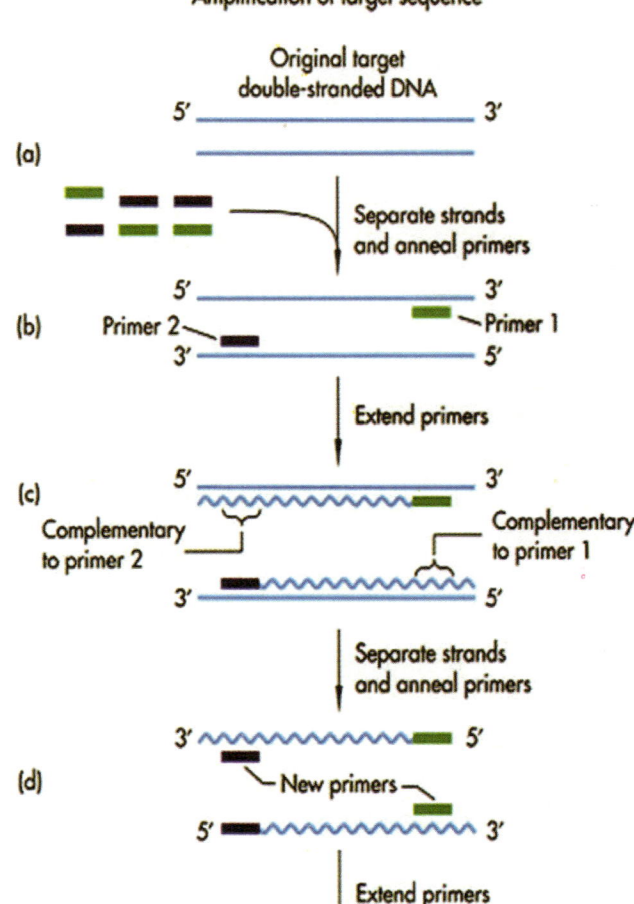

Fig. 10.11: PCR (a) Denaturation, (b) annealing, (c) amplification, (d) Repeat cycle

11

Infection

Definitions

Pathogenicity is the ability of the microbial **species** to produce the disease.

Term **virulence** is applied to the ability of a **strain** to cause disease. For example, *Staphylococcus aureus* has ability to cause wound infection. The actual isolate from a patient is the strain of the *Staphylococcus aureus,* and organism from another patient becomes different strain. Thus, virulence of these strains may vary.

Attenuation and exaltation: Decrease in the virulence of the organism is called attenuation. After attenuation, many strains of organisms can be used as live-attenuated vaccines. Attenuation can be achieved by various methods:

1. Repeat culture in artificial culture media
2. Passage in an unfavorable host
3. Growth under high temperature
4. Desiccation
5. Prolonged storage
6. Growth in presence of weak antiseptics

Exaltation is opposite to attenuation, it increases in virulence of an organism.

Infection: Lodgment and multiplication of a parasite on or in the tissues of the host, which may or may not result in disease (Fig. 11.1).

Primary infection: Initial infection with a parasite or organism is called primary infection.

Reinfection: Subsequent infection by the same parasite or organism is called reinfection.

Secondary infection: Infection by a new parasite in a host whose resistance is lowered by a pre-existing infectious disease. In AIDS patient, secondary infections with opportunistic fungus like *Cryptococcus neoformans* occur.

Focal infection: Infection at localized sites (e.g. tonsils, appendix) producing generalized effects.

Cross-infection: It is a new infection from an external source or from another host, in an individual already suffering from disease.

Nosocomial infection: It means cross-infection occurring in a hospital (infection, a patient gets during the hospital stay).

Iatrogenic infections: These are physician-induced infections resulting from investigative, therapeutic or other procedures. For example, if lumbar puncture is done by physician in a suspected case of meningitis but the patient is actually not suffering, the clinician carrying *Staphylococcus* on fingers leading to contamination during lumbar puncture so that the patient develops meningitis due to *Staphylococcus* (which came from physician's fingers).

Types of Infections Based on Source of Infection

- *Endogenous infection*: Source of infection is from the patient's own body, e.g. urinary tract infection caused by *E. coli* present in groin of the patient himself.
- *Exogenous infection* : Source of infection is external. If a patient has trauma, spores of *Clostridium tetani* entering from the soil cause infection.

Types of Infections Based on Clinical Effects

Inapparent infection (subclinical infection): Infection in which clinical effects are not apparent. If a person is in contact with a patient with common cold, the virus is entering in his body without showing symptoms is an example of inapparent infection.

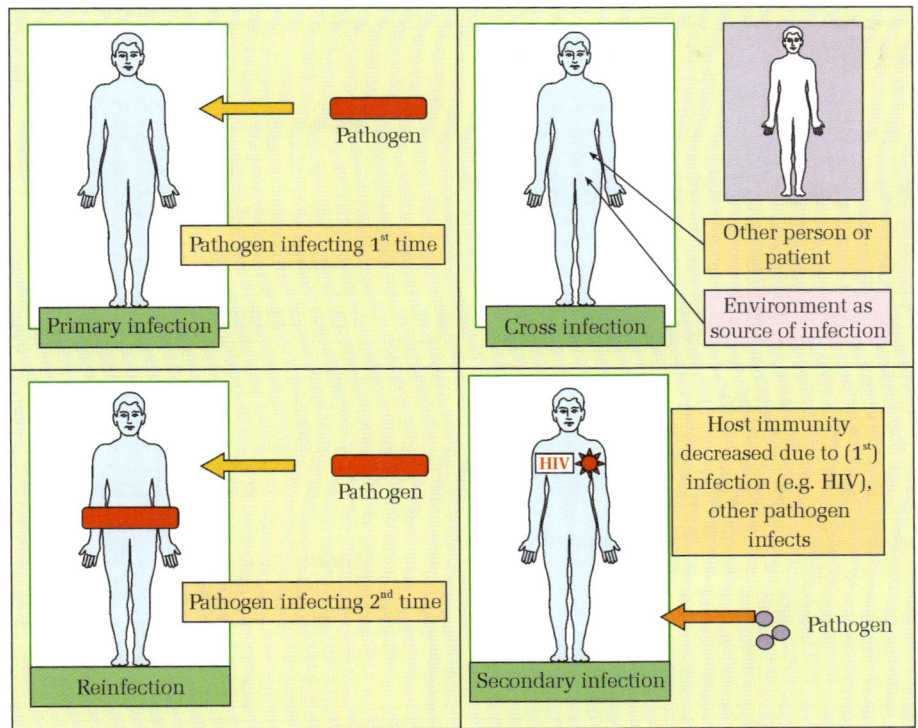

Fig. 11.1: Definitions of different types of infections

Latent infection: Following infection, the parasite remains latent in the tissues, proliferate and produce disease when host resistance is lowered (hidden infection). This type of infection is *Herpes simplex virus* in which virus remains latent in trigeminal ganglion, the virus may come on skin causing fever blisters.

Atypical infection: Typical characteristic clinical manifestations of the particular disease are not present. A small portion of patients with *Mycobacterium tuberculosis* may present with erythema nodosum which is atypical presentation of pulmonary tuberculosis.

Sources of Infection (Fig. 11.2)

1. Human Beings

- Carrier is a person who harbors organism without suffering any ill effect and sheds the organisms.
- Healthy carrier is one, who has never suffered from the disease.
- Convalescent carrier is a person who has recovered from the disease and carrying and shedding organism.
- Carrier could be temporary (<6 months) or chronic carrier (several years).
- Contact carrier is a person who acquires infection from a patient.
- Paradoxical carrier acquires infection from another carrier.

2. Animals

Animals may be the reservoir host which maintain parasite in nature.

Zoonosis: Infectious disease that is transmitted from animals to human beings and vice versa. Examples are bacteria (e.g. plague from rats), viruses (e.g. rabies from dogs), protozoa (e.g. toxoplasmosis from cats), helminths (e.g. hydatid disease from dogs) and fungi (e.g. zoophilic dermatophytes from dogs and cats).

Arthopod Vectors

Arthopod vectors may be mosquitoes, ticks, flies, mites, fleas and lice.

Diseases caused by vectors are called arthropod-borne diseases.

a. *Mechanical vectors* mean there is no development or multiplication of the infectious agent in the vector and the vector just transmits the agent mechanically, e.g. dysentery and typhoid by domestic fly.

b. *Biological vectors:* In this type of infection, the development or multiplication of the infectious agent takes place in the body of the vector, e.g. yellow fever and malaria by mosquitoes.

List of arthropod-borne diseases (Table 11.1)

- *Bacterial infections:* Plague (rat flea), typhus fever, endemic typhus, scrub typhus (mites), Lyme disease, relapsing fever.

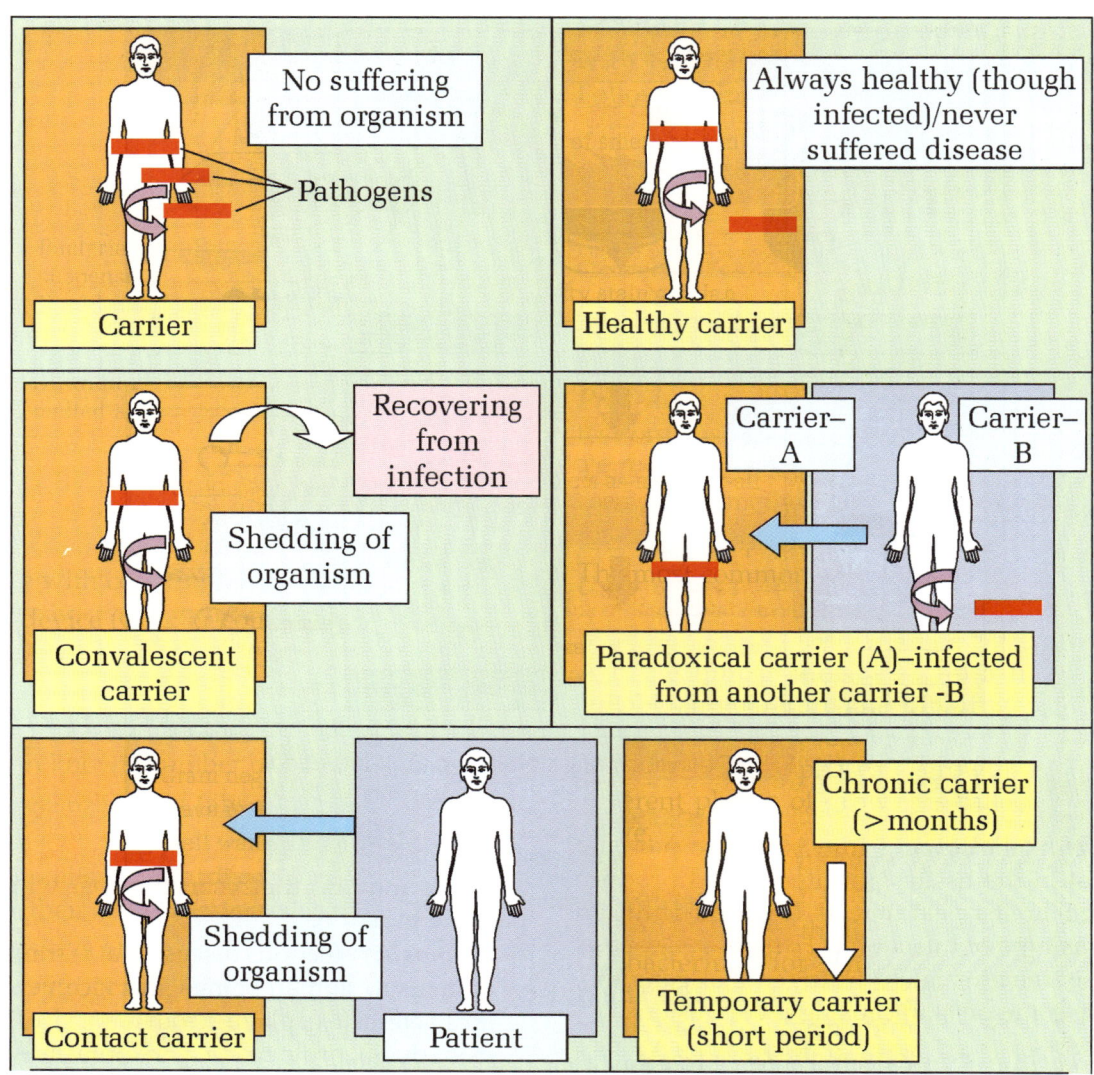

Fig. 11.2: Different types of carriers

TABLE 11.1: Arthropod-borne diseases with causative agent, vectors and list of diseases transmitted

Arthropod vector	Disease transmitted	Causative agent	Reservoirs
Soft ticks	African relapsing fever	*Borrelia duttonii*	Wild rodents, pigs
Hard ticks	Tick-borne typhus	*Rickettsia rickettsii*	Wild rodents, domestic
	Rockey mountain spotted fever		dogs, cats
	Looping ill	Flavivirus	Sheep, cattle
	Tularemia	*Francisella tularensis*	Rabbits, squirrels
	Colorado tick fever	Arbovirus	
	Omsk hemorrhagic fever	Flavivirus	
Lice	Epidemic typhus	*Rickettsia prowazekii*	Man
	Louse-borne relapsing fever	*Borrelia recurrentis*	Man
Rat flea	Flea-borne typhus	*Rickettsia mooseri*	Rats
	Plague	*Yersinia pestis*	Rats
Mites	Scrub typhus	*Rickettsia tsutsugamushi*	Rodents
	Rickettsial pox	*Rickettsia akari*	House mice
Tsetse fly	African trypanosomiasis	*Trypanosoma brucei*	Wild game
Reduviid bugs	American trypanosomiasis	*Trypanosoma brucei gambiense*	Man

- *Viral infections*: Arboviruses as dengue, chikungunya (*aedes aegypti*), yellow fever, Kyasanur forest disease.
- *Parasitic infections*: Malaria (female anepheline mosquito), leishmaniasis (sandfly), trypanosomiasis (tsetse fly), filariasis (phlebotomus mosquito).

Extrinsic incubation period: It is the time between entry of pathogen into vector and vector becoming infective. Insects can also be reservoir hosts, maintained by transovarial passage.

4. Soil

Clostridium tetani, Histoplasma capsulatum, Nocardia, parasites like roundworm and hookworm, fungi as zoophilic dermatophytes may be present in soil and they can infect.

5. Water-borne Diseases

a. *Bacterial infections*: *Vibrio cholerae, E. coli, Shigella,* typhoid fever.
b. *Viral infections*: Hepatitis A and E virus and poliovirus.
c. *Parasitic infections*: Guinea worm infestation—due to presence of aquatic vector (cyclops), amoebiasis, *Balantidium coli,* cryptosporidiosis, *Isospora.*

6. Food

External contamination may act as source of infection. For example, staphylococcal food poisoning (milk products), food poisoning due to *E. coli, Bacillus cereus* (Chinese fried rice), *Clostridium welchii.*

Pre-existent infection in meat or animal products, e.g. salmonellosis, *Taenia saginata* and *T. solium,* brucellosis may also result in infection.

Methods of Transmission of Infection

1. *Contact*: It may be direct contact as in sexually transmitted infections—syphilis and gonorrhea (contagious disease) or indirect contact as by fomites (inanimate objects), e.g. clothing, toys, pens, etc. Examples of diseases transmitted by contact are trachoma, diphtheria, herpes simplex, bacillary dysentery. The term infectious diseases denotes all modes of transmission.
2. *Inhalation*:
   a. *Droplet transmission*: Larger droplets (>10 μm size) travel for a short distance, settle down as dust particles. Examples of organisms transmitted by this mode are respiratory viruses and *Bordetella pertussis.*
   b. *Air-borne transmission*: If droplet is small (1–10 μm— droplet nucleus), it can travel a longer distance. It can infect any person it finds on its way. Organisms transmitted this route include TB bacilli, measles, chickenpox.
3. *Ingestion*: The infection may be:
   - Water-borne, e.g. cholera
   - Food-borne, e.g. food poisoning
   - Hand-borne, e.g. dysentery
4. *Inoculation*: For example, tetanus, rabies, *HIV, hepatitis B,* iatrogenic infections.
5. *Insects or vectors*: For example, arboviruses.
6. *Congenital (vertical) transmissions*: Pathogens cross placental barrier and infect fetus in utero, e.g. TORCH infections.
   TORCH: The causative agents of congenital infections are grouped together and called "TORCH" infections. In this 'T' means *Toxoplasma gondii,* ' R' means *rubella virus,* 'C' means *cytomegalovirus,* 'H' means *herpes simplex viruses, hepatitis virus, HIV* and 'O'means others which include syphilis, *parvo B virus.* If the mother has recent infection during pregnancy, then the chances of transmission of infections to fetus are more as compared to past infections in which chances are negligible. The percentage of transmission of infections in first trimester is less but if infection occurs, it is severe form because teratogenesis occurs; while chances of transmission are more in 3rd trimester but complications are less. As the immunoglobulin G is passively transmitted from mother to fetus, to diagnose congenital infections in newborns, antibody IgM is detected by serological tests, as ELISA. Some of these infections can be prevented by immunization of women of child-bearing age against *HBV, rubella virus.*
   Teratogenic infections: Intrauterine infections that lead to congenital malformation.
7. *Iatrogenic and laboratory infections*: These infections may occur during diagnostic or therapeutic procedures.

Microbial Pathogenicity

Pathogenicity is the ability of a microbial species to produce disease while virulence is the ability of a microbial strain to produce disease.

Exaltation is enhancement of virulence of microorganisms.

Attenuation is reduction of virulence of microorganisms and these strains can be used as attenuated vaccines. The different methods as passage through unfavorable hosts, repeated culture in artificial media, growth under high temperature or in presence of weak antiseptics, desiccation and prolonged storage in culture are used for attenuation.

Virulence Factors of Bacteria

1. Adhesions (Ligands)

Adhesions, which are proteins and antigenic in nature, could be fimbriae, pili or colonizing factors. Adhesions are responsible for tissue tropism and host-specific pathogenicity.

Important organisms having pili

- *Gonococci*—adhere to throat, genitourinary tract, rectum, eye
- *Meningococci*—adhere to nasopharynx
- *E. coli*—adhere to urinary epithelium
- *Vibrio cholerae*—adhesion to intestinal mucosa
- *Pseudomonas*—colonizes on wounds or lungs

Other adhesions

- *Lipoteichoic acid*—binds to fibrinectin
- *T. pallidum*—adhesins bind to fibrinectin
- *Bordetella pertussis*
- *Filamentous agglutinins*—adhere to glycoprotein of respiratory epithelial cells
- *Pertussis toxin*—adheres to glycolipids
- *Gonococci*—produce opa protein III
- *Staphylococcus* produces protein A
- *Pseudomonas* produces lectins

2. Invasiveness

It varies from bacterium to bacterium. For example, *Salmonella* and *Shigella* cause manifestations of diarrhea or dysentery respectively and these organisms have ability to invade intestinal epithelium, on the other hand, Cholera bacillus infects GIT and causes diarrhea by production of toxin. It does not carry invasiveness. Similarly *Clostridium perfringenes* causing gas gangrene has minimum invasiveness. Highly virulent bacteria have ability to cause generalized infections.

3. Toxigenicity

Bacteria produce exotoxin or endotoxin (Table 11.2).

Exotoxins: Bacteria excrete exotoxins extracellularly which diffuse in surrounding medium. They are acid-labile proteins. Toxins are mostly produced by Gram-positive bacilli except a few Gram-negative bacilli (e.g. *Vibrio cholerae, E. coli*). They can be separated by filteration. They have specific affinity for certain tissues and they possess enzymic action. As compared to endotoxins, they are highly antigenic in nature. They can be converted into toxoid which looses toxigenicity but retains antigenicity hence used for vaccination, e.g. tetanus toxoid. Each toxin possesses specific pharmacological action and it can be neutralized by antitoxins

TABLE 11.2: Differences between exotoxins and endotoxins

Exotoxins	Endotoxins
Proteins	Protein polysaccharide-lipid complex
Highly antigenic	Weakly antigenic
Action often enzymic	No enzymic actions
Heat labile	Heat stable
Actively secreted by cells, diffuse into surrounding medium	Form part of cell wall, do not diffuse into surrounding medium
Specific tissue affinity	No specific activity
Active in very minute doses	Active only in large doses
Can be separated from medium by filtration	Obtained by cell lysis
Action specifically neutralized by antibody	Neutralization by antibody ineffective
Can be toxoided	Cannot be toxoided

which are antibodies produced against (e.g. antitetanus serum).

Endotoxins: They are part of bacterial cell wall of Gram negative cell wall. They are heat-stable and not secreted in the medium. Endotoxins can be obtained by cell lysis. They have no specific pharmacological action and have no specific tissue affinity. They are weakly antigenic, hence not toxoided. They cannot be neutralized antitoxins (Fig. 11.3).

4. Plasmids (Extrachromosomal DNA)

Plasmids may bear genes coding for virulence characteristics, for example, *E. coli* (surface antigens and enterotoxin), *S. aureus* (enterotoxin), multidrug-resistant plasmids (e.g. *Salmonella*).

5. Communicability

It is ability of a parasite to spread from one host to another. It determines survival and distribution of the parasite in the community. The organisms especially infecting GIT or respiratory tract spread over large geographic area. Thus pandemic strain of an organism requires high degree of communicability and virulence.

6. Bacterial Appendages

i. Capsules (e.g. *Klebsiella, Haemophilus influenzae*) inhibit phagocytosis.
ii. Surface antigens, e.g. 'Vi' of *S. typhi*, 'K' antigen of *E. coli,* inhibit phagocytosis.

7. Presence of Bacteriophages

The bacteriophage is the virus which lives on bacteria and it carries genes for toxin production as seen in *Corynebacterium diphtheriae*. If infected with TOX phage, this bacteriophage carries the genes for toxin, *C.*

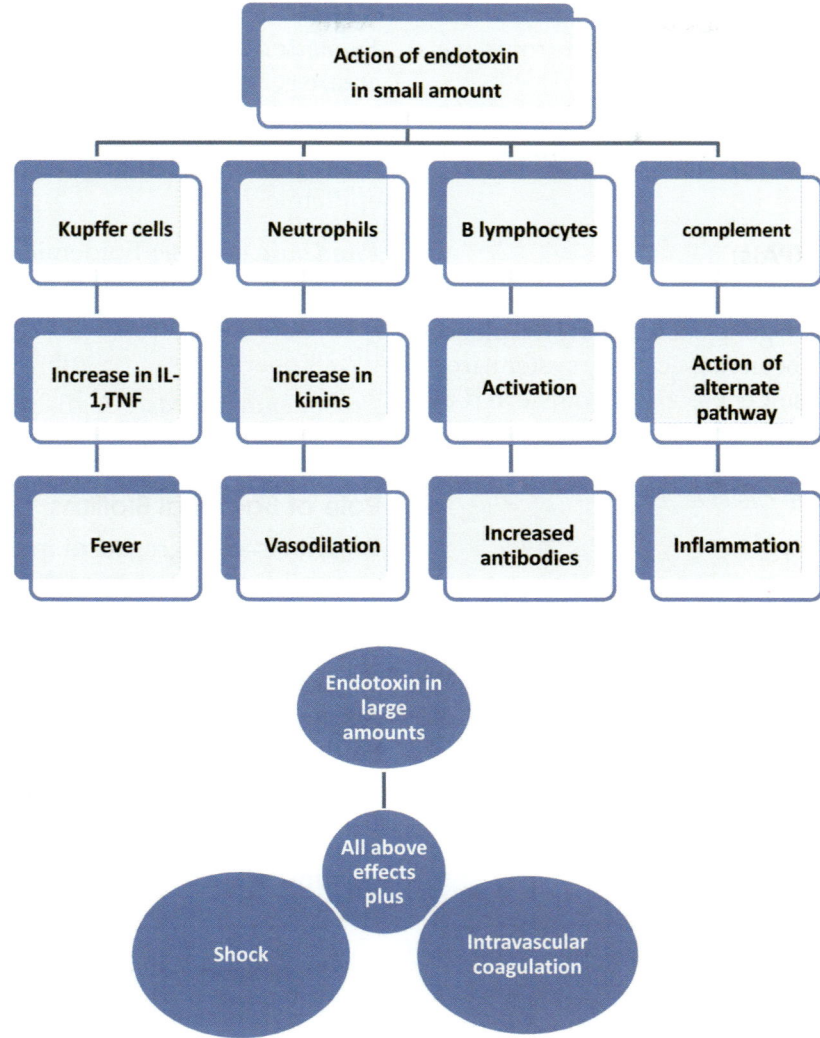

Fig. 11.3: Actions of endotoxin with small dose and large dose

diphtheriae will produce toxin, if the strain of diphtheria is made free from the TOX phage, the bacterium becomes nonpathogenic. The conversion of nonpathogenic strain to pathogenic by infection with bacteriophage is called lysogenic conversion.

Phage-coded toxins:
- Diphtheria toxin
- Cholera toxin
- Verocytotoxin of *E. coli*
- Botulinum toxin C and D

8. Other Bacterial Products (Other than Toxins)

- Coagulase forms fibrin barrier around bacteria thus preventing from phagocytic cells
- Fibrinolysins, hyaluronidase, DNAase, help in spreading infection in case of *Streptococcus*
- Leucocidins
- Haemolysins

9. Infecting Dose

Infective dose: Minimum infecting dose (MID)—minimum number of bacteria required to produce clinical evidence of infection. This also determines the virulence, for example *Shigella* has low infective dose of 100 bacilli while *Salmonella* has 10000 bacilli. If the infective dose of *Hepatitis B* virus and HIV is compared, the infective dose of Hepatitis B is low.

Minimum lethal dose (MLD): Minimum number of bacteria required to produce death of tested animal.

ID50 or LD50: Dose required to kill 50% of animals tested under standard conditions.

10. Route of Infection

- *Staphylococci*—survive by any route
- *Vibrio cholerae*—infective orally but not subcutaneously.

11. Other Virulence Factors of Bacteria (Table 11.3)

Other enzymes produced by it like hylouronidase, DNAase, also help in spread of infections.

IgA protease: It is produced by gonococci which have the ability to breakdown locally produced IgA antibody.

Pathogenicity Islands (PAIs)

Islands of genes located on chromosomal regions of some bacteria. The set of genes code many virulence factors such as toxins, adhesions, secretory system, iron uptake system, etc. These genes can be transferred as one unit from different sites within chromosome or to other bacteria. **PAIs** are studies in *Staphylococcus aureus, Salmonella, Shigella, Vibrio cholerae, E. coli.*

Bacterial Secretory System

This system helps bacteria in transfer of effector molecules as cholera toxin across cell membrane from cytoplasm to the exterior. Six such systems have been identified in Gram-negative bacteria.

Pathogens are selective in sites of localization and multiplication. They differ in ability to produce damage of different organs in different species.

- **Bacteremia** is circulation of bacteria in blood with or without symptoms.
- **Septicemia** means circulation and multiplication of bacteria in blood forming toxic products resulting in signs and symptoms.
- **Pyaemia** means septicemia with multiple abscesses in the internal organs

TABLE 11.3: Virulence factors of bacteria

Bacteria	Virulence factors
Staphylococcus aureus	Coagulase, protein A, enterotoxins
Streptococcus pyogenes	Protein M, DNAase, hyalouronidase, streptokinase
Streptococcus pneumoniae	Capsular polysaccharides
Enterococcus fecalis	Biofilm formation
Gonococci	IgA proteinase, pili, opacity associated proteins
Meningococci	Capsular polysaccharide
Bacillus anthracis	Capsule, edema factor, lethal factor
E. coli	Pili, enterotoxin, capsule k
Haemophilus influenzae	Capsular polysaccharide
Vibrio	Cholera toxin, motility
Salmonella	Invasiveness
Shigella	Invasiveness
Proteus	Urease
Staphylococcus epidermidis	Slime, biofilm

Spread of Infections in the Community

Endemic disease: Infection constantly present in a given area, e.g. typhoid fever is endemic in most parts of India.

Epidemic disease: Infections spread rapidly, involve many persons in an area at the same time, e.g. cholera epidemic.

Pandemic disease: Epidemic that spreads throughout the world, involving large numbers of people in a short period, e.g. influenza, cholera, plague, *HIV, SARS,* bird flu.

Prosodemic disease: A disease passing directly from one person to another is called prosodemic disease.

Role of Bacterial Biofilms

Biofilm is an aggregate of interactive bacteria attached to a solid surface or to each other and encased in exo-polysaccharide matrix. This is different from free living bacteria and planktonic bacteria in which interactions do not occur in same way. Biofilm is slimy coat that occur on solid surface and present throughout the nature. Usually a single species of bacteria aggregates to form biofilms, but more than one species may be involved. After the formation of biofilm, **quorum sensing molecules** are produced by bacteria in the biofilm, which result in **modification of metabolic pathway**.

Significance of Biofilms Formation

1. Bacteria in biofilms are protected from hosts defence mechanisms.
2. It also acts as barriers for antibiotics. Some of the bacteria in biofilms show marked resistance to antibiotic as compared with same strain of bacteria grown free living in broth.
3. Biofilms are important in infections that are persistant and difficult to treat.

Examples of Biofilms in Infections

- *Staphylococcus epidermidis, and Staphylococcus aureus* cause biofilms on venous catheters and cause infections of catheters which may lead to bacteremia.
- Eye infections caused by bacteria following use of contact lenses on which biofilms may be formed.
- *Streptococcus viridans* causes dental plaque.
- Infections of prosthetic joint infections.
- *Pseudomonas aeruginosa* causing airway infections in patients with cystic fibrosis.
- Scavenger receptors are a group of receptors that recognize modified low denisity lipoprotein by oxidation and acetylation.

12

Immunity

The term immunity is the resistance offered by host against harmful effects of organisms or their products. It is of two types: **Innate immunity** and **acquired immunity** (Fig. 12.1).

INNATE IMMUNITY (NATIVE IMMUNITY)

Definition: An individual is protected from infection with microorganisms by various ways which are present from birth and these mechanisms of protection do not depend upon prior exposure to any micro-organism. Such type of immunity is naturally present (natural immunity) and is not due to prior sensitization to an antigen either by an infection or vaccination.

- It is first defense (within hours) which comes in picture following entry of infective organism (Fig. 12.2).
- It presents from birth. Since it is not stimulated by specific antigens, innate immunity is generally non-specific.
- It is 'natural' or "innate" to the host, depending, in part, on genetics.

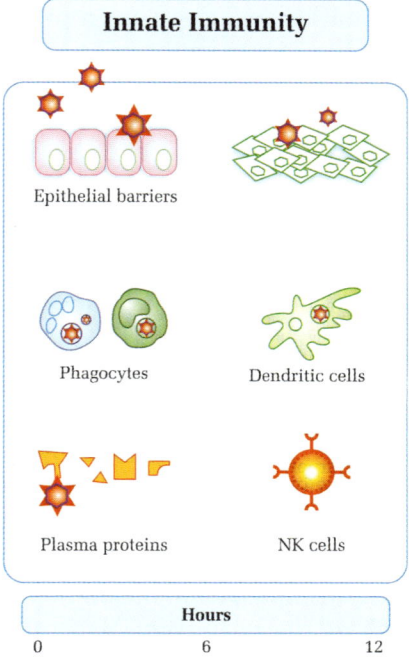

Innate Immunity

Epithelial barriers

Phagocytes

Dendritic cells

Plasma proteins

NK cells

Hours

0   6   12

Fig. 12.2: Innate immunity (appears early)

- Innate defense mechanisms are constitutive to the host, meaning they are continually ready to respond to invasion and do not require a period of time for induction.
- Innate immunity also plays a role in generation of an efficient and effective acquired immune response.

Determinants of Innate Immunity

Species

There are differences in susceptibility of different species to infective agents. Rat is resistant to diphtheria while guinea pig is highly susceptible. All human beings as one species are resistant to plant viruses.

Rabbit is susceptible to myxomatosis, human being is susceptible to leprosy, syphilis, and certain pathogens

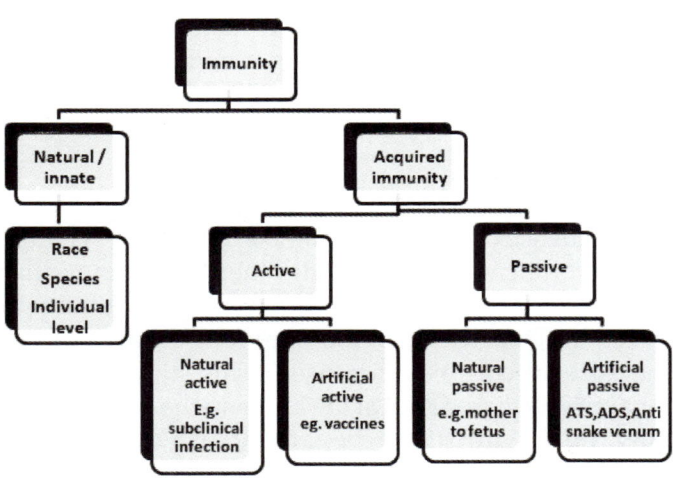

Fig. 12.1: Types of immunity

(e.g. canine distemper virus) do not infect humans. *Shigella* infects humans and baboons but not chimpanzees.

Sometimes genetic abnormality in a person is added advantage to host.

a. *Absence of specific tissue or cellular receptors for attachment (colonization) of the pathogen*: For example, different strains of enterotoxigenic *E. coli*, defined by different fimbrial antigens, colonize human infants, calves and piglets by recognizing species-specific carbohydrate receptors on enterocytes in the gastrointestinal tract. **Lack of a target site for a microbial toxin:** Most toxins produced by bacterial cells produce their toxic activity only after binding to susceptible cells or tissues in an animal. Certain animals may lack an appropriate target cell or specific cell receptor for the toxin to bind and may therefore, not be susceptible to the activity of the toxin. For example, injection of diphtheria toxin is unable to kill the rat as it lacks receptor for toxin. Hence, the unchanged toxin is excreted in the urine. If a sample of the rat urine (or pure diphtheria toxin) is injected into the guinea pig (guinea pig has receptor for toxin attachment), it dies of typical lesions caused by diphtheria toxin.

b. *Temperature of the host and ability of pathogen to grow*: Birds do not normally become infected with *Mycobacterium tuberculosis* because these strains of *M.tuberculosis* cannot grow at the high body temperature of birds. The anthrax bacillus (*Bacillus anthracis*) will not grow in the cold-blooded frogs (unless the frog is maintained at 37°C).

c. *Lack of the exact nutritional requirements to support the growth of the pathogen*: Naturally-requiring purine-dependent strains of *Salmonella typhi* grow only in hosts supplying purines. Mice and rats lack this growth factor. By injecting purines into these animals, the growth factor requirement for the bacterium is satisfied, the organisms become virulent.

Racial Immunity

Within a species, different races show variation in susceptibility or resistance to infections. Algerian sheep is resistant to anthrax to which other races are susceptible. In human beings, American negroes are more susceptible to tuberculosis than white race. Such differences could be due to socioeconomic status.

Races with sickle cell anemia in Mediterranean coast are immune to *P. falciparum* infection. Genetic abnormality of RBCs in these individuals gives the immunity as such cells cannot be infected with parasites. Persons with hereditary deficiency of glucose-6-phosphate dehydrogenase are less susceptible to *P. falciparum*.

Strain or Individual Immunity

Variations in resistance to infection have been noticed in different strains of mice. It is possible to breed, by selection, rabbit of low grade, intermediate and high resistance to experimental tuberculosis. Individual differences in levels of innate immunity are exhibited by studies of infection with *Mycobacterium tuberculosis* in homozygous and heterozygous twins. If one in homozygous pair develops tuberculosis, another person in homozygous pair is highly susceptible to tuberculosis as compared to same infection in heterozygous twins.

Factors Determining Individual Resistance

Sex

Level of innate immunity is linked to the presence and/or development of the sex organs. For example, mastitis and infectious diseases leading to abortion will obviously occur only in the female; orchitis would occur only in males. It could also be due to anatomical structure related to sex. Bladder infections are 14-times more common in females than males because of proximity of female urethra, and possibly the effects of sex hormones on infections. There is no major difference in susceptibility to infections in males as compared to females.

Age

People at two extremes of life are more susceptible to infections. Immune system of fetus is immature while immune responses in old age are on decline. Fetus in uterus is protected from maternal infections by placenta. Some pathogens may cross this barrier and cause congenital infections (rubella, cytomegalovirus).

In some infections, as chickenpox and poliomyelitis, the illness is more severe in adults than young children which is due to more active immune response which may cause greater tissue damage.

Stress

Stress is due to different factors that apparently have a real influence on health. Undue exertion, shock, change in environment, climatic change, nervous or muscular fatigue, etc. are factors which increase susceptibility to infection. During stress, the output of cortisone from the adrenal cortex is increased. This suppresses the inflammatory processes of the host and the overall effect may be harmful. There are also a number of relationships between stress-related hormones and the functioning of the immune defenses.

Hormonal Influences

Persons with diabetes mellitus, hypothyroidism, adrenal insufficiency are more susceptible to infections which may be related to activities of enzymes and hormones. Glucocorticosteroids are anti-inflammatory drugs which inhibit phagocytosis. Sometimes they have beneficial effect as they may interfere with toxic effects of bacterial endotoxins.

Diet and Malnutrition

Infections may be linked with vitamin and protein deficiencies. Many infectious diseases are more prevalent and infant mortality rates are highest in parts of the world where malnourishment is a problem. Cytokines and enzymes are proteins, protein energy malnutrition decreases humoral as well as cell-mediated immunity. Also there is decrease in phagocytic activity and leucopenia. Diets high in sucrose predispose individuals to dental caries.

Intercurrent Disease or Trauma

The normal defenses of an animal are impaired by organic diseases such as leukemia, Hodgkin's disease, diabetes, AIDS, etc. Frequently, inflammatory or immune responses are delayed or suppressed. Cold or influenza may predispose an individual to pneumonia. Smoking tobacco predisposes to infections of the respiratory tract. Burned tissue is readily infected by *Pseudomonas aeruginosa*.

Therapy Against Other Diseases

Modern therapeutic procedures used in some diseases can render an individual more susceptible to infection. Under these conditions not only pathogens, but also organisms of the normal flora and nonpathogens in the host's environment, may be able to initiate infection. Examples of therapeutic procedures that reduce the efficiency of the host's defenses are treatment with corticosteroids, cytotoxic drugs, antibiotics, or irradiation.

Mechanisms of Innate Immunity (Tables 12.1, 12.2 and Fig. 12.3)

1. Microbial Antagonism

It is the protection of the epithelial and mucosal surfaces afforded by an intact normal flora in a healthy animal. The ways that the normal flora protect the surfaces where they are colonized are:

- *Competitions with non-indigenous species for binding (colonization) sites. The normal flora are* highly-adapted to the tissues of their host.
- *Specific antagonism against non-indigenous species:* Members of the normal flora may produce very specific proteins called bacteriocins which kill or inhibit other (usually closely-related) species of bacteria.

TABLE 12.1: Innate immunity

Cellular, skin and mucosae, epithelial surfaces	Mechanical and chemical function
Phagocytic cells—PMNs and macrophages	Ingest bacteria and fungi
Proinflammatory cells (macrophages, masts cell, eosinophil, basophils, platelets)	Induce host defenses and inflammation
Natural killer cells	Kill viral infected cells and tumor cells
Antigen presenting cells (dendritic cells and macrophages)	Antigen recognition, processing and presentation to T cell, initiate adaptive immune responses
Humoral factors	
Antimicrobial peptides	Kill microorganisms
Complement	Induces opsonization, kills bacteria by lysis, causes chemotaxis, kills enveloped viruses
Cytokines	Soluble mediators of immune reaction both humoral and CMI
Chemokine	Attract leukocytes
Acute phase proteins	Enhance cellular and humoral defenses, enhances opsonization
Enzymes	Kill and digest organisms
Inflammation increased blood supply, increased vascular permeability, chemotaxis	Bring the phagocytic cells and antimicrobial proteins to the site of infection

- *Nonspecific antagonism against non-indigenous species:* The normal flora produce a variety of metabolites and end products that inhibit other microorganisms. **Commensal flora is protective in various ways:**
  1. It competes for nutrients.
  2. It produces byproducts (lactate, peroxides) that can inhibit the growth of other bacteria.
  3. It inhibits encroachment by competitive inhibition.
  4. It can produce inhibitory substances as lysozymes.
  5. Commensals from gut pose problem, if they go to other sites in body. They cause catheter-associated urinary tract infection.

2. Inflammation

Inflammation is a tissue reaction to infection or injury. Certain bacterial cells and/or their products (e.g. structural components or toxins) can induce an inflammatory response. The **characteristic symptoms** are **redness, swelling, heat** and **pain**. The redness is due to increased blood flow to the area of injury. The swelling (edema) is due to increased extravascular fluid and phagocytic infiltration to the damaged area. The heat is due to the increased blood flow and the action of pyrogens (fever-inducing agents). Inflammation increases the blood supply and temperature in the inflamed tissues, which favors maximal metabolic activity of the leukocytes, and lowers the pH slightly, which tends to inhibit the multiplication of many micro-organisms.

Some of the main events involved in the induction and maintenance of an inflammatory response during a microbial infection are summarized below.

- The inflammatory response is stimulated by pathogen invasion or tissue injury.
- Injured and dying cells release cytoplasmic constituents which lower the pH in the surrounding extracellular environment.
- The increased acidity activates an extracellular enzyme **kallikrein** which in turn activates **bradykinin**. Bradykinin binds to receptors on the capillary walls opening junctions between cells to allow leakage of plasma components collectively referred to as the **inflammatory exudates**.

Increased capillary permeability allows leukocytes to pass from the vessels into tissues (this process is called **diapedesis**). The first cells to appear, and the most dominant are neutrophils, which are actively phagocytic.

3. Mechanical Barriers and Surface Secretions

Epithelial surfaces

a. Skin: The ways skin acts as defense factor are:
- It acts as physical barrier preventing entry of foreign organism.
- Horney layers of skin have keratin which cannot be digested by microorganisms.
- Sebaceous secretions, sweat glands contain inhibitory substances to bacteria.
- Relatively dry skin and high salt in drying sweat are inhibitory or lethal to organisms. The ability of sebaceous secretions and sweat of skin varies with age. Some fungal infections of skin previously present in child disappear when it attains puberty when there is an increased sebaceous secretion.
- If the integrity of the epidermis is broken (by the bite of an insect, needle stick, abrasion, cut, etc.), invasive microbes may enter.

b. Respiratory tract: Inhaled particles are arrested in moist mucosa of nose. Mucosa of respiratory tract traps the particles while cilia propel the particles towards pharynx where particles are swallowed or coughed out. Cough reflex acts as important defense mechanism. Particles which manage to enter alveoli are trapped by phagocytes.

c. Intestinal tract: Saliva in mouth has inhibitory effects on bacteria. Some of the organisms may be swallowed which are destroyed by acidic pH of stomach. Normal bacterial flora of mouth inhibits the colonization of pathogens.

d. Conjunctiva: Tears have flushing action with which they remove bacteria and dust particles.

e. Genitourinary tract: Flushing of urine removes bacteria from urinary tract. The acidic pH of vagina is due to acids produced from fermentation of glycogen. Due to acidic pH, vagina is resistant to infection by pathogens. In males, semen is considered to have some antibacterial substances.

4. Antibacterial Substances in Blood

Antibacterial substances in blood are complement system, beta lysin, basic polypeptides like leukins secreted by lymphocytes, plakins secreted by platelets, etc. which have the antibacterial activity.

5. Fever

A rise in temperature following infection is a natural defense mechanism.

6. Acute Phase Proteins

CRP, α-1-acid glycoprotein, serum amyloid P enhance host resistance, their levels are increased after tissue injury, inflammatory lesion, or infection. Complement, mannose binding proteins, serum amyloid P help in opsonization and phagocytosis.

7. Antibacterial Substances in Tissues

Antibacterial substances in tissues, beta lysins, leukins extracted from WBCs, have antibacterial properties.

8. Cellular Factors in Innate Immunity

Phagocytic cells—microphages (PMNS) and macrophages (RE system): Bacteria are taken inside—phagosome (a vacuole), which fuses with lysosomes in cells to form phagolysosome, bacterium is killed. NK cells have activity against viruses (activated by interferon).

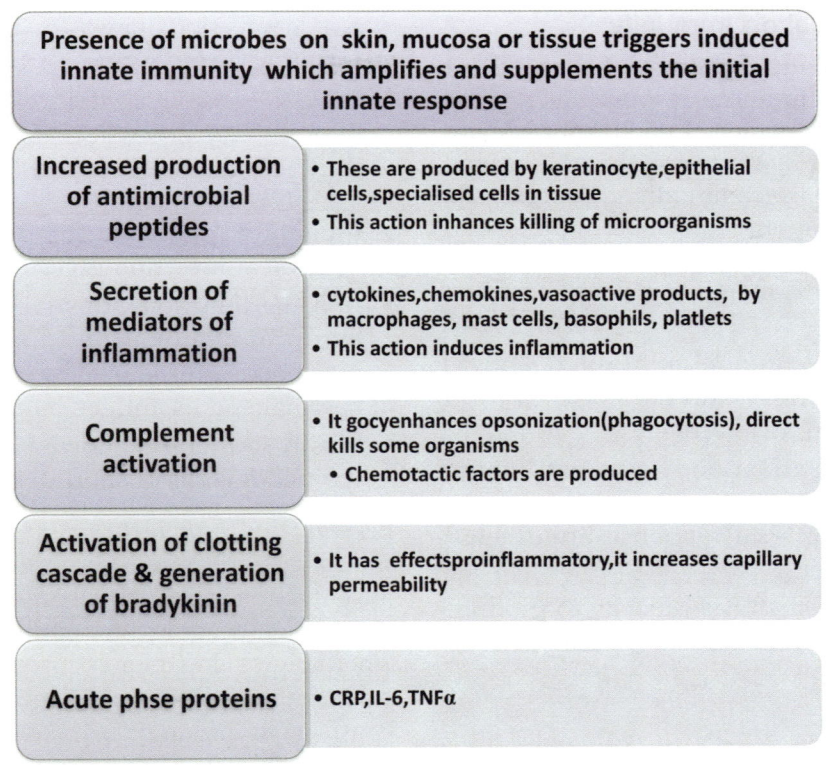

Presence of microbes on skin, mucosa or tissue triggers induced innate immunity which amplifies and supplements the initial innate response

| Increased production of antimicrobial peptides | • These are produced by keratinocyte,epithelial cells,specialised cells in tissue
• This action inhances killing of microorganisms |

| Secretion of mediators of inflammation | • cytokines,chemokines,vasoactive products, by macrophages, mast cells, basophils, platlets
• This action induces inflammation |

| Complement activation | • It gocyenhances opsonization(phagocytosis), direct kills some organisms
 • Chemotactic factors are produced |

| Activation of clotting cascade & generation of bradykinin | • It has effectsproinflammatory,it increases capillary permeability |

| Acute phse proteins | • CRP,IL-6,TNFα |

Fig. 12.3: Components of innate immune system

TABLE 12.2: Defenses on skin and mucosae

Component	Main function
Mechanical	
Keratinized epithelial cells of skin	Offer protection against microorganisms
Desquamation of epithelial cells	Removal of organisms with them
Unsaturated fatty acids in sweat, sebum	Inhibitory to bacteria
Dermicidin in sweat glands	Kill many bacteria
Ribonucleases on skin	Kill many bacteria
Epithelial cells joined by tight junctions	Protection from microorganisms
Mucus coated cells	Trap organisms and remove them
Coughing and sneezing	Remove particles
Flow of urine	Remove particles, clean urethra
Chemical and molecular components	
Low pH in stomach	Killing of bacteria
Antimicrobial peptides	Kill many bacteria
Defensins in skin, mucosae, intestine	Kill bacteria and fungi
Lipases in tears and intestinal cells	Kill bacteria and fungi
Mucopolysaccharide in saliva, mucus secretions	Inactivate bacteria
Enzymes	
Lysozyme in tears, sweat, saliva, serum	Hydrolyses bacterial cell wall
Amidase in skin and serum	Hydrolyses bacterial cell wall
Microbial antagonism	Competes for nutrients and produces bacteriocins
Antimicrobial peptides	
Defensins	Antibacterial
Cathelicidin	Antibacterial

ACQUIRED IMMUNITY OR ADAPTIVE IMMUNITY

The **resistance** an individual acquires during life following **contact** with an antigen which results in selective elimination of antigen (or organism) is called 'acquired immunity' (Fig. 12.4).

It is further classified as—**(A) active** and **(B) passive immunity.**

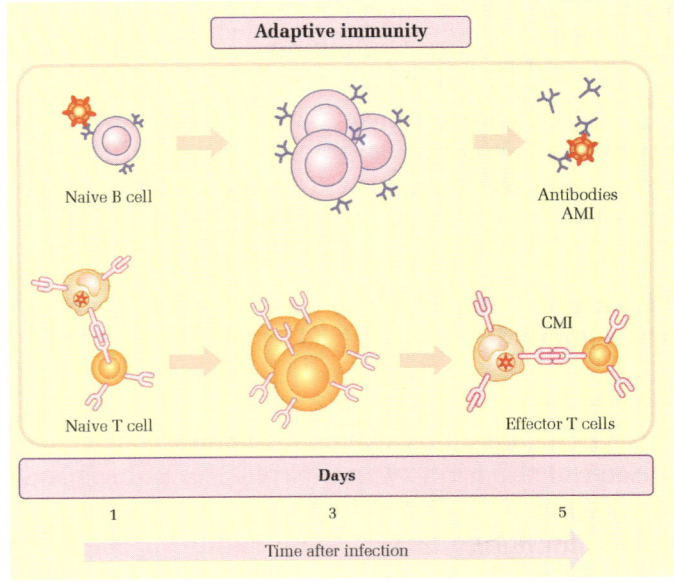

Fig. 12.4: Acquired immunity (appears late, 1–5 days)

Characteristics of Acquired Immunity

- *Antigen specificity*: First contact of antigen (or bacterium) produces immune response as well as memory by producing memory T and B lymphocytes specific to antigen (or against organism). If second encounter occurs with the same antigen or organism, protective immune response develops, but if second antigen or organism is different, there will be no response. The reason is memory is specific to first antigen.
- *Immunological memory*: As explained above, immunological memory develops so second response is fast and more effective.
- *Self/non-self recognization*: Body does not mount immune response against self-antigen because cells capable of mounting such response are deleted during embryonic life.
- *Diversity*: Immune system has capacity to produce numerous antibodies with different specificities.

Active Immunity

It develops as a result of antigenic stimulus.

Important Features of Active Immunity

- There is active participation of host's immune system to produce protective **antibodies** (**AMI**—antibody-mediated immunity or also called '**humoral immunity**') **or immune competent cells** (**CMI**—cell-mediated immunity) to deal with foreign antigen (or organism).
- During first contact with antigen, there is **latent period** as required by immune apparatus to recognize and process the antigen.
- Immunological **memory** develops against the antigen.
- Second response (following contact with same antigen second time) is prompt and powerful.
- It has **negative phase**. The level of immunity produced initially is lower than expected, if antibody to the antigen pre-exists in body which combines with antigen causing elimination of antigen–antibody complexes.

Active immunity is further classified as—natural active immunity and artificial active immunity.

Natural Active Immunity

This type of immunity develops by **natural contact** with antigen in the form of **inapparent (or subclinical) infection or clinical infection.**

- Such immunity may be **long lasting** particularly against viral infections. Sometimes it may be short duration.

- Single infection of measles gives lifelong immunity. In India, a single dose of BCG is given to protect against tuberculosis, repeated subclinical infections give immunity to the person. Similarly adults in developing countries get protected by unapparent infections in children.
- Immunity against **chickenpox** either by **inapparant or clinical infection gives lifelong** immunity.
- In some infections, this type of immunity is short lived. Immunity against influenza is short as new infection is caused by new strain of that virus which has changed its antigen by antigenic variation.
- Mostly immunity followed by bacterial infection as typhoid fever is of short duration only.

Premunition immunity or infection immunity: It is a special type of immunity in which immunity against the pathogen is present till original infection is present. The person becomes susceptible to the same infection when original infection is cured. This type of immunity is present in syphilis and a few parasitic diseases.

Artificial Active Immunity

Artificial active immunity is produced by **vaccines** (Table 12.3).

Vaccines are preparations of live or killed micro-organisms or their products used for immunization. **Live**-attenuated vaccines (immunizing agents) initiate an infection without causing disease, immunity produced by live vaccines parallels natural infection, though of lower order, immunity lasts for several years but boosters are required.

Examples of live vaccines: BCG, live OPV (Sabin), measles, mumps, rubella.

Killed vaccines: Killed vaccines are less immunogenic, protection lasts for short period, booster doses are necessary, given with an adjuvant to increase the immunogenicity of vaccine so that a good immune response is achieved. e.g. TAB, Polio (Salk) (IPV).

Killed vaccines give protection for a short period. They are poorly immunogenic. Minimum two doses are given. The 1st dose is called primary dose (priming to immune system), the subsequent doses are called booster doses.

Subunit vaccines: For example, Vi polysaccharide for typhoid, hepatitis B subunit vaccine.

Thus, factors stimulating active immunity are subclinical infections (one attack of measles gives long lasting immunity), live vaccines as BCG, OPV, MMR, killed vaccines as TAB, polio and subunit vaccine as hepatitis B vaccine, VI for typhoid.

TABLE 12.3: Different types of vaccines

Bacterial	BCG for tuberculosis	Typhoral for typhoid fever
Viral	MMR	Measles, mumps, rubella
	OPV (Salk)	Poliomyelitis
List of killed vaccines		
Bacterial	TAB	Typhoid
	Killed cholera vaccine	Cholera
Viral	Sabin IPV	Polio
	Rabies	Rabies
Toxoids	Tetanus toxoid, diphtheria toxoid	
Subunit vaccines	Hepatitis B subunit vaccine, subunit vaccine for rabies	

Passive Immunity

In passive immunity as per the name passive means no activity, here body's immune system is remaining passive and immunogenic preparation is given in readymade form. Though it has the disadvantage that it is not long lasting but in some conditions it is useful. If a patient is diagnosed as a case of diphtheria, it is important to give antibodies immediately in the form of antiserum as diphtheria antiserum which will immediately neutralize the toxin produced by this bacillus in human body. Here, if anyone thinks of giving DPT vaccine (active immunity) and waits for antibodies to form which take several days, the patient may die.

Characteristics of Passive Immunity

- Immunity is **readymade** without contact with antigen.
- **No latent period,** hence gives **immediate protection** hence used in some conditions for treatment and immunoprophylaxis.
- There is **no negative phase**. Antibodies being proteins, decrease with time due to metabolism and elimination.
- There is **no secondary response**, in fact, foreign antibodies removed rapidly.
- It is less effective in long term as compared to active immunity.

  Passive immunity is classified into natural passive and artificial passive immunity.

Natural Passive Immunity from Mother to Fetus

IgG is present in colostrum, also during embryonic life. IgG is transferred from mother to fetus which gives readymade antibodies for fetus. This logic is applied in prevention of neonatal tetanus by active immunization of mother with tetanus toxoid during pregnancy. Mother will form anti-tetanus antibodies which are passively transferred to fetus, protect the newborn from tetanus.

Artificial Passive Immunity

Immunity is passively transferred in the form of readymade antibodies.

The preparations used for this type of immunity are:
1. *Hyperimmune sera of animal origin* as equine hyper immune sera obtained from horses sensitized against pathogens. These sera carry the disadvantage of hypersensitivity (serum sickness like) but they are easily obtained and used only where human sera are not available. The examples are:
   - **Anti-gas gangrene serum**
   - **Anti-tetanus serum (ATS)**
   - **Anti-botulinum sera**
   - **Anti-snake venom**
2. Hyperimmune sera of human origin
3. *Convalescent sera*: Serum of patient recovering, i.e. in convalescent stage contains a large number of specific antibodies against that pathogen which can be used for passive immunization.
4. *Pooled human gamma globulins*: If sera of normal individuals are pooled, it contains gamma globulins (antibodies) against the organisms common in the particular area.

   Convalescent sera and pooled sera are used in treatment of viral infections, e.g. hepatitis A virus.

   Readymade antibodies given in some conditions to suppress the antibodies formation in that individual by a negative feedback mechanism. This concept applies to immunization of Rh negative women with anti-D serum (anti-Rh serum) to present immune response against Rh blood group antigen. It prevents hemolytic disease of newborn.

   Differences between active immunity and passive immunity are given in Table 12.4.

COMBINED IMMUNIZATION

Readymade antiserum is given to a nonimmune person to one side with toxoid vaccine on contralateral side.

TABLE 12.4: Differences between active immunity and passive immunity

Active involvement of person's immune system	Person's immune apparatus remains passive, thus does not play role
Takes some time for development of immunity as there is lag period	It is given as readymade immunity, there is no delay
Immunity long lasting	Immunity short lived as antibodies get catabolized being glycoproteins
Immunological memory is present, boosters are given, which produce prolonged response	Memory absent, immunity short lived
Induced by vaccines or antigen or infection	Readymade antibodies given
Used for prophylaxis or treatment of subacute or chronic infections	Used for giving immediate protection, can also be given for prophylaxis, e.g. anti-D globulin

Later, full course of immunization is completed. It is called combined immunization.

The concept of immunization with lymphocytes is called **'adoptive immunity'.** An extract of lymphocytes known as 'transfer factor' may be given.

Measurement of Immunity

The true value of immunity against an organism can be tested by challenging immunity of the person against that organism. The rough estimates can be made by serological tests (antigen–antibody reactions as ELISA, agglutination, precipitation). It is also ideally not an indicator of overall level of immunity as cellular immune response produced against challenging pathogen cannot be measured. Also antibodies would include those against all the components of the pathogen.

The **practical solution** is to measure the level of antibodies against particular antigen of pathogen (protective antigen) only.

In those conditions in which cell-mediated immune response (CMI) is required against the pathogen, skin tests for delayed hypersensitivity and *in vitro* tests of CMI can be used. For example, by lepromin test individuals who are able to mount CMI against leprosy can be identified (those individuals are allowed to work in a place where leprosy patients are admitted).

Herd Immunity

Definition: The level of resistance of a community or group of people to a particular disease. It means this concept of immunity is not at individual level but it is at community level or group of people.

It also implies group protection beyond that given by protection of immunized people. Thus it concerns the immunity or influence of herd structure on the transmission of infection. If herd immunity of a community is good, it prevents the spread of the disease in the community. It also decides the trends of the newly emerged pathogen in the community. Hence, if the herd immunity is lowered down, the infectious agent spreads over large area at a time. When an influenza viral strain is circulating in a community which had previous exposure to the same virus with some antigenic similarity to previous viral strain, then spread of virus in the community is checked. The influenza virus has the characteristic of changing its antigenicity. If the new virus is totally antigenically different from the previous viral strain, then there is rapid spread of virus and it may cause pandemic also.

Elements which contribute to herd immunity are:
- Occurrence of the clinical or subclinical infection in the population.
- Immunization increases the herd immunity, for example, in polio OPV increases the herd immunity.
- *Herd structure:* This is never constant, shows variation because of births, deaths, population, migration of population.
- The ongoing program of immunization keeps the herd immunity on increase.
- The structure of herd also includes presence and distribution of other animal hosts and vectors as well as socioeconomic factors which favor or inhibit the spread of infection.

If herd immunity is high, the chances of epidemic are low. If high level of immunity is achieved and maintained by immunization by such a level that the susceptible population is reduced to negligible, it may play an important role in irradication of the disease. This has happened in diphtheria and poliomyelitis in some countries.

Though it was thought, but it will not possible to detect herd immunity by serological tests.

Acute Phase Proteins

These are the proteins secreted by liver cells following antigenic stimulus. They are different from antibodies. The concentration of these proteins is increased during acute phase of infection or injury. The detection and quantitation of C-RP is possible with latex agglutination test. **Normal concentration in serum is up to 6 µg/mL.** Detection of acute phase proteins has **prognostic** significance than diagnostic. It has the **diagnostic** significance only when it is to be detected in CSF, the levels of which are raised during pyogenic meningitis while they are not increased in aseptic meningitis. The list of acute phase proteins is as follows:

Induced by IL-1,6 and TNF
Complement factor 3, haptoprotein, c-reactive protein, factor b, serum amyloid protein 'a' and p
Regulated by only IL-6, CRP
Albumin, fibrinogen, hemopexin, cysteine protease inhibitor

The receptors of adaptive immunity show specificity so that they recognize and react to particular pathogen. Innate immune system recognizes unique molecular patterns, i.e. pathogen associated molecular patterns (PAMPs) and the receptors for this are pattern recognizition receptors.

Toll-Like Receptors (Table 12.5)

Toll is transmembrane signal receptor protein and related molecules with role in innate immunity. Thus these are cell-associated or soluble receptors which recognize microbial molecules of specific pattern and signal the cells to produce immunostimulatory cytokines.

TABLE 12.5: Different receptors of innate immunity

Receptors of innate immunity	Target and effect of recognization
Complement	Microbial cell wall component-complement activation, opsonization
Mannose binding proteins	Cell wall of GNB-complement activation, opsonization
LPS receptor	Cell wall of GNB-delivery to cell membrane
Toll-like receptors	Microbial component induces innate immunity
NOD family receptors	Bacterial cell wall component induces innate immunity
Scavenger receptors	Gram-positive and negative bacteria induce phagocytosis

Ligands which bind to TLRs are important component of pathogen, LPS of GNBs, fungal zymogene, viral nucleic acid.

TLRs that recognize extracellular ligand are found on surface of cells, those recognize intracellular ligand as viral nucleic acids are localized in intracellular compartments.

TLR-4 is receptor for bacterial LPS, TLR-recognizes flagellar protein; TLR-3 recognizes RNA and TLR-9 recognizes DNA sequence.

13

Antigen

Definition

Antigen is a substance which when introduced parenterally into a host introduces the formation of antibodies and stimulates lymphocytes that are reactive against the antigens. It has two characteristics—immunogenicity and specificity.

Antigenicity **(immunogenicity)** is the ability to produce or mount an immune response and specificity means the antigen specifically reacts with specific antibody (exception are cross-reacting antigens). This is also called immunological reactivity.

- Originally, the term antigen was applied for any molecule that induces B cell to produce antibody. The term is now more widely used for **molecules that specifically recognized by antigen receptors of B cells or T cells.**
- Antigens are broadly defined as molecules that initiate adaptive immune responses—immunogen.
- Antigens are not just component of foreign proteins such as pathogens; self molecules can serve as antigens.
- Antibodies are specific for the epitopes rather than antigen.
- Antibodies keep watch on extracellular spaces and so only recognize and target extracellular antigens or pathogens. Intracellular pathogens may escape antibody damage.
- Antigen presenting cells (APCs) not only display antigenic peptide-MHC complexes on the surface, but also express costimulatory molecules that are necessary for initing immune responses.
- Costimulatory signals are unregulated by presence of antigens.

The smallest unit **(determinant)** of antigen is called **epitope**.

Classification of Antigens

1. **(a) Complete antigens** which are able to induce antibodies formation and react with antibodies. **(b) Haptens** are substances which are incapable of inducing antibodies formation by themselves, but react with antibodies.

   Hapten can become immunogenic on combining with large molecule, carrier. Haptens are low molecular weight substances, usually nonprotein. They can react with their antibody. Many chemicals and drugs act as haptens. Certain haptens can produce type IV hypersensitivity.

   Complete haptens are relatively large, combine with antibodies and visible reaction occurs, while **simple haptens** are low molecular simple chemicals, with low valency hence may not produce visible reaction with antibody. Examples of haptens are capsular polysaccharides of Pneumococcus, substances causing allergic contact dermatitis, peptide hormones and steroid hormones.

2. Other classification is **T cell dependent and T cell independent antigens.**

3. *Particulate antigen and soluble antigen*: Particulate antigen forms clumps with its antibody and soluble antigens form precipitate when they react with their specific antibodies. The examples of particulate antigens are RBCs, yeast cells. A soluble antigen can be combined with carrier and detected by passive agglutination.

Determinant of Antigenicity

a. *Size*: Very large molecules are highly antigenic, while molecules with low molecular weight less than 5000 are not antigenic.

b. *Chemical nature*: Proteins are better antigenic than polysaccharides. Lipid and nucleic acid are less antigenic and antigenicity is enhanced by combination of proteins. Proteins are easily broken down as small peptides inside the antigen presenting cells, i.e. macrophages, hence they are better antigens. Heteropolymers are more immunogenic than homopolymers. Though lipids are not good antigens, if they are attached to a carrier as bovine serum albumin or protein **keyhole limpent hemocynin (KLH),** antibodies against lipids can be produced.

Protein antigens:

- They are more immunogenic
- T cell dependent antigen
- No tolerance
- Induce production of all types of antibodies
- Memory response is present
- Antigen requires processing by antigen presenting cell
- They are quickly catabolized

Carbohydrate antigen:

- Less immunogenic
- T cell independent
- Induces formation of IgM and IgG only
- No memory response
- Antigen presenting cell not required.
- Antigens slowly catabolized

c. *Susceptibility to tissue enzymes*: Only substances which are metabolized and susceptible to action of tissue enzyme, behave as antigens, as in initial step of immune reaction consist of antigen processing by antigen processing cells (APCs) which breakdown antigen into small peptide and present it to helper T (TH) cell.

d. *Foreignness*: Only antigens which are foreign to the individual induce an immune response. (If antigens are not foreign, they will be recognized as self-antigen. During embryonic life, cells capable of mounting immune response against self-antigens are removed.)

Antigenic Specificity

a. *Species specificity*: Tissue of all individual in species contain species-specific antigens. There is some degree of cross-reaction between antigens from related species.

b. *Autospecificity*: Autologous or self-antigens are non-antigenic. Because of their contact with immune system during embryonic life, tolerance is developed. Some antigens are not exposed to immune apparatus during embryonic life, e.g. lens proteins (because they are an intact capsule). When injury to lens occurs, lens protein will be released and body will mount an immune response.

c. *Organ specificity*: Some organs, such as brain, kidney and lens protein of different species, share the same antigen.

d. *Heterogenic (heterophilic specificity)*: The same or closely related antigens may sometimes occur in different biological species, class and kingdom. This property is used in diagnostic serological reactions. Weil-Felix reaction for typhus fever, Paul-Bunnell test for infectious mononucleosis and cold agglutination test for primary atypical pneumonia are examples of heterophile tests.

Biological Classes of Antigens

T cell independent (TI) antigens stimulate antibody production by B cells without participation of T cells and T cell dependent (TD) antigens require T cell participation to generate an immune response.

T cell independent antigens consist of repetitive epitopes, as in case of polysaccharides of pneumococcal capsule. The immune response is dose dependent, there is no memory and there is no antigen processing by antigen presenting cells. Antibodies produced against them remain in serum for longer period.

T cell independent antigen can be converted into T cell dependent antigen by binding to certain proteins and thus the immune response against them can be increased. This concept is followed in immunization against *Haemophilus influenzae*. The capsular antigen 'b' is antigenic and it is combined with killed diphtheria, increasing immunogenicity.

Examples of Antigens

Foreign Antigens

1. *Microorganisms* contain many antigens; hence a microorganism is a **mosaic antigen.** Cell wall protein, flagellar protein, pilin, capsular polysaccharides, exotoxins which are present on bacterial cell are examples of foreign proteins to human beings.
2. *Drugs*: For example, sedermoid (changes immunogenicity of platelets and body mounts immune response against platelets leading to purpura).
3. *Environmental*: For example, dust, pollen grains (produce allergy).
4. *Isoantigens*: For example, blood group antigens (ABO, Rh).
5. *Autoantigens (immune response against these antigens results in autoimmunity)*: Lens protein, thyroglobulin.
6. *Heterophile antigens*: (Also called as cross-reacting antigens.) For example, streptococcal protein and myocardium, heterophile antigens of *Rickettsia* and nonmotile strains of *Proteus* OX-19, OX-K, OX-2.

MHC

Gorer's work on the antigens responsible for allograft rejection in inbred mice led to discovery of the **major histocompatibility complex (MHC).** He identified two blood group systems in mice: antigen 1 was common to all the strains, antigen 2 was found only in some strains and was responsible for allograft rejection. This was called **H-2 antigen (H for histocompatibility).**

Histocompatibility antigens (HLA) are cell surface antigens that induce an immune response leading to rejection of allograft. The H-2 antigen system was found to be major histocompatibility antigen for mice which is coded by closely linked multiallelic clusters of genes called **major histocompatibility complex (MHC).** The name **'histocompatibility complex'** was given as its discovery was based on transplantation experiments. The major antigen which decides histocompatibility in human beings is **'alloantigens'**present on the surface of leukocytes called human leukocytic antigen (HLA), **major histocompatibility antigens.**

HLA Complex (Fig. 13.1)

The HLA complex gene is located on short arm of chromosome 6. The complex has 3 separate clusters of genes.

- Class I having A, B, C loci
- Class II or D region with DP, DQ, DR loci
- Class III. It contains genes for complement components C2, C4, properdin factor-B of alternate complement pathway, heat shock proteins, TNF-α, β.

HLA molecules: HLA molecules have two glycoprotein chains anchored on surface membrane of cells.

HLA loci are multiallelic, i.e. gene present on locus can be one of several alternative forms (alleles). Each allele determines a distinct antigen.

There are 24 alleles at HLA-A locus, 50 at HLA-B. HLA is very pleomorphic.

Class I Antigens (A, B, C) (Fig. 13.2)

- It has one heavy peptide chain (a chain) noncovalently attached to a smaller chain 2 microglobulin or beta chain. The amino acid sequence on beta chain is constant (coded by gene on chromosome 15).
- The association of β2 microglobulin with a chain is necessary for expression of MHCA I on the cell surface. (In a rare instance, though MHC is synthesized but not expressed on cell surface.) In **Daudi cells** (a type of B cell tumor cell), such situation occurs.
- There are three domains, i.e. α1, α2, α3 in alpha chain which protrude from cell surface. Apart from these, there is small length of transmembrane C terminus reaching into cytoplasm.
- **Alpha 1 and alpha 2 are folded to form a groove.** The amino acid sequence in this **region is highly variable.**
- Antigen processed by macrophages lodges in this groove of HLA class I molecule present on the macrophage and presented to CD8 cells.
- HLA class I antigens are found on the surface of all nucleated cells.
- HLA class I antigens are involved in graft rejection, cell-mediated cytolysis.

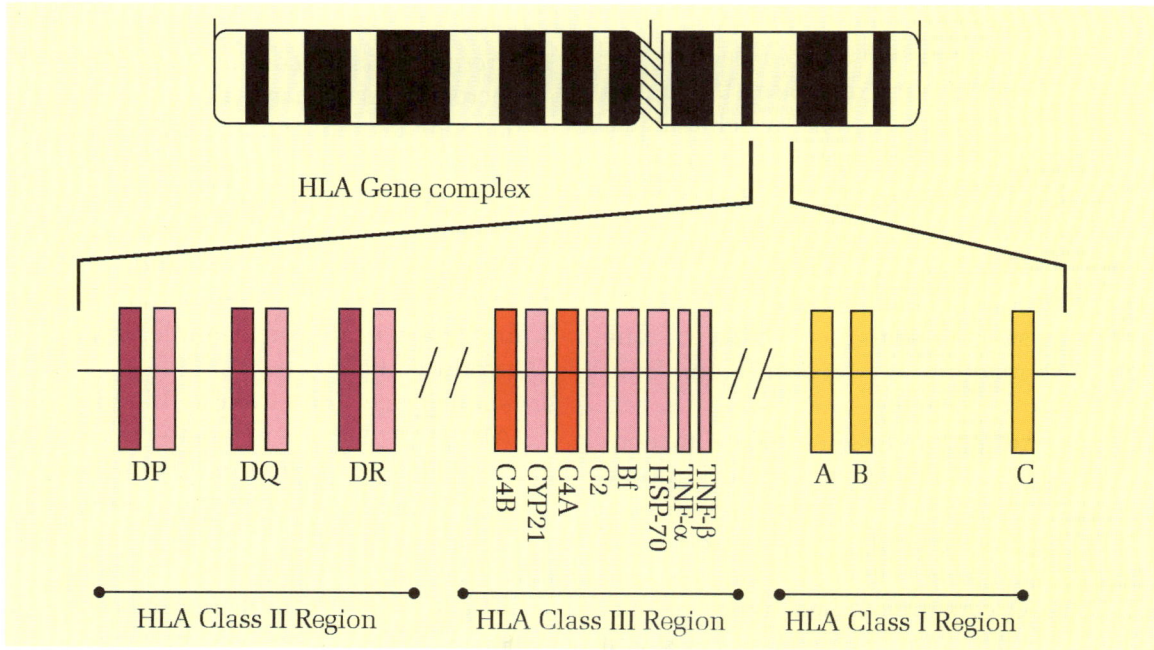

Fig. 13.1: Complex of HLA

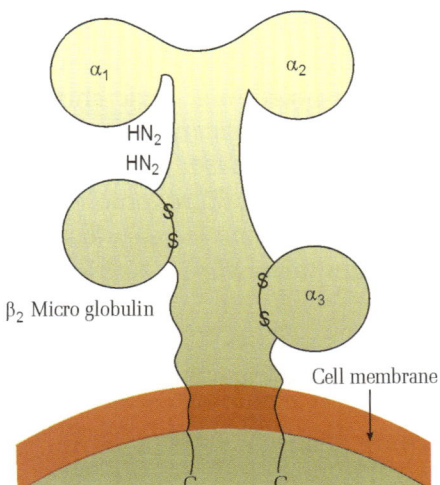

Fig. 13.2: HLA class I molecule

HLA Class II Molecules (Fig. 13.3)

- *Structure*: There are alpha and beta chains, each having 2 domains, proximal constant and distal variable. **Distal domains, i.e. alpha 1 and beta 1 chains, form a groove** in which antigenic peptide lies and presented by macrophages to CD4 cells.
- MHC class II antigens are present on cells of immune system: T cell, B cell, macrophage, dendritic cell.
- Class II molecules are principally responsible for graft versus host response, mixed lymphocytic reaction (MLR).
- **Immune response genes** (IR genes) which regulate immune response of a person are situated on class II region (probably DR locus).

Class III Molecules

These are also heterologus. They code for complement components, heat shock proteins and TNF-α.

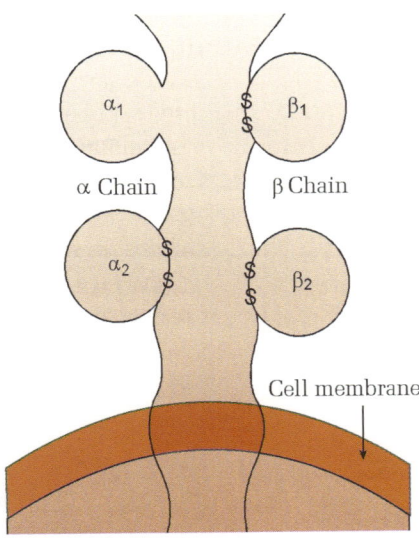

Fig. 13.3: HLA class II molecule

MHC Restriction

CD4 cells will take antigen only when the antigen presenting cell is presenting antigens associated with Class II, while CD 8 cells will take antigen from cells having the same class I molecule. Thus **CD 4 is class II restricted while CD8 is class I restricted.**

Detection of HLA antigen is done by microcytotoxicity testing. Among the donors of similar HLA types, the exact match is identified by mixed lymphocytic reaction (MLR).

Transplants between members of a highly imbred strains of animals always accepted. The exception is seen, if donor is male (XY) and recipient is female. Grafted tissue has additional antigens determined by 'Y' chromosome which are absent in female recipient (XX). Interesting thing is graft from female to male will be accepted as male has X chromosome also. This **sex-linked histoincompatibility is called 'Eichward-Silmer effect.**

TABLE 13.1: HLA and disease association

Disorder	HLA allele
Ankylosing spondylitis	B27
Graves' disease	DR3
SLE	DR2
Reiter's syndrome	B27
Insulin dependent diabetes mellitus	DQw
Juvenile rheumatic disease	Dw14, Dw4,

Applications of HLA typing

- *Transplantation*: The compatibility between recipient and potential donor is done before transplantation.
- *Paternity testing*: HLA typing is useful in case of disputed parity.
- Prediction of disease because of HLA and disease association.

EPITOPE

The smallest unit of antigenicity is called **epitope.** Antigens are large molecules but only restricted portions are involved in immune mechanisms. Such areas which determine the specific immune response and react with antibody are the epitopes, which is the basic recognition unit. The number of antigenic determinants on antigen may vary with its size and complexity. Antigenic determinant is composed of structures present on the surface of molecules and can be constructed in the following ways:

a. Within a single segment of primary sequence— **sequential epitopes**

b. Assembled from residues far apart in primary sequence but brought together on surface by folding of molecule into its native confrontation—**conformational epitopes**.

Majority of antigenic structures recognized by antibodies depend on tertiary configuration of antigen (**conformational**) while T cell epitopes are defined by primary structure (**sequential**).

The properties of epitopes are:
- Size: 25–35A
- Molecular weight: 400–1000 Daltons
- The determinant group on protein antigens is penta- or hexapeptide. Roughly it is made up of 5 amino acids.

Valency of antigens and antibodies: Number of antigenic determinents on antigens which react with antibodies is the valency of antigen. (Similarly antibodies have valencies.) Functional valencies are areas on the surface of antigenic molecule reacting with antibodies while total valencies are functional and nonfunctional valencies. Antibodies may be polyvalent, one molecule of which may react with many molecules of antigens.

SUPERANTIGENS

Normally when antigen is presented by antigen presenting cell to TCR of T cells, it lies in the groove formed by MHC class II, but the superantigen attaches to the side of MHC molecule. The superantigens do not require initial processing by APC and T cell. They activate a large number of T cells with release of cytokines, leading to shock (Fig. 13.4).

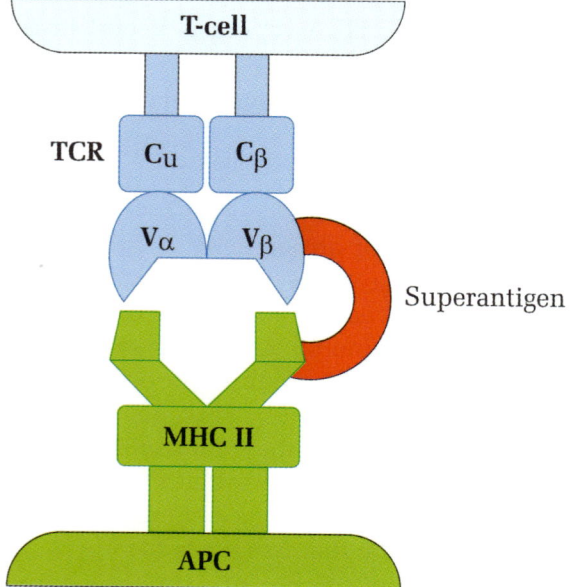

Fig. 13.4: Presentation of superantigen

Human Diseases Associated with Superantigens

- *Staphylococcus aureus:* Superantigen—enterotoxin, diseases: Food poisoning, toxic shock syndrome, multiple sclerosis, *Staphylococcus* exfoliative toxin causing exfoliative disease.
- *Group A streptococci:* Pyrogenic exotoxins cause shock, psoriasis, rheumatic heart disease.
- *Mycobacterium tuberculosis:* Not identified, tuberculosis.
- *HIV:* Negative regulatory factor—AIDS.
- *Rabies virus:* Nucleocapsid is superantigen—causes rabies.
- *Epstein-Barr virus:* Superantigen not identified—causes B cell lymphoma.
- *Yersinia pseudotuberculosis*
- *Mycoplasma:* Arthritis
- Mouse mammary tumor virus

Superantigens are capable of activating up to 20% of peripheral T cells pool, whereas conventional antigens activate <1 in 10000.

HETEROPHILE ANTIGEN OR HETEROGENIC SPECIFICITY OR HETEROPHILE SPECIFICITY (Table 13.2)

Two antigens when share some antigenic determinant they are called hetrophile antigens (*Hetero* means different, *philia* means loving). Such antigens may be present on tissues or cells or organs of different species. This property is utilized in preparation of diagnostic tests. For example, *Rickettsia* and non-motile strains of *Proteus*, i.e. **OX19, OX2 and OXK** share antigen. If a person is suffering from rickettsial infection, the antibodies produced against this bacterium (here cross-reacting antigen) cross-react with *Proteus*, hence *Proteus*

TABLE 13.2: Examples of heterophile antigens

EB virus	Human fetal thymus (also crossreacts with RBCs of certain species which is basis of Paul-Bunnell test)
Streptococci	Cardiac muscle (meromyosin)
Klebsiella	HLA-B-27 (possible basis of ankylosing spondylitis)
Mycobacterium	65KDa heat shock protein—tuberculosis?
Neisseria meningitidis	Embryogenic brain
Mycoplasma pneumoniae	RBCs
Plasmodia	Tymosin-α1
Trypanosoma cruzi	Heart, nerve
CMV	Glycoproteins, HLA, Ig
Schistosome	Albumin

antigens are used in diagnostic tests instead of rickettsial own antigens. The reason why rickettsial own antigens are not used for diagnosis of rickettisial fevers is that these bacteria are dangerous to handle and can produce fatal infection in laboratory person during handling for antigen preparation. Other examples of heterophile antigens include, **Epstein-Barr virus** causes infectious mononucleosis, shares antigenicity with **sheep** and **OX RBCs**. This property is used in Paul-Bunnell test for diagnosis of Epstein-Barr viral infection.

In primary atypical pneumonia, antibodies produced against *Mycoplasma* cross-react with **'O' RBCs**. This property is used in 'Cold agglutination test' for the diagnosis of primary atypical pneumonia.

Forssman antigen: Other example of heterophile antigen is **Forssman antigen**. Forssman observed that injection of guinea pig tissue into rabbit stimulated production of a hemolysin for sheep RBCs. It is present on many cells, particularly RBCs of animals, e.g. horse, cat, and sheep. Certain bacteria with this antigen are *Streptococcus pneumoniae*, some strains of *Salmonella*.

TABLE 13.3: Differences between T cell dependent and T cell independent antigens

Property	T cell dependent	T cell independent
T cell involvement	Yes	No
Antigen interaction	Involves tertiary complexes of T cell receptors	Involves binary complexes of membrane Ig and IgA
Antigen processing by macrophages	Yes	No
Degradability	Easily degradable	Type 2 easily degradable
Chemical nature	Mostly soluble proteins	Type 1 LPS, type 2 protein and poly-saccharide
Complement activation	No	Type 2 causes complement activation,
Isotopic switching	No	Type 1 no, type 2 limited
Immunological memory	Yes	No
Polyclonal activation	Yes	No
Effect on antibody production	Full range	IgM, IgG3

Flowchart 13.1: Definitions of epitope and paratope

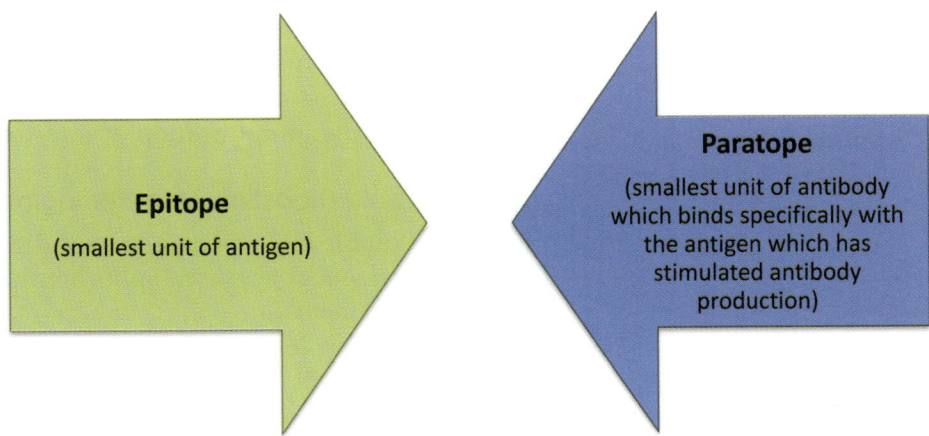

Epitope
(smallest unit of antigen)

Paratope
(smallest unit of antibody which binds specifically with the antigen which has stimulated antibody production)

14

Antibodies

INTRODUCTION

Circulating antibodies (also called immunoglobulins) are soluble glycoproteins that recognize and bind antigen specifically.

They are substances which are formed in response to antigen and react with antigen in specific and observable manner. They are formed in sera, body fluids or on cell membrane.

Antibodies are present on B cell membrane and secreted by plasma cells. Secreted antibodies circulate in blood, remove antigen or neutralize it by various ways as phagocytosis, opsonization, and antibody dependent cell-mediated cytotoxicity.

All antibodies except IgD are bifunctional. They recognize and bind antigen and promote killing or removal of antigen.

PROPERTIES OF ANTIBODIES

- **Fractionation of immune** sera by half saturation with ammonium sulphate separates serum proteins into soluble albumins and insoluble globulins. Serum globulins can be separated into pseudoglobulins (water soluble) and euglobulins (water insoluble). **Most antibodies are euglobulins.**

- Based on sedimentation studies, most antibodies are sedimented at **7S** (MW 150000–180000).

- Immunoglobulins constitute 20–25% of total serum proteins.

- Based on electophoretic mobility, Tiselius separated serum proteins into albumin and alpha, beta and gamma globulins (Fig. 14.1). **The antibody activity was associated with gamma globulin fraction.** Most antibodies are found in **these gamma globulin fractions** and **named immunoglobulins.**

In 1964, WHO expert committee proposed the term 'immunoglobulin' which was internationally accepted

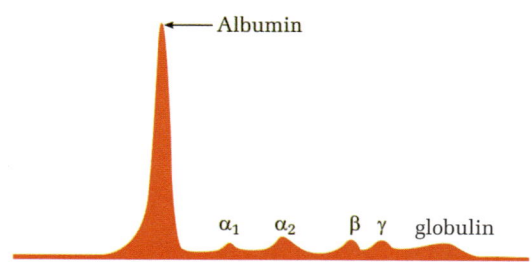

Fig. 14.1: Migration of proteins

for 'proteins of animal origin endowed with known antibody activity and for certain other proteins related to them by chemical structure. Besides antibody globulins the definition includes abnormal proteins found in myeloma, macroglobulinemia, cryoglobulinemia and naturally occurring subunits of immunoglobulins. Immunoglobulin is structural and chemical concept while antibody is functional concept.

Immune sera contain high quantities of antibodies following immunization or infection.

Papain Digestion of Immunoglobulin (Fig. 14.2)

- Rabbit IgG to egg albumin digested by papain in presence of cysteine splits immunoglobulin into two fragments.

- An insoluble fraction which crystallizes in cold is called **'Fc'** (for crystallisable).

- Soluble fraction which is unable to precipitate with egg albumin but can bind is called **Fab** (antigen binding) site.

- Each molecule of immunoglobulin is split by papain in three parts, one Fc and two Fab with sedimentation coefficient of 3.5S.

Pepsin Digestion of Immunoglobulin (Fig. 14.2)

When IgG is treated with pepsin, 5S fragment is obtained which is composed of two Fab fragments hold

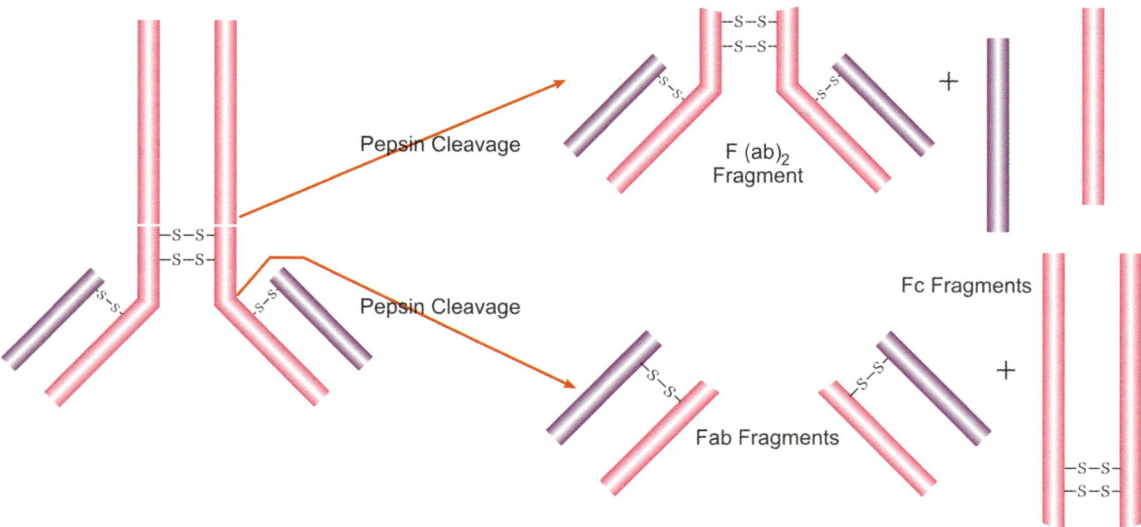

Fig. 14.2: Digestion of immunoglobulin with enzymes

together. It is bivalent and precipitates with antigen. This fragment is called F (ab') 2. Fc fragment is digested by pepsin in small fragments. Chemical treatment with mercaptoethanol cleaves disulphide bonds into four subunit structures.

ANTIBODY STRUCTURE

Immunoglobulin Chains (Table 14.1)

- Antibodies or immuoglobulins are glycoproteins having 4 polypeptide chains.
- Two identical heavy (large) chains (H) having molecular weight more than 50 kDa are present.
- Two identical light chains (small) (L) having molecular weight more than 25 kDa are present.
- Nature of heavy chain present in immunoglobulin determines the class of immunoglobulin. The 5 types of immunoglobulins are IgA, IgG, IgD, IgE, and IgM. They have alpha (α), gamma (γ), delta (δ), epsilon (ϵ) and mu (μ) heavy chains, respectively.

Light Chains

- Two types of light chains are either kappa (κ) or lambda (λ). The names are derived from scientists Korngold and Lapari who described them.
- Each molecule of immunoglobulin has either kappa or lambda chains, never both.

Light chains have molecular weight 25000 and **larger chain—heavy chains (H)** have molecular weight 50000.

'L' chain is attached to "H' chain by disulphide bond. Two H chains joined together by S – S bound.

Constant, Variable and Hypervariable Regions

110 amino acids are present at one terminus called 'N' terminus. The amino acid sequence at 'N' terminus is quite variable hence it is called **variable** region—variable light chain **'VL'** and variable heavy chain **'VH'**. Antigen combing site **(Fab) is at amino terminus composed of both 'H' and 'L' chains.**

'Fc' fragment is composed of **carboxyterminal portion** of 'H' chains (CH). It does not possess antigenic binding activity; it has **other functions such as complement fixation, placental transfer, skin fixation and catabolic rate.** In 'L' chain, the two regions are of equal length, the variable region constitute one-fifth of the chain at amino terminus. The infinite range of the antibody specificity depends on amino acid sequences at variable region of 'H' and 'L' chains which form the antigen combing sites.

Hypervariable region: The highly variable zones numbering three in L chains and four H chains are known as **hypervariable** region (**hot spot**) and involved with the formation of antigen binding sites. The hypervariable regions form the area of antibody molecule complementary in structure to antigenic determinants or epitopes and hence also known as **complementarity determining regions (CDRs).**

Variable sequences are less in some areas known as **'framework region'.**

Immunoglobulin Domains

The polypeptide chains are folded by disulfide bonds into globular region called **domains**. The domains of heavy chains are labeled as **CH-1, CH-2, CH-3, CH-4,** which are domains in constant regions and VH is there

TABLE 14.1: Properties of immunoglobulins

Property	IgG	IgA	IgM	IgD	IgE
Sedimentation coefficient (S)	7	7	19	7	8
Molecular weight	150,000	160,000	900,000	180,000	190,000
Serum concentration (mg/mL)	12	2	1.2	0.03	0.00004
Half life (days)	23	6	5	2–8	1–5
Daily production (mg/kg)	34	24	3.3	0.4	0.0023
Intravascular distribution (%)	45	42	80	75	50
Carbohydrate %	3	8	12	13	12
Complement fixation classical alternative	++––	––+	+++––	––––	––––
Placental transport	+	––	––	––	––
Present in milk	+	+	––	–	––
Selective secretion by seromucous glands	–	+	––	––––	––
Heat stability (56°C)	+	+	+	+	––

IgA may occur in 7S, 9S, 11S forms

in variable region. The domains of light chain are labeled as **CL,** and **VL** of constant and variable regions, respectively.

Constant Region Domains

The presence of CH1 and CL domains appears to increase the number of stable VH and VL. This contribute to diversity.

Hinge Region

Area between CH1 and CH2 domains is called hinge region. The gamma, delta, alpha heavy chains have hinge regions while others do not have.

Antigen-binding sites of antibodies (paratope) are specific for three dimensional shape (conformation) of their target-epitope or antigenic determinant.

Classes (five) of immunoglobulins distinguished by heavy chain are IgG, IgM, IgA, IgE and IgD having γ, μ, α, ε, δ heavy chains. Collectively there are nine isotypes, i.e. IgG1, IgG2, IgG3, IgG4, IgM, IgA, IgD and IgE.

IgG (Fig. 14.3)

- It is major serum Ig constituting 80% of total immunoglobulins.
- It is distributed equally between intravascular and extravascular compartments.
- This immunoglobulin contains less carbohydrates.
- Half-life is 23 days.
- Valency –2.
- Number of basic 4-polypeptide chains—monomer.
- It is monomeric with two light and two heavy chains.
- Normal serum concentration 8–16 mg per mL.

- It has molecular weight 150,000–160,000.
- The heavy chain exists in 4 different formats, there are 4 subclasses IgG1–IgG4. IgG1 and IgG3 are involved in complement activation, immunological response to bacterial capsule is IgG2.

Functions

- It crosses placenta and gives passive protection to fetus.
- It is the second immunoglobulin that appears following antigenic contact.
- It acts as **opsonin,** hence enhances phagocytosis.
- It neutralizes viruses and toxins.
- Antigen binding site binds to organism and Fc binds to receptor on phagocyte thus ensuring killing by phagocyte.
- It has four subclasses IgG1, IgG2, IgG3 and IgG4 with γ1, γ2, γ3, γ4 H chains. These subclasses differ in their ability to fix complement.
- It is involved in antibody dependent cell mediated cytotoxicity **(ADCC)** which kill viral infected cells.
- It protects body fluids.
- Passively given anti-D immunoglobulin prevents hemolytic disease of newborn by negative feedback mechanism.
- Passive immunity produced by human immunoglobulin gives protection against Hepatitis B following exposure. Immunoglobulins against diphtheria, tetanus, and rabies are used to treat these infections.
- It plays role in CFT test, precipitation test, and neutralization tests.
- It plays a role in type II and type III hypersensitivity reactions.

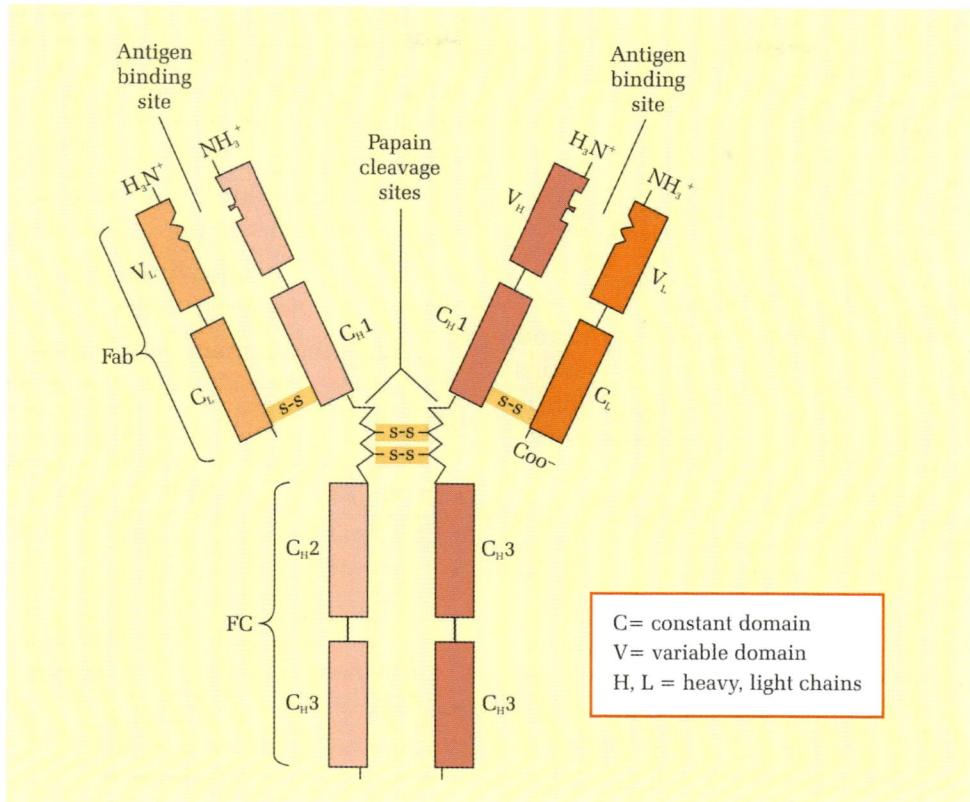

Fig. 14.3: Structure of IgG

IgM (Fig. 14.4)

- Because of its molecular weight (9,00,000–10,00,000), it is called **'millionaire' molecule.**
- It is a **pentamer containing** 10 H and 10 L chains—five subunits of monomers joined by joining J-chain.
- It constitutes 5–8% of serum Ig.
- Normal level 0.5–2 mg per mL.

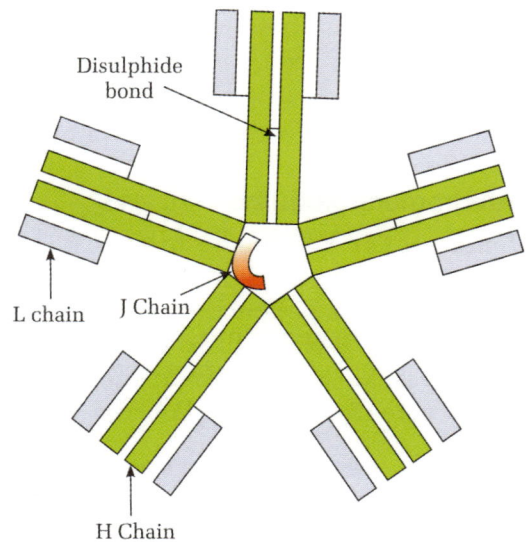

Fig. 14.4: Structure of IgM

- Half-life is five days.
- 80% of total IgM is intravascular, protects from septicemia and bacteremia.
- It is not transported across placenta hence detection of IgM is used in diagnosis of congenital infection.
- Earliest Ig synthesized by fetus.
- It is short lived, disappears earlier than IgG, inactivates complement.
- Most active in agglutination, CFT (IgM 500–1000 times more effective than IgG in opsonization).
- It is 100 times more effective in bactericidal action, 20 times in bacterial agglutination.
- IgM is 500–1000 times more efficient in oposonization as compared to IgG.
- It is less effective in neutralization of toxins, and viruses.
- It takes part in opsonization.
- Neutralizes toxins, and viruses.
- Eighty percent of total IgM is in intravascular compartment.
- It is the first immunoglobulin which appears after infection.
- Presence of IgM in serum indicates recent infection.
- Some antibodies as isohemagglutinins, antibodies to typhoid 'O' antigen, rheumatoid factor, reaginic antibodies in syphilis are of IgM class.

There are two subclasses of IgM.

Its valency is ten, which is observed with small haptens. With bigger antigen, valence falls to 5 due to steric hindrance. Treatment with 0.12 mL 2% mercapto-ethanol selectively destroys IgM and not IgG which is used to differentiate between IgM and IgG.

IgA (Fig. 14.5)

- It is second most common Ig in serum.
- It occurs in two forms, i.e. **monomeric** form and **dimeric form**. Monomeric form has two heavy chains and two light chains. As this immunoglobulin is present in secretions giving local protection, it is also called secretory IgA.
- Secretory IgA is present in saliva, secretions of lungs, gastrointestinal system, secretions of genitourinary system, tears where it occurs in diameric form. It has a joining **J chain** which is cysteine-rich polypeptide. This J chain joins two monomeric molecules together making it diameric molecule.
- It has additional polypeptide called **secretory piece or 'S'** attached to IgA molecule during transport through cells. This secretory piece protects the IgA from proteolytic enzymes present, which would otherwise cause degradation of this molecule.
- SIgA synthesized by plasma cells situated near mucosal or glandular epithelium.
- It constitutes 10–13% of serum Igs.
- Normal serum level is 0.6–4.2 mg per mL.
- Half-life is 6–8 days.

Functions of IgA

- It is produced by plasma cells near mucosal or glandular cells.
- It has some role in stimulating alternative complement pathway.
- It also helps in phagocytosis.

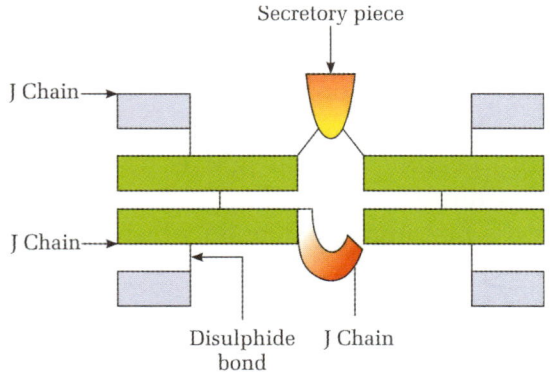

Fig. 14.5: Structure of IgA

- SIgA concentrated in secretions and on mucus surfaces forming antibody 'paste'.
- It plays important role in local immunity against respiratory and intestinal pathogens.
- IgA functions to inhibit adherence of microorganism to surface of mucosal cells.
- It activates alternate complement pathway.
- It promotes phagocytosis and intracellular killing.
  IgA1—predominant serum IgA
  IgA2—predominant secretory–mucosal.

IgE

- It has 8s molecule, molecular weight about 190000.
- Its half-life is 2 days.
- It is heat labile, inactivated at 56°C for 1 hour.
- It has affinity to mast cells and basophils with which it attaches and produces effects of type I hyper-sensitivity. It binds with these cells of same species only, hence it is called **homocytotropic** antibody.
- It takes part in type I hypersensitivity and also in Prausnitz-Kustner reaction.
- Normal serum levels are a few nanograms which are increased during allergic reactions.
- High levels of this Igs are associated with intestinal worm infestations in children.
- IgE mainly produced in the linings of respiratory and GIT.
- As it mediates type I hypersensitivity, it is called **reagin antibody.**

IgD

- Structurally, it resembles IgG.
- Concentration—3 mg per 100 mL of serum.
- Mostly intravascular.
- Half-life is 3 days.
- It occurs on the surface of unstimulated B lympho-cytes and serves as recognition receptor for antigen.

Abnormal Immunoglobulins

Bence-Jones proteins: They are formed in multiple myeloma. These are the light chains of immuno-globulins either kappa or lambda. In one patient, only one form is present. It is identified in urine by heating urine at 50°C (causes coagulation of proteins) further heating at 70°C re-dissolves the proteins.

Waldenstrom's macroglobulinemia: Plasma cells producing IgM are involved. There is excess production of 'M' proteins and their light chains (Bence-Jones proteins).

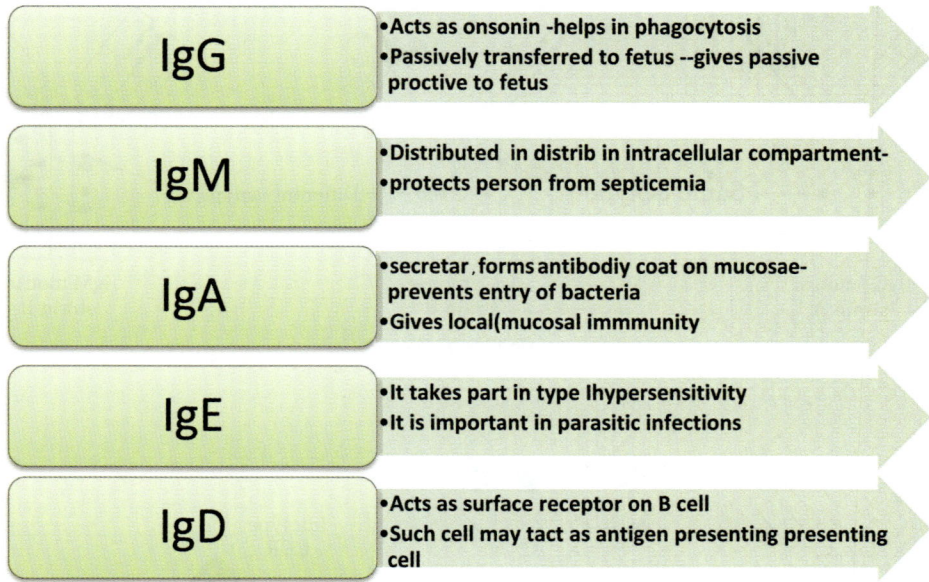

Fig. 14.6: Important function of immunoglobulins

Heavy chain disease: It is lymphoid tumor and there is overproduction of Fc parts of heavy chains. Four types of diseases are known based on 'H' chain—α chain disease **(Seligmanri's disease)**, γ chain disease **(Franklin disease)**, μ chain disease, δ chain disease.

Cryoglobulinemia: There is formation of a precipitate on cooling the serum and it dissolves on heating. This condition may be associated with myelomas but rarely seen in normal individuals.

IMMUNOGLOBULIN SPECIFICITIES (Fig. 14.7)

Isotypic Variation or Isotypic Specificities

- The genes for isotypic specificities are present in all the healthy individuals within the species. For example, the genes for A1, A2, and A3 and lambda chains are all present in human genome and these are the different isotypes. Thus isotypic specificity is one which distinguishes between different classes and subclasses of immunoglobulins in a given species. Isotypic markers on 'H' distinguishes different 'H' chain classes.
- *Allotypic specificities:* This is the genetic variation between individuals in a species. It is not found in all people hence allotypic. Allotypes occur as variants of heavy chain constant region. Thus allotypic specificities are those which distinguish between immunoglobulin of the same class between different groups of people within the species. The allotypic markers in humans are 'Gm' on gamma heavy chain, 'Am' on alpha heavy chain, 'Km' and 'Inv' on kappa light chains. More than 20 'Gm' on IgG, 2 'Km' on

IgD, and IgE and 2 'Am' on IgA have been identified. Allotypic markers are used in testing paternity and population genetics.

Idiotypic Specificities

- Variations in the hypervariable domains produce different idiotypes. This antigenic specificity is specific to each immunoglobulin molecule.
- It is genetic variation in constant region of Ig classes and subclasses within a species. Different species inherit different constant region genes, hence express different isotypes.
- Each individual genetic determinant of variable region (paratope) is called **idiotope.** The sum of idiotopes on Ig molecule is **idiotype.** Idiotype is actual binding site.

  Antibody may be formed against idiotopes are anti-idiotype antibodies. The network of idiotype and anti-idiotype can control immune response.

COLD ANTIBODIES

Autoantibodies against erythrocytes are demonstrable in autoimmune hemolytic anemias. Serologically, two groups of autoimmune hemolytic anemia described, i.e. warm antibodies and cold antibodies, respectively. Such antibodies are thought to be due to crossreacting antigens on the bacteria and red cells (heterophile).

Definition: Cold antibodies are complete agglutinating antibodies belong to class IgM and agglutinate RBCs at 4°C but not at 37°C. This was first described in paroxysmal nocturnal cold hemoglobulinuria. In most of cases, they are specific for 'Ii' blood group system.

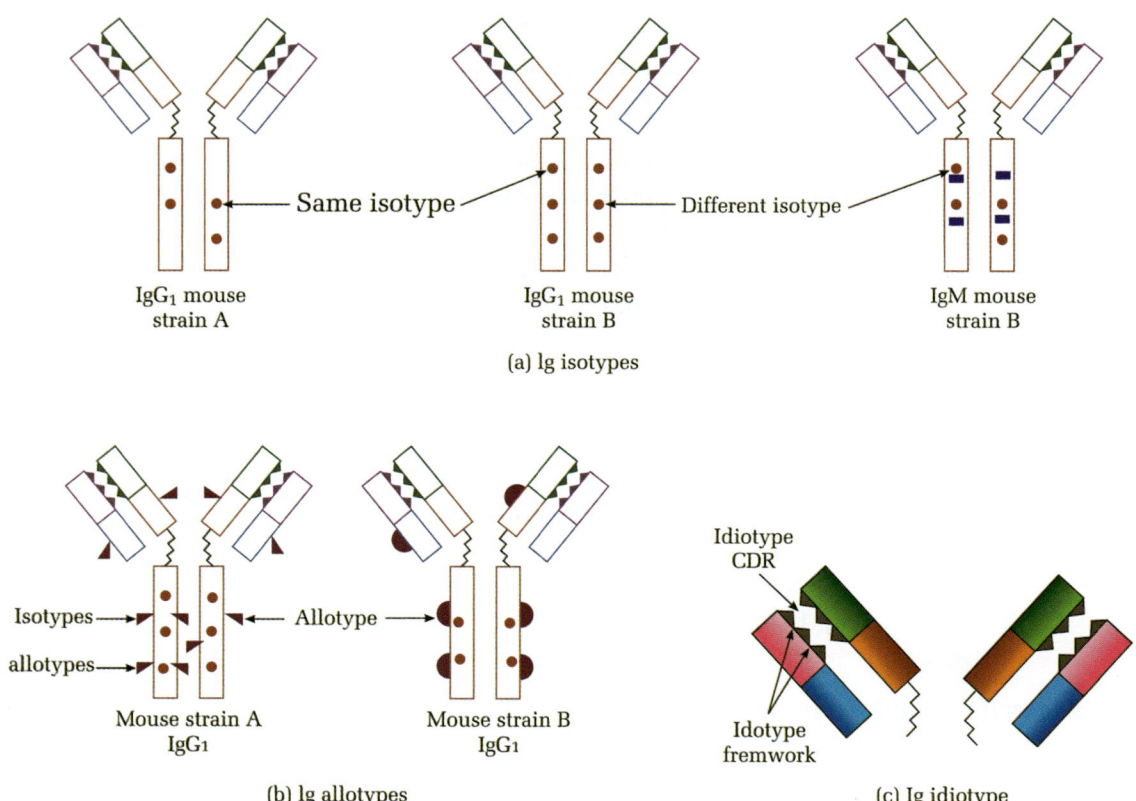

Isotypes → ←— Allotype →

allotypes →

Fig. 14.7: Antibody specificities

Conditions in which cold agglutinins seen: This condition is associated with syphilis which is rare now, but it may be seen in primary atypical pneumonia caused by *Mycoplasma pneumoniae,* rarely with trypanosomiasis and black water fever. **Anti-Ii-gM antibodies** also occur as cold agglutinins in some viral infections and diseases of reticulendothelial system.

Detection of cold agglutinins: Cold agglutinins are detected by agglutination test, significant titer is **1:32.** The patient's serum is serially diluted and mixed with equal volumes of 0.2% washed human "O" group RBCs and the reaction is observed after incubation at 4°C.

Precautions for the test: Patients blood sample should not be refrigerated before separation of serum as the agglutinins are readily absorbed by homologus RBCs at low temperature.

Other cold antibodies: IgM, IgG antibodies associated with blood group systems other than ABO and Rh systems are occasionally encountered in compatibility testing. These include: Anti-M and anti-N IgM reacting antibodies belonging to MN system.

The reaction of cold antibody with RBC takes place in body in peripheral circulation (particularly in winter) where the temperature in capillaries in exposed part of skin may fall. This causes peripheral necrosis due to aggregation and microthrombus formation in small

vessels, in severe cases, anemia also occurs due to complement-mediated destruction of RBCs in periphery.

GENETIC REARRANGEMENT OF ANTIBODY (MECHANISM OF DIVERSITY)

Antibody Diversity

- The host possesses the capacity to produce enormous number of structurally distinct antibodies. Each antibody produced has distinct specificity. Large number of antibodies that bind to different antigens or pathogens produces '**antibody diversity**'.
- The total collection of antibodies with different specificities is called '**antibody repertoire**'.
- During B cell development, diversity of antigen binding variable region of IgG is generated by set of IgG genes.
- Genes which code for variable region and constant region are 'V' and 'C'.
- Genetic rearrangement occurs in variable region, constant region remains constant.
- In 'V' region, there are three segments—V, D, and J.
- For heavy chain, first rearrangement of D segment to J occurs, followed by second rearrangement between V gene and newly formed D–J sequence, the C segment is aligned to V–D–J complex to generate functional IgG heavy chain gene (V–D—J–C).

- Similar rearrangements occur for light chain V region except there are two segments involved, i.e. V and J.
- Light chain rearrangements occur at later stages. A functional kappa or lambda chain is regenerated by rearrangement of V segment to J segment, ultimately producing an intact Ig molecule composed of heavy chains and light chains.

Class Switching

Class switching combines rearranged VDJ genes with different heavy chain constant region genes so that same antigen receptor (surface immunoglobulin) can activate a variety of effect or functions.

Following antigenic stimulation, the heavy chain VDJ unit can join any constant light chain gene segment and express antibody class. This process is called **class switching.** Class switching depends upon interplay of following factors: Switch region or site switch recombinase cytokine signals.

Antibodies Kill Bacteria by Three Ways

- Antibodies are soluble protein, they coat bacteria, act as opsonins and promote phagocytosis (opsonization).
- Antibodies combine with bacteria as antigen, immune complex is formed which stimulates complement system. Activated complements C7, 8, 9 act as **membrane attack complex** and drill bacterial wall.
- Antibodies may bind to bacteria with Fab receptors and bind to phagocytic cell and other cells which destroy bacteria (Fig. 14.8).

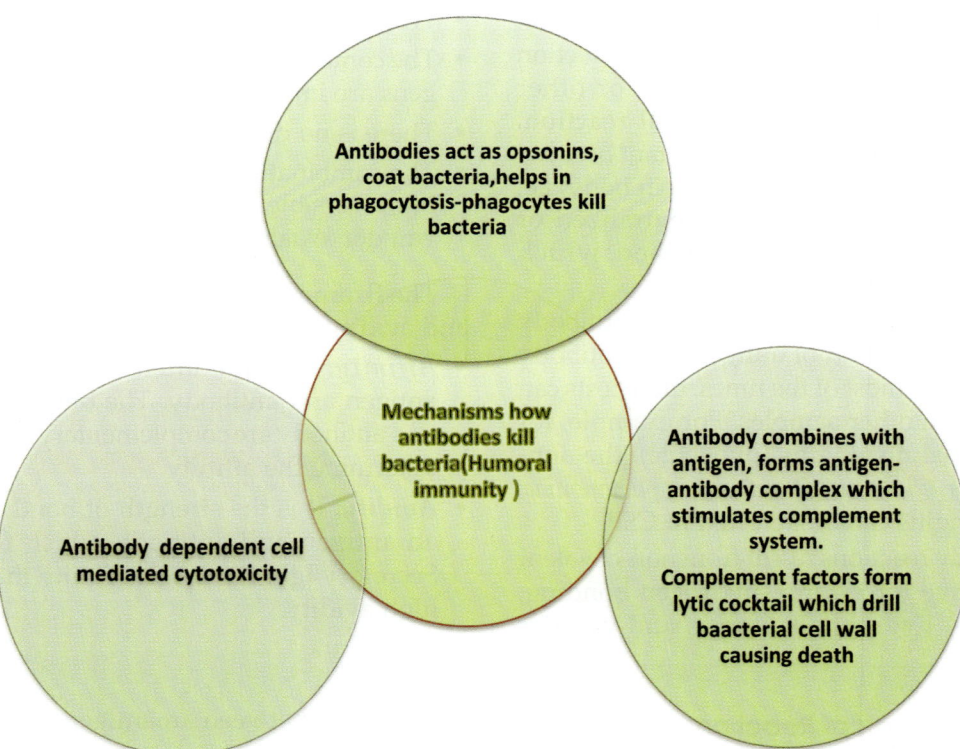

Fig. 14.8: Mechanisms of killing bacteria by antibody (humoral immunity)

15

Serological Reactions (Antigen–Antibody Reactions)

Definition of Serological Reactions

When an antigen combines with the specific antibody (antibody that is specific for antigen) *in vitro*, a reaction occurs which is observable, thus helpful in detection of antigen or antibody in patients serum or other suitable samples. This is called **serological reaction.** (The word *in vitro* in the definition is important because if an antigen reacts with specific antibody in body, i.e. *in vivo*, the antigen will be killed or neutralized or antigen–antibody complexes are formed which stimulate complement system).

These reactions are used for the detection of antibody or antigen. Though detection of antigen and antibody is performed on serum most of the times, these tests can also be performed on other samples. For example, for diagnosis of bacterial meningitis (pyogenic), the antigens as *Haemophilus influenzae, Streptococcus pneumoniae,* which cause meningitis can be detected in CSF.

Antigen–antibody reactions result from non-covalent bonds. The attractive forces are—hydrogen bonding, electrostatic bonds, hydrophobic forces and van der Waals forces.

Applications of Serological Reactions

1. Detection of antibody against pathogen is an indirect evidence of infection with that organism. For example, ELISA test is used for the diagnosis of HIV infection.
2. These tests may be important in sero-epidemiological survey.
3. These reactions can be used for quantitation of antigen or antibodies. Reaction differs in body, i.e. *in vivo* and from that *in vitro*.

General features of serological reactions

- The reaction is specific; it means antigen combines with its specific antibody (or vice versa). Only in some cases, crossreactions occur as two antigens are partially similar (e.g. heterophile).
- Whole molecule takes part in reactions.
- The combination occurs at surface; hence surface antigens are important for the detection of antibodies.
- There is no denaturation of antigen or antibody.
- The combination formed during the reaction is firm but reversible. No covalent bonds are formed, weak van der Waals forces act in combination.

The **firmness of combination** depends upon affinity and avidity.

- *Affinity*: It is the intensity of attraction between antigen and antibody. The binding sites of antigen and antibody are complementary to each other which determine the affinity.
- *Avidity*: It is the strength of bond formed between an antigen and antibody which form a complex. Secretory IgM has lower affinity than IgG but it has high avidity.

Stages

The reaction between an antigen and antibody occurs in *three* steps.

- *Primary stage*: The initial reaction between antigen and antibodies occurs at low temperature, the reaction is reversible. This reaction can be detected by estimating free or bound antigen or antibody.
- *Secondary stage*: Demonstrable effects occur. This includes agglutination, precipitation, and complement fixation.

Antibody involved in agglutination was called 'agglutinin', while antibody which takes part in precipitation was known as 'precipitin'. The corresponding antigens were known as 'agglutinogen' and 'precipitinogen', respectively.

- *Tertiary stage:* Some reactions between antigen and its specific antibody initiate neutralization of toxin or destruction of organism outside the body.

Measurement of Antigens and Antibody

Antigens and antibodies can be measured commonly as **titer** or **units.** It may also be measured in terms of mass (e.g. **mg of nitrogen**).

Some Terms Used in Serological Tests

- *Titer:* It is the reciprocal of highest dilution of the patient's serum which shows positive reaction in the test with observable manner. For example, VDRL test is used to detect antibodies in patient's serum for the diagnosis of syphilis. Serial dilutions of serum, like 1:2, 1:4, 1:8, 1:16, are performed. For preparing 1:2 dilution, take 0.5 mL of patient's serum and equally 0.5 mL of diluent, i.e. normal saline. If test is positive with 1:8 dilution but negative with 1:16, the titer would be 1:8.
- *Significant titer:* The value of titer in positive test is equal to or greater than significant test value of that test; it is called significant titer. These values are already known for each test. In VDRL test, if patient's serum is showing titer 1:4 (for this test, the significant titer is 1:8), here the 1:4 titer of patient's serum is considered insignificant.
- *Sensitivity of the test:* The ability of the test to detect very minute amount of antigen or antibody (which is to be detected). It detects true negatives.
- *Specificity of the test:* Ability of the test to detect reactions between homologous antigens and antibodies only. If the test is highly specific, false positive reactions are absent or minimum.
- *Paired sera:* Patient's serum is collected twice, the first sample is collected in early phase of infection while second sample is collected after 8–10 days. Compare the titers of these two sera and if there is increase (fourfold) in titre as compared to first serum, it suggests active infection.

Types of Serological Test

Types of serological tests used in diagnostic micro-biology laboratory are:
- Agglutination tests
- Precipitation tests
- Complement fixation test
- Immunofluorencence tests (direct and indirect)
- Enzyme-linked immunosorbent assay (ELISA)
- Radioimmunoassay (RIA)
- Immunochromatographic tests
- Neutralization test
- Staphylococcal coagglutination test
- *Other tests:* Flow cytometry, RAST.

TABLE 15.1: Sensitivity of serological tests

Serological test	Sensitivity microgram antibody/mL
Agglutination	
Direct agglutination	0.3
Passive agglutination	0.006–0.06
Precipitation in fluids	20–200
Immunoelectrophoresis	20–200
Rocket electrophoresis	2
ELISA	0.00001–0.01
Immunofluorescence	1
RIA	0.0006–0.006
Flow cytometry	0.0006–0.06

AGGLUTINATION TESTS (REACTION)

Definition

If a particulate antigen reacts with its antibody at suitable temperature, pH and in presence of electro-lytes, particles are clumped or agglutinated.

Classification of Agglutination Reactions
(Flowchart 15.1)

- Slide agglutination tests which are further classified as **direct agglutination** and **indirect agglutination** tests.
- Tube agglutination tests are further classified as **homologous** and **heterophile** agglutination tests.

Slide Agglutination Tests

a. *Direct agglutination test:* Antigen and antibody reacts with each other forming clumps. Simplest example of this method is blood grouping test. But in microbiology, direct agglutination test is done on isolates as *Salmonella, Vibrio, Shigella* grown on culture media. A few colonies grown on agar are emulsified in normal saline which act as an antigen, readymade antiserum is added to it and observed for clumps formation.
b. *Indirect agglutination tests:* Here antigen is coated on inert substances, which by themselves do not take part in reaction but just carry antigen absorbed on it and give visible reaction. Indirect tests are also called **passive agglutination tests.** The examples of these tests are as follows.

Latex agglutination test: Latex particle carry antigen and visible reaction is seen in the form of clumps of latex particles (Fig. 15.1).
1. *ASO test:* It is performed for detection of anti-streptolysin 'O' antibody in patient's serum with post-streptococcal infection. Serial dilutions of patient's serum are taken on latex slide like, 1:2, 1:4, and 1:8 (doubling dilutions). If highest dilution giving test positive is 1:2, concentration of ASO is calculated as:

Flowchart 15.1: Different types of agglutination tests

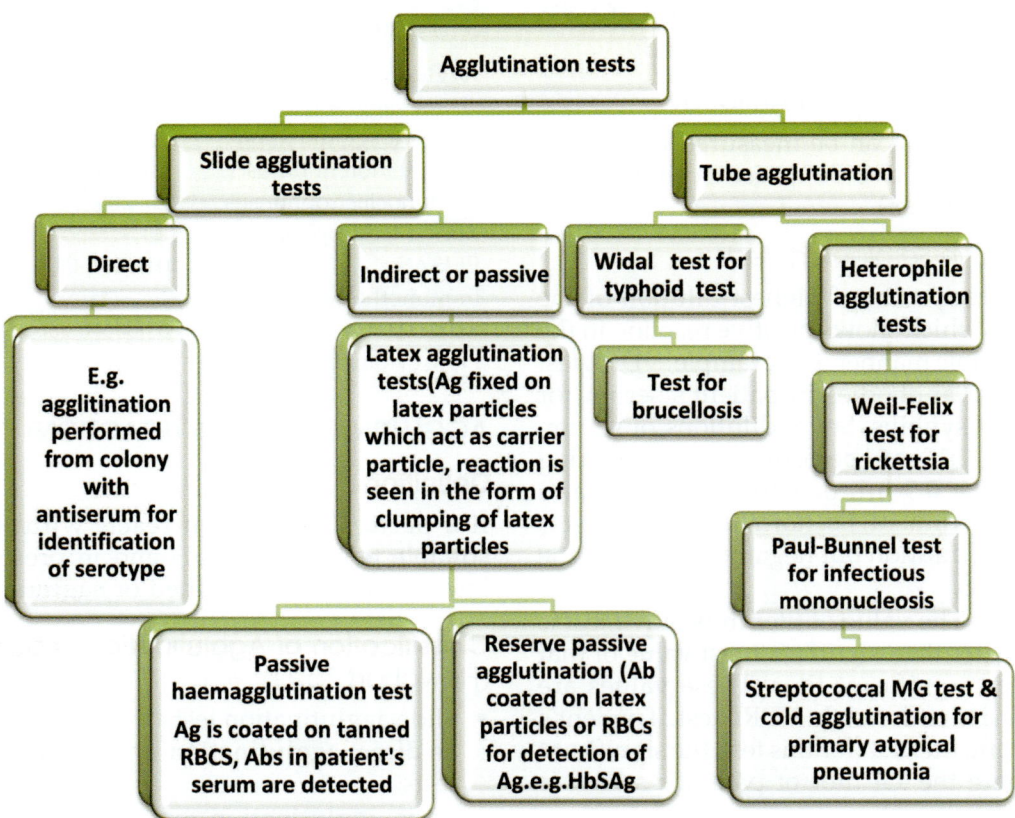

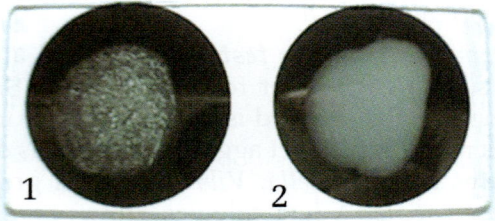

Fig. 15.1: Latex agglutination test

ASO (IU/mL) = highest dilution of the test × sensitivity of the reagent which is 200 IU/mL, hence it would be 2 × 200 = 400 IU/mL.

2. *RA test*: It detects antibody against human immuno-globulin (anti-IgG) which is called 'RA' factor, IgG is coated on latex particle. In rheumatoid arthritis, antibodies against normal immunoglobulins are produced. This test is used for diagnosis of rheumatoid arthritis. Like ASO test, this test can also be quantified.

3. *CRP (C-reactive protein)* is also based on the principle of latex test.

Other Slide Agglutination Tests

Rose-Waaler test: Hemagglutination was performed for the diagnosis of rheumatoid arthritis. Here, instead

of latex particle, tanned RBCs are coated with antigen and visible reaction is seen in the form of clumping of RBCs.

TPHA test (*Treponema pallidum* haemagglutination test): This is specific test for diagnosis of syphilis. *Treponema pallidum* (Nichol's strain) is coated on the surface of tanned RBCs acts as antigen.

Other particles which can be used to coat antigen are **gelatin and carbon particles.**

Tube Agglutination Tests

Widal test: It is performed for the serodiagnosis of typhoid fever. This test checks whether antibodies against, *S. typhi*, *S. paratyphi A* and *S. paratyphi B* are present in patient's serum. This test is positive in the second week of infection.

Febrile agglutination tests: Widal test is included in the panel of tests called **febrile agglutination tests** which include other agglutination tests as for brucellosis, Paul-Bunnell test for diagnosis of infectious mononucleosis, Weil-Felix test for rickettsial fevers, Streptococcus MG test and test for leptospirosis.

Note: Nowadays many manufacturers are coming with slide agglutination tests for Widal.

Test	Widal test	Standard agglutination test for brucellosis	Weil-Felix test	Paul-Bunnell test	Streptococcus MG test	Cold agglutination test
Diagnostic titer	TH 1:200 TO:1:100	>1:200	1:1000	1:200	1:20	1:32

TABLE 15.2: Heterophile agglutination tests

Heterophile Agglutination Tests (Table 15.2)

If two antigens share some antigenic similarity, they are called heterophile antigens. In such case, one antigen can be used for the detection of antibodies against second antigen, then the reactions are called 'heterophile agglutination tests'.

Examples of heterophile agglutination tests are:
- *Weil-Felix test*: Antigens from nonmotile strains of *Proteus mirabilis* OX19, OX2 and OX-K are used for the detection of antibodies against rickettsial infections.
- *Streptococcal MG test*: *Streptococcus MG* strains are used as an antigen for the diagnosis of primary atypical pneumonia in which antibodies against *Mycoplasma pneumoniae* are detected.
- *Paul-Bunnell test* is used for diagnosis of infectious mononucleosis.
- *Cold agglutination tests* are used for the diagnosis of primary atypical pneumonia caused by *Mycoplasma pneumoniae*.

Coombs' Test or Antiglobulin Test

- This test is used for detection of incomplete antibodies. Such type of antibodies may be produced following infection. These antibodies do not react in an observable manner, hence diagnosis of such infection by detection of antibodies makes difficult. The problem is solved by using **Coombs' serum** which is antibody produced against normal immunoglobulin (by injection of normal serum into rabbits, normal serum contains IgG, rabbit will produce antibody against IgG).
- For example, if a patient is suspected to be suffering from brucellosis, antibrucella antibodies will be produced in patient's serum which is incomplete antibody, it is detected by adding Coombs' serum.
- Like Widal test, serial dilutions of patients serum are produced which are added to brucella antigens in tubes. If it is incubated no results will be seen. If Coombs' serum is added to these tubes observable clumping is seen.
- Initially this test was basically developed for the detection of incomplete antibodies produced in Rh incompatibility.

- If sera containing incomplete anti-Rh antibodies are mixed with Rh+ red cell, the antibody coats the red cell but agglutination is not seen. When such RBCs (sensitized RBCs) are washed free of all unattached proteins and treated with antiglobulin or Coombs' serum, the cells will agglutinate.

Types of Tests: Direct and Indirect Test (Fig. 15.2)

Direct Coombs' test: In the first step antigen coated RBCs are mixed with patient's serum. If patient's serum has antibodies they will react with RBC's but no clumping is seen. Hence, in the second step Coomb's antiserum is added that brings visible reaction.[7]

Indirect test: In this, sensitization is done *in vitro*. Hence it is performed in two steps (Fig. 15.2). It detects anti-Rh antibodies.

PRECIPITATION

Definition

When a **soluble** antigen reacts with a specific antibody at suitable temperature (37°C) and pH (7.4), it results in formation of insoluble precipitate.

Flocculation: It is a type of precipitation in which the precipitate formed due to antigen–antibody reactions remains suspended instead of sedimentation, e.g. VDRL test.

Precipitation reactions are used for the detection and quantitation of antigen, detection of antibody; they are also used for standardization of toxins and antitoxins.

Mechanism

Zone Phenomena

In a mixture of antigen and antibodies, the antibody has two valencies, while antigen is multivalent. It means one molecule of antigen is capable attaching with two antibody molecules. In a given mixture of antigen and antibody, if all the valencies of antigens are satisfied and there no antigen or antibody left out, a proper lattice is formed and reaction become visible. Thus, precipitation occurs when both antigen and antibodies are present in optimum proportions and a 'lattice' is

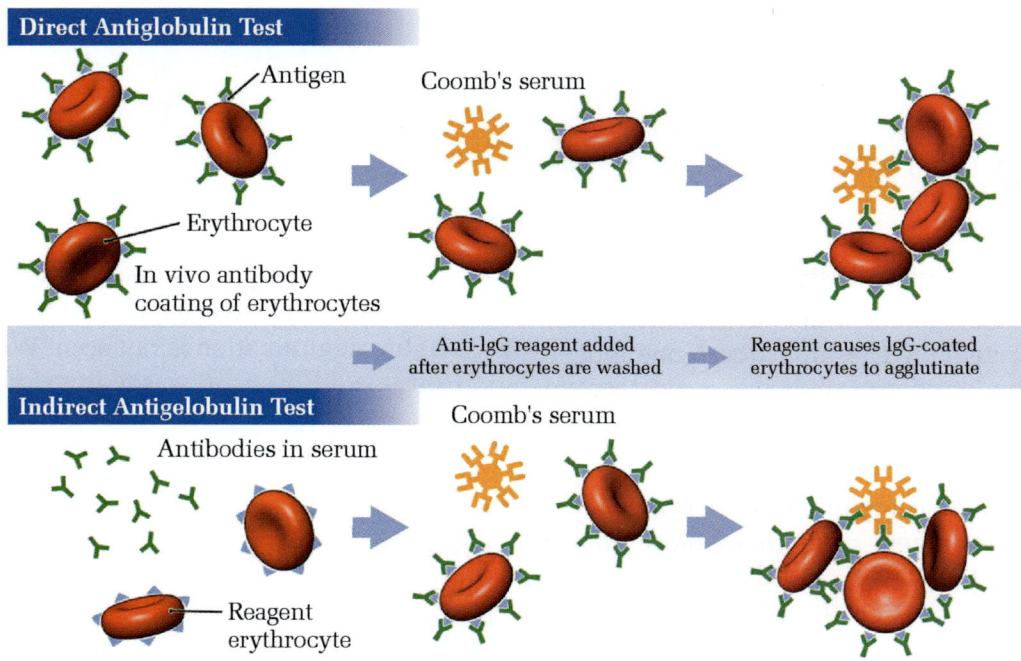

Fig. 15.2: Coombs' tests

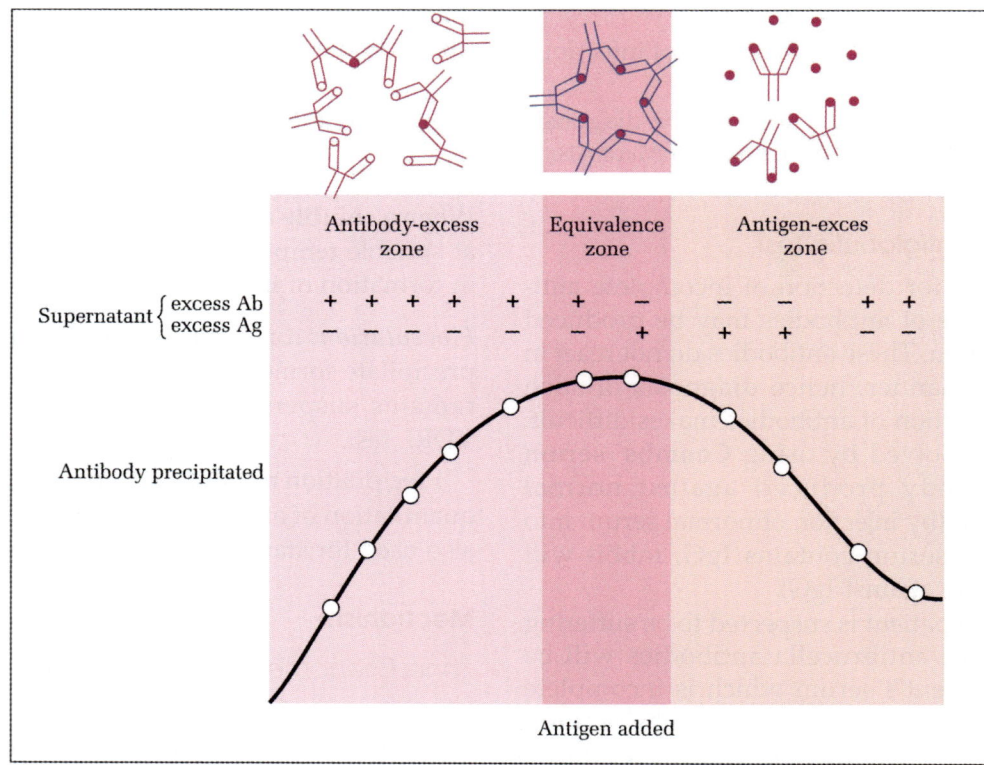

Fig. 15.3: Lattice hypothesis

formed. This is called **lattice hypothesis** (Fig. 15.3). If antibody is in excess, precipitation will not occur readily and abundantly. This is called **prozone phenomenon.** On the other hand, in a mixture, if antigen is present in excess amount, some molecules will be used to satisfy valencies of antibody while some antigens are left out, here also proper precipitation will not occur, this is called **post-zone phenomenon** (Fig. 15.3)

If increasing concentrations of antigens are added in test tube to fixed amount of antiserum, precipitation occurs rapidly and abundantly in one of the middle test tubes where both antigen and antibodies are present in equivalent proportions. In first few tubes, reaction will not occur as antibody is in excess, this is prozone. Similarly, in some of the later tubes, antigen is in excess (postzone), reaction will not occur.

Clinical significance of prozone phenomena: In case of secondary syphilis, very high titres of antibodies may be present in serum, the VDRL test with undiluted serum may give negative test, but if test is performed with diluted serum it will appear positive.

Different Precipitation Reactions (Figs 15.4–15.5)

Ring test: If antigen solution is layered over antibody solution, they will form a precipitation where they meet in optimum proportion and a ring will be formed.

Uses:
- Detection of C-reactive protein.
- Ascoli's thermoprecipitation test
- Grouping of *Streptococcus pyogenes* by Lancefield technique.

Slide flocculation test: A drop of patient's serum and a drop of antigen taken on VDRL tile, which is mixed, the result is formation of floccules.

Tube flocculation test: This test is performed in test tube instead of VDRL tile. **Kahn test** for syphilis is tube flocculation test.

Immunodiffusion Tests

As the reaction is performed in gel a band of precipitation occurs which can be stained. The different tests are described as follows.

Simple Immunodiffusion

On a clean glass slide, 1% agarose solution is poured. When the gel sets, two wells are punched. In one well, known antibody is taken, in another, patient's serum is taken. The slide is incubated. If the band of precipitation occurs, it means that antigen is present in patient's serum (Fig. 15.6).

Following terms are used in immunodiffusion test. The understanding of the simple rules given here will make understanding of the tests easy.
- Single diffusion means only one component of serological test either antigen or antibody diffuses.
- Double diffusion means both diffuse.
- Diffusion in one dimension means diffusion in one plane (one dimension, i.e. horizontal or vertical) while two dimension mean horizontal as well as diffusion in downward.

Single diffusion in one dimension (Oudin procedure) (Fig. 15.4b): Antibody is mixed in agar gel in a test tube and antigen solution is poured on it, antigen only diffuses in downward direction and where they meet in optimum quantity precipitation bands are formed. Different antigens may form different bands.

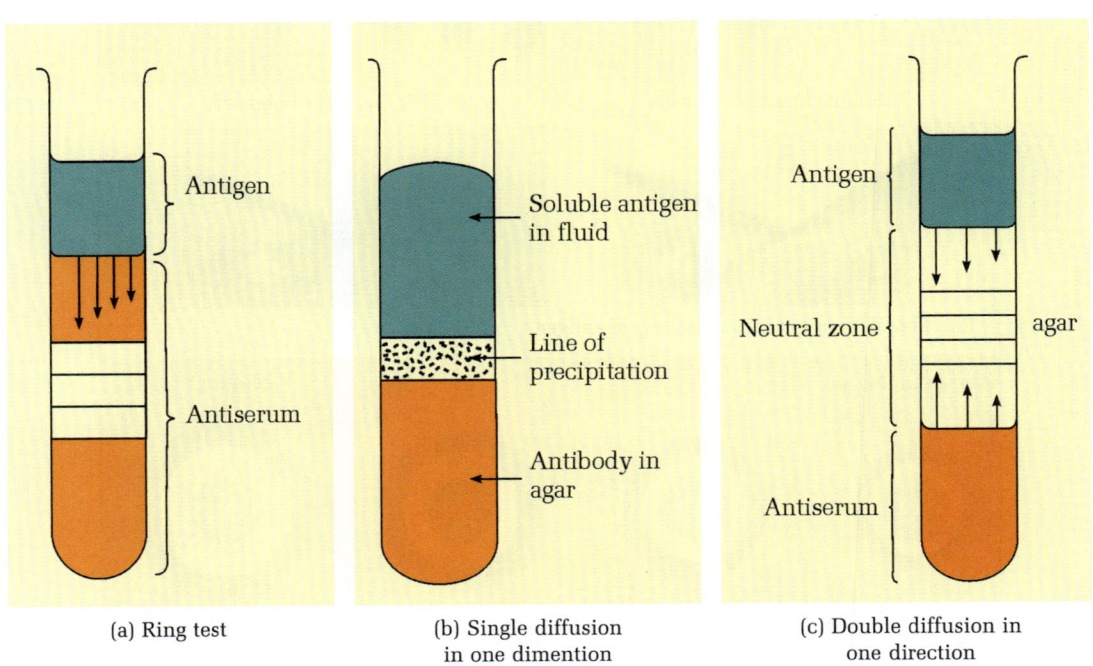

(a) Ring test   (b) Single diffusion in one dimention   (c) Double diffusion in one direction

Fig. 15.4: Different precipitation tests

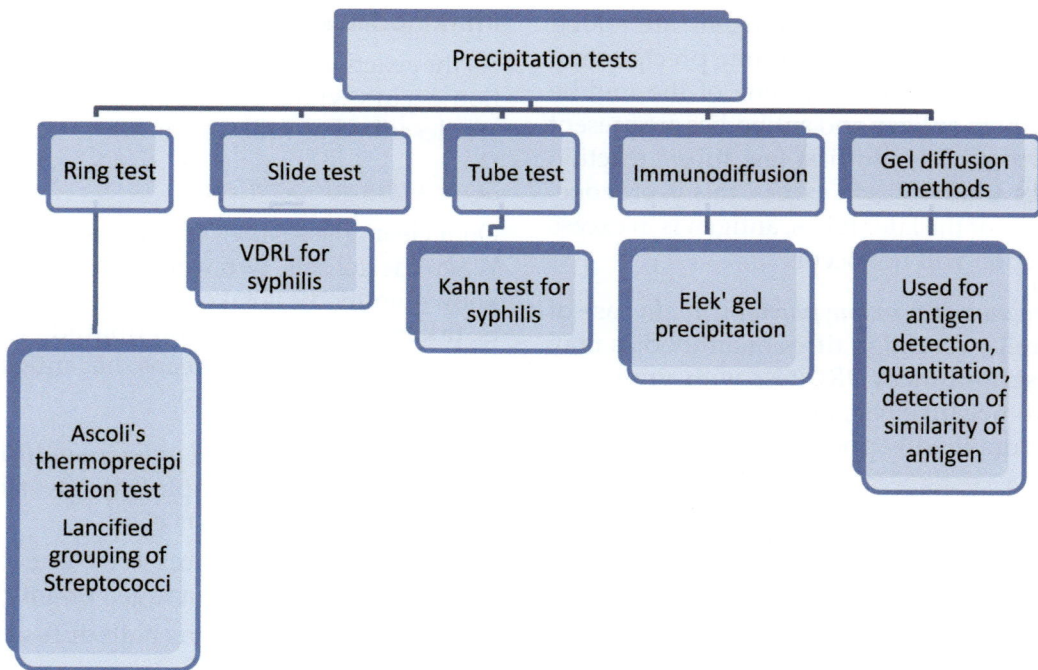

Fig. 15.5: Precipitation tests

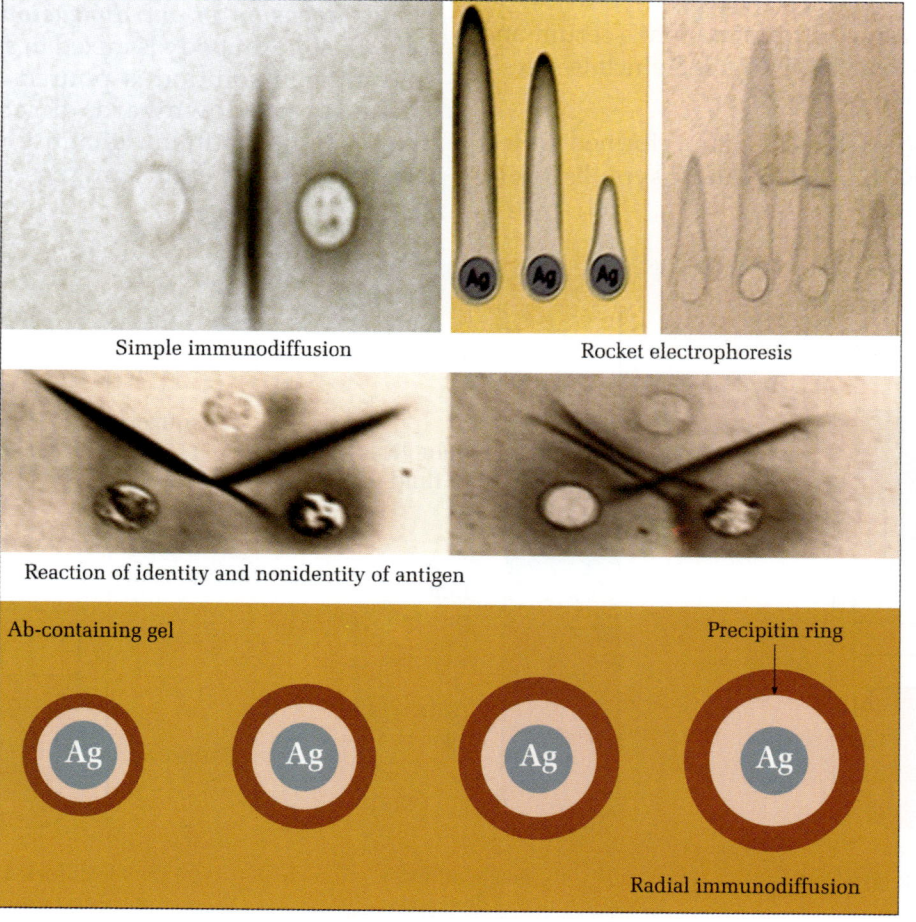

Fig. 15.6: Precipitation tests

Double diffusion in one dimension (Oakly–Fulthorpe) (Fig. 15.•e): Agar gel with antibody is at the bottom of a test tube. Over this a layer of plain agar is poured. Above this layer of antigen is made. Both antigen and antibody move towards each other (double diffusion in only one direction) and form a band of precipitation.

Use: It is used to determine antigens in mixture.

Single diffusion in two dimensions (radial immuno-diffusion—RID) (Fig. 15.6): Antibodies are mixed in agar. This is taken on glass slide. When agar gets solidified, wells are cut in agar and known concentrations of antigen are taken in some of the wells. Remaining wells will contain unknown antigens. Only antigen diffuses radially, react with antibodies in agar, forms rings and the diameter of ring formed is proportional to antigen concentrations. By comparing rings of unknown with known concentration, quantitation is performed.

Uses:
• Quantitation of immunoglobulins, complements and other proteins in blood.
• For quantitation of antigen in body fluids.

Double diffusion in two dimensions (Ouchterlony procedure): Agar gel is poured on a broad slide. Well are made on it. Antiserum is taken in central well. Different antigens are taken in remaining wells. If two adjacent antigens are identical, line of precipitations formed by these two antigens will unite, if they are not identical, they will not unite; while if they crossreact (partial identity), a spur is formed (Fig. 15.6).

Uses: To detect antigen, to compare antigens, diagnosis of various infectious diseases as Elek's gel precipitation test for diphtheria.

Immunoelectrophoresis (Fig. 15.7)

The test is performed in two steps. Agar gel is poured on glass slide. One hole is punched in it, in which antigen is added, trough is also cut below. The antigen is separated by electrophoresis. In the second step, antiserum is added to trough. Both antigen and antibodies will diffuse in two directions form bands of precipitations.

Uses:
• To analyze normal human serum.
• Detection of abnormal immunoglobulins is possible like multiple myeloma protein.

To detect multiple myeloma proteins, in antigen well normal serum is taken, electrophoresis is performed to separate normal immunoglobulins, in the second step patients serum is added. If patient's serum contains myeloma proteins, a band of precipitation will be formed.

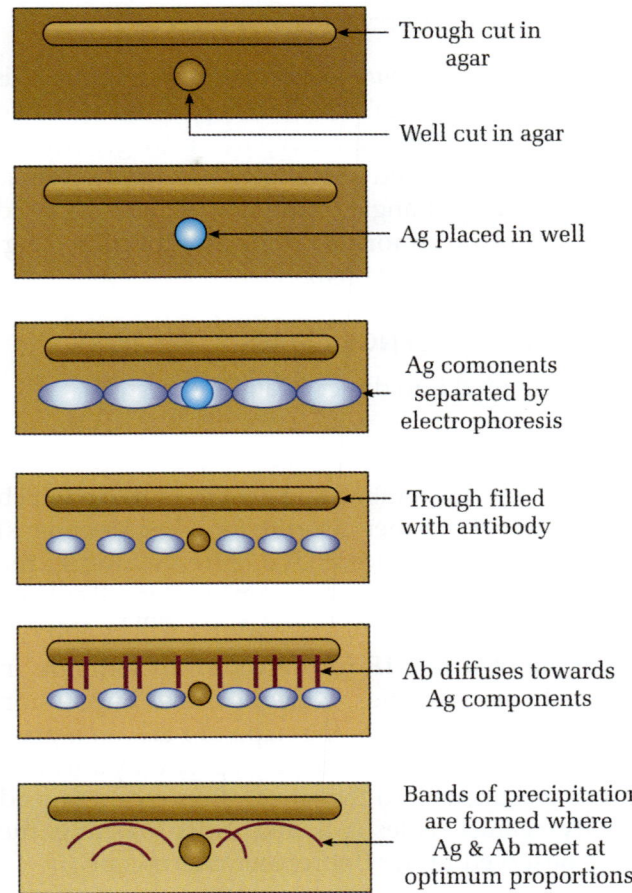

Fig. 15.7: Immunoelectrophoresis

Labels:
- Trough cut in agar
- Well cut in agar
- Ag placed in well
- Ag comonents separated by electrophoresis
- Trough filled with antibody
- Ab diffuses towards Ag components
- Bands of precipitation are formed where Ag & Ab meet at optimum proportions

Electroimmunodiffusion: The formation of precipitin lines can be speeded up by electrically driving antigen and antibody with diffusion with various methods.

Countercurrent immunoelectrophoresis: In this test, two wells are made on a slide with agar gel, in one hole antigen is taken while in another antibodies (antiserum contains antobodies) are taken. Electric current is applied so that the movement of antigen and antibodies towards each other is accelerated.

Uses: Detection of *Cryptococcus* antigen in CSF, similarly pneumococcal antigen can be detected. Hepatitis B surface antigen can be detected in patient serum; various antigens can be detected in body fluids.

Rocket electrophoresis (one dimensional single electrophoresis) (Fig. 15.6): Agar gel containing antibody is poured on a slide, wells are cut, and cathode side is filled with known and unknown antigens and electrophoresis is carried out. Result is formation of rocket-shaped bands. Comparing the height of the band with that of known antigen, quantitation can be done.

Uses: Quantitation of proteins or antigens.

Two/dimensional immunqelectrophoresis: Antibody is incorporated in agar gel. This test is performed in two steps. In first step, antigen is separated by gel electrophoresis, in the second step, again electrophoresis is carried out at right angle to the first. The test is used for detection of abnormal immunoglobulins (e.g. multiple myeloma proteins).

IMMUNOFLUORESCENCE (IF) TESTS (Fig. 15.8)

They are divided into direct IF and indirect IF.

Direct IF Test

In direct IF test, the antibody against the antigen which is to be detected in patients serum (or other specimens) is tagged with fluorescent dye. After washing, the slide is observed under fluorescent microscope. If antigen is present in the specimen, fluorescence will be seen.

Example of **direct IF for detection of antigen:** In suspected case of rabies, collect corneal impression smears or scrapings from the nape of neck on a glass slide (being near to brain, chances of positivity are more in these specimens). To the smear, fluorescent tagged antibody against rabies is added. After washing, the slide is observed under fluorescent microscope.

Uses of Direct Immunofluorescence

- It is used for detection rabies antigen; this test is used for antemortem diagnosis of rabies.
- Detection of *Herpes simplex* antigen on brain biopsy for diagnosis of herpetic encephalitis.

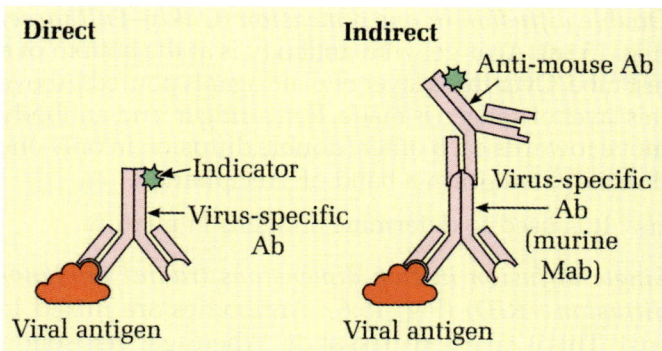

Fig. 15.8: Direct and indirect immunofluorescence test

- Detection of streptococcal antigen in nasopharyngeal secretions for diagnosis of sore throat.
- Detection of *Chlamydia* antigen in clinical specimens.

Indirect Immunofluorescence Test

Already antigen coated slide is taken, patient's serum (diluted serum) is added to the slide. After washing, second antibody against normal immunoglobulin tagged with fluorescent dye is added. The slide is observed under fluorescent microscope. Indirect immunofluorescence is used for the detection of antibodies against pathogens. For example, detection of specific antibodies against syphilis (FTA-ABS-fluorescent treponemal antibody absorption test).

ENZYME IMMUNE ASSAYS (EIA) (Fig. 15.9)

Antigen or antibodies are conjugated with enzyme, in presence of suitable substrate antibody or antigens are detected. Enzyme immune assay includes all tests

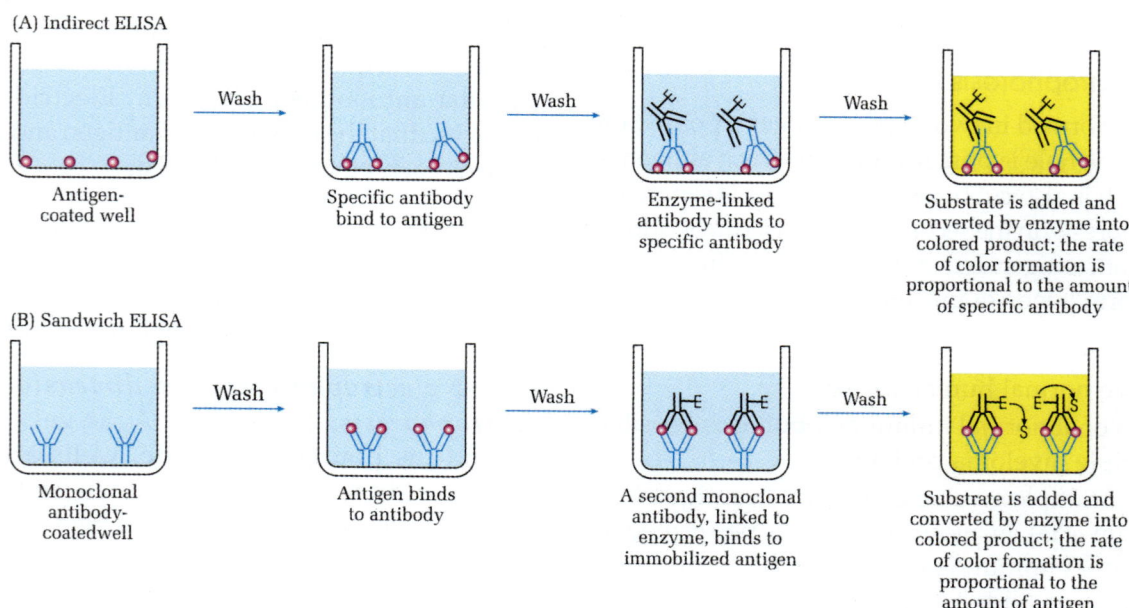

Fig. 15.9: ELISA

which measure enzyme-labeled antigen or antibody or hapten.

a. *Homologus EIA*: All reagents are added simultaneously in a single step. Separation of bound and free fractions of antibody (or antigen) is not required. An example is enzyme multiplied immunoassay technology (EMIT). Such assays are used for detection of hapten, e.g. cocaine in serum.

b. *Heterologus assay*: Separation of free and bound fragments is done by absorption of either antigen or antibody on solid surface, with reagents are added stepwise.

Main type of **heterogenous EIA** is **ELISA (enzyme linked immunesorbent assay).**

ENZYME-LINKED IMMUNOSORBENT ASSAY (ELISA)

It is called immunosorbent test because an absorbing material specific for one of the components of reaction (antigen or antibody) is present in the test.

The absorbing material may be cellulose or a solid phase as polystyrene, polyvinyl or polycarbonate tubes or microwells. The test is done usually in a 96 well microtitre plates (Fig. 15.10).

Sandwich ELISA (Fig. 15.9)

- Antibody against antigen to be detected is attached to solid surface as ELISA microtitre plate.
- Antigen present in the specimen binds to the fixed antibody.
- After washing which removes unattached substances, second antibody directed against different epitope of antigen conjugated with enzyme (e.g. Horseradish peroxide) is added to the reaction mixture on plate. This binds to antigen which is captured on plate.

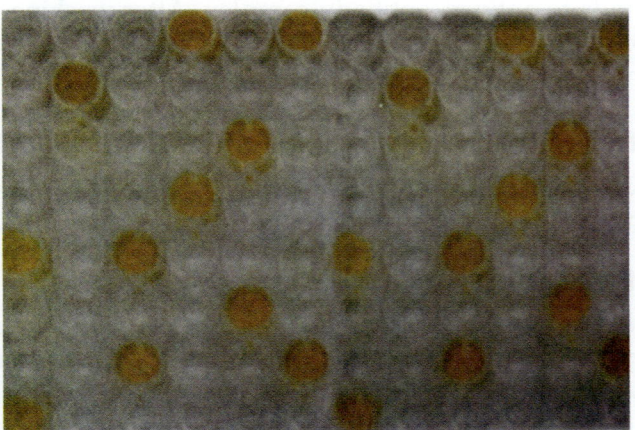

Fig. 15.10: ELISA microtitre plate (96 wells) with positive results

- After a wash, a chromogenic substrate is added. The chromogenic substance produces color.
- The enzyme hydrolyses the substrate which shows a color change, the color can be seen by naked eye or read by spectrophotometrically.

The antigen in positive test sandwiched between first antibody and enzyme-linked second antibody, hence it is known as sandwich ELISA.

Enzymes used in ELISA and substrates

Horseradish peroxidase	Hydrogen peroxide
Urease	Urea
β-galactosidase	ONPG
Alkaline phosphatase	Pnpp

Sandwich ELISA is used for detection of:

- Rotavirus in stool sample
- HbsAg in serum for diagnosis of HBV
- Detection of p24 antigen of HIV during window period
- Detection of *Chlamydia* antigen from corneal scraping of patient of trachoma.

Previously used ELISA required additional instrument as ELISA washer, time required was minimum 2–3 hours, controls should be used, many samples tested at a time on 96 well ELISA microtitre plate and also trained staff required. Nowadays simple, membrane based enzyme immunoassays (EIAs) are available which are rapid, results available within minutes. They have provided with inbuilt controls, no machinery required.

Indirect ELISA

It is used for detection of HIV antibodies (Fig. 15.9).

- Antigen is attached to solid phase (microtitre plate)
- Patient's serum is added, if specific antibodies against attached antigen are present, they get attached to antigen firmly. In washing step, unattached antibodies are removed (other antibodies which are not specific to antigen, also normal Igs get washed away).
- Antibody which is anti-IgG (produced in experiment animal by injecting normal pooled sera) is tagged with enzyme is added.
- Chromogenic mixture added. Change of color observed (membrane EIA) or read spectrophotometrically.

Competitive ELISA (Fig. 15.11)

Both unknown antigen and the known standard antigen added simultaneously which compete for antibodies

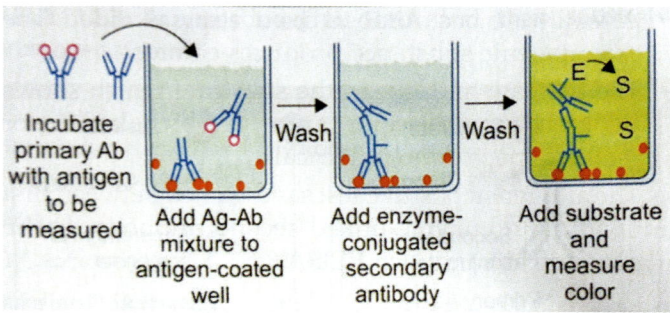

Fig. 15.11: Competitive ELISA for detection of antigen

which are fixed. High concentration of antigen in serum generates less color.

- Antibody is first inoculated in a solution with sample containing antigen.
- The antigen–antibody mixture formed is added to an antigen coated microtitre well.
- The more antigen present in the sample, less free antibody will be available to bind to antigen coated wells.
- Addition of enzyme conjugated second antibody specific for isotype of primary antibody is used to determine amount of primary antibody bound to well. Higher the concentration of antigen in original sample, the lower is the absorbance.
- Normally it is used for detection of hepten.

Other modifications of ELISA as **capture ELISA** are more specific.

Cylinder or Cassette ELISA

One or few samples can be tested at a time. Each specimen is added to disposable cassette. The advantages of this type of ELISA are—the test is rapid (10–15 minutes), no need of ELISA washer or reader which are otherwise required in ELISA and results are visible with naked eye making the test simple.

Uses of ELISA

Viral Infections

- Detection of antibodies against *Herpes simplex virus*.
- Detection of specific IgM antibodies for diagnosis of congenital cytomegalovirus infection.
- Detection of specific antibodies against *E-B virus*.
- Detection of antibodies against mumps.
- Detection IgM specific antibody against measles.
- Detection of hepatitis D antibodies.
- Detection of p24 antigen in window period.
- Detection of hepatitis B surface antigen.
- Detection of HBS antibodies in *HBV*.
- Detection of HCV antibodies. Detection of IgM antibodies against hepatitis A virus.

EIAs can be used for detection of hormones, HCG and toxin.

Bacterial Infections

- Detection of antibodies against *Chlamydia trachomatis*
- Diagnosis of Lyme disease by antibody detection
- To detect antibodies to *Yersinia pestis*
- Detection of genus specific antibodies of *Leptospira*
- To detect virulence marker antigens of *Shigella* in stool sample (VMA)
- Detection of antibodies against *Rickettsia*
- To detect antibodies against pneumococci
- Detection of *Chlamydia* antigen in corneal scrapings
- To detect antibodies against gonococci
- Detection of antibodies against Mycoplasma
- Detection of antibodies against anthrax bacillus
- Detection of *Salmonella* antigen in first week of fever
- Detection of *Bordetella* antibodies
- Detection of antibodies against *Brucella*
- Detection of antibodies against *Treponema pallidum*

RADIOALLERGOSORBENT TEST (RAST)

This test measures antigen specific IgE in a radio-immunoassay where the legend is a labeled anti-IgE Ab. It is identical to standard RIA except, antigen (allergen) is covalently bound to a cellulose disk rather than non-covalently to a radiolabeled plate.

Dipstick Comb Immunoassays to Detect Antigen

A plastic comb is used for testing 6 samples and controls, also comb can be cut into pieces to detect few samples. (Each specimen required one comb.) The specific antibody is fixed to one end of comb which is dipped in specimen. If specific antigen is present in specimen, it is captured. After washing, the comb is dipped in colloidal gold antibody conjugate, which binds to antigen–antibody complex. After washing, a pink dot is produced. Based on same principle, tests for antibodies are also available.

NEUTRALIZATION TESTS: VIRAL NEUTRALIZATION TESTS

Neutralization of animal viruses can be demonstrated in **three systems—animals, egg and tissue cultures.**

Plaque Inhibition Assay

Neutralization of bacteriophages can be demonstrated by **plaque inhibition test.** Bacteriophages are viruses which live on specific bacteria and produce visible pocks by lysis of bacteria. A lawn culture of bacterium is performed. On this, bacteriophages is applied. Patient's serum is added. If serum contains antibodies

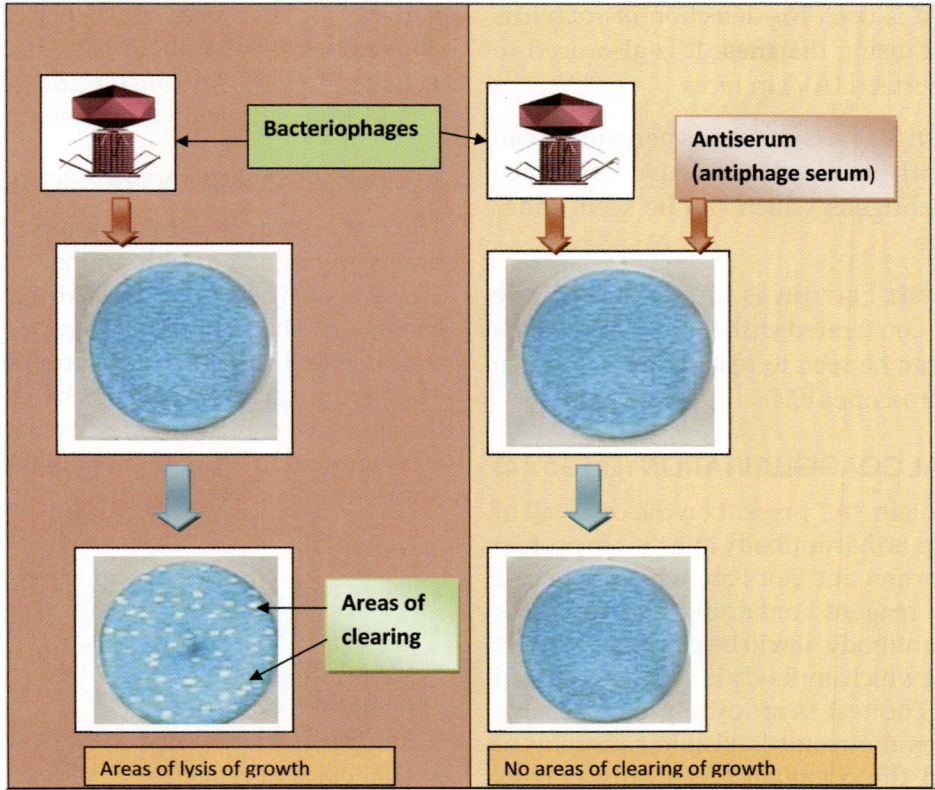

Fig. 15.12: Viral neutralization tests

against viruses plaque formation is inhibited plaque formation by neutralization of viruses (i.e. bacteriophages) (Fig. 15.12).

Toxin Neutralization Tests

Bacterial toxins are good antigens and induce formation of antibodies (antitoxins). **Toxin neutralization** can be tested *in vivo* and *in vitro*.

Tests in animals consist of injecting it with toxin-antitoxin mixtures and estimating least amount of antitoxin that prevents death or disease in the animals. For diphtheria toxin, toxin neutralization tests can be done by rabbit skin test.

Schick test is based on the ability of circulating antitoxin to neutralize diphtheria toxin given intradermally, and indicates immunity or susceptibility to the disease. 0.2 mL diphtheria toxin (1/50 MLD) injected intradermally in man, no reaction will be seen at the site of injection, if person contains circulating antitoxin. *In vitro* test depends on the inhibition of some demonstrable toxic effect.

Neutralization in vitro
- *Agar gel precipitation test*: Detects production of toxin by *C. diphtheriae*.
- *Nagler reaction*: *Cl. welchii* toxin neutralized by antitoxin when organism is grown in serum or egg yolk medium containing antitoxin (Fig. 15.13). When

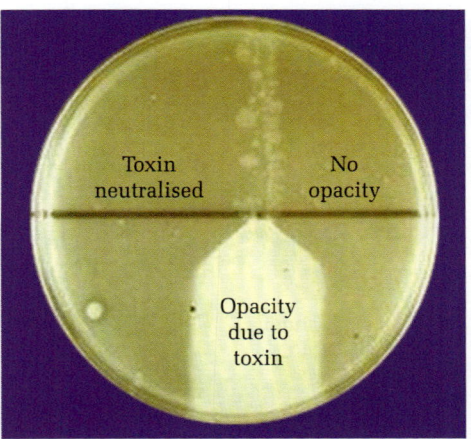

Fig. 15.13: Nagler's reaction (toxin neutralization)

organism is grown on medium, it produces toxin, which in turn produces opacity. If antitoxin is applied on half of medium, there will be no opacity on that half of medium.
- Anti-streptolysin 'O' test, in which antitoxin in the patient's sera neutralizes the hemolytic activity of the streptococcal 'O'.

Immunoelectron microscopy: When viral particles are mixed with specific antisera and the preparation is observed under the electron microscope, they are seen to be clumped. IEM is used for detection of rotavirus and other viruses causing diarrhea. It is also used to detect hepatitis A virus (HAV) in feces.

Immunoenzyme test: Stable enzymes as peroxidase can be conjugated with antibody and used to trace intracellular viral antigens which can be seen under electron microscope.

Immunoferritin test: Ferritin is an electron-dense substance. It can be conjugated with antibody and such labeled conjugate can be seen to react with an antigen under electron microscope (EM).

STAPHYLOCOCCAL COAGGLUTINATION (Fig. 15.14)

The property of protein "A" present on the cell wall of *Staphylococcus aureus* is that antibody attaches to protein 'A' through 'Fc' portion and not Fab, which is free. If serum is added to reagent containing *Staphylococcus aureus* coated with antibody, it will be possible to detect the antigen (against which antibody is already attached to the organism). The test is an example of passive agglutination test as the result is visible clumping of staphylococci and the *Staphylococcus* only carries antibody for the detection of its antigen and does not take part in the reaction.

Uses of Tests

• Test is used to detect antibody coated bacteria in urine, in case of upper urinary tract infection.

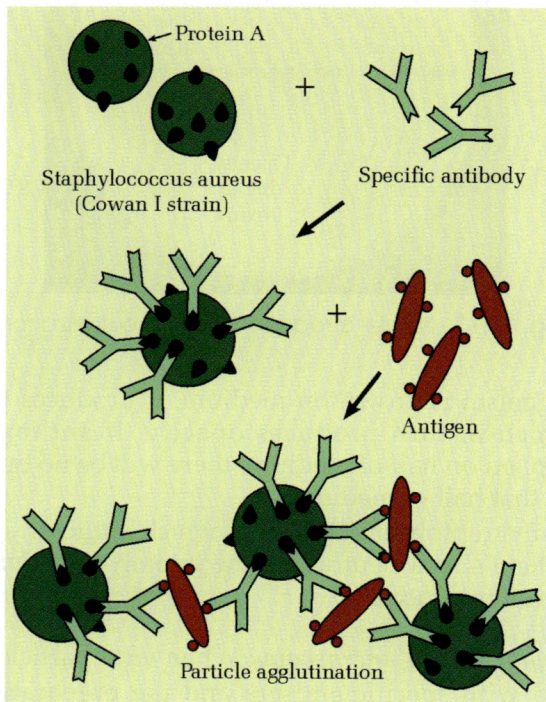

Fig. 15.14: Staphylococcus coagglutination test

• It can be also used to detect capsular antigen of pneumococci, meningococci, *Haemophilus* in CSF.
• Detection of *Salmonella* antigen in 1st week of infection is done by this method.

IMMUNOCHROMATOGRAPHIC TESTS (Fig. 15.15)

The test system is a small cassette containing a membrane impregnated with antibody against hepatitis B Surface antigen (anti-HBsAb) colloidal gold dye conjugate. The membrane is exposed at windows on the cassette. The test serum is dropped into the window. The serum travels upstream by capillary action and formation of control and test bands are observed. The adavantages of this test are simplicity, reliability, economy.

Uses

• Diagnosis of *malaria*
• Diagnosis of *HIV*
• Diagnosis of *hepatitis B virus*
• Diagnosis of *dengue*
• Diagnosis of *leptospira*
• Diagnosis of *rotavirus*

COMPLEMENT FIXATION TEST (Fig. 15.16)

When an antigen combines with antibody, antigen—antibody complex is formed. These complexes have the ability to 'fix' complement and this property is used in this test.

Procedure

In the first step, known antigen is taken (against which antibodies are suspected in patient's serum), serum is added in presence of complement. If antibodies are present in patient's serum, they will form antigen–antibody complexes which will fix complement. Hence complement is utilized in the first step. Complement is

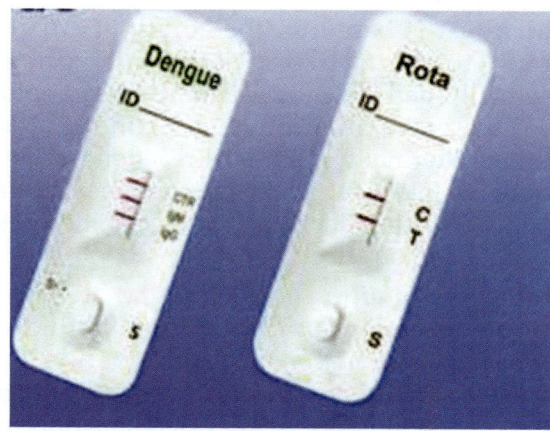

Fig. 15.15: Immunochromatography

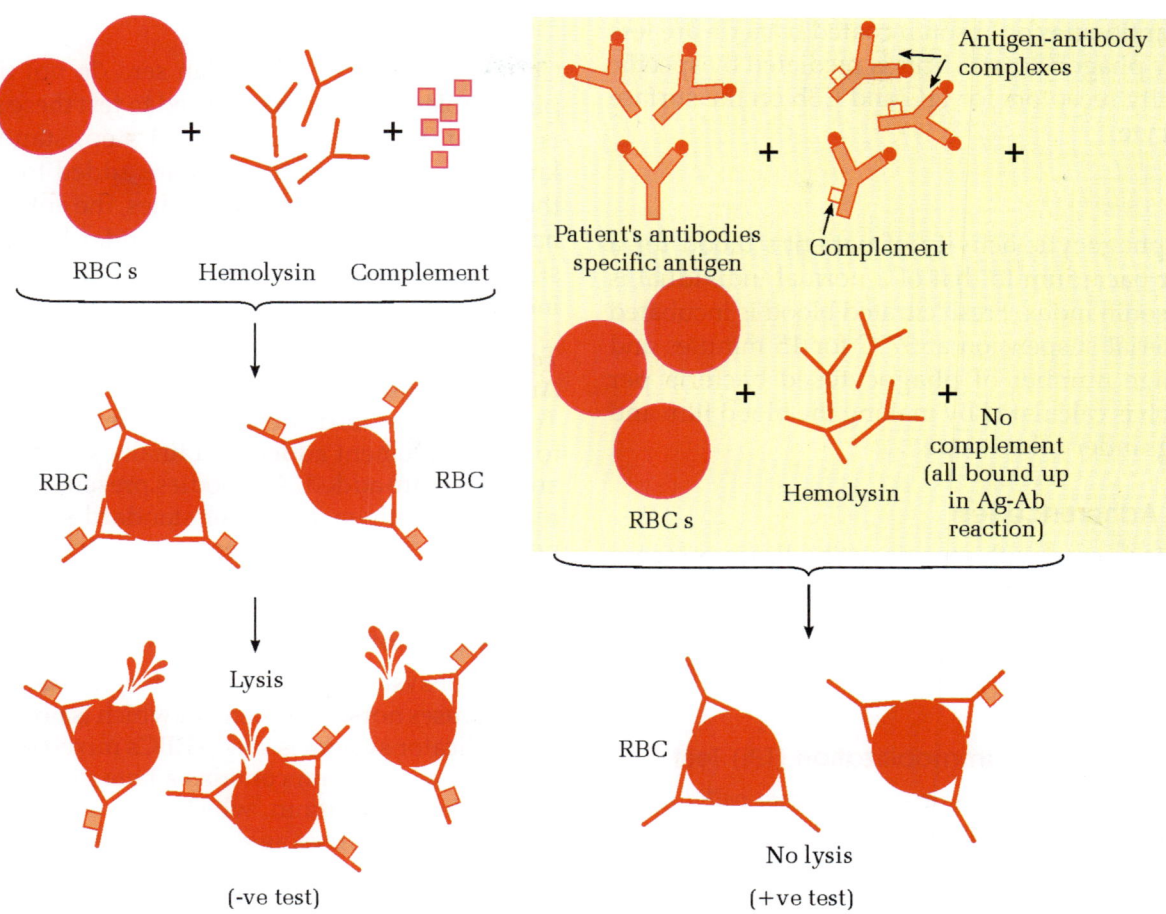

Fig. 15.16: Complement fixation test

not available in the second step, in which another antigen and antibody system in the form of RBCs and antibody against RBCs called **'amboceptor'** is added. This acts as **indicator system,** because if complement is present in second step (if not utilized in first step); in presence of complement, there is lysis RBCs. Thus positive test, i.e. presence of antibodies in patients serum means there will be no hemolysis at the end of second step.

1. Antigen + Antibody (Patient's serum in which antibodies are suspected) + complement: Complement fixed
2. (Step 1) + Hemolytic system → No hemolysis (Positive test)

Antigen + no antibodies + complement → complement not fixed + Hemolytic system → Hemolysis (**Negative test).**

- The antigen may be soluble or particulate. The antiserum should be heated at 56°C for 30 minutes to destroy complement activity of patient's serum and to remove nonspecific inhibitors of complement present in some sera.
- This test detects as little as 0.04 mg of antibody nitrogen and 0.1 mg of antigen.

It has two steps with five reagents, i.e. antigen, antibodies, complement, sheep erythrocytes and amboceptor (rabbit Abs to sheep RBC), each reagent standardized separately. Guinea pig serum freshly drawn or preserved in lyophilized or freeze dried state or with special preservatives (Richardsons's method). It acts as a source of complement as it contains all complement components.

Uses of CFT

Diagnosis of arboviruses, CMV, herpes zoster, leptospirosis, wassermain reaction for syphilis and diagnosis of *Chlamydia.*

Other Comple ment Dependent Serological Tests

Opsonization

It is a process by which a particulate antigen (microbial cell) becomes more susceptible to phagocytosis by combination with opsonin (antibodies-like substance or other component of serum).

There is a synergism between antibodies and complement for opsonization (in complement deficient animals, antibodies or opsonin coated bacteria are less effectively phagocytosed). This is mediated by specific high affinity receptors for IgG and C3b on the surface of phagocyte.

Opsonin Index

Ratio of phagocytic activity of patient's blood for a particular bacterium to that of a normal individual is called opsonin index. Fresh citrated blood is incubated with bacterial suspension at 37°C for 15 minutes and the average number of phagocytosed bacteria per polymorph is calculated by making the blood film and observing under microscope.

Immune Adherence Test

Some bacteria react with specific antibodies in presence of complement and particulate materials such as RBCs, platelets, bacteria are aggregated and adhere to the cells. It is used for 'Treponema pallidum particle agglutination' (TPPA) test.

Treponema Pallidum Immobilization (TPI) Test

Test serum (antibodies against Treponema pallidum) is mixed in presence of complement with live suspension of Treponema pallidum maintained in laboratory. On incubation, the specific antitreponemal antibodies inhibit the motility of the Treponema.

Cytolytic Tests

When bacteria are mixed with its specific antibodies in presence of complement, they are lysed, e.g. vibriocidal antibodies tests for measurement of anticholera antibodies.

Indirect CFT

Certain avian and mammalian sera do not fix guinea pig complement. This test is used to test these sera. Test is set up in duplicate. After 1st step, standard sera known to fix the complement are added to one set. If the test serum contained antibodies, the antigen would have been used up in 1st step. Standard serum added subsequently will not fix complement. Hemolysis indicates positive result.

Test is set up in duplicate antibodies are in 1st step: Antigen, test serum + Complement are added (human). To one set standard anti-serum against antigen known to fix complement added and finally sheep RBCs with antibodies are added. Antibodies present in test serum, react with antigen, hence for standard serum, there is no antigen and complement causes lysis of RBCs in presence of antibodies.

Conglutination Complement Absorption Test

It used for systems which do not fix guinea pig complement. It uses horse complement which is nonhemolytic. The indicator system is sheep RBCs mixed with bovine serum. Bovine serum contains a beta globulin component called conglutinin, which acts as an antibody to complement. It causes agglutination of sensitized sheep RBCs **(conglutination),** if they have combined with complement. If horse complement has been used up by antigen–antibody reaction in the 1st step, agglutination of sensitized cells will not occur.

FLOW CYTOMETRY (Fig. 15.17)

It performs quantative analysis and separation of cells labeled with fluorescent antibody when they pass a laser beam. Its newer version called FACS, i.e.

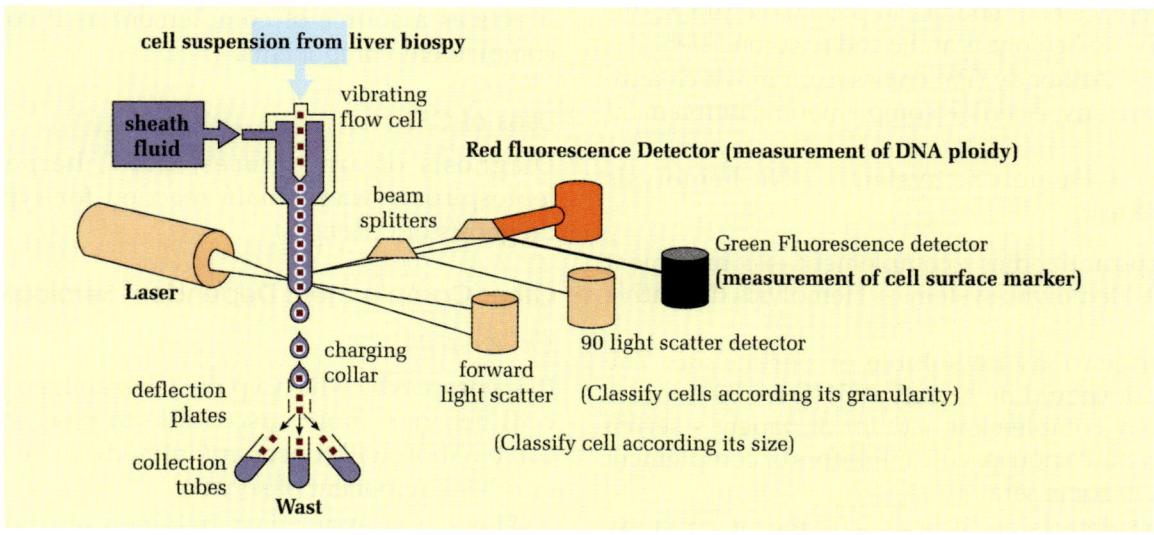

Fig. 15.17: Flow cytometry

fluorescent-activated cell sorter. In this cell labeled with specific antibody and tagged with fluorescent dye is passed through an ultrasonic controlled nozzle. This nozzle generates microdroplets and allows only one cell to go out at a time. The cells from nozzle pass through a beam of laser which excites the fluorescent dye resulting in emission of a light of specific wavelengths.

During this flow, following things happen:
a. Laser beam is deflected each time the cell crosses.
b. A fluorescent light is emitted.

Both the events are recorded by computer which generates a graph of data indicating the number of cells at Y axis and fluorescence emitted by them on X axis.

Using electromagnetic field, the outflowing cells are collected into separate containers. This device does two things:
1. Analysis—detecting cells which are emitting fluorescence.
2. Collecting cells separately:
   • The instrument is capable of sorting cell population into different containers depending on their fluorescence profile. This is called as **cell sorting.**
   • Each cell is measured by size (forward light scatter) and granularity (90° light scanner) as well as for red and green fluorescence, to detect two different surface markers. A three-dimensional plate shows a whole lymphocyte population and CD8 population obtained by cell sorting stained with anti-CD 8.
   • *Uses:* This test is used in HIV patients to find out CD4 count, CD8 count, CD4/CD8 ratio—these values are used to monitor the antiretroviral therapy. This test can also be used for the diagnosis and treatment of cancers.

Chemiluminescence

During antigen–antibody reaction, a light is produced from a substance used in the system which generates energy. It is automated method and measures light and quantifies antibody.

The versions of ELISA using chemiluminescence uses luxogenic substance (light generating substance) as substrate. Oxidation of compound lumonol by H_2O_2 and horseradish peroxide produces light. The light generated during luxogenic reactions may be determined by its ability to expose photographic film. Quantitative measurement of light emission is made by luminometer.

RADIOIMMUNOASSAY (Fig. 15.18a and b)

It is competitive assay. Fixed amount of antibodies and radiolabeled antigen are mixed with test antigen, both antigens compete for binding sites on antibodies. The level of test antigen (called analyte or ligand) is determined. After the reaction, the antigen is separated into free and bound fractions and radioactivity is measured. Concentration of test antigen can be calculated from the ratio of bound and total antigen lebels, using a standard dose response curve. The **standard dose response curve (calibrating curve)** is obtained by running the reaction with fixed amounts of antibody and labeled antigen, and varying known

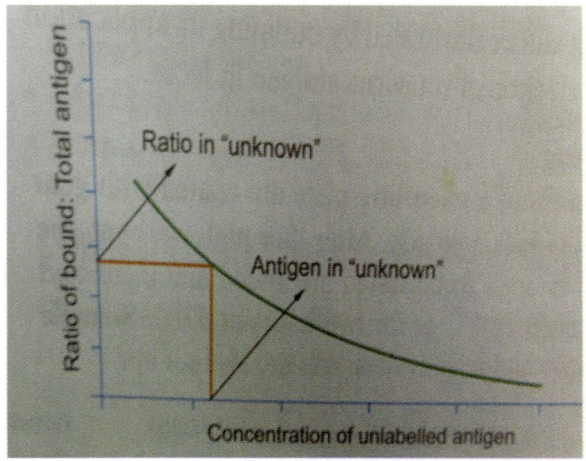

Fig. 15.18a: Radioimmunoassay—standard curve

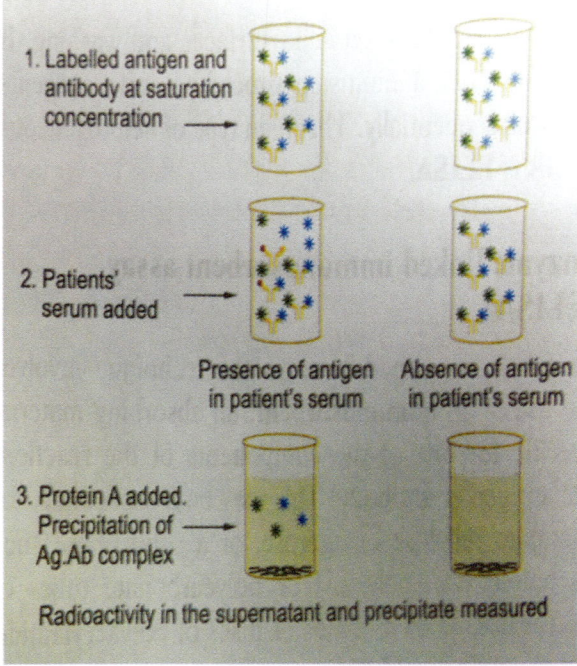

Fig. 15.18b: Radioimmunoassay procedure

amounts of unlabeled antigen. The ratios of bound: total labels (B:T ratio) plotted against analyte concentrations give the standard response curve. Quantitation of test antigen is done from B:T ratio of the test by interpolation from standard curve. RIA is rarely used in microbiology. It is used for quantitation of hormones as insulin and drugs.

ELISPOT TEST

It is a modification of ELISA which detects and quantifies cells producing antibodies (plasma cells) or cytokines.

Microtitre well is coated with capture antibody specific for the cytokine.

Cell suspension is added to the wells and incubated. Sensitized cells capable of producing cytokines attach to wells.

The cytokines released are bound by capture antibodies in the vicinity of secreting cells with production of a ring of antigen–antibody complexes around each cell that is producing the cytokine of interest.

After washing, an enzyme labeled anticytokine antibody is added.

After washing, a chromogenic substance is added. The colored product precipitates and forms a spot only on the area of well where cytokine secreting cells are deposited.

The number of colored spots represents the number of cytokine producing cells present in added suspension.

16

Complement

COMPLEMENT SYSTEM

The complement system consists of a tightly regulated network of proteins that play an important role in host defense and inflammation. Complement activation results in opsonization of pathogens and their removal by phagocytes, as well as cell lysis.

Introduction

Complement was first discovered in the 1890s when it was found to aid or "complement" the killing of bacteria by heat-stable antibodies present in normal serum.

Pfeiffer observed that cholera vibrios were lysed when injected intraperitoneally into specifically immunized guinea pigs (**bacteriolysis** *in vivo*). It was called '**Pfeiffer phenomenon'**.

Research on complement began when Jules Bordet at the Institute Pasteur in Paris showed sheep antiserum to the bacterium *Vibrio cholerae* caused lysis of the bacteria and that heating the antiserum destroyed its bacteriolytic activity. Surprisingly, the ability to lyse the bacteria was restored to the heated serum by adding fresh serum that contained no antibodies directed against the bacterium and was unable to kill the bacterium by itself. Bordet correctly identified that bacteriolytic activity requires two different substances; first, the specific antibacterial antibodies, which survive the heating process, and a second, heat-sensitive component called '**alexine'** responsible for the lytic activity.

- Bordet devised a simple test for the lytic activity, the easily detected lysis of antibody-coated red blood cells, called hemolysis.
- Paul Ehrlich in Berlin independently carried out similar experiments and coined the term complement, defining it as **"the activity of blood serum that completes the action of antibody."** In ensuing years,

it was discovered that the action of complement was the result of interactions of a large and complex group of proteins.

- The complement system consists of more than 30 proteins that are either present as soluble proteins in the blood or are present as membrane associated proteins.

Not only is complement involved in immunity but is also involved in tissue regeneration, tumor growth and human pathological states such as atypical hemolytic uremic syndrome, age-related macular degeneration, etc.

Properties of the Complement

- The proteins of complement system are present in normal sera.
- Once the complement system is stimulated, it acts like clotting systems.
- The system constitutes a group of biological effector mechanisms including fibrinolytic system and kinin system.
- Amplification of these actions occurs at each stage because each enzyme activates many succeeding components. Also each step has own control mechanism so that exaggerated response will not occur.
- Complement proteins constitute 5% of total serum proteins which include at least 20 different proteins.
- Complement as a whole is heat labile though some of the individual factors if separated and tested may appear resistant. The serum is deprived of its complement activity by heating at 56°C for half hour in water bath.
- Complement is not stimulated in presence of antigen or antibody alone but when antigen combines with its antibody, the immune complex is formed and it has the ability to stimulate the complement system.

- Complement system is a system of **soluble factors** in normal serum which are activated by antigen–antibody interactions and once stimulated they **'complement'** the other immune responses hence the name.
- This system is one of the major evolved defence systems to eliminate the pathogens.
- Complement system is central to development of inflammatory reaction.
- **Amplification** of these actions occurs at each stage because each enzyme activates many succeeding components. Also each step has **own control mechanism** so that exaggerated response will not occur.
- Initially, it was thought that, once the complement system gets activated it takes part in **innate immunity** (nonspecific immunity).
- The **classical pathway** links **adaptive immune system** through antibodies as antigen–antibody complex stimulates **classical system**. The **alternate pathway** is independent of antibody, gives **innate immunity**.
- The **lectin pathway** is most recently described which is also **antibody independent**. All three pathways share few things as:
  1. **Involve activation of C3** which is most abundant and most important complement protein.
  2. Once stimulated this system acts in **'cascade' manner (proteolytic cascade)** and mediates important consequences which are important in immune responses.
  3. The complement system **mediates biological effector** functions and interacts with other complex systems like blood clotting system and adaptive (acquired) immune responses. The complement system **complements or completes the action of antibodies.**
- Complement system is central to development of inflammatory reaction.
- It forms one of the major evolved defense systems of body.
- The lectin pathway is most recently described, it also bypasses antibody for its activation.
- Systems comprise a **proteolytic cascade** in which complexes of complement proteins create enzymes which breakdown complement proteins in some order to create new enzymes, thereby amplifying activation cascade.
- All pathways **converge terminally** causing membrane damage and lytic killing of pathogens.

- The immune defense and pathological effects of complement activation are mediated by fragments and complexes generated during activation which are:
  1. The small chemotactic and **proinflammatory fragments C3a, C5a;**
  2. The large opsonic fragments C3b, C4b and **lytic membrane attack complex**.
- The site of complement is present in Fc part of immunoglobulin and it is expressed only when antigen–antibody complex is formed.

Surface Binding is Key

- **IgM is the most efficient activator**. A transition occurs when IgM binds to surface of bacterium which allows complement activation. **The molecule is converted to a form which exposes its binding sites for C1.**
- The first component of complement pathway is **C1 consists of** a large, **6 headed recognition unit termed C1q and two molecules each of C1r and C1s, the enzymatic** units of the complex. The assembly of complex is dependent on calcium.
- The activation occurs only if several of the head groups of C1q are bound to antibody.
- C1q in the complex binds through its globular head groups to Fc regions of immobilized antibody and undergoes changes in shape which triggers auto-catalytic activation of C1r, activated C1r activates C1s.
- Since C1 activation occurs only when several of the six head groups of C1q bound to antibody, only surfaces that are densely coated with antibody will trigger the process. This limitation reduces the risk of inappropriate activation on host tissue.

Components of Complement System

The proteins of complement system include complement components, properdin system and control proteins. The complement component is made of factors from C1 to C9 of which C1 is not a single factor but complex of C1q, C1r, C1s making 11 proteins. Other complement proteins include components of alternative pathway and regulatory proteins.

COMPLEMENT PATHWAYS

Complement activation is known to occur through **three different** (complement cascade) **pathways: alternate, classical** and lectin involving proteins that mostly exist as inactive zymogens which then sequentially cleaved and activated. **All the pathways converge at C3 which is the most abundant complement protein found in the blood.** Steps are same in all the pathways means stages after C3 activation resulting in the formation of the activation products, C3a, C3b, C5a and the membrane attack complex (C5b-9).

Classical Pathway

- Complement activation by the classical pathway commonly begins with the formation of soluble antigen–antibody complexes (immune complexes) or with the binding of antibody to antigen on a suitable target, such as a bacterial cell.
- IgM and certain subclasses of IgG (human IgG1, IgG2, and IgG3) can activate the classical complement pathway. The initial stage of activation involves C1, C2, C3, and C4, which are present in plasma in functionally inactive forms. Because the components were named in order of their discovery and before their functional roles had been determined, the numbers in their names do not always reflect the order in which they react.
- The formation of an antigen–antibody complex induces conformational changes in the Fc portion of the IgM molecule that expose a binding site for the C1 component of the complement system.
- C1 in serum is a macromolecular complex consisting of C1q and two molecules each of C1r and C1s, held together in a complex (C1qrs) stabilized by Ca^{2+} ions.
- First binding portion of C1 is C1q which is a hexamer with six globular heads, each acts as a binding site. For effective activation, C1q attaches to antibody with at least two of the globular binding sites. As IgM is pentamer, one molecule of it needed to initiate the cycle. Thus IgM stimulates the complement system more efficiently than IgG.
- The activated C1s is esterase enzyme in nature, one molecule of which cleave many molecules of next component, i.e. C4 which is broken down into a larger portion C4a and C4b of which, C4a quits while C4b remains attached to the membrane, means, it is in the cascade.
- C1, 4b in presence of Mg breaks C2 into C2a and C2b of which C2a remains with C1, 4b forming C1, 4b, 2a which has enzymatic action and it is the C3 convertase in the classical pathway. The C2b is released into the medium.
- C3 convertase splits C3 into C3a and C3b, C3b is anaphylatoxin and leaves the cycle while the C3a forms complex with C1q, 4b, 2a and the result is formation of 'C1, 4b, 2a, 3b' which has enzymatic action and it is the C5 converter.
- The C5 converter (C1, 4b, 2a, 3b) breaks C5 into C5a which is also anaphylatoxin and quits while C5b joins the cascade.

- After this C6, C7 join together and there is formation of trimolecular complex C5–C7, part of which binds to the cell membrane of organism or in this model, it binds to the RBC and the complex prepares cell membrane for the lysis by C8 and C9 which join subsequently.
- Most C5–C7 quit and bind to the nearby cell, i.e. bystander cell which was not in picture previously and it was not sensitized with the antigen–antibody complex rendering them to susceptible to the lysis by C8 and C9. The unbound C5–C7 is chemotactic. Ultimately, the lysis of the cell occurs by production of holes on the cell wall by the complement complex (MAC—membrane attack complex), hence cell lysis and cell death occurs. Other stimuli which may activate the classical pathway are other antigen–antibody complexes, aggregated immunoglobulins and DNA, CRP.

Alternate Complement Pathway (Fig. 16.1)

Alternative pathway by **Properdin system** was first demonstrated by **Pillemer** (1954), the activator of that system was **'zymosan'**, a polysaccharide form of yeast cell wall.

The steps of classical and alternative pathways are same after C3 gets activated. In classical pathway, the C1q, 4b, 2a is the C3 convertase. The activation of C3 without prior activation of C1, 2 and C4 is called alternative pathway.

One example of alternative pathway is properdin system. It can be get activated by bacterial endotoxins, IgA and IgD and cobra venom and nephritic factor 'A' present in patients with glomerulonephritis.

The C3b is continuously produced in the circulation in small quantities in free form which is rapidly cleared by factors H and I. The bound C3b is protected from inactivation and it interacts with serum protein called B factor to form Mg dependent **C3b,B complex.** This complex is again broken down by factor D into Ba, Bb, of which Ba is released in the medium and Bb remains bound to C3 forming **C3b, Bb which has esterase activity.** The enzyme C3b, Bb is extremely labile and the function of properdin system is to stabilize it. This is C3 convertase which activates C3, after that cascade starts.

C3 Covertase of Lectin Pathway (Fig. 16.1)

This pathway is activated by binding of mannose binding lectin (MBL) which is similar to C1q, mannose containing polysaccharides present on cell wall of many bacteria and fungi. It results in activation and complexing of MBL with MBL associated proteases

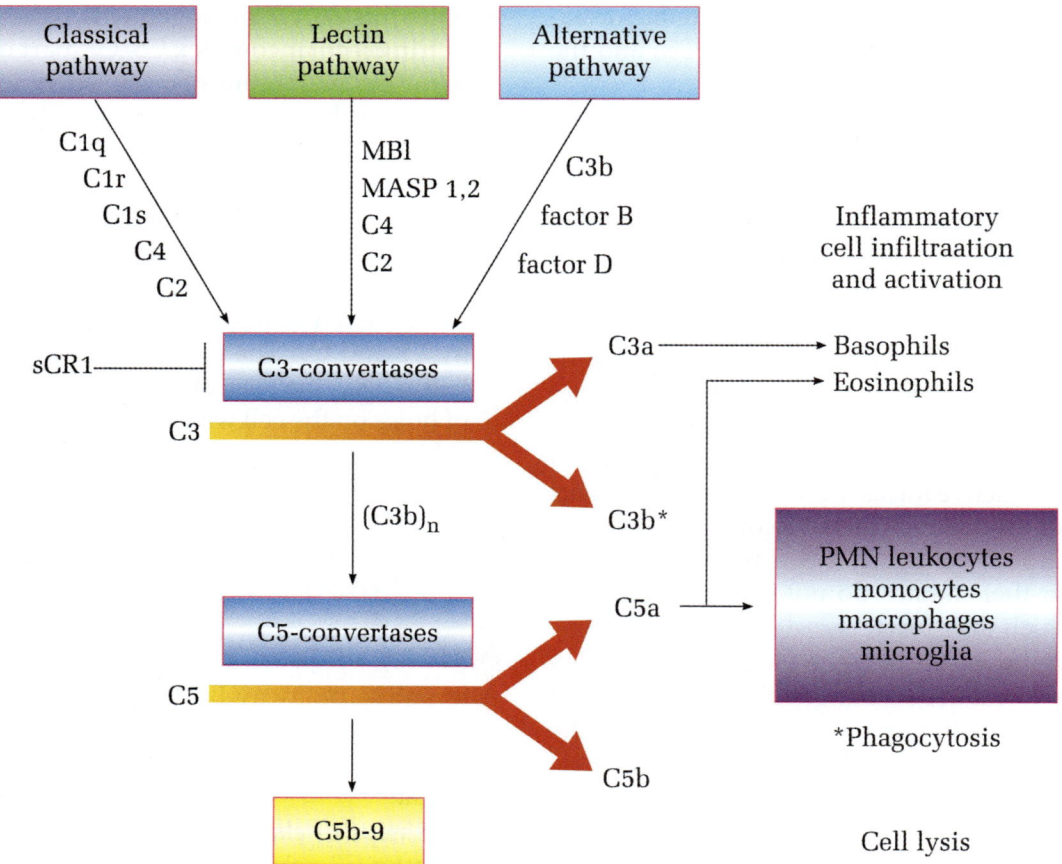

Fig. 16.1: Complement pathology

MASP1 and MASP2 which cleave C4 and C2 to generate C4b2a which is the C3 convertase.

The complement activity in serum is measured by finding out the highest dilution of serum lysing sheep RBCs in presence of its antibody. The other method is radioimmunoassay and ELISA.

Hereditary Angioneurotic Edema

Deficiency of complement C1 inhibitor is associated with hereditary angioneurotic edema. The decrease in C1 inhibitor leads to excessive stimulation of auto-catalytic C1 and the breakdown of C4 and C2 is unchecked specially C2 kinins are released. The patient presents with repeated episodes of angioedema of subcutaneous tissue or mucosa of gastrointestinal or respiratory system. If larynx or trachea is affected, the condition may turn fatal and prophylaxis with epsilon aminocaproic acid is useful. The condition may be treated with infusion of fresh plasma which provides C1 inhinitor (Table 16.1).

SUMMARY OF ACTIONS OF COMPLEMENT ACTIVATION (BIOLOGICAL EFFECTS) (Fig. 16.2)

1. Role in Inflammation and Chemotaxis

- Increase in vascular permeability
- Smooth muscle contraction
- Chemotaxis (C3a, C5a—chemotatic factors).
- Inflammation
- Mast cell degranulation and further increase in inflammation and chemotaxis
- C2 kinins are vasoactive amines and increase the capillary permeability.

TABLE 16.1: Clinical syndromes associated with deficiencies

Group	Deficiency	Syndrome
C1 inhibitors	C1 inhibitors	Hereditary angioneurotic edema
	C1, C2, C4	SLE and other collagen disorders
	C3 and its regulatory protein	Severe recurrent pyogenic infections
	C5 to C8	Bacteremia mainly with Gram-negative diplococci, toxoplasmosis

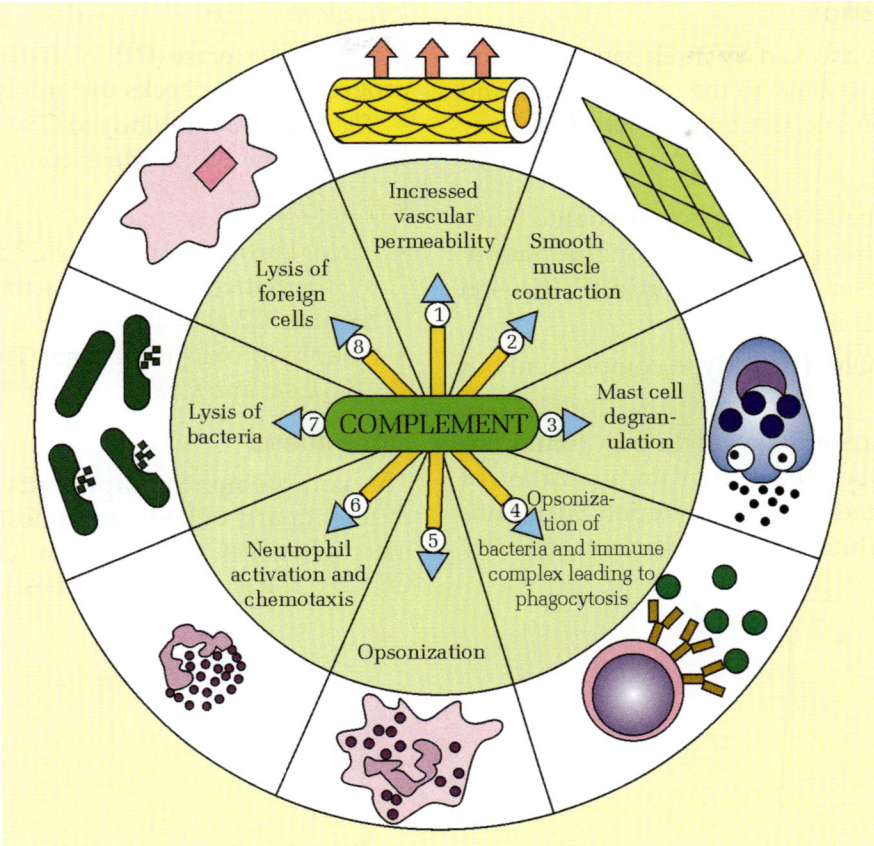

Fig. 16.2: Functions of complement

2. Role of Complement in Defense Mechanisms (Effector Mechanisms)

- It coats microorganisms and makes them susceptible to the phagocytosis **(opsonization)**.
- Lysis of bacteria in protective immune mechanisms. The cells vary in their susceptibility of damage by complement, Gram-negative bacteria are generally sensitive to killing without lysis.
- Complement lyses some organisms themselves.
- Complement activates antimicrobial system of phagocytes.
- Activation of complement produces anaphylatoxins which are chemotactic for polymorphs.
- Activation of complement produces by products which promote inflammatory response.
- Complement also kills enveloped viruses.

3. Role of Complement in Hypersensitivity

- Opsonization of immune complexes.
- Breakdowns of immune complexes is done so that complexes are removed from the circulation and carried to spleen and liver.

- Lysis of RBCs and other cells in type II hypersensitivity leading to hemolytic disease and purpura.
- The complement also plays role in paroxysmal nocturnal hemamoglobinuria and angioneurotic edema.

4. Role of Complement in Other Systems

- During coagulation of blood, the C3 is activated by prothrombin releases platelet activating factor, thus increases the consumption of prothrombin.
- Complement also takes part in coagulation process.

5. Role of Complement in Endotoxic Shock

In endotoxin shock, there is massive C3 fixation and platelets adherence. A large number of platelets lyse and release their contents causing disseminated intravascular coagulation, and thrombocytopenia. Gram-negative septicemia and dengue may have same pathogenesis.

6. Complement in Serological Tests

Complement is important in immune adherence test, complement fixation test, *Treponema pallidum* immobilization, *Treponema pallidum* immune adherence test.

Regulation of Activation

The overactivation is checked by inhibitors which are of two types; inhibitors bind to the complements and prevent further action and inactivators which destroy complements.

Conglutination: If cells (or particles) coated with complement form clumping called 'conglutination' which is due to presence of **'conglutinin' (K)**—an unusual protein in bovine serum.

Conglutinin resembles antibody to complement but actually not.

Antibodies with action like conglutinin **(immunoconglutinin, IK)** can be produced by immunization of animal with complement coated material. Such antibodies may be seen in human beings as an autoantibody to complement.

Inhibitors

Inhibitor of esterase (C1SINH) does not prevent normal progression but checks the autolytic activation.

The 'S' protein: It binds to C5–C7 and modulates the action of membrane attack complex.

Inactivators

- Factor I provides control of C3 activation particularly by alternative pathway. Factor H acts with factor I, regulate C3 activation.
- Anaphylotoxin inhibitors: This protein degrades C3a, C4a, and C5a.

Biosynthesis

The complement components are synthesized in different parts of body, e.g. intestinal epithelium (C1), macrophages (C1, C4), spleen (C5, C8) and liver (C3, C6, C9). The site for C7 synthesis is not known.

17

Structure and Functions of Immune System

IMMUNE APPARATUS (Fig. 17.1)

The immune apparatus consists of:

- **Cells:** The immune system consists of lymph reticular cell like T lymphocyte, B lymphocyte; cells of reticuloendothelial system as macrophages, monocytes; mast cell, basophils, antigen presenting cells, phagocytic cells (apart from macrophages and monocytes) as PMNs, eosinophil. Cells are derived from pluripotent stem cells in bone marrow.
- **Soluble substances** as antibodies, complement, acute phase proteins help in phagocytosis.
- Soluble mediators of immune reactions called **cytokines.**
- Immune cells organized into different organs like primary lymphoid organs, secondary lymphoid organs.

- Natural defense system as epithelial barriers, phagocytes, opsonins.
- **T lymphocytes** further divided into the helper T cell (TH) which helps B cells to produce antibodies, Tc is cytotoxic T lymphocyte which forms cell-mediated immune responses, kill intracellular organisms as TB bacilli and viruses by mechanisms called **cell-mediated immunity** (CMI); they also secrete set of cytokines which control immune responses.
- Monocytes in blood and macrophages in tissues perform the function of taking antigen, processing and presenting to the immune system. These cells also have phagocytic functions.
- **B lymphocyte** forms antibodies which kill organisms by helping phagocyte or stimulating complement system and antibody-dependent cell-mediated

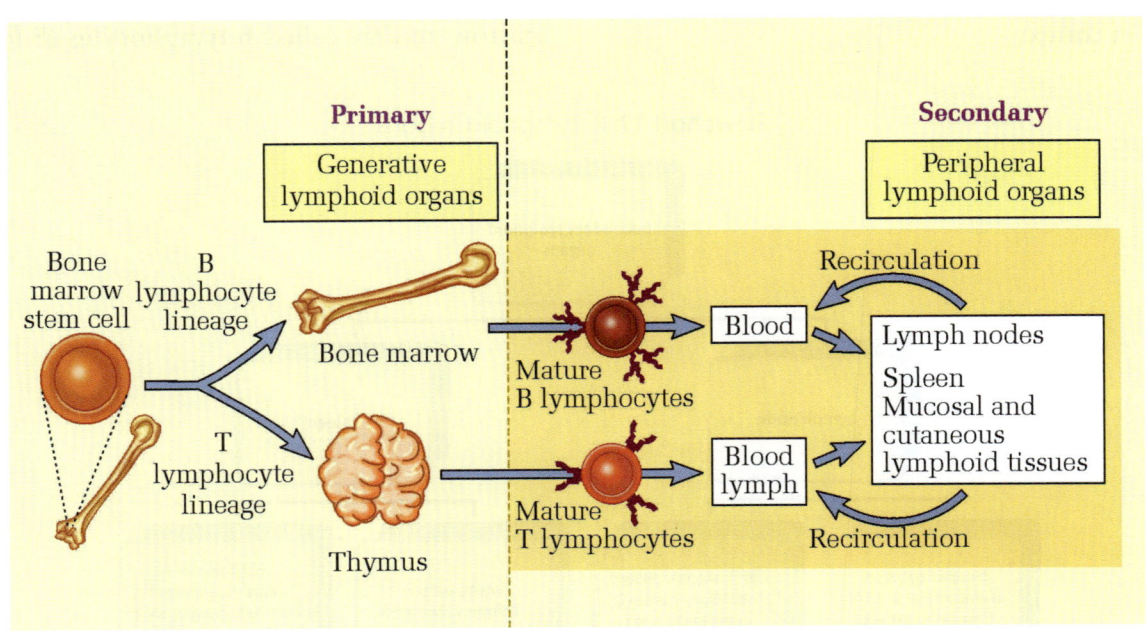

Fig. 17.1: Structure of immune system

cytotoxicity. The mechanisms by which B cells or antibody take part in killing is called antibody-mediated immune (AMI) response.

Hematopoiesis: Cells involved in immune system originate from hematopoietic stem cells.

T and B lymphocytes before coming in contact with antigen are called **'Naïve cells'**.

Thymus and bone marrow where lymphocytes become mature are called **primary lymphoid organs,** while spleen, lymph node and mucosa associated immune system form the secondary lymphoid organs.

LYMPHOID TISSUES AND ORGANS

The lymphoid organs based upon functions are called primary lymphoid organs and secondary lymphoid organs (Flowchart 17.1).

Primary (Central) Lymphoid Organs

These are the organs where precursor lymphocytes proliferate, develop, differentiate, educated and become immunologically competent. It includes thymus and bone marrow, where T lymphocytes mature while fetal liver and bone marrow are the sites where B cells mature.

1. Thymus

It is the first lymphoid organ to develop.

Structure

- It has 2 lobes. It is surrounded by capsule.
- Septa originate from capsule, penetrate the gland.
- Septa divide gland into lobules and further as cortex and medulla. Actively proliferating lymphocytes are present in cortex.

- *Medulla*: It consists of mature lymphocytes; epithelial cells. Hassal's corpuscles are whorl like clumps of epithelial cells.

Functions of thymus

- Production of thymic lymphocyte is the main function of thymus.
- It is major organ in body where lymphocytes proliferate in body.
- It causes differentation of T lymphocytes. The precursor lymphocytes enter thymus, which mature and acquire new antigens (**thymic** antigens) are called T cell (**thymus-dependent cells**). Thus, in this organ, T lymphocyte become trained and become **immunologically competent cells.**
- Cells capable of mounting immune responses against self antigens are destroyed (Clonal delection). Small proportion of T cell become memory cells.

Clinical significance

- **Deficient CMI** seen in congenital aplasia of thymus (**DiGeorge syndrome**) and in 'nude mice'.
- **Runt disease:** Deficient CMI is seen in lymphopenia, 'Runt disease' seen in neonatally athymectomized mice.
- **Post-thymectomy:** T cell-dependent areas of lymph node and spleen get depleted in thymectomized neonate. It also affects immune response to thymus-dependent antigens, response to other antigens is normal.

2. Bone Marrow

Some lymphoid cells develop and mature in bone marrow and are called **B lymphocytes** (B for bursa of

Flowchart 17.1: Lymphoid organs

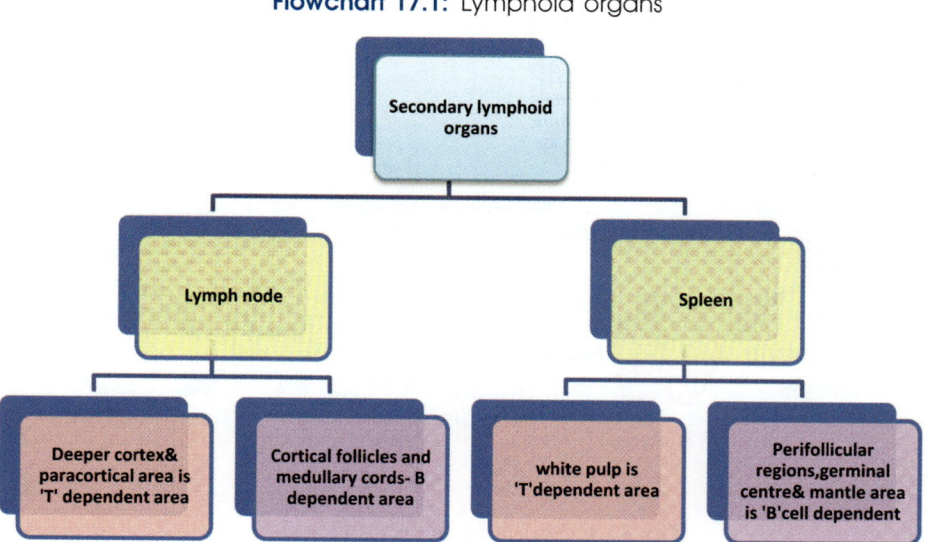

Fabricius in birds and bone marrow in humans). **Bone marrow** is also the site of proliferations of stem cells and the **origin of pre B cells** which mature to become B lymphocytes.

Immature B cells proliferate and differentiate in bone marrow. Stromal cells secrete cytokines required for the development of B cell. B cells develop their immuno-globulin receptors by DNA rearrangements. Before leaving, B cells acquire IgM on the surface. B cells are transformed into plasma cells, capable of producing antibodies.

Secondary or Peripheral Lymphoid Organs

These organs act as the sites of interaction of mature lymphocytes with antigen.

a. Lymph Node

Structure of lymph node
- It is divided into outer cortex and inner medulla.
- **Cortex:** It contains lymphoid cells which form primary lymphoid follicles.
- **Germinal centers (secondary follicles)** develop inside primary follicles after antigenic stimulus. Dendritic macrophages which act as antigen presenting cells are also present in follicles.
- **Medulla:** Lymphocytes, plasma cells, macrophages are arranged as branching bands called **medullary cords.**
- Between cortical follicles and medullary cords, there is intermediate zone made of lymphocytes and interdigitating cells which form the **paracortical area.**

The T lymphocytes are found predominantly in deeper cortex or paracortical area called **T cell-dependent area**. The cortical follicles and medullary cords are **B dependent** area. Lymph node acts as a filter for lymph. It phagocytoses foreign particles including microorganisms. It also acts as the site for proliferation of T and B cells (Fig. 17.2a).

b. Spleen

It acts as a filter for trapping circulating blood-borne particles. It is also major site of antibody synthesis. The external lymphoid area consisting of perifollicular region, germinal center and mantle layer is the **B dependent area** while the **white pulp is T dependent area** (Fig. 17.2b).

Clinical significance: Spleen traps antigens; it acts as a site where effective opsonization takes place. Hence, splenectomy makes the individual susceptible to bacterial infections (**sepsis** or **septicemia**) as *Streptococcus pneumoniae, Haemophilus influenzae*. Therefore, vaccines are indicated before splenectomy.

Marginal zone B cells are thought to protect against **polysaccharide antigens**. They respond to **T independent antigen** and they form main protective response against polysaccharide antigens.

They also produce '**natural antibodies**'.

Together with B1 cells, they are called '**innate-like B cells**'.

c. Mucosa Associated Lymphoid Tissue (MALT) (Local Immunity)

Lymphocytes producing local IgA are present throughout the mucosal lining of GIT, respiratory, and GUT. The lymphoid follicles lining the gut are called **gut associated lymphoid tissue** while the lymphoid tissue lining respiratory tract is called '**bronchus associated lymphoid tissue**' (**BALT**). The '**GALT**'

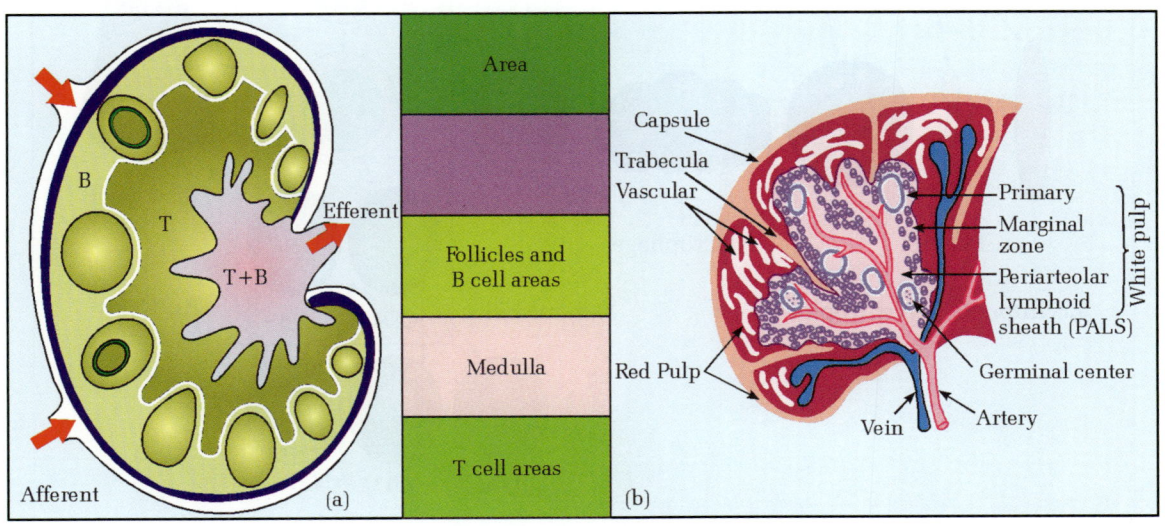

Fig. 17.2: (a) Lymph node, (b) spleen

consists of tonsils, appendix, and Payer's patches of intestine and lamina propria of intestine, while the **'MALT'** consists of mixture of B cells, T cells, and phagocytic cells. 'MALT' gives local immunity mainly by producing locally IgA.

MALT in intestinal mucosa

MALT is composed of different layers.

- Submucosa consists of **Payer's patches;** each is a nodule of lymphoid follicles.
- **Lamina propria** has collection of lymphocytes and macrophages.
- Epithelial layer has specialized lymphocytes and 'M' (modified epithelial cells) cells.
- **Intraepithelial lymphocytes (IELs)** are the γδ T cells which may encounter the antigen (deal with lipid antigen).
- **'M' cells:** These are specialized epithelial cells with deep invaginations of pockets in basolateral side that contains B cells, T cells, and macrophages.
- Enteric pathogens, as *Salmonella, Shigella* enter through 'M' cells. M cells pick up the pathogens by endocytosis, transport in vesicle. They deliver antigen to the basolateral pockets where appropriate cells are stimulated.
- Secretory IgA forms a mucosal paste, prevents entry of pathogens.

LOCAL IMMUNITY

An infection which is localized and which can be controlled by blocking the entry of pathogen is known as 'local immunity'. For example, oral polio vaccine produces local IgA mediated mucosal immunity (small quantities of other immunoglobulins are also produced).

Cells involved in Immunity (Fig. 17.3)

Most of the cells of immune system originate from **hematopoietic stem cells** in fetal liver and in postnatal bone marrow (mainly in vertebral column, sternum, ribs, femur and tibia).

The cells belong to different categories, it is heterogeneous collection to perform various functions as:

1. Phagocytosis
2. Antigen presentation

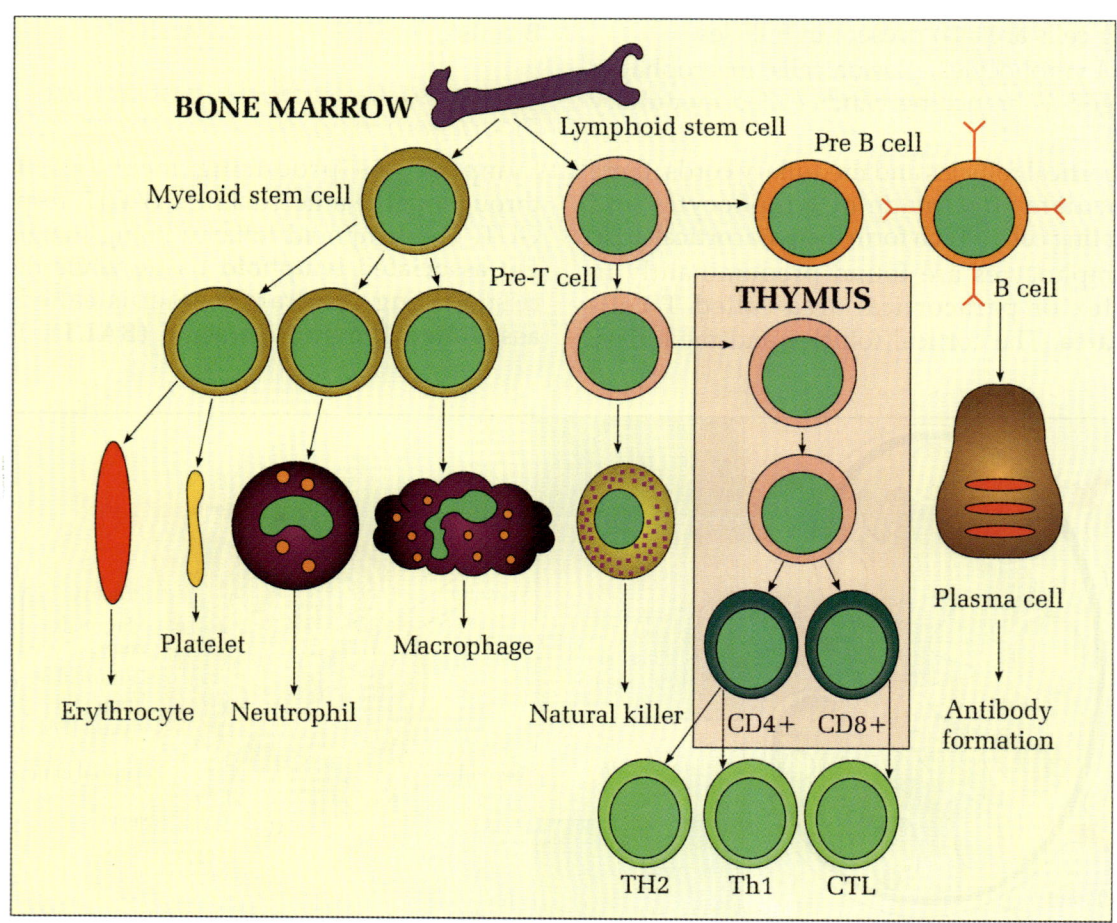

Fig. 17.3: Cells of immune system

3. Lysis of virally infected cells secretion of specific antibodies which kill microorganisms by various methods as complement-mediated lysis, help in **cytotoxicity (ADCC)** or **neutralization.**

Cells can divided into three functional categories (Flowchart 17.2 and Fig. 17.3):

   I. Cells which produce innate immunity

  II. Cells which produce acquired immune responses.

 III. One separate function group of cells is **antigen presenting cells (APCs)** which **link** innate and adaptive immune responses. These cells take up antigens, process it so that antigen is recognized by T cells. They produce cytokines. APC enhance innate immune cells function. They are also important in activation of T cells.

- These functional groups of cells work together

- Though innate and acquired immune responses are different, they may be produced by common cells, e.g. monocytes and macrophages whose main function is phagocytosis but they also act as antigen presenting cells.

- Innate system represents an ancient defense mechanism which recognized conserved patterns, characteristics of a variety of pathogens, and it forms firstline of defense. Microorganisms have **pathogen associated molecular pattern (PAMP)** which are recognized by **pattern reorganization receptors (PRRs) of innate system.**

Cells of innate system include:

- Monocyte/macrophage
- Polymorphonuclear granulocytes

Flowchart 17.2: Cells of immune system

FUNCTIONS OF IMMUNE CELLS

neutrophil
- phagocytosis

eosinophil
- it has basic membrane protein which can act on worms, hence it takes part in immunity against helminths

basophil& mast cells
- take part in type I hypersensitivity

monocyte(in blood)
macrophage in tissue
- phagocytosis
  it also takes part in antigen taking , processing

lymphocyte
- T LYMPHOCYTE
  - Th
    helper cell which stimulates B cell to form antibodies & Tc cell which form CMI AGAINST virus infected cells
  - Tc cell forms CMI
- b LYMPHOCYTE

- NK cells
- Mast cells
- Platelets

ADAPTIVE IMMUNE RESPONSE

Adaptive immune response is more recently evolved.

Adaptive immune system cells are lymphocytes—T lymphocytes which recognize antigen through highly specific T cell receptors (TCR) and B lymphocytes which produce antibodies (recognize antigen through surface immunoglobulins).

As cells of immune system develop, they acquire functional molecules which are important for their function. These specific functional molecules are known as **'lineage markers'**, as they identify **cell lineage**, for example:

1. *Myeloid cells*—monocytes and polymorphs
2. *Lymphoid cells*—T and B cells.

Myeloid Cells

Phagocytes belong to two cell lineages:
     I. Mononuclear phagocytes—**monocytes or macrophages**
     II. Polymorphonuclear granulocytes (PMNs)

I. Mononuclear Phagocytes

Mononuclear phagocytes consist of circulating cells in **blood (monocytes)** and **macrophages (tissue macrophages)** that differentiate from monocytes and live in **various organs** (spleen, liver, kidney, lungs where they show distinct morphology).

Blood Monocytes

Myeloid progenitor in bone marrow differentiate into **pro-monocytes** and then into **circulating monocytes**. Monocytes and polymorphs develop from **common precursor cell**, the **CFU-granulocyte macrophage cells (CFU-GMs).**

- **Myelopoiesis** (development of myeloid cells) starts in bone marrow of fetus at about 6 weeks of gestations. They mature under influence of colony-stimulating factors (CSFs) and other cytokines.
- Monocytes develop from CFU-granulocyte macrophages (CFU-GMs) cells.
- These cells initially give rise to proliferating monoblasts.
- Monoblasts further develop into promonocytes and finally into mature monocytes which serve as replacement pool for tissue macrophages.
- Common precursor of monocyte, neutrophils express MHC class II molecules, but only monocytes continue to express it in significant amount. Monocytes can present antigen to T cells but neutrophils cannot.

Monocytes
- Large 8–10 μ
- They have horseshoe nucleus.
- They contain primary azurophilic (blue staining) granules.
- They possess muffled membranes, Golgi complex and intracytoplasmic lysosomes (peroxidases, hydrolases).

II. Polymorphonuclear Granulocytes (PMNs)

Three different types of **polymorphonuclear granulocytes** (called **polymorphs** or **granulocytes**)—mainly neutrophil (PMNs), eosinophils and basophils.

Non-differentiated hemopoietic cell marker CD34 is lost in mature monocytes and neutrophils.

Neutrophils
- These cells are released at a rate of **7 millions/ minute** from bone marrow.
- By chemotaxis and diapedesis, they reach the site of infection.
- Patients with genetic defect have low levels of PMNs which make them susceptible for infections.
- Enzymes and other antibacterial substances are store in two types of granules:
  a. Primary or azurophilic: Liposomes containing acid hydrolyses, muramydase (lysozyme), antimicrobial proteins (defensins, cathelicidians, serocidins).
  b. Secondary specific to neutrophils—lactoferrin, lysozyme.

Lysosomes fuse with vacuoles containing microorganisms (phagosome) and forms phagolysosmes.

Pathogen combines with antibody to form immune complexes which activate neutrophils by binding through **Fc receptors**. Neutrophils release granules and cytotoxic substances extracellularly.

Eosinophils
- They comprise 2–5% of blood leukocytes.
- They have bilobed nucleus and cytoplasmic granules which stain with acidic dye eosin.
- Though phagocytosis is not their primary function, they are capable of phagocytosis and killing of microorganisms.
- The granules in mature eosinophils are membrane bound organelles with crystalloid core that differs from surrounding matrix.

The **crystalloid core contains** the **major basic proteins** which are:
- It is a potent toxin to helmintic worms.
- Induces histamine release from mast cells.

- Activates neutrophils and platelets.
- Produces bronchospasm in allergic persons.

Other proteins found in granule matrix are:
- Eosinophilic cationic protein (**ECP**), and
- Eosinophil-derived neutrotoxins (**EDN**)

Release of granules is the only way in which eosinophils can kill large pathogen as parasite.

Basophils (in blood) and mast cells (in the tissues)
These cells are characterized by basophilic (blue) staining. These cells contain the pharmacological mediators causing the adverse symptoms of IgE mediated allergy. These mediators may be released from the granules during allergic reactions. Some of the mediators are preformed (primary mediators) while some are formed after activation (secondary mediators).

> Lymphocytes and other WBC have many surface antigens or markers called as leukocyte differentiation antigens. A particular leukocyte differentiation antigen has given a CD (cluster of differentiation) number on basis of its reaction with monoclonal antibodies. A marker may reflect stage of development and different functional properties. Surface antigens of different cells are:
>
> CD4 – Helper cell
> CD8 – Cytotoxic cell
> CD19 – B cell
> CD3 – Present on T cell and forms a CD–TCR complex

Cells of Lymphoreticular System

This system consists of **structural cells** (fibroblasts, reticulum cells, endothelial system) and those cells that serve special immunological functions which are **lymphocytes, macrophages and plasma cells.**

Lymphocytes constitute 20–45% of leukocyte population in peripheral blood while they form predominant population in lymphoid organs.
- According to **size,** they are classified as small (5–8 μ), medium (8–12 μ), and large (12–15 μ). Most of lymphocytes are of smaller type.
- Depending upon the lifespan, there are short lived (2 weeks) and long lived (3 years or more). Short lived are effectors cells, while long lived are memory cells. Human body contains 10^{12} lymphocytes out of which 10^9 are renewed daily.
- **Lymphocyte recirculation:** Constantly the lympho-cytes circulate from peripheral lymphoid organs, central lymphoid organs, lymphatic tissue hence contact with antigen anywhere causes response at all the sites where lymphocytes lie.

Functionally, there are two important subsets, i.e. **T** lymphocyte and **B** lymphocyte, within each subset there are memory cells.

T LYMPHOCYTES (T CELL)

Development of T Cell (Flowchart 17.3)

Precursor T cells originate in thymus, fetal liver and bone marrow migrate to thymus during embryonic life.

Within thymus, **T** cell progenitor undergoes differentiation under the influence of local hormones; **T** cells differentiate into committed T cells with a specific T cell receptor (**TCR**).

Cells during maturation stage are **Pro-T cells, Pre-T cells, and CD4 or CD8 T cells.**

Within each lobe of thymus, the lymphoid cells are arranged into:
- Outer tightly packed **cortex** contains relatively immature proliferating thymocytes and
- Inner **medulla** containing more mature cells, forming a differential gradient from cortex to medulla.

The main blood vessels called high endothelial venules (**HEVs**) situated at corticomedullary junction of thymic lobules regulate the cell traffic in thymus.

Through these venules (HEVs), **T cell progenitors formed in fetal liver and bone marrow enter** and migrate towards cortex.

In the **cortex,** they undergo **proliferation and development** which lead to generation of **mature T** cells through corticomedullary gradient of migration.

Epithelial cells network in lobules play important function in **differentiation and selection processes of pre-thymic cells to mature T cells.**

Mature T cells leave the thymus through the same venules (**HEVs**).
- **Nurse cells of cortex** sustain proliferation of progenitor T cells, mainly through IL-7 production.
- **Cortical thymic epithelial cells (TECs)** are responsible for **positive selection (the first stage of thymic education)** of maturing lymphocytes **allowing survival of cells** that recognize self MHC I and II molecules with associated peptides via TCRs of intermediate affinity.
- **Medullary TECs** display organs-specific self-peptides.

Positive selection
- It takes place in thymus. Those maturing lymphocytes are allowed to survive which recognize self MHC I and MHC II molecules with associated peptides through TCRs of intermediate sensitivity.
- T cells with TCRs showing **high, low receptors affinity** for self-MHC undergoes **apoptosis** (programmed cell death).

Flowchart 17.3: Development and maturation of T cell

T cell precursors from yolk sac, fetal, liver & bone marrow move to thymus

↓

On entering thymus **Pro-T cells** acquire CD2 (cells capable of reacting with self antigens are functionally deleted or by – negative selection)

↓

Pro-T cells synthesize CD3 in cytoplasm- become **'Pre-T cell'** (surface markers -CD-7,CD-2)

↓

Synthesize TCR, MHC restriction develops

↓

Immature T cells in thymus have TCR on surface and CD7,2,3,1,4,8

↓

T cells mature , lose CD1 & develop into 'CD8-4' + or 'CD8+4'-

↓

CD4+8- TCR αβ cells are supressor/Tc- cytotoxic T cells, CD8-4+ cells are helper/ inducer cells

Negative selection
- Out of positively selected T cells, some cells have TCRs that do not recognize self components other than self MHC. Such cells are deleted by negative selection.
- Only T cells that fail to recognize self-antigens are allowed to proceed to further development.
- T cell at this stage of maturation (CD4 + CD8 + TCR10) go on to express TCR at high density and **lose either CD4 or CD8** to become **'single positive' mature T cells.**

Negative selection may also occur outside thymus, in peripheral lymphoid tissue.

The probable mechanisms of peripheral negative selection are:

- Downregulation of TCR and CD3 so that cells are unable to interact with autoantigens.
- Anergy may occur due to absence of co-stimulatory signals, followed by apoptosis.
- **Treg** function.

T Cell Receptor (TCR)

- This receptor present on the surface of T cell which takes antigen from **'antigen presenting cell'**. It is made of glycoprotein chains and it forms complex with CD3 (TCR-CD3 complex).
- The glycoprotein chains of TCR are αβ or γδ. **Majority of T cells have αβ TCR.**
- Part of TCR present within membrane is called transmembrane portion while tail part of it extends into cytoplasm.
- Two chains held together by disulphide bond.
- Like immunoglobulin's, TCR contains four encoded regions V (variable), D (diversity), J (joining) and constant (C) region. **Reassortment of these regions is responsible for their diversity.**

TCR—T cells become positive for the expression of other surface molecules, i.e. CD4, CD8 and co-receptors. T cells at this stage possess functional TCR.

T cells undergo **positive** and **negative selection** so that only those cells which are nonself-antigen specific are retained (while cells capable of mounting immune response against self-antigens are removed or made functionally inactive). Foreign antigens can be recognized only in context of self-MHC (self-MHC restricted). 90% T cells die in thymus.

When cells undergo further maturation, they loose their expression of either CD4 or CD8 and become single positive cells which now express TCR/CD3 complex and become **either CD4+ or CD8+** (small group of T cells with both CD4+ve, CD8+ve exist). Only small number of cells escape and enter in periphery.

Subsets of T Cells and Effector Functions

Proliferating **CD4 cells** can become one of the effector cells and regulatory cells. Cells are further differentiated into **TH1, TH2,** and **TH17** or regulatory T cells **(Treg)** (Fig. 17.4).

Three major subpopulations of αβ T cells are:
1. **Helpers T cells (TH)** express the CD4 marker (**CD4+ T cells**) and mainly help or induce immune responses are divided into two main subsets (**TH1, TH2**).

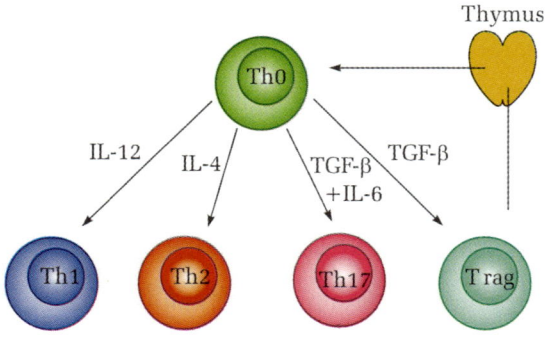

Fig. 17.4: Different subsets of TH cell

2. **Regulatory T cells (Treg)** that express CD4 marker (**CD4+ T cell**)) and regulate immune responses.
3. **Cytotoxic T cells (Tc)** that express CD8 marker (**CD8+**) also called **cytotoxic T lymphocytes (CTLs).**

A small proportion of αβ T cells neither express CD4 nor CD8, these '**double negative T cells**' might have regulatory function.

In contrast, while most circulating γβ cells are double negative, most γβ T cells in tissues express CD8.

TH1: In an environment of INF γ, TH1 cells predominate and these cells either activate macrophages or stimulate T cells to produce **IL-2 and INFγ**. In either of the conditions, they promote bacterial clearance either by activated macrophages or antibody mediated opsonization (coating of antigens with opsonin as antibodies which promotes phagocytosis). Main function of TH1 is promotion of cell-mediated immunity (CMI).

In an environment where IL-4 predominant, TH2 cells predominate.

TH2 cells produce IL-4, 5, 6, 10.
- Activate mast cells, eosinophils and cause production of IgE.
- These cells have many functions associated with cytotoxicity and local inflammatory reactions.
- They help cytotoxic T cell precursors develop into effecter cells to kill virally infected cells and activate macrophages infected with *Mycobacterium tuberculosis*, enhancing intracellular killing by production of INFγ. They are important in defense against intracellular pathogens including viruses, bacteria, protozoa.
- They are effective at stimulating B cells to produce antibodies of some IgG subclasses and especially IgE, thus primarily to protect against free living, extracellular microorganisms (humoral immunity).

TH17: These cells are similar to subsets of TH1.
- Induction of TH17 from TH0 cell is dependent on TGFβ and not IL-12, INF-α.
- They are related to regulatory cells. They produce **IL-17** and **IL-22.**
- They appear to be important in **maintaining the integrity of mucosal cells**, thus in protection against entry of microorganisms in the body.
- They cause recruitment of neutrophils and macrophages at the site of infection.
- The measurement of a single cell secreting a particular cytokine or antibody can be done by using enzyme-linked method, **ELISPOT.**

Treg cells regulate immune responses. They are two types (Table 17.1):
1. Naturally occurring Treg cells

TABLE 17.1: Treg cells—types

Naturally occurring Treg cells	Inducible Treg cells
• Express CD25 • Constitute about 5–10% of CD4+ T cells • Do not proliferate in response to antigenic stimulus • Produce suppressive effects through cell contact (i.e. with APC, TH1 or TH2 cells)	• Express CD25 • Can develop from peripheral CD25–, CD4+ T cells • Produce their effect through IL-10

2. **Inducible Treg cells**—following activation by specific antigens.

γδ T cells

- These cells are frequent in (GUT) mucosal epithelia (most intraepithelial cells are γδ T cells and express CD8 marker not found in circulating cells) and minor population (5%) of circulating T cells.
- Thus these cells form population of cells called **'intraepithelial lymphocytes' (IEL).**
- They have specific repertoire of TCRs biased towards certain bacterial or viral antigens (super antigens).
- Human blood γδ cells have specificity for low molecular mass mycobacterial products.
- Some γδ cells may recognize antigens directly.
- They may deal with lipid antigens.

They recognize unconventional antigens as heat shock proteins, phospholipids, phosphoproteins.

TH1

TH activates macrophage or B cells. B cells produce antibodies which cause opsonization. Activated macrophage kills bacteria.

Main functions of helper cells (inducer cells) (Table 17.2)

- Help in activation of B cells which mature into plasma cells and produce antibodies.
- TH1 cytokines activate cytotoxic activity.
- TH2 help in production of cytokines which stimulate eosinophils.
- TH2 cytokines regulate antibody responses.
- TH17 cells which produce cytokines that cause recruitment of neutrophils and macrophages at the site of infection.

Cytotoxic T cells—Tc—CD8 effector cells: CD8 cells differentiate into effectors cells which proceed to kill the target, these are cytotoxic cells. The primary method of killing is through cytotoxic granules which contain **perforins** (Fig. 17.5).

Differences between T helper cells and cytotoxic T cells are given in Table 17.3.

TABLE 17.2: Cytokines production and principle functions of TH1 and TH2 cells

	TH1	TH2
Cytokines production		
IL-2	+	—
INF-β	++	—
TNF-β	++	—
GM-CSF	++	+
IL-3	++	++
IL-4	–	++
IL-5	–	++
IL10	–	++
IL-13	–	++
Humoral immunity		
Help for total antibody production	+	++
Help for IgG production	—	++
Eosinophil and mast cell production	—	++
Cell-mediated immunity		
Macrophage activation	++	—
Delayed hypersensitivity	++	—
Tc cell activation	++	—

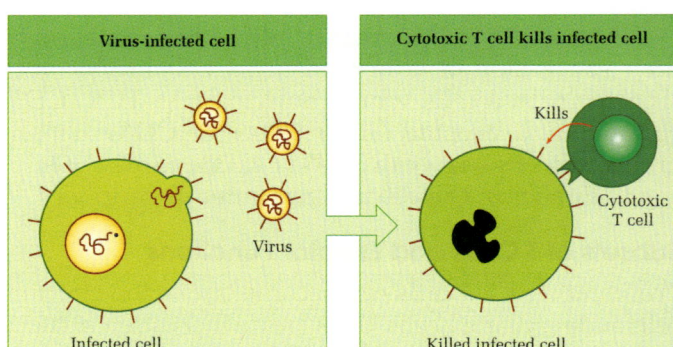

Fig. 17.5: Cytotoxic T cell

TABLE 17.3: Differences between T helper cells and cytotoxic T cells

Helper cell	Cytotoxic cell
Carries CD4	Carries CD8
Helps Tc cells or B cell	Cytotoxic
MHC class II restricted	MHC class I restricted
Can stimulate macrophage to kill intracellular pathogens	Themselves kill intracellular pathogens or virus infected cells or tumor cells

B CELL

B cell production: Certain cells of lymphoid series remain in bone marrow. The bone marrow derived lymphocytes are called as B lymphocytes or B cells. They are called

B cells, as in birds they are derived from bursa of Fabricius, in humans they are of bone marrow origin.

About 5–15% of circulating lymphocytes are B cells which have surface immunoglobulin, transmembrane molecule, which are continuously produced and inserted into B cell membrane, where they act as specific antigen receptors.

Most human B cells express IgM and IgD. B cells with IgG, IgA, IgE may be present at specific locations in the body (IgA in intestinal mucosa). About 10% of circulating B cells possess IgG, IgA, or IgE.

Immunoglobulins associated with other accessory molecules on B cells form '**B cell antigen receptor complex' (BCR)**.

The heterodimers form complexes with trans-membrane components of immunoglobulin receptors and they are involved in **cellular activation**.

BCR interaction with specific antigen triggers immunoreceptors tyrosine based activation motifs **(ITAM)** phosphorylation which regulated downstream cascade of intracellular events leading to changes in genes expressions.

Other markers on B cells are:
- MHC class II
- Complement receptors for C3b(CD35), C3d(CD21)
- CD19, and CD20 are main markers used to identify B cells.
- CD40 is involved in T and B cell interactions CD19/CD21 interactions with complement, associated with antigen, play a role in antigen-induced activation of B cells.

Number of B cell: 30% of circulating lymphocytes are B cells. Approximately 10^9 are produced daily.

Location: They are found in the germinal centers of lymph nodes, in white pulp of spleen and in MALT

Maturation: B cell precursors during embryonic life proliferate and develop in fetal liver. They migrate to bone marrow where they mature.
- The B lymphocyte **precursors 'Pro-B cells'** develop in fetal liver in embryonic life and bone marrow afterwards.
- Pro-B cell synthesizes '**mu' chains;** this polypeptide is confined within the cell.
- **Pre-B** cells are the next stage beginning with of an early stage in which 'mu' and surrogate light chains are synthesized and the 'mu' surrogate light chain monomer is displayed on the cell surface.
- The **final pre-B cell** occurs when alpha and lambda light chains are synthesized and they replace the surrogate chains.

- **Immature B cells** then synthesize and display IgM monomers on their surfaces.
- Immature B cells migrate to periphery, undergo '**immunoglobulin's class switching'** so that apart from IgM alone, cells express other immunoglobulins (IgG, IgA, IgE) on their surface; means IgD and other immunoglobulin.
- Each mature B cell displays both IgM and IgD of identical specificity on their surface.
- On contact with antigen, mature B cell undergoes '**clonal proliferation'.** Majority of the cells become **plasma cells** which produce antibodies and small proportion of B cells become memory B cells.
- **Plasma cells** represent the end cell in the differention of lineage cells and function as factories synthesizing and secreting immunoglobulins (Fig. 17.6).

CD5 B-1 cells and marginal zone B cells produce natural antibodies.

CD5 B-1 cells:
- Many of the first B cells that appear during ontogeny express **CD5** (a marker originally found on T cells).
- These cells are present in peritoneal cavity of mice
- They express their immunoglobulins from un-mutated or minimally mutated germ line genes and produce IgM (some IgG, IgA).
- These so-called **natural antibodies** are of **low avidity**, but, unusually they are polyreactive and found at high concentrations in adult serum.

CD5 B cells:
- Respond well to TI antigens.
- They may be involved in antigen presentation and processing.
- Probably play role in both tolerance and reaction.

Functions proposed for natural antibodies are:
- First line of defense against microorganisms
- Clearance of **damaged self cells components**.
- Regulatory 'idiotypic' interactions within immune system.

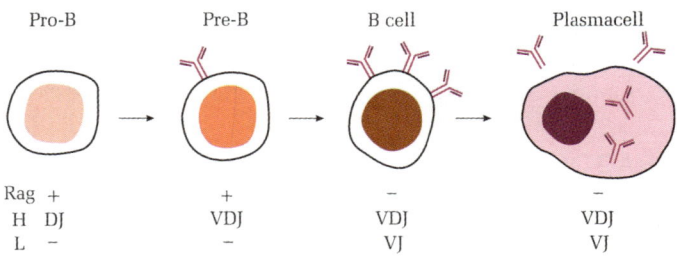

Fig. 17.6: Key stages in B cell development and differentiation

They react against autoantigens including:

- DNA
- Fc of IgG
- Phospholipids
- Cytoskeleton components
- Marginal zone B cells are thought to protect against polysaccharide capsules. These cells accumulate slowly in marginal zone of spleen—a process takes 1–2 years. They respond to **thymus independent antigens (TI).**
- They give main protection **against polysaccharide antigen.** They produce **natural antibodies** and together with B1 cells are called '**innate-like B cells'.**

Function of B Cells

They mature into antibodies producing cells which produce antibodies. The antibodies on the surface of the B cells act as rerceptor and accept the antigen.

- B cell acts as antigen presenting cells, especially in secondary immune respone.
- B cells give constimulatory signals to T cells so that T cells get activate.

The stages of B cell development show change in the gene activity within the cell and its ability to synthesize, display, and secrete immunoglobulins.

PLASMA CELLS

Antigenically stimulated B cell undergoes blast formation and form plasma cell. They are oval cells, size double that of lymphocyte. **Nucleus** is small **oval eccentrically** placed with radially arranged chromatin giving **'cart wheel' apperance.** They have lifespan of 2–3 years. It is antibody producing cell. **Plasma cell produces antibody of single immunoglobulin class with single specificity and allotype.** The exception takes place in **primary immune** response in which due to class switch, **initially IgM is produced followed by IgG.**

All blood cells originate from stem cell and develop into four major cell lineages

Erythroid precursors	Differentiate into RBCs
Megakaryocyte	Differentiate into platelets
Myeloid precursors	Differentiate into neutrophils, monocytes, eosinophils, basophils
Lymphoid cell precursors	Differentiate into T cell and B cell

PHAGOCYTOSIS

Engulfment of organisms and killing inside a cell which acts as phagocytic cell is called phagoctosis. If the antigen or the organism is coated with soluble sub-

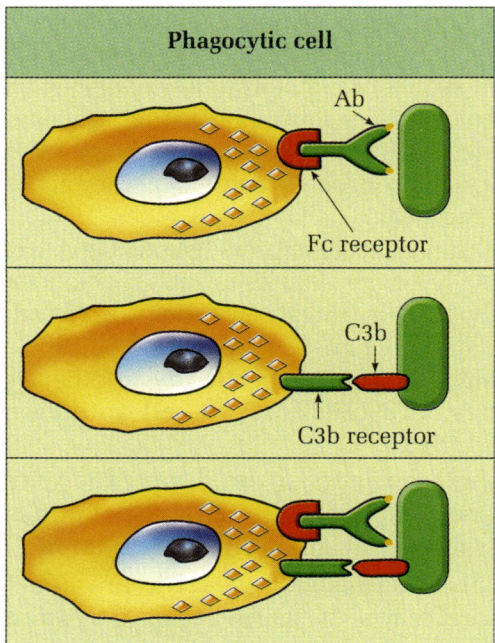

Fig. 17.7: Opsonization

stances as complement or antibodies which make the phagocytosis easy is called as **opsonization** (from Latin, *opsonin* means to prepare victuals for) (Fig. 17.7).

Macrophages are important cells involved in phagocytosis.

Development of macrophages: Haemopoietic stem cell (HSC) develops into colony forming unit (CFU) which gives rise to granulocytes, erythrocytes, monocytes and macrophages (CFU-GEMM), maturation of these cells occur under the influence of the cytokine, i.e. CSF and IL-1, 3, 5, 6 derived from stromal cells of bone marrow. Phagocytes form the innate or nonspecific immune mechanisms which act as first line of defense against organisms. Apart from monocytes and macrophages, other cells as polymorphs and dendritic cells have the function of phagocytosis.

Types of Phagocytes

The phagocytes are the mononuclear macrophages (of blood and tissues) and polymophonuclear microphages. The mononuclear cells developed from stem cell come out as monocytes in circulation. They leave the circulation to go to the different tissues and get converted **tissue** macrophages. The macrophages in lungs are called alveolar macrophages; those in liver are called Kupffer cells.

Macrophages

Lifespan: Monocytes have short half-life span of three days while macrophages survive for several months.

Morphology: Large round to oval cells with kidney-shaped nucleus and abundant cytoplasm. Size of macrophages: 15–20 μ, size of microphages: 12–15 μ.

Surface Receptors of Macrophages

- Receptor for the Fc portion of antibody
- Receptors for complements
- Receptors for cytokines
- M1 marker, protein similar to receptor for C3, i.e. CR3.

Activated macrophages show following characteristics:
- Macrophages get activated following cytokines, interferon secreted by helper T cell or by complement.
- Immunity produced by activated macrophage is nonspecific, not against a particular pathogen.
- It may be specific in some cases as **antibody-dependent cell-mediated cytotoxicity (ADCC).**
- **ADCC** is important in immunity against cancer and graft rejection.
- Cells increase in size, become **more competent** for phagocytosis and get adhered to glass surface in a faster way.
- Activated macrophages release biologically active substances as:
  a. **Interlukin-1** mainly stimulates T cells to produce interlukin-2 which on other hand causes activation of T cells.
  b. **Interleukin-1** also acts as **endogenous pyrogen** and it along with tumor necrosis factor acts as **cachectin.**
  c. **Colony-stimulating factor (CSF)** a cytokine which causes stimulation of pluripotent stem cells.
  d. Hydrolytic enzymes, binding protein (fibronectin).

Activation: Activation of macrophages take place under the influence of IL-2 produced by activated TH cell.

Cytokine Produced by Marophages: TNF, CSF, IL-1

Functions (Fig. 17.8)
- Phagocytosis and opsonization of foreign particles or organisms.
- Whenever any antigen or organism enters our body, macrophages act as **antigen-presenting cell,** they breakdown the antigen into small peptides which lie in groove formed by MHC class II, and the antigen is presented to the T cells (function of antigen presenting and **antigen processing cell).**
- By secreting its cytokines, it stimulates T cell to produce cytokines which cause differentiation and proliferation of B lymphocytes which form antibodies and Tc has cytotoxic action.

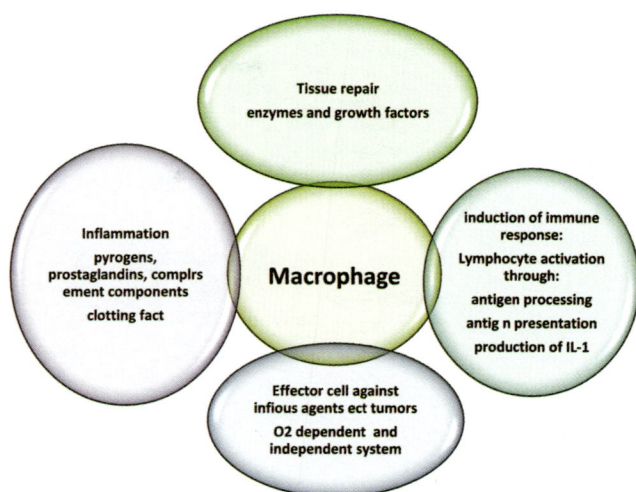

Fig. 17.8: The central role of macrophage

- The cell has receptor for Fc portion of antibody. The Fab of antibody attaches to the antigen while Fc attaches to macrophages linking antigen towards the macrophage.
- In an effort to kill intracellular bacteria as MTB, these cells get converted into epitheloid cells and giant cells.
- IL-1 secreted by it, stimulates TH cells.
- Microbicidal activities which are O_2 dependent: H_2O_2, O_2^-, NO, OH.
- Microbicidal activity which are O_2 independent: Lysozymes, acid hydrolases, cationic proteins.
- *Tissue damage:* H_2O_2, acid hydrolases, C3a, TNF alpha damage tissues.
- *Tumoricidal activity:* Cytotoxic activity, H_2O_2, NO, TNF alpha, proteases.
- *Inflammation and fever:* IL-1, 6, TNF alpha.

Mechanism of Phagocytosis (Fig. 17.9)

It consists of different steps as chemotaxis to the site of infection, movement of phagocyte out of blood vessel, ingestion and killing.

i. *Chemotaxis:* Various factors act as chemotactic agents so that phagocytes are invited to the site of infection. These include active members of complement system, i.e. C2a, C5a. Also lymphokine secreted by T cells acts as chemotactic agents. Then the phagocyte starts movement toward the site of infection, it comes out of blood vessel by diapedesis.

ii. *Traping an antigen or engulfment:* Once the contact is made with foreign particle, macrophage traps the particle by producing pseudopodia like structures, engulfs the foreign particles. The engulfed particles initially lodge in a vacuole called as phagosome. It fuses with liposomal granules to form phgolysosme.

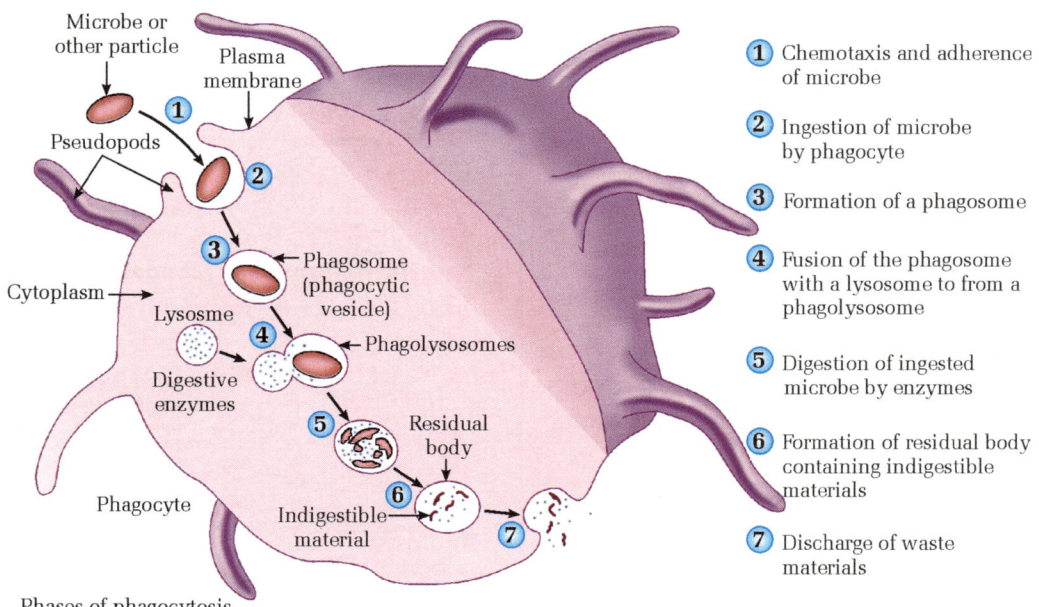

Phases of phagocytosis

Fig. 17.9: Phagocytosis

① Chemotaxis and adherence of microbe

② Ingestion of microbe by phagocyte

③ Formation of a phagosome

④ Fusion of the phagosome with a lysosome to from a phagolysosome

⑤ Digestion of ingested microbe by enzymes

⑥ Formation of residual body containing indigestible materials

⑦ Discharge of waste materials

iii. Damaging the bacteria (organisms): Variety of enzymes come out of granules such as proteases, peroxides, lipases, and nucleases. The oxygen radicals which include superoxide radicals, H_2O_2; hydroxyl radicals are toxic which kill the organisms. Other nitrogen intermediates as nitrous oxide, nitrogen dioxide, nitric oxide have also antimicrobial activity.

Mononuclear macrophages develop into special macrophages. Different macrophages in different tissues are:

Tissues	Macrophages
Blood	Monocytes
Tissue macrophages	Histocytes
Lung	Alveolar macrophages
Liver	Kupffer cells
Bone	Osteoclasts
Kidney	Mesangial cells

Microphages

These are small polymophoneuclear leukocytes present in the blood; they include neutrophils, eosinophils, and basophils of which the neutrophil acts as phagocytic cell. The cell contains bactericidal substances. The life-span of these cells is short; it is 2 days in blood, a few hours in tissues.

The stimuli for production, mechanisms of damage and other characteristics of macrophages and polymorphs are summerised in Table 17.4.

Differences between T cell, B cell and macrophage are given in Table 17.5.

The mechanisms of damage caused to organisms is summarized in Table 17.6.

ANTIGEN PRESENTING CELLS (APCS)

The basic immune responses include antibody-mediated immunity (AMI) or humoral immunity and cell-mediated immunity (CMI). The soluble mediators called cytokines released by helper T cells (TH) activate these immune responses. But it is essential to present antigen to TH cells. The cells which take up antigen and present to TH cells are known as 'antigen presenting cells (APC)'.

As TH cells are **MHC class II restricted,** they will accept antigen only if it is presented by APC with self-MHC class II on their surface. **The antigen presenting cells include dendritic cells, macrophages, and B cells** (in secondary immune response, **Langerhans cells** and microphages).

DENDRITIC CELLS

- They are bone marrow-derived cells of different origin other than from those lymphocytes or macrophages.
- **Function:** These cells are major **profession antigen presenting cells (APCs)** presenting antigen to T cells in immune response.
- They express MHC class II on surface (**MHC class II restricted**).
- Also express B7, CD23 which are co-stimulatory signals for stimulation of T cells (TH).
- **Morphology:** Show pleomorphism, cells with small central body with long processes.
- **Distribution:** They are present in peripheral lymphoid organs (germinal area) of spleen and lymph nodes and peripheral blood.

TABLE 17.4: Comparision of macrophages and microphages

	PMN	Macrophage
Site of production	Bone marrow	Bone marrow
Duration in marrow	14 days	54 hours
Duration in blood	7–10 hours	20–40 hours
Average lifespan	4 days	Months to years
Principal killing mechanism	Oxidative and nonoxidative	Oxidative nitric oxides, cytokines
Activated by	TNFα, INFγ, GM-CSF, microbial products	TNFα, INFγ, GM-CSF, microbial products (e.g. LPS)
Major secretory products	Lysozyme	Many, over 80, main are lysozymes, cytokines-IL-1, TNFα
Important deficiencies	CGD, myeloperoxidase Chédiak-Higashi	Lipid storage diseases

TABLE 17.5: Differences between T cell, B cell and macrophage

Property	T cell	B cell	Macrophage
CD3 receptor	+	—	—
Surface immunoglobulins	—	+	—
Receptors for FC piece of IgG	—	+	
EAC rosette (CD3 receptor), CR2 receptor, EBV virus	—	+	—
SRBC rosette (CD2); Measles receptor)	+	—	—
Thymus specific antigens	+	—	—
Numerous microvilli on the surface	—	+	—
Phagocytic action	—	—	+
Adherence to glass	—	—	+
Blast formation with			
Anti-CD-3	+	—	—
Anti-IgG	—	+	—
PHA	+	—	—
Concavalin	+	—	—
Endotoxin	—	+	

TABLE 17.6: Cytotoxic molecules of different cells

Host component	Cytotoxic molecules	Effective against
Liver cells, macrophages	Complement (C1-3)	Bacteria, fungi
	Complement (C5-9)	Neisseria
		Streptococci
Macrophages	Reactive oxygen	Bacteria, fungi, malaria
Neutrophils	intermediates	
Eosinophils	(plus peroxidases)	
Macrophages	Lysozyme	Gram-positive bacteria
	Interferon α, β	Viruses
	TNF α	Viruses, bacteria
	Reactive nitrogen	Malaria
	Intermediates	Leishmania
Neutrophils	Defensins	Bacteria, fungi
	Cathepsins	Bacteria, fungi
	Lactoferrin	Bacteria, yeasts, schistosomes
Eosinophil	Cationic proteins	
T lymphocyte	Cytokines	Virues
	Perforins	Some bacteria,
	Granzymes	fungi, protozoa
NK cells	Perforins	Viruses
	Granyzymes	

B cells: B cell acts as antigen presenting cell during secondary immune response (immune response following 2nd contact with the same antigen or organism).

Langerhan's cells: These cells are present on skin. They act as antigen presenting cells for the antigens entering dermis.

Dendritic cells: They are derived from stem cell, mainly act as antigen presenting cells, with little or no phagocytic activity. These cells are present in peripheral lymphoid organs, and in skin. They take the antigen entering through skin or epithelial surfaces.

NATURAL KILLER CELLS, LAK CELLS (NULL CELLS)

The blood lymphocytes are mostly T cells and B cells and they have the receptors present on them but there is small population of lymphocytes which is neither T nor B lymphocytes which are called as **null cells.** Morphologically, these cells are **large granular lympho-cytes** with double the size of small lymphocytes. The Null cells are of three types: Natural killer cells, killer cells, and lymphokine-activated cells.

NK cells: These cells make a small population of lymphocytes (15%). These cells are called NK cells as they have no conventional receptors those present on the surface of T or B cell. The markers present on the surface of NK cells are CD16, CD56; they are also present in spleen. These cells do not require antibody and their action is nonspecific. The cells are naturally present in blood and contain more granular cytoplasm than T or B cells. (Fig. 17.10).

Comparision between NK cells and Tc cell

- Cytotoxic Tc cells are MHC-I resticted, while NK cells are not MHC restricted.

- Tc cells have memory while NK cells do not have memory.

- Surface markers of Tc cells are CD3, CD8 while surface markers of NK cells are CD16, CD56.

Mechanism of Action of NK Cell (Fig. 17.10)

NK cells first bind to the receptors present on the surface of target cells. The target cell is modified first so that it is programmed for the death. The NK cell release many cytolytic factors which include perforins, TNFα, and natural killer cytotoxin. The perforin drills cell wall of microorganisms and causes release of cell contents and death. TNFα enters cells and causes their **apoptosis (programmed cell death).**

Functions (Fig. 17.11)

- The cells are believed to play a role against tumor cells. They perform constant immune surveillance and cause mop up operation, if there is overgrowth of cells.

- NK cells kill virus-infected cells also.

- They also act on cells with intracellular bacteria.

- The cells secrete INFα and IL-1 which play role in regulation of immune responses.

- Killer cells possess receptors for the Fc portion of IgG, lyse or kill target sensitized by IgG antibodies. These cells are responsible for ADCC which is antibody-dependent cell-mediated cytotoxicity (ADCC). The Fab part of antibody attaches to the antigen and Fc part attaches to NK cells making a bridge of antigens and cell, cell damage is produced independent of complement.

Some microorganisms are killed by reactive oxygen and nitrogen:

- *Staphylococcus aureus*
- *E. coli*
- *Serratia*
- *C. albicans*
- *Aspergillus* sp.
- *Plasmodium* sp.
- *Leishmania* sp.

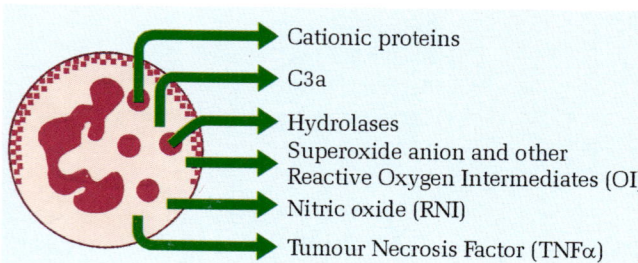

Fig. 17.10: NK cell

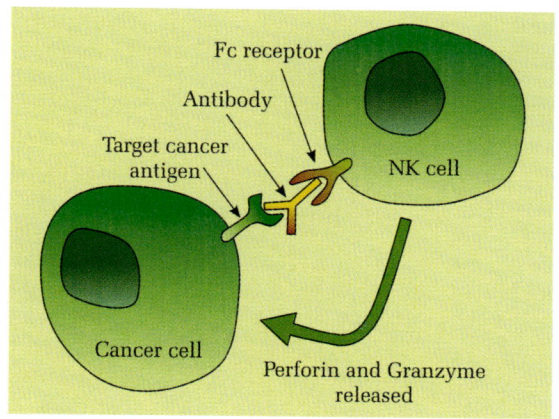

Fig. 17.11: NK cell function against cancer cell

18

Immune Response

When a host reacts specifically against a particular antigen, how it reacts is called immune response.

In infectious disease, the purpose of immune response is to get protection from microorganisms. But if an antigen is in other form, like nonliving allergen, it may cause some injury to host by hypersensitivity. Occasionally, the response against some antigenic stimuli may lead to a state of specific non-reactivity called **tolerance.**

IMMUNE RESPONSE (Flowchart 18.1)

Immune responses may be nonspecific as **innate immune responses** (e.g. phagocytosis) as discussed earlier and **acquired immune responses**.

Types of Acquired Immune Responses

1. **Acquired immune responses** can be driven by **antibodies** produced by B cells—called **humoral response** (**humoral immunity**) or

2. They may be driven by cells (effectors) as **cytotoxic cell (Tc)** called **cellular responses or cell-mediated immunity (CMI).**

   - Humoral responses and cellular responses may be produced following infection, but usually one of them dominates.
   - Nature of antigen drives these responses and, therefore, determines the nature of immune response, either humoral or cellular.

Types of Immune Responses

- Humoral (antibody mediated)
- Cellular (cell mediated)

They may develop together, though at times one or the other may predominate.

Antibody-mediated Immunity (AMI): Scope or Functions of AMI

- It provides primary defense against most extra-cellular bacterial pathogens.

- It helps in defense against viruses that infect through the respiratory or intestinal tracts. These viruses are neutralized by antibodies (Fig. 18.1). These viruses, e.g. influenza viruses, are neutralized by antibodies by combining with their surface antigens like hemagglutinin and neuraminidase. The local immunity given by IgA protects mucosal surfaces.

- AMI prevents recurrences of virus infections.

- Spread of the viruses is also prevented by antibody, e.g. hemagglutinin (HA) and neuraminidases (NA) are present on the surface of influenza virus. HA helps in attachment while NA helps in cell to cell spread. Antibody against HA is neutralizing while antibody against NA prevents spread of the virus from one cell to another.

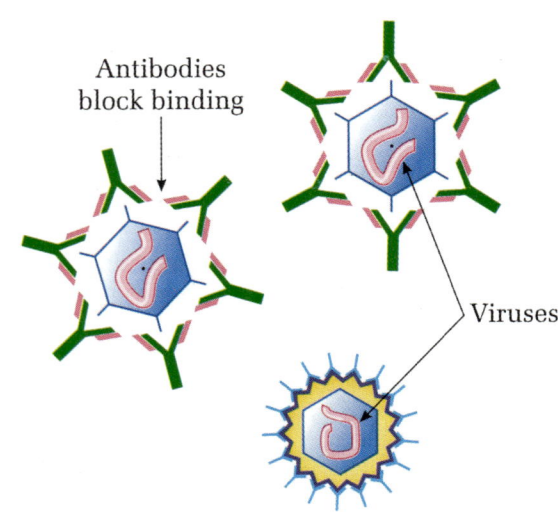

Antibodies block binding

Viruses

Fig. 18.1: Neutralization

Flowchart 18.1: Immune response

Entry of microorganism
Recognization by dendritic cells through pattern recognition receptors

Uptake of antigen (microorganism) by dendritic cell,
migration of dendritic cell to lymph nodes and
maturation into antigen presenting cell

Expression of costimulatory molecules on dendritic cell
(B7, also known as CD80/CD86)

Processing of antigen by dendritic cells, load antigenic peptide in the
groove present on surface MHC class II molecule)

Presentation of 'antigen peptide-MHC complex' to T helper cells

TH cell requires two signals, i.e. antigen presentation and costimulatory
molecule present on antigen presenting cell (B7)

TH cell secretes cytokines which stimulate B cell and cytotoxic Tc cell

For dealing with extracellular organism as bacterium, antibody formed by
B cells (humoral immunity) takes the lead

For intracellular organisms as viruses, cytotoxic cells
take lead—cell-mediated immunity (CMI)

Effector functions of antibody or Tc cell

Elimination of antigen

- AMI takes part in the pathogenesis of types I, II and III hypersensitivity reactions and certain auto-immune diseases. In type I, IgE takes part while in type II and III hypersentivities, IgG takes part.
- In hyperacute rejection of graft, AMI takes part along with CMI.

Scope of Cell-Mediated Immunity (CMI) or Functions of CMI

- CMI protects against fungi, viruses and facultative intracellular bacterial pathogens as antibodies cannot reach there. CMI causes damage to infected cells directly.
- CMI participates in the rejection of homografts and graft-versus-host reaction.
- Natural killer cells perform the function of immuno-logical surveillance and immunity against cancer.
- CMI mediates pathogenesis of delayed (type IV) hypersensitivity and certain autoimmune diseases.

HUMORAL IMMUNE RESPONSE

The process of production of antibodies consists of afferent limb, efferent limb and central functions.

Afferent limb: The entry of antigen, its spread in the tissues and its contact with appropriate immune-competent cells, e.g. antigen presenting cell (APC) is the afferent limb of AMI.

Central functions: The processing of antigen by antigen processing cells or antigen presenting cell and the regulation of antibody forming process is the central function. **Antigen is processed by antigen presenting cell (APCs).**

Antigen is presented to the TH cells in association with MHC class II. Stimulation of cytokines by TH activate B cell to produce antibodies. These events take place in central limb of immune response.

Afferent Limb and Central Functions

Antigen presentation, processing, activation of T cells:

- **Antigen presentation** involves the degradation of antigen into peptide fragments, which may bound to MHC class I or class II molecules.
- It plays a central role in starting appropriate immune responses and maintaining them.

Antigen presentation occurs in lymphoid organs which result in T cells proliferation. But antigen presen-tation may occur in limited amount in tissues (causes release of cytokines).

Which cells act as antigen presenting cells depend upon how and where the first contact of antigen to immune system takes place. Activation of naïve T cells following first contact with antigen on the surface of antigen presenting cells is called **priming.**

T cells only recognize antigen peptides attached to MHC molecules.

Antigen Processing Pathways

1. *Endocytic pathway:* Extracellular antigens as bacteria or their products are processed by this pathway. Antigen processing cells, as macrophages, dendritic cells, process the antigens, antigenic peptides lodge in MHC groove and present antigens to TH cells.

2. *Cytosolic pathway:* Intracellular organisms, as viruses, TB bacilli , tumor antigens, are processed by cytosolic pathway. After this, antigens are presented along self-MHC class I molecule.

In lymphoid organs three main types of APCs are present which include:

1. **Dendritic cells (DCs)** which are most efficient to present antigen to naïve T cells
2. Macrophages and
3. B cells

Dendritic cells are present in larger amount in T cell dependent areas of lymph nodes and spleen. They are most effective APCs in activation of naïve T cells.

Dendritic cells pick up antigens by **pinocytosis** in **peripheral tissues** and **migrate to lymph nodes** where they express antigens and **initiate T cells activation.**

A small proportion of dendritic cells arrive in the lymph nodes though high venules (HEV) which have acquired antigen from lymph or transfer from other cells.

Macrophages and B cells are less effective than DCs at antigen presentation. Macrophages ingest micro-organisms, kill them in phagocytosis.

In **secondary immune response** (when concentration of antigen is low and other APCs cannot capture enough antigen), **B cells act as major antigen presenting cells** through their high affinity IgM and IgD receptors.

Antigen Processing

It involves degradation of antigen into peptides by action of proteases present in APCs. Only minority of peptide fragments are able to bind to particular MHC molecule.

Summary of key intercellular signals in T cells activation:
Binding between APCs and T cells occurs through adhesion molecules.

Antigen specific activation

- The specificity of reaction between antigenic peptide in MHC groove and TCR is basis of specificity of reaction and it ensures prolonged cell to cell contact. The bond formed between TCR and MHC/peptide has low affinity, interaction of other molecules of CD4 cells makes the binding more strong. These molecules increase sensitivity of T cell by its target antigen by approximately 100-fold.
- A second signal known as 'co-stimulatory signal' is necessary for T cells activation otherwise tolerance may develop.
- Most important **comolecules are B7s which include B-7-1(CD-80) and B 7-2 (CD-86).**
- B-7 co-receptors bind to CD28 and its homolog CTLA-4 (CD-152).
- CD28 stimulation prolongs and augments production of IL-2 and other cytokines and prevents induction of tolerance.

IL-2 drives the T cell division

Stimulation of CD28 increases production of IL2 and other cytokines. T cell activation leads to production of IL-2 and IL-2 receptors so that T cell can act on itself and surround cells.
Antigen presentation is not a unidirectional process.

Activated T cells produce:
- INFγ, granulocyte macrophages colony stimulation factors(GM-CSF) and
- Express CD154 (which binds to co-stimulatory molecule)

Activated APCs produce:
- IL-1, IL-6, TNF-α
- They express more MHC molecules, Fc receptors and co-stimulatory molecules.

Effects of activation of lymphocytes are:
1. Cell proliferation
2. Cell differentiation into effectors.

Fate of lymphocyte varies, some cells are short lived, some become long lived; memory cells.

Activation of Tcell requires:
Antigenic stimulus and
1. Co-stimulatory molecule or signals.
2. Signal transduction

Signal transduction: It is required for TH cell activation. CD + reacts with CD3 complex of TH cell which then pass on signals to TH activation.

Differentiation of TH cells:
- Binding of IL-2 binds to IL-R (receptor for IL-2) present on the surface of TH cells. Induction and proliferation of TH cells take place.
- TH cells become **blast cells** which then differentiate into effector T cells and memory cells. Effector cells further differentiate into TH1 and TH2 cells.

- **TH1 cells** produce IL-2, INFγ, and TNFβ.
- **TH2 cells** produce IL-4, 5, 6, 10, and 13 which activate B cells to produce antibodies (AMI or HI).
- Effector cells are cytotoxic T cells (Tc), NK cells, macrophages, neutrophils.
- Out of these effector cells, production of Tc is specific response.

Tc cells require three signals:
1. Antigen specific signal: Binding of TCR-CD3 complex to naïve Tc to MHC class I molecule.
2. Co-stimulatory signals: CD28 reacts with B7 present on target cells (e.g. viral infected cell).
3. IL-2 acts on high affinity IL-R (receptor for IL-2) on cytotoxic T cells.
4. Tc produces **performins and granzymes**.

Activation of B cells

Thymus-dependent antigens (TD) are taken and processed by APCs, presented to TH cells. Activated TH cells activate B cells (through cytokines). Thymus independent antigens (TI) stimulate B cells directly.

Antigen presentation of B cells to TH cells: Antigen is recognized by B cells with the help of surface immunoglobulin receptors. B cells process antigen and present to TH cells. It generates two signals.

Signal induction

Naïve B cells are in resting stage, the activation of which requires three signals.
The activation of resting B cells requires three signals.
1. Cross-linking of immunoglobulin molecules present on surface of B cells.
2. Signal 2 is generated by binding of B cell (CD40) with CD40B of TH cell.
3. Signal 3 is provided by cytokines secreted by activated TH cells which bind their receptors on B cells.

Signal transduction

B cell receptors (BCR) generate signals. The transmission of this signal is required for B cell activation. Antigen causes cross-linking of surface Igs which produce signals for B cells activation.

Proliferation and differentiation of B cells: It takes plane under the influence of cytokines produced by TH cells. The activated B cells differentiate into **centroblasts** which further transform into nondividing cells called **centerocytes** with membrane Ig. 'Somatic hypermutations' occur randomly, some Ig molecules with high affinity and some Ig molecules with low affinity are produced. **The centerocytes with low affinity Ig undergo apoptosis.** The **cells with high affinity Ig survive** undergo a process of **enhancement of affinity** of membrane Ig called as 'affinity maturation'.

Class switch over: Centerocytes bind to follicular dendritic cells undergo maturation and then class switch.
Early part immune response produces IgM. As the maturation progresses, other classes of Igs are produced by same B cell by class switch over. Centerocytes receive a positive signal from TH in the form of cytokine. Different cytokines induce production of different classes of Ig by switching mechanism.

Differentiation of centerocytes into plasma cells: After the class switch, the selected centerocytes further differentiate into effector cells (plasma cells) and memory cells.

Affinity maturation

Following primary immune response, antibodies with average affinity are produced. But it increases during process of activation. Clones of high affinity are produced which are selected, the process being called 'affinity maturation'. Individual B cells do not usually change their overall specifity; the affinity of antibody produced by a clone may be altered.

Affinity maturation is achieved by:

1. **Somatic hypermutation of region** including the recombined VDJ gene segment which encode variable domain of heavy chain.
2. IL-2 promotes B cell division, INFγ promotes affinity maturation and class switching to IgG2a which acts as opsonin and fixes complement.

Efferent Limb

It includes the production of antibody, its distribution in tissues and body fluids and the manifestations of its effects. Antibodies kill bacteria by opsonization or activating complement system or by cytotoxicity (ADCC). Antibodies can neutralize viruses.

Kinetics of Antibody Production

Antibody production follows a characteristic pattern consisting of lag phase, log phase, plateau or steady state and phase of decline.

- *Lag phase*: Following antigen entry till the formation of antibodies is lag phase. The reason why the antibody production requires time is, the antigen being new, it is recognized, processed and presented to TH cells which stimulate B cell to produce antibodies. This phase is important in clinical microbiology especially in the diagnosis of infections. For example, in typhoid fever, antibodies are formed in the second week of infection hence Widal test which detects antibodies, is positive in second week of infection and not in the first week. The 'window period' in HIV infection is also due to lag phase. Window period is time between infection till detection of antibodies.
- *Log phase*: Once antigen is recognized and immune system is stimulated, there is exponential production of antibodies.
- *Steady state*: Antibodies are chemically glycoproteins, their catabolism starts after their production hence after the log phase, a phase of steady state is reached.
- *Phase of decline*: Due to increased catabolism, antibody titer falls.

PRIMARY IMMUNE RESPONSE (Fig. 18.2)

First contact of immune system to an antigen (priming dose) leads to primary immune response, while subsequent contact with the same antigen leads **to secondary immune response**.

- The responding cell in primary response is naïve B cell (not exposed to Ag).
- The lag period following antigenic stimulation is 4–7 days.
- The time of peak response is 7–10 days; the magnitude of peak antibody response depends upon the antigen.
- The IgM predominates in early response.
- The antibody developed has low affinity.
- Both thymus-dependent and thymus-independent antigens produce primary response.

SECONDARY IMMUNE RESPONSE (Fig. 18.3)

If the person comes in contact with the same antigen again, the immune respose produced is called secondary response. The secondary respose is fast, exaggerated manner because the memory cells exist which retain memory of antigen. Hence, there is no lag period, antibody formed is mainly IgG. Antibodies titer is high.

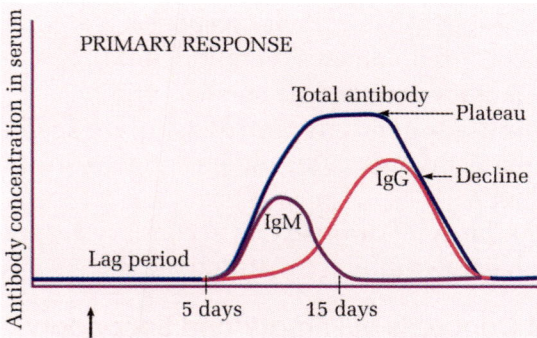

Fig. 18.2: Primary immune response

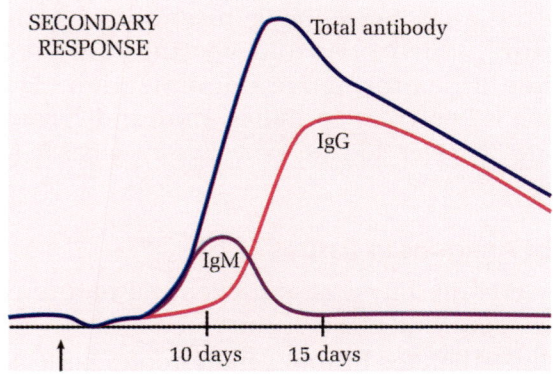

Fig. 18.3: Secondary immune response

TABLE 18.1: Differences between primary and secondary immune responses

Primary immune response	Secondary immune response
Responding naïve B-cell	Responding cell is memory B-cell
Lag period following antigenic administration is generally 4–7 days	Lag period is very short, it is 1–3 days
Slow, sluggish, and short lived	Prompt, powerful, prolonged
Long lag phase as antigen is first time coming in contact with immune system hence there is no memory	Lag phase is short, negligible as the antigen had prior contact and there is immunological memory
Antibody titer is low, they do not last long IgM is the predominant antibody formed	High antibody titre, lasts for a long time
More specific, less avid	IgG is the predominant antibody formed less specific, more avid

The characteristics of secondary response are:
- The responding cell is memory B cell.
- The lag period following antigenic contact is short; it is **1–3 days**.
- The time of peak antibody response is 3–5 days.
- The magnitude of antibody response is **100–1000** times higher than primary response.
- The IgG predominates (very little IgM).
- The antibody formed has higher affinity.
- Thymus-dependent antigens give secondary response; thymus-independent antigens do not have memory.
- The affinity of antibody in secondary response is much greater (affinity maturation).

Use of Concepts of Primary and Secondary Immune Response in Vaccination (Table 18.1)

A single injection of an antigen acts as sensitizing or priming dose. Effective levels of antibodies are produced after subsequent injections of antigens. Therefore, killed or toxoid vaccines are given in multiple doses for active immunization. The 1st injection is known as "priming" dose and subsequent ones are "booster" doses. With live vaccines, a single dose is sufficient.

Fate of Antigens in Tissues

It depends on: Physical and chemical nature of the antigen, dose, and route of entry.
- Antigens entered by intravenous route gets localized in the spleen, liver, bone marrow, kidneys and lungs.
- Antigens are broken down by the reticuloendothelial cells and excreted in the urine, about 70–80%, thus being eliminated in 1–2 days.
- Antigens entering subcutaneously are localized in the draining lymph nodes, only small amounts being found in the spleen.
- Particulate antigens are removed from circulation in 2 phases, namely the non-immune phase and the phase of immune elimination.
- Removal soluble antigen takes place in three steps, i.e. phase of **equilibrium**, metabolism and immune elimination.

Phagocytes engulf antigen and remove it (non-immune phase) while specific removal of antigen by antibody (opsonization) is phase of immune elimination.
- Antigen–antibody (Ag–Ab) complex formed in the phase of elimination may cause tissue damage leading to 'immune complex diseases' such as serum sickness.
- Protein antigen is eliminated within days or weeks whereas polysaccharide antigens persist for months or years.

Immune response to an antigen is brought about by three types of cells
- Antigen is captured by antigen-presenting cells (APCs). Antigen is broken down into small peptides which occupy groove of MHC class II molecule.
- APC give antigenic peptide to TH cells. TCR present on the surface of TH cell will take the antigen only if it is presented along with MHC class II (TH cells are MHC class II restricted).
- APC produces IL-1. The combination of TCR with the antigen and IL-1 stimulates TH cells.
- Another stimulus in the form of co-stimulatory molecule B7 is also required for T cell activation.
- IL-2, 4, 5, 6 are produced by TH cells cause growth and differentiation of B cells to plasma cells which start production of antibodies.
- If antigen is intracellular like virus, cell-mediate immunity takes part in immunity. CD8 cells are activated when they come in contact with antigen presented by APC along with class I MHC molecule, they are stimulated by IL-2 produced by TH cells.
- Activated Tc cells release cytotoxins which form holes on antigen (viral infected cell or tumor cell) by releasing perforin.

Signal transduction: After generation of signal, its transduction is initiated at CD4 molecule which interacts with CD3 complex which in turn transmit the signal leading to TH activation.

Differentiation of TH cells: Activated TH cells secrete IL-2 under the influence of which TH cells proliferate and differentiate into effecter cells and memory cells. Effector cells are further divided into TH1 and TH2 cells. Memory T cells are in resting stage but after antigenic stimulus they become activated and differentiated into effector cells.

FACTORS INFLUENCING ANTIBODIES PRODUCTION

Regulation of Immune Response

- The quality and quantity of immune response is determined by various factors including form, dose, route of inoculation of antigen.
- Antigen presenting cells
- Genetic background of person
- History of previous dose of antigen
- Any concurrent infection

Genetic Factors

The immune response is under genetic control. The terms '**responder**' and '**non-responder**' are used for individuals who are capable or not of responding to a particular antigen.

MHC class II region has immune regulatory (ir) genes which determine person's immune response.

Age

The embryo is immunologically immature. Production of antibodies starts only with the development and differentiation of lymphoid organs. Immune system continues to develop as infants grow. Antibody production starts after 3–6 months of age and full competence is acquired only about 5–7 years for IgG and 10–15 years for IgA. Peoples at extremes of life are susceptible for infections. Premature infants are susceptible for sepsis because of their immature immune system.

Nutritional Status

Proteins are glycoproteins and other enzymes as well as cytokines required in immunity are proteins, hence in malnutrition, immune system is suppressed. It affects CMI also. Protein calorie malnutrition suppresses both humoral and cellular immune responses. Deficiency of amino acids and vitamins has negative effect on decrease antibodies production. Children with protein energy malnutrition in India suffer from measles.

Route of Administration

Response is better following parenteral administration of antigen than through oral or nasal routes. It may also influence the type of antibody produced. For production of IgA antibodies which give local protection, the oral or nasal route is most suitable. Hence, vaccines against infections of GIT and respiratory tract are useful in preventing infections. Oral polio vaccine produces good local immunity. Inhalation of pollen induces IgE synthesis, whereas the same antigen given parenterally induces IgG synthesis. With some antigens, it may determine whether tolerance or antibody response develops.

Size and the Numbers of Doses

Antibody response is dose dependent. Antibody production only occurs if antigen dose more than critical dose. Increase in dose enhances the intensity of response. If antigenic dose exceeds a particular level increase in response is not seen but may even inhibit it or induce tolerance. Very high dose of antigen suddenly sometimes causes '**immune paralysis**' name given by Felton.

Antigen

- Intracellur antigen, as viruses, induces CMI, extracellular antigen as bacteria AMI is important.
- *Dose*: It should be over a threshold level to mount an immune response. Very high dose causes tolerance.
- *Route of administration*:
  - Antigens given subcutaneously or intradermally initiate good response.
  - Antigen given by intravenous route or oral route or as aerosol may cause tolerance or immune deviation from one type of CD+ cell to other.

Multiple antigens: If two or more antigens are administered simultaneously, the effects may vary. Antibodies may be produced against different antigens, as though they were given separately or antibody response to one or the other may be enhanced or the response to one or the other may be diminished (antigenic competition).

As bacteria have different antigens present on them, the response to different antigens varies. Following infection with *Salmonella*, antibodies against flagellar '**H**' antigen are more as compared to cell wall antigen-'**O**', because '**H**' is comparatively strong immunogen.

Regulation by APC

- If antigen is presented by non-professional APC, it is unable to give co-stimulatory signal, tolerance or deviation may result.
- Dendritic cells or macrophages produce IL-12 and TGF beta which can drive conversion of naïve CD4 cells to T cells into regulatory T cells which act as suppressor.

Treg cells regulate immune response and prevent tolerance. They can also suppress virus specific responses.

NK cell secrete INF2 which plays important role in immune response against viruses.

Regulation by Antibody

- Some vaccines are given only after one year of age because passively transferred antibody takes 6 months to clear which would otherwise result into inadequate immune response.

- In case Rh incompatibility, anti-D antibody to fetal antigen given to mother will remove antigen, i.e. Rh (RBCs).
- Passively transferred antibody binds to antigen in competition with B cells (antibody blocking).
- Antibody may form immune complex which can augment or inhibit immune response.

Genetic Factors

MHC genes or MHC-related genes control immune response.

Adjuvants

Adjuvant refers to any substance that enhances the immunogenicity of an antigen. They may confer immunogenicity on non-antigenic substances, increase the concentration and persistence of the circulating antibodies, induce or enhance the degree of cellular immunity. Substances that can be used as adjuvants include:

1. Fruend's incomplete adjuvant which is an antigen incorporated in water phase of water in oil emulsion.
2. Fruend's complete adjuvant which is combination of Fruend's incomplete adjuvant and killed TB bacilli.
3. Aluminium phosphate, aluminium hydroxide.

Types of Adjuvant

Depot: Fruend's incomplete adjuvant (water in oil), aluminium hydroxide and aluminium phosphate (repository adjuvants) form depot from which antigen is slowly released.

Bacterial: Fruend's complete adjuvant (Fruend's incomplete Ag+ killed *Mycobacterium tuberculosis*, *Mycobacterium vaccae*.

- **BCG**
- Killed *Pertussis* bacillus
- *Propionobacterium acne*

Chemicals: Bentonite, calcium alginate, silica particles Adjuvants suitable for laboratory animals are:

- Fruend's complete adjuvant which is given with soluble antigen to raise antisera against it.
- Bacterial endotoxin
- Fungal polysaccharide

Mechanisms of Action of Adjuvant

- *Depot formation*: Adjuvant forms a depot with antigen which is released slowly so that prolonged antigenic stimulus is given to immune system.
- Increased antigenic uptake by macrophages
- Activation of macrophages
- Stimulate CMI

Immunosuppressive Agents

In transplantation, in order to prevent rejection, recepient's immunity should be dampened. For this reason, immunosuppressant is required. Immunosuppressive agents include X-ray irradiation, radiomimetic drugs, corticosteroids, antimetabolites and antilymphocytic serum.

1. *X-ray irradiation* is more toxic to multiplying cells, they improve the graft survival.

   Whole body irradiation: Irradiation is given in such dose that it will kill the body cells(sub-lethal dose). If irradiation is given before 24 hours of antigen exposure, antibody production is inhibited and if irradiation is given 2–3 hours before exposure to an antigen, the antibody response is enhanced.

2. *Radiomimetic drugs*: These are alkylating drugs as cyclophosphamide, nitrogen mustard. Cyclophosphamide suppresses antibody response (selectively inhibits B cell response).

3. *Corticosteroids*:
   - They cause depletion of lymphocytes from blood and lymphoid tissues.
   - They have anti-inflammatory action
   - They decrease responsiveness of both T and B cells.

4. *Antimetabolites*: They inhibit nucleic acid synthesis, inhibit cell division and differentiation of immune cells. Antimetabolites are:
   - Folic acid antagonists—methotrexate.
   - Purine analogues-6 mercaptourine, azithioprine.
   - Uracil

6. *Cyclosporine*: It selectively inhibits T cell activity.

7. *Antilymphocytic serum*: It prevents graft rejection. It is effective against T lymphocytes.

Effect of antibody: The humoral immune response can be inhibited by passive administration of homologous antibody. The action appears by a feedback mechanism. Primary response is more susceptible to inhibition than the secondary response.

Anti-D immunoglobulin given to Rh-mothers acts by negative feedback mechanism.

MONOCLONAL ANTIBODIES (Figs 18.4 and 18.5)

Definition: Antibodies produced by a single clone and directed against a single antigenic determinant are called as monoclonal antibodies.

(Georges Kohler and Cesar Milstein developed the hybridoma technology).

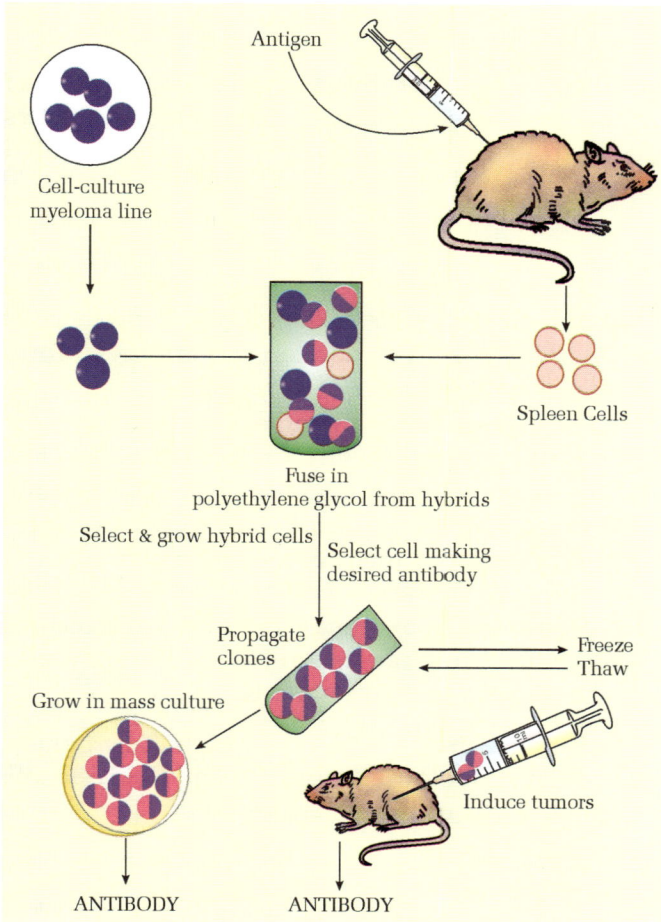

Fig. 18.4: Hybridoma technology for production of monoclonal antibodies

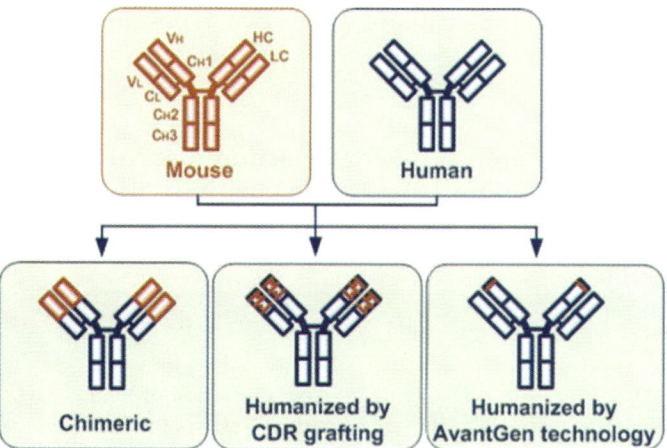

Fig. 18.5: Monoclonal antibodies

Production of Antibodies by Hybridoma Technology

Methodology

A hybridoma, which can be considered as a harry cell, is produced by the injection of a specific antigen into a mouse, procuring the antigen-specific plasma cells

(antibody-producing cell) from the mouse's spleen and the subsequent fusion of this cell with a cancerous immune cell called a myeloma cell.

The hybrid cell, which is thus produced, can be cloned to produce many identical daughter clones. These daughter clones then secrete the immune cell product. Since these antibodies come from only one type of cell (the hybridoma cell), they are called monoclonal antibodies.

The advantage of this process is that it can combine the qualities of the two different types of cells; the ability to grow continually, and to produce large amounts of pure antibody.

Hypoxanthine aminopetrin thymidine (HAT) medium is used for preparation of monoclonal antibodies.

Laboratory animals (e.g. mice) are first exposed to an antigen to which we are interested in isolating an antibody against.

Once splenocytes are isolated from the mammal, the B cells are fused with immortalized myeloma cells which lack the HGPRT (hypoxanthine-guanine phosphoribosyl transferase) gene using polyethylene glycol or the Sendai virus.

Fused cells are incubated in the HAT medium. Myeloma cells die, as they cannot produce nucleotides by the de novo or salvage medium blocks the pathway that allows for nucleotide synthesis. Unfused cells die.

Unfused B cells have a short lifespan. Only the B cell-myeloma hybrids survive, since the HGPRT gene coming from the B cells is functional. These cells produce antibodies (a property of B cells) and are immortal (a property of myeloma cells).

As mouse monoclonal antibodies can induce immune response, they are not suitable for human use. Also Fc portion of mouse could not initiate effector defense mechanisms. Various modifications were done. Cleaved Fab fragments could be coupled to various active substances as toxins, enzymes, and cytotoxic drugs. Mouse monoclonal antibodies have been humanized by genetic manipulations to make chimeric antibodies.

Antibiotic Engineering

Chimeric antibodies: Genes are desired and constructed in such a manner that variable region gene is taken from mouse and constant region from human. New genes link nucleotide sequences coding nonantibody proteins with sequences that encode antibody variable regions specific for particular antigens. These molecular hybrids called as chimeras. They can deliver toxin to tumor cells only without affecting normal cells, so that tumor cells will be destructed. This antibody produced is called as "**immunotoxin**".

Uses of Monoclonal Antibodies (Table 18.2)

In vitro Diagnostic

- Leukocyte detection
- Lymphocyte subsets detection
- HLA antigen detection
- Viral detection, subtyping, e.g. influenza virus, parasitic identification
- Hormone detection
- Detection of carcinoembryogenic antigens
- Typing of leukemias

Immunohistochemical Application in Tissue Sections

- Detecting pregnancy
- Diagnosing pathogenic microorganisms.
- Measuring drug levels in blood.

(Radiolabeled monoclonal antibodies can be used *in vivo* to detect or locate tumor antigens, e.g. MAb to breast cancer cells labeled with Iodine-131).

Therapeutic

Antitumor therapy, immunosuppression, treatment GHV, fertility control: antiHSG antibodies.

CELL-MEDIATED IMMUNITY

Tc-Mediated Cytotoxicity

Cell-mediated cytotoxicity is function of cytotoxic Tc cells and also the function of other cells as macrophages, NK cells, and K cells. The type of receptor binding with cells involved in cytotoxicity is viral antigen expressed on the surface of host cell recognized by MHC class I of Tc cells.

Virus antigen is expressed on the surface of virus infected cells. Antibody binds to these antigen. Its Fc portion binds with Fc receptors present on cytotoxic cells (Tc or NK). It causes antibody-mediated cell cytotoxicity. The lysis is due to several factors as perforins, lymphotoxins, TNFα and natural killer, cytotoxic factor. Perforin resembles with action of membrane attack complex of complement. TNFα enters and destroys cell by programmed cell death called 'apoptosis'.

Mechanisms of Cell-Mediated Toxigenicity

- Cytotoxic lymphoid cell releases **perforins** and various enzymes near the target cell. In presence of Ca⁺⁺, there is polymerization of perforin to form channels on the surface of target cells.
- Degradative enzymes and other toxic substances of Tc enter the target through the new channels formed.
- **TNFα** from Tc cells, macrophages, **INF gamma either** from Tc cells or nearby macrophages trigger the target cells via their receptors. Susceptible cells die. There is increased activity of target cell cyclo-oxygenase and lipoxygenase pathway which causes intracellular free radicals release. There are also changes in the protein synthesis.

The mechanisms by which monocyte–macrophage series may contribute to cytotoxicity of myeloid cells are:

- Cationic protein
- Hydrolases
- Superoxide ions
- Reactive oxygen intermediates, nitric oxides
- TNF alpha

Tests for Detection of CMI

The tests can be classified into two types, *in vivo* test and *in vitro* tests

In vivo Test

Skin tests are useful for detection of CMI *in vivo*. These tests detect the hypersensitivity to common antigens which body comes in contact. Tuberculin PPD,

TABLE 18.2: Some monoclonal antibodies in clinical use (immunotherapy)

Monoclonal antibody	Nature of antibody	Target	Use
Muromonab	Mouse mAB	T cell CD3, a T cell antigen	Acute rejection of liver, heart, kidney transplant
Inflixibmab (Remicade)	Human–mouse chimeric	Tumor necrosis factor α	Rheumatoid arthritis Crohn's disease
Rituximab	Human mouse chimeric antibody	CD-20, a B cell antigen	Refractory nonHodgkin's lymphoma
Palivizumab	Human–mouse children chimeric antibody	F protein of respiratory syncytial virus	RSV infections in children
Gemtuzumab	Humanized	CD33 an adhesion molecule (many cells of myeloid lineage)	Acute myeloid leukemia

dinitrochlorobenzene (DNB) or dinitrofluorobenzene are used as antigens in testing the hypersensity. Normal people respond by showing delayed type of response. Absence of the reactions indicates cellular immunodeficiency.

In Vitro Tests

MIF test: Sub quantitative measurement of CMI is possible by this test. Human WBCs stimulated by antigen are incubated in capillary tube, in culture chambers containing culture fluid. In presence of antigen, the WBCs are prevented from migration while in absence of the antigen the WBCs migrate out to the open end of capillary tube in fan-like pattern.

Lymphocyte blast formation test: If a lymphocyte is stimulated by some antigens as concavalin or phytohemagglutinin, it is converted into blast cell. During blast formation of lymphocytes, there is increase in the DNA synthesis. Increase in the DNA synthesis can be measured by incorporation of tritiated thymidine.

Enumeration of T cell, B cell and subpopulations: Fluorescent-activated cell sorter is used to count the number of each cell type. Cells are mixed with monoclonal antibodies tagged with fluorescent dye as rhodamine. The number of cells that fluorose is registered by passing those single cells through a laser light beam. The total number of B cells can be counted by using fluorescent labeled antibodies against all immunoglobulin classes (B cell receptor). Monoclonal antibodies directed against T cell markers allow counting of T cells, and their subpopulation. The CD4, CD8 cell ratio is counted; in normal persons, it is 1.5 or more but becomes lesser than 1 in persons with AIDS.

Rosette formation: T lymphocytes when mixed with sheep RBCs, the RBCs attach to the T cell forming a structure called **E-rosette formation**. The rosette is a T lymphocyte to which three or more sheep RBCs are attached. The T cells can be counted by counting the rosettes. This test is useful to detect T cell hence it detects CMI of the host.

Transfer Factor

The first transfer of CMI was detected by injection of the extract of leukocytes of a person sensitized with an antigen. The extract contains soluble substances called as transfer factor. Transfer of this factor from one person to another person would transfer CMI to the antigen which sensitized the donor and immune response as that of donor. Transfer factor acts probably by stimulating the release of lymphokines from sensitized T cells. This transferred immunity is specific to the antigen which has sensitized the donor. The immunity which is transferred is systemic. TF is low molecular weight (2000–4000 Da) nucleopeptide which is not antigenic and the action of which is unknown. It is resistant to the action of DNAse, RNAse, and trypsin.

Uses of Transfer Factor

- It may be useful in disseminated diseases associated with deficiency of CMI as TB, lepromatous leprosy.
- Treatment of cancers as malignant melanoma.
- Treatment of congenital immunodeficiency disorders as T cell deficiencies.

Induction of Cell-Mediated Immunity (CMI)

- Antigenic nature is important factor for induction of CMI.
- Intracellular organisms as **Mycobacterium tuberculosis, Mycobacterium leprae, viruses** are best inducers of CMI as these are intracellular organism where antibodies cannot reach.
- Killed vaccines and other non-living antigens if combined with Freund adjuvant, induce CMI.
- Antigens coming contact with skin and causing delayed type of hypersensitivity (**skin allergens**).
- Induce CMI to produce those allergic reactions.
- Helper T cells after activation due to antigen produce cytokines which stimulate macrophages. Activated macrophages kill intracellular organisms, thus induce CMI.
- CMI is also induced by **viral infected cells, tumor cells,** foreign antigen present in **allografts** stimulate Tc cells producing CMI.

CYTOKINES

These are biologically active substances secreted by monocytes, lymphocytes, and other immune and non-immune cells which are actively involved in innate immunity, adaptive, i.e. acquired immunity, and inflammatiom. Cytokines are the proteins of low molecular weight which regulate important biological processes—cell growth, cell activation, inflammation, immunity, tissue repair, fibrosis and morphogenesis. Cytokines are peptide mediators or intercellular messengers. They are hormone-like substances active in small concentrations.

They are currently used as biological response modifier **or immunomodulators**. They are synthesized as and when needed in immune responses. Many cytokines are produced by many cells and act on many cells means, they are pleiotropic and in many instances they have similar actions which is due the nature of receptors. They **differ from hormones** that they are not produced by specific cells or glands and many cytokines are produced by many cells.

Autocrine effect: Acting on the same cell which has produced that cytokine.

Paracrine effect: Acting on adjacent cell

Endocrine effect: Acting on cell present at distant site.

Cytokines usually work together and there are many interactions among themselves.

Cytokine Interactions

- *Pleiotropy effect*: Same cytokine may have different actions on different cells.
- *Rudimentary effect*: Different cytokines may produce same effect on acting a cell.
- *Synergy*: Two cytokines may work with each other in such a way that they increase working of each other.
- *Antagonism effect*: It may occur when two cytokines produce oppositive effects.

Biologically active substances released by an activated T cell were called **lymphokines.** Similar substances secreted by monocytes were called monokines. All the lymphokines show multiple effects and multiple effects were produced by same lymphokines, hence the term lymphokine was considered unsuitable. Thereafter, term interleukin was introduced for the products of lynphokine which have effect on other cells. Later on, it was found that these sets of interferons, growth factors and others have same biological effects, hence all substances were grouped into cytokine. But while describing the many cytokines, their original names retained.

Categories

Cytokines Affecting Macrophages

- Macrophage chemotactic factors cause accumulation of the cells at the site where antigen-mediated release takes place.
- Migration of inhibiting factor inhibits migration of phagocytic cells and localizes circulating and tissue monocytes at the site of infection.
- *Interferon γ*: This is macrophage-activating factor so that macrophage becomes activated such that it can kill organisms.
- INF-α—it has antiviral activity.
- Interferon-β, and INF-γ are produced by fibroblasts, and inhibit replication of viruses.

Cytotoxic Cytokines

TNF-α produced by monocytes and macrophages causes lysis of tumor cells; along with IL-1 it acts in causing cachexia. It resembles IL-1 and has many biological activities as manifestation of endotoxic shock, it is also strong immunomodulator.

Other Cytokines

TGF-β: It has the ability to transfer fibroblasts, also acts as growth factor for fibroblasts, causes wound healing.

Interferons (INF): There are three classes, INF-α produced by WBCs, INF-β produced by fibroblasts, INF-γ gamma produced by activated T cells. INF-γ causes immunological effects as it causes activation of macrophage, enhances function of PMNs.

Interleukin-1 (leukocyte-activating factor or B cell-activating factor): It is secreted by macrophages and monocytes but can be produced by most nuclear cells. It is a stable polypeptide, activity up to 56°C and pH between 3 and 11. It occurs in two forms, i.e. IL1 α and IL1 β.

Immunological effects of IL1 are:
- It stimulates T cells to produce IL2 and other cytokines.
- It stimulates B cell proliferation and helps in synthesis of antibodies.
- It is called endogenous pyrogen.
- Together with TNF-α, it causes many hematological changes in septic shock and also enhances initial meningeal inflammation in bacterial meningitis.
- It stimulates neutrophils chemotaxis and phagocytes.
- It mediates many metabolic, physiological, inflammatory and hematological effects.

IL2
- It is produced by activated T cells.
- It is important immunomodulator of immune response.
- It acts as T cell growth factor.
- It causes growth and differentiation of T and B cells.
- It also stimulates Tc and NK cells. In its presence, large granular lymphocytes are converted into lymphokine-activated killer cells (LAK cells).

IL3
- It acts as growth factor for bone marrow stem cells. Its main function is that, it stimulates multiple lineage hemopoiesis hence called as **multiple colony stimulatory factors (CSF).**
- It produces class switching within B cell.

IL4

- It is produced mainly by TH cells and macrophages.
- Stimulates development of TH2.
- Stimulates T cells to produce other cytokines.
- It is required for TH.
- It activates resting B cells and acts as B cell growth factor and B cell differentiation factor.
- It enhances action of cytotoxic Tc.
- It promotes synthesis of IgE.

IL5: Produced by T cell, it promotes the growth and differentiation of B cells and eosinophil. It enhances synthesis of IgA.

IL6: It is produced by T cell, B cell, and macrophages, which stimulates the production acute phase proteins in liver.

IL7: Produced by spleen and bone marrow stromal cells, it acts as T cell and B cell growth factor.

IL8: Produced by macrophage mainly, it acts as neutrophil chemotactic factor.

IL9: Produced by T cell and helps in growth and proliferation.

IL10, 11, 12 affect lymphocytes.

IL10 is produced by activated macrophages and TH2 cells, it inhibits the production of interferon γ by TH-1 cells which shifts immune response to TH2 type. IL-11 inhibits acute phase proteins. IL-12 produced by T cells which activates NK cells. IL-13 produced by T cells inhibits functions of mononuclear cells.

Cytokines Based Therapies in Clinical Use (Table 18.3)

- INF-α 2a: *HBV*, hairy cell leukemia, kaposis sarcoma
- INF-α 2b: *Hepatitis C virus*, melanoma
- INF-β 1a, 1b: Multiple sclerosis

TABLE 18.3: Uses of cytokines

Organisms	Cytokine
Hepatitis A virus	INF-α (usually given with ribavirin)
HBV	INF-α (used if mutants develop during long therapy with lamivudine)
HIV	INF-α, IL-2 (given intermittently)
MTB	INF-γ (aerosolized treatment given on trial basis)
M. leprae	INF-γ, IL-2 (bacterial number reduced when given in the lesions in experimental animals)
Aspergillosis	INF-γ (given to patients with chronic granulomatous disease)

- INF-γ 1b: Chronic granulomatous disease
- Monoclonal antibody against TNF-α receptor: Rheumatoid disease, Crohns's disease.

Cytokines Related Diseases

- Septic shock
- Overproduction of proinflammatory cytokine as TNF-α and IL-1β occurs. Cytokine imbalance causes high body temperature, respiratory rate, WBC count, followed by capillary leakage, tissue injury, and lethal organ failure.
- **Toxic shock syndrome** is due to superantigens as TSST1 production by staphylococci, pyrogenic exotoxin from *Streptococcus pyogenes*, Mycoplasma arthritis supernant (MAS): Induce high levels of IL-1, TNF-α.

Viruses use following anti-cytokine strategies:
- *Production of homologs*: E-B virus produces IL-10 homolog, HSV-6 produces IL-6 homolog, CMV chemokine receptor homolog.
- Production of soluble cytokines binding proteins.
- Homologs of cytokines receptors.
- Interference with cytokine production.
- Interference with intracellular signaling.
- Induction of cytokines inhibitors in cells.

IMMUNOLOGICAL TOLERANCE

Contact with antigen produces immulogical unresponsiveness instead of mounting a immune response. Any antigen that comes into contact with the immunological system during embryonic life would be recognized as a self-antigen, this is called '**specific immunological tolerance**.

Immunological tolerance is state of unresponsive to particular antigen which is primarily established in T and B lymphocytes. The breakdown of tolerance results in autoimmunity.

Central Tolerance

Central tolerance refers to mechanisms of tolerance acting during lymphocyte development in the thymus or bone marrow. It is mostly due to the elimination or inactivation of those T and B cells that recognize self-antigens. These cells are destroyed or inactivated after they have expressed receptors for self-antigens and before they develop into fully immunocompetent lymphocytes. Deletion of self-reactive cells at an early stage in their development has been termed 'clonal abortion' or 'clonal deletion'. In early fetal life, self-reactive lymphocytes that are part of the developing immune system are deleted when exposed to self-antigens. As mentioned above, new immunologically competent cells are generated throughout life and these must be continuously deleted or inactivated also.

Peripheral Tolerance

It refers to many different mechanisms which develop and maintain T cells tolerance outside the thymus.

1. The **mechanisms** include prevention of contact between autoreactive T cells and their target antigens (immunological ignorance). The self-reactive cells (T cell) might never encounter the self-antigen.

2. Peripheral deletion of autoreactive T cells by activation induced death or cytokine withdrawal, the incapacity of T cells to mount immune response upon recognition of self-antigen which is called immunological ignorance.

3. Suppression of immune responses by regulatory cells.

B Cell Tolerance

- Clonal deletion of autoreactive B cells occurs mostly in bone marrow.

- Rearrangement of autoreactive B cells called **B cell anergy.**

- Suppression of immune responses by **regulatory T cells.**

- Antibody production by class switch depends upon stimulation by T cells, hence tolerance of T cells affects class switch and B cells that recognize that antigen remain tolerant.

- *Anergy*: Immunological unresponsiveness to antigenic stimulus. APC may bind to antigen without co-stimulatory signals.

- Self-reactive T cells may react with APC carrying self-antigen undergo full activation but produce nonpathogenic cytokines, hence tolerance occurs.

- *Apoptosis by ACID*: APC present antigen to T cells causing upregulation **Fas island** which then reacts with death receptors, leading apoptosis.

- Treg cells may downregulate self-regulatory T cells.

- *Phenotypic skewing*: After presentation of self antigen by APC's, wrong set of cytokines are released.

- Tolerance can occur in an embryo, newborns or adults; tolerance may be total or partial, short-lived or long-lasting.

- Tolerance can be induced in adults interrupted by immunosuppressive agents.

- Physical state of the antigen is important—soluble antigens and haptens are more tolerogenic than particulate antigens.

- Tolerance can be overcome spontaneously or by injection of crossreacting immunogens.

Mechanisms of Tolerance (Flowchart 18.2)

Clonal deletion: During the embryonic life, clones of immune cells are produced which would mount response against self-antigens. Such clones are deleted in the embryonic life.

Clonal anergy: Clones capable of mounting immune response are might be present but remain inert.

Suppression: In this mechanism, the clones of immune cells that recognize self-antigens are preserved but expression of immune responses following antigen presentation might be suppressed.

Flowchart 18.2: Mechanisms of tolerence

Clonal deletion: Clones of lymphocyte potentially capable of mounting response against cell antigens are eliminated. This clonal deletion is thought to occur in thymus during T cell maturation. Even the newly developed cells do not leave as they are forbidden self reactive clones. Clonal deletion may be seen in B cell but it is slow.

Suppressed T cells

The response of lymphocytes in a clone may be actively inhibited by suppressor T cell.

Clonal anergy

Functional inactivation of T cell. Specific clones may be present but they may have received signals through the receptor system and thus may be less responsive to antigen. Function inactivation has also been observed when an antigen is presented to cells without co-stimulatory signals or molecules.

Types of Tolerance

Natural Tolerance

This develops during embryonic life. The antigen coming contact with immune system during embryonic life is recognized as self-antigen; hence body doesn't mount immune response against the exposed antigens. Naturally occurring tolerance seen in congenital rubella, cytomegalovirus infections in which there is persistent viremia with a decreased ability for the production of neutralizing antibodies [persistent tolerance infection]. When tolerance is interrupted by an induction of antibody or an injection of sensitized lymphocytes, disease results.

- *Acquired tolerance*: This is developed when a particular antigen induces tolerance.
- *Artificial tolerance* can be induced by injection of antisera, cytotoxic drugs.
- *Split tolerance*: Tolerance of either AMI or CMI without affecting other.

The degree of tolerance depends upon following factors (Fig. 18.6):

- *Dose dependent*: Higher doses or small doses produce tolerance, while intermediate doses cause immune reaction.
- *Species of animals*: Rabbits and mice are easily tolerogenic than guinea pigs.

- *Route of administration*: The route which causes equilibrium of antigen between extravascular and intravascular compartments is more capable of inducing tolerance. Higher the degree of immunocompetence of host, the more difficult it is to induce tolerance.

Acquired Tolerance

Tolerance in later life may occur under special situations. Higher doses of antigens may induce tolerance.

Specific Immunological Tolerance

In specific immunological tolerance, immune response is absent against a particular group. It may be due to clonal deletion or production of tolerant immunocompetent cells by antigen itself.

Naturally occurring tolerance is observed in some vertical transmission of viruses from mother to fetus without any pathological effect, e.g congenital rubella viruses multiply in fetus without any disease. But this tolerance is lost by giving antibody, the fetus suffers from disease.

THEORIES OF ANTIBODIES FORMATION OR IMMUNE RESPONSE (Fig. 18.7)

Instructive theories: These suggest that an immunocompetent cell is capable of synthesizing antibody of any specificity.

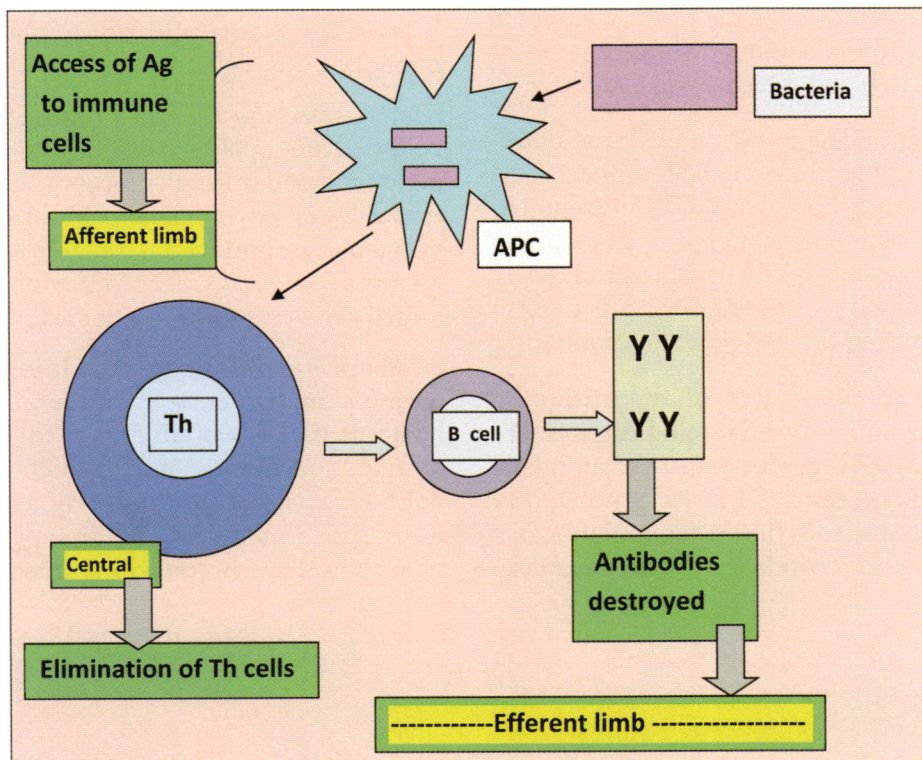

Fig. 18.6: Different levels of immune response where tolerance can be achieved

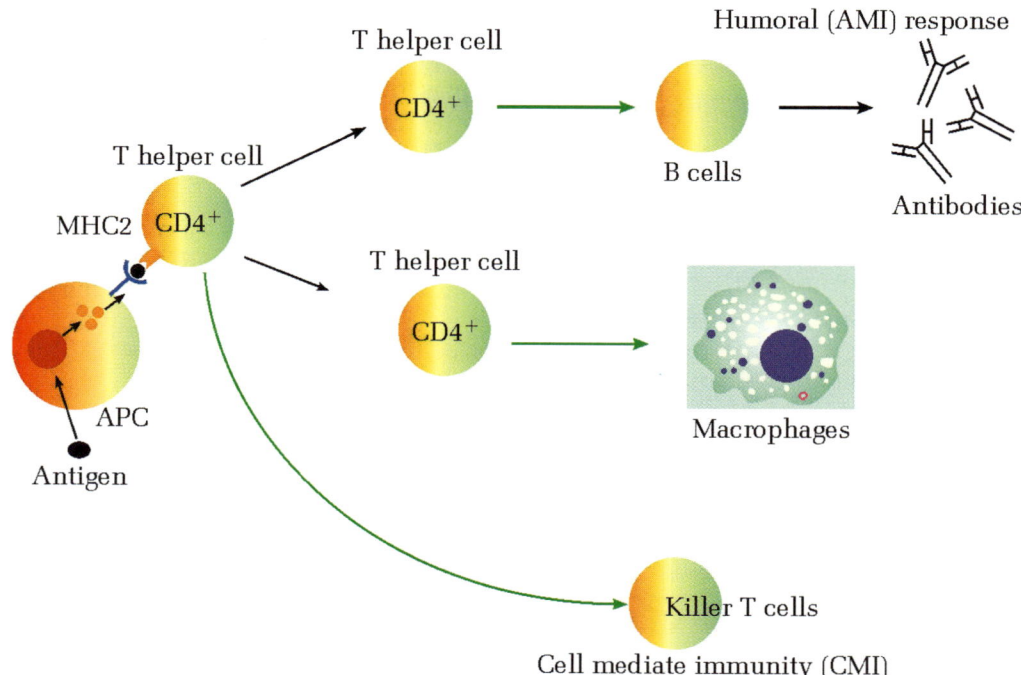

Fig. 18.7: Immune response

Selective theories: These suggest that immunocompetent cells have only a restricted immunological range.

Side chain theory: Ehrlich proposed side chain theory. It was proposed that cells bearing receptors with capacity to react with substances having complementary side chains. Foreign antigens enter and combine with these cellular receptors. The overproduction causes spillage of receptors in blood which act like antibodies.

Direct template theory: The antigen/antigenic determinant enters the antibody forming cells and acts as a template against which antibody molecules are synthesized which can combine with complementary sites on antigen. Pauling suggested specificity is determined by the folding of the antibody polypeptide chains to form a tertiary structure fitting the antigenic determinant.

Indirect template theory: Entry of the antigenic determinant into the antibody producing cell induces in it a heritable change. A 'genocopy' of the antigenic determinant is thus incorporated in its genome and transmitted to its progeny cells (indirect template). This explained specificity and secondary immune response.

Natural selection theory: A million of globulin (Ab) molecules were formed in embryonic life, which covered full range of antigenic specificities—called 'natural antibodies'. Antigen combined selectively with the globulin that had the nearest complementary 'fit'. Here selection was postulated at the antibody molecule level. This theory did not explain immunological memory of the cells.

Clonal selection theory: Proposed by Burnet (1957), cells that are capable of reacting with different antigens are developed during embryonic life. Out of these, the forbidden clones of cells capable of reaction against self-antigens are removed. Contact of cells with antigen results in activation and proliferation to generate clones which can synthesize antibodies.

Network hypothesis (Jerne): Idiotype of antibody is amino acid sequence at antigen combining site and adjacent part of variable part. Idiotype can act as an antigen and can induce production of anti-idiotypic antibody. Part of this antibody again acts as antigen leading to formation of anti-idiotypic antibody. Network of such antibodies controls antibody formation.

19

Autoimmunity

DEFINITION

Autoimmunity is a condition in which structural or functional damage is produced by the action of immunologically competent cells or antibodies against the normal components of the body. Auto means self, immunity means immune response. It, however, instead of causing protective immune responses, causes damage. Normally, body does not mount immune response against self antigens, as immunoreactive cells capable of mounting immune responses are eliminated in embryonic life (forbidden clones).

Ehrlich (1910) postulated the concept of **horror auto-toxicus.** He observed that goats produced antibodies against RBCs of other goats but not against their own RBCs.

Diseases of autoimmune origin mostly show following characteristics:

- Levels of normal immunoglobulins are raised.
- Autoantibodies are formed which can be demonstrated, e.g. by immunofluorescence test.
- Immunoglobulins or antibodies get deposited at certain sites where there is high turbulence of blood as glomerular basement membrane.
- Lymphocytes and plasma cells infiltrate the sites of their deposition.
- Incidence is higher in females and there may be a genetic factor which predisposes for autoimmunity.
- More than one lesion of autoimmune origin present in body.
- Course is chronic, get some benefit from corticosteroids or other immunosuppressive agents.

MECHANISMS (Flowchart 19.1)

Sequestered Antigen or Hidden Antigens

There are certain antigens to which there is no access to antibody forming cells (privileged sites) during embryonic life, e.g. lens and uveal tract of eye, sperm, CNS tissue and thymoglobulin.

They are not recognized as self-antigen by immune system. When these are released in circulation after birth due to injury, they elicit an immune response. Following injury to lens, lens protein is released which is considered by immune system as non-self, hence immune response is mounted against lens proteins which damages lens of the injured as well as noninjured side (phecoanaphylaxis). Similar patho-genesis is applied to orchitis following mumps. Mumps causes damage to seminiferous tubules, sperms are released, body will mount immune response causing orchitis. (This is **'sequestration in time'** because sperms are not developed during embryonic life hence they are not exposed to immune apparatus before.)

Tolerance against these antigens is not developed during embryonic life as antigens are not exposed to immune system.

Spermatozoa are not formed during embryonic life, they develop after puberty. Therefore, spermatozoa antigen is not exposed to immune system during embryonic life. As tolerance is not developed against spermatozoa in embryonic life, antibodies produced against them produce damage.

Altered Antigen or Neoantigens

Tissue antigens may be altered by drugs, injury or disease or due to somatic mutation or by chemical influences, so that it is no longer recognised as "self", e.g. in rheumatoid arthritis, denaturation of gamma globulin occurs. During viral infections, new cell surface antigens called neoantigens appear, which induce antibodies production active against other molecules.

Example: Drug combines with platelet changing its surface, hence antigenic structure of our own platelets is changed, and body mounts a response against platelets, leading to purpura, e.g. chemical (2-mercaptoethanol).

Flowchart 19.1: Mechanisms of autoimmmunity

sequestrated or hidden antigen

•1.Lens antigen of eye-- injury to eye releases antigen, damages other eye also (phaecoanaphylaxis)

2.Sperms- released after damage to seminiferous tubules , leading mumps orchitic

Neoantigens

•Physicial agents changing normal antigenicity of cell or tissues

•Photosensitivity cold allergy

•chemicals -drugs cause contact dernititis

•Drug induced anemia, leucopenias, thrombocytopenic purpura sedormid perpura

•Biological agents altering antigenecity

•Neuraminidase of influenza virus causes change in cell antigen , they act on RBCs releasing T natigen

Cross reacting antigens (molucular mimcry)

Immune response against one antigen causes damage of human tissue.

e.g. gacute rheumatic fever(Streptococcal AG cross react with myocardium

In glomerulonephritis antibodies get deposited on glomerular basement membrane

Breakdown of tolerance, release of cells capable of mounting immune response against self antigens

T cell & B cell defects

Genetic factors

Exposure of cryptic epitopes: During antigen processing, there are some nondominant epitopes which remain sequestrated. If due to injury they are released, it may lead to autoimmunity.

Heterophile or Crossreacting Foreign Antigens (Molecular Mimcry)

Infectious agents, as *Streptococcus*, cause production of antibodies against itself. As myocardial proteins of human have some similarity with *Streptococcus* (myocardium contains determinants similar to components of the host's body—heterophile Ag), antibodies formed in response to a microorganism may damage the tissues that share the crossreacting determinants, e.g. M protein in rheumatic heart disease. (This is also called a molecular mimicry coxsackie virus and myocardium, *Mycobacterium tuberculosis* and joint membranes.)

Anti-rabies neural vaccines produced in animals may cause reaction in human beings due to some similarity between human and animal brain.

Emergence of Forbidden Clones

Clone means group of immune cells. Normally, there are some groups of immune cells which can cause danger to us because they have ability to cause damage to our cell but they are locked. When general mechanism of immune response breaks down due to genetic mutation, or immunological tolerance stops, these (hidden clone which otherwise no permission) forbidden clones of immunocompetent cells emerge, which are capable of evolving immunological response against "self" antigens.

Polyclonal B Cell Activation

An antigen generally activates only its corresponding B cell, certain stimuli nonspecifically stimulate on multiple B cell clones, e.g. EBV infecion, other stimuli may be chemical (2-mercaptoethanol), bacterial products (PPD, lipopolysaccharides), antibiotics (nystatin) and infections with some bacteria (*Mycoplasma*) and parasites (malaria).

Defects in T and B Cells (Altered Function)

Epstein-Barr virus is a potent stimulator of B cell and may lead to overproduction of antibodies, but these antibodies are nonspecific hence can mount a response. The activation of B cell may be the result of genetically determined, intrinsic B cell abnormalities or loss of T suppressor cell influence.

Breakdown of Immunological Homeostasis

Loss of Treg cell-mediated suppression of self-reactive cells leads to emergence of Forbidden clones of immunocompetent cells capable of mounting immune response against self-antigens.

Some T and B cell defects may cause autoimmune mechanisms.

Shared B cell epitopes between *Yesinia enterocolytica* and extracellular domain of thyroid-stimulating hormone receptors exist.

Stimulation of Autoreactive Cells by Foreign Antigens

Lipopolysaccharide or EB virus cause direct B cell stimulation and some of the clones of activated cells will produce autoantibodies, though in absence of T cell help, these are normally of low titer and low affinity. However, an activated B cell might pick up and process its cognate autoantigen and present it to a naïve autoreactive T cell.

Cytokine dysregulation, inappropriate MHC expression and failure of suppression may induce autoimmunity.

Pre-*existing defects in target organs may increase susceptibility to autoimmunity.* For example, rheumatoid arthritis in which the agalacto IgG glycoform is abnormally abundant. The post-translational modification of arginine to citrulline, producing new neoantigen is a mechanism by which autoimmunity may occur.

Genetic Factors

They are usually not sufficient to cause the disease without additional stimulus. In some autoimmune disorders, single HLA gene appears to determine susceptibility to diseases, e.g. HLA-B27 and ankylosing spondylitis. Haplotype B8, DR3 is common in both organ specific and systemic autoimmune disorders. For type I diabetes, DQ2/8 heterozoites have greater risk of developing the disease. Genes of MHC including HLA-A1, B8, and DR3 have been linked with SLE.

Waste Disposal Hypothesis

SLE and similar other disorders are caused due to failure of clearance of apoptosis cells, i.e. due to decreased macrophage 'scavenger' functions. After the cell death due to apoptosis, cellular material is accumulated on the surface of cell. Antigen normally buried deep within cell is exposed. In healthy persons, these cell debris are effectively cleared.

CLASSIFICATION OF AUTOIMMUNE DISEASES

Based on the site of involvement and nature of lesions, autoimmune diseases may be classified as:
- Hemolytic autoimmune diseases
- Localized (organ specific)
- Systemic (non-organ specific)
- Transitory diseases

Mechanism of Damage in Autoimmune Response

The actual mechanism of damage caused by localized disorders is type II hypersensitivity reaction and in systemic disorders (non-organ specific) damage is due to type III hypersensitivity.

Autoimmune hemolytic anemia: Autoantibodies against erythrocytes are two types, 'cold' and 'warm' antibodies. Warm antibodies are seen in patients taking drugs like sulphonamides, antibiotics, and alpha-methyldopa.

Autoimmune thrombocytopenia: Antibodies against platelets are produced, e.g. idiopathic thrombo-cytopenic purpura.

Localized Autoimmune Diseases (Table 19.1)

- *Autoimmune disease of thyroid gland:* Hashimoto's disease (antibodies against thymoglobulin, acinar colloid, microsomal antigen, thyroid cell surface component).
- *Autoimmune diseases of the skin:* There is auto-immune response against intercellular cement substance, e.g. pemphigus vulgaris and Addison's disease.

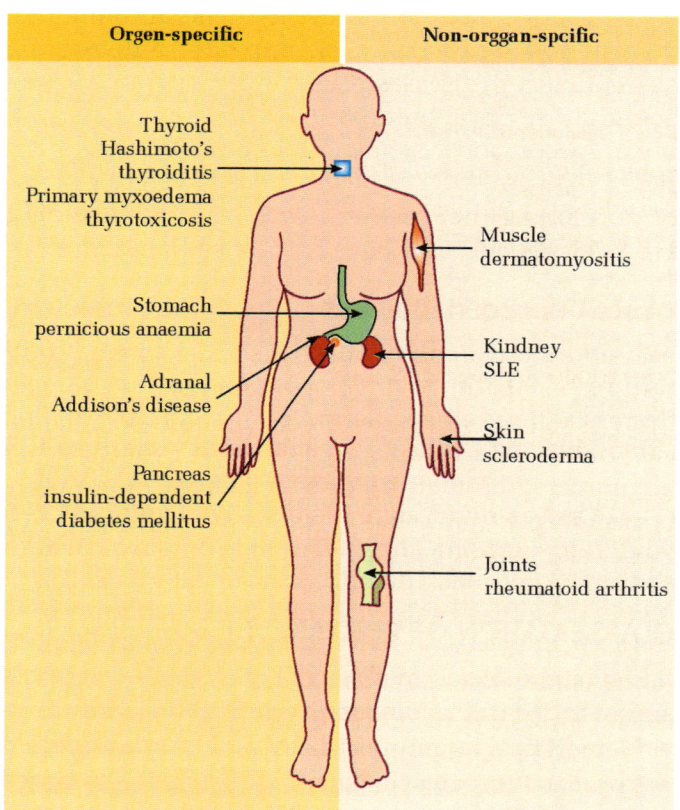

Fig. 19.1: Two types of autoimmune disease

- *Thyrotoxicosis (Graves' disease):* Antibodies to thymoglobulin are present. Long-acting thyroid stimulator is an antibody to thyroid membrane protein. It combines with surface membrane of thyroid cells which leads to excessive hormone secretion.
- *Addison's disease:* Circulating antibodies against zona glomerulosa are produced.
- *Autoimmune orchitis:* Circulating antibodies against sperms are produced. This condition follows mumps infection which by damaging membranes of seminiferous tubules releases sperms.
- *Myasthenia gravis:* Antibody against acetylcholine receptors at myoneural junction is produced which prevents binding of acetylcholine to acetylcholine receptors. Patients present with excess fatigability.
- *Autoimmune diseases of eye:* Autoimmune response following cataract surgery produces an autoimmune response against lens proteins called '**pheco-anaphylaxis**'.
- Injury to one eye may release lens proteins in circulation which are exposed to immune system leading to formation of autoantibodies which damage other eye. This is called **sympathetic ophthalmia**.
- *Pernicious anemia:* Antibodies against partial cells are produced causing atrophic gastritis, achlorhydria. Antibody against intrinsic factor is also produced which prevents absorption of vitamin B_{12} intrinsic complex, reducing uptake of vitamin B_{12}.
- *Autoimmune diseases of CNS:* Neuroparalysis following rabies vaccine produced in animal cross-reacts with human nervous tissue. Idiopathic neuritis (Guillain-Barré syndrome) may be autoimmune response against peripheral nervous tissue.
- *Hashimoto's disease:* Enlargement of thyroid gland, hypothyroidism, and myxedema is seen. Antibodies against different substances thymoglobulin, a second acinar colloid, microsomal antigen and a thyroid cell surface component are produced.

Cold antibodies: Cold agglutinating antibodies belong to IgM class. They agglutinate erythrocytes at 4°C but not at 37°C. These antibodies are associated with paroxysmal cold hemoglobinurea, primary atypical pneumonia, tryapanosomiasis and black water fever.

Warm antibodies: They are incomplete, non-agglutinating antibodies of class IgG, shown by coating erythrocytes in direct Coombs' test. These are seen in patients taking drugs like sulphonamides, antibiotics, and alpha-methyldopa.

TABLE 19.1: List of localized autoimmune diseases

Disease	Autoantibodies produced
Myasthenia gravis (thyrotoxicosis)	Antiacetylcholine antibodies
Graves' disease	Antibodies to thyroglobulin and to microsomal Ags
Hashimoto's thyroiditis	Antibody anti-insulin receptor
Pernicious anemia	Antibody to gastric parietal
Addison's disease	Antibody to adrenal cells (B8, DR3)
Autoimmune orchitis associated mumps	Antibody to sperm
Pemphigus vulgaris,	Antibodies against intercellular cement substance
Bullous pemphigoid, Dermatitis herpetiformis Systemic lupus erythematosus (SLE)	Antinuclear (anti-DNA) antibodies Anti-RNP, antilymphocyte antibodies Anti-RBC, anti-neuronal cell antibodies Antiplatelet antibodies Antibodies to gamma globulin Anti-smith antibodies, anti-ss, antibodies, antidouble-stranded antibodies
Goodpasture's syndrome	Antibasement membrane antibodies
Autoimmune hemolytic anemia	Anti-red blood cell antibodies
Idiopathic thrombocytopenic purpura	Antiplatelet antibodies
Chronic active hepatitis	Antinuclear and antihepatocyte antibodies
Sympathetic ophthalmia	Antibodies to uveal or retinal tissue
Type 1 or juvenile diabetes	Insulin-dependent (B8, DR3/4) antibodies

Systemic Autoimmune Diseases

Systemic Lupus Erythematosus

- Chronic multi-system disease with remissions and exacerbations.
- Autoantibodies against cell nuclei, intracytoplasmic constituents, immunoglobulins and other organ specific antigens are produced.
- **LE phenomenon** is seen.
- LE cell is neutrophil with pale, **homogenous body (LE body).** LE body is damaged nucleus of a leukocyte.
- Immunofluorescent tests detect **antinuclear antibodies.**
- Specific antibodies detected for diagnosis: **Anti-DNA antibodies**—ss (single-stranded), ds (double-stranded).

- Detection of **anti-Sm antibodies**—by ELISA (specific test).
- Lupus band test: The test detects deposits of immunoglobulins and complement proteins in skin. It is based upon direct immunofluorescence test.

Rheumatoid Arthritis

- It is systemic polyarthritis with muscle wasting and subcutaneous nodules.
- It is associated with serositis, myocarditis, and vasculitis.
- Most commonly found in women.
- Presence of circulating autoantibody, 19S IgM type called as **rheumatoid factor** (RF or RA), an antibody against the Fc fraction of the Ig (anti-antibody).
- RF reacts with autologous, isologous heterologous immunoglobulins.

Methods of detection of RA factor: RA factor is detected by latex agglutination (**LA**) tests. Before this, **Rose-Waaler test** was used in which tanned RBCs were coated with immunoglobulin. If patient's serum contains RA factor, clumping of RBCs occur (passive hemagglutination test).

RA factor detection may be negative only in 15% cases.
- ***Detection of anticitrullinated peptide antibodies (ACPA):*** It is an autoantibody to citrullin protein. Though the test is highly specific, its sensitivity is only 67%.

Polyarteritis Nodosa

- It is necrotizing angitis involving medium-sized arteries.
- It may be fatal due to coronary thrombosis, cerebral hemorrhage or gastrointestinal bleeding.
- It may be a component of serum sickness.
- The autoantibody responsible is not found.

Sjögren's Syndrome

- It is a **triad** of conjunctivitis sicca, dryness of mouth, with or without salivary gland involvement and rheumatoid arthritis.
- It occurs in association of other collagen disorders.
- Antinuclear antibodies and rheumatoid factor commonly found in the sera.

Pathogenesis (Mechanisms)

Type 2 cytotoxic reactions: In autoimmune hemolytic anemia, autoantibody and complement destroys red cells and in Goodpasture's syndrome, fixation of anti-basement membrane antibody and complement to the glomerular basement membrane causes inflammation.

Type 3 toxic complex reaction (immune complex disease): In SLE, deposition of circulating immune complexes in tissues (glomerular basement membrane) lead to tissue injury. Myasthenia gravis, Graves' disease and certain forms of diabetes mellitus are also included in this group.

TREATMENT OF AUTOIMMUNE DISORDERS

a. Metabolic control.
b. Uses of anti-inflammatory drugs.
c. Uses of immunosuppressors.
d. If organ dysfunction occurs, grafting can be done.
e. *Future strategies*: Anti-IL-2R antibodies which are involved in maturation of lymphocytes.

Some of the Diagnostically Useful Autoantibodies

- Antibodies to cyclic citrullinated peptide (CCP) are more specific than rheumatoid factor in rheumatoid arthritis.
- Presence of anti-nuclear antibodies is one of the revised ACR criteria for SLE but is non-specific. In contrast, anti-dsDNA antibodies are highly specific for SLE (70%). Anti-Sm antibodies are found in 10% of Caucasian and 30% of Afro-Caribbean SLE patients; like ds DNA antibodies; they have high specificities for SLE.
- Individuals testing positive to both insulin and glutamic acid decarboxylase have high risk of developing type I diabetes mellitus.

Prognosis and disease subtype:

- In rheumatoid arthritis, CCP antibodies are associated with poor prognosis and predict erosive disease.
- SLE
- Presence of specific autoantibodies is associated with specific disease manifestations.
- **Anti-La antibodies** are associated with features of **Sjögren's syndrome, anticardiolipin antibodies** and **anti-beta2 glycoprotein I** antibodies with **thrombosis** and **miscarriage; anti-ds DNA antibodies** with **glomerulonephritis; anti-RNP** with **pulmonary hypertension** and **anti-Ro** with **photosensitivity.**
- *Disease monitoring*:
  - **Anti-ds DNA antibodies** can be used as a measure of disease activity in **SLE**. A rising titer of **anti-ds DNA** antibodies is associated with **disease progress**, especially if accompanied by a falling C3 level and should prompt the clinician to monitor patient more frequently.
  - Similarly, a **rise in titer of ANCA** may indicate impending **relapse in AAV**. However, the association between **ANCA** is much **less robust** than between **anti-ds DNA antibody titer** and **lupus activity.**

20

Hypersensitivity

Definition

If a host is sensitized to an antigen (during first contact with antigen) and again comes in contact with the same antigen, injury occurs. Thus hypersentivity means injury in a sensitized host following contact with the same antigen. The sensitized host reacts in an exaggerated manner.

Hypersensitivity reactions are called allergic reactions, while some authors use the term allergy to only type I hypersensitivity.

CLASSIFICATIONS

There are two classifications:

a. Classification based upon the time required to manifest the consequences of hypersensitivity after the second contact with same antigen.

1. *Immediate type*: Clinical manifestations occur within 24–72 hours after the second contact.

2. *Delayed type of hypersentivity*: Manifestations occur after 72 hours of second contact. It is mediated by CMI (cell mediated).

b. *Coombs and Gel classification*: This is based on the immunological mechanism of hypersensitivity test. The *four* types are:

1. Anaphylaxis and atopy
2. Cytolytic and cytotoxic
3. Immune complex diseases
4. Delayed type which includes contact dermatitis type, tuberculin type and granulomatous.

A fifth type of hypersensitivity is added.

TYPE I HYPERSENSITIVITY

Examples of type I hypersensitivity are anaphylaxis, atopy, allergic rhinitis, bronchial asthama, atopic dermatitis.

Mediators: IgE, histamine and other substances released by mast cells and basophils.

1. Anaphylaxis (Ana—means no, Phylaxis—Protection)

Pathogenesis or Mechanism of Anaphylaxis (Fig. 20.1)

First contact with allergen: Human mast cells and basophils have receptors present on their surface for attachment to immunoglobulin IgE. During first contact with antigen, antibodies of type IgE are overproduced, some of which come out and attach to the surface receptors present on mast cells and basophils. This is sensitizing dose (priming dose).

Second contact: If host comes in contact with the same antigen again (shocking dose), the antigen binds to the IgE which are already bound to mast cells and basophils. As the antigen binds to two adjacent IgE molecules, it causes cross-linking, bridges the gap between adjacent molecules, that results in presence of cations, increase in permeability of mast cells and basophils. Pharmacological mediators from mast cells and basophils released which ultimately increase capillary permeability. Internal chemicals of these cells

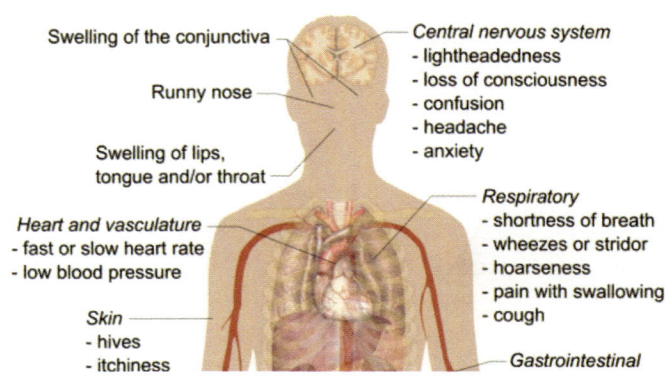

Fig. 20.1: Anaphylaxis

are released some of which are formed during second contact (hence called **secondary mediators**) while some are already present in cells, called as **primary mediators.** As this type of reaction is mediated by **IgE,** it is called **reagin dependent** (Fig. 20.2).

IgE is sensitive to heat. It is inactivated at 56°C in 2–4 hours. It does not pass through placenta.

Primary mediators: These are histamine, serotonin, eosinophil chemotectic factors (ECF), neutrophil chemotactic factors (NCF), enzyme mediators as proteases, hydrolyses.

Secondary mediators: These include slow reactive substance, of anaphylaxis (SRS), prostaglandins, leukotrienes and platelet-activating factor (PAF) (Table 20.1).

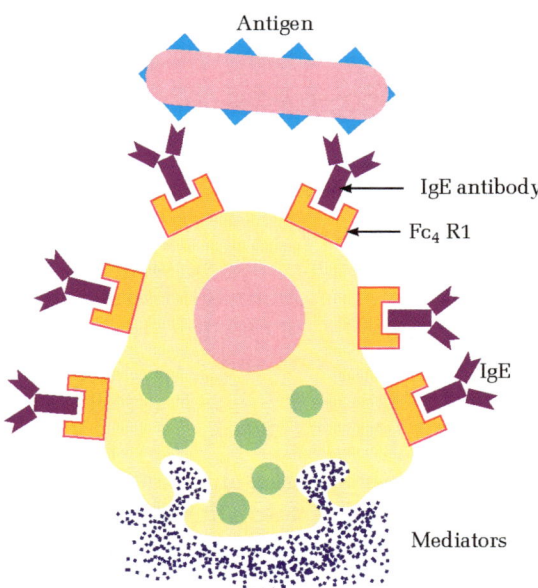

Fig. 20.2: Sensitized mast cell

Other mediators of anaphylaxis: Biologically active substances, as anaphylatoxins, are released by complement activation and bradykinin, other kinins formed from plasma kininogen.

Increase in capillary permeability, vasodilatation, smooth muscle contraction are responsible for the clinical manifestations of anaphylaxis.

Anaphylaxis is the systemic reaction and many systems may be involved but involvement of one system is predominant. The main organ affected is called target organ. It may be lung, or heart or cardio-respiratory system.

Antigens which can cause anaphylaxis: **Penicillin, foreign serum.**

Clinical features are tingling, flushing of face, fall in BP and if not treated urgently, it causes the death. Therefore, if penicillin is given, it is first tested on arms and always a syringe filled with adrenaline should be kept ready.

The inflammatory agents released cause the following:
- Dilatation of blood vessels—local redness (erythema) and shock.
- Increased capillary permeability—swelling of local tissues (edema), shock.
- Constriction of bronchial airways—wheezing and difficulty in breathing.
- Stimulation of mucus secretion—congestion of airways.
- Stimulation of nerve endings—itching and pain in the skin.

Differences between anaphylaxis and other type I reaction, i.e. atopy
- There is no hereditary tendency in anaphylaxis.
- Manifestations occur in sensitized persons within minutes.

TABLE 20.1: Mediators of type I hypersensitivity		
Pharmacological primary mediators		
	Histamine	Vasodilatation, increased capillary permeability, bronchoconstriction
	Heparin	Anticoagulant
	Tryptase	Activates C3
	β glucosamidinase	Spilts glucosamine
	ECF	Eosinophils chemotaxis
	NCF	Neutrophils chemotaxis
	Platelet activating factor	Mediator release
Pharmacological secondary mediators		
Lipoxygenase pathway	Leukotrienes C4 and D4	Vasoactive, bronchoconstriction, chemotaxis/chemokinesis
	Leukotriene B4	Chemokinesis
Cyclo-oxygenase pathway	Prostaglandins, thromboxanes	Affect bronchial muscles, platelets aggregation and vasodilatation

- The same antigen acts as sensitizing and shocking dose.
- Systemic manifestations occur which may be fatal.

Sensitization is effective by parenteral route. Antigens as well as haptens act as allergens. The clinical manifestations of anaphylaxis are same with any antigen (but reaction is specific means sensitizing dose, the person will react only if exposed to the same antigen) but clinical features are different in different animals. A particular organ is more targeted depending upon species and it is called as **shock organ**.

The clinical features include edema, fall in BP, and fall in temperature, thrombocytopenia, leucopenia, decreased coagulability of blood. In guinea pig, shocking organ is lung. Fatal paralysis is rare in human beings.

Clinical features in humans are itching of scalp, and tongue, breathlessness due to bronchospasm, nausea, vomiting, abdominal pain, hypotension, unconsciousness, and rarely death may occur.

Types of allergens: Antibiotic therapy, sting bite.

Cutaneous anaphylaxis: This test is used for testing the antigen responsible for atopy or testing for hypersensitivity. If person had previous contact with the antigen and he is exposed to same antigen intradermally, there is formation of **'wheel-flair response'**, i.e. central area of edema and flare, i.e. redness or hyperemia due to increased capillary permeability.

Passive cutaneous anaphylaxis is used to detect human IgG antibody which is **heterocytotropic,** means capable of fixing cells of other species but not used for the detection of human IgE which is **homocytotropic,** i.e. capable of fixing to cells of same species.

A small dose of antibody is injected intradermally into a normal animal. If the same antigen with Evans blue dye is injected intravenously 4–24 hours afterwards, there will be immediate bluing at the site of injection of dye. This is due to vasodilatation and increase in capillary permeability.

Anaphylaxis in vitro: Female guinea pig is sensitized with an antigen. Its intestinal or uterine muscles are taken out and held in a bath of Ringer's solution. If the specific antigen (as previous) is added to the bath, the muscles contract vigorously. This is called as '**Schultz-Dale phenomenon**'. The reaction is specific; hence if the antigen given to guinea pig and the antigen added to the bath are similar, the reaction takes place.

Anaphylactoid reaction: Certain substances as peptone, trypsin are given intravenously, they stimulate a non-specific mechanism which causes complement activation with release of anaphylatoxins. The result is a clinical condition similar to anaphylactic shock which is known as '**anaphylactoid reaction'**.

2. Atopy (Means Strangeness)

- It is naturally occurring familial hypersensitivity of human beings, e.g asthma, hay fever.
- *Antigens*: Inhalants (house dust, pollen grains), or ingestants (milk protein, egg, mushroom, nuts) or contact allergen act as antigens.
- Predisposition is **genetically** determined.
- The sensitivity to a particular allergy is not inherited but the tendency to overproduce **IgE which spills in blood** is inherited. Thus father may be allergic to one antigen, child may be sensitive to another allergen, this tendency is passed on to the son.
- **Symptoms** depend upon the mode of entry of antigen. The clinical features are conjunctivitis, gastrointestinal symptoms, and dermatitis, if allergen is entering through conjunctiva, or GIT or skin. Rarely clinical features occur at different site from that of the site of entry.

3. Allergic Rhinitis

It is known as **hay fever**. It results from inhalation of air-borne allergens and subsequent reaction with sensitized mast cells in conjunctiva and nasal mucosa.

Localized effects of increased capillary permeability and vasodilation occur. The patient presents with watery discharge from nose, conjunctiva, upper respiratory tract, sneezing and coughing.

4. Asthama

It is an example of organ specific hypersensitivity. The reaction develops in respiratory tract instead of nose. Air borne allergens, as pollens, dust, mite, fumes, viral antigens, are common triggering factors; other are cold, excercies. Increased contraction of smooth muscles produces bronchoconstriction. Increased secretions, edema add to pathogenicity. Eosinophils are capable of causing damage by releasing toxic enzymes.

5. Atopic Dermatitis (Allergic Eczema)

It is inflammation of skin associated with a family history of atopy.

Common allergens associated with type I hypersensitivity:
- *Proteins*: Foreign serum, vaccines
- *Foods*: Nuts, egg, milk, peas, beans, seafood
- *Drugs*: Penicillin, sulfonamide, local anesthetic, salicylates
- *Insects*: Bee venom, ant venom, dust mite
- *Others*: Animal hairs, latex, pollen grains.

Detection of Type I Hypersensitivity (Fig. 20.3)

i. *Skin prick test*: Patient is exposed to small dose of antigen which is injected at different sites.

Development of local wheel and flare response at the inoculation site within 30 minutes indicates that the person is allergic to that antigen.

ii. *Skin test*

- The skin response takes 5–15 minutes to develop and may persist for 30 minutes or more.
- **Technique of skin test:** Allergen is injected in small amount (0.02 mL by intradermal route. If raised wheal is produced with well-defined edge after 25 minutes, it indicates a positive test. Test result is compared with positive control (histamine) and negative control (saline injection).
- Positive test suggests that patient has **specific IgE antibodies on mast cells in skin**. It **indirectly** implies that bronchial or nasal discharge will also be positive. Blood tests are less sensitive than skin tests.
- Approximately **one-third of skin test positive** individuals exposed to allergen **do not** experience symptoms.
- All injections for skin test have potential to cause anaphylaxis hence for safety measure **prick test is performed before skin test.**

iii. *Patch test*: Allergen in small amount (10 µg) is placed on gauze pad (2.5 cm²) which is kept over denuded skin area and biopsy is taken after 24 and 48 hours. A **positive test** induces:
- Macroscopic eczema
- Spongiosis of epidermis (hallmark of eczema)
- An infiltrate of cells into dermis.

iv. *Radioimmunosorbent test (RIST)*: It detects total serum IgE. The test is based on the principle of radio-immunoassay in which patient's serum is added to agarose beads or disks coated with anti-IgE.

v. *Radioallergosorbent test (RAST)*: This test quantifies allergen specific IgE. The allergen is coated to solid support, patient's serum is added. Allergen specific IgE binds to allergen. Radiolebeled anti-IgE is added and radioactivity is measured.

Treatment

- ***Epinephrine (adrenaline)*:** It stimulates cAMP in mast cells by binding to adrenergic receptors on mast cells.
- ***Antihistamines*:** Block H1 and H2 receptors on target cells.
- ***Steroids*:** Cortisone reduces histamine levels by blocking conversion of histidine to histamine, prevents degranulation of mast cells by increasing cyclic-AMP.

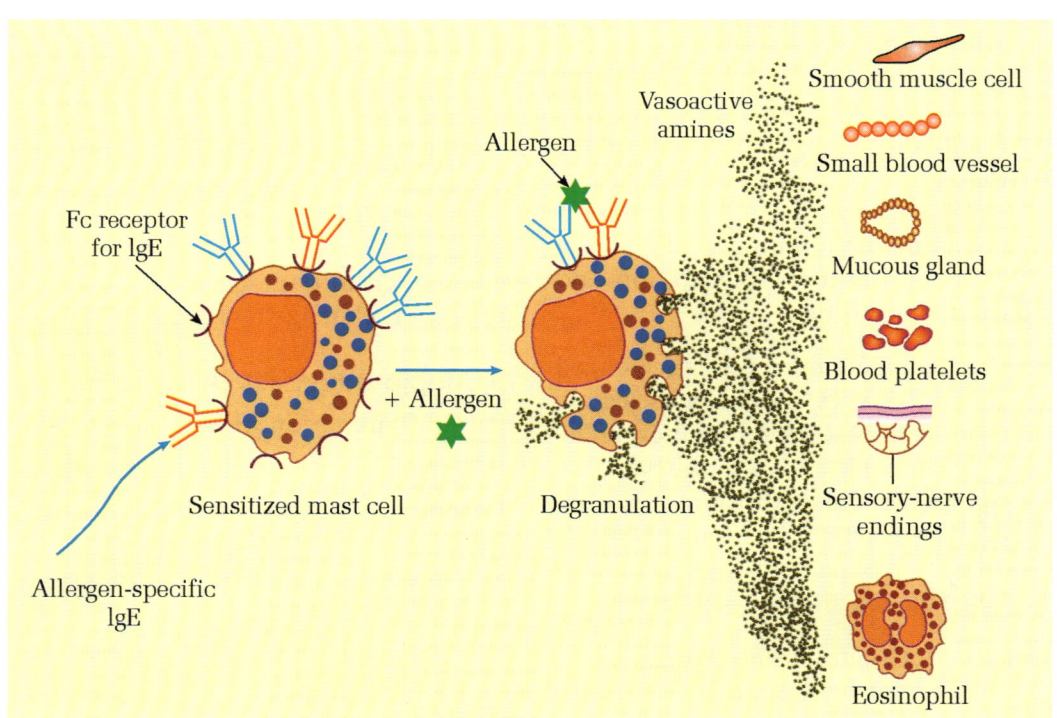

Fig. 20.3: Type I hypersensitivity

- Sodium cromolyn blocks Ca++ influx in mast cells.
- Specific desensitization is used in the treatment of allergy.
- **Immunotherapy with (or hyposensitization) allergen** is started between **1 and 10 µg** and increased to **10 µg** allergen per dose. Response to immunotherapy is due to **shift of TH2 response to TH1**.
- *Allergen-specific immunotherapy*: Peptides from primary sequence of allergen, approximately 20 amino acids are used for therapy.
- **Modified recombinant antigens** that have decreased affinity for IgE are used.
- **DNA vaccines** are being designed to change immune response.

Other forms of immune based therapies: Humanized monoclonal anti-IgE.

Desensitization: It is achieved by giving series of small injections of the antigens, the dose of which is gradually increased. Another method is depot therapy (injection of allergen in an oil adjuvant. The sentization is due to IgG which acts as blocking antibody which competes with IgE.

Prausnitz-Küstner reaction (PK reaction)
- It was the original method for the detection of atopic IgE antibodies.
- Human IgE is **'homocytotropic'** which can fix to the surface of human cells only.

- Prausnitz-Küstner observed that serum of Küstner who had atopy to some fish antigen, if injected in Prausntz intracutaneously and after 24 hours intracutaneous injection of a small amount of cooked fish antigen is given to the same site, a **"wheel and flair"** appeared at that site within few minutes.

TYPE II CYTOLYTIC OR CYTOTOXIC REACTIONS (ANTIBODY-DEPENDENT CYTOTOXICITY) (Fig. 20.4)

Examples
  i. AB and Rh blood group reactions
  ii. Autoimmune diseases such as hemolytic diseases of newborns
  iii. Idiopathic thrombocytopenic purpura
  iv. Drug reactions

Comparison of type II and type III reactions
- Type II reactions are mediated by IgG and IgM (and IgA) antibodies.
- These **antibodies bind** specifically to **specific cells or component of extracellular matrix**. Hence, the **damage is restricted** to specific cells or tissues bearing the antigen.
- Type II differs from type III reaction in which the antibody is directed against soluble antigens in serum lead to formation of circulating immune complexes.

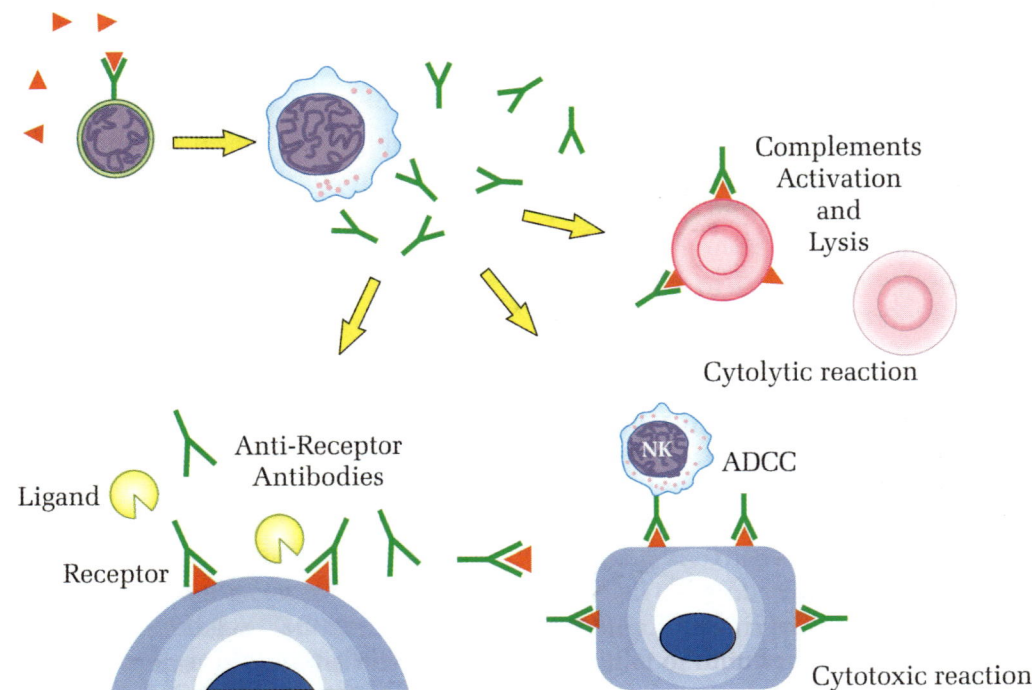

Fig. 20.4: Type II hypersensitivity

Mechanisms of Tissue Damage

- Antibodies directed against specific cells or tissues are produced.
- **Antibodies attach** to **antigens on specific cells** or tissues **by Fab portion** and by their **Fc portion**. Antibodies **attach** to various **effectors cells** as macrophages, neutrophils, eosinophils, NK cells **via FcRs** present on effector cells.
- Antibody attached to antigen **stimulates complement system**, some components of complement system as C3a, C5a attract cells to the site of inflammation. By stimulation of classical and alternate pathways, **membrane attack complex** is formed which damages the specific cells or organs.
- How effector cells, neutrophils, macrophages, and eosinophils, damage the specific cells or organs?
- Neutrophils damage target specific cells by **phagocytosis** or if target cells are large, neutrophils get **frustrated** and **exocytosis** releasing toxins extracellularly causing damage to target cells or organs.
- Phagocytic cells engulf RBCs (**erythophagocytosis**)
- **NK cells, granulocytes, macrophages, platelets have FcR** for antibody, so bind to target cells through antibody bridge or with their complement receptors they bind to target cells and cause **damage by complement mediated lysis or release of toxins from effector cells.**

Type II Reactions Against Blood Cells and Platelets

Examples

1. Incompatible blood transfusion where recipient becomes sensitized with antigens on the surface of donor's RBCs leads to transfusion reactions.
2. Hemolytic disease of newborn where pregnant women become sensitized to fetal RBCs.
3. Autoimmune hemolytic anemia.
   a. *Transfusion reactions*: **Antibodies to ABO group system** are more important as they are strong immunogenic.
   b. *Hemolytic disease of newborn* due to **Rh incompatibilities,** as mother become sensitized to Rh antigen present on fetus RBCs, forms antibodies which damage fetus RBCs (second pregnancy) by **complement-mediated lysis.** Only antibodies to Rh system cause damage as they are IgG in nature hence transfer placenta. **Antibodies ABC blood group antigens are IgM in nature** which **do not pass placenta**, hence do not cause hemolytic disease of newborn. Other blood group antigens are less important as they are less immunogenic.

   c. **Autoimmune hemolytic anemia arises spontaneously or drug induced.**

Fc receptor-mediated erythrophagocytosis or complement-mediated damage of RBCs occurs. There is accelerated clearance of sensitized RBCs by spleen macrophages.

Cold reactive antibodies are present in **high titer** and they are of **IgM** in nature which **fixes complement** strongly. Mostly they are specific for **Ii** system. Autoantibodies against RBCs may be produced following infection with microorganisms as *Mycoplasma pneumoniae* which share antigenic epitope with RBCs.

Drug induced reactions to blood components (against RBCs, platelets)

- **Sedormid purpura** (destruction of platelets due to change in antigenicity of platelets).
- Drug-induced antibodies bind to RBCs and damage RBCs by complement-mediated lysis.
- **Drug (α methyldopa)** induces formation of anti-RBC antibodies.
- **Idiopathic thrombolytic purpura (ITP):** This condition occurs following—**bacterial or viral infections** or in course of autoimmune disorders as **SLE** or due to **drugs** and damage occurs by **increased phagocytosis** of sensitized platelets by splenic macrophages.

Other Type II Reactions in Tissues

- Antibodies against basement membranes (collagen type IV) produce nephritis. **Goodpasture's syndrome** usually results in severe necrosis of glomerulus with fibrin deposition along with lung hemorrhage.
- **Pemphigus** is caused by **autoantibodies to intracellular adhesion molecule** leading to breakdown of epidermis with separation of superficial layers of skin and blisters formation.
- **Myasthenia gravis:** Autoantibodies to acetylcholine receptors cause muscle weakness. Autoantibody and complement increase turnover of receptors and cause partial blocking of acetylcholine binding.

Common Diseases of Type II Hypersensitivity

Transfusion Reaction

Hemolysis: Mismatch of ABO blood group severely destroys RBCs of donors due to presence of iso-antibodies against A, B, O antigens present on RBCs. This antibody is of IgM type. The antibody in presence of complement causes massive intravascular hemolysis.

Hemolytic disease of newborn: Mother Rh⁻; first baby Rh⁺ (Ab), second baby Rh⁺: Maternal antibodies specific to fetal RBCs cross the placenta and destroy RBCs. Such type of reaction occurs when mother is Rh negative, she is presensitized and mounts a response against Rh positive RBCs of fetus. Fetal RBCs get destroyed.

Autoimmune Hemolytic Anemia and Other Type II Drug Reactions

Foreign antigen or hapten: Penicillin binds to RBC, changes its antigenicity and hemolytic anemia occurs. Quinin changes the antigenicity of platelets causing thrombocytopenic purpura. Similar mechanism causes agranulocytosis due to pyramidone.

Antibody-mediated cellular dysfunction: Auto-antibodies bind and distrub function of self antigens. Antireceptor antibodies may cause inhibition of receptors causing host injury, e.g. myasthenia gravis antibody-mediated cellular dysfunction is basis of damage in Goodpasture syndrome, pernicious anemia and myocarditis in Chagas disease.

Goodpasture's syndrome: In this syndrome, auto-antibodies against glomerular basement membrane of kidneys and basement membrane of lungs occur which invite complement. Due to complement activation, C5a is produced which is chemotactic to leukocytes. These cells produce enzyme proteinase which act on kidneys and lungs.

Rheumatic fever: Antibodies produced against *Streptococcus pyogenes* cause damage as they crossreact with cardiac tissue. The damage takes place due to complement activation.

TYPE III HYPERSENSITIVITY (Fig. 20.5)

It is called immune complex disease.

Mechanism of Pathogenesis

When an antigen combines with an antibody it forms immune complex. Naturally, this occurs routinely but they are cleared by body by various methods. If large-sized immune complexes are not cleared by body, they may get deposited at certain sites causing immune

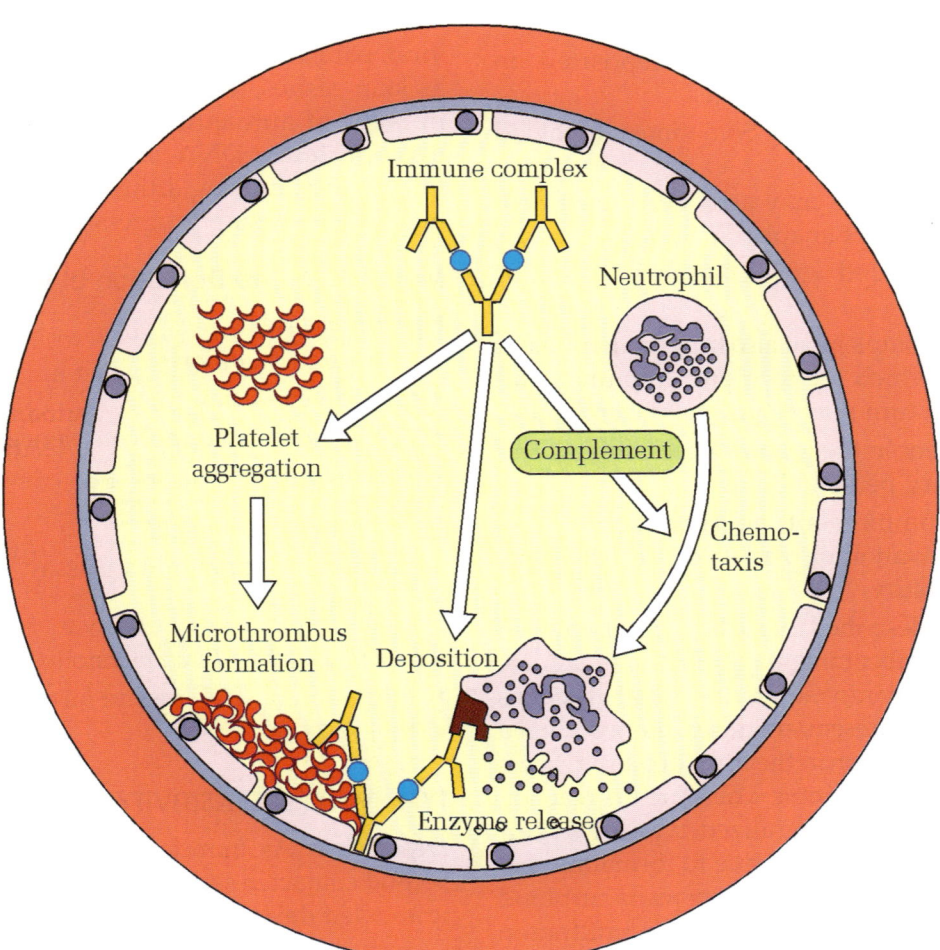

Fig. 20.5: Type III hypersensitivity

complex disease. The sites, where these complexes are deposited are those where there is 'turbulence' of blood, as glomerular basement membrane. Immune complexes cause inflammation as seen in glomerulonephritis (GN).

Types of Immune Complex Diseases

Systemic: Immune complexes are circulating in blood, deposited at many sites in body, as seen in many collegen disorders. Example of systemic disease is serum sickness.

Localized: Locally immune complexes are produced which cause local damage by causing inflammation, as seen in allergic alveolitis. **The example of localized disease in experimental animal is called Arthus reaction.**

Mediators of type III hypersensity are IgM complements. (Hence it is humoral mediated.)

Arthus Reaction

This is an experimental example of localized immune complex disease. The similar clinical example is antigen entering through respiratory tract and causing **extrinsic allergic alveolitis.**

- Antigen–antibody complexes are deposited on endothelium of small blood vessels.
- They lead to acute vasculitis. Sometimes the blood supply is hampered.
- The immune complexes may activate complement which causes release of anaphylatoxins.
- Histamine is released with change in vascular permeability.
- The activation of complement also triggers chemotaxis of polymorphs which try to ingulf immune complexes, which on turn release proteolytic enzymes.
- Substances present in the granules are released, this increases capillary permeability.
- Activation of complement, aggregation of polymorphs, and activation of platlets cause inflammation and tissue injury.

The reaction first described by Arthus. He discovered that after repeated subcutaneous injections of soluble antigens—horse serum into rabbits, the initial injections had no effect but with subsequent doses, there occurred a local reaction, the reaction in the form of hemorrhagic necrosis, edema and induration. Thus Arthus reaction is local manifestation of generalized type III hypersensitivity. The tissue damage is due to formation and deposition of immune complexes on walls of blood vessels that increase capillary permeability, infiltration of site with polymorphs and platelets which aggregate and cause microthrombi, leading to further damage.

Serum Sickness

These reactions occur due to injection of foreign sera, hyperimmune sera produced in horses. Manifestations produced are systemic. As presently, antisera prepared in human volunteers are used, this type of reactions are not common.

Immune complexes formation causes damage in other infective and non-infective conditions. These include following:

Infectious:
- Malaria
- Hepatitis B leading to skin rash and arthralgia
- Infectious mononucleosis
- Trypanosomiasis
- Meningitis

Noninfectious:
- Systemic lupus erythematosus
- Rheumatoid arthritis

Drug reactions: Allergies to penicillin and sulphonamide.

Complexes of antibodies against various bacterial, viral, parasitic antigens have shown to cause reactions as skin rashes, arthritis, and glomerulonephritis. A number of autoantibodies against self-proteins, as glycoproteins, DNA, may accumulate in synovial membranes, causing arthritis or glomerular basement membrane causing progressive damage.

Methods for the Detection of Immune Complexes

Physical methods:
- Ultracentrifugation
- Cryoprecipitation
- Precipitation with polyethyleneglycol
- Nephelometry

Reaction with complement:
- Solid phase radioimmunoassay
- C1q binding test

Interactions with cell receptors:
- Inhibition of EAC rosette formation
- Raji cell test

TYPE IV HYPERSENSITIVITY (Fig. 20.6)

Definition: As manifestations occur late following second contact in sensitized host with the same antigen, it is called delayed hypersensitivity reaction.

Mediators: Cytokines, T lymphocytes, and macrophages are mediators of this reaction.

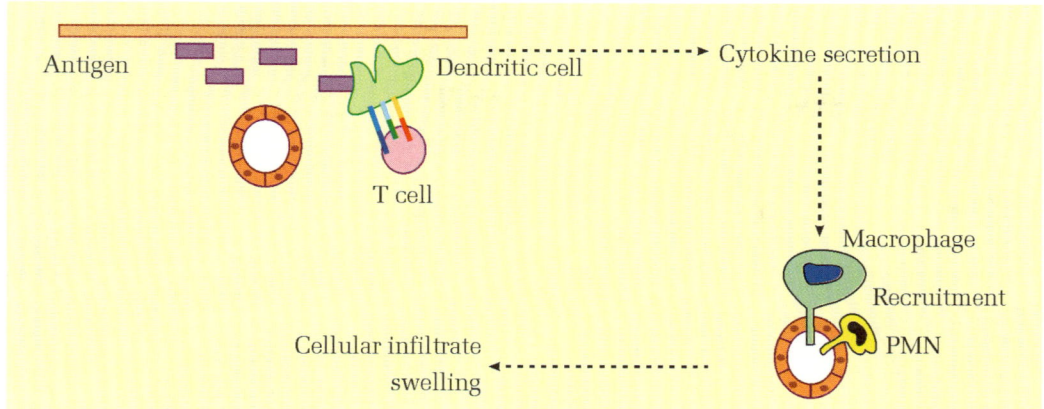

Fig. 20.6: Mechanism of type IV hypersensitivity

The reaction is not mediated by antibody but **sensitized T cells,** thus it is a cell-mediated reaction as comparison to other hypersensitivity reactions, which are antibody mediated.

Antigens: Blind substances as **incomplete antigen,** combine with proteins present in skin become complete antigens.

Reaction: Contact of antigen with sensitized T cells, release cytokines by T cells which cause infiltration of various cells as macrophages, tissue cells, and leukocytes at the site of reaction causing **induration**.
- TH1 cell secretes INFγ and IL-2. These cytokines activate macrophages and other lymphocytes.
- TH2 cell releases IL-4, IL-5, GM-CSF. It leads to influx of eosinophils and tissue damage.
- Killing of target cells is mediated by Tc cells.

Type IV Reaction: Immunopathogenesis

After 1st contact with antigen, APCs process antigens, present to T helper cells which are differentiated into T_{DTH}. Most T_{DTH} are derived from **TH1 cells** (occasionally **CD8+ T cells)** and **CD4+TH17** also act as T_{DTH} **cells**.

T_{DTH} on subsequent contact with antigen secrete cytokines which attract and cause recruitment of cells (e.g. macrophages) at the site of delayed type hypersensitivity (DTH) reaction.

Cytokines released from T_{DTH} and their functions are as follows:

INFγ activates resting macrophages, activated macrophages are able to deal with intracellular antigen by many **mechanisms** as:
- Increased expression on cell surface so that macrophages act as good APCs.
- Increase receptors for TNF.
- Increased levels of oxygen radicals and nitric oxide.

- IL: Its autocrine effect stimulates proliferation of T_{DTH} cells.
- MIF (migration inhibition factor)—inhibits migration of macrophages from the site of DTH.
- MCAF (monocyte chemotactic and activating factor) due to which monocytes from blood migrate to DTH site and get converted into tissue macrophages.

Passive transfer of this type of hypersensitivity is not possible by transfer of antiserum from one person to another as it is cell mediated; passive transfer was considered possible by transfer of transfer factor, which probably contained cytokines. Type IV reaction is seen in three formats, i.e. **contact dermatitis type, tuberculin type, chronic granuloma formation.**

I. Contact Dermatitis Type

- Antigens responsible for this reaction are—drugs like penicillin, sulphonamides, metals as nickel, chemicals as soaps, dyes, formaldehyde.
- These antigens are **haptens** and combining with skin proteins become antigenic. Contact dermatitis reaction shows macules, papules to small vesicles which breakdown with oozing material as seen in acute eczematous reaction of skin.
- Identification of allergen is possible by **patch test,** in which suspected antigen in small amount is applied to skin under a dressing and local reaction is observed.

II. Tuberculin Type (Infection) (Fig. 20.7)

Small dose of tuberculin antigen (1–5 TU) is injected intradermally, if person is sensitized already due previous infection or previous contact, after 48 hours, induration of size more than 10 mm size is seen along with erythema. Locally there is infiltration of lymphocytes, mononuclear cells and macrophages. Lepra reaction is also an example of this type of reaction.

This type of reaction is also seen in other chronic or subacute infections.

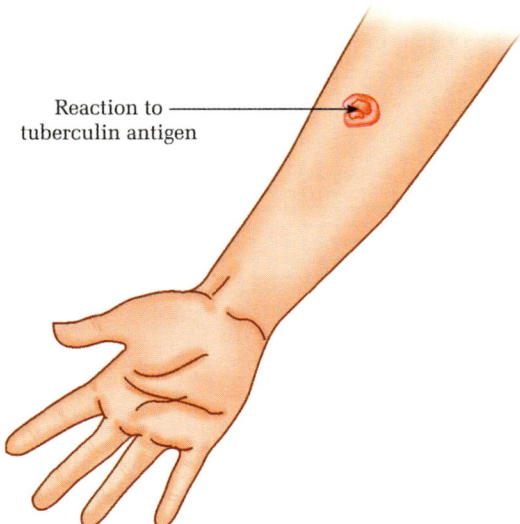

Reaction to tuberculin antigen

Fig. 20.7: Tuberculin reaction

III. Granulomatous Reaction

An antigen survives inside macrophages giving persistant stimulus causing granuloma. Macrophages take the initiative to kill the bacilli and activate T cells by producing IL-1. T cell produces IL-2 which activates macrophages to kill antigen, in presence of cytokines and in an attempt to cure epitheloid cells and giant cells are formed. Thus tubercle formation is an example of type IV hypersentivity.

Intracellular pathogens and contact allergens that produce type IV hypersensitivity reactions are as follows.

Intracellular bacteria:
- *Mycobacterium tuberculosis*
- *Mycobacterium leprae*
- *Brucella abortus*
- *Listeria monocytogenes*

Fungi:
- *Candida albicans*
- Cryptococcus neoformans
- Histoplasma capsulatum
- *Pneumocystis carinii*

Parasite: *Leishmania donovani.*

Contact allergens:
- Hair dyes
- Picrylchloride
- Nickel salts

Examples of infections in which tissue damage is due to hypersensitivity reactions (Table 20.2).

TABLE 20.2: Examples of immune complex diseases in infections

	Principle mechanism	Examples
Type I		Helminth Ruptured hydatid cyst
Type II		Virus infected cells Malaria infected RBCs Autoantibodies in *Mycoplasma* Streptococci *Trpanosoma cruzi*
Type III	Immune complexes Complement PMN	In tissues Allergic alveolitis *Actinomyces* In blood vessels Glomerulonephritis Malaria Streptococci Hepatitis B Syphilis

TYPE V HYPERSENSITIVITY (Fig. 20.8)

In this type of hypersensitivity, the antibody enhances the activity of cell, e.g. **long-acting thyroid stimulator (LATS)** is antibody against some protein of thyroid tissue which excessively stimulate thyroid hormone.

Graves' diseases

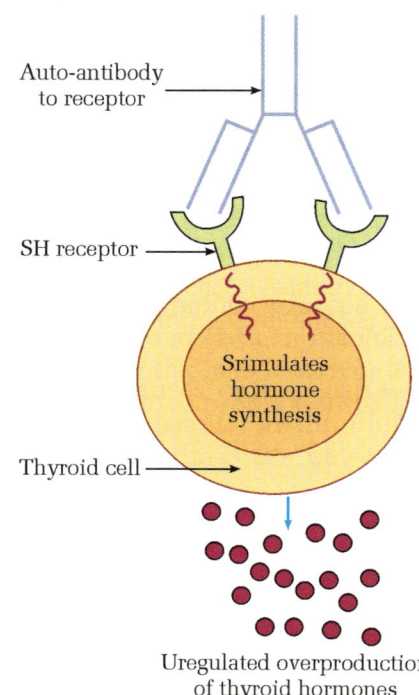

Auto-antibody to receptor

SH receptor

Srimulates hormone synthesis

Thyroid cell

Uregulated overproduction of thyroid hormones

Fig. 20.8: Type V hypersensitivity

TABLE 20.3: Some examples of allergic diseases

Disease	Agent	Predisposing cause
Farmer's lung	Thermophilic *Actinomyces*	Contaminated hay or grains
Bagassosis		Contaminated bagasse
Domestic hypersensitivity	*Bacillus subtilis*	Contaminated walls
Malt worker's disease	*Aspergillus* spp	Moldy barley
Tobacco worker's disease		Moldy tobacco
Sauna worker's disease	*Aurobasidium*	Contaminated sauna water
Humidifier's lung	*Aurobasidium, Graphicum* species	Contaminated humidifiers
Maple bark disease	*Cryptostroma corticale*	Maple bark
Cheese worker's disease	*Penicillium casei*	Moldy cheese
Wood worker's lung	*Alternaria, Penicillium* species	Wood pulp
Furrier's lung	Animal furrs	Animals pelts

SWARTZMAN'S REACTION

It is not a hypersensitivity reaction, but clinicaly it has some resemblance with hypersensitivity.

Culture filtrate of *Salmonella typhi* injected intradermally in rabbit
↓
Same filtrate given intravenously
↓
Hemorrhagic necrosis at the original site of subcutaneous injection
↓
Two doses need not be the same, thus there is no immunological specificity

Probably the mechanism which causes purpuric rash in meningococcemia is responsible for this type of reaction.

Allergens causing hypersensitivity pneumonitis: The mechanism of damage is exactly not known whether it is type IV or type III disease (Table 20.3).

Humoral amplification system: These are nonimmune mechanisms which include inflammation, complement, coagulation, fibrinolytic and kininogenic systems have impact on pathogenesis and clinical features of hypersensitivity.

21

Transplantation

Transplantation is indicated, if tissue or organ is affected or malfunctioning. Tissue or organ is transplanted for restoration of function. Donor is the individual from whom transplant is obtained while recipient is the individual to whom transplant is applied.

CLASSIFICATION OF TRANSPLANTS

a. Classification based on organ or tissue transplanted, e.g. kidney or liver transplant.

b. Classification based on anatomical site of origin and the place in the recipient where it is placed. **Orthotopic grafts** are placed in anatomically normal sites in the recipient, e.g. kidney from donor is placed in the recipient at the same site.

   Heterotopic grafts are placed in anatomically abnormal sites, e.g. if thyroid from the recipient is placed subcutaneously in right arm of recipient.

c. Transplants may be fresh tissue and organs or stored tissue and organs.

d. **Vital grafts,** also called live graft as kidney, heart, etc. **Static or structural** grafts—bone, artery grafts which laid down tissue, form the scaffolding on which new tissue is formed.

e. Classification based on genetic relationship between donor and recipient (Fig. 21.1):

   • *Autograft*: It is grafted on individual himself, e.g. skin graft of the same person grafted at other site.

   • *Isograft*: It is graft taken from one individual. It is placed on another individual of the same species. with same genetic make up, e.g. graft between identical twins or highly inbred strains of animals.

   • *Allograft*: Grafts between genetically non-identical members of same species, e.g. blood transfusion, other examples of allograft include fetus in uterus. Tumor may also considered as allograft.

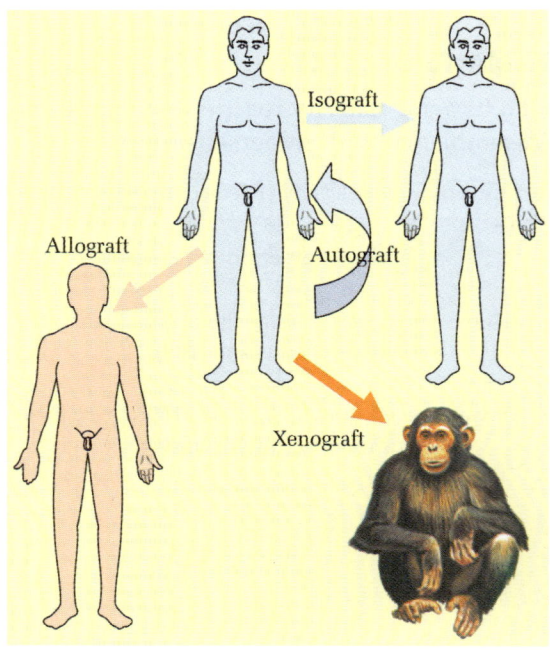

Fig. 21.1: Types of grafts

• *Xenograft*: Transplant between members of different species, e.g. transplant from monkey is taken for restoration of functions in humans.

IMMUNOLOGY OF TRANSPLANTATION

Allograft Rejection

First Set Response

If graft is taken from genetically identical members of the same species the graft is initially accepted. Vascularization occurs; it functions normally for initial few days. About after 2–3 days, lymphocytes and macrophages proliferate, blood supply is diminished, necrosis starts and the graft sloughs off by 10th day. This process of rejection is called **primary set response**.

Immunological process behind primary set response:
After allogenic transplant, the HLA antigens of the
donor are foreign to the recipient hence the recipient's
antigen presenting cells process the antigen and present
to the immune system of the recipient and recipient
mounts cell-mediated responses causing necrosis of the
graft and the graft is rejected.

The graft from female to male will be accepted as
male has 'X' chromosome also as female. This sex-linked
histocompatibility is called **'Eichwald-Silmser'** effect.

Second Set Response or Second Set Rejection

If a graft is taken from the same donor from which first
graft was taken and it was rejected, for the second time
vascularization occurs, but necrosis starts early and
graft sloughs off within a week. In the second set
response, the donor has memory of antigens of previous
graft hence the rejection is rapid as compared to first
set response. This response is specific because if the
second graft is taken from another donor the rejection
like primary set occurs as this is recognized again as a
new antigen and second set rejection was specific to
antigens of first donor.

In contrast to first set response which is exclusively
cell mediated (T cells), the second set response is
brought about by CMI and AMI also. The antibodies
can be detected by serological tests.

Immunological Enhancement

If antibodies act opposite to cell-mediated immunity,
it may inhibit graft rejection, a phenomenon called
'immunological enhancement' which acts by following
ways:

- *Afferent inhibition*: Antibodies may combine with
  released graft antigen so that it cannot initiate an
  immune response.
- *Central inhibition*: Antibodies by combination with
  immune cells prevent the cells to act against antigen
  by negative feedback.
- *Efferent inhibition*: Antibodies may coat the surface
  of cells in graft so that sensitized lymphocytes are
  kept away.

Hyperacute Rejection or White Graft Response

If graft is applied on an animal possessing high titers
of antibodies directed against antigens present on donor
cells or tissues, the graft will not be vascularized,
remains pale and rejected within few hours. This is
called **'hyperacute rejection'**. This type of rejection is
seen in human kidney transplantation when recipient
has high titers of antibodies agaist donor cells due
to previous transplantation or repeated blood transfusions.

Rejections of graft is due to reaction of host to grafted
tissue (host versus graft reaction—HVC).

Immunological Responses in Graft Rejection (Mechanisms of Graft Rejection) (Flowchart 21.1)

- *Cyototoxicity*: The donor's antigens sensitize the
  cytotoxic cells which damage the graft cells by
  cytotoxicity.
- *ADCC (antibody dependent cell-mediated cytotoxicity)*: The Fab part of antibody attaches to the
  antigen and the Fc part attaches to the receptor
  present on Tc cells making access of Tc to antigens
  on donor tissues, which is damaged.

Flowchart 21.1: Mechanism of graft rejection

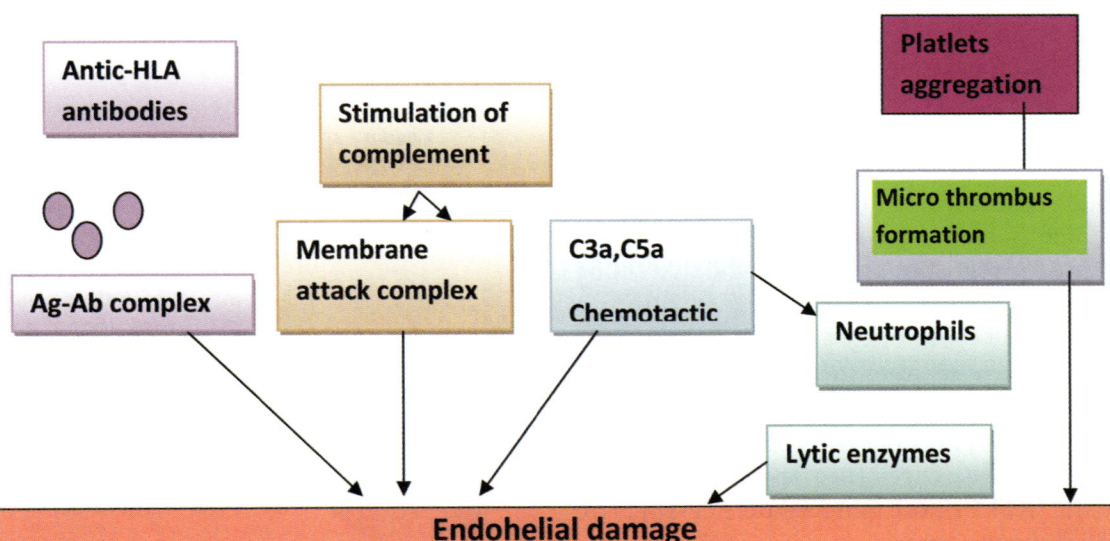

- Antigen combines with antibody forming antigen–antibody complexes which activate complement system causing damage.
- The immune complexes formed invite platelets which adhere to endothelium and cause damage to endothelium leading to necrosis.
- Along with Tc, NK cells also take part in the damage process.

Factors Favoring Allograft Survival

1. **HLA compatibility:** If the donor and the recipient have same HLA antigens, the graft may be accepted. The HLA typing is done by microcytotoxicity test while tissue matching is done by mixed lymphocytic reaction or culture.
2. **Immunosuppression:** If immune responses are dampened by immunosuppressing agents, the rejection reactions will be lowered down. The immunosuppressing drugs include steroids, azathioprine, cyclosporine, repamycin, and FK-506.
3. **Privileged sites:** There appears to be certain privileged sites where graft may be accepted, e.g. cartilage where immune cells cannot go, testes where lymphatic drainage is not effective and cornea because of lack of vascularity.

HLA typing methods: Microcytotoxicity test, restriction fragment length polymorphism (RFLP) with southern blotting, polymerase chain reaction (PCR).

Histocompatibility

HLA Typing

HLA typing is done for detecting the HLA type. It is done by **'microcytotoxicity test'**. By this, we can identify HLA type of donor. For example, if that recipient is HLA B8 type, he will accept graft of a person having same HLA type. To check HLA type of donor, in microtitre plate, a known monoclonal antibody directed against particular HLA type is taken to which added donor's blood, complement and tryphan blue dye. If the donor's blood contains same HLA type against which antibody is coated, antigen–antibody complex is formed which fixes the complement available and this system causes lysis of lymphocytes, the dye stains only dead cells so we can find whether donor's lymphocytes are killed or not by staining.

Serological typing is not possible for HLA-DR antigen; they are detected by mixed leukocyte reaction **(MLR)**, and prime lymphocyte typing **(PLT)**. The genetic methods are restriction fragment length polymorphism **(RFLP)** and **gene sequence-specific oligonucleotide probe typing**.

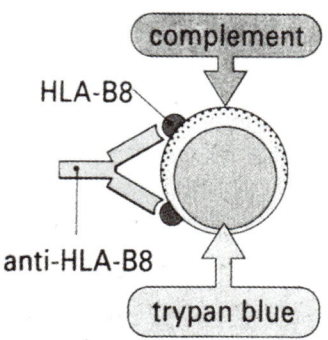

If a set of donors is identified by HLA typing, the exact match among these is identified by tissue matching.

Tissue Matching (Flowchart 21.2)

The donor's lymphocytes are killed, HLA antigens of which act as antigen. The recipient's lymphocytes are exposed to killed donor's lymphocytes in culture which undergo **blast formation,** which is seen by Giemsa staining. The intensity of blast formation is equivalent to disparity of HLA antigens of donor and the recipient.

Graft versus Host Reaction

Normally during the rejection of graft the antigens of donor's are considered as foreign and the recipient's cytotoxic cells take part in causing damage. If reverse occurs, the graft may mount an immune response against the host which shows the clinical features of reaction.

Prerequisites of this reaction are:

- The recipient contains the novel antigens which are absent on donor.
- Tc cells should be present in the graft which cause damage.

Flowchart 21.2: Tissue matching by microcytotoxicity

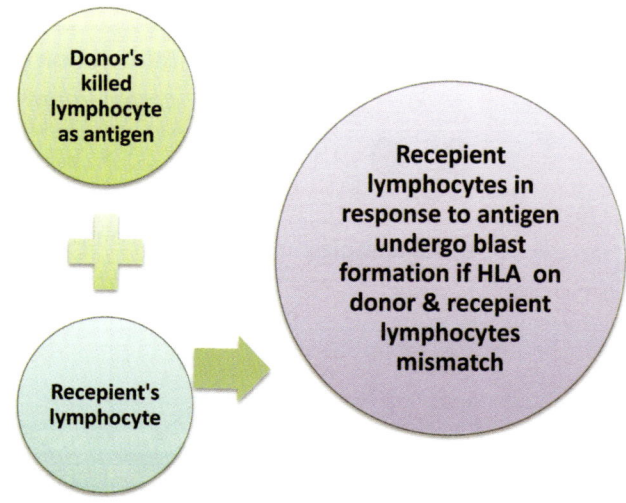

- The graft must be accepted otherwise it cannot mount the response.
- Thus GVR is predominantly CMI of donor tissue.

Examples of GVH

Graft in a recipient whose immune response is dampened by tolerance.

F1 hybrid receiving graft from any of the parent strain.

Clinical features are fever, rash, weight loss, retardation of growth, emaciation, anemia, hepatosplenomegaly and death. This is called Runt disease.

IMMUNOLOGY OF MALIGNANCY

Clinical evidence of immune response against tumors:
- Instances of spontaneous regression
- Removal of primary tumor leads to regression of metastasis
- Higher prevalence observed at autopsy
- Lymphocyte, plasma cells and macrophages provide histological evidence
- High incidence in immunodeficiency states.

Tumour Antigens (Table 21.1)

TSTA or TATA: The specific antigens present on tumor cells which cause rejection of the tumor, if it is transplanted in a synergic animal, are called tumor specific transplantation antigens (TSTA) or tumor associated transplantation antigens **(TATA).**

If the tumor is caused by chemicals, the TATA are tumor-specific while in tumor induced by viruses it is virus-specific.

Oncofetal Antigens

This type of antigen is present in embryonic life or present in tumor but not in human adults. **Alpha-fetoprotein** is an alpha globulin secreted by normal embryonic hepatocytes, the amount of it decreases after birth such that it is almost not detectable in adult blood. High levels of alpha-fetoprotein are found in hepatoma while carcinoembryonic antigen (CEA) is seen in colonic cancer.

Differentiation antigens are those, whose levels are raised in certain cancers helping the diagnosis of the cancers.

Immune Response in Malignancy

Both antibodies-mediated immunity and cell-mediated immunity are involved in tumor immunology. Delayed hypersensitivity is demonstrable by skin test. Anti-TSTA antibodies are demonstrable by indirect membrane immunofluorescence.

Mechanism of lapses
- Fast rate of proliferation
- Circulating tumor antigens acting as smokescreen
- Tumor antigens covered by antigenically neutral substance
- Immunological enhancement
- Low immunogenicity of tumors
- Blocking activity of antigen, antibody, antigen–antibody.

Immunotherapy of Cancer

Passive immunotherapy: Antisera, monoclonal antibody or chimeric antibodies called as 'immunotoxins' which are antibodies carrying gene for production of diphtheria toxin and Fab sites so that they only attach to tumor cells.

Specific active immunotherapy: Tumor cells were initially tried as **'tumor vaccine.'** Newer preparations containing modified tumor cell membrane antigens which are more antigenic, induce better response.

Nonspecific active immunotherapy: The various preparations used:
- Combination of BCG or inactivated *Corynebacterium parvum* (act as good immunomodulators) with tumor cells were tried in treatment of leukemia, malignant myeloma.
- Intradermal BCG after mastectomy used for treating breast cancer.
- Dinitrochlorobenzene used for treatment of skin cancers as squamous cell carcinoma.
- Certain polymers, as glucans, levamisole, induce CMI.
- **Specific adoptive immunotherapy:** Lymphocytes, immune rRNA, lymphokine activated killer cells (LAKs)

TABLE 21.1: TATAs used as tumor markers for diagnosis of cancers

Oncofetal proteins	Cancers
Alpha-fetoprotein (AFP)	Hepatoma, testicular carcinoma
Carcinoembryonic antigen (CEA)	Gastrointestinal cancers, lung cancer, ovarian cancer
Secreted tumor antigens	
CA125	Ovarian cancers
CA19-9	Various carcinomas
Prostate specific antigen	Prostate cancer
Beta 2 microglobulin	Multiple myeloma
Hormones	
Beta subunit of chorionic gonadotropin	Choriocarcinoma, hydatiform mole

Immunodiagnostic Tests

I. Analysis of blood for oncofetal antigens, alpha-fetoprotein in hepatoma and carcinoembryonic antigen in cancer colon.

II. GM1 monosialoganglioside—pancreatic carcinoma and colorectal carcinoma.

III. Localization of tumor by scanning after injection of radiolabeled monoclonal antibodies.

Immunological Surveillance

The immune system continuously performs survey of body for the presence of abnormal cells which are destroyed when recognized. The immune response to a tumor is thought to be an early event leading to destruction of the majority of tumors before the tumors present clinically. It is also proposed that immune system plays a role in delaying the growth or causing regression of tumors. According to this hypothesis, tumor formation occurs when it escapes the surveillance. The decreased surveillance happens due to immunodeficiency conditions. The mechanisms how tumors escape the immune surveillance may be due change of surface antigens, production of blocking antibodies. The CMI probably plays role in immune surveillance of which natural killer (NK) cell is more important. The evidences which show the role of immune surveillance, are:

1. Postmortem data suggest that there would be more tumors than clinically apparent.

2. Many tumors show the infiltration of lymphocytes.

3. Spontaneous regression of tumors occurs.

4. Tumors occur at the extremes of age when the immune responses are weak.

But other evidences which go against the concept are: In conditions of immunodeficiency or immuno-suppression, the spectrum of tumors arise is limited and viruses are causing most of them hence it was suggested that the immune surveillance may be important in controlling spread of oncogenic viruses.

22

Immunohematology

INTRODUCTION

Landsteiner (1900) discovered blood groups A and B. He cross-tested his own serum and his five colleagues with their RBCs. Based on agglutination, he designated group "O" to cells which did not give agglutination with any of the serum samples tested, while cells agglutinating in the two different patterns were called groups "A" and "B", respectively. The fourth group designated as AB was discovered by his student. Landsteiner, in the year 1930 was awarded Nobel Prize for his work.

ABO BLOOD GROUP SYSTEM

Blood groups are identified based on presence or absence of antigens **"A"** and **"B"** on RBCs. RBCs of blood group **"A"** carry A antigen on surface while his serum contains anti-B antibodies. RBCs of blood group B carry B antigen, serum of person with blood group B contain anti-A antibodies. On group AB, the antigen present is AB, while **'O' group RBCs carry no antigen.** These persons have no antibodies and anti-A and anti-B antibodies, respectively.

Natural Isoantibodies (Saline Agglutinating Antibodies) versus Immune Isoantibodies (Albumin Agglutinating Antibodies)

Natural isoantibodies: Antibodies against these blood groups are isoantibodies or natural antibodies as they arose without antigenic stimuli, under genetic control. They are saline agglutinating antibodies, IgM in nature which agglutinate RBCs in presence of saline, optimally at temperature between 4°C and 18°C.

Immune isoantibodies (albumin agglutinating antibodies) may develop due to ABO incompatible blood transfusion or pregnancies which agglutinate RBCs at 37°C in presence of albumin. Immune isoantibodies may cause severe transfusion reactions.

H antigen or H substance: It is a precursor for formation of A, B antigens and present in all RBCs of all blood groups. It is not significant as it does not cause reactions.

Bombay or OH blood: In a rare situation some person may not carry the antigens A, B and also antigen H. This is known as "**Bombay or OH group**. Sera of such persons are incompatible with all red blood cells except of those with the rare blood group.

Serum of this person contains antibodies to all antigens.

Distribution of ABO antigens on RBCs and iso-antibodies in the serum

Blood group	Antigen on RBC	Isoantibodies in serum
A	A	Anti-B
B	B	Anti-A
A B	AB	None
O	O None	Anti-A and Anti-B

RH BLOOD GROUP SYSTEM

History

Levine and Stertons work: A new type of antibody was demonstrated in the serum of a woman who had history of severe reactions after transfusion of her husband's ABO-compatible blood and she had recently delivered a stillborn infant with hemolytic disease. They suggested that some antigen inherited by the fetus from his father acted as sensitizing antigen and the name **anti-Rh factor antibody** was given to the new antibody developed in woman.

Landsteiner and Winer work: They identified a new type of antigen in RBCs of the majority of person's sera, an antigen which reacted with rabbit antiserum to Rhesus monkey RBCs; hence they called the antigen as "**Rhesus or Rh factor**".

Levine and colleagues proved that Rh sensitization as the cause of hemolytic disease in newborn.

At present, the Rh blood group system consists of 50 defined blood group antigens of which antigen D, C, c, E, and e are more important. **The term Rh factor refers to the D antigen only which is more immuno-genic.**

Rh typing: Of all the Rh antigens, antigen-D is most antigenic. Hence if mismatch occurs, majority of cases occur due to presence or absence of **antigen D (Rho)** when tested with anti-D (anti-Rh) antibodies which was the basis of Rh typing.

Distribution of Rh positives vary with different races, 93% of Indian are Rh positive compared with Europeans (85% Rh positive, 15% Rh negative).

Du subtype: Du is a variant of D. D cells may not be agglutinated with anti-D sera, but such cells adsorb antibodies which can be detected by direct Coombs' test. Practically for blood donation Du cells are considered as Rh positive. The Rh antibodies are not natural antibodies but they are produced due to mismatch Rh incompatible transfusion or pregnancy.

OTHER BLOOD GROUP SYSTEMS

Lewis blood group system consists of Le a and Le b. These antigens are present in plasma or saliva.

MN system: Initially three blood groups identified, i.e. N, MN; S antigen was later added (presently total 28 antigen types).

PREVENTION OF TRANSFUSION REACTIONS

These can be prevented by proper selection of donor by crossmatching. Ideally, the donor and recipient should have same **ABO** group, **O** group could be given to person with any **ABO** group as RBCs lack **A** and **B**. Therefore, the group **O** is considered as **universal donor.**

Dangerous O group: Mostly anti-A or anti-B antibodies present in serum of **O** group are not harmful because they become ineffective as they get diluted within recipient's plasma, but some **O** group plasma may contain high quantity of isoantibodies, damage to recipient's cells may occur, this is known as 'dangerous **O** group'.

Universal recipients: These are persons with **AB group** as isoantibodies are absent in plasma.

AB donors are rare, in such cases group A blood is safer than B as anti-A antibody is comparatively more potent.

Importance of Rh compatibility: Rh positive person can be safe even if the donor is Rh negative (as their sera already contain anti-Rh antibodies). **If recipient is Rh negative, then Rh compatibility is necessary** as these recipients get sensitized with Rh antigen which causes trouble in subsequent transfusions. It is particularly important, **if recipient is Rh negative woman** as she carries the risk of hemolytic disease in newborn, if child is Rh negative.

Importance of crossmatching: To ensure that donor's blood is compatible with recipient' blood, it is necessary to perform crossmatching. Rapid crossmatching is done by slide agglutination reaction between RBCs and serum.

Major crossmatching: Ordinarily **major** crossmatching is done by testing donor RBCs against recipient's serum. **Minor crossmatching** is done by testing recipient's RBCs against donor's serum.

HAEMOLYTIC DISEASE OF NEWBORN

Hemolytic disease occurs mostly when **mother is Rh negative** while **child is Rh positive**. During 1st pregnancy, fetus RBCs enter maternal circulation and induce Rh antibodies. During subsequent pregnancy, anti-Rh antibodies (**IgG class**) pass to fetus and damage RBCs. Mother being Rh negative, and antibodies are developed only after exposure to Rh antigen and take time to generate anti-Rh IgG antibodies which can cross placenta, therefore maternal antibodies do not lyse RBCs during 1st Rh incompatible pregnancy. Administration of anti-Rh antibodies can be given to mother so that by negative feedback mechanism, antibodies formation in mother is inhibited.

Erythroblastosis Fetalis

This clinical condition is known as hemolytic disease of newborn. Severity varies from patient to patient. It varies between mild accentuation of physiological jaundice or erythroblastosis fetalis or intrauterine death due to hydrops fetalis.

Incidence of hemolytic disease of newborn is less than expected because:

- **Immunological unresponsiveness (no responders)** of many individuals to Rh antigen.
- **ABO incompatibilities:** Hemolytic disease will occur, if same ABO group is present in donor and recipient blood compatibility while if both compatibility co-exist, Rh sensitization of mother due to fetus RBCs antigen is rare. Fetal cells entering circulation are destroyed rapidly by mother's ABO antibodies before they can induce Rh antibodies.

Zygocity of father with respect to Rh antigen plays a role as if father is homozygous, all his children will be Rh positive and if he **is heterozygous half** his children will be Rh negative.

Detection of Rh Antibodies

Most of the anti-Rh antibodies produced are IgG class and small proportion of IgM class (as they do not cross the placenta, they are clinically insignificant). The IgG antibodies are incomplete antibodies which can be detected by following methods:

- Indirect Coombs' test
- Agglutination with 20% bovine serum albumin as medium
- Using RBCs washed with enzymes as trypsin, pepcin, ficin or bromeli.

Identification of Rh Incompatibility

Rh typing should be done as routine antenatal examination. When fetal complications are expected, **intrauterine** infusion of Rh-negative **blood** may be indicated.

- RBCs injected in peritoneal cavity of fetus will enter blood and will live normally.
- Premature delivery with transfusion is done in some cases.

ABO Hemolytic Disease

Persons with antigen A or B possess anti-B or anti-A antibodies which are being **IgM** in nature and do not cross placenta. But person with blood group O has antibodies which are IgG in nature and may cause hemolytic disease. The disease is mild.

Transfusion Reactions

These are complications of blood transfusion which are of two types—**immunological** and **nonimmunological.**

Immunological Complications

a. *Acute hemolytic reactions*: As RBCs may undergo intravascular hemolysis or they are phagocytosed leading to extavascular lysis. These reactions are rare and occur due to mismatched blood transfusion.

Patients develop fever, chills, rigors, chest pain, hemorrhage, tachycardia, dyspnea, and hypotension or renal injury. If this reaction is suspected, transfusion is suddenly stopped.

b. *Delayed hemolytic reactions*: They may follow mismatched blood transfusion, reaction resembles acute hemolytic reaction but mild.

- *Febrile reaction* due to release of inflammatory substances released by WBCs present in stored blood.
- *Allergic reactions*: Recipient having preformed antibodies to substances present in donor's blood.
- **Post-transfusion thrombocytopenia** due to platelets with human platelet antigen-1a.

Nonimmunological Complications

This includes transfusion **transmitted infections.**

Viral infections
- HIV
- Hepatitis B, C,D
- CMV
- Human T lymphotropic virus

Bacteria
- *Leptospira interrogenes*
- *Borellia* species

Parasites
- *Plasmodium* species
- *Babesia* species
- *Leishmania donovani*
- *Toxoplasma gondii*
- *Trypanosome cruzi*

'T' antigen and Thomsen-Friedenreich phenomenon:
- *T antigen*: Normally all RBCs have this antigen but it is masked and anti-T antibodies are present in human sera.
- If a suspension of RBCs gets contaminated with certain bacteria (e.g. *Pseudomonas aeruginosa*), 'T' antigen is unmasked hence RBCs can cause agglutination with all blood group sera. This is called **Thomsen-Friedenreich phenomenon.**

23

Immunodeficiency

DEFINITION

The conditions in which the defense mechanisms of body are compromised which may lead to increased susceptibility to infections or sometimes increased susceptibility to malignancy.

Immunodeficiency is classified as **primary or secondary**.

Primary immunodeficiency is due to abnormalities in development of immune mechanisms while secondary immunodeficiency is consequence of disease, drugs, nutritional deficiency, metabolic disorders or other conditions which affect immunity.

Deficiency may be specific immunodeficiency as humoral, cellular immunodeficiency or it may be non-specific as deficiency of complement, phagocytic cells.

Primary immunodeficiency disorders are classified as those affecting B cells or T cells or both. There may be overlap between B cell and T cell systems.

DISORDERS OF SPECIFIC IMMUNITY

1. *Humoral immunodeficiency*:
   I. X-linked agammaglobulinemia
   II. Transient hypogammaglobulinemia of infancy
   III. Common variable immunodeficiency
   IV. Selective Ig deficiencies
   V. Immunodeficiency with hyper-IgM
   VI. Transcobalmin II deficiency

2. *Cellular immunodeficiency (T cell defects)*:
   - Thymic hypoplasia (DiGeorge's syndrome)
   - Chronic mucocutaneous candidiasis
   - Purine nucleoside phosphorylase (PNP) deficiency

3. *Combined immunodeficiency*:
   a. Ataxia telangiectasia
   b. Wiskott–Aldrich syndrome
   c. Immunodeficiency with thymoma

d. Immunodeficiency with short limbed dwarfism
e. Severe combined immunodeficiency which include Swiss type immunodeficiency, reticular dysgenesis of de Vaal, adenosine deaminase deficiency
f. Cellular immunodeficiency with abnormal immuno-globulin synthesis—Nezelof's syndrome
g. Episodic lymphopenia with lymphocytotoxin

1. Humoral Immunodeficiency

i. *X-linked agammaglobulinemia*: It is called 'Bruton disease' because Bruton first time described it.
   It is the first immunodeficiency to be described.
- Manifestations occur 6 months after birth in the form of recurrent infections with pyogenic bacteria as pneumococci, streptococci, meningococci, *Pseudomonas and Haemophilus influenzae*.
- Immunity to viral infections is normal.
- All types of immunoglobulins are depleted.
- Atrophy of tonsils and adenoids is observed.
- There is depletion of cells in B dependent area of lymph node.
- Number of B cells in circulation is decreased.
- Even after antigenic stimulation, antibodies formation does not occur.
- CMI is intact; delayed hypersensitivity is present. Allograft rejection is normal as CMI is normal.
- Arthritis, hemolytic anemia and atopic manifestations may occur.

Treatment: Immunoglobulin levels are maintained by injections of 300 mg of gamma globulins per kg body weight as starting dose and 100 mg per kg monthly dose.

ii. *Transient hypogammaglobulinemia of infancy*:
- There is delay in initiation of normal IgG synthesis.
- Recurrent otitis media and other respiratory infections occur.

- Spontaneous recovery is seen in 18–30 months.
- Both sexes involved.

iii. *Common variable immunodeficiency*: B cells present in peripheral blood are normal, but there is defect in development and differentiation (into plasma cells and secretory Igs)
- Late onset hypogammaglobulinemia.
- Giardiasis is common.
- Manifests at 15–35 years.
- Recurrent pyogenic infections, autoimmune diseases are seen.
- Malabsorption is seen.
- B cell number is normal but do not differentiate in plasma cells.
- There is increased suppressor T cell activity, and decreased helper T cell activity.

iv. *Selective Ig deficiencies*:
- IgA deficiency—0.2% of population affected, respiratory infection is common, and steatorrhea, atopic manifestations are seen in patients.
- IgM deficiency leads to septicemia.
- *IgG deficiency*: It causes chronic progressive bronchiectasis.

v. *Immunodeficiency (IDD) with hyper-IgM and low IgA and IgG*: It presents as infections, thrombocytopenia, neutropenia, hemolytic anemia, renal lesions.
     There is defect in isotypic class switch.

vi. *Transcobalamin II deficiency* presents as megaloblastic anemia, villous atrophy.

2. Cellular Immunodeficiency

***Thymic hypoplasia (DiGeorge's syndrome)*:**
- Developmental defect of 3rd and 4th pharyngeal pouches occurs.
- Hypoplasia of thymus and parathyroid glands occurs, neonatal tetany may occur.
- In lymph nodes or spleen—deficient thymus dependent areas are seen.
- T cells in circulation are reduced.
- Fatal viral, fungal, bacterial infections may occur.

***Chronic mucocutaneous candidiasis*:** Abnormal immunologic response to *Candida albicans* is seen in these patients. There may be severe candidiasis of skin, nails, mucosa along with endocrinopathies. Deficient CMI to Candida and antibodies to Candida present in high titer are the features present.

***Purine nucleoside phosphorylase (PNP) deficiency*:**
- PNP—purines, hypoxanthine, uric acid

- It is autosomal recessive trait.
- Recurrent infections (pneumonia, diarrhea, candidiasis, anemia) are seen.
- Low serum uric acid is observed.

3. Combined Immunodeficiencies

A. *Ataxia telangiectasia*:
- Hereditary, autosomal recessive condition.
- Immunodeficiency (IDD) with cerebellar ataxia, telangiectasia, ovarian dysgenesis, chromosomal abnormalities are seen.
- Telangiectasia present on conjunctiva, face.
- Death is due to infection or malignancies.
- IgA, IgE deficiencies are common.

B. *Wiskott-Aldrich syndrome*:
- X-linked—eczema, thrombocytopenic purpura, recurrent infections occur.
- Boys are affected.
- Fatal in 1st decade of life.
- Progressive deterioration of CMI may occur.

C. *Immunodeficiency with thymoma*:
- It is benign thymic tumor.
- Impaired CMI and agammaglobulinemia present
- Aplastic anemia

D. *Immunodeficiency with short-limbed dwarfism*: The defects are inherited as autosomal recessive which include:
- Short-limbed dwarfism
- Thymic defects
- Dysplasia of ectoderm
     Susceptibility to infections is increased.

E. *Severe combined immunodeficiencies*:
- There is severe deficiency of both CMI and humoral immunity. It is an autosomal recessive defect in immunocompetent cells of fetal liver and bone marrow. Various patterns are seen.
- **Swiss type agammaglobulinemia:** Agammaglobulinemia with lymphocytopenia and severe defects in CMI seen.
- Reticular dysgenesis of de Vaal in which defect in hemopoietic stem cell in bone marrow shows aplasia and there is lymphopenia, neutropenia, thrombocytopenia, and anemia.

Adenosine deaminase (ADA) deficiency
- There may be mild abnormality of B or T cell function or abnormality is absent.
- This is the first immunodeficiency which has relation to enzyme deficiency.
- ADA is required in purine metabolic pathway.

F. Cellular immunodeficiency with abnormal immuno-globulin synthesis (Nezelofs syndrome):
- CMI is depressed.
- Immunoglobulins selectively increased, decreased or normal.
- Thymus is small, peripheral lymphoid tissues are hypoplastic.
- Autoimmune processes as hemolytic anemia are common.

G. Episodic lymphopenia with lymphocytotoxin:
- It is a familial disease.
- It is characterized by episodes of profound T cell dysfunction due to production of circulating complement-dependent lymphocytotoxin.
- The toxin acts as antilymphocyte antibody
- Immunological memory is absent.

PRIMARY IMMUNODEFICIENCY OF NONSPECIFIC IMMUNITY

Disorders of phagocytosis
a. Chronic granulomatous disease
b. Myeloperoxidase deficiency
c. Chediak-Higashi syndrome
d. Leukocyte G6PD deficiency
e. Job's syndrome
f. Tuftsin deficiency
g. Lazy leukocyte syndrome
h. Shwachman's syndrome

Deficiencies of complement
1. *Complement component deficiencies*: C3, C6, C7, C8- SLE, infections
2. *Complement inhibitor deficiencies*: C1 inhibitor.

Disorders of Phagocytosis

a. Chronic granulomatous disease:
- It is a familial disease with chronic progress which may be fatal.
- Recurrent infections with organisms with low virulence occur hence chronic suppurative granulo-matous lesions on skin along with hepatosplenomegaly with involvement of lymph nodes are seen.
- Humoral and cellular immunity is normal.
- Recurrent infections are common.
- WBCs of patients are not able to kill catalase-positive bacteria such as *Staphylococcus, E. coli.* These organisms multiply intracellularly.
- *The reasons are*:
  1. Decreased oxygen consumption
  2. Decreased hexose monophosphate pathway activity.

3. Decreased production of hydrogen peroxide.
4. Delayed granulation rupture and defective release of myeloperoxidase.
- Leukocytes fail to reduce nitro blue tetrazolium during phagocytosis (NTB).

b. Myeloperoxidase deficiency: It is a rare disorder in which leukocytes are deficient in the enzyme myeloxidase. Patients may develop recurrent infections with *C. albicans.*

c. Chediak-Higashi syndrome: Polymorphonuclear leukocytes of the patients have abnormally large lysosomes which do not fuse easily with phagosome. Hence; these leukocytes have reduced phagocytic activity. Patients develop from severe pyogenic infections.

d. Leukocyte G6PD deficiency: Leukocytes lack the enzyme glucose-6 -phosphates hence show diminished bactericidal activity. Patients are susceptible to microbial infections.

e. Job's syndrome:
- The mechanism causing this immunodeficiency is not clear.
- Commonest presentation is formation of multiple, large staphylococcal 'cold abscesses' on skin or in other organs. There is minimum inflammation.

f. Tuftsin deficiency: Tuftsin is an enzyme which stimulates phagocytosis; hence recurrent systemic bacterial infections are common. The enzyme **tuftsin** (leukokinin) is a small **tetrapeptide (Thr –Ly-Pro-Arg).**

g. Lazy leukocyte syndrome: Peripheral neutropenia is seen even if bone marrow shows normal counts, hence recurrent bacterial infections with stomatitis, otitis and pharyngitis are seen.

h. Shwachman's syndrome: There are neutropenia, pancreatic insufficiency, bone marrow dysfunction, short stature and skeletal abnormalities.

Disorders of Complement

1. **Complement component deficiencies:** Genetic deficiency of many complement components have been detected in man. Deficiency of C1r and C4 is associated with systemic lupus erythematosus. Deficiency of C3 is severe abnormality which results in increased susceptibility to pyogenic infections. Deficiencies of C6–C8 are associated with neisserial infections. Most of the complement component deficiency disorders are autosomal recessive traits except that of properdin which is X-linked recessive disorder.

2. *Complement inhibitor deficiencies*: Genetic deficiency of C1q inhibitor leads to hereditary angioneurotic edema. It is transmitted as autosomal dominant trait. There is uncontrolled activation of C1 that leads to excessive release of substances. In C1 inhibitor deficiency, complement pathway as well as other pathways as clotting, fibrinolytic, kinin are also affected. Activation of factor XII (Hageman factor) leads to formation of bradykinin and C2 kinin. Kinins cause contraction of endothelial cells of venules, form gaps which allow plasma leakage leading to edema.

Conditions causing secondary immunodeficiencies:
1. HIV
2. CLL
3. Nephritic syndrome
4. Protein losing enteropathies
5. Multiple myeloma
6. Hodgkin's disease
7. Leprosy
8. Aging
9. Immunosuppressive agents

24

Staphylococcus

HISTORY

- A summary of history of staphylococci was provided by AC Baird-parks.
- Sir Alexander Ogston demonstrated in 1880 that a cluster forming coccus was the cause of certain pyogenic abscesses in man.
- He named the organism *Staphylococcus* in 1882.
- Gram-positive cocci are classified into two families—**Micrococcaceae** and **Streptococcaceae.**
- Members of family Micrococcaceae are catalase-positive, while members of the family Streptococcaceae are catalase-negative.
- *Staphylococcus* belongs to family **Micrococcaceae** which include four genera:
  1. Staphylococcus
  2. Micrococcus
  3. Stomatococcus
  4. Planococcus.
- **Stomatococcus** and **Planococcus** are not pathogenic to man.
- **Micrococci** are skin commensals, usually do not cause human infection, they are of size 1–1.8 µ, arranged in tetrads. They give oxidative O-F test positive.
- **Staphylococci:** They are special cocci, grow easily on media. Some of the species are members of normal flora of skin, mucosa, others cause suppuration, abscess formation and septicemia. They easily develop resistance making them difficult to treat.

CLASSIFICATION OF STAPHYLOCOCCI

Based on the production of enzyme coagulase:

- ***Coagulase-positive:*** *Staphylococcus aureus* (*S. intemedius* and *S. hyicus* are tube coagulase-positive which are animal species.)
- ***Coagulase-negative staphylococci (CoNS):*** *Staphylococcus epidermidis* and *Staphylococcus saprophyticus* account to most of the infections caused by CoNS.
- ***Other CoNS are:*** *Staphylococcus haemolyticus, S. lugdunensis, S. schleiferi, S. capitis, S. homonis* and *S. warnerii.*

  S. lugdunensis, S. schleiferi may give slide coagulase-positive, but tube coagulase negative. *S. aureus* is VP positive and *S. intermedius* and *S. hycus* are VP negative (among these two, *S. intermedius* may give PYR test positive).

Old Classification based on the Pigment Production
(Fig. 24.1)

- *Staphylococcus aureus* produces golden yellow pigment.
- *Staphylococcus albus* produces white pigment.
- *Staphylococcus citrus* produces lemon yellow pigment.

TABLE 24.1: Tests used for differentiation of staphylococci and micrococci

	Staphylococci	*Micrococci*
Sensitivity to lysostaphin	Resistant	Sensitive
Modified oxidase test	Negative	Positive
Anaerobic breakdown of mannitol	Positive	Negative
Bacitracin	Resistant	Sensitive
Sensitivity to lysozyme	Resistant	Some strains are sensitive

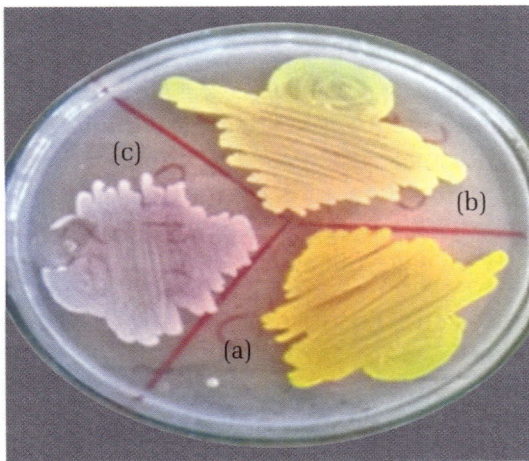

Fig. 24.1: (a) *S. aureus*, (b) *S. citrus*, (c) *S. albus*

As later on, the focus was on the basis of coagulase as a factor for pathogenicity, it was found that coagulase positive *Staphylococcus aureus* may produce pigment, the color of which may vary from golden yellow, white, lemon yellow, orange and also some strains may not even produce any pigment, the classification based on pigment production is not in use.

STAPHYLOCOCCUS AUREUS

Morphology

- These are Gram-positive cocci arranged in clusters (**grape-like clusters**, coccus means berry hence the name) as cell division occurs haphazardly in three planes which are perpendicular to each other (Fig. 24.2). In liquid media, short chains may appear but unlike streptococci, **staphylococci rarely form chains containing more than four members.**
- The size of each coccus is about 1μ.
- Non-motile, **non-sporing, non-capsulated.**
- Many strains may have capsule.

Cultural Characteristics

- Growth requirements are simple; it grows on ordinary or simple media.

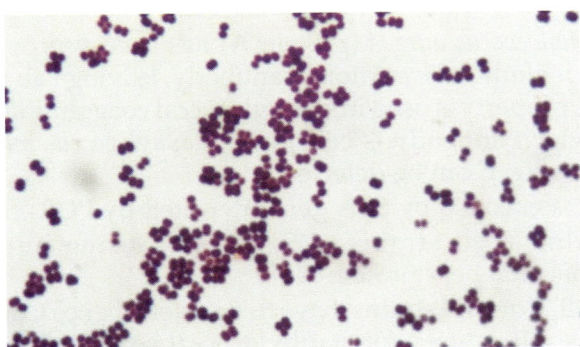

Fig. 24.2: Gram-positive cocci in clusters

- Optimum temperature is 37°C (10–42°C).
- pH—7.4–7.6.
- It is aerobic and facultative anaerobic.

A. Simple medium or ordinary medium
Nutrient agar:
- Nutrient agar plate: After 24 hours incubation, 2–4 mm circular convex, smooth, shiny opaque colonies produced which are easily emulsifiable. It may or may not produce non-diffusible pigment, the color of which is usually golden yellow. The pigment is of lipoprotein (carotene) in nature.
- Micrococci form regular packets of four (tetrads) or eight cocci. Their colony can be red or orange yellow.
- Nutrient agar slope: The confluent growth presents characteristic "**oil paint**" appearance.

B. Enriched medium

Blood agar: β hemolysis is produced by most strains, which is enhanced by incubation under 20–25°C (Fig. 24.3).

Selective media for *S. aureus* are listed below which are only used to grow this bacterium from stool sample from a case of **food poisoning**.
- **Salt-milk agar,** salt broth (contains 8–10% sodium chloride, polymyxin)
- **Ludlam's medium** (lithium chloride and tellurite added)
- **Mannitol salt agar:** Yellow colonies produced. It is selective as well as indicator medium used for screening *methicillin-resistant Staphylococcus aureus (MRSA)* from nose to find out carrier which may act as source of outbreak (Fig. 24.4).
- **Blood potassium tellurite medium:** It produces black colonies as it reduces potassium tellurite to metallic tellurium (normally blood potassium tellurite is a selective medium used to grow *Corynebacterium diphtheriae* from a case of pharyngitis).

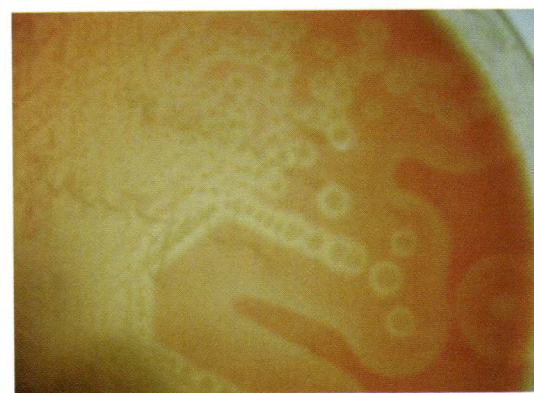

Fig. 24.3: Blood agar showing golden yellow, beta hemolytic colonies

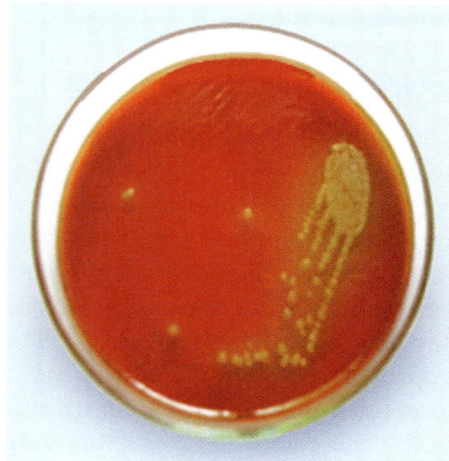

Fig. 24.4: Mannitol salt agar with growth of *Staph aureus*

C. Enrichment broth: Salt cooked meat broth used for stool sample in case of food poisoning.

D. Media to increase pigment production are 1% glycerol monoacetate, milk agar. Pigment production is enhanced by incubating culture plate at room temperature.

Pigment is not produced during anaerobic growth or in liquid culture.

Note: Initially pigment production by this bacterium was correlated with virulence but now it is proved that other factors are responsible for pathogenicity.

MacConkey agar is usually not used for Gram-positive cocci but *Staphylococcus aureus* may give pinpoint pink colonies.

Biochemical Reactions of *S. aureus*

- **Catalase positive:** This test differentiates it from streptococci which are catalase negative.
- **Coagulase test is positive:** This test differentiates *Staphylococcus aureus* from *Staphylococcus epidermidis* and *Staphylococcus saprophyticus*.
- **It ferments mannitol:** This test differentiates *Staphylococcus* from *Micrococcus* (which may cause confusion in diagnosis).
- **DNase positive:** For the detection of thermonuclease (DNase), medium with toludine blue is used. From broth suspension of organism (which was boiled for 15 minutes), one drop is taken on DNase agar, the plate is incubated at 30°C to 2–4 hours. Formation of pink halo around the drop is positive test. The agar contains toludine blue DNA complex (blue color), the enzyme acts on it producing pink occurs.
- It reduces nitrates to nitrites.
- It liquefies gelatin.
- Indole is negative.

- MR, VP, citrate, urease are positive.
- **Phosphatase:** Organism is grown on phenophthalein diphosphate agar. *Staphylococcus aureus* breaks down phenophthalein diphosphate releasing phenophthalein. If plate is exposed to ammonia, under the alkaline condition, pink color is formed.
- It is lipolytic on egg-yolk media, hence produces opacity on egg-yolk agar.

Characteristic Features of Pathogenic Strains of *S. aureus*

- Beta hemolysis
- Production of golden yellow pigment.
- Catalase, coagulase positive
- DNase positive
- Phosphatase positive
- Liquefies gelatin
- Mannitol fermentation
- Reduce potassium tellurite to metallic tellurium, hence produce black colonies.

Resistance

They remain live for 36 months. Comparatively heat resistent, killed by 62°C for 30 minutes. They may grow in presence of 10–15% NaCl. They are highly sensitive to crystal violet (1:500,000). They are sensitive to lysostaphin or resistant to lysozyme.

Virulence Factors of *Staphylococcus aureus*

Antigens

- Capsular polysaccharide is present in some strains only, it inhibits phagocytosis.
- Peptidoglycan can cause complement activation, and can stimulate IL-1 production which acts endogenous pyrogen and causes fever. It has chemotactic activity, endotoxin activity and activates complement.
- Teichoic acid helps in adhesion and protects from opsonization. It is antigenic; antibodies against it detected by gel diffusion and is found in endocarditis.

Protein-A (SpA)

Staphylococcus aureus (protein-A) has special property that it binds to Fc portion of antibody, leaving Fab free. This property is used in staphylococcal coagglutination in which antibody is coated on *Staphylococcus aureus* and antigen can be detected.

- It is encoded by **SpA gene (detected by PCR)**.
- Almost all strains of *S. aureus* causing human infection bear protein-A.
- All 'Cowan I strains' have this protein; hence **Cowan I strain** is used for **staphylococcal coagglutination test.**

- **Biological properties:** Antiphagocytic, anticomplementary, antichemotactic
- **Mediates 'co-agglutination reaction'.**

Microcapsule

Some strains possess microcapsule made up of polysaccharide which inhibits phagocytosis. This is important in abscess formation.

Adhesions

- Fibronectin-binding adhesion
- Collagen-binding adhesion
- Clumping factor or bound coagulase, which is a fibrinogen-binding adhesion, mediates slide coagulase.

Clumping Factor

It is surface protein; also called bound coagulase. When suspension of organism from colony in normal saline is mixed with plasma on a slide, it forms clumps. This test is used as one of the tests for identification of *S. aureus*.

Toxins

Cytolytic toxins
Hemolysin—α, β, γ and δ.

- *Alpha toxin:* It is important in pathogenicity, it is toxic to macrophages and lysozymes. It is lethal leukocidal and dermonecrotic. It is inactivated at 70°C but regain activity paradoxically at 100°C as it combines a heat labile inactivator which gets denatured at 100°C.
- *Beta toxin:* It shows **hot cold phenomena,** hemolysis begins at 37°C and evident only on chilling. It lyses human RBCs, rabbit RBCs but not sheep RBCs.
- *Gamma toxin:* Antigenic antibodies against it are produced in deep infections which can detected by latex agglutination test.
- Delta toxin has effect on RBCs, platelets.
  Leukocidin damages polymorphs and macrophages.

Leukocidins/Panton Valentine Toxin

- It acts synergistically with 'γ hemolysin' (synergohymenotropic toxins) which damages RBCs, leukocytes and macrophages.
- **MRSA strains** which are **community acquired (CA-MRSA)** (cause community-acquired infections) express this toxin, while hospital-acquired MRSA (HA-MRSA) stains do not have this toxin (Table 24.2).
- It has two components, coded by mobile bacteriophage.
- It can kill leukocytes of humans and rabbits.
- It causes desquamation of skin by dissolving mucopolysaccharide matrix of epidermis.

TABLE 24.2: Differences between community-acquired MRSA and hospital-acquired MRSA

CA-MRSA	HA-MRSA
Staphylococcal cassette chromosome mec (SCCmec) type IV	SCC types I, II, III are associated with HA-MRSA
More transmissible	Less transmissible
Less resistant to other antibiotics	Resistance to many antibiotics
Outbreaks restricted to some geographical area in USA and some parts of Europe	Worldwide
More virulent	Less virulent
Presence of PVL	Absent PVL
No underlying risk factors in patients as present in HA-MRSA	Presence of underlying predisposing factor

Enterotoxin

It causes for manifestations of food poisoning. Toxin is present in meat, fish, milk and milk products cooked and left at room temperature after contamination. Eight antigenic types of toxin A, B, C1-3, D, E and H are seen. Type A is responsible for most cases. Intective dose is 1 μg. The toxin acts on neural receptors present in GIT. Toxin detection is done by ELISA and latex agglutination.

Staphylococcus food poisoning is due to consumption of **preformed toxin** (toxin secreted in food before consumption) in food hence, it has **short incubation period.** More than one patient is involved, and organism can be isolated from food also.

- Carriers act as source of infection.
- Food items responsible for food poisoning are milk, milk products, bakery products, custards or processed meat.
- Some cases of pseudomembranous colitis following use of antibiotics are due to enterotoxin.
- Treatment is supportive which involves correction of fluid loss and electrolytes imbalance.

Toxic Shock Syndrome Toxin (TSST-1)

It is enterotoxin F. It does not cause food poisioning.

Super antigen: It is presented by antigen presenting cells in a different way hence causes excessive stimulation of T cells that leads to excess production of cytokines. Due to this, patient has multiple organ failure and shock. This condition was common among females using absorbent tampons through which oxygen enters inside and bacteria multiply and produce toxins. This condition is also seen in male following other infections. The gene for the toxin is found in 20% of *Staphylococcus* isolates including MRSA. Most of the strains which produce this toxin belong to phage **group I.**

Exfoliative Toxin

It is also called as epidermolytic toxin or staphylococcal scalded skin (SSS) toxin. It is responsible for staphylococcal scalded skin syndrome.

The mild forms of the disease known as pemphigus neonatorum and impetigo.

Ritter's disease is severe form in newborn and toxic epidermal necrosis in older patients.

Enzymes

- *Coagulase*: It clots human plasma. It acts with coagulase-reacting factor (CRF) present in plasma, binds to prothrombin and converts fibrinogen into fibrin.
- Lipases (lipid hydrolases) breakdown lipids.
- Hyaluronidase breaksdown intracellular cement substance.
- Nucleases lyse nucleic acids which come along their way.
- Fibrinolysins have fibrinolytic activity.

Pyrogenic exotoxins A, B and C are identified, but their role in pathogenesis is not known.

Type 'C pyrogenic exotoxin' is produced by *Staphylococcus* strains producing toxic shock syndrome.

Coagulase: The bacterium produces two types of coagulases, i.e. slide (bound coagulase) and free coagulase. Bound coagulase is detected by slide coagulase test while free coagulase is detected by tube coagulase test. Free coagulase acts with coagulase reacting factor present in plasma, binds to prothrombin and converts fibrinogen to fibrin, which forms clumps. It is antigenic in nature and 8 antigenic types are known, type 'A' is commonest type produced by most pathogenic strains of *S. aureus*.

The differences between these are as follows:

Free coagulase	Bound coagulase (clumping factor)
Heat labile	Heat stable
Requires the help of coagulase reacting factor to give test positive	Action independent
It has 8 antigenic types	Only one antigenic type
Secreted into medium	It is constituent of cell wall, bound to it

Panton–Valentine Leukocidin

It has two components, coded by mobile phage. It can kill WBC of humans and rabbits. This toxin is an important factor for community acquired MRSA, i.e. *CA-MRSA*. It causes desquamation of skin by dissolving mucopolysaccharide matrix of the epidermis (Table 20.2).

Pathogenesis

These organisms are members of normal flora of human skin and respiratory tract especially *S. epidermidis*. 10–30% of normal individuals carry staphylococci in nose. These organisms are also found on clothing, bed linen, and other fomites. Infection may be endogenous or exogenous. The pathogenic property is the combined effect of extracellular factors, and toxins together.

Pathogenicity

- Peptidoglycan activates alternative pathway complement.
- Teichoic acids help in adhesion to mucosal cells. They also cause complement activation.
- Protein 'A' binds to 'Fc' portion of antibody and, therefore, decreases opsonization. Protein 'A' released into surrounding medium, binds free antibodies.
- Catalase converts H_2O_2 into water thus counteracts the neutrophil's ability to kill bacteria.
- Coagulase converts fibrinogen into fibrin and fibrin surrounding the bacteria protects them from phagocytosis.
- Several pore-forming toxins damage phagocytes, vascular endothelium, myocardial cells, neurons, renal endothelial cells.

Staphylococci have cell wall associated proteins called 'Microbial surface components recognizing adhesive matrix proteins which help them to colonize skin and mucosa. Fibronectin-binding proteins present on them helps in invasion through skin, mucosa. It also help to attach to fibronectin present in wound. The bacteria have also MSCRAMs for collagen binding proteins. Collagen binding proteins (CBPs) are important component of bones, connective tissue, joints. Other MSCRAMs called clumping factors A and B are present for fibrinogen binding.

Leukocidin damages phagocytic cells. It contributes to pus producing lesions (pyogenic).

Other pyogenic bactereia are *Streptococcus pyogenes, Streptococcus pneumoniae, E. coli, Klebsiella sp., Proteus sp., Pseudomonas aeruginosa.*

Diseases

Diseases caused by staphylococci are divided into infections—which may be **superficial or deep and toxin-mediated diseases.**

Survival of staphylococci depends upon infective dose, site involved, the speed with which host mounts immune response. When inoculum is small and host is competent, infections are halted.

- Staphylococci form a localized collection of pus called **abscess.**
- **Abscess in skin is called boil or furuncle.**
- Multiple interconnecting abscesses are called **carbuncles.** Carbuncles are larger multiloculated skin lesions which may lead to bacteremia.
- Spread in subcutaneous or submucosal tissue causes diffuse inflammation called **cellulitis.**

The formation of abscess is a complex process involving host and bacteria. Early events may be fast, with development of acute inflammation. Chemotactic factors from bacteria and those derived from complements invite neutrophils which may kill some of the bacteria but some of them survive. The lysed neutrophils release large amounts of lysozymes and cause further damage.

The protein 'A' is a cell wall component of a strains of staphylococci and it is a bacterial surface protein, that has been characterized among a group of adhesions called microbial surface *components* recognizing adhesive matrix molecules called **MSCRAMs**.

The combinatioin of MSCRAMs and intense host response to bacteria results in the area being surrounded by fibrin. The centre of abscess is necrotic, contain debris which contains dead epithelial cells, dead neutrophils, bacteria, edema fluid. There is great fight between bacteria and neutrophils. Usually neutrophils always win.

Superficial and Deep Infections (Flowchart 24.1)

1. **Skin infections** (Fig. 24.5) include boils, folliculitis, carbuncle, furuncle, secondary infection of wounds, burns, impetigo, cellulitis and hidradenitis suppurativa (recurrent infection in areas rich in sebaceous glands).

Flowchart 24.1: Sources for staphylococcal infections and their acquization or modes of infection

Infected lesions	• Dried pus from infected wound or burn, coughed sputum by person with pneumonia • Mode of infection is by direct contact
Healthy carriers	• Carriers have Staphylococci in nose, hands. Carriers shed bacteria in skin squames and cloth fibers
Endogenus infections	• Patient himself has Staphylococci in nose or at other sites from where bacteria go to other sites and cause infections. e.g. Staphylococcus aureus in nose carried by fingers of the patient producing stye
Environment(exogenous infections)	• It does not form spores but remain alive in a dormant state for several months when dried in pus , sputum, beddings or cloths and surfaces as floor
Animals	• Milk from dairy cow with mastitis causing Staphylococcus food poisioning. Mode of infection is feco-oral/ ingestion

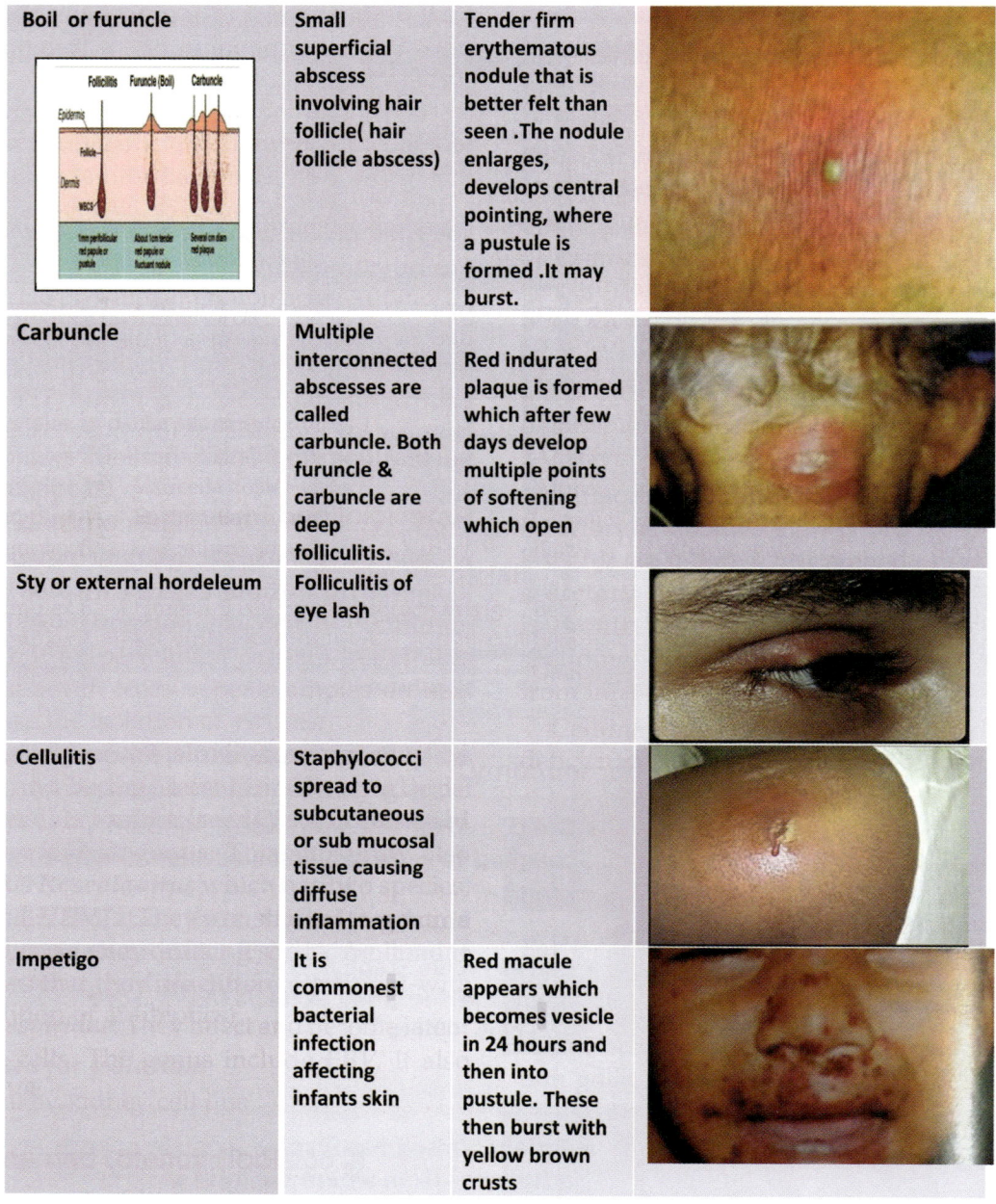

Boil or furuncle	Small superficial abscess involving hair follicle(hair follicle abscess)	Tender firm erythematous nodule that is better felt than seen .The nodule enlarges, develops central pointing, where a pustule is formed .It may burst.	
Carbuncle	Multiple interconnected abscesses are called carbuncle. Both furuncle & carbuncle are deep folliculitis.	Red indurated plaque is formed which after few days develop multiple points of softening which open	
Sty or external hordeleum	Folliculitis of eye lash		
Cellulitis	Staphylococci spread to subcutaneous or sub mucosal tissue causing diffuse inflammation		
Impetigo	It is commonest bacterial infection affecting infants skin	Red macule appears which becomes vesicle in 24 hours and then into pustule. These then burst with yellow brown crusts	

Fig. 24.5: Skin infections produced by *Staphylococcus aureus*

2. **Respiratory infections** are tonsillitis, sinusitis, otitis, lung abscess, empyema, pneumonia.
3. **CNS infections** are meningitis, brain abscess.
4. **Musculoskeletal infections** include pyogenic arthritis, osteomyelitis, bursitis and botryomycosis (a condition resembling mycetoma).
5. Urinary tract infections.
6. Other infections are bacteremia, septicemia, endocarditis, and pericarditis, renal abscess, polymyositis, breast abscess.

Other manifestations include:
- Respiratory tract infections, ventricular associated pneumonia.

- Septic pulmonary emboli.
- Pneumatocele is seen in neonate due to shaggy thin-walled cavities in lungs, the condition is common in neonates.
- PSOS abscess.
- Epidural abscess.

Food Poisoning

- It causes toxic type of food poisoning as preformed toxin in food is consumed by patients.

- As preformed toxin is consumed by patients, clinical incubation period is short (1–6 hours).

- Types of food responsible for it are meat, fish, milk, milk products which are cooked and left at room temperature for enough time so that staphylococci multiply and produce toxin before food is consumed.

Patient presents with fever, hypotension, vomiting, diarrhea and erythematous rash.

Staphylococcal Scalded Skin Syndrome (SSSS)

It is because of exfoliative toxin which causes separation of layers of epidermis from underlying tissue. Two types of toxin, thermostable (ETB) and thermolabile, are known, the toxin producing strains belong to phage group II.

The illness is common in newborns and children. There may be localized tender blister or bullae formation or exfoliation and separation outer epidermis layer.

Resistance to Penicillin

Three types of resistance is seen.
1. *Production of beta lactamases*: It is plasmid mediated, transmitted by **transduction or conjugation.** Four types of penicillases are produced A to D. Hospital strains form **type A.** This enzyme is induced in presence of antibiotic.
2. *Changes in surface receptor*: It is due to altered **PB2-penicillin binding protein-2.** The change is chromosomal, the resistant gene is **mec A gene** which forms a part of **staphylococcal cassette chromosome (SCCmec).** This resistance also extends to penicillinase resistant penicillins as methicillin and cloxacillin. The genetic material is transmitted to *Staphylococcus aureus* from *S. seiuri.*

   The resistance is expressed at 30°C rather than 37°C. At 37°C, methicillin is unstable, therefore, oxacillin disc was used as surrogate marker for detection of MRSA. Cefoxitin is better representative, presently it is used for screening of MRSA. The gene for resistance can be detected by PCR.
3. Third type of resistance seen is due to development of **tolerance**.

STAPHYLOCOCCUS EPIDERMIDIS

It produces slime layer with which it colonizes medical devices and cause infection which may lead to **septicemia.** It is present on normal skin. It is common cause of stich abscess. It may cause prosthetic wall endocarditis, cystitis especially in drug addicts.

Staphylococcus saprophyticus can cause urinary tract infection in sexually active young women.

Novobiocin test differentiates between *S. epidermidis* and *S. saphrophyticus* (resistant) shedders.

Epidemiology

Most common sources of infection are carriers and patients. About 10–30% of healthy persons carry staphylococci as commensals in nose and about 10% on perineum and hair. Carriage occurs early in life. Acquisition of *S. aureus* infection may be exogenous or endogenous (from a carriage site or minor lesion elsewhere in body.

Laboratory Diagnosis of Staphylococcal Infections

Specimen Collection

Depending upon the sites of infection, specimens collected are:
- Swab or aspirates from wound infections, burn infections, and osteomyelitis.
- Blood if septicemia is suspected, it is collected in glucose broth, which after 48 hours of incubation is subcultured on nutrient agar and blood agar.
- Stool and food samples are collected from cases of food poisoning.
- Other source of infection in a patient suffering from **TSS.**
- Swabs from anterior part of nose: This sample is only collected for detection of carriers.

Gram staining: It shows pus cells and Gram-positive cocci in clusters, some cocci in pairs or short chains.

Culture: Nutrient agar is used for pigment production.

BA: It shows colonies with betahemolysis.

MSA: Mannitol salt agar is used for stool sample and nasal swab, looked for yellow colonies.

Ludluam's medium: This is selective medium used for food poisoning.

Biochemical tests: Catalase test differentiates *Staphylococcus* from *Streptococcus*.

Coagulase test is positive for *Staphylococcus aureus*.

If results of slide and tube coagulase (Fig. 24.6) are not sure, other tests performed—DNase, phosphatase test.

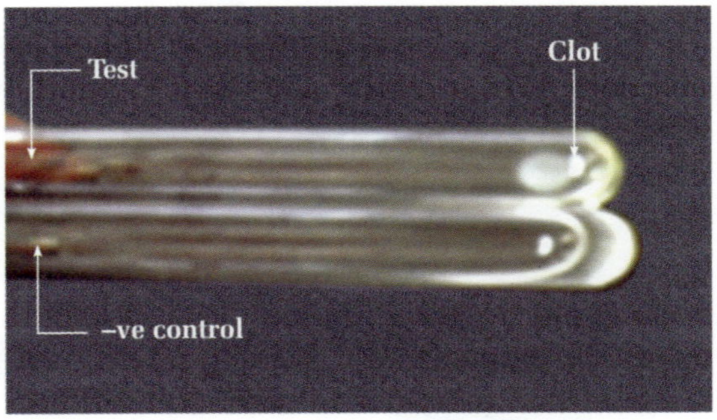

Fig. 24.6: Tube coagulase test

Serological Diagnosis

Deep seated staphylococcal infections can be diagnosed by detection of antibodies in patient's serum.

1. **Antibodies against teichoic acids** are useful.
2. **Anti-staphylolysin 'O' titer** is also detected in patient's serum. Titer more than 2 is significant.

Antibacterial susceptibility testing is done by Kirby Bauer's disc diffusion test. The following antibiotics are tested and reported on Müeller Hinton agar. Antibiotics tested are penicillin, erythromycin, gentamicin, vancomycin, netilimicin and chloramphenicol. Cefoxitin disc is tested for MRSA screening.

Laboratory Diagnosis of Staphylococcus Aureus Food Poisoning

It produces toxic type of food poisoning as, food containing preformed toxin is consumed by patient. As preformed toxin is ingested along with food, clinical **incubation is short, 6–8 hours** and manifestations are vomiting and loose motions.

Types of food responsible are milk **or milk product, ice-cream.**

If more than one person has consumed the same food, more than one patient may suffer from food poisoning and it is an outbreak. In this case, to prove that food was responsible, one needs to isolate organism from patient's samples and the common food and the strain of *Staphylococcus aureus* should be the same. Strains from patients are matched with strains isolated from food by any one of the typing method as bacteriophage typing or genotypic method as RFLP. (Flowchart 24.2)

Sample collection: Samples collected are stool samples, vomitus and food.

Flowchart 24.2: Identification of staphylococci

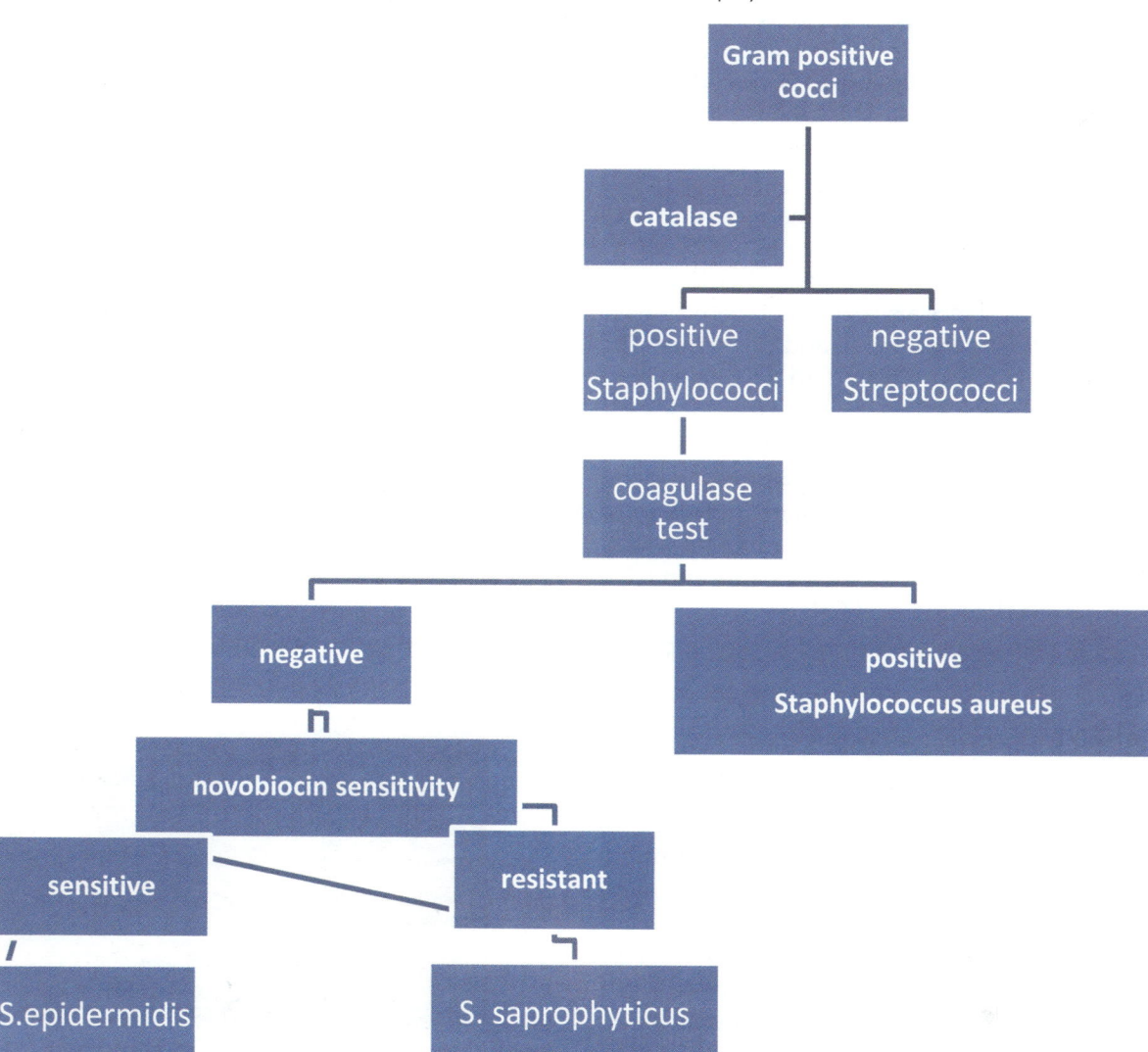

Transportation: Part of each specimen transported in enrichment medium as salt meat broth. Rest samples transported in sterile container to perform Gram staining.

Processing

Gram staining of stool sample will show predominantly Gram-positive cocci in clusters with no pus cells.

Importance of Gram staining: Predominance of cocci and absence of pus cells give clue for food poisoning due to *Staphylococcus*, and provisional report may be given to start treatment.

Samples are inoculated on following media:

- **Nutrient agar** for pigment production
- **Blood agar** for demonstration of **betahemolysis.**
- **Ludlam's or salt milk agar** which are selective media which inhibit the growth of commensals present in stool samples.

Processing from the Growth

a. **Repeat Gram staining** and confirm the morphology.
b. Perform biochemical tests
   - Catalase: Positive
   - Coagulase test positive
   - Other test: Phosphatase test positive, urease positive, indole negative, MR, VP, citrate positive, and mannitol fermentation positive
c. **Put up antibiotic sensitivity** by Kirby-Bauer disk diffusion against antibiotic disks.

   Remember: Main line of treatment is fluids and electrolytes but antibiotic sensitivity pattern called as antibiogram is useful in investigating the outbreak. If **antibiogram** of isolates from patient's stool samples and the isolate from food are similar, it acts as typing method and confirms the food as the source of infection.
d. **Typing methods** are used for staphylococci to find out source of infections in outbreaks having some common source. If the isolates from patient's and sources match each other by typing method, it means, that is the common source of infection. (Flowchart 24.2)
e. **Phage typing** is done for staphylococci which has epidemiological value. It is done at Maulana Azad Medical College, New Delhi.

   Other typing methods include molecular typing as **pulsed field gel electrophoresis**
f. **Serological test on food:** Passive latex agglutination test can be done for enterotoxins A, B, C.

g. Direct detection of toxin in food is possible by molecular methods (DNA probes).
h. Multiplex PCR for toxin detection is sensitive method.

Rapidec Staph test: This test is useful for identification of *Staphylococcus aureus* from blood culture. It detects enzyme produced by *Staphylococcus aureus*. It reacts with substance to form a complex which lyses a substrate to release fluorogen. The fluorogen is detected by fluorescence under UV light. This test is useful in identification of *S. aureus*, *S. epidermidis* and *S. saprophyticus* in **two hours.**

   Diagnosis of coagulase negative staphylococci is done by novobiocin testing, *S. saprophyticus* is resistant to novobiocin antibiotic, and the test is done by placing the disk of novobiocin as it is done for antibiotic susceptibility testing on MHA.

Treatment of Staphylococcus Infections

Isolates sensitive to penicillin—penicillin G is drug of choice, for patient allergic to penicillin, cefazoline is drug of choice.

Methicillin Resistant *Staphylococcus aureus* (MRSA)

Methods of Demonstration of MRSA

Screening methods: Phenotypic tests using oxacillin disk diffusion or oxacillin screen agar, Müeller-Hinton agar with 4% NaCl and 6 μg of oxacillin may be used for detection of methicillin resistance.

Cefoxitin disk diffusion test (Cefoxotin acts as surrogate marker of methicillin) is now recommended.

Genotypic method: The **gene *mec* A** is detected by **PCR.** Most of the clinical laboratories detect resistance by this method. **Another phenotypic** test for detection of **PB2a is available.**

HAI: *MRSA* may cause hospital-acquired infections which become difficult to treat as these strains do not respond to penicillins, cephalosporins.

Source: Anterior part of nose or fingers of health personnel may act as the source of infection and they are screened for *MRSA*.

Screening for MRSA: A wet swab from anterior part of nose is taken from all health personnel and finger impressions are taken on mannitol salt agar. If yellow colored colonies are produced, they are suggestive of *Staphylococcus aureus*; which are then tested for *MRSA* by phenotypic methods. The treatment of the source limits the spread of infection.

- *Typing methods*: Identification of *Staphylococcus aureus* to a **subspecies level** called as typing method. It helps to find out the source of infection by matching bacteriophage types of isolates from clinical specimens and from foods or vomitus. Hence, it helps to identify the source of infection during outbreak.

- *Phenotypic method* (Fig. 24.7):
  - **Bacteriophage typing** and **antibiogram** (compare sensitive pattern of isolates).
  - Test strain is inoculated as lawn culture on nutrient agar plate.
  - A bacteriophage is spot inoculated on the plate. Standard known strains of bacteriophages are used.
  - Area of clearing is observed. Strain is typed by a number of bacteriophages which cause areas of clearing. For example, if areas of clearing are seen where phages 29, 52a, 71 are applied then bacteriophage type is 29, 52a, 71.

  - Phage typing is done by Maulana Azad Medical College, New Delhi.
  - Phage **types 80 and 81 are most common isolates** in food poisoning.

- *Genotypic methods*: Pulsed field gel electrophoresis (PFGE) assessing gene of staphylococcal surface protein 'A' **(spa typing)** is popular for MRSA typing.

Study of international MRSA transmission and evolution is done by **SSCmec typing**.

Control Measures

- Person positive for *MRSA* in nose should apply mupirocin ointment for 5–7 days (Fusidic acid ointment). Resistant cases are treated with oral rifampicin.
- Screening of staff and keeping carriers away from work till lesions heal.
- Strict aseptic precautions in theatres.
- Wash with antiseptic solution (Ecoshield) is advised.
- Proper handwashing should be done.

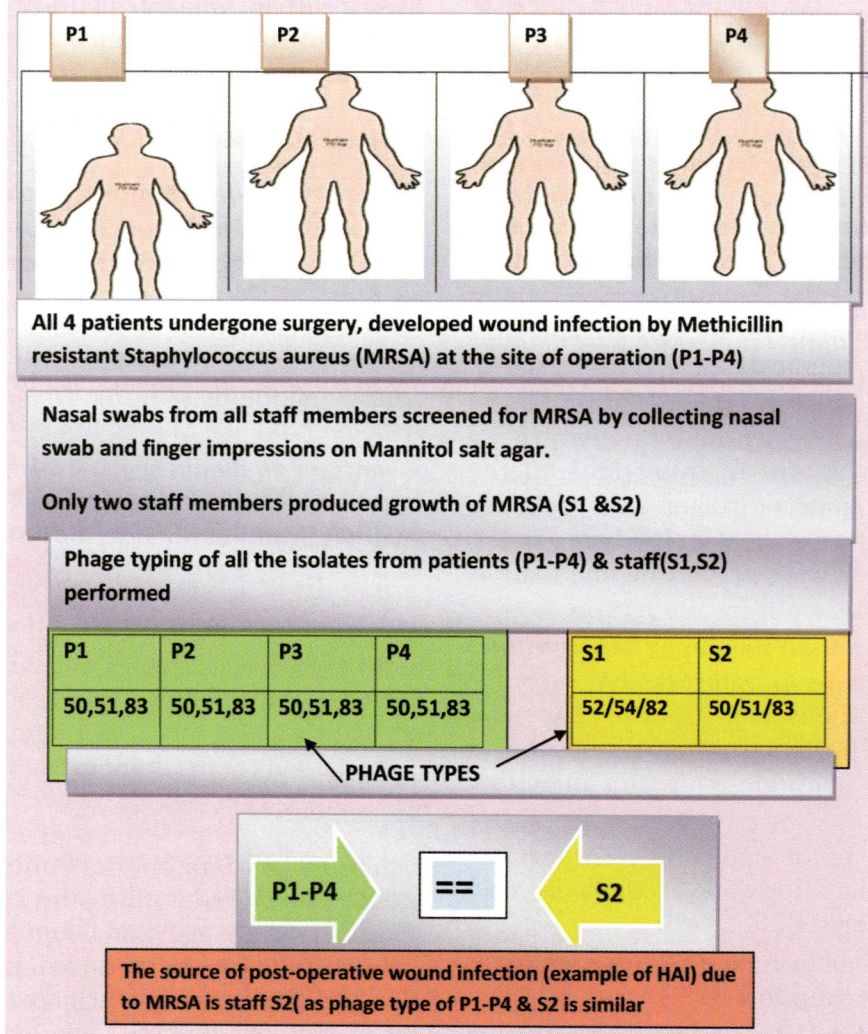

Fig. 24.7: Role of phage typing in investigating staphylococcal outbreak

- Personal hygiene is recommended as nail clipping.
- Isolation of patients with open lesions and their treatment.

Prevention of medical interventions as insertion of intravenous catheters is effective in prevention of control of MRSA. (This method is called 'bundling'.) MRSA causes rapidly spreading outbreaks. Phage type 80/81 is common.

Treatment Options for MRSA

Vancomycin is given; other drugs for MRSA are—TMP-SMZ, linezolid, daptomycin, quinpristin, dalfopristin, ciprofloxacin, levofloxacin, teicoplanin. Adjuvent drugs used are gentamicin, rifampin, and fusidic acid.

Empirical therapy: If *MRSA* status of individual is not yet established, vancomycin with or without amino-glycoside is given. Vancomycin is given if the condition is serious (e.g. cardiac implant therapy).

EMRSA: Many strains of *Staphylococcus aureus* produce outbreaks in hospitals hence called as *epidemically methicillin resistant Staphylococcus aureus.* Strains may be resistant to gentamicin also, they are called as *GMRSA.*

VRSA and VISA:

- Injudicious use of vancomycin may lead to development of resistance to this antibiotic.
- It may be low grade resistance known as 'VISA (vancomycin intermediate resistance) or high grade resistance (VRSA—vancomycin resistant *Staphylococcus aureus*).
- VRSA is mediated by van-A gene.
- VISA is due to increase in cell wall thickness of bacteria.
- Van-A gene is acquired by conjugation (a method of gene transfer between two bacteria).
- This gene is taken by *Staphylococcus aureus* from *Enterococcus fecalis.*

Teatment to *VISA* (vancomycin intermediate sensitive strains): **Telavanin**—it is parenteral derivative of vancomycin, given for treatment (If MIC is 2 µg/mL or less, of intermediate susceptible, if MIC is 4–8 µg, and resistance if MIC is 16 µg/mL).

Recently a novel cephalosporin, **ceftaroline**, has been approved for treatment of skin and soft tissue infections produced by *MRSA* but it is not yet indicated for septicemia.

An experimental bivalent vaccine against *Staphylococcus aureus* is reported to be safe and immunogenic for approximately 40 weeks in patients with end-stage renal disease undergoing hemodialysis. The vaccine called **StaphVAX** is composed of *S. aureus* types 5 and 8 capsular polysaccharide conjugated to nontoxic recombinant *Pseudomonas aeruginosa* exotoxin. The pharmaceutical company Nabi has developed a trivalent **staphylococcal polysaccharide conjugate vaccine** called TriStaph™. It contains the two main capsular types, 5 and 8, found in the outer coating of more than 80% of *S. aureus* strains, conjugated to non-toxic recombinant *Pseudomonas* exotoxin.

Toxic Shock Syndrome

- Toxic shock syndrome toxin (TST). It has two subtypes—TST-1 and TST-2.
- *TST-1:* Enterotoxin F or pyrogenic exotoxin C is most common type of TST-1.
- Toxin causes excessive stimulation of T cells which release cytokines.
- *Clinical features:* Fever, vomiting, diarrhea, hypotension, pain in abdomen, erythematous rash are followed by involvement of organs as liver, kidney, GIT, CNS.
- *Diagnosis:* TST is detected by latex agglutination, ELISA, PCR.
- *Treatment:* Clindamycin along with semisynthetic penicillin is given.

Tests used for identification of common staphylococcal species (undergraduate students are desirable to know only that sensitivity to novobiocin disk is used to differentiate *S. epidermidis* and *S. saprophyticus*) are given in Table 24.3.

TABLE 24.3: Differentiation of staphylococcal species

Test	S. aureus	S. epidermidis	S. saprophyticus	S. lugdunesis
Tube coagulase test	+v	—	—	—
Clumping factor	+	—	—	+
Heat stable thermonuclease	+	—	—	—
Phosphatise test	+	+(v)	—	—
Novobiocin test	+	S	R	S
Urease	V	+	+	V
PYR	—	—	—	+
Ornithine decarboxylate	—	—	—	+

Note: PYR (pyrrolidonyl beta-naphthylamide, S—sensitive, R—resistant, V—different strains give variable results)

25

Streptococci

HISTORY

- Billroth in 1874 demonstrated streptococci in erysipelas and wound infection.
- Pasteur (1879) demonstrated them in blood of patient with puerperal sepsis.
- Organism was isolated in pure form by Fechleisen (1883).
- Rosenbach (1884) isolated cocci from human suppurative lesion and gave name *Streptococcus pyogenes.*
- Lancefield classification came into existence in 1933.
- Todd described the method of titration of antistreptolysin-O (ASO).

CLASSIFICATION OF STREPTOCOCCI

Depending upon O$_2$ requirement, streptococci are classified as (Flowchart 25.1):

1. *Obligate anaerobes*: *Peptostreptococcus sp.*
2. *Aerobic and facultative anaerobes*: Aerobes and facultative anaerobic *streptococci* are classified based upon type of hemolysis produced on blood agar.

A. Alpha-hemolytic Streptococci

These are viridans group: *Str. mutans, Str. sanguis, Str. mitis, Str. milleri, Str. salivarius.* Usually they are nonpathogenic, they occur as commensal in throat. They may cause dental caries and infective endocarditis.

- Incomplete lysis of RBCs with reduction of Hb and formation of green pigment is called **alpha hemolysis.**
- It has been proved that the factor causing greenish discoloration is hydrogen peroxide which oxidizes hemoglobin to green methemoglobin.

B. Beta-hemolytic Streptococci

Complete disruption of RBCs with clearing of blood agar around bacterial growth is called beta hemolysis (Fig. 25.1).

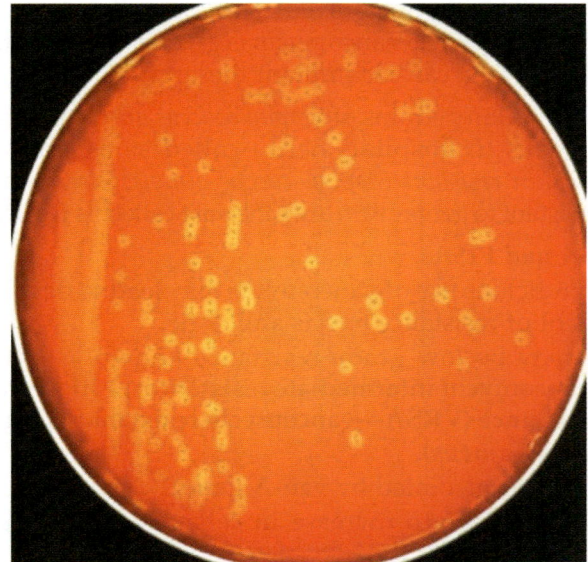

Fig. 25.1: Beta-hemolytic colonies of *Streptococcus pyogenes*

Based upon serological grouping which identifies carbohydrate antigen in cell wall, beta-hemolytic streptococci are further classified into Lancefield groups 'A' to 'V' except I and J.

Group 'A' beta-hemolytic Streptococcus is called *Streptococcus pyogenes* **(GAS).**

TABLE 25.1: Differences between alpha hemolysis and beta hemolysis

Alpha hemolysis	Beta hemolysis
Greenish discoloration	Clear zone
It is partial hemolysis (few RBCs are intact)	All RBCs in that zone are lysed
Zone of hemolysis is small 1–2 mm	Large zone of hemolysis
Margins are not clear—indefinite	Margins are sharp, clearly defined

Flowchart 25.1: Classification of streptococci

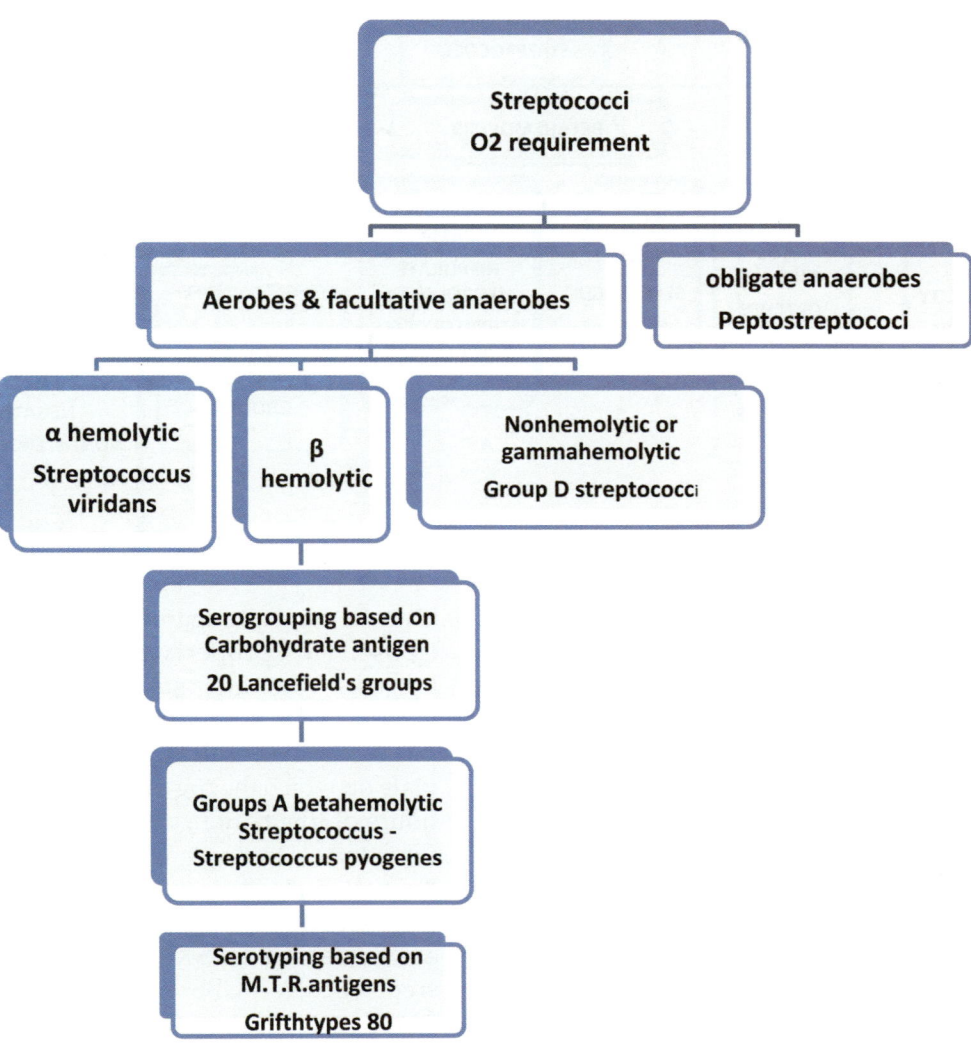

S. pyogenes based on 'M' protein is further classified as 80 Griffith types (1, 2, 3, etc. up to 80). Further classifications are based on 'T' and 'R' antigens.

Group B. *Str. agalactiae* (bovine mastitis)
Group C. *Str. equisimilis*

Gamma-hemolytic or Non-hemolytic Streptococci

a. *Enterococcus group*: St. fecalis, St. faecium, St. durans.
b. *Nonenterococcus group*: St. bovis and St. equinus.
   Gamma hemolysis is misnomer as there is no hemolysis.

MORPHOLOGY (Flowchart 25.2)

- These are Gram-positive cocci arranged in chains (Fig. 25.2).
- They are spherical cocci, 0.5–1μ in diameter.
- Chain formation is due to cocci dividing in one plane only and daughter cells fail to separate (Streptos = twisted). Longer chains are formed when grown in liquid medium.

The length of chain is inversely proportional to adequacy of medium. Prior to division, the individual cocci become elongated on axis of chain, eventually dividing to form pairs. When individual pairs do not separate which results in formation of chains. Factors which increase chain formation are conditions which impair growth (unfavorable medium, cold, antimicrobials, etc.) and presence of antibodies which react with cell wall.

- Non-motile, non-sporing, capsulated.
- Capsule made up of hyaluronic acid is seen in some strains from Group A and C, while polysaccharide capsule is seen in Group B and D.

Cultural Characteristics

- Cocci are aerobic and facultative anaerobic, grow better in presence of 5–10% CO_2, which also promotes hemolysis.
- Optimum temperature is 37°C (range 22–44°C).

Flowchart 25.2: Identification of streptococci

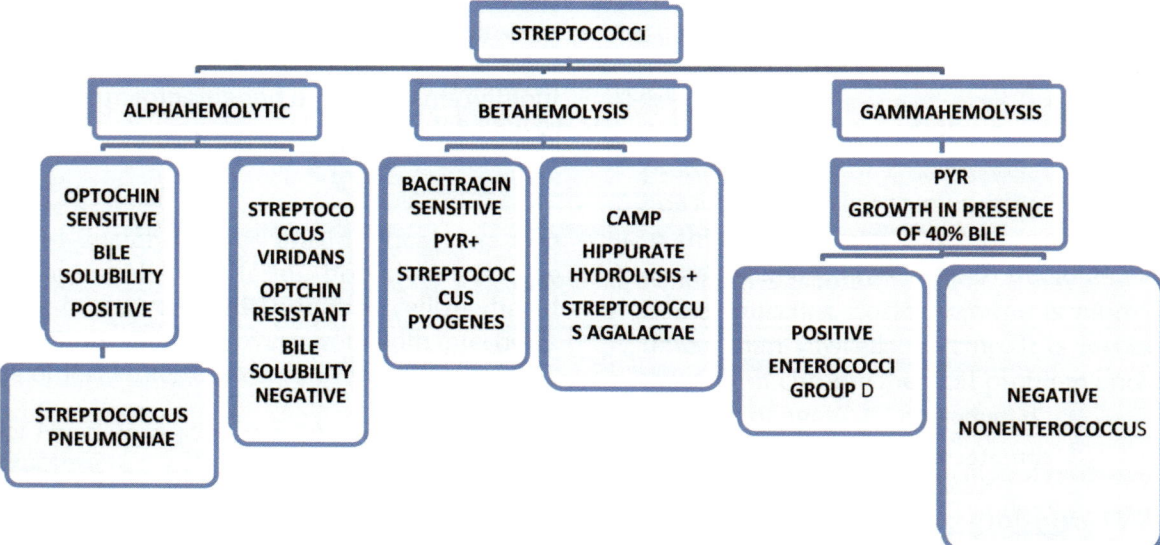

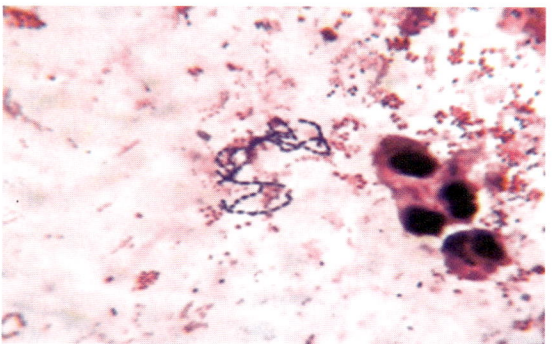

Fig. 25.2: Gram-positive cocci in chains

- **They are exacting in nutritive requirements,** hence they do not grow on simple media as nutrient agar.
- They grow in media containing fermentable carbohydrates or enriched with blood or serum.
- Blood agar after 48 hours of incubation produces 0.5– 1 mm, circular, low convex, **transparent colonies with β-hemolysis.** Virulent strains form granular **(matt)** colonies, avirulent strain may form **glossy colonies.** Organisms with 'M' protein produce 'matt' colonies while those with loss of 'M' protein produce 'glossy colonies'.
- Mucoid colonies are produced by strains which produce capsule.
- Growth in liquid medium (glucose broth) occurs as granular turbidity with powdery deposit.
- **Selective medium:** Crystal violet blood agar which inhibits growth of staphylococci is selective medium.
- **Transport medium: Pike's medium.**

Biochemical Tests

- *Catalase negative:* This test differentiates between *Staphylococcus aureus* and streptococci.

- They ferment all sugars (with acid and **no** gas) except ribose. This property differentiates *Streptococcus pyogenes* from other streptococci.
- **Bacitracin sensitivity (Maxted's observation):** Bacitracin disk with 0.04 mg is placed on blood agar plate on which the organism is inoculated. After 18–24 hours of incubation, zone of inhibition is produced (Fig. 25.3).
- *Trimethoprim-sulfamethoxazole (SXT) sensitivity test:* Group 'A' β-hemolytic streptococci (GAS) are resistant to SXT and bacitracin (Group B sreptococcus—'GBS' is resistant to both).
- *PYR test:* Hydrolysis of pyrrolidonyl naphthylamide **(PYR)** test is positive.
- *Streptozyme test:* It is passive hemagglutination test. It is sensitive and specific test.

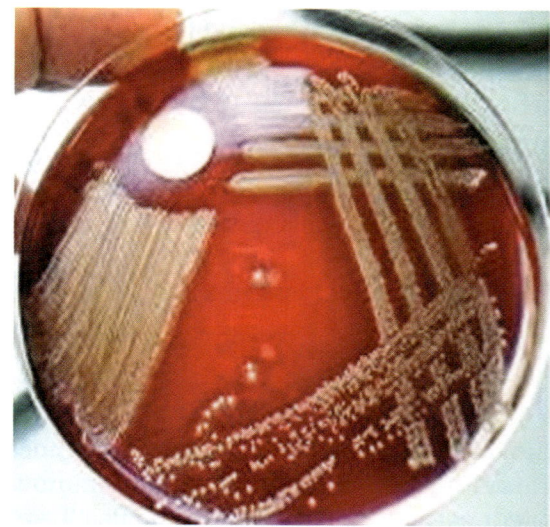

Fig. 25.3: Bacitracin sensitivity test

Grouping

The biochemical identification of Group A *Streptococcus* is further confirmed by Lancefield grouping in which beta hemolytic streptococci are grouped serologically based on carbohydrate-C antigen. The extracted antigen is tested with the commercially available antisera. Methods for testing are precipitation, gel diffusion, latex agglutination, immunofluorescence and ELISA.

Typing

It is done by either phenotypic method **(Griffith typing)** or by genotypic method (emm typing).

Griffith typing is based on 'M' protein. It can be extracted by Lancefield's acid extraction method and typing is done with type specific antisera.

emm typing: It is genotypic method in which gene coding for **'M' (emm)** is used for typing. Certain strains which are nontypable with Griffith typing are typed by this method. Total **124 emm genotypes** have been identified.

Resistance

- *Streptococcus pyogenes* is resistant to crystal violet.
- Crystal violet (1 mg/L), nalidixic acid (15 mg/L) and colistin sulfate (10 mg/L) are used in selective medium for streptococci.
- They are sensitive to many antibiotics (including penicillin), drug resistance is not seen.

Antigens (Table 25.2)

- **Capsular hyaluronic** acid when present, inhibits phagocytosis
- **Capsule binds to hyaluronic acid binding protein CD44 present on human epithelial cells.**
- **Outer layer** is made up of protein and lipoteichoic acid.
- **Group-specific carbohydrate antigen:** This **forms middle layer of cell wall.** It is cell wall antigen, serogrouping is based on the type of "C" antigen present.
- The antigen (extract) and its antibodies are taken in a capillary tube which shows precipitation reaction.

TABLE 25.2: Antigenic similarity which may cause damage due to autoimmune diseases (molecular mimicry)

Hyaluronic acid	Synovial membrane
Cell wall protein	Myocardium
Group A carbohydrate	Cardiac valves
Cytoplasmic membrane antigen	Vascular intima
Peptidoglycans	Skin antigens

- The pattern of 'O' antigen determine the sero group.
- This antigen plays role in pathogenesis of non-suppurative sequelae of Streptococcus because of antigenic similarity with heart and kidney. Streptococci are grown in liquid medium, Todd Hewitt Broth and the antigen is extracted by various methods as autoclaving (Rantz and Randall's method), enzyme produced by *Streptomyces albus* (Maxted's acid exraction method) or treatment with formamide (Fuller method), or with HCl (Lancefield method). The extract (antigen) and the antiserum are allowed to react in a capillary tube, the precipitation reaction is performed.
- **Inner layer** of peptidoglycan (mucopeptide).
- **Type specific antigens:** M, T, R proteins.

'M' protein (80 types): It is an important virulence factor, resists phagocytosis, promotes adherence, enhances virulence. **Anti-M antibody is protective.** It is present on surface and forms outer layer of cell wall. Typing is based on M antigen, thus helps in classification into "M" types. **There are 80 'M' types, as they are many, a person may have repeated infection due to different "M" types.** The 'M' protein and other cell wall antigens play role in pathogenesis of rheumatic fever.

A component of selective "M" type induces antibodies that react with cardiac muscle. **Conserved antigenic domains on "M" proteins may be virulence determinant in pathogenesis of rheumatic fever.**

- **Pili:** They help in adhesion to epithelial cells. They project outside. They are partially made up of 'M'protein and partially lipoteichoic acid.
- 'M' associated proteins.
- **'F' factors:** Fibronectin-binding protein help in adhesion.

'T' protein and *'R' protein:* Play no role in virulence but help in typing of bacteria.

Serum opacity factor: Many strain of these bacteria produces this factor, the culture supernatants of which produce opacity on agar gel containing horse serum.

GAS (Group A Streptococcus) cannot penetrate intact skin. In pharyngeal infection, the organism binds to mucosa using adhesions on bacterial surface so that they are not swept away by fluid secretions. **LTA binds to human fibronectin,** coat the bacteria. Protein 'M' is important adhesion molecule, attaches to the keratinized wall, the main cell type present in the outer layers of skin.

Toxins and Enzymes

Hemolysins (streptolysins O and S; Table 25.3)

- **Streptolysin 'O':** It is protein in nature, oxygen labile; it is hemolytic in reduced state, hence detected by hemolysis seen in pour plate method or hemolysis detected in anaerobic state. It lyses red cells and also acts on neutrophils, platelets. It is antigenic. **Anti-streptolysin 'O'** is antibody produced against it, detected by latex agglutination (ASO titer 160–200 units).
- **Streptolysin 'S':** Oxygen stable, responsible **for beta hemolysis** seen on the surface of blood agar, leucocidal, not antigenic.
- Group A, C, G produce this hemolysis.
- The name is derived from the fact that it can be extracted from intact cells with serum. No streptolysins have been described but this action is inhibited by serum lipoproteins.

Streptokinase (fibrinolysin)
It converts human fibrinogen into plasmin by activating plasminogen which is active proteolytic enzyme which digests fibrin, and other proteins. This property is used in treatment of pulmonary embolism to break it. It is partially responsible for the spread of streptococcal infection. It is also used in treatment of coronary artery and venous disease.

Erythrogenic toxin A, B, C
This is antigenic, soluble, and destroyed by boiling for 1 hour. It is pyrogenic, cytotoxic, suppresses RE system, increases susceptibility to endotoxin. Rash of scarlet fever (acute pharyngitis with extensive erythematous rash) is due to this toxin production. Toxin is detected by **Dick test**. Intradermal injection of this toxin produces erythematous reaction. Blanching of rash after injection of convalescent serum (which contains antibodies against this toxin) is called as **Schultz-Charlton reaction**. The rash is due to hypersensitivity reaction. The toxin production is controlled by a bacteriophage.

Intradermal injection of this toxin in susceptible host causes erythematous rash. Dick observed this effect. Hence, name erythrogenic toxin or Dick toxin is given to this toxin.

Deoxyribonuclease or streptodornase
There are four types **A, B, C, and D.** Type D is more antigenic. This enzyme degrades DNA, helps in spread of the infection by liquefying pus. It liquefies exudates and facilitates removal of pus and necrotic tissue, antimicrobials gain access and infected surfaces recover quickly. An anti-DNase develops after infection especially after skin infection (normal limit 100 units).

Hyaluronidase
It splits hyaluronic acid, the ground substance of connective tissue. It is also called as spreading factor. It is antigenic and following infection, antibodies are produced against it. Strains with 'M' type 4 and 22 produce this enzyme in larger quantity.

Lipoproteinase (serum opacity factor)
It destroys proteins.

Other enzymes
produced by *Streptococcus pyogenes* are NADase, proteinase, neuraminidase.

Streptococcal toxic shock syndrome
Erythrogenic toxin or pyrogenic: Three antigenic types A, B and C exist. It is produced by a strain carrying a phage. This toxin is associated with streptococcal toxic shock syndrome and scarlet fever. Toxins act as **superantigen**. Mechanism of action is similar to staphylococcal toxic shock syndrome toxin.

PATHOGENESIS AND PATHOLOGY OF STREPTOCOCCUS PYOGENES

Diseases are divided into two groups, i.e. diseases attributed to invasion and sequelae of infections.

Diseases attributed to invasion by *Streptococcus pyogenes.*

The portal of entry determines the clinical presentation. Infection is diffuse and rapidly spreading and extends along the lymphatics, it can extend to bloodstream.

Adhesion
- It allows the organisms to multiply without being washed away by secretions.

TABLE 25.3: Differences between hemolysin 'O' and hemolysin 'S'

Hemolysin O	Hemolysin S
Oxygen labile hence called 'O'	Oxygen stable, soluble in serum hence called 'S'
Inactive in oxidised form and active in presence of reducing agent	
The activity is seen on blood agar with pour plate method or hemolysis is seen surrounding colonies below the surface	It is responsible for hemolysis seen on surface of blood agar
It is antigenic, antibodies produced against it is called as ASO, which can be used for diagnosis of streptococcal infection	It is a protein but not antigenic
In experimental animals, it is cardiotoxic	In experimental animals, it is nephrotoxic

- **Lipoteichoic acids** attach to fibronectin, a host protein that coats epithelial cells of oropharynx.
- Another protein **'F' protein**, a fibronectin binding protein found in many strains also takes part in adhesions.

Multiplication: In order to multiply, streptococci must avoid the attack of phagocytic cells. 'M' protein is a rod-shaped molecule that projects from surface of bacterial cell. 'M' protein binds to fibrinogen; fibrin and their degradation products form a dense coating on surface of bacteria that blocks complement deposition. 'M' protein bearing streptococci are poorly opsonized.

'M' protein binds to factor 'H', a protein that inhibits cleavage of complement protein C3; without cleavage of C3, complement cannot be activated.

The antibody produced against 'M' protein helps in opsonization of bacteria. The antibody to 'M' protein though protective, it is type specific. Streptococci have many 'M' types and every time new 'M' type infects, it escapes the defences.

Streptokinase binds to host plasminogen to form complexes that catalyze the conversion plasminogen to plasmin, which degrades fibrin and other proteins.

Hyaluronic acid capsule is also antiphagocytic agent. Group 'A' streptococci have hyalouronidase. The bacteria shut down the production of this enzyme when they encounter epithelial surface.

The pyrogenic exotoxins suppress antibody production. They stimulate monocyte to produce IL-1.

Pathogenicity (Fig. 25.4 and Flowchart 25.3)

Sore throat is a condition in which there is inflammation of mucosa of throat.

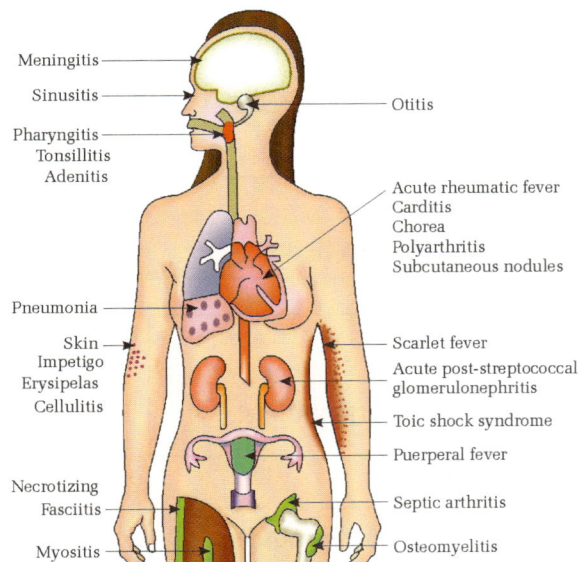

Fig. 25.4: Infections produced by *S. pyogenes*

Mode of infection is through respiratory tract, by inhalation of droplets.

Organisms causing sore throat (pharyngitis) are:
Bacteria: *Streptococcus pyogenes*, *Corynebacterium diphtheriae*, *Staphylococcus aureus*, *Haemophilus influenzae*, *Streptococcus pneumoniae*, *Mycoplasma pneumoniae*, *Borrelia vincentii*.

Viral agents: *Herpes simplex 1 virus*, *Ebstein-Barr virus*, *cytomegalovirus*, *adenovirus*, *influenza* and *parainfluenza viruses*.

Fungal agent: *Candida albicans*

Pharyngitis:
- Abrupt onset of fever, sorethroat, malaise, headache develop 2–4 days after exposure.
- Post-pharyngeal wall becomes red, tonsils get enlarged, show grayish-white exudate on their surface. Pus may accumulate in crypts.
- Cervical lymphadenopathy develops.
- Occasionally, tonsillar abscess is formed.

Impetigo: Infection of superficial layers of skin which results in crusty lesions called impetigo. It is caused by higher number of serotypes. It is skin infection of children, discrete superficial spots of 2–5 mm appear which heal without scar.

Common sites affected are face and legs. Red papules appear, become vesicles, pustules which breakdown and coalesce which give **honeycomb-like crusts**. Lesions are painless.

Subcutaneous Infections

Erysipelas: The bacterium enters through skin and there is massive browny edema and rapidly spreading margin of infection. **Lower number serotypes which cause throat infections cause erysipelas.**
- Superficial lymphatics are involved.
- A form of cellulitis, with bright red, swollen and indurated **peau de'orange** texture of skin due to superficial lymphatics are involved.
- Most common areas affected are face, lower extremities.

Cellulitis: It is an acute rapidly spreading infection of skin and subcutaneous tissue. It follows mild trauma, burn, wound or surgical incision. Pain, tenderness, swelling, and redness occur. The lesion is not raised and the line between normal and infected tissue is clear as compared to erysipelas.

It also causes secondary infection of burn and wound.

Necrotizing fasciitis: It is an extensive and rapidly spreading necrosis of skin, fascia, and tissues. The

Flowchart 25.3: Pathogenesis of rheumatic heart disease

```
            ┌──────────────────────────────┐
            │ Streptococcus pyogenes        │
            │ infection                     │
            └──────────────┬───────────────┘
                           │
                           ▼
            ┌──────────────────────────────┐      ┌──────────────────────────┐
            │ 'M' protein of bacterium acts │      │ Immune response to        │
            │ as virulence factor           │      │ Streptococcal antigen     │
            └───────────────────────────────┘      └────────────┬─────────────┘
                                                                 │
                   ┌──────────────┐                              ▼
                   │ Mimic        │                  ┌───────────────────────┐
                   └──────┬───────┘                  │ Autoimmune            │
                          │                          └──────┬──────────┬─────┘
                          ▼                                 │          │
            ┌──────────────────────────────┐                │          │
            │ Endogenous membrane protein   │◄───────────────┘          │
            │ in heart, skin, connective    │                           ▼
            │ tissue                        │             ┌──────────────────────────┐
            └──────────────────────────────┘             │ Inflammatory response    │
                                                          └────────────┬─────────────┘
   ┌──────────────────────────────┐                                    │
   │ Changes in vascular           │◄───────────────────────────────────┘
   │ permeability                  │
   │                               │
   │ High macrophage, PMN activity │──────────────────────────┐
   └────┬──────────────┬───────────┘                          │
        │              │                                      │
        ▼              ▼                                      ▼
   ┌─────────┐   ┌──────────────────┐          ┌──────────────────────────┐
   │Arteritis│   │ Destruction of   │          │ Destruction of joints    │
   └─────────┘   │ subcutaneous     │          └──────────────────────────┘
                 │ tissue           │
                 └──────────────────┘
        ┌──────────────┐
        │ Pancarditis  │───────────────────────────────┐
        └──┬────────┬──┘                                │
           │        │                                   ▼
           ▼        ▼                      ┌──────────────────────────┐
  ┌──────────────┐ ┌──────────────────┐    │ Decreased ventricular     │
  │ Endocarditis │ │ Acute swelling of│    │ filling capacity          │
  │              │ │ heart tissue     │    └────────────┬─────────────┘
  │ Pericarditis │ └──────────────────┘                 │
  └──────────────┘                                       ▼
                                             ┌──────────────────────────┐
                                             │ Congestive heart failure  │
                                             └──────────────────────────┘
```

```
   ┌──────────────────────────────┐
   │ Inflammation, changes in      │──────────────────────┐
   │ vascular permeability         │                      │
   └────┬──────────────────┬───────┘                      ▼
        │                  │              ┌──────────────────────────┐
        ▼                  │              │ Destruction of            │
   ┌──────────┐            │              │ subcutaneous tissue       │
   │ Arteritis│            │              └────────────┬─────────────┘
   └────┬─────┘            │                           │
        │                  │                           ▼
        ▼                  │              ┌──────────────────────────┐
   ┌──────────────────┐    │              │ Erythema marginatum       │
   │ Sydenham' chorea │    │              └──────────────────────────┘
   └──────────────────┘    │
                           ▼
             ┌──────────────────────────┐
             │ Granulomatous nodules in  │
             │ heart tissue             │───────────┐
             └──────────────────────────┘           │
                                                     ▼
                                        ┌──────────────────────────┐
                                        │ Ascoff's nodules          │
                                        └──────────────────────────┘
```

group A Streptococcus causes this condition. The condition may be caused by mixed aerobes and anaerobes. Streptococcus **'M' type-1** producing pyrogenic exotoxin 'A' may alone cause this condition. (The bacteria are called as **flesh eating bacteria.**) Necrosis of subcutaneous tissue, muscle tissue may be associated with systemic illness—a toxic shock syndrome characterized by disseminated intravascular coagulation and multiorgan failure. *S. pyogenes* can be isolated from the site and antibodies can be detected in serum.

In case of skin infections, the response to ASO is not high, **anti-DNase and anti-hyaluronidase are more useful in retrospective diagnosis of streptococcal skin infections.**

Streptococcal pyoderma: It presents with severe ulcerative skin lesions. It is local infection of superficial layers of skin.
- It affects exposed area of face, arms, legs.
- Infection is by contact. Bacteria enter skin through small defects.
- Vesicles appear which later on get filled with pus.

Bacteremia and septicemia: This develops following the infection of trauma, surgical wound or following cellulitis.

Respiratory tract infections: Primary site involved is throat causing **sore throat**. It causes pharyngitis and tonsillitis. The bacteria attach to epithelial cells by lipoteichoic acid and surface pili, the fibronectin serves as receptor for streptococci. From throat, the bacteria may spread to surrounding tissues causing otitis, mastoiditis, Ludwig's angina, suppurative adenitis and quincy. Lower number serotypes cause pharyngitis.

Scarlet fever is uncommon but presents with sore throat and erythematous rash.
- Toxins SPE-A, B, C are responsible for this condition.
- Rash with sandpaper feel is observed.

- Strawberry tongue (enlarged papillae on coated tongue).
- Rash in skin fold (Pastina's illness).

Genital infections: It causes puerperal sepsis; most of the infections are endogenous. Streptococci enter in uterus after the delivery, cause puerperal sepsis which is a septicemia originating from infected wound.

Deep infections are bone and joint infections, lymphadenitis, septicemia, acute endocarditis, abscess in internal organs (e.g. brain, liver, kidney).

Non-suppurative Complications (Table 25.4)

1. *Heart*: Acute rheumatic fever (ARF) is the most serious sequela of *Streptococcus pyogenes* as it affects heart muscles and valves. Certain strains of Group A streptococci contain **membrane antigen** which cross-reacts with human heart tissue antigen. Sera from patients with rheumatic heart disease show these antibodies in high titers.

Rheumatic fever affects heart muscle and valves. Membrane antigen of streptococci resembles with heart tissue.

Rheumatic fever occurs 1–4 weeks after pharyngitis. Severity of pharyngitis is correlated with severity of rheumatic fever. Rheumatic disease is one of the most important causes of heart disease in developing countries. Typical symptoms and signs include fever, malaise, migratory or fleeting polyarthritis and there is inflammation of all parts of heart, i.e. endocardium, myocardium, and pericardium. The carditis leads to thickening of heart valves and small perivascular granulomas in myocardium. These are called as **Aschoff's nodules**. Myocardium is finally replaced by scar tissue. ESR rate and serum transaminase levels are increased which along with ECG are used to estimate the damage.

TABLE 25.4: Comparision of acute rheumatic fever and glomerulonephritis

	Acute rheumatic fever	Glomerulonephritis
Site of infection	Throat	Throat or skin
Prior sensitization	Required	Not necessary
Serotype *Streptococcus pyogenes*	Any	Pyoderma type 2, 49, 37, 59, 61 and pharyngitis types 1 and 12
Complement	Level unaffected	Level affected
Immune response	Marked	Moderate
Genetic predisposition	Present	Not known
Penicillin prophylaxis	Essential	Not required
Progress	Progressive or static	Spontaneous resolution may occur
Repeated attacks	Common	Absent

The pathogenesis of acute rheumatic fever is not known. Three theories are autoimmune theory, damage due to cell-mediated autoimmune response or cytotoxic theory.

a. *Autoimmune theory*: Various autoantigens involved in pathogenicity of acute rhematic fevor are myosin, tropomysin, laminin, keratin in humam tissue and group 'A' antigen in cell wall in addition to epitopes of same variants of surface 'M' proteins.

b. *Cytotoxic action*: Streptococcal toxins, as SPE and enzymes (streptolysin-O) are probably directly cytotoxic to human cardiac tissue leading to the damage.

c. *Cell-mediated autoimmunity*: Current research in the pathogenesis of acute rheumatic fever is focussed on cellular autoimmunity rather than humoral autoimmune responses.

Various streptococcal preparations, including fragments of 'M' proteins containing crossreactive epitopes, stimulate cytotoxic T cells that react against cardiac myocytes.

Streptococcal superantigens including **pyrogenic exotoxin** and several other molecules stimulate T cell proliferation when bound to MHC on antigen presenting cells. They react with conserved regions of TCR V domain. As a result, many lymphocytes are activated. This may cause **breakdown of tolerance and result in autoimmunity.**

Clinical presentation:
- Heart, joints, skin and brain are affected.
- The classical lesion is formation of **Aschoff nodules**—there is degeneration of heart valves and formation of inflammatory myocardial lesions.
- Clinical diagnosis is based on modified Jone's criteria (Table 25.5).

Importance of penicillin prophylaxis: Rheumatic fever causes slight damage but repeated infection increases the damage. Hence, it is important to protect such patients from repeated infections with *Streptococcus pyogenes* by penicillin prophylaxis.

2. *Acute glomerulonephritis (AGN)*: This sometimes develops 1–4 weeks after *Streptococcus pyogenes* skin infections (pyoderma, impetigo) or pharyngitis. Some strains are particularly **nephritogenic**, principally **'M' types 2, 42, 49, 56, 57 and 60 (skin)**. 'M' types associated with throat infections and glomerulonephritis are **4, 12, and 25.**

Other nonsuppurative complications produced by *Streptococcus pyogenes* are reactive arthritis and pediatric autoimmune neuropsychiatric disorders.

TABLE 25.5: Revised Jones criteria for acute rheumatic fever

Criteria	Manifestations
Major manifestations	Subcutaneous nodules Pancarditis
—	Arthritis (migrating, polyarthritis) Chorea (CNS manifestations) Erythema marginatum (skin lesions)
Minor manifestations	*Clinical*: Fever, arthralgia *Laboratory*: Raised ESR, CRP protein *ECG*: Prolonged P-R interval
Evidence of previous streptococcal infection	Raised ASO titre, or +ve throat culture, or rapid test for GAS or recent scarlet fever
Rheumatic fever is diagnosed if	Two major manifestations or one major and two minor manifestations plus evidence of past streptococcal infection

***Clinical features of post-streptococcal glomerulo-nephritis are*:**
- Hematuria leading to coffee-colored urine.
- Edema of face extremities.
- Renal impairment leading to circulatory congestion.

Immunopathogenesis: Glomerulonephritis is initiated by antigen–antibody complexes on glomerular basement membrane. The most important **antigens** are thought to be **SpeB** and a **nephritis associated plasmin factor**. In acute nephritis, the patient has blood and protein in urine, edema, high blood pressure, and urea nitrogen retention; serum complements levels are low. A patient may die, some develop chronic glomerulonephritis with kidney failure, and majority may recover.

Epidemiology

The person harboring the organism becomes the source of infection. He may have clinical or subclinical infection or he may be carrier shedding organisms in droplets from nasopharyngeal secretions or skin. The nasal discharge of person harboring cocci is the most dangerous source of infection. Overcrowding is an important factor in transmission of infection.

LABORATORY DIAGNOSIS

Specimens
- Nasopharyngeal secretions taken by sterile cotton swab
- Pus is collected in pyogenic infections
- Blood in glucose broth in cases of septicemia
- CSF in case of meningitis

- Vaginal swab for puerperal sepsis
- Serum for serological test, for diagnosis of acute rheumatic fever or acute glomerulonephritis.

Laboratory Diagnosis of Sore Throat

Specimens: Nasopharyngeal secretions taken by sterile cotton swabs (Fig. 25.5).

Transport: Transport the swabs in **Pike's medium** or **Stuart's transport** medium.

Pike's medium contain blood agar, crystal violet (1:100000) and sodium azide (1:16,000).

Processing of Specimens

Microscopy: Gram staining is done from the smear prepared from the secretions. It shows pus cells with Gram-positive cocci in chains.

Fluorescent microscopy: Direct immunofluorescence (DIF) is used for detection of bacteria in the nasopharyngeal secretions.

Procedure

- Nasopharyngeal secretion collected by cotton swab is rolled on clean glass slide.
- Antistreptococcal antibody tagged with fluorescent dye is added to the slide.
- The slide is then washed so that if antigen is present in the specimen will attach to the antibody hence it will not wash out (if antigen is not present everything will wash out).
- The slide is observed under fluorescent microscope which shows fluorescence.

Culture

- **Bacitracin** antibiotic identification disk **(0.04 mg)** may be placed on the blood agar which is inoculated with the specimen. Zone of inhibition is taken as sensitive.

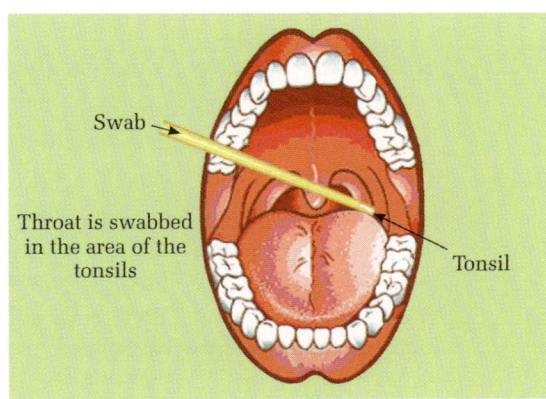

Fig. 25.5: Throat swab collection

- Similarly, for rapid identification **1 µg benzyl penicillin** disk is used for identification of growth as *Streptococcus pyogenes*.
- **Blood agar:** After overnight incubation, BA shows small, transparent, circular, low convex colonies with **beta hemolysis**. Growth and hemolysis is enhanced by 5–10%CO_2.
- **Selective medium:** Crystal violet blood agar inhibits the growth of other organisms.
- Sheep blood agar supplemented with **trimethoprim-sulfamethoxazole** to suppress growth of commensals may also be used.

Biochemical Tests

- Catalase test is negative.
- Blood agar with **bacitracin** disk shows zone of inhibition surrounding the bacitracin disk (bacitracin sensitive).
- **PYR test positive:** The enzyme L-*pyroglutamyl-beta-naphthylamide* (PYR) hydrolyses the substrate L-pyrrolidonyl-beta-naphthylamide to produce beta-naphthylamine which combines with cinnamaldehyde and produces bright red color.
- Fermentation of ribose is negative.

Detection of antigen in serum is done by latex agglutination **(LA)** and **ELISA** test. The sensitivity of ELISA varies from 60 to 90% depending on the prevalence of the disease in community and the test is 98–99% specific.

Direct immunofluorescence is also sensitive and specific for the detection of antigen.

Detection of Antibody

Pharyngitis is followed by rise in titers of antibodies against all antigens, whereas patients with pyoderma only show rise in anti-DNase. Serological tests are helpful for the detection of infection in patient, in which Group A Streptococcus is not isolated but who presents with sequelae suggestive of rheumatic fever or glomerulonephritis. Serum obtained as long as 2 months after infection shows antibody.

- **ASO test:** Detected by latex agglutination test. Titer more than or equal to 200 indicates streptococcal infection.
- **Anti-DNase test:** Significant titer is 1:300
- **Streptozyme** is passive slide hemagglutination test. Streptococcal antigen is coated on RBCs. This is used for detection of antibodies. It has high sensitivity and specificity.

A nucleic acid probe detects DNA in the sample.

MALDI is used for rapid identification of the bacterium.

Newer Rapid Tests (RADTs)

- **These tests are performed on throat swab.** They are based on detection of carbohydrate antigen of cell wall.
- **Latex agglutination** methods were relatively insensitive.
- **EIA** techniques offer increased sensitivity and a more sharply defined end point.
- RADTs are **optical immunoassay** and **chemiluminescent DNA probes.**
- Rapid tests have high **specificity (90%)** but lower sensitivity (70%). The sensitivity is increased with chemiluminescent assay.

TREATMENT OF STREPTOCOCAL INFECTIONS

- *Pharyngitis:* Benzathine penicillin, and penicillin G are used.
- *Erysipelas:* For mild to moderate, procaine penicillin is used and for severe cases penicillin G is used.
- *Necrotising fasciitis:* Surgical debridement is done and penicillin G plus clindamycin are given.
- *Pneumonia or empyema:* Treatment is surgical drainage and penicillin plus clindamycin.
- *Toxic shock syndrome:* Penicillin plus clindamycin, plus IV immunoglobulins are given.

GROUP B STREPTOCOCCI (GBS)—*STREPTOCOCCUS AGALACTIAE*

- It is identified by **Hippurate test** and **CAMP** test which are positive; and may produce orange pigment.
- It causes β-hemolysis (some strains cause α-hemolysis). **Penicillin and gentamicin** identification disks are used as these are sensitive to penicillin and resistant to gentamicin.

They are resistant to both bacitracin and SXT.

- *CAMP test:* This test detects production of a CAMP factor which enhances action of staphylococcal hemolysin (Fig. 25.6).
- Inoculate a β-hemolysis producing strain of *Staphylococcus aureus* across a blood agar plate containing 5% sheep blood. Then inoculate a single streak of *Streptococcus agalactiae* perpendicular to that of Staphylococcus, leaving about 1 cm space between two streaks. Incubate for 24 hours at 37°C in presence of air or air with 10% CO_2. An area of increased hemolysis appears at the junction of two streaks.
- **Predisposing factors** for infections in nonpregnant individuals include: Diabetes, cancer, advanced age, liver cirrhosis, patients on steroid, HIV infections. In these groups, respiratory infections, skin and soft tissue infections, and genitourinary infections occur.

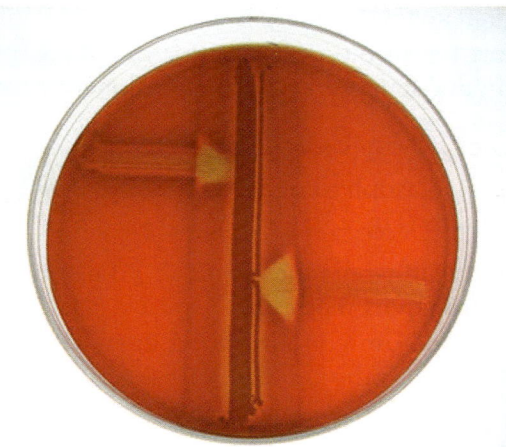

Fig. 25.6: CAMP test

- *Pathogenicity:* This species causes mainly neonatal infections which may be early onset or late onset.
  Early onset: It may cause fatal infections as neonatal meningitis and neonatal septicemia. Infections present within one week of birth and these are acquired in birth canal (Table 25.6).
  Late onset infections: These develop two weeks after birth, infections are hospital acquired (Table 25.6).

Intravenous ampicillin given to mothers who are colonized and are in labor prevents colonization of infants and subsequent disease.

GROUP C STREPTOCOCCI

This group includes four animal pathogens—*S. equi, S. equisimilis, S. dysgalactiae, S. zooepidemicus. S. equisimilis* may cause pharyngitis, skin infections, osteomyelitis, endocarditis, and septicemia. Streptokinase which is used for thrombolytic therapy is obtained from *S. equisimilis*. It ferments ribose.

GROUP G STREPTOCOCCI

They may sometimes cause pharyngitis, sinusitis, bacteremia, and endocarditis.

TABLE 25.6: Early onset and late onset group B streptococcal disease

Characteristic	Early onset disease	Late onset disease
Age of onset	0–6 days of life	7–90 days after birth
Mode of infection	During or before birth, from colonized maternal genital tract	Contact with colonized mother and nursing person
Clinical features	Pneumonia or respiratory distress, meningitis	Bacteremia and meningitis (most common)
Serotypes	Ia, III, V, II, Ib	III

GROUP D STREPTOCOCCI

They include—Enterococcal group (faecal streptococci) and non-enterococcal group (*Stre. bovis, equinus*).

Enterococci

Common species which cause human infections are *E. faecalis, E. faecium,* and *E. durans.*

Tests used for the identification of enterococci are as follows:

- Growth in presence of:
  - 40% bile
  - 6.5% NaCl
  - pH 9.6
  - 45°C
- 0.1% methylene blue milk
- *Morphology*: Pairs of oval cocci, at an angle to each other show 'spectacular arrangement'.
- Colonies usually nonhemolytic but may show alpha or beta hemolysis.
- **PYR test positive.**

Heat tolerence test: They are relative heat resistant. They survive 60°C for 30 minutes.

Penicillin resistance is common and it is due to production of beta-lactamase or **altered penicillin binding proteins (*E. faecalis*).**

Treatment

Penicillin, or combination of penicillin with gentamicin and if resistant to penicillin, Vancomycin is given.

Vancomycin resistant enterococci (VRE): They show resistance to vancomycin also, in this condition linazolid or quinpristin or dalfopristin is given.

VRE is mediated by Van gene which alters the target site for vancomycin present in the cell wall (D-alanyl-D-alanine side chain of peptidoglycan). Van gene has 5 genotypes. Strains with Van A gene show high level of resistance to both the glycopeptides, i.e. vancomycin and teicoplanin, strains with Van B gene show low level of resistance to vancomycin but are sensitive to teicoplanin. *E. gallinarum* and *E. casseliflavus* possess Van C genes which show resistance to both.

Pathogenicity

- Urinary tract infections
- Wound infections
- Septicemia
- Endocaridits
- Meningitis
- Biliary tract infections
- Peritonitis
- Intra-abdominal abscess
- Surgical wound infection

Nonenterococcal Group (*Streptococcus bovis, Streptococcus eqinus*)

These are generally sensitive to penicillin. They are PYR negative and they cause infections as UTI, endocarditis in patients with neoplasms of GIT, i.e. carcinoma or polyp.

Antibiotic resistance: The vancomycin resistance is more commom in ***E. faecium*** but is also seen in strains of ***E. faecalis.*** Because the resistance is plasmid mediated which may carry genes for resistance to other antibiotics as aminoglycoside, ampicillin; newer drugs as daptomycin, linezolid, quinpristin, dalfopristin and tigecycline are used for treatment of **VRE.**

TABLE 25.7: Differences between *Staphylococcus aureus* and *Streptococcus pyogenes*

	S. aureus	Streptococcus pyogenes
Morphology	Gram-positive cocci in clusters	Gram-positive cocci in chains
Capsule	If present, polysaccharide	Capsule made up of hyaluronic acid
Nature of infections	Localized infections Do not produce streptokinase, streptodornase but produce fibrin which tries to seal the lesion hence localized infections	Spreading infections Streptokinase, streptodornase, hyaluronidase breakdown intracellular substances hence infections are generalized
Nature of pus	Thick	Thin pus produced
Recurrent infection	Not commom	Recurrent infections may occur
Catalase	Positive	Negative
Normal flora	It may be normal flora of skin	It is not normal flora of skin
Drug resistance	MRSA—resistant to penicillins, cephalosporins	Drug resistance to penicillin is not seen

Streptococcal Species and Characteristics

	Lancefield group	Hemolysis	Habit	Lab. test	Diseases
St. pyogenes	A	Beta	Throat, skin	Bacitracin sensitive PYR+, ribose not fermented	Upper respiratory tract infection, pyoderma, rheumatic fever, glomerulonephritis
St. agalactiae	B	Beta	Female genital tract	CAMP test, + Hippurate + hydrolysis	Neonatal meningitis, septicemia
Str. equisimilis	C	Beta	Throat	Fermentation of ribose and trehalose	Pharyngitis, endocarditis
Str. angiosus	A, C, F, G, untypable	Beta (alpha, gamma)	Throat, colon, female genital tract	Gr. A strains bacitracin-resistant, PYR –ve	Pyogenic infections
Enterococcus spp. E. faecalis and other	D	Gamma (alpha, beta)	Colon	Growth in 6.5%NaCl	Urinary tract infections, endocarditis, suppurative infections
Nonenterococcal Group D species E. bovis	D	Gamma	Colon	No growth in 6.5% NaCl	Endocarditis
Viridians streptococci	Not typed	Alpha	Mouth, colon, female genital tract	Optochin-R Species classification on basis of biochemical tests	Endocarditis (Str. sanguis), dental caries (St. mutans)

ALPHA-HEMOLYTIC STREPTOCOCCI (STREPTOCOCCUS VIRIDANS)

Alpha-hemolytic sreptococci occur as commensals in throat and they are non-pathogenic. Rarely they produce infections as endocarditis and dental caries. *Str sanguis* mostly causes endocarditis while **Str. mutans** causes **dental caries.** It breaks sugar into acid and dextran, acid damages dextrin, binds debris, epithelial calls, mucus and bacteria to tooth causing plaques which form caries.

GROUP F STREPTOCOCCI

They are called as minute streptococci. They grow poorly on blood agar. They may cause suppurative lesions.

STREPTOCOCCUS MG

Streptococcus MG is α-hemolytic agent in this group which is used in heterophile agglutination test for detection of antibodies against *Mycoplasma pneumoniae*.

TABLE 25.8: Differences between *S. pyogenes* and *S. agalactiae*

Characteristic	S. pyogenes	S. agalactiae
Lancefield group	A	B
Bacitracin sensitivity	Sensitive	Resistant
PYR test	Positive	Negative
CAMP test	Negative	Positive
Hippurate hydrolysis	Negative	Positive
Colony morphology	0.5–1 mm, pinpoint transparent colonies	Larger, mucoid colonies

Streptococci-like Bacteria

These are *Aerococcus, Gemella, Lactococcus, Pedicoccus and Leuconstoc*. They are present on mucosal surfaces and may cause infections in immuno-suppressed patients. They may cause wound infection septicemia, endocarditis.

Nutritionally Deficient Streptococci or Satellite, Thio Requiring, Nutritionally Variant, Pyridoxal Dependent, Vitamin B₁₂ Dependent or Symbiotic Streptococci

- Once they were considered as members of viridians streptococci but now two distinct species identified.

- *Abiotrophia* (*defectiva and adiacens*).
- They may cause endocarditis.
- They do not routinely grow on blood agar or chocolate agar; pyridoxal can be added to medium or can be supplied by other bacteria.
- The satellite procedure uses one organism to support the growth of other organism.
- In the center, a streak of *Staphylococcus aureus* (provides pyridoxal) is made. Suspected Streptococcus is streaked perpendicular to central streak. After incubation, larger colonies are seen near central staphylococcal streak as compared to peripheral colonies.

26

Pneumococcus (*S. pneumoniae*)

HISTORY

- The organism was identified concurrently in old world and new world, Pasteur in France, Stenberg in USA.
- Initially, the name Diplococcus was given; in 1974 it is renamed as *Streptococcus pneumoniae*.
- Griffith in 1920 demonstrated transfer of genetic material by a process called transformation.

Morphology

- These are Gram-positive capsulated diplococci (Fig. 26.1)
- *Size*: 1 μm (0.6–0.8) diameter
- Arranged in pairs with broad ends close
- *Shape*: Smear from clinical sample shows 'lanceolate' shape (flame-shaped)
- Non-motile, non-sporing
- *Capsule demonstration*: Negative staining with India ink or Nigrosin: Capsule is seen as clear halo around the pair of cocci.

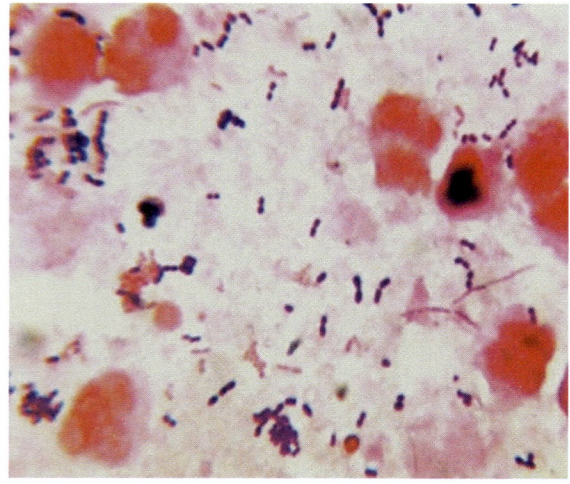

Fig. 26.1: Gram-positive cocci in pairs suggestive of *Streptococcus pneumoniae* (×1000)

Quellung Test (Fig. 26.2)

The sample containing pneumococci is mixed with its specific antiserum which contains antibodies against capsular antigen; the capsule is seen as refractive halo around cocci. **The capsule swells** and bacteria agglutinate by crosslinking of antibodies. This reaction is used for rapid identification of pneumococci in sputum or in culture. The polyvalent antiserum which contains antibodies to all capsular antigenic types is used. It is a rapid microscopic test for determination whether a patient is infected or not with this organism.

Culture

- Cocci are fastidious in growth requirements.
- They are aerobe and facultative anaerobe.
- Their growth is enhanced by 5–10% CO_2.
- Optimum temperature for growth is 37°C (range 25°–42°C).
- Optimum pH for growth is 7.8 (6.5–8.3).

Media

- Cocci grow well on enriched media like blood agar, chocolate agar.

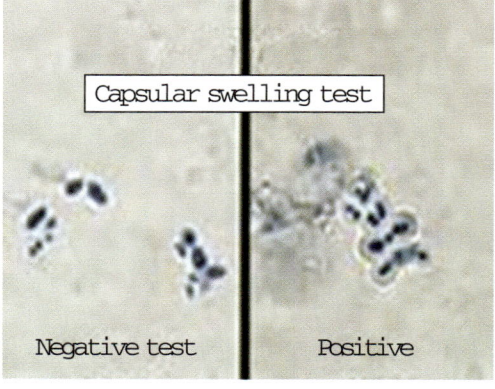

Fig. 26.2: Quellung test

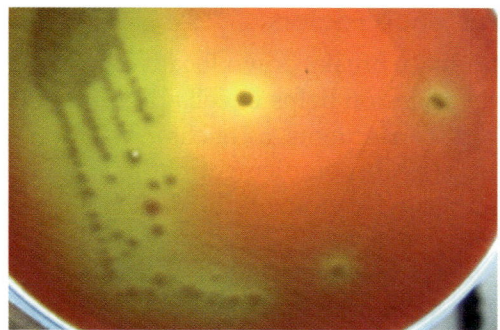

Fig. 26.3: α-hemolytic colonies on blood agar

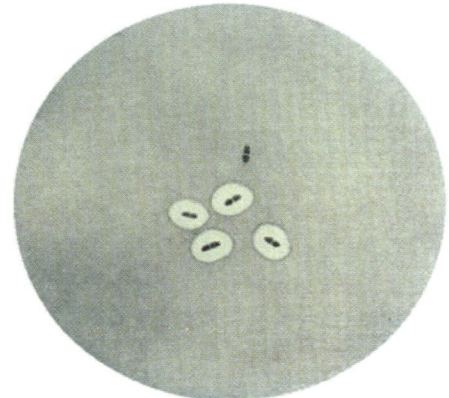

Fig. 26.4: Capsulated *St. pneumoniae*

- Colonies on **blood agar** after 18–24 hours are small transparent, **α-hemolytic** (Fig. 26.3). Further incubation of blood agar plate causes central umbonation with raised edges resembling "**draughtsman** "or "carrom coin" like appearance.
- After prolonged incubation, autolysis of bacteria within the flat colonies result in typical subsidence in the center that gives 'draughtman' colonies.
- Some isolates may produce abundant capsule hence produce mucoid colonies (Fig. 26.4).

Biochemical Tests (Table 26.1)

- **Fermentation** is tested in Hiss serum slope, it ferments **inulin.** This test differentiates it from *Streptococcus viridans.*
- Catalase and oxidase tests are negative.
- **Bile solubility test positive** (Fig. 26.5): This test is performed in two ways:
  1. 2% solution of NA deoxycholate or OX bile (10%) is poured on some colonies of this organism on blood agar, autolysis occurs and clearing of colony occurs.
  2. The organism is grown in glucose broth. It is divided into two test tubes. To one test tube, add solution of bile and another test tube with suspension of the organism, acts as control.
- **Optochin sensitivity test** (Fig. 26.6) is also used for identification and differentiation of *Streptococcus pneumoniae* from *Streptococcus viridans.* The optochin disk **(5 μg)** is placed on blood agar or chocolate agar plate, which is inoculated with the organism. Zone of inhibition is measured around the disk and if it is **more than 14 mm,** the test is positive (at least 5).
- **Growth in liquid medium:** Uniform turbidity with deposit is seen in liquid medium as nutrient broth.

Resistance

Thay are easily destroyed by heat. They are sensitive to most of antibiotics.

Antigens

- **Capsular polysaccharide** is soluble in the surrounding medium hence also called **specific soluble substance (SSS).** It inhibits phagocytosis. It is type specific. On the basis of capsular antigen, typing is done and this is immunologically distinct for each of more than 80 serotypes. Typing is done by precipitation reaction. Other methods for typing are agglutination, and Quellung reaction.

TABLE 26.1: Differences between *Streptococcus viridans* and pneumococci

	Streptococcus pneumoniae	*Streptococcus viridans*
Morphology	Lanceolate or flame-shaped	Round cocci
Shape	Cocci in pairs	Cocci in chains
Arrangement	Pairs	Chains
Capsule	Capsulated	Non-capsulated
Quellung reaction	Positive	Negative
Cultural characteristics	Draughtsman like colonies	No special appearance
Tests for identification		
Inulin fermentation	Positive	Negative
Optochin sensitivity	Positive	Resistance
Bile solubility test	Positive	Negative
Animal pathogenicity	Pathogenic to mice	Non-pathogenic to mice

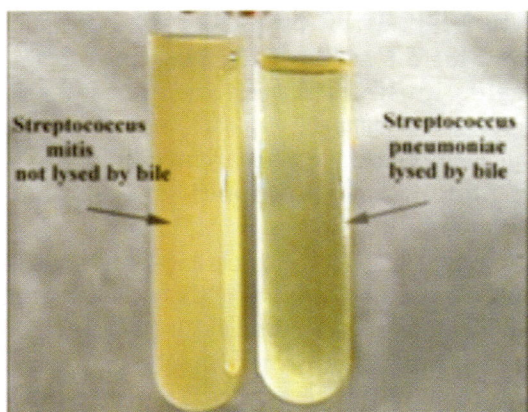

Fig. 26.5: Bile solubility test

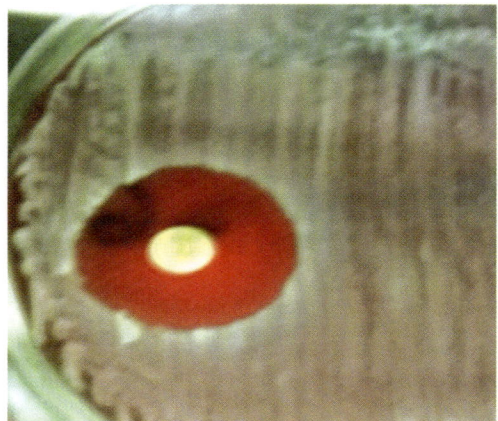

Fig. 26.6: Optochin test

- Pneumococci isolated from pneumonia belong to types I, II, III and IV.
- Other antigens are **protein** in the cell wall and somatic 'C' carbohydrate antigen. These are species-specific antigens.
- One more antigen lipoteichoic acid is **Forssman antigen**.
- **CRP:** It is an abnormal protein that precipitates carbohydrate 'C' of cell wall hence also called **C reactive protein. C reactive protein (CRP)** appears in acute phase sera of cases of pneumonia and other infections. It is not antibody formed in presence of streptococcal infection. It is produced in liver. It is detected by Latex agglutination test. It has more prognostic value than diagnostic value.

It has **prognostic value**, hence used in rheumatic fever and other conditions as index to access prognosis.

Only condition in which it helps in **diagnosis of infection** is detection of CRP in CSF, its presence indicates pyogenic meningitis and absence indicates aseptic meningitis.

Somatic 'M' protein acts as virulence factor.

Other Virulence Factors

- IgA protease breaks down locally produced IgA.
- Protein adhesion helps in cell adhesion.
- Cell wall constituents, as teichoic acid and peptidoglycan, activate complement pathway.
- Pneumolysin is cytotoxic and activates complement pathway.
- *Autolysin*: It breaks down own peptidoglycan leading to cell lysis. It is an amidase enzyme and activity is increased in presence of surface active agents as bile salts. It is responsible for the property (bile solubility).
- Pneumococcal surface protein-**A (PsPA)** and surface protein-**C (PsPC).**
  - **A (PsPA)** prevents complement activation.
  - **C (PsPC)** binds to factor 'H' of complement system and accelerates breakdown of C3 component.
- PsPA prevents complement activation while PsPC activates breakdown of C3.
- Pneumococcal **iron aquization (Pia-A) and iron uptake A(Piu-A).**
- Hyaluronidase, neuraminidase, enolase, penicillin binding protein.

Smooth to rough variation is seen in pneumococci. Capsulated forms of pneumococci—smooth forms are virulent but non-capsulated forms are avirulent. Repeated subculture of this organism may lead to smooth to rough variation. 'R' forms are auto-agglutinable, avirulent, noncapsulated and form rough colonies. In vitro, rough forms may be converted to smooth forms by **transformation** of DNA of smooth form inside the cell (Griffith experiment).

Pathogenicity

Source of Infection—Carrier

Modes of transmission are inhalation of droplets, droplet nuclei. In adults, capsular types 1–8 are responsible for most of the cases of pneumonia and more than half of the fatalities. In chidren, types 6, 14, 19, and 23 are frequent causes.

Loss of natural resistance: As 40–70% of human beings at some time carry pneumococci, the normal respiratory mucosa, they must possess great natural resistance to disease. The factors which predispose to infection are as follows:

- Viral or other respiratory tract infections damage surface cells, abnormal accumulation of mucus (due to allergy) protect organisms from phagocytosis and respiratory tract infection causes irritation, damage cilia.

- *Alcohol or drug intoxication*: It depresses phagocytosis, depresses cough reflex, and facilitates aspiration of foreign material.
- Abnormal circulatory dynamics (pulmonary congestion, heart failure).
- Malnutrition, sickle cell anemia, hyposplenism, complements deficiency.

Infections Caused by S. pneumoniae

Respiratory infections:
- Lobar pneumonia or bronchopneumonia
- Acute tracheobronchitis
- Empyema
- Acute exacerbation of chronic bronchitis
- Meningitis
- Bacteremia

After entry of cocci by respiratory tract, the person carries them in throat becoming carriers or if resistance is low, cocci cause pneumonia. Cocci penetrate bronchial mucosa and spread along peribronchial tissues and lymphatics. Serotypes 1–8 cause pneumonia in dults while, serotypes 6, 14, 19, and 23 cause infection in children.

Branchopneumonia is secondary infection by cocci in a person suffering from viral infection.

Other Infections

Suppurative complications are conjunctivitis, mastoiditis, suppurative arthritis, otitis media, sinusitis, pericarditis and empyema. Osteomyelitis, endocarditis and rarely brain abscess are other complications.

Epidemiology

Patients with respiratory tract infection or carriers act as source of infection. Mode of infection is through droplets or droplet nuclei. Crowding helps to spread infections. Pharyngeal carriage is common. Disease occurs when resistance is lowered. In adults, types 1–8 are common. In children, types 6, 14 and 19 are common.

Laboratory Diagnosis of Pneumonia

Samples: Sputum, larynegal swab (children)
- **Lobar pneumonia:** Sample collected is sputum in a sterile container.
- **Gross examination:** Rusty sputum.

Microscopic examination
- **Gram stain** shows Gram-positive cocci in pairs and pus cells.
- **Quellung reaction:** Sample mixed with polyvalent anti-capsular antiserum with methylene blue; capsular swelling occurs, which increases refractiveness.

Culture: **Homogenized** sputum is inoculated on blood agar and chocolate agar and incubated overnight, at 37°C and in presence 5–10% CO_2 in a candle jar. Further incubation gives typical colony morphology.

Colony morphology: Typical colonies which are tiny, alpha hemolytic and on further incubation they show 'draughtsman' appearance.
- Gentamicin (5 µg/mL) blood agar is used as selective medium.
- **Quantitative culture** on sputum is helpful to differentiate between infection of lower respiratory tract and only carriage in throat. **Colonies more than 10^6 suggest infection.**

Biochemical: Inulin +ve, bile solubility +ve, optochin: Sensitive. **OP sensitivity** is tested by placing optochin disk on inoculation plate-chocolate agar which is incubated and zone of inhibition is measured (positive test >14 mm positive).

Animal pathogenicity: Intraperitoneal inoculation in mice causes death in 1–3 days. Pneumococci can be isolated from peritoneal exudates and heart blood.

Blood culture: In acute stage of pneumonia, blood culture may be positive.

Laboratory Diagnosis of Pneumococcal Meningitis

Sample: CSF is collected by lumbar puncture, under all aseptic precautions in sterile container.

Transport: CSF is immediately transported to the laboratory. CSF is never refrigerated. If there is delay in transport, keep in incubator, if incubator is not available, keep it at room temperature.

It would be best option to collect CSF in 3 sterile tubes which are used for different tests (morphology, biochemistry and culture and antigen detection), or if collected in one tube, it is divided into 3 parts.

Gross appearance: CSF will be opalescent, hazy, turbid, and blood-tinged.

First portion is centrifuged and centrifuged deposit used for wet mount and Gram stain. Supernatant is used for (capsular) **antigen detection "SSS" by Latex agglutination**. Second portion used for culture and third portion is kept as it is for later use or inoculated in nutrient broth which is incubated, it acts as back up medium.

Biochemical tests: Proteins will be raised, CSF glucose will be reduced, CRP test on CSF will be positive. (CRP- is positive in pyogenic meningitis).

Microscopy

Wet mount: It shows pus cells.

- *Negative staining*: It is done by India ink or nigrosin. For this, on a clean glass slide, take one drop of CSF and one drop of reagent, put a coverslip and observe under high power microscope for capsulated diplococci.
- *Gram staining*: It shows Gram-negative pus cells and Gram-positive cocci (lanceolate in pairs) of size approximately 0.6–0.8 microns; they are nonsporing. **Direct immunofluorescence can** be performed, it is a sensitive test.

Culture

Following media are used and they are incubated in incubator at 37°C in Candle jar—the jar with media is placed in incubator (Candle jar gives 5–10% CO_2).

- **Blood agar and chocolate agar**—small translucent, **alpha hemolytic** colonies will be produced. If plates are incubated further typical draughtsman appearance will be seen on chocolate agar.
- **Liquid medium used as a backup—nutrient broth**. Uniform turbidity with deposit is seen in liquid medium as nutrient broth.

Biochemical tests: Catalase test is negative.

- **Fermentation** is tested in Hiss serum slope. It ferments **inulin** which differentiates it from *Streptococcus viridans*
- Bile solubility test positive.
- **Optochin sensitivity test**: Zone of inhibition is measured around the disk and if it is more than 14 mm, the test is positive.

Antigen Detection

Capsular antigen is detected by Latex agglutination test, ELISA, counter immunoelectrophoresis, or staphylococcal coagglutination test.

Antibody tests are of not much helpful, these tests are agglutination.

The alteration of penicillin binding proteins present on bacterial surface is the mechanism behind resistance. Such resistant strains may be multiple drug resistant (MDR).

Biomarkers

CRP is biomarker which can be tested by latex agglutination test. Another biomarker is **procacitin;** the levels of which are raised in '**invasive pneumococcal disease**'.

Molecular Method

Multiplex PCR is useful for detection of a few organisms in fluid. It is also helpful in diagnosis of infection in patients on antibiotics.

Animal pathogenicity test (nowadays it is not performed routinely): A suspension of bacterium is prepared in saline and it is given intraperitoneally in mice. In autopsy, fluid from peritoneal cavity will show Gram-positive diplococci. Other specimen which may show bacteria is blood smear of the animal.

Rapid test for detection of pneumococcal antigen in urine: Recently, an immunochromatographic test, the '**NOW S. pneumoniae urinary antigen test'** (Binax, Inc., Portland, Maine), has been developed; the test is simple to perform, detects the polysaccharide cell wall antigen common to all *S. pneumoniae* strains, and provides results within 15 min.

Prophylaxis

Various vaccines against pneumococci include:

- Purified capsular PS vaccine (14 serotypes), **Pneumovac.**
- A polysaccharide vaccine containing 23 types **(PPSV-23)** is another vaccine. It is not useful in children below 3 years.
- Conjugate vaccine: **polysaccharide conjugated to diphtheria CRM197 protein.** It consists of polysaccharide of 7 serotypes of Pneumococcus. It includes main childhood serotypes such as 6B, 9V, 14, 19F, 23F and 18 C.
- A 13 valent conjugate **vaccine (PCV-13).**

Antibiotic sensitivity: It is done on Müeller-Hinton agar with 5% sheep blood. The antibodies tested are penicillin, vancomycin, cephalosporin, erythromycin; clindamycin. Pencillin resistance is reported in pneumococci.

Treatment

Penicillin G is drug of choice. Cephalosporins, as ceftraixone, can be used as alternate drug. Penicillin resistance, though rare, is increasingly reported. In such cases, macrolides as erythromycin is given.

Multidrug resistant strains have been reported.

Penicillin resistance is due to **alteration of penicillin binding protein (PBP) to PBPaB.**

27

Neisseria

HISTORY

- The term **"gonorrhea" (flow of seeds)** was first introduced by Galen (AD 130).
- The organism was described by Neisser and cultured in 1882 by Leistikow and Loffler.

The family Neisseriaceae contain following genera: *Neisseria, Branhamella, Kingella, Moraxella* and *Acinetobacter.* The genus Neisseria has two species—*N. gonorrheae* which causes gonorrhea and *N. meningitidis* which causes pyogenic meningitis.

NEISSERIA GONORRHEAE

Morphology

- They are Gram-negative cocci (Fig. 27.1), often arranged in pairs (diplococci).
- Cocci are **bean (reniform or pear) shaped,** the adjacent sides are concave.
- The line of the long axis of cocci is **parallel** to the line joining two cocci in pairs.
- These diplococci are **mostly intracellular** seen inside the pus cells; some are seen outside the pus cells which are extracellular.
- Size of these organisms approximately 0.6–0.8 μ. Pili are present on the surface of cocci.

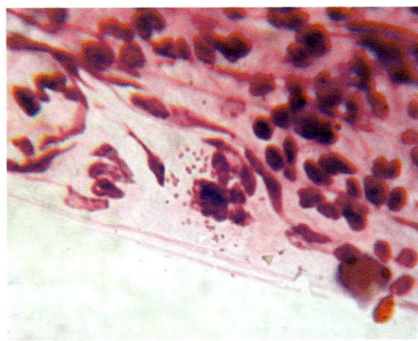

Fig. 27.1: Intracellular Gram-negative diplococci

Cultural Characteristics

- They are fastidious, exacting growth requirements.
- Meningococci and goncocci are difficult to cultivate, primarily because of their sensitivity to toxic fatty acids and trace metals present in peptone and agar. The inhibitory effect may be eliminated by adding to medium blood, serum, starch, charcol.
- It grows on enriched media.
- It is aerobe but can grow anaerobically.
- 5–10% CO_2 is required for their growth.
- Optimum temperature 35–36°C.
- Optimum pH 7.2–7.6.
- Humidity is provided by placing a gauge piece soaked in saline.

Transport Media

1. Stuart's transport medium
2. Amies transport medium
3. *Commercial media*: JEMBECC or GONOPACK system.

Media Used for Culture

Chocolate agar is preferred over blood agar, rather it is recommended (Fig. 27.2).

Selective media

- *Thayer-Martin (TM) medium*: Thayer-Martin medium, a chocolate medium with isovitalex and it also contains vancomycin, colistin and nystatin to prevent the growth of Gram-positive cocci, Gram-negative bacilli and yeasts, respectively. The growth rate is slow on this medium and 4% of gonococci are inhibited by vancomycin hence **Modified New York City medium** is preferred.
- *Modified New York City medium*: This transparent medium contains lysed horse blood, horse plasma, yeast dialysate, and same antibiotics as in Modified

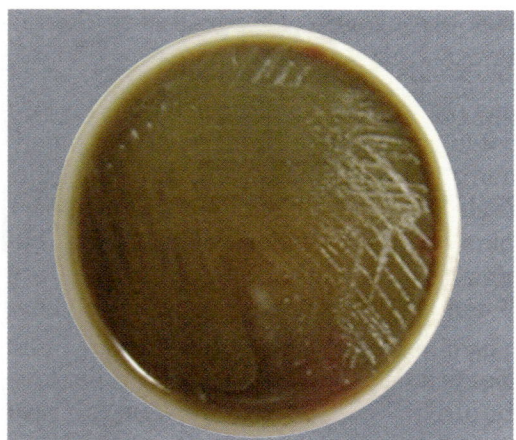

Fig. 27.2: Growth of gonococci on CA

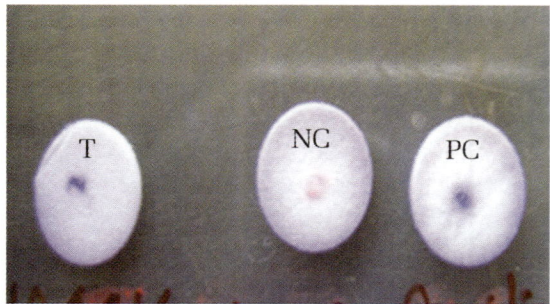

Fig. 27.3: Oxidase test with positive and negative control

Thayer-Martin medium. Within 24 hours, greyish small, circular, low convex, translucent colonies are formed. Some granularity may be observed.

On the basis of colony and autoagglutinating ability, some strains of gonococci can be correlated with virulence. The colonies are classified as:

- Types T1 and T2: They form small brown colonies, when colonies are emulsified in saline, clumps are produced without addition of antiserum to colony suspension. This is called **autoagglutination.**
- T1 and T2 colonies are **autoagglutinable,** and the **virulence** of these strains is **more,** they have pili on their surface.
- T3 and T4 form smooth large granular nonpigmented colonies, the organisms of these strains **do not cause invasive disease.**
- Fresh isolates from acute cases show T1 and T2 colonies. On subculture, colonies change to T3, and T4 morphologically. T1, and T2 types are known as P+, P++ respectively while T3, and T4 are known as P.

Modified Thayer-Martin medium contains additional trimethoprim to inhibit swarming of proteus. It is also called selective medium.

Biochemical Tests

- Catalase positive
- Oxidase positive (Fig. 27.3)
- Glucose is utilized without formation of gas. Fermentation is tested in serum slopes.

Other species normally colonize mucosal surfaces of oropharynx and nasopharynx and occasionally anogenital mucosal membranes.

Sensitivity

They are sensitive to heat, drying. They are sensitive to penicillins but they may produce β-lactamase.

Penicillinase producing gonococci (PPNU) produced plasmid coded β lactamase. Such plasmids are transferred horizontally. Chromosomally resistant *N. gonorrhoeae* (CMRAG) show resistance to penicillin and tetracycline. Tetracycline resistance (TRNG) is mediated by plasmid. ONNG stains are resistant to quinolone.

Virulence Factors

- **IgA protease** causes lysis of locally produced IgA antibody.
- **Fimbria or pili** help in attachment to the epithelial surfaces and help to prevent phagocytosis.
- **Capsular polysaccharide** helps to survive the bacteria inside phagocytes.
- **Outer membrane proteins**-I, II, III are **called por proteins**, I and III help in adhesion while **protein III** is responsible for the **clumping of bacteria in the sample,** i.e. urethral discharge. **Por (porin protein)** prevents phagolysosome fusion following phagocytosis and thereby promotes intracellular survival.
- **Liposaccharide:** It has some endotoxic effect.
- **Opa (opacity associated protein)** mediates firm attachment to epithelial cells and subsequent invasion into cells.

It also causes clumping of cocci seen in smear from urethal discharge. Strains of cocci having this protein may form opaque colonies. Based on porion proteins, there are two major serotypes—Por B, IA (associated with local and disseminated disease) and Por B, IB causes genital disease.

- Lip (H8) protein is surface exposed protein.
- H-8 lipoprotein (outer protein).
- Tbp-1 and 2 (transferrin binding protein) help in iron uptake.
- Ferric binding protein (Fbp) is expressed in infection when available iron supply is reduced.
- Lactoferrin binding protein (LBP).

Typing methods: Serotyping is based on porin protein IA and 32 protein-IB.

Pathogenicity

Disease in men (gonorrhea): The name gonorrhea means flow of seeds (bacteria appear as seed-like in a Gram's staining).

It is sexually transmitted disease. It is **only human disease,** there are no animal reservoirs.

Most infections among men are acute and symptomatic with purulent discharge and dysuria (painful urination) after 2–5 days incubation period.

Bacteria have the capacity to invade intact mucous membranes or skin with abrasions. Adherence to mucosal epithelium is with help of pili. Penetration into and multiplication occurs before passing through mucosal epithelial cells. They establish infection in the subepithelial layer, penetrate through intracellular spaces and reach subepithelial tissues and cause urethritis.

Series of Events After Infection

Pili and other proteins help in attachment to mucosal surfaces. The pili and surface protein are highly changeable. Genital secretions contain IgA and IgG. Gonococci produce **IgA protease.** They attach to nonciliated cells of fallopian tubes. Ciliary activity slows down, ciliated cells die and sloughed from epithelial surface. This step does not require intact organisms and can be caused by peptidoglycan and LPS. Microvilli of nonciliated cells act like pseudopods, engulf bacteria. Gonococci are transported to the base of nonciliated cells where bacteria laiden vacuoles fuse with basement membrane. The phagocytic vacuoles discharge gonococci into subepithelial connective tissue.

Organisms cause local inflammation or enter blood vessels to cause disseminated disease.

There is sloughing of ciliated cells. The inflammatory response in urethra is probably responsible for pain (dysuria) and urethral discharge. However, symptoms do not differ from other urethral infections. The pain is severe and discharge is thick greenish yellow.

Complications (Gonorrhea)

Disease in Males

- **Urethritis**
- **Epididymitis**
- **Prostatitis**
- Various discharging sinuses are formed which open outside. This is called **'water can perineum'. (periurethral tissue involved).**
- There may be stricture formation in urethra.
- Conjunctivitis may occur due to autoinfection by contaminated fingers.

- If persons are involved in anal sex, proctitis may occur.
- Most common presentation in male is acute urethritis a few days after unprotected intercourse. Dysuria and purulent penile discharge are the signs and symptoms.

Asymptomatic carriage is rare in males.
Bacteremia and lesions at other site may also occur. Higher risks of disseminated disease are present in patients with late **complement deficiencies.**

The two bacterial agents primarily responsible for urethritis among men are *N. gonorrhoeae* and *Chlamydia trachomatis.*

Disease in Women

- Vaginal mucosa is resistant to infection and its acidic pH also inhibits infection. Vulvovaginitis occur in prepubertal girls.
- Clinical disease is less severe in females. Some of the infected females become asymptomatic carriers who also act as source of infection.
- Cervicitis, vaginitis
- Infection of Bartholin glands, endometrium, and fallopian tube leads to pelvic inflammatory disease (PID) which is one of the causes of infertility.
- Peritoneal spread occurs occasionally producing perihepatic inflammation **(Fitz-Hugh-Curtis syndrome).**
- Ectopic pregnancy is another complication in this infection.
- Disseminated gonococcal infection (DGI) leads to arthritis.

Disseminated Gonococcal Infection (DGI)

It is result of gonococcal bacteremia and may present as:
- Skin lesions
- Petechiae (small, purplish, hemorrhagic spots)
- Pustules on extremities
- Arthralgias (pain in joints)
- Tenosynovitis (inflammation of tendon sheath)
- Septic arthritis
- *Occasional complications*: Hepatitis; rarely endocarditis or meningitis

Nonvenereal Disease

- Infection of neonates while passing through birth canal leads to ophthalmitis called ophthalmia neonatorum.
- The time honoured method of preventing **ophthalmia neonatorum (Crede's method)** consists of dropping 1% silver nitrate solution into infant's eyes immediately after birth. Ophthalmic ointment containing penicillin may be used.

- Gonococcal bacteremia may occur causing hemorrhagic rash, tensoynovitis, suppurative arthritis of knees, ankles and wrists.

Epidemiology—Gonorrhea

The incidence of gonorrhea has declined in developed countries. But still it remains major public health problem worldwide. There were still 362000 new cases reported in USA. The incidence is difficult to calculate because of limited surveillance and diagnostic facilities.

The infectivity of organism is such that the chance of acquiring infection from a single exposure to infected partner is 20–30% for men and even higher for women.

Gonorrhea can be reduced by:
- Avoiding multiple sexual partners
- Early diagnosis and treatment
- Finding of cases and contacts through education and screening the population at risk
- Use of condoms provides partial protection.

Laboratory Diagnosis

Samples collected are:
- **Urethral discharge or morning drop secretion:** After cleaning meatus with a gauze soaked in saline, sample is collected by loop or taken on slide.
- If discharge is not present, sample after **prostatic massage** is collected.
- **Early morning urine drop** may also be collected for diagnosis. It is centrifuged.
- From females, endocervical swabs, vaginal swabs, and exudate from urethra are collected.
- In both the sexes, anal swab, and in disseminated disease **blood culture** is done.

These specimens are collected **by Dacron swab** because cotton swabs absorb material and they are inhibitory substances present in it.

Transport medium: Stuart's medium: It is recommended to inoculate the media at the site where sample is collected (bedside inoculation).
- **Gram stain:** Small, Gram-negative diplococci mostly inside polymorph nuclear leukocytes (PMNs) are seen. Adjacent sides of cocci are concave and cocci are bean-shaped.
- **Direct immunofluorescence** is used to detect bacteria directly in specimens, increases the sensitivity and helps in early diagnosis.
- **Culture:** Gonococci are susceptible to drying and cooling, so immediate culture of specimen on to prewarmed selective (e.g. modified Thayer-Martin, Martin-Lewis agar) and non-selective media

(chocolate agar) with moisture and atmosphere containing 5 to 10% carbon dioxide in a candle jar is preferred. Moisture is provided by keeping a gauge piece soaked in saline which in turn placed in incubator. Optimum temperature is 35–36°C and optimum pH is 7.2–7.4.
- Chocolate agar is preferred over blood agar, rather it is recommended.

Growth identified by morphology and biochemical characteristics.

Morphology: Smear is again prepared from colonies. Gram-negative cocci often arranged in pairs are seen.

Biochemical characteristics:
- Catalase positive, **oxidase positive.**
- Fermentation of glucose with acid production occurs. Maltose and sucrose are not fermented. Sugars can be tested by rapid carbohydrate utilization tests.
- **New superoxol test** used for rapid identification.

New superoxol test: Superoxol (30% of H_2O_2)— *N. gonorrheae* produces immediate brisk bubbling when colony picked from medium is touched to the solution of H_2O_2 on a glass slide.

Immunoserological identification: Particulate agglutination tests are available which are performed on suspension from colonies on primary isolation plates.

Tests for the direct detection of antigen are:
- ELISA
- Immunochromatography
- Direct immunofluorescence

Commercial molecular assays are:
- **DNA probes:** Detection of ribosomal RNA by DNA probe with identification based on **chemiluminescence.**
- PCR.

MALDI-TOF has ability for rapid diagnosis and identification.

Antibiotic susceptibility testing can be performed on chocolate agar. The antibiotics tested are penicillin, erythromycin, ciprofloxacin, spectinomycin, doxycycline, tetracycline, ceftriaxone. Acidometric tests for penicillinase or beta lactamase production are done. Another method is using the nitrocefin disk.

Serological reactions: Using polyvalent antigen antibodies can be detected in patient's serum. They are not useful for routine diagnostic purposes. The tests are ELISA and hemagglutination.

Gonococcal urethritis is a seriously **under reported sexually-transmitted disease.**

Treatment

Antibiotics which can be used are penicillin, erythromycin, ciprofloxacin, doxycycline, ofloxacin, tetracycline, ceftriaxone, cefipime. **Ceftriaxone is the drug of choice.**

Although third generation cephalosporins are drugs of choice, some strains of gonococci with reduced susceptibility to ceftiaxone and cefixime are reported as resistant strains. The mechanism may be altered penicillin binding protein-2.

Drug Resistance in Gonococci

- Penicillinase producing gonococci (PPNG) produce plasmid coded β lactamase. Such plasmids are transferred horizontally by conjugation.
- Chromosome-mediated resistant *N. gonorrhoeae (CMRNG)* shows mutational resistance to penicillin and tetracycline. It is due to that resulting in decreased permabilily of cell to antibiotics. Tetracycline resistance (TRNG) is mediated by plasmids. QNIG strains are resistant to quinolone.

CDC recommends a single intramuscular dose of **ceftriaxone (250 mg)** or **400 mg oral cefixime;** additional 1 g erythromycin to be given in combined infection with Chlamydia. Azithromycin is helpful in pregnancy.

ATYPICAL NEISSERIA

N. gonorrhoeae, SSP kochii, is suggested as unusual neisseria isolated from conjunctival cultures in Egypt. These isolates do not react with monoclonal antibodies used in serological classification of gonococci.

NEISSERIA MENINGITIDIS (Meningococcus)

History

- Epidemic cerebrospinal fever (meningococcal meningitis) was first described by Vieusseaux in 1805.
- Weichselbaum isolated meningococcus from CSF and etiological relationship between organism and disease was established.

Morphology

- These are encapsulated small, Gram-negative diplococci (Fig. 27.4) with adjacent sides flattened. The long axis of cocci is at right angles to a line joining two cocci in pair (**half moon-shaped**). Smears prepared from cultures show more rounded forms.
- Size: 0.6–0.8 μ
- They are present inside the polymorphs. Some cocci are seen outside the polymorphs.

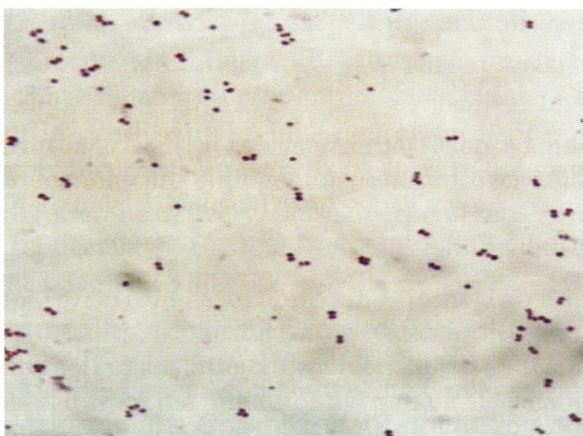

Fig. 27.4: Gram-negative diplococci

- Non-sporing, non-motile.
- Capsule is not ordinarily evident in smears.

It is second most common cause (after *S. pneumoniae*) of community-acquired meningitis in previously healthy adults.

Cultural Characteristics

- These are fastidious organisms, having exacting growth requirements. Growth occurs on enriched media only.
- Growth is enhanced by 5–10% CO_2 and moisture is required for the growth. A gauge piece soaked in saline is kept in the same incubator which will provide humidity.
- *Optimum temperature*: 35–36°C.
- *Optimum pH*: 7.4–7.6.

Media Used

- *Enriched media:* Blood agar; chocolate agar, of which chocolate agar is preferred for the growth.
- *Selective media:* Thayer-Martin medium is used to isolate the organisms from a site where there are commensals, e.g. carrier in throat.
- Modified Thayer-Martin medium (with vancomycin, colistin and nystatin) is also used as selective medium.

They do not grow on ordinary media; require blood agar or chocolate agar

- Blood agar—small colonies of size 1–2 mm are produced which are round, gray, translucent and after 48 hours, they become opaque.
- No hemolysis is seen on blood agar.
- Colonies are slightly bigger on chocolate agar.
- Inoculation on nutrient agar is used for differentiating from commensals as *N. meningitidis* will not grow on nutrient agar.

Biochemical Characteristics

- Catalase positive
- Oxidase positive
- Glucose and maltose are fermented with acid; no gas. Lactose and sucrose are not fermented.

Antigenic Properties and Classification

- Based on polysaccharide capsule, they are classified into serogroups A, B, C, D, X, Y, Z, W135, 29E, H, I, J, K, L.
- *Serogroup*: A, B, C, 29E, W-135, Y cause the most (90%) of the infections.
- Polyvalent vaccine containing serogroups A, C, Y and W135 are effective in people older than 2 years of age for immunoprophylaxis as an adjunct to chemoprophylaxis. Five classes of outer membrane proteins classify meningococci into 20 serotypes, 2 and 15 cause epidemics.
- Serogroup B is only weakly immunogenic and protection must be acquired naturally from exposure to cross-reacting antigens.
  Group A is associated with epidemics.
  Group C causes localized outbreaks.
  Group B causes both epidemics and outbreaks.

Resistance

They are easily killed by heat, antiseptics, they die in 1–2 hour in pus outside body. They have plasmid coding for β lactamase production.

Virulence Factors

- Capsular polysaccharide—inhibits phagocytosis.
- Pili help in adhesion to epithelial surfaces.
- Endotoxin is released during multiplication. It is an important toxin responsible for the manifestations of Waterhouse-Friderichsen syndrome.
- IgA protease breaks down IgA antibody.
- Outer membrane proteins help in attachment.
- Outer membrane also contains lipopolysaccharides which induce formation of IL-1 and TNF-α which are responsible for the serious complications as shock and hemorrhage.

Pathogenicity (Flowchart 27.1)

Meningococci enter through the nasopharynx. Other modes of entry in CNS are probably—spread along perineural sheath of olfactory nerve, through cribriform plate to subarachnoid space or through bloodstream or conjunctiva. Infection is usually asymptomatic.

Pathogenesis

Human beings are the only natural hosts. Person-to-person transmission takes place by aerosols in crowded conditions. Close contact with infectious person (e.g. family members, day care centers, military barracks, prisons, and other institutional settings) helps in spread of infection. Meningococci commonly colonize nasopharynx of healthy individuals; highest oral and nasopharyngeal carriage rates are seen in school-age children, young adults and lower socioeconomic groups. Outer membrane proteins and pili help in adhesion to epithelial surfaces. Following colonization of the nasopharynx, protective humoral immunity develops against the same or closely related organisms of the same serogroup, but not against other serogroups. Bacteremia results in seeding the organisms in meninges. Pili can bind to CD **46 protein** expressed on choroid plexus and meningeal epithelial cells. Both bacterial growth and inflammatory response occur within CSF, where levels of endotoxin, IL-6, TNF, IL-2a and IL10 exceed the plasma cocentration.

Diseases Associated with Neisseria meningitidis

- *Meningitis*: Affects young children. It presents with fever, headache, vomiting and neck stiffness.
- *Septicemia (meningococcemia) with or without meningitis*: Patient with septicemia may present as fever, chills, and hemorrhages. Petechial rash may or may not be present. Patients with **deficiency of complement (C5–C9)** are more prone for septicemia. The cocci may infect joints, adrenals, eyes, ears and lungs through bactermia.
  Endotoxin may be released from bacteria by autolysis which acts on vascular endothelium causing hemorrhagic rash. Pathogenesis is due to **Schwartzman like phenomenon.**
- **Waterhouse-Friderichsen syndrome:** Fulminant meningococcemia is characterized by shock, disseminated intravascular coagulation, and multisystem failure.
- Meningoencephalitis
- *Post-meningococcal disease*: It results from deposition of immune complexes. The manifestations are arthritis, rash, iritis, and polyserositis.
- Pneumonia
  Bactericidal activity of the complement system is required for clearance of the organism.

Epidemiology of Meningococcal Meningitis

- More than 50% cases occur in first 5 years of life. Peak prevalence is seen in first year of life. With increase in age, asymptomatic carriage gives immunity. Epidemics occur worldwide.

Flowchart 27.1: Pathogenesis of bacterial meningitis

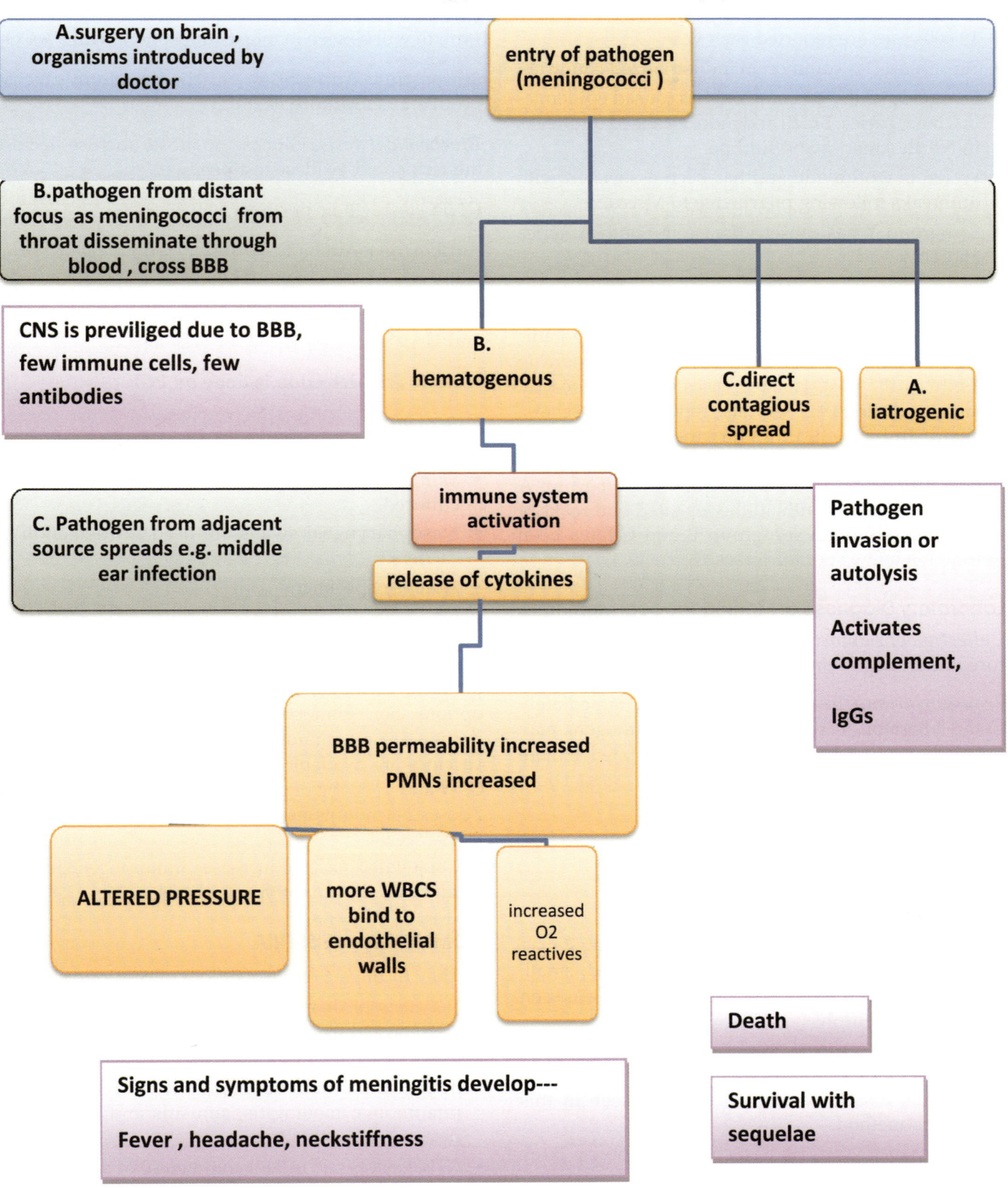

- Serogroup A is most prevalent in sub-Saharan Africa (African meningitis belt) and Middle East where 10,000 cases are reported each year.
- Serogroup-B is common in industrialized countries.
- Serogroup-C (ST-11 complex) has caused epidemics in China, Africa, Brazil and more localized outbreaks in North America and Europe.
- W-135 is worldwide and has been associated with outbreaks following pilgrimage to Mecca.
- Serogroup Y has caused disease in South America and USA.

Indian Scenario

Meningococcal disease is endemic in Delhi and sporadic cases of meningococcal meningitis have been occurring in Delhi in the past. Isolated cases of meningococcal meningitis during 1985 were also reported from several states of India including Haryana, Uttar Pradesh, Rajasthan, Sikkim, Gujarat, Jammu and Kashmir, West Bengal, Chandigarh, Kerala and Orissa. **Serogroup A** has been associated with all the repeated outbreaks of meningitis, although serogroup B and C have been detected in a few sporadic cases.

Laboratory Diagnosis of Meningococcal Meningitis

Collection of sample: CSF is collected by lumbar puncture under aseptic precautions in a sterile container.

Transportation: CSF must be transported immediately to the laboratory because the delicate pathogens may lose their viability, hence it is never refrigerated. If there is some delay, keep CSF in incubator or at room temperature.

Gross examination: CSF will be turbid.

Processing

1st portion: Centrifuge.
- **Gram stain** is done from centrifuged deposit: It may show intra- and extracellular encapsulated, small, Gram-negative diplococci (most of cocci are seen inside polymorphs).
- Centrifuged preparation is also used to prepare **methylene blue mount** which determines the cell type and also intracellular cocci are seen in this staining method.
- *Supernatant*: Antigen detection is done by latex agglutination or CIE, ELISA.

2nd portion: It is used for culture on blood agar and chocolate agar.

Colonies: Transparent, non-pigmented non-hemolytic colonies are formed on blood agar and enhanced growth will be seen in moist atmosphere with 5% CO_2.

3rd portion: Add CSF in enriched medium glucose broth and subculture next day.

Biochemical tests: Glucose, maltose, sucrose, lactose are fermented, oxidase test positive.

ONPG test will be positive.

Antibiogram: Antibiotic sensitivity is done against penicillin, cefotaxime, chloramphenicol, and sulphonamide.

Detection of antibodies: It can be done by ELISA, CFT, and HAI.

Nucleic acid detection is done by PCR.

Other cultures
- *Blood culture*: Effective in case of meningococcemia.
- *Skin scrapings*: Meningococcus may be seen and cultured.
- Nasopharyngeal swabs are used for detection of carriers.
- Autopsy specimens.

Treatment and Prophylaxis

Intravenous penicillin G is drug of choice. Chloramphenicol, ceftriaxone, ceftazidime are other treatment options. For chemoprophylaxis, rifampin and minocycline are recommended. Bivalent and polyvalent vaccines are available containing capsular groups A, C, W and Y. 50 mg of each antigen per dose is given in 2 doses 2–3 months apart. It gives good protection (79%) for 3–5 years.

Conjugated vaccine increases immunogenicity and it can be used even for young children.

COMMENSAL NEISSERIA

- They form part of normal flora of respiratory tract.
- Very few of them (*M. flavescens* and *M. catarrhalis*) are reported from cases of meningitis.
- *Branhamella catarrhalis* (formerly *N. catarrhalis*) causes opportunistic infections as laryngitis, bronchopneumonia, meningitis, sinusitis and middle ear disease.
- *N. lactamica* is a virulent commensal of throat which may cause confusion because of its resemblance with meningococci
- It gives ONPG test positive.

TABLE 27.1: Differences between Neisseria species

Species	Colonies	Growth on NA	Growth at 22°C	Glucose fermentation	Maltose fermentation	Sucrose fermentation	Serological classification
N. meningitidis	Round, smooth, shiny, creamish	–ve	–ve	A	A	–ve	13 groups
N. gononorrhoeae	Same as above, smaller, opalescent	–ve	–ve	A	–ve	–ve	Antigenically heterogenous
N. flavescens	Resembles meningococcus but pigmented yellow	+	+/–	–ve	–ve	–ve	Antigenically distinct homo-genous
N. sicca	Small, opaque, dry, brittle	+	+	A	A	A	Autoagglutinable
N. catarrhalis (Branhamella catarrhalis)	Variable smooth or opaque	+	+	–ve	–ve	–ve	Autoagglutinable

28

Corynebacterium Diphtheriae

HISTORY

- Diphtheria was not initially clearly differentiated from other respiratory illness. In the epidemic in South France, it was first differentiated from respiratory illness.
- Bretonneau first recognized the disease and gave name diphtheria.
- Kleb described (1883) chain forming cocci and bacilli in sections of membrane.
- Next year Loffler first isolated bacillus in pure culture. Hence the bacterium is also called as **Klebs-Loffler bacillus.**
- Roux and Yersin (1888) discovered diphtheria exotoxin and established its pathogenic effects.

Corynebacteria are Gram-positive, non-acid-fast, non-motile rods with irregular staining and sometimes with granules. They frequently show club-shaped swellings and hence the name (coryne-club). Diphtheria the disease name is derived from tough, leathery pseudomembrane formed in the disease (diptheros—leather). Apart from *C. diphtheriae*, other members of the family include *C. ulcerans, C. minutissimum, C. tenius* and diphtheroids.

Morphology

- It is Gram-positive slender rod, but tend to get decolorize easily.
- These bacilli show club-shaped swellings at one or both ends, the club-shaped swelling is due to presence of granules. The granule appears more dark than the rest of the bacillus. Due to presence of granules, bacteria may show irregular staining.
- *Size*: 3–6 × 0.6–0.8 µ. It may be pleomorphic.
- Chinese letters/cuneiform arrangement is due to incomplete separation of daughter cells after binary fission (bacilli form obtuse angle). Bacilli are present in pairs or small groups. They appear at various angles to each other, showing arrangement like letter V, L.
- **Diphtheroid** may give similar morphology but they have very **few metachromatic** granules and their arrangement is pallisidal.
- *Granules* (Figs 28.1 and 28.2)**:** They are stained with Loffler's methylene blue, as bluish purple, hence called **metachromatic granules** (other names for granules are volutin granules or Babes-Earnest granules); granules are also seen in *C. xerosis* and *Gardnerella vaginalis*.

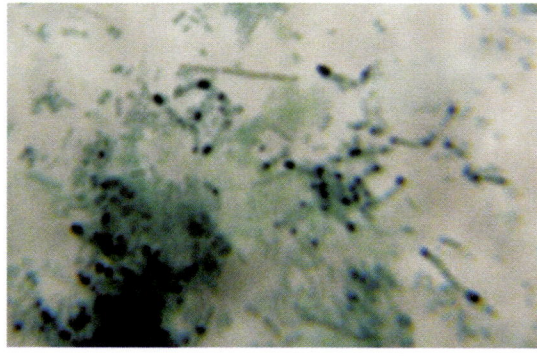

Fig. 28.1: Albert's smear showing metachromatic granules

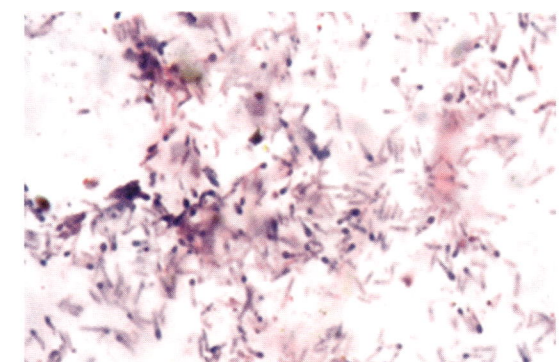

Fig. 28.2: Gram staining showing Gram-positive bacilli with granules

- **Special staining** commonly used for the demonstration of granules is Albert's staining in which the bacillus appears greenish. The granules take dark black color.
- Other stains for granules are Ponder's stains, Neisser's stain.

Cultural Characteristics

- Growth is scanty on ordinary media.
- It is aerobe and facultative anaerobe.
- Optimum temperature is 37°C (range 15–40°C), pH –7.2.
- *Transport medium*: As bacteria sustain drying, **Ames transport** medium is used for transport of clinical specimen.
- *Plating media*: Media enriched with blood, serum or eggs are required for proper growth, as bacilli are fastidius.
- **Loffler's serum slope** is an enriched medium, colonies can be seen within 6–8 hours before other bacteria grow, hence though it is not a selective medium but it helps to pick up the growth of this pathogen. Loffler's serum slope supports formation of granules; colonies are small, circular, white, opaque disks.
- **Blood potassium tellurite medium (BPT)** (McLeod's) is a selective medium, in which the organism reduces potassium tellurite to tellurium, which is black, hence colonies are black (Fig. 28.3).
- *Modified Tinsdale medium*: Sometimes diphtheroids may confuse morphologically with *C. diphtheriae* hence **modified Tinsdale medium** is used which shows black colonies surrounded by brown halo, which is absent in case of diphtheroids. The halo surrounding the colony is due to cystinase activity.

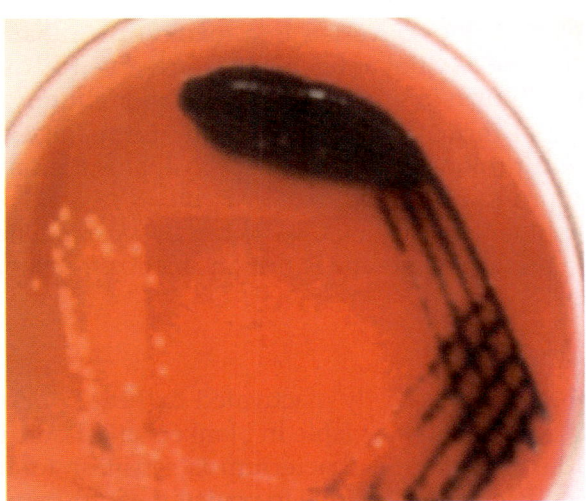

Fig. 28.3: BPT showing black colonies

Biotyping based on colony morphology on BPT (Table 28.1): Initially, the pathogenicity was correlated with different types of colonies produced on BPT, but now it is proved that the virulence is due to the production of toxin, still biotypes described which produce infections with varying severity.

- *Gravis*: After 18 hours of incubation on BPT, the colonies produced are of size 1–2 mm. They have grayish-black center, pale translucent periphery and crenating edge. In 2–3 days, flat colony with raised dark center, crenated edge with radial striation appears which gives appearance of '**daisy head**'.
- *Intermedius*: This biotype after 18 hours produces colonies of size about 1 mm which have dull granular center, glistening periphery, and lighter ring near edge giving the appearance of '**frog's egg**'.
- *Mitis*: Size of colonies variable, in 2–3 days, become flat, with a central elevation '**poached egg colony**'.

Biochemical Tests

- *C. diphtheriae* ferments sugars with production of acid (no gas) glucose, galactose, maltose, dextrin but not lactose, mannitol, sucrose. Hiss serum water medium used for fermentation test.
- It does not hydrolyse urea or form phosphatase.
- Proteolytic activity is absent.
- *Pyrizinamide test*: *C. diphtheriae, C. ulcerans, C. pseudo-tuberculosis* produce this enzyme, which breaks down pyrizinamide (positive test).

Antigens

- A deep-seated antigen found in *C. diphtheriae* (and *Mycobacterium tuberculosis*)
- A heat-labile protein antigen
- A heat-stable carbohydrate antigen.

Toxin (Flowchart 28.1)

Virulence is associated with exotoxin production. Toxin has A and B fragments, both are necessary for toxic action. When released by bacterium, toxin is inactive as active site on fragment 'A' is masked. Proteases cause activation. 'A' has enzymatic action while 'B' is responsible for binding to cells. Antibody produced against fragment 'B' prevents binding of bacilli to human cells. Hence, protective.

It is protein which can be crystallized. Toxin is highly potent. Lethal dose for experimental animal (gninea pig –250 gm) is 0.0001 mg. Fraction 'A' has molecular weight 24000 and 'B' has 38,000. The toxin is labile. prolonged storage, incubation at 37°C for 4–6 weeks, treatment with formalin (0.2–0.4%) and acidic pH removes its toxicity and converts toxin in toxoid which

Flowchart 28.1: Pathogenesis of diphtheria

Diphtheria toxin possibly assists colonization of bacteria in throat or skin by killing epithelial cells & neutrophils

In upper respiratory tract a bacteria cause inflammation , produce exudate and necrosis of epithelial cells of faucial mucosa

Bacteria multiply locally, do not penetrate mucosa, bacteremia is absent

The toxin is produced locally enters blood and circulates
toxin has special affinity for heart muscles, peripheral nervous system& adrenal glands

Toxemia occurs due to toxin
Diphtheria is toxamic disease

Mechanical complications are because of pseudomembrane formation while systemis manifestations are due to toxin production

is used for immunization. **Park-Williams strain** is used for toxin preparation.

The toxin production depends on **optimum iron concentration (0.1 mg/litre),** but higher levels may inhibit toxin synthesis. **All three biotypes can produce toxin** (100% of gravis, 90–95% strains of intermedius and 80–85% of mitis type strains). Similar toxin may also be produced by *C. ulcerans* and *C. pseudo-tuberculosis*. Toxin is converted into **toxoid** by contact with formalin, acidic pH and prolonged storage.

Genes for toxin production are present on a bacteriophage—beta phage. Non-pathogenic strains lack beta phage. But non-toxigenic strain can be made toxigenic by infection with beta phage this is called as 'lysogenic conversion'. Toxin production is influenced by concentration of iron in the medium.

Diphtheria toxin probably assists the organism to colonize of throat or skin by killing epithelial cells or neutrophils. The toxin binds to specific receptors on host cells and enter by receptor-mediated endocytosis. 'A' separated from 'B' and it inserts and passes through lysosomal membrane into cytoplasm.

Mechanism of Action of Toxin (Fig. 28.4)

- Toxin inhibits protein synthesis. Fragment 'A' inhibits polypeptide chain elongation in presence of NAD by inactivating the elongation factor EF-2.
- Toxin mainly affects myocardium, adrenals, and nerve endings.

Toxin can be converted into toxoid (toxin that has lost toxigenicity but antigenicity is preserved). Toxoid gives antitoxin immunity (not infection immunity).

Toxoid formation is promoted by formalin, acidic pH and prolonged storage. Park-Williams 8 strain is used for production of toxoid vaccine.

Diphtheria is a toxemia. Toxin causes systemic effects while pseudomembrane is responsible for mechanical effects.

Resistance

The bacterium is easily inactivated by heat (1 minute at 100°C). It remains viable in blankets and floor dust for 13–14 weeks. The bacterium is sensitive to antiseptics. Bacilli are sensitive to penicillin, erythromycin and broad-spectrum antibiotics. Bacilli show more

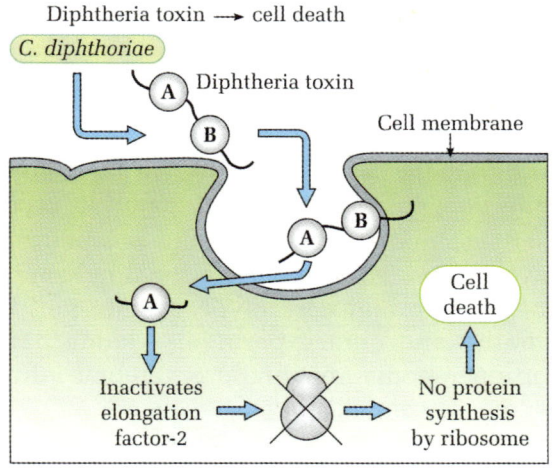

Diphtheria toxin → cell death

C. diphthoriae

Diphtheria toxin

Cell membrane

Cell death

Inactivates elongation factor-2 ⇒ ⊗ ⇒ No protein synthesis by ribosome

Fig. 28.4: Mechanism of action of diphtheria toxin

resistance to action of light, desiccation, freezing than most non-sporing bacilli.

Typing

- Biotyping is based on growth on (McLeod's) blood potassium tellurite medium.
- *Serotyping*: Gravis has 13, intermedius has 4, and mitis has 40 serotypes.
- 15 bacteriophage types described, 1 and 3 are mitis, 4, 6 intermedius.
- Serotyping is based on mycolic acid antigens and heat stable polysachharide antigen.
- *Other typing methods*: DNA typing (RFLP), hybridization with DNA probes.

Pathogenicity

Diphtheria is an important pediatric disease.

Source of infection: Patients, carriers (nose, throat) act as source of infection to others.

Mode of infection: Infection spreads by droplet infection, fomites are less important. Toys and pencils may act as source of infection.

In cows, infection of udder may occur, infection in this case transmitted by milkers. The infection may spread through the milk of infected cows.

Incubation period is 3–4 days.

Primary Sites of Infection

Primary sites of infection order are faucial, laryngeal, nasal, otitic, conjunctival, genital—vulval, vaginal, prepucial. Cutaneous infections are secondary infections on pre-existing skin lesions. Cutaneous infections are common with non-toxigenic strains. Diphtheric whitlow or ulcer may occur.

- *Faucial diphtheria*: It is varies from mild to severe form. It is the commenest presentation of diphtheria.

- *Malignant or hypertoxic*: There is severe toxemia with marked adenitis (bull neck). Death is due to acute circulatory failure. Paralytic sequelae are seen in some patients.
- *Septic*: Ulceration, cellulitis, and gangrene around pseudomemberane may occur.
- *Hemorrhagic*: There may be bleeding from edge of membrane, epistaxis, purpura, conjunctival hemorrhage and generalized bleeding tendency.

Anterior nasal diphtheria: The onset of anterior nasal diphtheria is indistinguishable from that of the common cold and is usually characterized by a mucopurulent nasal discharge (containing both mucus and pus) which may become blood-tinged. A white membrane usually forms on the nasal septum. The disease is usually fairly mild because of apparent poor systemic absorption of toxin in this location, and it can be terminated rapidly by diphtheria antitoxin and antibiotic therapy.

Pharyngeal and tonsillar diphtheria: The **most common sites** of diphtheria infection are the **pharynx** and the **tonsils**. Infection at these sites is usually associated with substantial systemic absorption of toxin. The onset of pharyngitis is insidious. Early symptoms include malaise, sore throat, anorexia, and low-grade fever.

Within 2–3 days, a bluish-white membrane forms and extends, varying in size from covering a small patch on the tonsils to covering most of the soft palate. Often by the time, a physician is contacted, the membrane is grayish green or black, if bleeding has occurred. There is a minimal amount of mucosal erythema surrounding the membrane. The pseudomembrane is firmly adherent to the tissue, and forcible attempts to remove it cause bleeding (Fig. 28.5).

Extensive pseudomembrane formation may result in respiratory obstruction. While some patients may recover at this point without treatment, others may develop severe disease. Fever is usually not high, even though the patient may appear quite toxic. Patients with severe disease may develop marked edema of the submandibular areas and the anterior neck along with lymphadenopathy, giving a characteristic **"bull neck"** appearance (Fig. 28.6). If enough toxin is absorbed, the patient may develop severe prostration, striking pallor, rapid pulse, stupor, and coma, and may even die within 6 to 10 days.

Laryngeal diphtheria: Laryngeal diphtheria can be either an extension of the pharyngeal form or can involve only this site. Symptoms include fever, hoarseness, and a barking cough. The membrane can lead to airway obstruction, coma, and death.

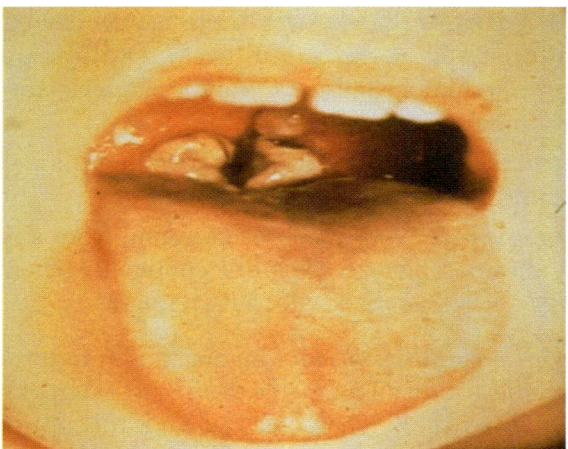

Fig. 28.5: Pseudomembrane seen in diphtheria

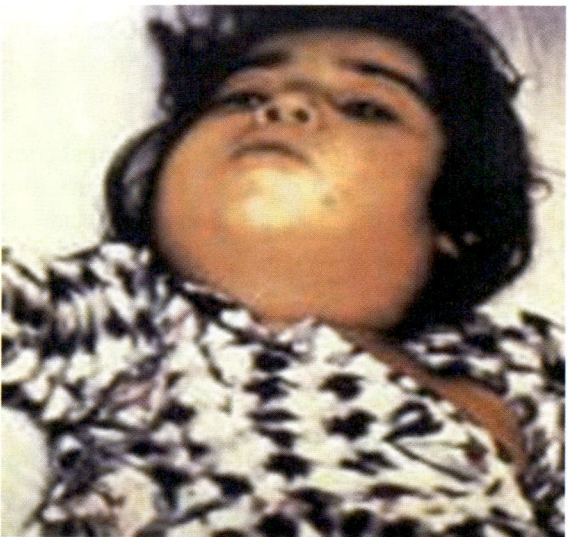

Fig. 28.6: Bull neck appearance

Cutaneous (skin) diphtheria: Skin infections are quite common in the tropics and are probably responsible for the high levels of natural immunity found in these populations. Skin infections may be manifested by a scaling rash or by ulcers with clearly demarcated edges and membrane, but any chronic skin lesion may harbour *C. diphtheriae* along with other organisms. Generally, the organisms isolated from cases in the United States were nontoxigenic. The severity of the skin disease with toxigenic strains appears to be more than from other sites.

After entry, bacteria multiply in local tissue. The toxin secreted by bacteria is responsible for tissue necrosis locally. The fibrinous exudate together with disintegrated epithelial cells, RBCs, WBCs and bacteria form—'**pseudomembrane**' characteristic of diphtheria. It does not contain epithelial cells. If any attempt is made to remove pseudomembrane, capillaries tear and bleeding occurs.

Complications

- Pseudomembrane obstructs airways, causes asphyxia for which emergency tracheostomy is needed.
- Acute circulatory failure (cardiac or peripheral).
- Post-diphtheric paralysis: It is seen in 3rd or 4th week of infection, palatine and ciliary paralysis occurs.

Other systemic complications are polyneuropathy and myocarditis. There are demyelinating conditions present with cranial nere involvement, peripheral neuropathy and ciliary paralysis—some patients develop pneumonia, renal failure, cerebral infraction and pulmonary embolism.

Non-toxigenic strains may cause infection even in immunized individuals, as toxoid gives antitoxin immunity and not anti-infection immunity.

- Non-toxigenic strains may cause pharyngitis and cutaneous abscess. Some strains may also cause endo-carditis, arthritis, septic rhinitis and osteomyelitis. *C. diphtheriae biotype belfanti* may be involved in the process of **atrophic rhinitis** called **ozona.**

Most of the vaccine preventable diseases showed a decline after introduction of Expanded Program of Immunization in 1978 and Universal Immunization Program in 1985. It is still endemic in our country. The last decade has seen resurgence of diphtheria in both developed and developing countries where it was previously well controlled.

Epidemiology—Diphtheria

Diphtheria almost disappeared from developed countries following mass immunization. It is still endemic in many regions of world. About 50000 cases occurred in Soviet Union during 1990–1996. Other countries that have experienced recent outbreaks are China, Ecuador, Algeria, and southeast Asia. In the year 2003, total 896 cases reported by WHO.

Infection is restricted to human beings. Cases and carriers act as source of infection. The most common mode of spread is by aerosolized droplets or direct contact with skin lesions. Unimmunized children less than 15 years old are most likely to contract disease.

Bacteria persist longer in skin lesions than tonsils and nose. Cutaneous disease is more contagious. Untreated person remains infectious for about 2 weeks.

Laboratory Diagnosis

Aims of laboratory diagnosis are:
1. Confirmation of clinical diagnosis.
2. For initiation of control measures.
3. Epidemiological purpose.

CDC case definitions: These are based on both a clinical syndrome (upper respiratory tract infection with sore throat, fever, and adherent membrane on tonsils, pharynx and/or nose) and laboratory criteria (isolation of bacteria from lesions or histopathological diagnosis).

Case is '**confirmed**' either by laboratory or epidemiologically linked to a laboratory confirmed case.

'**Probable case**' is one which is neither confirmed by laboratory or cannot be epidemiologically linked to a confirmed case.

Both asymptomatic patients and patients with respiratory findings without pseudomembrane are classified as carriers.

Confirmed diagnosis consists of isolation of the bacillus and demonstration of toxigenicity.

Specimen collection: Two swabs from lesions on tonsils and posterior pharyngeal wall are collected under vision, using tongue depressor.

Transport: Swabs are transported in Ame's transport medium. If there is delay in transportation of swabs, viability of pathogen can be preserved by moisteining it with sterile serum.

Microscopy: Gram staining, Albert's staining and Leishman's staining (to differentiate from streptococcal or Staphylococcus sore throat and Vincent's angina) are performed on smears.

- Gram-stained smear shows Gram-positive bacilli with dark-colored club-shaped swelling.
- Albert-stained smear shows green bacillary body and granules dark greenish black.

Importance of primary staining: Based upon primary staining, provisional report can be given to the clinicians who can start specific treatment which is life saving.

Direct immunofluorescence: It helps in rapid diagnosis of the condition.

Direct detection of toxin in clinical specimen is possible by **PCR**. This test is developed at **CDC Atlanta**.
- Tox gene is detected by PCR.
- ELISA and immunochromatography are used for toxin detection.

Culture

- *Loffler's serum slope*: Growth may appear within 6–8 hours (given negative after 24 hrs).
- *Blood potassium tellurite agar (Hoyle's or BPT)*: It contains 0.04% potassium telurate as selective agent. It is a selective medium, incubated at least for 2 days before considered negative. This medium is important in isolation of bacilli from contacts, carriers, convalescents. Black colonies are produced on BPT.
- *Modified Tinsdale medium*: Colonies of *C. diphtheriae* on this medium are black surrounded by brownish halo. This colony morphology is helpful in differentiating it from diphtheroids which may produce blackish colonies, but without halo.

Virulence Tests

As toxin is correlated with virulence, its detection is important and it is done by in-vivo tests and in-vitro tests.

Toxigenicity Tests

In vivo Tests

Subcutaneous test: A colony is picked up from Loffler's slope and it is emulsified in 2.4 mL of broth, 0.8 mL of it is injected subcutaneously into 2 guinea pigs or rabbits. One of the animals is protected with 500 units of antidiphtheric serum 18–24 hours previously; if strain is virulent, the unprotected animal dies (Flowchart 28.2).

Intracutaneous test: 0.1 mL is injected intracutaneously in test and control animal each. Control receives 500 units of antitoxin on previous day. The other animal receives 50 units of antitoxin intraperitonealy 4 hours after skin test. This is given to prevent death. Test animal shows inflammatory reaction at the site of injection leading to necrosis within 48–72 hours while there will be no change in control animal. Many strains can be tested as there is no death of animal (advantage—no wasteful of animal) (Flowchart 28.3).

In vitro Test

Elek's gel precipitation test (Fig. 28.7): Elek's test, also known as the immunodiffusion technique, is an *in vitro* virulence test performed upon *Corynebacterium diphtheriae*. It is used to test for toxigenicity of *C. diphtheriae*.

A filter paper strip impregnated with diphtheria antitoxin is buried just beneath the surface of a special agar plate (20% horse serum agar) before the agar hardens. Strains to be tested, known positive and negative toxigenic strains are streaked on the agar's surface in a line across the plate and at a right angle to the antitoxin paper strip. After 24–48 hours of incubation at 37°C, plates are examined with transmitted light for the presence of fine precipitation lines at a 45-degree angle to the streaks. The presence of precipitation lines indicates that the strain produced toxin that react with the antitoxin.

Flowchart 28.2: Demonstration of toxin by *in vivo* test

Growth of C.diphtheriae emulsified in 2-4 ml of broth

Control animal protected with 500ml of antitoxin

Unprotected animal

0.8ml subcutaneously

Animal survives as toxin is neutralized by anti-toxin

Animal dies due to toxemia neutralized by anti-toxin

Flowchart 28.3: *In vivo* test (intracutaneous test) for toxin detection

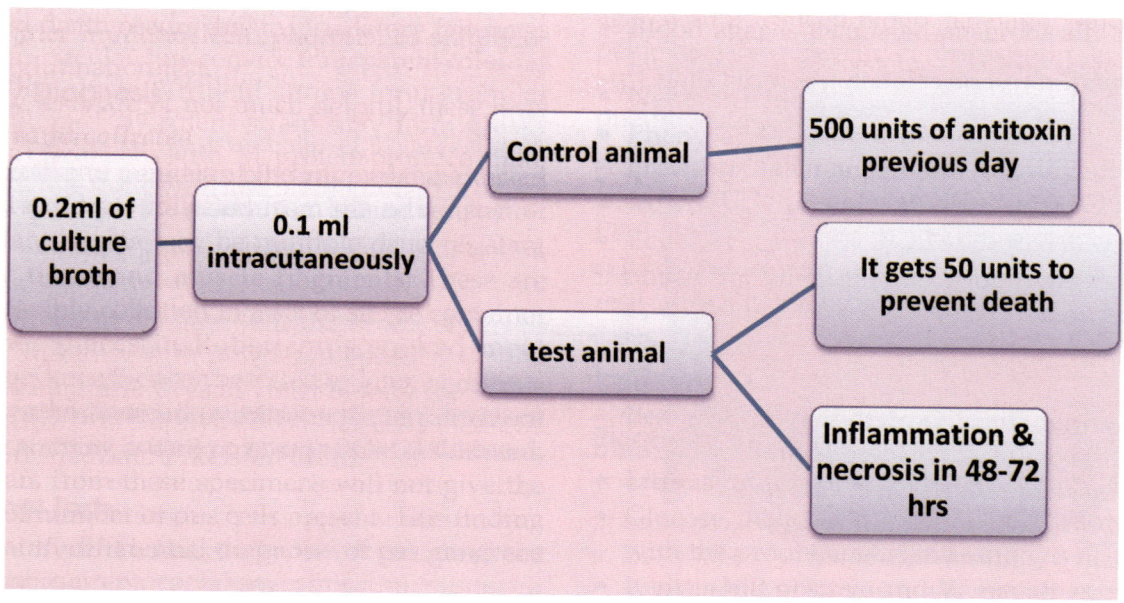

0.2ml of culture broth

0.1 ml intracutaneously

Control animal

500 units of antitoxin previous day

test animal

It gets 50 units to prevent death

Inflammation & necrosis in 48-72 hrs

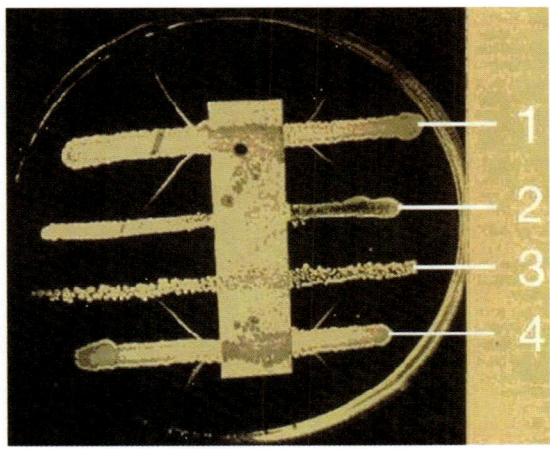

1. (+ve) control, 2. (–ve) control and 4 test strains

Fig. 28.7: Elek's gel precipitation test

Modified Elek's gel precipitation test (WHO): This test uses filter paper disks with 10 IU of antitoxin per disk. Precipitation is seen in 24 hours.

Tissue Culture Test

The strain is inoculated in agar overlay of cell culture monolayers; toxin diffuses into cells and kills them.

Other **newer** methods for detection are **thin paper chromatography** and **gas liquid chromatography**. They analyse fatty acids produced by bacteria.

- Commercial kits as API Coryne strip can be used for identification.
- Rapid diagnosis is also possible with MALDI-TOF).

Prophylaxis

- *Active immunization:* Diphtheria Pertussis Tetanus vaccine is used.
- *Passive immunization:* Antidiphtheric serum is used.
- *Combined immunization:* Passive immunization is followed by active immunization.

Active Immunization

a. *Formal toxoid:* It is prepared by incubating the toxin with formalin at pH 7.4–7.6 for 3–4 weeks at 37°C days, until toxicity is lost.
b. *Adsorbed toxoid:* Purified toxoid adsorbed on to aluminium phosphate or hydroxide. It is more immunogenic than formol toxoid. It is given by intramuscular injections as subcutaneous injections may be painful.

DPT vaccine

- This triple vaccine contains tetanus toxoid and killed Pertussis bacillus (acts as an adjuvant) along with DT.

- Young children—dose is 10–25 Lf units; smaller doses, 1/2 Lf units used for older children and adults to minimize adverse reactions.
- *Immunization schedule of DPT:* 3 primary doses are given at intervals of 4, 6, 10 weeks, followed by 4th dose, a year afterwards.
- Further booster dose given at school entry.

Other combined vaccines are:
DaPT: It contains DT, TT and a cellular pertussis (ap).

DT: It contains DT and TT.

dT: It contains TT and adult dose diphtheria (2 Lf) toxoid (d). It is given to adults more than 12 years. Three doses are given at 0, 1 month and 1 year.

As vaccine produces antitoxin immunity and cutaneous disease is due to mostly non-toxigenic strains increase of cutaneous disease is observed.

Passive Immunization

In emergency cases, passive immunization is given as treatment. It consists of subcutaneous administration of 500–1000 units of antitoxin (anti-diphtheric serum—ADS). Anitoxin which is prepared in horses may cause hypersensitivity.

Combined Immunization

First dose of adsorbed toxoid is given on one arm, while ADS is given on the other arm, followed by full course of active immunization. Ideally all cases that receive ADS prophylactically should receive combined immunization.

Treatment

Specific treatment consists of antitoxin and dose is 20,000 to 1,00,000 units for serious cases, half the dose is given intravenously.

Penicillin is given as supplementary to antitoxin. Antitoxin is not recommended for cutaneous cases as nontoxigenic strains cause cutaneous infections.

CORYNEBACTERIUM ULCERANS

It causes disease in cows, human infection may be due to consumption of contaminated milk. It causes diphtheria-like lesions. It produces two types of toxins, one resembling *C. diphtheriae* and another resembling *C. pseudotuberculosis.* It liquefies gelatin, and ferments trehalose. Erythromycin is used for the treatment.

Arcanobacterium (previously known *Corynebacterium haemolyticum*): It can cause pharyngitis and skin ulcers. *C. jakeium* can cause cutaneous and blood infection and it is multiple drug resistant. It responds to vancomycin.

TABLE 28.1: Differences between three biotypes of *Corynebacterium diphtheriae*

	Gravis	Mitis	Intermedius
Length of bacilli	Short	Long forms	Long curved
Staining	Uniform	Irregular	Pleomorphic
Blood agar	Hemolysis may be or may not be produced	Nonhemolytic	Hemolytic
BPT	1–2 mm, gray colony with raised center, crenated edge Colony appearance—'Daisy head' like colonies	1 mm, gray black colonies with granular centre, glistening periphery, lighter ring near edge 'Frog's egg' like colonies	Circular, black, convex, smooth colonies 'Poached egg' like colonies
Consistency of colony	Not easily emulsifiable in normal saline	Intermediate between gravis and mitis type	Easily emulsifiable
Glycogen fermentation	Positive	Negative	Negative
Starch fermentation	Positive	Negative	Negative
Virulence	High	Moderate	Mild
Complication	Paralysis	Hemorrhages	Obstructive complications and hemorrhages

Corynebacteria Causing Superficial Skin Infections

Localized lesion of stratum corneum affecting axilla and groin caused by *C. minutissimum* is called **erythrasma**.

C. Tenuis

Causes pigmented nodules surrounding axillary and pubic hair shafts; the condition is called **'trichomycosis'**.

Corynebacteria of veterinary importance

Preisz-Nocard bacillus (*C. pseudotuberculosis*). It causes pseudotuberculosis in sheep and lymphadenitis in horses. *C. renale* causes **cystitis** in cattle. *C. equi* causes **pneumonia** in **foals.**

DIPHTHEROIDS

They may resemble *C. diphtheriae*, they are commensals in throat, conjunctiva, skin. They are differentiated morphologically from *C. diphtheriae* by **pallisidal** arrangement with few or no metachromatic granules. On modified Tinsdale medium, they produce black colonies without brown halo. Nonvirulent *C. pseudo-diphtheriticum* is found in throat while *C. xerosis* is found in conjunctival sac.

Other corniform bacilli: *Propionibacterium acnes* often isolated from acne lesions but its role is not sure.

CORYNEBACTERIUM PARVUM

Corynebacterium parvum is used as **immunomodulator.**

29

Bacillus Anthracis

Bacillus species are Gram-positive bacilli (Fig. 29.1) with nonbulging spores (*Clostridia* are also Gram-positive bacilli but they have spores which bulge out of bacillary body).

BACILLUS ANTHRACIS

This organism has **historical importance** because:

- It is the first pathogenic organism to be observed under microscope.
- It is the first bacterium to be isolated in pure form.
- Robert Koch postulated his hypothesis by working on this bacillus.
- Pasteur developed first bacterial vaccine by using Anthrax bacillus (Fig. 29.2).
- It was the first communicable disease shown to be transmitted by infected blood.

Morphology

- They are Gram-positive bacilli, 3–10 μ × 1–1.6 μ.
- Ends of bacilli are truncated or concave, somewhat swollen.

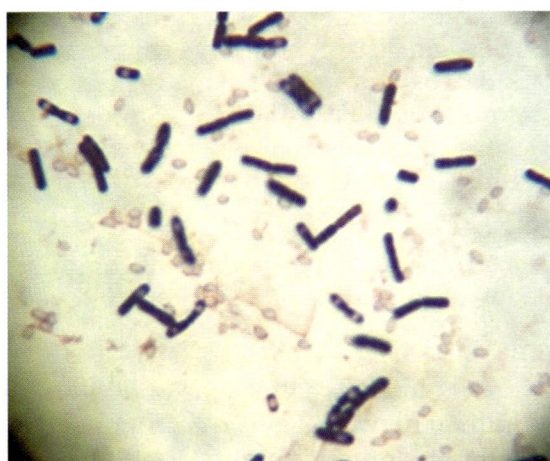

Fig. 29.1: Gram-positive bacilli

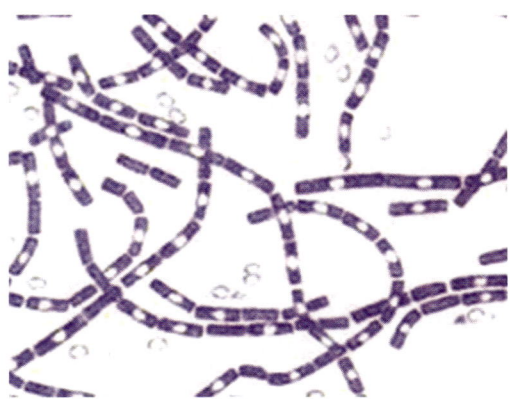

Fig. 29.2: Anthrax bacillus

- *Arrangement of bacilli*: Single, in pairs or short chains.
- They are capsulated, **capsule** produced only under 10–25% CO_2 in media containing serum, starch, charcoal, and albumin or in presence of bicarbonate. The capsule surrounds the chain of bacilli. The capsule is polypeptide in nature.
- Capsular gene is present on plasmid, PXO_2.
- In cultures—long chains of bacilli with swollen ends give **'bamboo stick' appearance.**
- Spores are central, oval, with same width as bacilli, **nonbulging spores** are produced under adverse conditions. Spores are formed in soil and in cultures. Sporulation can be induced by distilled water or 2% NaCl.
- Giemsa-stained smear shows red capsule around purple bacilli.
- Lipid granules are produced which are stained by Sudan black.

MacFadyean's Reaction

Blood smear is stained with polychrome methylene blue for a few minutes. It is observed under microscope. Amorphous material will be seen around the bacilli (capsular material).

Cultural Characteristics

- It is aerobe, facultative anaerobe.
- Optimum temperature is 35–37°C (for sporulation 25–30°C).
- It grows on ordinary media.
- On agar plates, round, 2–3 mm, raised, dull, opaque, grayish-white colonies with irregular edge are produced (Fig. 29.3). Virulent bacilli form smooth colonies while avirulent bacilli form rough colonies.
- *Under microscope*: **Medusa head appearance** (Fig. 29.4) is seen, if edge of colony is focussed, while the **Frosted glass appearance** is seen when colony is observed under microscope.
- *BA*: On this medium, no hemolysis is seen.
- In presence of penicillin, the bacteria become large, spherical, form chains on the surface of medium resembling 'string of pearls'. **String of pearls** reaction on blood agar with penicillin—differentiates it from *B. cereus*.

  Gray colonies have rough texture, comma-shaped outgrowths project from colonies (weavy margin with small projections) (Medusa head, "curled hair")
- **Selective medium: PLET medium** (contains polymyxin B, lysozyme, ethylenediaminetetraacetic acid and thallus acetate) is selective medium.
- Gelatin stab culture shows **'inverted fir tree'** appearance with liquefaction starting from top (Fig. 29.5).
- In liquid medium, it produces floccular deposits with little or no turbidity.

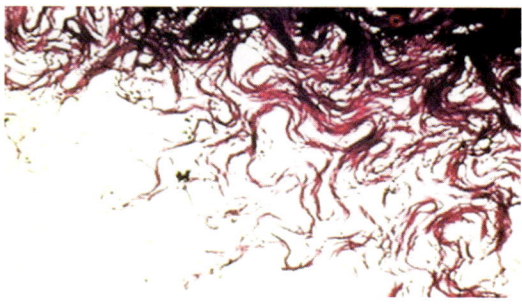

Fig. 29.3: Edge of colony

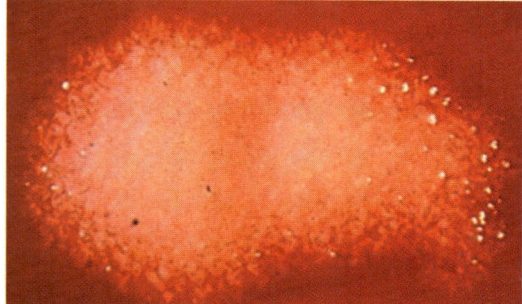

Fig. 29.4: Medusa head-like colony

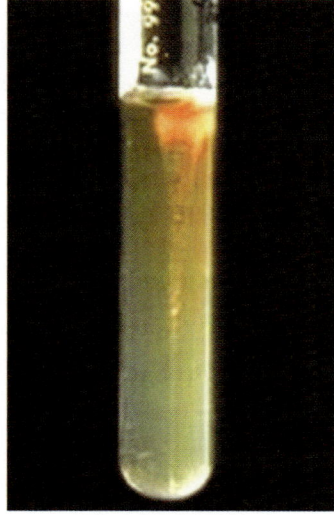

Fig. 29.5: 'Inverted fir tree' apperance

Biochemical Reactions

- Glucose, maltose, and sucrose are fermented with production of acid, no gas.
- Nitrates are reduced to nitrites.
- Catalase positive.
- *B. arthracis* is suceptible to gamma phage.

Resistance

- Vegetative bacilli get easily destroyed (60°C for 30 min).
- Spores highly resistant (dry heat 140°C for 1–3 hours, boiling for 10 minutes).
- Spores survive in infected soil up to 60 years.
- 'Duckering' is a process used for disinfection of animal products. Two percent formaldehyde at 30–40°C for 20 minutes is used for wool and 0.25% at 60°C for 6 hours is used for animal hairs and bristles.
- It is susceptible to sulphonamides, penicillin, erythromycin, streptomycin, tetracycline, and chloramphenicol.

Virulence Factors

Capsule inhibits phagocytosis. Exotoxin produced consists of edema factor, protective antigen factor, and lethal factor. Toxin as a whole shows toxic effects. Separate plasmids control capsule and toxin production. If bacteria loose plasmids, they will loose virulence. This is probably logic behind live-attenuated vaccine produced by Pasteur.

Mode of infection: Bacteria enter through skin by inoculation or inhalation or ingestion.

Pathogenesis of Anthrax (Flowchart 29.1)

- Endospores introduced into the body by abrasion, inhalation, or ingestion are phagocytosed by macrophages and carried to regional lymph nodes. Endospores germinate inside the macrophages and become vegetative bacteria. The vegetative bacteria are then released from the macrophages, multiply in the lymphatic system, and enter the bloodstream, causing massive septicemia.

- Once they have been released from the macrophages, there is no evidence that an immune response is initiated against vegetative bacilli.
- Anthrax bacilli express virulence factors, including toxin and capsule.
- The resulting toxemia has systemic effects that lead to the death of the host.
- The major virulence factors of *B. anthracis* are encoded on two virulence plasmids, pXO1 and pXO2.

- The toxin-bearing plasmid, pXO1, is 184.5 kilobasepairs (kbp) in size and codes for the genes that makeup the secreted exotoxins.
- The toxin-gene complex is composed of protective antigen, lethal factor, and edema factor. The three exotoxin components combine to form two binary toxins.
- Edema toxin consists of edema factor, which is a calmodulin-dependent adenylate cyclase and protective antigen, the binding moiety that permits entry of the toxin into the host cell. Increased cellular levels of cyclic-AMP upset water homeostasis and are believed to be responsible for the massive edema seen in cutaneous anthrax.

Flowchart 29.1: Pathogenicity of anthrax

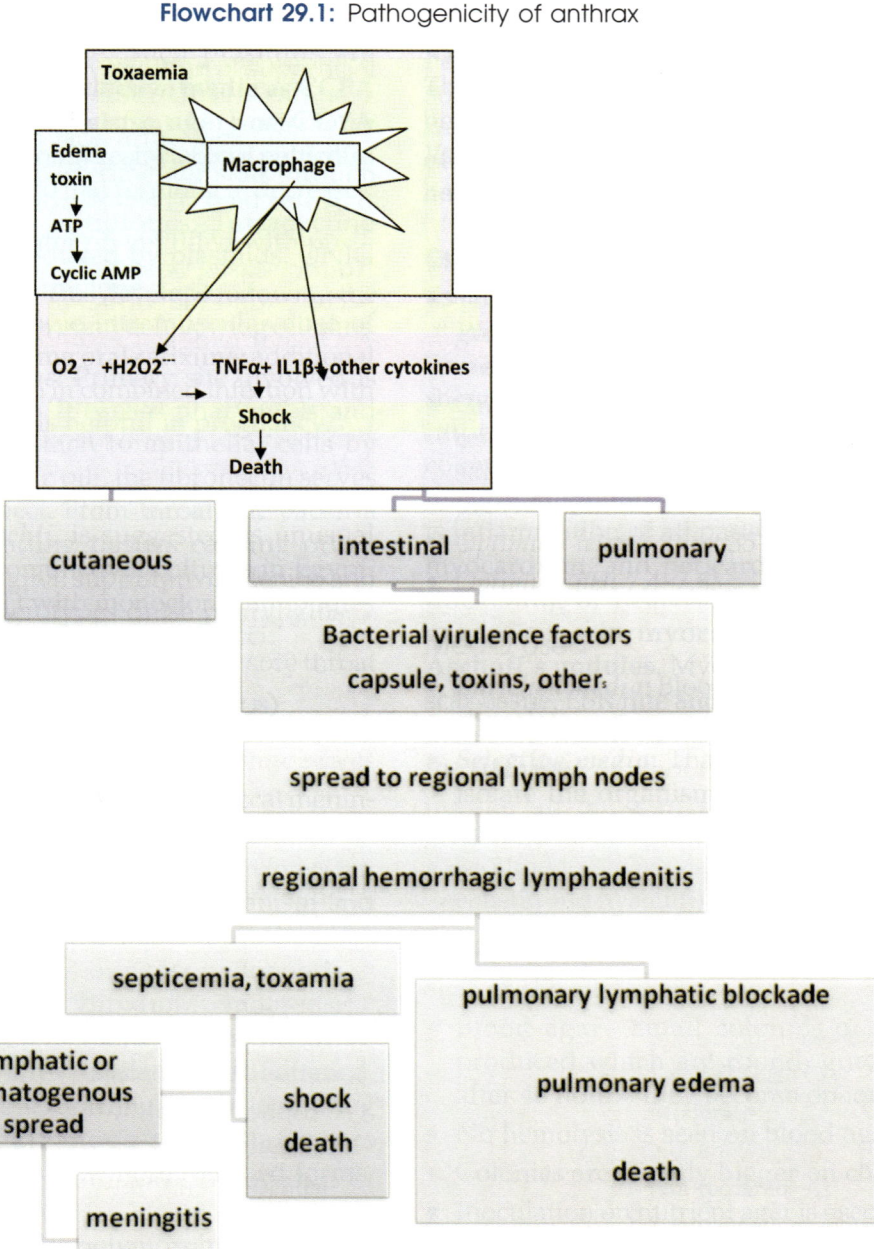

- Edema toxin inhibits neutrophil function in vitro, and neutrophil function is impaired in patients with cutaneous anthrax infection.
- Lethal toxin consists of lethal factor, which is a zinc metalloprotease that inactivates mitogen-activated protein kinase *in vitro*, and protective antigen, which acts as the binding domain.

Lethal toxin stimulates the macrophages to release tumor necrosis factor and interleukin-1 which are partly responsible for sudden death in systemic anthrax.

1. Cutaneous Anthrax (Fig. 29.7)

- Cutaneous anthrax accounts for 95% of all anthrax infections.
- The name **anthrax (from the Greek for coal)** refers to the typical black eschar that is seen on affected areas.
- Patients often have a history of occupational contact with animals or animal products. The most common areas of exposure are the head, neck, and extremities, although any area can be involved.
- Pathogenic endospores are introduced subcutaneously through a cut or abrasion. There are a few case reports of transmission by insect bites; presumably after the insect fed on an infected carcass.
- The primary skin lesion is usually a nondescript, painless, pruritic papule that appears three to five days after the introduction of endospores. In 24 to 36 hours, the lesion forms a vesicle that undergoes central necrosis and drying, leaving a characteristic **black eschar** surrounded by edema and a number of purplish vesicles.
- The edema is usually more extensive on the head or neck than on the trunk or extremities.
- The common description **"malignant pustule"** is actually a misnomer, because the cutaneous lesion is not purulent and is characteristically painless.
- A painful, pustular eschar in a febrile patient indicates a secondary infection, most often with Staphylococcus or Streptococcus.

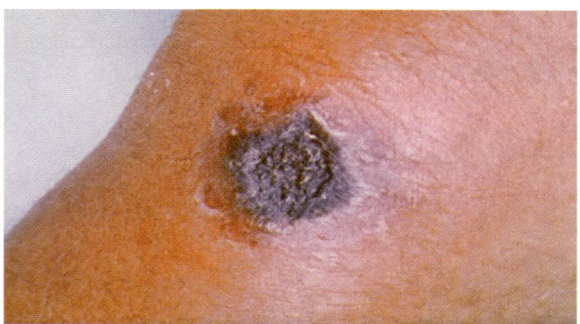

Fig. 29.7: Cutaneous anthrax

- Although cutaneous anthrax can be self-limiting, antibiotic treatment is recommended. Lesions resolve without complications or scarring in 80 to 90% of cases.
- **Malignant edema** is a rare complication characterized by severe edema, induration, multiple bullae, and symptoms of shock. Malignant edema involving the neck and thoracic region often leads to breathing difficulties that require corticosteroid therapy or intubation.
- Histologic examination of anthrax skin lesions shows necrosis and massive edema with lymphocytic infiltrates. There is no liquefaction or abscess formation, indicating that the lesions are not suppurative. Focal points of hemorrhage are evident, with some thrombosis. Gram's staining reveals bacilli in the subcutaneous tissue.

2. Gastrointestinal Anthrax

It can be fatal. The symptoms appear two to five days after the ingestion of endospore-contaminated meat from diseased animals. Therefore, multiple cases can occur within individual households.

- On pathological examination, bacilli can be seen microscopically in the mucosal and submucosal lymphatic tissue, and there is gross evidence of mesenteric lymphadenitis.
- Ulceration always seen. It is not known whether ulceration occurs only at sites of bacterial infection or is distributed more diffusely as a result of the action of anthrax toxin.
- Microscopic examination of affected tissues reveals massive edema and mucosal necrosis at infected sites.
- Associated symptoms include fever and diffuse abdominal pain with rebound tenderness. There are reports of both constipation and diarrhea; the stools are either melenic or blood-tinged. Because of ulceration of the gastrointestinal mucosa, patients often vomit material that is blood-tinged.
- Ascites develops with concomitant reduction in abdominal pain two to four days after the onset of symptoms. Morbidity is due to blood loss, fluid and electrolyte imbalance, and subsequent shock. Death results from intestinal perforation or anthrax toxemia.
- Oropharyngeal anthrax is less common than the gastrointestinal form. It is also associated with the ingestion of contaminated meat. Initial symptoms include cervical edema and local lymphadenopathy, which cause dysphagia and respiratory difficulties.

3. Pulmonary Anthrax

Inhalation anthrax

- The incubation period may be as long as 6 weeks.
- There is **mediastinal hemorrhagic necrosis and edema.** Substernal pain is important feature and there is pronounced mediastinal widening evident on chest radiograph.
- **Hemorrhagic pleural effusion** may occur.
- **Sepsis** occurs with spread to gastrointestinal tract leading to **bowel ulceration** or to **meninges** leading to **meningitis.**

4. Meningitis

It may complicate any type of anthrax when bacteremia spreads to CNS. The pathologic sign of meningitis is termed as cardinal's cap characterized by dark red extensive hemorrhaging beneath the lining of skull.

Heavy contamination of soil exists in enzootic foci. In an attempt to test anthrax spores as biological warfare bomb, heavy contamination of Gruinard island off the northwest cost of Scotland occurred in 1942–1943. Even by 1979, spores could be detected there. The area was decontaminated by 5% formaldehyde spread. By 1987, the area declared as anthrax-free.

Epidemiology of Anthrax

Anthrax is a zoonotic disease that primarily affects herbivores such as cattle, sheep, goats and deer, which become infected by ingesting contaminated vegetation, water, or soil; humans are generally incidental hosts.

Anthrax is most common in agricultural regions in Central and South America, sub-Saharan Africa, Central and Southwestern Asia, and Southern and Eastern Europe. Anthrax is now rare in the United States and Canada; however, sporadic outbreaks occur every year in livestock and wild herbivores in these countries. The most commonly reported form (95–99%) of anthrax in humans worldwide is cutaneous anthrax.

Outbreaks of cutaneous and gastrointestinal anthrax have been associated with handling infected animals, and butchering and consuming meat from those animals. Such outbreaks are primarily reported from endemic areas in Asia and Africa. Travelers to endemic areas have acquired cutaneous anthrax through either direct or indirect contact with carcasses of animals that died from anthrax. Cases of cutaneous, gastrointestinal, and inhalation anthrax have been reported among people who have handled or played drums made with contaminated goat hides **(Hide porter's disease)** from countries endemic for anthrax or who have been present at events where those drums have been played.

Inhalation of spores present in wool may also initiate disease (wool sorter's disease).

Severe soft tissue infections, including cases with sepsis and systemic infection, have been reported in drug users in northern Europe and are suspected to be due to use of heroin contaminated with *B. anthracis spores*. No associated cases have been identified in people who had not deliberately taken heroin.

Spores may be used in biological war fare.

The bioterrorism events in USA after fall of 2001 resulted in 22 cases of anthrax, five cases of inhalation anthrax died.

Prophylaxis

It involves improvement of factory hygiene, proper disposal of infected carcasses and vaccination. Vaccine was first demonstrated by Pasteur which consisted of attenuated bacilli. Spore vaccines have been developed (**Sterne**, Carbazoo, Mazucchi)—used in animals. In humans, alum precipitated toxoid—used in occupationally exposed persons.

Vaccine: AVA Biothrax is made from supernatant of cell free culture of nocapsulated but toxigenic strain of *B. antharcis*. There is need for better vaccines due to possible use for biological warfare.

Laboratory Diagnosis of Anthrax

Caution: Processing should be done in biosafety cabinet.

Samples collected: Swabs, pus or fluids (cutaneous), blood (septicemia), sputum (pulmonary) are the samples required.

Microscopy

- These are **Gram-positive bacilli**, **capsulated**, long chains of bacilli with swollen ends with bamboo **stick appearance.**
- **Demonstration of capsule is done by India ink.**
- **Direct immunofluorescence is used for direct detection in sample.**
- *M'Fadyean's reaction*: Blood films containing anthrax bacilli are stained with polychrome methylene blue for a few minutes. Amorphus material is deposited around bacilli which is capsular material.

Culture

- On agar plates, opaque, grayish-white colonies with frosted glass appearance are produced.
- String of pearl's reaction seen on blood agar with penicillin.

Animal inoculation: Sample is inoculated intraperitoneally in white mice.

Tissue can be applied to shaven skin of guinea pig.

Serological test : CFT, gel diffusion, **ELISA** tests detect antibodies to PA.

Definite diagnosis requires:
1. Lysis by specific bacteriophage
2. Capsular detection by fluorescent method
3. Detection of genes by PCR

   PCR is highly sensitive and specific test.

CDC Guidelines for Diagnosis

- Presumptive; identification based on marphology and culture (any Gram-positive bacillus with morphology and cultural properites similar to anthrax bacilli).
- Confirmation is done by lysis by gamma phage and direct immunofluorescence. Further confirmation is done by PCR.

Diagnosis of Anthrax in Animals

Caution: Autopsy is not to be performed, as organisms may contaminate soil.

Specimens
- Ear of animal
- Swabs soaked in blood
- Blood smears

Diagnosis is done by demonstration of bacilli by MacFadyean reaction and culture.

If sample for culture is putrid, diagnosis can be done by demonstration of antigen in tissue by 'Ascolis thermoprecipitation test'.

Ascolis Thermoprecipitation Test

In a test tube, antiserum against anthrax bacillus is taken. Animal tissue is boiled and extract is poured in the test tube containing antiserum. The reaction is seen in the form of ring when antigen in tissue and antiserum react.

Treatment

The antibiotics used against anthrax are doxycycline, ciprofloxacin, penicillin, and streptomycin.

Anthrax immunoglobulins: Human monoclonal antibodies having affinity for 'PA' are produced.

Prevention

It includes general control measures as disposal of animal carcasses by deep burial or burning, decontamination of animal products and use of personal protective equipment. Two types of vaccines used.

  i. The original **Pasteur's vaccine** is of historical importance which was anthrax bacillus live-attenuated by growth at 42–43°C.
  ii. Live-attenuated non-capsulated spore vaccine **(Stern vaccine)** is used in animals.
  iii. The '**Mazzuchi vaccine'** contained spores of attenuated **Carbazoo strain.**

Alum precipated toxoid vaccine prepared from protective antigen is effective for human use.

Three doses are given intramuscularly at first day, 6 weeks and 6 months. Booster is given after one layers.

BACILLUS CEREUS

Bacillus cereus causes toxin type of food poisoning, when food is stored at warm temperature, spores germinate, bacilli are formed which form toxin. It causes two types of clinical presentations, i.e. **emetic type** and **diarrheal type** (Table 29.1 and Flowchart 29.2). Diarrhea type of poisoning has incubation of 8–16 hours and various types of food, as meat, vegetables, are responsible for food poisoning. The emetic type of food poisoning has short incubation period, it is associated with consumption of cooked fried rice from Chienese restaurants.

Diarrheal type is caused by serotypes 2, 6, 8, 9, 10 or 12 while rice associated food poisonings are caused by 1, 3, 5 serotypes.

Other infections caused by *B. cereus* are ocular disease (keratitis, panophthalmitis) following trauma which may cause blindness.

Endocarditis: Mengitis, osteomyelitis, pneumonia.

The bacillus is generaly motile, non-capsulated and not susceptible to gamma phage. On egg containing medium, the bacterium produces opacity due to production of lecithin. A special selective medium–mannitol–egg yolk–phenol red–polymyxin agar medium **(MYPA)** is used for isolation. Another medium (PEMBA) contains polymyxin B, egg yolk and mannitol.

Diagnosis is made by isolation of bacteria from stool samples of patients and food. Egg yolk agar to which mannitol, polymyxin B added (MYPA) is used for culture.

Treatment: It is sensitive to clindamycin, vancomycin, erythromycin and aminoglycoside. It is resistant to trimethckprim and penicillin by producing β lactamase.

TABLE 29.1: Different types of food poisioning caused by *B. cereus*

Diarrheal type	Emetic type
Clinical incubation period is 8–16 hours	1–5 hours
Meat, vegetables are responsible	Chienese fried rice is responsible
It is caused by serotypes 2, 6, 8, 9, 10 or 12	It is caused by serotypes 1, 3, 5
Organisms are not present in large numbers in fecal specimens of patients	Organisms are present in large number in cooked rice and fecal samples
It produces enterotoxin similar to heat-labile toxin of ETEC	Toxin resembles with that of Staphylococcus food poisioning

Flowchart 29.2: Various types food poisonings caused by *B. cereus*

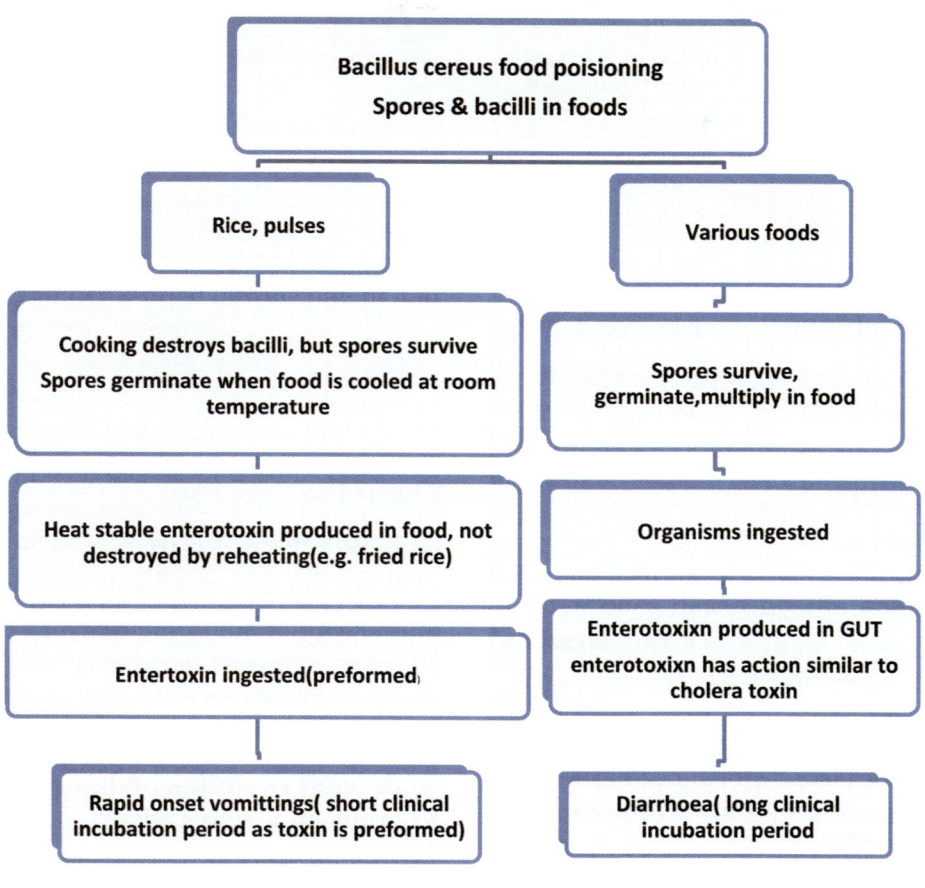

Direct toxin detection is done by immunofluorescence.

TABLE 29.2: Differences between anthrax and anthracoid bacilli

Property	Anthrax	Anthracoid bacilli
Capsule	Present	Absent
Motility	Non-motile	Motile
Length of chain	Long	Short
MacFadyean reaction	Positive	Negative
Growth on nutrient agar	Typical medusa head-like colony	No typical characteristic growth
Growth at 45°C	Doesn't grow	Grows
Growth on penicillin agar	Positive	Negative
Ascoli's thermoprecipitation test	Positive	Negative
Susceptibility to gamma phage	Susceptible	Non-susceptible
Pathogenicity to guinea pig	Pathogenic	Non-pathogenic
Gelatin liquefaction	Slow	Rapid
Salicin fermentation	Positive	Negative
Growth in liquid medium as broth	No turbidity	Turbidity is seen
Hemolysis	Absent or weak	Present

Sterilization test—bacilli
B. stearothermophilus—autoclave
B. globigi (red pigmented variant of *B. subtilis*)—ethylene oxide sterilizers
B. pumilis—ionizing radiations

B. cereus is important cause of endophthalmitis. It can also cause systemic infections as endocarditis, meningitis, osteomyelitis, pneumonia. Presence of medical device or intravenous drug abuse predisposes to these inections.

30

Clostridia

GENERAL FEATURES

- *Morphology*: Clostridia are Gram-positive bacilli, with bulging spore (Fig. 30.1), all are motile, except *C. perfringens* and *C. tetani* type VI.
- *Reservoirs of organism*: Many species are present in soil which cause exogenous infections.
- Some species form normal flora of intestine which may cause endogenous infections.
- *Anaerobic conditions*: Some are strict anaerobes as *C. novyi*, while some may be aerotolerant (*C. histolyticum*).
- *Sporulation*: Some sporulate profusely (*C. sporogenes*); some do inconsistently (*C. perfringens*).
- *Resistance of spores*: Spores of *Cl. tetani* mostly destroyed by boiling for 5 minutes except some strains form heat resistant spores. Spores of *Cl. perfringens* are killed by boiling for 5–10 minutes except strains of type 'A' survive for several hours. All spores are killed by autoclaving at 121°C for 10 minutes. Spores are resistant to phenolic disinfectants, halogens are effective sporidicidal; acqueous solution of iodine, 2% gluteraldehyde can kill the spores.

Major diseases: Gas gangrene, food poisoning and tetanus are diseases caused by them.

SPORES

- Spores bulge the bacillary body which, therefore, may be spindle-shaped, hence the name *Clostridium* (closter means spindle-shaped).
- Central or equatorial spore giving the bacillus a spindle shape (*Cl. bifermentans*).
- Sub terminal spore, the bacillus appearing club shaped (*Cl. perfringens*).
- Oval and terminal, resembling tennis racket (*Cl. tertium*).
- Spherical and terminal, giving a drumstick appearance (*Cl. tetani*).

Clostridial infections

A. The gas gangrene group	
1. Established pathogens	*Cl. perfringens*
	Cl. septicum
	Cl. novyi
2. Less pathogenic	*Cl. histolyticum*
	Cl. fallax
3. Doubtful pathogens	*Cl. bifermentans*
	Cl. sporogens
B. Tetanus	*Cl. tetani.*
C. Food poisoning	
Gastroenteritis	*Cl. perfringens* (Type A)
Necrotizing enteritis	*Cl. perfringens* (Type C)
Botulism	*Cl. botulinum*
Acute colitis	*Cl. difficile*

CLOSTRIDIUM PERFRINGENS (Cl. welchii)

It is normal flora of the large intestine of human being and animals. The spores are commonly found in soil, dust and air.

C. perfringens type 'A' occurs normally in number of 10^4/gm wet weight of feces in large intestine of man and animals. The classical *C. perfringens* of **gas gangrene belongs to type A1.**

Morphology

- It is plump, Gram-positive bacillus with straight, parallel sides and truncated ends showing "box car" appearance.
- *Size*: 4–6 μm × 1 μm, occurring singly or in chains.
- Capsulated and non-motile.
- It may be pleomorphic, filamentous and involution forms are common.

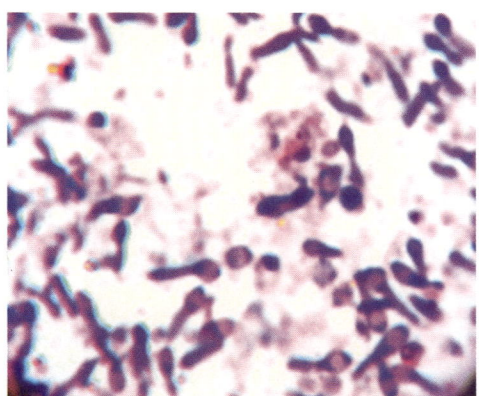

Fig. 30.1: Gram-positive bacilli with bulging subterminal spores

- Spores are central or subterminal, rarely seen in lesions. Primary smear from lesion doesn't show spores; this is a characteristic finding (Fig. 30.1).

Cultural Characteristics

- Anaerobe, but also grows under microaerophilic conditions.
- pH range 5.5–8.0. Temperature range 20°C–50°C, optimum is 37°C, 45°C is optimal for many strains.
- *Generation time*: 10 minutes
- As this organism grows fast in RCM as compared to other bacteria, inoculation into RCM and incubation for 4–6 hours at 45°C (before other organisms grow) makes enrichment for *C. perfringens*.
- *Growth in RCM*: Meat turns pink (**saccharolytic action**), but not digested, with acid reaction and a sour odor.
- *Litmus milk*: Litmus milk medium containing lactose is inoculated with the organism and incubated at 37°C for 18–24 hours. *C. perfringens* ferments lactose with production of acid and gas. The pH of the medium becomes acid, hence coagulation of casein occurs. The gas produced in the reaction causes disruption of clot, small fragments of which get attached to glass giving '**stormy fermentation**' (Fig. 30.2).
- *On blood agar 'target hemolysis' is seen*: There is a narrow zone of complete hemolysis due to theta toxin and a much wider zone of incomplete hemolysis due to the alpha toxin (double zone of hemolyis).
- *Egg yolk agar*: Opacity is produced surrounding the colonies due to lecithinase.

Nagler Reaction

The princle of the test is toxin neutralization test (Fig. 30.3).

The test is performed on media containing human serum or egg yolk.

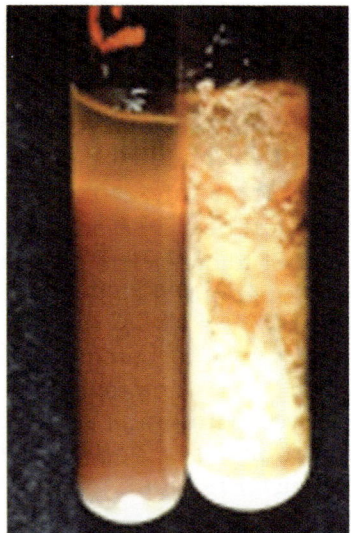

Fig. 30.2: Stormy fermentation

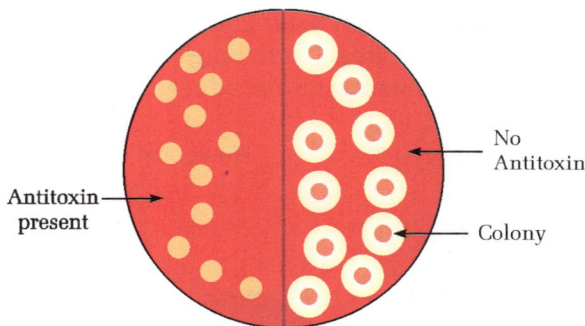

Fig. 30.3: Nagler's reaction

The zone of opacity around the colonies is due to production of the toxin which causes breakdown of lecithin into phosphorylcholine and diglyceride, with deposition of lipids. The action of the toxin is neutralized by specific antiserum. Hence, it inhibits opacity formation.

Procedure
- A plate of good quality digest agar containing egg yolk (5%) is taken.
- On one-half of plate, spread 2–3 drops of *C. perfringens* antitoxin (Prolab or Pragma) and allow to dry.
- Seed the test organism, stroking from the antitoxin free side to antitoxin bearing half and incubate anaerobically at 37°C.
- On section of plate not containing antitoxin *C. perfringens* colonies show a surrounding zone of opacity, whereas colonies on other half of plate show no opacity.
- Parallel stroke cultures of different strains or isolates can be tested on one plate. (Medium containing 5% Fildes peptic digest of sheep blood and 20% human serum can be used in place of egg yolk agar.) (Other lecithinase-forming bacteria—*Cl. novyi*, *Cl. bifermentans*.)

Biochemical Reactions

- Glucose, maltose, lactose and sucrose are fermented with the production of acid and gas.
- MR positive and VP negative. Indole negative, the bacterium produces abundant H_2S.
- Most strains reduce nitrates to nitrites.
- Reverse CAMP test positive (Fig. 30.4).
- Spore test or heat tolerance test: *Cl. perfringens* can tolerate high temperature (45°C) for 4–6 hours when cultured in RCM.

Resistance

Spores are destroyed within 5 minutes by boiling but, food poisoning strains of type A and certain type C strains resist boiling for 1–3 hours. Autoclaving at 121°C for 15 minutes kills bacteria.

Classification

They are classified into types 'A 'to 'E' (typing method– neutralization) based on the toxins produced by them. **Toxins:** 12 distinct toxins, enzymes and biologically active soluble substances are produced.

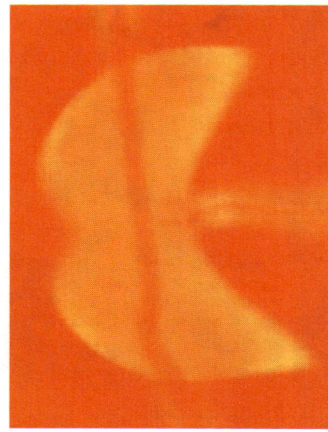

Fig. 30.4: Reverse CAMP test

Toxins and Virulence Factors

Four '**major toxins**', **alpha, beta, epsilon and iota**, are responsible for pathogenicity.

- *Alpha (α) toxin* (phospholipidase): It has lecithinase effect, it is produced by all types of *Cl. perfringens* (Abundantly by type 'A' strains) (Flowchart 30.1).

Flowchart 30.1: Role of α toxin (PLO—phospholipase)

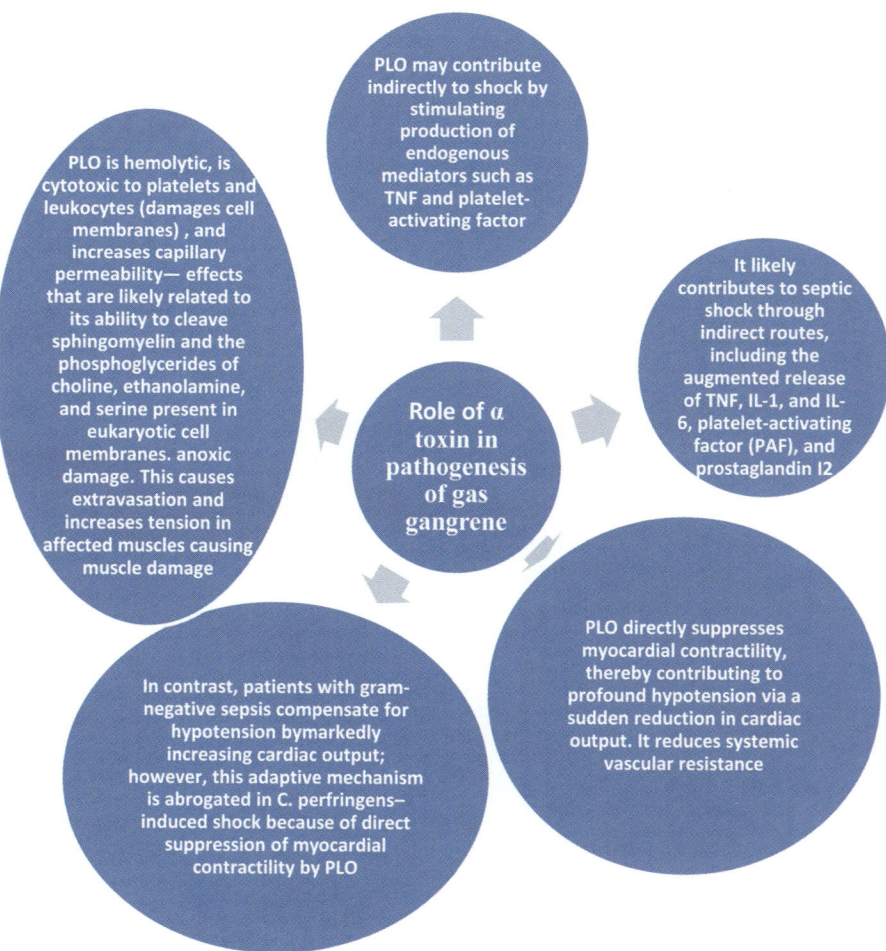

When *Cl. perfringens* is grown on medium, due to action of alpha toxin (lecithinase), opacity surrounding the colonies is produced.

- Beta, epsilon and iota are lethal and have necrotizing property.
- Gamma and eta have minor lethal action.
- Delta toxin is lethal and hemolytic.
- Theta toxin is oxygen labile, lethal and general cytolytic.
- Kappa toxin is collagenase.
- Lambda toxin is proteinase and gelatinase.
- mu toxin is a hyaluronidase.
- nu toxin is deoxyribonuclease.

Enzymes

- Enzymes destroying blood group substances neuraminidase.
- Hemagglutinin is active against human RBCs.
- *Bursting factor*: It acts on muscles and produce myonecrosis seen in gas gangrene.
- *Circulating factor*: It makes capillaries more active against adrenaline.

Pathogenicity (Flowchart 30.2, Table 30.1)

- *Gas gangrene*: **Type 'A' 1** is the predominant agent.
- *Food poisoning* **(Type 'A'2):** It is caused by cold or warmed up meat dish. Incubation period is 8–24 hours. Isolates from patients with food poisoning produce enterotoxin having mechanism of action like heat labile toxin of *E. coli*. Patient has abdominal pain, diarrhea and vomiting (Flowchart 30.3). It is a self-limited illness. Recovery takes place in 24–48 hours. Diagnosis is done by isolating heat resistant *Cl. perfringens* Type A from the feces and food.
- *Gangrenous appendicitis*: It is caused by *Cl. perfringens* type A (and occasionally Type D).
- *Necrotizing enteritis* **(enteritis necroticans or pigbel):** *Cl. perfrigens* **type 'C'** strains cause this condition. Pig meat along with trypsin inhibitors like sweet potatos are responsible for this condition.
- *Biliary tract infection (rare and serious)*: These are acute emphysematous cholecystitis, which may lead to septicemia.
- **Endogenous gas gangrene** of intra-abdominal origin (complication of abdominal surgery): The infection is endogenous as bacteria from own intestine cause it.

Flowchart 30.2: Pathogenesis of gas gangrene

Injury to arteries causes reduced blood supply to muscles causing necrosis

Extavasation of blood increase pressure on capillaries which reduces blood supply

Chemical changes, hypoxia causes energy deficit, lactic acid accumulation, fall in pH

Metabolic acidosis causes vasoconstriction, peripheral blood pooling ,cell membrane dysfunction,failure of Na pump, intracellular lysosomes release.

Histologically clostridial myonecrosis is remarkable for absence of acute inflammatory cells in the area and accumulation of cells within blood vessel

Flowchart 30.3: *Clostridium perfringens* food poisoning

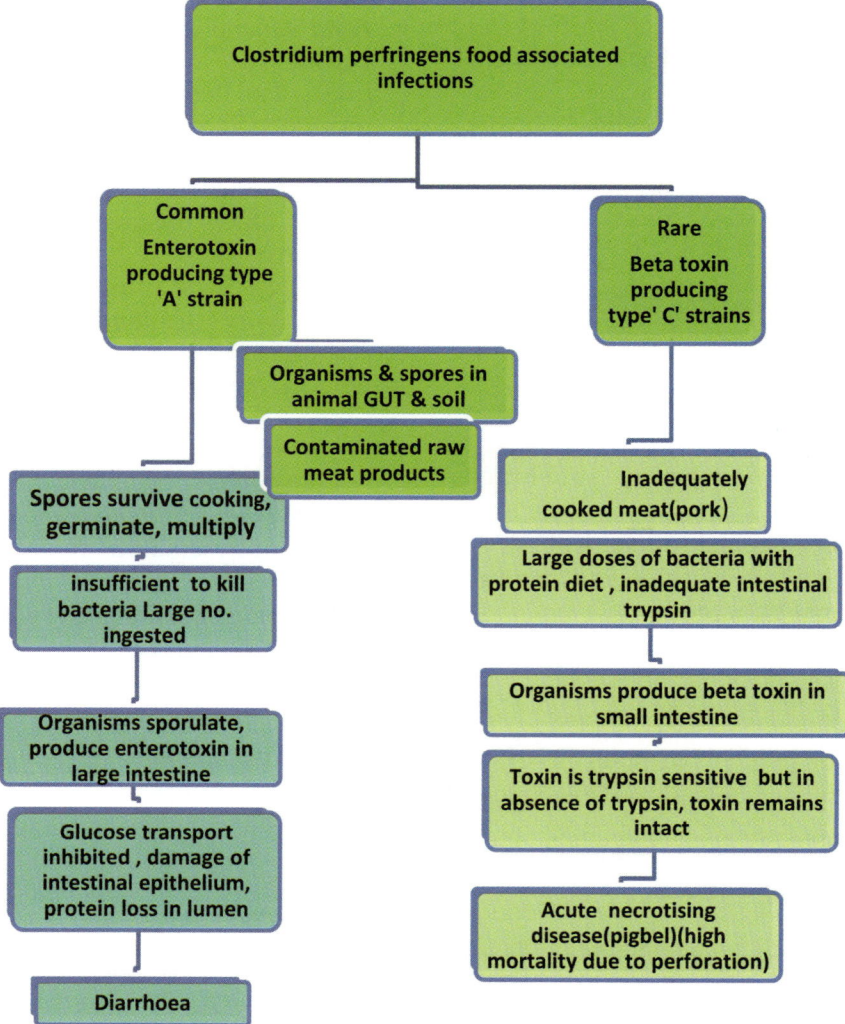

- **Brain abscess and meningitis.**
- **Panophthalmitis** may occur after eye injury.
- **Thoracic infections** follow penetrating wounds of thorax, battle casualties.

- **Urogenital infections** follow surgical procedure, such as nephrectomy.
- **Infection** of uterus is associated with septic abortion. Septicemia is common.

CLOSTRIDIUM NOVYI

It has 4 types A, B, C, and D which are differentiated on the basis of toxins they produce. Types A and occasionally B are associated with gas gangrene.

Morphology

- These are large Gram-positive rods of size 5–8 × 0.8–1μ.
- They have rounded ends.
- They are motile by peritrichous flagella.
- Spores are oval, central or subterminal.

Cultural Characteristics

Type 'A' is strict anaerobic. All types grow in RCM. Special media are required for surface growth. Colonies are

TABLE 30.1: Diseases associated with different serotypes

Type	Diseases association
A 1	Gas gangrene Puerperal infection Septicemia
A 2	Food poisoning
B	Lamb dysentery
C	Struck in sheep Enteritis in other animals Enteritis necroticans in man
D	Enterotoxemia of sheep Pulpy kidney disease
E	Doubtful pathogen of sheep and cattle

raised, opaque, sometimes dome-shaped and circular in young cultures. It may produce hemolysis. On egg yolk media, epsilon, theta toxins produce zone of opacity.

Biochemical Tests

Type 'A' is saccharolytic and mildly proteolytic, ferments maltose and inositol. Changes produced in litmus milk medium are slight. H_2S positive, nitrates are reduced to nitrites. Type 'A' strains are Indole negative. Gelatin liquifaction is positive.

Animal Pathogenicity

An intramuscular injection of 0.2 mL of culture of type A into thighs of guinea pigs may cause massive gas gangrene with minimum gas production.

CLOSTRIDIUM SEPTICUM

It occurs in soil as well as intestine of humans and animals.

Morphology

- It is a large Gram-positive bacillus with rounded ends.
- It is of size 3–20 × 0.6–1 μ.
- It may be pleomorphic, short forms which are swollen (**'citron bodies'**) and large filament form may occur.
- It is actively motile with peritrichous flagella.
- Spores are readily formed, oval, central or subterminal.

Cultural Characteristics

- It is obligatory anaerobe. Grows on ordinary media.
- BA: It produces transparent colonies with irregular edge. After further incubation, colonies become opaque. A narrow zone of hemolysis may be present.

Biochemical Reactions

It ferments glucose, maltose, and lactose, while sucrose and mannitol are not fermented. Slight acid production in litmus medium may produce clotting. It is indole negative, produces H_2S, nitrates are reduced to nitrites. It does not produce phospholipase or lipase.

An intamuscular injection in guinea pig produces gas gangrene.

CLOSTRIDIUM HISTOLYTICUM

It is long slender Gram-positive rod, it is aerotolerent, proteolytic in RCM. In meat medium, it causes digestion of meat particles. It may be associated with gas gangrene.

Gas Gangrene (Clostridial Myonecrosis)

Muscle necrosis following severe wounds which favor entry of spores in wounds leading to toxemia is called as gas gangrene. There is edematous swelling (due to gases formed by bacteria). The infection spreads so rapidly that amputation may be required. Wound infections and cellulitis are not considered, as gas gangrene. It is only when muscles are involved and patients show signs and symptoms of toxemia, the term gas gangrene is used.

1. Established pathogens	*Cl. perfringens*
	Cl. septicum
	Cl. novyi
2. Less pathogenic	*Cl. histolyticum*
	Cl. fallax
3. Doubtful pathogens	*Cl. bifermentans*
	Cl. sporogens

Organisms causing gas gangrene: *C. perfringens* (60%), *C. novyi* (20–40%), *C. septicum* (20–40%) and *C. histolyticum.*

Pathogenicity

Predisposing factors: Gas gangrene generally follows road accidents or injury involving crushing of large muscle masses, rarely, it follows surgical operations.

Modes of Infection

Exogenous: Clostridia enter the wounds with impure foreign particles such as soil, road dust, and bit of clothing or shrapnel.

Endogenous: These organisms may be present in the perineum and contaminate the wound causing endogenous gas gangrene.

Three types of anaerobic wound infections are:
1. **Simple wound contamination** with no invasions of the tissue, it causes delay in wound healing.
2. *Anaerobic cellulitis*: Invasion of fascial planes with minimal toxin production and no invasion of muscle tissues.
3. *Anaerobic myositis or gas gangrene*: Clostridial infection of muscle tissues takes place and there is abundant formation of exotoxins, which cause systemic illness, and toxemia.

Myonecrosis and toxemia are characteristics of gas gangrene. Simple wound infection and cellulitis are not considered as gas gangrene.

Mechanisms of developing low redox potential in the tissues favoring gas gangrene formation
- *Low oxygen tension*: Ionized calcium salts and silicic acid in the soil cause necrosis.
- *Anoxia of the muscle*: It is due to crushing tissue or tearing of the arteries.

- *Reduction of blood supply*: Extravasations of blood increases pressure on the capillaries, reducing blood supply.
- **Fall in pH and oxidation reduction potential.**
- Breakdown of carbohydrates and liberation of amino acids from proteins occur favoring anaerobic growth.
- Reduction of:
  1. Hemoglobin and myohemoglobin
  2. Pyruvate to lactate
- Reduction of capacity of hemoglobin and myohemoglobin to carry oxygen
- Aerobic oxidation stops.

The clostridia are locally invasive but produce powerful exotoxins.

Role of toxins

- Alpha toxin damages cell membrane, causes increased capillary permeability, leads to increased muscle tensions causing anoxia.
- Kappa toxin is a collagenase, breaks down collagen.
- Lambda toxin is proteinase.
- Mu toxin is hyaluronidase.
- Nu toxin is deoxyribonuclease.

These toxins dissolve the tissues making conditions more favorable for invasion by organisms.

Incubation period: It is 7 hours to six weeks after wounding, average 10–48 hours with *Cl. perfringens*, 2–3 days with *Cl. septicum* and 5–6 days with *Cl. novyi*.

Clinical features: Pain, tenderness and edema of the affected part with systemic signs of toxemia are present. There is thin watery discharge, which later becomes profuse and serosanguinous. Accumulation of gas (crepitus) occurs. Profound toxemia and prostration develop and death occurs due to circulatory failure.

Laboratory Diagnosis

Specimens to be collected

1. **Swabs** from the muscles at the edge of the affected area and exudates collected from the active part of lesions.
2. **Necrotic tissue and muscle fragments**: These are also preferably collected in a set of sterile container and other pieces in Robertson's cooked meat medium.

Specimens collected in sterile container are more suitable for staining as other pieces in RCM get diluted, hence smears from these specimens will not give the exact idea of number of pus cells present. This finding is important in differential diagnosis of gas gangrene from anaerobic streptococcal myostitis.

Gram Stain

Importance of Gram staining

- In case of **gas gangrene,** the findings will be **scanty or absence of pus cells and polymicrobial flora** as apart from Clostridia, other facultative bacteria also enter in the tissue causing infection.
- A clinical condition which simulates with gas gangrene is **anaerobic streptococcal myositis**. In this condition, the Gram-stained smear will show many pus cells along with predominantly Gram-positive cocci and not the polymicrobial flora.

The **modes of treatment** for these two conditions are different.

- In gas gangrene, immediately antigas gangrene serum is given and amputation may be required to save patient.
- Anaerobic streptococcal myositis responds well to antibiotics.

As the treatment as well as **prognosis** is different, immediately provisional report can be given based upon the findings of Gram staining.

Clostridium perfringens appears as **Gram-positive, plump bacilli with truncated end giving 'box car' apperance.** Usually it does not show spores in the smears prepared from samples. If spores are present, they are bulging subterminal or central.

Clostridium novyi has central or subterminal bulging spore while *C. septicum* shows short bacilli with swollen spore giving appearance called '**citron bodies**'.

Direct immunofluorescence test helps in early detection of *C. perfringens*.

Aerobic and Anaerobic Culture

- **Blood cultures** are often positive in *Cl. perfringens* and *Cl. septicum* infections.
- **Blood agar** is incubated anaerobically in McIntosh Jar or in gas pack system—look for '**target hemolysis.**
- **Neomycin blood** agar is used as a selective medium.
- Pheny ethyl alcohol blood agar will support the growth of other anaerobes.
- **RCM**—look for **saccharolytic** effect (pinkish RCM).
- **Egg yolk agar** is also used to demonstrate Lecithinase effect (Fig. 30.5), i.e. opacity surrounding the colonies of *C. perfringens*.

The isolates are identified based on their morphological, cultural, biochemical and toxigenic characters.

Biochemical Tests

- **Litmus milk agar** shows **stormy fermentation**.
- Glucose, maltose, lactose and sucrose are fermented with the production of acid and gas.
- It gives MR positive and VP negative,

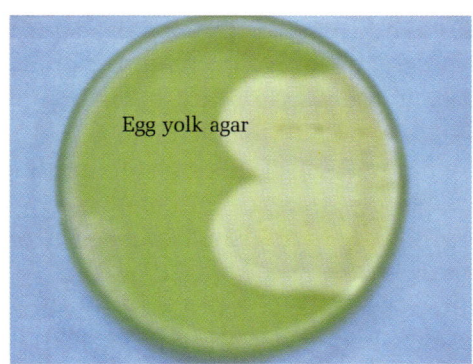

Fig. 30.5: Lecithinase effect

- Indole negative, produces abundant H_2S.
- Most strains reduce nitrates to nitrites.

Gas liquid chromatography is used in special laboratories which analyse the unsaturated fatty acids produced by different species.

Prophylaxis and Therapy

- Surgery
- Hyperbaric oxygen
  - *Prophylaxis*: Antibiotics are used in combination with surgical methods.
    Antibiotics: Clindamycin is used, if patients are allergic to it, chloramphenicol, doxycycline, metronidazole, imipenem are used.
  - Passive immunization with anti gas gangrene serum (10,000 IU *Cl. perfringens,* 10,000 IU *Cl. novyi* and 5,000 IU *Cl. septicum* antitoxin given IM or in emergencies IV).

CLOSTRIDIUM TETANI

It is causative organism of tetanus.

Morphology

Gram-positive, slender bacillus, 4–8 μm × 0.5 μm in size.

Spores: Spherical, terminal, and bulging giving **drumstick appearance** (Fig. 30.6).

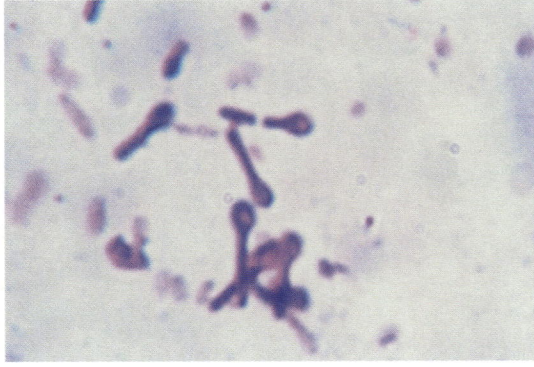

Fig. 30.6: Drumstick apperance (*Cl. tetani*)

Cultural Characteristics

- It is obligatory anaerobe.
- It grows at 37°C and pH 7.4.
- It has tendency to swarm on surface of agar.

Fildes technique: Swarming helps to isolate *Cl. tetani* from other bacteria. If agar slant is taken, the water condensed at the bottom of medium is inoculated. (mixture) *Cl. tetani* only swarms, reaches top of slant from where it can be isolated. Other bacteria in that mixture will not reach top of slant.

- *RCM*: Meat is not digested but turns black on prolonged incubation (proteolytic action)
- Blood agar shows α hemolysis initially and later β due to production of tetanolysin.

Biochemicals

- Slight proteolytic property (meat particles in RCM turn black), no saccharolytic property.
- Sugars not fermented.
- Indole positive, MR and VP are negative.
- H_2S is not formed.
- Gelatin liquefaction occurs slowly from top that gives 'fir tree' appearance.
- Nitrates not reduced.
- Serotyping is done by agglutination test. Only type VI is nonflagellated, non-motile. All serotypes produce same toxin.

Toxins (Flowchart 30.4)

- **Tetanolysin** is heat-labile, oxygen-labile hemolysin, active against RBCs of many animal species. Its pathogenic role is unknown. Hemolysis seen on blood agar is due to action of this toxin.
- **Tetanospasmin** is oxygen stable, relatively heat labile, plasmid coded toxin and responsible for clinical manifestations of tetanus. It is protein in nature, antigenic and specially neutralized by antitoxin. It is toxoided and the Tetanus toxoid produced is used in vaccination, either as DPT or TT. All clinical features are due to action of tetanospasmin.
- **Neurotoxin:** Its role not known.

Pathogenicity

Spores implanted in wound germinate and multiply in favourable condition. Germination of spores and formation of vegetative bacteria are favored by—(1) necrotic tissue, (2) Ca salts, (3) associated pyogenic infections.

- Toxin produced locally is absorbed by motor nerve endings and transported to CNS along the axis cylinders of peripheral nerves

Flowchart 30.4: Mechanisms of action of tetanus toxin

```
┌─────────────────────────────────────┐
│          Tetanospamin                │
│       A-B two chain toxin            │
└─────────────────────────────────────┘
              ↓
┌─────────────────────────────────────┐
│ Complete toxin attaches to peripheral│
│ nerve endings in the region of wound │
└─────────────────────────────────────┘
              ↓
┌─────────────────────────────────────┐
│ Toxin transmitted to cranial nerve   │
│ nuclei either through intraspinal    │
│ transmission or  among involved motor│
│ neurons  or blood stream delivery to │
│ other neuromuscular junctions        │
└─────────────────────────────────────┘
              ↓
┌─────────────────────────────────────┐
│ Toxin inhibits neurotransmitter      │
│ release  & normal inhibitary input   │
│ causing lower motor neuron  to       │
│ increase resting muscle tone         │
│ producing reflex spasms              │
└─────────────────────────────────────┘
              ↓
┌─────────────────────────────────────┐
│ Several types of neurotransmittors   │
│ are blocked , including GABA         │
└─────────────────────────────────────┘
```

- Toxin is specifically and strongly fixed by ganglio-sides of gray matter of the nervous tissue
- Actions of toxin
  - Toxin **acts presynaptically (blocks release of GABA and glycine), blocks synaptic inhibition in the spinal cord**
  - Spinal inhibition is lost which causes uncontrolled spread of impulses generated in the nervous system.
  - Muscle rigidity and spasms of muscles develop.
  - Simultaneous contraction of agonists and anta-gonists occur in absence of reciprocal inhibition.

TETANUS

- It is an important complication of septic abortion. It may follow unsterile injections.
- Incubation period is 6–12 days.
- Experiment tetanus may be of following types:
  - *Local*: Spasm at the site of injection of toxin
  - *Ascending type*: From local site, it spreads to spinal cord.
  - *Descending type*: It is similar to natural tetanus.
- **Toxic muscle spasm** at the site of infection occurs followed by involvement of whole muscular system.
- Muscles of face and jaw are affected first as there is short distance for toxin to reach the presynaptic terminals. The first symptom to appear is **lock jaw or 'trismus '**due to increased masseter tone.

- 'Rises' sardonicus' is abnormal spasm of facial muscles that appears to produce grinning.
- Lock jaw is followed by muscular pain, stiffness, backache and default in swallowing.
- Initially painful muscle spasms are **localized** to the affected limb.
- **Generalized spasms** cause **descending spastic paralyses**.
- 'Opisthotonus' (abnormal body position) occurs when whole body is involved (Fig. 30.7).
- Deep tendon reflexes are exaggerated.
- Hands, feet are spared also there is no mental retardation.
- Change of blood pressure (low or high), tachycardia, sweating, increased tracheal secretions and renal failure may occur due to affection of autonomous system.
- Respiratory muscle spasm may cause airway obstruction.

Other forms of tetanus are **'tetanus neonatorum'**, **septic abortion** and **otogenic tetanus.**

Epidemiology

Tetanus bacilli may colonize human intestine. They may also found in animal feces and soil which cause most of the infections. Hence wound contaminated with soil needs attention. Tetanus spores are found in gardens, sport fields, roads, plaster on articles and hospital duct. Spores may contaminate surgical catgut and dressings. People in underdeveloped countries are more suscep-tible for infections due to poor hygiene, lack of shoes, neglect of wounds and inadequate immunization.

Some local customs which predisopose to tetanus are:
- Treatment of umbilical stump with primitive applica-tions that include animal dung.
- Tying of umbilical cords with primitive ligatures.
- Ear-piercing and other operations performed with unsterile instruments.

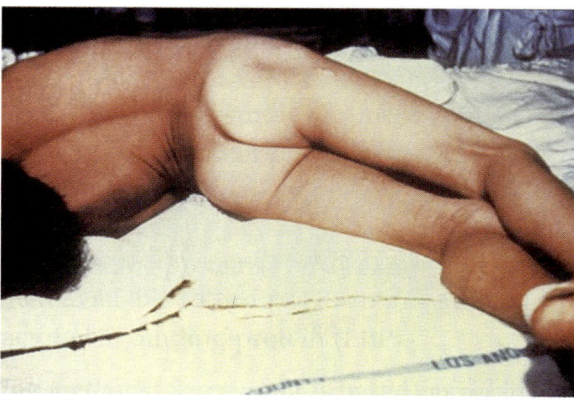

Fig . 30.7: Opisthotonus

Laboratory Diagnosis

Tetanus is usually a clinical diagnosis, the role of laboratory is to confirm diagnosis.

- *Specimen*: Excised bits of tissue from the depths of wounds and exudate from wound are collected.
- *Transport media*: Stuart's transport medium, or thioglycolate broth, or RCM is used.
- **Microscopy** is unreliable and demonstration of drumstick bacilli is not diagnostic of tetanus.
- Diagnosis by culture which is most reliable but not sufficient as demonstration of toxin by the isolated organism is important. This is done by toxigenicity testing.
- *RCM*: It shows slight proteolytic activity and becomes turbid.
- **Blood agar** shows beta-hemolysis and it also shows swarming.
- **Agar stab culture** shows 'fir tree' appearance.

Toxigenicity Testing

- **Test for demonstration of tetanolysin on horse blood agar.** It is similar to Nagler's reaction: Instead of opacity, hemolysis is observed.

   Antitoxin is spread on half plate of 4% horse blood agar. The organism inoculated on both sides. The plate is incubated for 48 hours. There will be **no hemolysis around the colonies** on the half of plate with antitoxin because the toxin produced by the organism will be neutralized by antitoxin. This method is used to demonstrate the activity of **tetanolysin.** But as the pathogenicity is because of tetanospasmin, this test is not much helpful.

- *In vitro* **test of toxingenicity of tetanospasmin:** Two healthy mice are inoculated with 0.2 mL broth solution into root of tail; one of them is protected with 1000 U of antitoxin, which acts as control animal. The test animal develops stiffness of tail, rigidity of leg of the side of inoculation, followed by oppositive side legs, trunk and forelimbs. This action is due to the production of tetanospasmin, hence the test is reliable.

Prophylaxis and Treatment (Table 30.2)

- Protect from noise and light.

- Maintain airway by tracheostomy with intermittent positive pressure respiration.
- TIG (tetanus immunoglobulin): 10,000 IU suitably diluted and given by slow IV infusion followed, if needed by 5000 IU later.
- Penicillin or metronidazole is given for one week.

Passive Immunization

Anti-tetanus serum (ATS): 1500 IU—SC/IM.

Disadvantages
1. Half-life is only 7 days.
2. Hypersensitivity may occur.
3. Immune elimination is common.

   It is given after trial dose—0.5 mL subcutaneously, syringe loaded with adrenaline (1/1000) must be kept ready.

Human anti-tetanus immunoglobulin (TIG): It is effective in smaller doses (250 units), longer half-life (3–5 weeks).

Disadvantage is nonavailability.

Active Immunization

It is the effective way by which tetanus following unnoticed injuries can be prevented.

   The control can be achieved by injections of **formol toxoid—plain toxoid or adsorbed** on aluminum hydroxide or phosphate.

   Triple vaccine along with diphtheria toxoid and killed Pertussis bacillus is in the form of DPT.

Toxoids: Three doses are given at the interval of 4–6 weeks between 1st and 2nd doses and 6 months between 2nd and 3rd doses. Immunity lasts for 10 years. Boosters given after 10 years.

   Course of immunization is as per National Immunization Programme. Booster dose given if wounding occurs 3 years or more after full course of immunization.

Combined Immunization

It is done by administering TIG to non-immune individual at one site along with first dose of toxoid at the contralateral site, followed by second and third doses at monthly intervals.

TABLE 30.2: Management of different types of wounds			
Wound type	Immune	Partially immune	Non-immune
Clean	1 dose of toxoid	1 dose of toxoid	3 doses of toxoid
Contaminated	1 dose of toxoid	1 dose of toxoid + TIG + antibiotics	3 doses of toxoid + TIG + antibiotics
Infected	1 dose toxoid + antibiotics	1 dose of toxoid + TIG + antibiotics	3 doses of toxoids + TIG + antibiotics

CLOSTRIDIUM BOTULINUM

Cl. botulinum causes botulism. The name botulism is derived from sausage. It causes severe form of food poisoning.

Morphology

- It is a Gram-positive bacillus, 5 μm × 1 μm in size.
- It is non-capsulated, motile by peritrichate flagella.
- Spores are subterminal, oval, bulging.

Cultural Characteristics

It is a strict anaerobe. The optimum temperature is 35°C (+ or – 1–5°C).

It grows on common media and colonies are large, irregular, translucent. In a medium containing alkaline glucose gelatin at 20–25°C, spores are definitely produced.

Classification

There are 8 types (A, B, C1, C2, D, E, F, G) based on the type of toxin produced.

The bacillus produces powerful exotoxin. The special characteristics of toxin are:

1. It is not released during the life of bacillus.
2. It is produced intracellularly.
3. It appears in the medium only after the death of cell and autolysis of bacterial cell. Gene for toxin production is present on bacteriophage.

It is most toxic substance known. Lethal dose for human beings is 1–2 μg and for mice is 0.0000000033 mg. The toxin is heat-labile but spores are heat resistant.

Action of toxin: It blocks the release of acetylcholine at synapses at neuromuscular junctions. It acts presynaptically. Toxins of all types are neurotoxic except C2 which is a cytotoxin (enterotoxin).

> Its action is at presynaptic neuromuscular junction terminals to break protein complex (snap) binding site of acetylcholine containing vesicles, thereby preventing acetylcholine release. It blocks the autonomic postganglionic terminals from releasing acetylcholine. It is available in lyophilized form in vials for use. It is used for treating the **wrinkles, spasticity, blepharoplasm, myoclonus, strabismus.**

Pathogenicity

All the clinical features are due to toxin production as bacteria are non-invasive and without toxin they are non-infectious.

Food Poisoning (Food-Borne Botulism)

Type of culprit food: Preserved foods like meat and meat products, fish, canned vegetables are responsible for food poisoning.

Type of poisoning: It causes **toxic type of food poisoning** as preformed toxin in the food is consumed. Human infections are due to types **A, B, E** and rarely F. (G has caused death in few patients).

Incubation period is 12–36 hours.

Clinical features: 3D—diplopia, dysarthria, and dysphagia.

They include vomiting, ocular paralysis, difficulty in swallowing, speaking, breathing followed by coma, the death is due to circulatory failure. Symmetric descending paralysis is seen. There is no sensory involvement. In early disease, deep reflexes are intact. Blurring of vision, non-reactive pupils suggest botulism.

Wound botulism: A rare condition resulting from wound infection, mostly all cases are due to **type A** (other types are B and E).

Infant botulism: It is seen in infants below 6 months, **honey** has been incriminated as culprit food. It is toxico-infection, spores are ingested, they germinate, establish and produce toxin.

Iatrogenic botulism develops from injection of botulism toxin.

Clinical features are lethargy, altered cry, loss of head control (floppy neck), poor feeding, weakened voice, ptosis and neackness **(floppy child syndrome).**

Laboratory Diagnosis

- Isolation of organism from contaminated food and stool sample.
- Demonstrate toxin in food and feces.

Control measures include use of home canning food. Active immunization consists of two doses of toxoids (given to laboratory persons). Polyvalent antiserum (against types A, B, E) is given immediately to save the life.

CLOSTRIDIUM DIFFICILE

It is a Gram-positive anaerobic bacillus. It is found as normal flora—ultimate opportunistic pathogen.

It was difficult to determine cause as the organism is ubiquitous. It was also difficult to culture it (hence the name difficile).

This bacterium causes **antibiotic associated colitis or pseudomembranous colitis.**

Many antibiotics cause this condition. These are clindamycin, lincomycin, tetracycline, chloramphenicol, and ampicillin. These antibiotics kill the drugs sensitive flora and allow multiplication of *C. difficile*. The condition is due to active multiplication of *Cl. difficile* and its production of an enterotoxin and a cytotoxin. Enterotoxin causes diarrhea while cytotoxin causes damage to gut mucosa causing acute colitis with or without membrane formation.

Predisposing factors are old age, gastrointestinal surgery, central tube feeding, antacid use, use of proton pump inhibitors, cancer patient.

Diagnosis

- *Stool culture*: It is done on **selective media as CCFA** (cefoxitin, cycloserine fructose agar) or **CCYA** (cefoxitin cycloserine egg yolk agar). Stool culture is highly sensitive and specific. Only isolation is not sufficient as *C. difficile* can colonize GIT. Test for toxin demonstration is more useful.

- **Stool culture** is done on human diploid cell culture or **Hep2 cell** culture for demonstration of **cytopathic effects** of toxin. **Stool culture is the most sensitive test. Most specific tests are cell culture, cytotoxin tests on stool and pseudomembrane seen on colonoscopy or sigmoidoscopy**. The toxin is specially neutralized by *Cl. sordelli* antitoxin.

- *C. difficile* antigen detected by latex **agglutination test and ELISA.**

- **DNA probe** can also detect the toxin.

Treatment

The antibiotic which has caused this condition should be stopped. Metronidazole is the drug of choice. Vancomycin can also be used.

Nonsporing Anaerobes

Definition

Obligate anaerobic bacteria are those bacteria that grow in the absence of free O_2 but fail to multiply in the presence of O_2 on the surface of nutritionally adequate solid media. Degree of anaerobiasis required for growth vary with each anaerobe.

Habitat

They are widespread in soil, marshes, lake and rivers, sediments, sewage, food and animals. In humans, they are normal inhabitants of mouth and nasopharynx, GIT specially colon, small intestine, orifices of genitourinary tracts.

NORMAL ANAEROBIC FLORA OF HUMAN BODY

Gram-negative cocci: Mouth, nasopharynx, gut, vagina.

Gram-negative bacilli
1. *Bacteroides fragilis:* GUT
2. *Prevotella melaninogenica:* Mouth, nasopharynx, vagina, GUT
3. *Fusobacterium sp:* Mouth, GUT

Gram-positive bacilli
1. *Lactobacillus (Doderlein's bacilli):* GUT, vagina
2. *Actinomyces:* Mouth, oropharynx
3. *Propionibacterium:* Skin

These organisms usually set up an infection when resistance is low and in presence of damaged and necrotic tissue is their normal habitat.

Infections are polymicrobial: Aerobic infection may be associated.

Classification

Gram-positive Bacilli

- *Lactobacilli*
- *Bifidobacterium*
- *Eubacterium*
- *Propionibacterium*
- *Actinomyces*
- *Mobiluncus*

Gram-positive Cocci

- *Peptococcus*
- *Peptostreptococcus*

Gram-negative Bacilli

- *Bacteroides*
- *Fusobacterium*
- *Prevotella*
- *Porphyromonas*
- *Leptotrichia*

Gram-negative cocci: *Veillonella*

Introduction

Anaerobic bacteria are present at almost all sites of body as normal flora. They are present in very larger number as compared to aerobes. The number of anaerobes in human intestine varies from 10^4–10^5/gm of fecal matter in small intestine and 10^{11}/gm of fecal matter in large intestine. Saliva also contain 10^8/mL of anaerobes.

Anaerobic cocci: They are further divided into Gram-positive and Gram-negative cocci.

Peptostreptococcus: Gram-positive cocci are arranged in pairs or chains.

Tests used for the differentiation of peptococcal species are susceptibility to substance, SPS (sodium polyanethol sulfonate), kanamycin and sugar fermentation tests.

- They cause skin, soft tissue infections and brain abscess.

- The only species *P. niger*—the cocci are arranged singly, in pairs or in small clusters but not in chains.
- Form normal flora of mouth, intestine and vagina.
- It produces black colonies on blood agar. They produce H_2S.

Infections caused by them are mixed with other anaerobic cocci, *Clostridium perfringens* and facultative Gram-negative bacteria.
- Puerperal sepsis
- Gangrenous appendicitis
- Osteomyelitis
- Urinary tract infection
- Abscesses in the brain, lung.

Peptostreptococcus
- The cocci arranged in pairs and short chains.
- The infections are mixed which are accompanied with other bacteria.
- Form normal flora of skin, mouth, and intestine.
- Puerperal sepsis, skin and soft tissue infections, brain abscess.
- *Pst. anaerobius* is most pathogenic followed by
- *Pst. asaccharolyticus, Pst. magnus, Pst. tetradius. Ps. prevoti.*
- *Pst. anaerobius responsible for puerperal sepsis.*
- *Pst. magnus:* It causes brain abscess.

Gram-negative cocci
- **Veillonella** are Gram-negative cocci arranged in pairs, short chains and groups. It is a normal commensal of mouth, intestine and genital tract. They are usually nonpathogenic.
- Mostly anaerobic cocci are sensitive to penicillin, choramphenicol, and metronidazole and resistant to gentamicin and streptomycin.

Anaerobic Gram-Positive Bacilli

Medically important genera are *Eubacterium, Propionibacterium, Lactobacillus, Mobiluncus* and *Bifidobacterium.* (*Actinomyces* is discussed in different chapters).

Eubacterium

They form normal flora of mouth and intestine.

Rarely some species as *E. brachy, E. timidum, and E. nodatum* cause periodontitis.

E. lentum is recovered from non-oral specimens.

Propionibacterium

- They are anaerobic diphtheroids related to *Corynebacterium diphtheriae.*
- They are skin commensals.
- *P. acnes* is contaminant of specimens as blood, CSF.

Lactobacillus (Doderlein's Bacillus)

- Gram-positive bacilli which may show bipolar and barred staining characteristics.
- They are saprophytic organisms, ferment cheese, milk and produce lactic acid from sugars, grow best at pH <5.
- They synthesize vitamin B_{12}, and vitamin K.
- Their role in pathogenesis of dental carries is postulated. They ferment sucrose and other carbohydrates, produce acidic pH, damages enamel and dentin.
- Acidic pH of vagina is due to fermentation of glycogen by Lactobacillus which acts as innate mechanism of immunity by preventing entry of pathogens.
- Spores of lactobacilli are used as probiotics.

Mobiluncus

Gram-positive or variable, motile bacilli.

They are isolated (*M. mulieris, M. curtisii*) from vagina from cases of bacterial vaginosis.

Bifidobacterium

- Non-motile pleomorphic rods frequently show branching. Their ends appear bifurgited, hence name *Bifidobacterium.*
- They form normal flora of mouth, gut; mostly non-pathogenic.

Anaerobic Gram-Negative Bacilli

Bacteroides

- Most common species of anaerobes causing human infection belongs to this genus.
- They are Gram-negative pleomorphic rods, may show coccobacillary forms. They are non-motile bacilli.
- They are strict anaerobes.
- Grow well in media as brain heart infusion agar in anaerobic conditions with 5–10% CO_2.
- They are normal inhabitants of intestinal, respiratory and female genital tract.
- Most pathogenic species is *B. fragilis.*
- Virulence factors—capsular polysaccharide, lipopolysaccharide, enterotoxin.
- *B. fragilis* is frequently isolated from blood, pleural fluid, peritoneal fluid, CSF, brain abscess, wound and urogenital infections.
- It causes peritonitis leading to pelvic inflammatory disease (PID).
- *Bacteroides species* are **sensitive to metronidazole** and usually to **clindamycin, chloramphenicol**.
- *B. melanogenicus* is susceptible to penicillin while *B. fragilis is resistant to penicillin.*

Fusobacterium

- These are thin, spindle-shaped bacilli having pointed ends.
- **F. nucleatum:** It is commansal of mouth, causes oral and pleuropulmonary infections.
- **F. necrophorum:** It causes liver abscess, abdominal infections and **Lemierre's disease (thrombophlebitis)**.

Prevotella

- Previously these bacteria were classified under *Bacteroides*.
- The moderately **saccharolytic species** inhibited by **20% bile** are included in the genus *Prevotella*.
- Various species in this genus are *P. melanogenica*, *P. buccalis*, *P. denticola* and others.
- Species can be organized into *two* groups:
  - **Pigmented (e.g. P. melaninogenica)**—produces pigmented colonies (black to brown). The color is not due to melanin pigment as previously thought, but to a hemin derivative.
  - It shows characteristic fluorescence under UV lamp.
- Infections caused by *Prevotella species* include—lung abscess, liver abscess, mastoiditis, intestinal lesions and lesions on gums and inside mouth.
- **Non-pigmented group:** For example, *P. denticola*, *P. buccalis*.

Porphyromonas

- Two important species are *P. gingivalis* and *P. endodomant*.
- Asaccharolytic pigmented strains are classified into new genus—*Porphyromonas*.

Leptotrichia buccalis

- Once it was called **Fusobacterium fusiformis**.
- Long spindle-shaped bacillus with pointed ends.
- It forms part of normal flora of mouth but may cause necrotizing lesions in mouth.
- It is held responsible for a condition known as' **Vincent's angina'** in which pharyngeal mucosa is inflamed with formation of grayish membrane which peels esily, smear shows larger number of fusiform bacilli

It resembles to diphtheria due to production of pseudomembrane.

Predisposing Factors for Anaerobic Infections due to Non-sporing Anaerobes

- Trauma
- Dead tissue

- Impaired blood supply
- Presence of other organisms—*E. coli* in abdominal wound may encourage growth of *B. fragilis*
- Presence of foreign bodies
- Diabetes mellitus
- Malignancy
- Prolonged antibiotic therapy
- *Synergistic infection*: **Meleny's gangrene**—*Staphylococcus aureus* and anaerobic streptococci cause infection.

Factors which give clue of presence of anaerobic infections are:

- Polymicrobial flora grown and seen in microscope.
- Foul smelling.
- Infection at a site where anaerobes act as commensals.
- Discharging sinuses—discharging sulfur granules.
- Routine culture is negative but pus cells and bacteria are seen in primary smear.
- Pronounced cellulitis.
- Fever not marked.
- Precipitating factors as trauma, tissue necrosis, impaired circulation, presence of foreign body.

General Guidelines for Laboratory Diagnosis

- Collection of a specimen of pus and not a swab
- Prompt transport
- Use of specific anaerobic transport media (PRAS media)
- Enrichment culture in RCM, thioglycollate broth
- Direct culture on appropriate anaerobic culture media whenever possible.

Proper Method of Sample Collection

- Pus is aspirated with the help of sterile needle syringe aspiration and a sterile rubber cock is attached to the needle and sample is transported as such to the laboratory.
- Pus sample or fluids can be collected in sterile airtight small bottles.
- Specimens can also be transported in—**Robertson's cooked meat medium.**
- Commercially available system is prereduced anaerobically sterilized media (**PRAS**)—these contain tubes gassed out with nitrogen and tightly fitted with butyl stoppers.

Acceptable samples
- Aspirated pus
- Tissue obtained by biopsy, surgically removed or autopsy
- Body fluids other than urine
- Sulfur granules in actinomycosis

Unacceptable samples: Any swab, expectorated or induced sputum, bronchial washing, bronchoalveolar lavage fluids, gastric content, small bowel content and voided urine are unsuitable samples.

Transport of Samples
- Rubber-stoppered collection tubes or vials which are gassed out with O_2 free CO_2 and N_2 and containing agar with O_2 tension indicator.
- A plastic collection device with its own anaerobic transport medium. For example, Gas Pak pouch, Anaerobic pouch, Bio bag.

Macroscopic examination: Foul smelling pus, with UV light brick-red fluorescence is suggestive of *P. melaninogenica* (Fig. 31.1).

Gram stain: It gives idea of organisms as some show typical morphology, e.g. *Fusobacterium* is fusiform or spindle shaped.

Culture is done on blood agar, phenylethyl alcohol blood agar (PEA) and kanamycin–vancomycin blood agar (KVB).

Selective Media
- Bacteroides bile esculin agar (BBE)
- Kanamycin–vancomycin laked BA (KVLB)

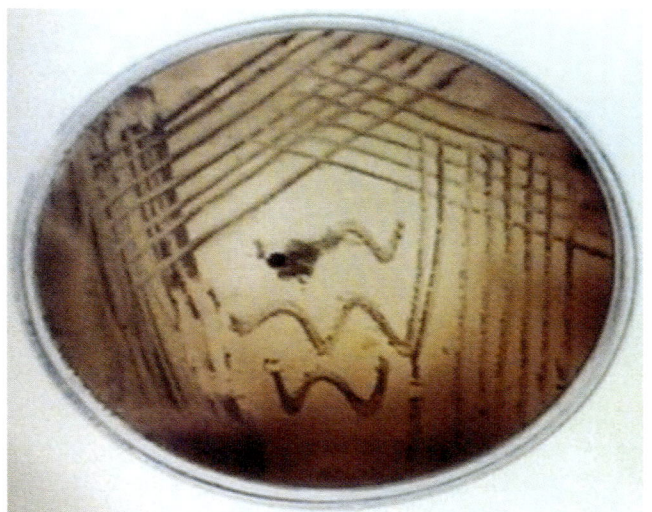

Fig. 31.1: Pigmented colonies of *P. melaninogenica*

- Phenylethyl alcohol sheep BA
- Liquid medium as thioglycollate medium

Identification disks of anaerobes, i.e. **gentamicin and metronidazole,** are placed on primary plates, i.e. blood agar. When the plates are incubated anaerobically, and if the isolate is sensitive to metronidazole and resistant to gentamicin, it suggests the growth of an anaerobe.

Once the organism is identified by "**G**" and "**Metro** "disk, further identification is done by biochemical tests.

Aero tolerance: Subculture is done on chocolate agar which is exposed to air and incubated at 30°C under 5% CO_2 for 24 hours to see the growth. An anaerobic bacterium does not show any growth on aero tolerance plate.

Gas liquid chromatography: It is used for the detection of anaerobes based on the analysis of fatty acids produced.

Treatment

Penicillin, clindamycin, and metronidazole are antibiotics used against anaerobes.

Common Anaerobic Infections and Bacteria Responsible (Table 31.1)
- *CNS:* Brain abcess—*B. fragilis. Peptostreptococcus.*
- *Ear, nose, and throat:* Chronic sinusitis, otitis media, and mastoiditis, orbital cellulitis—*Fusobacterium.*
- *Mouth and jaw:* Ulcerative gingivitis, dental abscess, cellulitis, abscess, sinus of jaw—*Fusobacterium, Spirochaetes* and *Actinomyces.*
- *Female genital tract infections:* Wound infection following genital surgery, puerperal sepsis, tubo-ovarian abscess, bartholins abscess, septic abortion—*P. melaninogenica,* anaerobic cocci, *B. fragilis.*
- *Skin and soft tissue infection:* Infected sebaceous cyst, breast and axillary abscess, cellulitis, diabetic ulcer, gangrene—anaerobic cocci, *P. melaninogenica, B. fragilis.*
- *Respiratory:* Aspiration pneumonia, lung abscess, bronchiectasis, empyema—*Fusobacterium spp, P. melaninogenica,* anaerobic cocci, *B.fragilis.*
- *Abdominal:* Subphrenic and hepatic abscess, appendicitis, peritonitis, and ischiorectal abscess—*B. fragilis*
- *Pelvic inflammatory disease:* *Peptostreptococci sp., B. fragilis, Prevotella sp.*

TABLE 31.1: Association between diseases and different species of anaerobes

Gram-negative bacilli

Fusobacterium species	*F. nucleatum*
Colonize human mucosal surfaces, considered as commensals of upper respiratory tract and gastrointestinal tract They tend to form filamentous rods with pointed ends (fusiform or spindle shaped)	It is frequently isolated from mixed infections of head and neck including dental abscesses, CNS infections *F. necrophorum* It may produce occasionally infections caused by *N. nucleatum* It causes Lemieere's disease syndrome (thrombophebitis)
Leptotrichia buccalis Commensal in oral cavity	Together with other bacteria, it causes Vincent's gingivitis
Bacteroides, Porphyromonas and Prevotella species A. The asaccharolytic, pigmented species are classified in the genus *Porphyromonas*, *P. gingivalis* causes periodontal infections B. Moderately saccharolytic species which are inhibited by 20% bile, present in oral cavity are in the genus *Prevotella* C. Bacteroides genus is restricted to *B. fragilis* and related species that are saccharolytic and grow in 20% bile	These species cause most common nonclostridial infections *B. fragilis* causes intra-abdominal infection and soft tissue infections below waist This group accounts to 25% of infections They also cause head, neck infections and bacteremia *Prevotella* and *Porphyromonas* cause soft tissue infections, abscesses in various parts of body
Gram-positive anaerobic cocci They form part of normal flora of mouth, GIT, skin	*Peptostreptococci* species They are isolated from abscess and other pyogenic infections
Gram-negative cocci Veillonella species is found in mouth and other sites	They are able to use some of the lactic acid produced by other bacteria and regularly from component of dental plaque
Gram-positive rods *Actinomyces spp. A. israelii* *Propionibacterium propionicum* *Bifidobacterium*	*Propionibacterium propionicum* causes infection of tear duct in lacrimal caniculitis *Eubacterium* spp. cause infections around intrauterine devices, periodontal infections *Bifidobacterium* causes dental caries, pulmonary infections

32

Enterobacteriaceae

Members of this family form normal flora of intestine. Though they are commensals in intestine, they have the ability to cause infections at other sites as urinary tract infection, wound infection, septicemia. This family also includes enteric pathogens, *Salmonella and Shigella*.

Characteristics of Organism in the Family Enterobacteriaceae

- Gram-negative bacilli
- Non-sporing
- Non-acid fast
- Bacilli are motile or non-motile
- Capsulated or non-capsulated
- They ferment at least glucose with production of acid with gas or without gas
- All reduce nitrates to nitrites
- All are oxidase negative

With introduction of modified technology, the classifications proposed for Enterobacteria as:

- Bergeys's mannual
- Edward's and Ewing's classification.
- Farmer and Kelly classification. There are only minute changes with basic concept to divide the family into tribe, genus and species.

Classification (Based on Growth on MacConkey's Agar)

I. Lactose Fermenter (LF) (Coliforms)

They form pink colonies on MacConkey's medium.

  i. *E. coli*

  ii. *Klebsiella*

These are called **"Coliforms"**.

II. Nonlactose Fermenter (NLF)

They form colorless colonies on MacConkey's medium.

  i. *Salmonella*

  ii. *Shigella*

These are major intestinal pathogens.

III. Late Lactose Fermenter

Shigella sonnei called as **"paracolons"** bacilli. Classification based upon DNA base composition classifies the family into major subdivision, tribes or groups.

Ewing's Classification

Family is clasified into tribe, genus, species—genera under each tribe share common properties.

Tribe I. Escherichiae
Genus: *Escherichia coli, E. blattae, E. fergusonii, Shigella*

Tribe II. Edwardsielleae
Genus: *Edwardsilla tarda*

Tribe III. Salmonellae
Genus: 1. *Salmonella*, 2. *Arizona*

Tribe IV. Citrobactereae
Genus: *Citrobacter freundii, Citrobacter koseri*

Tribe V. Klebsielleae
Genus:

1. *Klebsiella pneumoniae, K. oxytoca, K. ozanae, K. rhinoscleromatis*
2. *Enterobacter*
3. *Hafnia*
4. *Serratia*
5. *Pantoea*

Tribe VI. Proteeae
Genus:
1. *Proteus mirabilis, Proteus vulgaris, Proteus myxofaciens, Proteus peeneri*
2. *Morganella*
3. *Providencia*

Tribe VII. Yersinieae
Genus: *Yersinia*

Tribe VIII. Erwinieae
Genus: *Erwinia*

ESCHERICHIA COLI

(Escherich-described colon bacillus under name Bacterium coli commune).

Species: E. coli, E. furgusonii, E. hermanii, E. vulneris, and E. blattae (gut of cockroaches).

E. coli living only in human and animal intestine is voided in feces remains viable for few days only, this property is useful for testing of water samples.

Morphology

- These are Gram-negative straight rods 1–3 × 0.4–0.7 µm, arranged single or in pairs (Fig. 32.1).
- Sluggishly motile by peritrichate flagella.
- Non-capsulated (many pathogenic strains have polysaccharide capsule).
- Some strains are fimbriated.
- Spores not produced.

Cultural Characteristics

- Aerobe and facultative anaerobe, optimum temperature: 37°C.
- BA: It has simple growth requirements, good growth is seen on ordinary media. Colonies are large, thick, grayish white, flat, moist, and smooth.
- Lactose-fermenting (pink) flat colonies are produced on MacConkey's medium (Fig. 32.2).

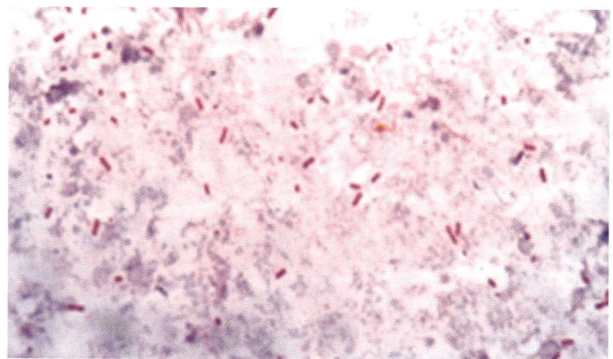

Fig. 32.1: Gram-negative bacilli

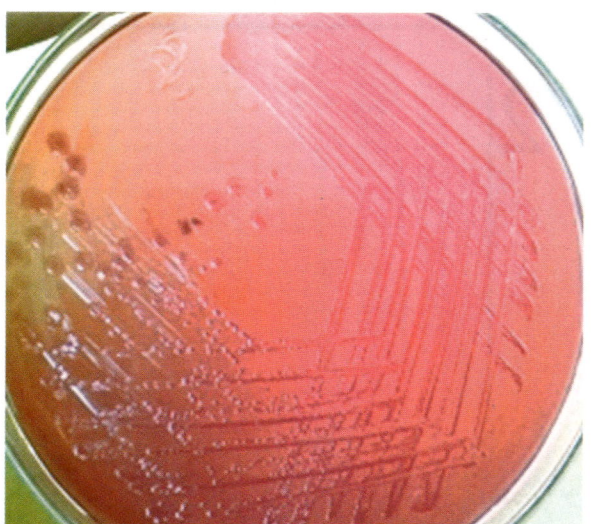

Fig. 32.2: Lactose-fermenting colonies of *E. coli* on MC agar

- Due to repeated subcultures—smooth to rough variation occurs (S-R), which indicates loss of surface antigens. Rough **(R) (autoagglutinable)** and smooth(s) forms of colonies are seen on blood agar and MacConkey agar.

  Some pathogenic strains having polysaccharide capsule may show mucoid forms.

  Most of isolates from clinical infections produce betahemolysis on BA, selective media used for *Salmonella* and *Shigella* inhibit the growth of *E. coli*. It produces yellow colonies on CLED medium.
- In liquid media, general turbidity with heavy deposit is produced.

Biochemical Tests (Flowcharts 32.1 and 32.2)

- Catalase positive, oxidase negative.
- Glucose, lactose, mannitol and maltose fermented with acid and gas. Sucrose is not fermented by typical strains.
- IMViC tests: Indole positive, methyl red positive, Voges-Proskauer negative, citrate not utilized.
- TSI gives A/A with gas reaction.
- H_2S, urease negative, gelatin not liquified and growth on media containing KCN is negative.

Antigenic Structure

- *Somatic antigen (O-170 types):* Normal colon strains usually belong to earlier 'O' groups (1, 2, 3, 4, etc.); **enteropathogenic strains** belong to later **groups (26, 55, 86, 111, etc.).**
- *Capsular antigen:* K-100 types (2 groups of K antigens—I and II). It covers 'O' antigen, hence *E. coli* **isolate with K** antigen is **not agglutinated with 'O'** antiserum.

Flowchart 32.1: Identification of common Gram-negative pathogens

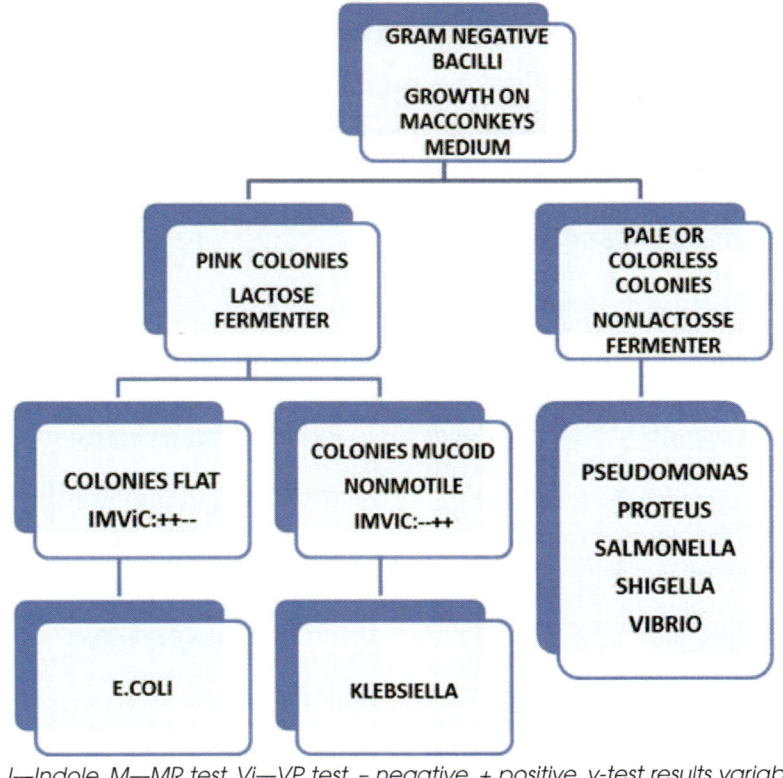

I—Indole, M—MR test, Vi—VP test, – negative, + positive, v-test results variable

80% of *E. coli* strains that cause neonatal meningitis and 40% of stains which cause neonatal septicemia without meningitis express **K1 antigen.**

Strains having **K1** or **K5** are **more virulent than other strains with different 'K' antigen because** they share structural **identity with host cells.**

'K' inhibits phagocytosis, thus acts as virulence factor. **Early serogroups (0, 1, 2, 3, 4, 5, etc.)** are present in colon. They may **cause UTI.** Late serogroups contain enteropathogenic strains.

- Flagellar antigen 'H', there are total—**75 types.**

Virulence Factors of *E. coli*

Surface Antigens

a. Lipopolysaccharide 'O' antigen. It is endotoxin and protects from phagocytosis and from action of complement.

b. Envelope 'K' antigen is antiphagocytic. **KL antigen** is present on those strains of *E. coli* which cause **neonatal meningitis and septicemia. K-88** antigen is found in strains causing **enteritis** in pigs, and **K-99** is found in strains causing enteritis in calves and lambs.

c. Toxins produced by *E. coli* are:
  1. Enterotoxins by diarrheagenic *E. coli.* They are heat stable and verotoxin.

2. Hemolysins
3. Siderophores which help iron uptakes
4. Cytotoxic necrotizing toxin which is toxic to bladder and kidney cells.

Fimbrial Antigens (Pilus)

- It helps in adhesion and colonization, a step towards infection.
- *Colonization factor antigen (CFA):* It is expressed by enterotoxigenic *E. coli.*
- *Mannose resistant fimbriae:* They hemagglutinate with RBCs that are not inhibited by mannose. Uropathogenic strains of *E.coli* have such fimbria, e.g. M, S, F1C, Dr fimbriae.
- *P fimbriae:* They bind to P blood group substance present on human uroepithelial cells and human RBCs.

d. *Toxins:* Enterotoxins: Heat-labile toxin (LT), heat-stable toxin (ST) and verotoxin or shiga-like toxin (SLT) are produced.

Toxins

Heat-labile toxin: It has A (A1 and A2) and B subunits.

Mode of action: Toxin binds to Gm1 gangliosides on intestinal epithelial cell by B subunit. 'A' unit is

Flowchart 32.2: Identification of common Gram-negative pathogens

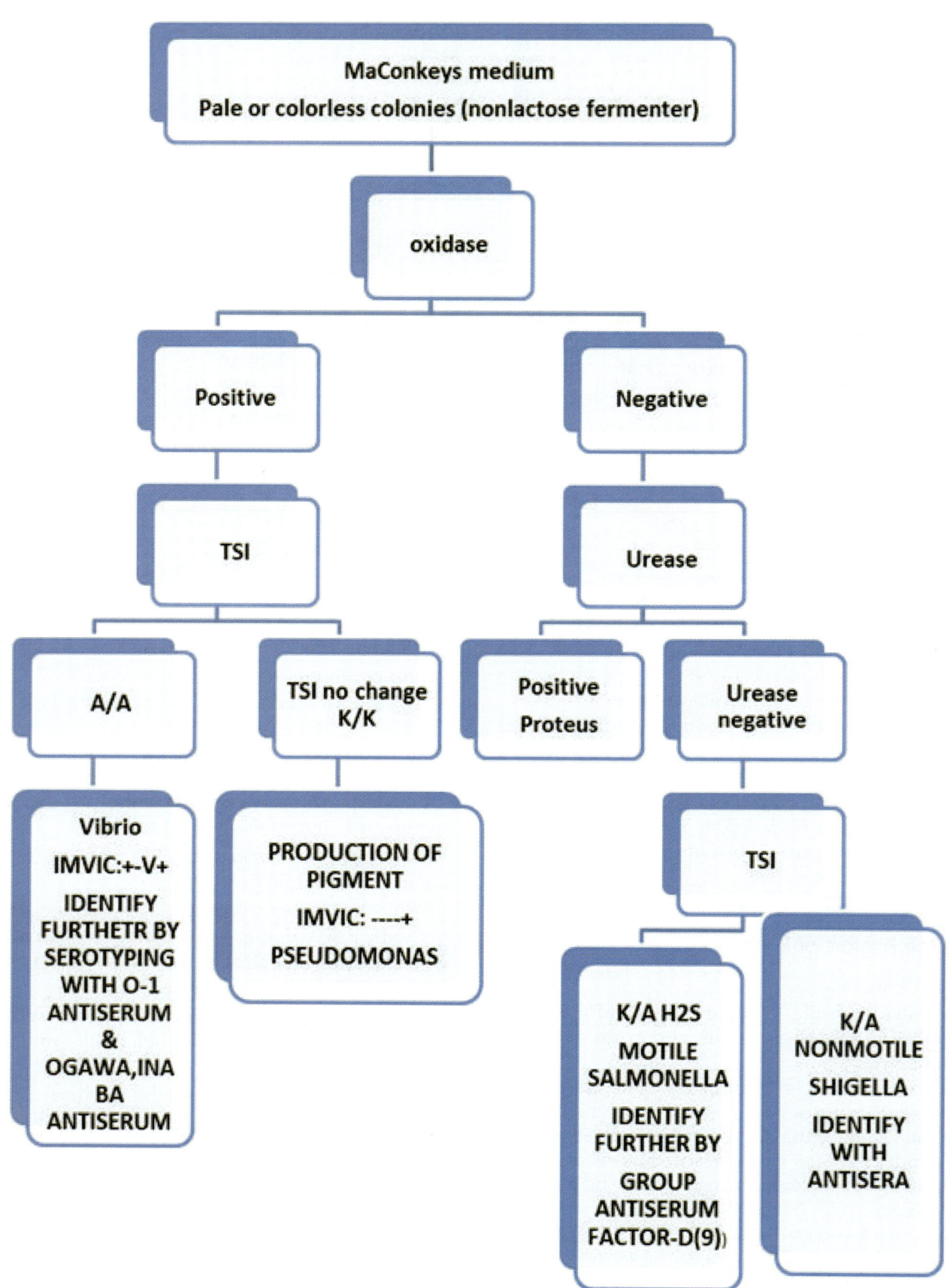

activated, it produces two fragments—A1 and A2. A1 activates adenyl cyclase—form cAMP—causes outpouring of water and electrolytes. Test used for detection of toxin is rabbit ileal loop test.

Heat-stable toxin: ***STa*** **(ST-I) and** ***STb*** **(ST-II) genes are carried on plasmids.** Test used for the detection is **infant mouse intragastric test.**

STa:
- Heat-stable toxins are of 2 types—STa (or ST I) and STb (or ST II)
- STa acts by stimulation of cyclic-GMP pathway.
- If the toxin is given to infant mice, it acts rapidly and causes accumulation fluid in intestine of mice within 4 hours.
- It is detected by mouse intragastric test, ST ELISA and gene probe.

STb: Its action is unknown.

Verotoxin (VT) or shiga-like toxin (SLT): It is similar to toxin of *S. dysenteriae* type I. The toxin produces cytopathic effects on Vero cell culture. Hence it is called as verotoxin. It shows enterotoxigenicity in rabbit ileal loops and genes appeared to be **phage coded.**

Pathogenicity

Infections produced by *E. coli* are:
- Urinary tract infection.
- Diarrhea
- Neonatal meningitis
- Septicemia
- *Peritonitis*: It may be primary peritonitis which occurs spontaneously or secondary peritonitis which usually follows perforation leading to spillage of organisms from intestinal flora
- *Visceral abscess*: Hepatic abscess, subdiaphragmatic abscess, perinephric abscess.
- Infection in perianal area.
- Ventilator-associated pneumonia which is health-associated infection.
- Osteomyelitis—soft tissue infections.
- Endovascular infection.
- Systemic inflammatory response syndrome.

Diarrheagenic E. coli
- *Enteropathogenic E. coli (EPEC)*
- *Enterotoxigenic E. coli (ETEC)*
- *Enteroinvasive E. coli or verotoxigenic E. coli (EIEC/VTEC)*
- *Enterohaemorrhagic E. coli (EHEC)*
- *Enteraggregative E. coli (EAC)*

EPEC

It is associated with diarrhea in infants and children. It may occur as epidemics. *EPEC* also causes sporadic cases of diarrhea in adults. Pathogenesis is not known. EPEC is non-invasive and non-toxic. Initial colonization and adherence occurs which leads to effacement of microvilli by plasmid coded 'bundle forming pilus. There is formation of **cup-like actin rich pedestals**. It doesn't ferment sorbitol. **It is detected by adhesion to HEP2 cell.**

Accurate identification is possible by detecting **'eae' gene by PCR.**

ETEC (Fig. 32.3)

It causes **'travelers' diarrhea**. It occurs in persons travelling from developed countries to developing countries. Serotypes which cause diarrhea are 6, 8, 15, 25, 27, 167. A strain of *E. coli* may produce heat labile (LT) or heat stable toxin (ST) or both. A large dose of *E. coli* (10^6–10^{10}) is required to produce the disease (Table 32.1).

Before toxin acts, the strain should adhere to intestinal mucosa by fimbria or colonization factor antigens (CFA I, II, III, IV). Diagnosis is done by isolation and detection of toxins.

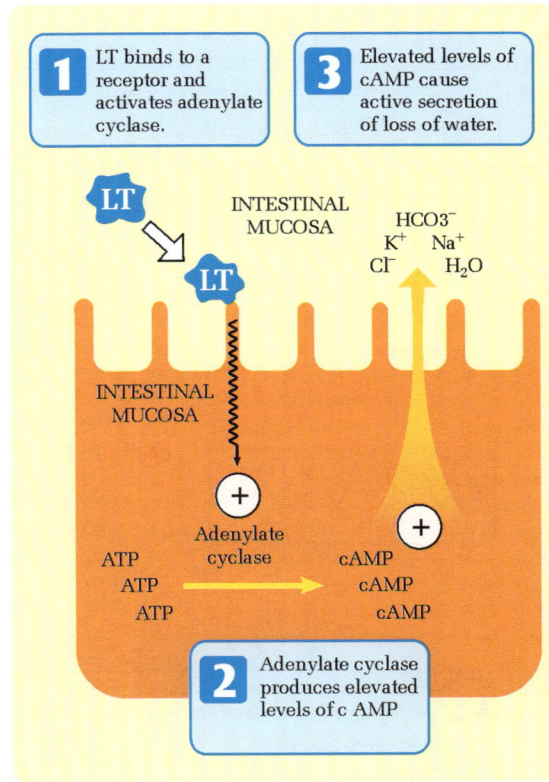

Fig. 32.3: Mechanism of action of heat-labile toxin of ETEC

TABLE 32.1: Differences between heat-labile toxin (LT) and heat stable toxin (ST) of ETEC

Assay	LT	ST
In vivo tests		
Ligated rabbit ileal loop		
Read at 6 hrs	+ OR–	+
Read at 18 hrs	+	–
Infant mouse intragastric test (4 hrs)	–	+
Adult rabbit skin (vascular permeability factor) test	+	—
In vitro tests		
Tissue culture tests		
Rounding of Y1 mouse adrenal cells	+	–
Elongation of CHO cells	+	–
ELISA	+	ST-ELISA
Passive agglutination test	+	–
Precipitation test (Eiken test)	+	–
Genetic tests (probes)	+	+

EIEC

Many strains are non-motile and non-lactose fermenting. Clinical features vary from mild diarrhea to dysentery. Many strain's 'O' antigen crossreact with *Shigella*. They resemble shigellae. They do not ferment lactose or ferment it late and give Lysine decarboxylase test negative. These strains were previously in the group called Alkalescens–Dispar group or (*S. alkalescens. S. dispar* Strains O28ac, O112ac, O124, O136, O143, O152, O154). They are now called as enteroinvasive *E. coli* having capacity to invade intestinal mucosa. The invasion is mediated by plasmid coded (virulence marker antigens) 'VMA' antigens.

Diagnosis is done by **Sereny test, VMA** (virulence marker antigens—these are outer membrane protein present on cell wall of this Gram-negative bacillus) detection **by ELISA**, and detection of invasion **of HeLa cells.**

Molecular methods for diagnosis of EIEC is detection of invasion **plasmid antigen (ipaH) and aerobactin expresion (iuc).**

EHEC

Common serotypes is "O157:H7". Other serotypes include—**O26:H11, O6, O103.0–111, P113.**

The infective dose is very small, organisms $<10^2$ can initiate infection.

Pathogenesis

Shiga-like toxin is produced.

Toxin acts by inhibiting protein synthesis. Its shigella-like toxin acts by inhibition of 28S subunit and 60 S subunit of 605 ribosome.

Shiga-like toxins are of **two types—Stx1 and Stx2 of which Stx2 is more commonly associated with HUS.**

The toxin has affinity for endothelial cells which causes capillary microangiopathy. The result is haemorrhagic colitis (HC) which presents as gross bloody diarrhoea, abdominal pain and faecal leukocytes.

Hemorrhagic Uremia Syndrome

There is injury to small blood vessels of kidney, brain.

Clinical presentation is:
- Bloody diarrhea, thrombocytopenia
- Renal failure
- Encephalopathy
- Fever is absent

Hemolytic Uremic Syndrome (HUS) (Fig. 32.4)
- Injury to small bood vessels of brain and kidney.
- Bloody diarrhea, thrombocytopenia, renal failure and encephalopathy without fever.

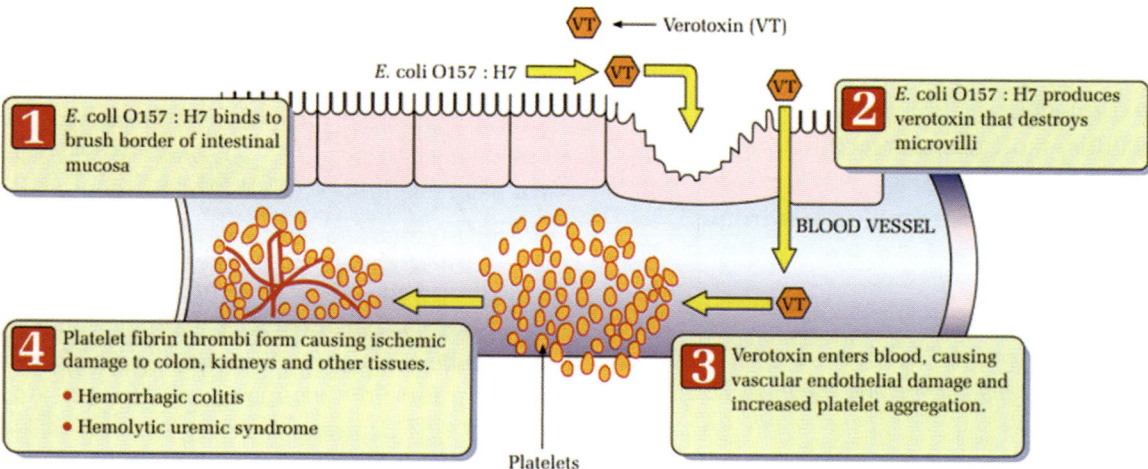

Fig. 32.4: Mechanism of production of HUS

Laboratory Diagnosis (Table 32.2)

- *Sorbitol MacConkey medium:* It doesn't ferment sorbitol. Pale colonies are produced.
- *Rainbow agar:* **O157** strains cause **black colonies** as they do not produce glucuronidase.
- *Toxin detection:*
  - Most standard method is demonstration of cytotoxicity *in vivo* cell lines.
  - Detection of toxin in feces by ELISA or rapid tests
  - PCR is highly sensitive method for toxin detection.

Contaminated food as lettuce, spinach, sprouts and undercooked ground beaf acts as source of infection. Infective dose is very small (>12 bacilli).

EAEC

They appear aggregated in 'stacked brick' formation on HEP2 cells. EAEC adhere to intestine with the help of adhesion fimbria-1. They cause diarrhea in developing countries. They may cause shortening of villi, hemorrhagic necrosis and mild diarrhea. These strains form enteroaggregative heat-stable toxin 1 (EAST 1).

E. coli O104:H4: It is an enteroaggregative strain of E. coli which caused outbreaks in Germany. It produces Shiga-like toxin and can cause HUS.

Diffusely-adherent E. coli (DAEC)

- These are strains which have ability to adhere to HEp-2 cells in a diffuse pattern.
- They express diffuse adherence fimbriae which contribute to pathogenesis.
- DAEC causes diarrhea in children aged 2–6 years.

Many strains of E. coli produce β lactamases as ESBL and MBL.

Laboratory Diagnosis of E. coli Diarrhea

EPEC diarrhea is diagnosed by fecal culture on MacConkey medium and identification of serotype, shown by slide agglutination with group specific 'O' antigen as there are specific types which cause diarrhea.

ETEC: It is diagnosed by culture and detection of enterotoxin by various methods.

Detection of heat-labile toxin (LT): It is done by demonstrating rounding of Y1 mouse adrenal cells, elongation of CHO (Chinese hamster ovary) cells. The toxin may be detected by ELISA, passive agglutination or gene probes. **Detection of heat-stable toxin (ST)** is done by infant mouse intragastric tests or the toxin is detected by ELISA or gene probes.

TABLE 32.2: Biochemical tests of family Enterobacteriaceae

	E. coli	Shigella-1	Edwardsella	Klebsiella	Enterobacter	Serratia	Hafnia	Citrobacter	Salmonella(2)	Proteus	Morganella	Providencia
Motility	+	–	+	–	+	+	+	+	+	+	+	+
Gas from glucose	+	—	+	+	+	d	+	+	+	d	+	+
Acid from lactose	+	—	—	+	+	—	—	+	—	–	–	–
Acid from sucrose	d	—	—	+	+	+	—	d	—	d	—	d
Growth in KCN	—	—	—	+	+	+	+	+	d	+	+	+
Indole	+	d	+	—	–	—	—	d	–	d	+	+
MR	+	+	+	–	—	—	—	+	+	+	+	+
VP	—	—	—	+	+	+	+	—	—	—	—	—
Citrate	—	—	—	+	+	+	+	+	+	d	d	d
H$_2$S	–	—	+	—	–	—	—	+	+	+	–	—
Urease	—	—	–	+	d	–	—	—	—	+	+	d
Phenyl deaminase test (PPA)	—	—	—	—	—	—	—	—	—	+	+	+
Arginine dehydrolase	d	—	—	—	d	—	—	d	+			
Lysine decarboxylase	+	—	+	d	d	+	+	—	+	—	—	—
Ornithine decarboxylase	d	D	+	–	+	+	+	d	+	+	+	—

Exception: (1) *Sh. sonnei* is late lactose and sucrose fermenter, (2) *S. typhi* is anaerogenic, it does not produce gas

D = strains or species give variable results

EIEC: **Invasiveness is detected by Sereny's test** (instillation of suspension of bacterium in eyes of guinea pig causes conjunctivitis and keratitis) or by cell penetration of HeLa or Hep2 cells. **The VMA is detected by ELISA test.**

EHEC: Isolation of bacillus, demonstration of VT (cytotoxic effects on Vero or HeLa cells; DNA probes), and use of sorbitol MacConkey agar (colorless colonies) are the tests used for the diagnosis.

ESCHERICHIA ALBERTII

It is a new species found in Bangladesh which has caused many cases of diarrhea in children. It is indole negative and it ferments mannitol.

> **Other causes of traveller's diarrhea are:** *Enteroaggregative E. coli, Shigella, Salmonella, Campylobacter jejuni, Aeromonas, Plesiomonas, Vibrio cholerae, rota virus, Norwalk virus, Entamoeba histolytica, Giardia, Cryptosporidium, Cyclospora.*

KLEBSIELLA

The genus includes four species, i.e. *Klebsiella pneumoniae, Klebsiella oxytoca, Klebsiella ozanae, Klebsiella rhinoscleromatis.*

KLEBSIELLA PNEUMONIAE

Morphology

- They are Gram-negative short, plump, straight bacilli
- Non-motile
- Capsulated

Cultural Characteristic (Fig. 32.5)

- It grows well on ordinary media.
- It forms large, dome-shaped mucoid colonies.
- *On MacConkey's agar (MCA)*: Lactose-fermenting (pink) mucoid colonies are produced.

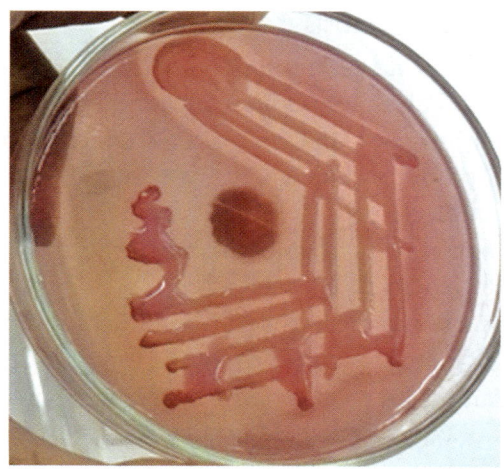

Fig. 32.5: MCA showing pink mucoid growth of *Klebsiella*

Antigenic Structure

It has capsular antigen, somatic 'O' antigen; typing is based on capsular antigen, other typing methods are antibiogram, biotyping, klebocin (bacteriocin) typing, phage typing. Klebsiella are classified into more than 80 serotypes based on capsular K antigen.

Biochemical Reactions (Table 32.3)

- It is catalase positive, oxidase negative.
- It ferments sugars with formation of acid and gas or acid.
- *IMViC tests*: Indole, methyl red—negative; Voges-Proskauer and citrate—positive.
- *Urease test*: Positive.

Diseases Caused by *Klebsiella*

It is common cause of nosocomial infections.

- *Pneumonia*: This illness is serious with high case fatality in persons with medical problems (DM, alcoholism, chronic lung disease). Massive mucoid inflammatory exudate occurs and it may be lobar or lobular pneumonia. Necrosis and abscess formation may occur. Serotypes 1, 2, 3 are more common.

TABLE 32.3: Biochemical tests of Klebsiella species

	Kl. pneumoniae	Kl. ozaenae	Kl. rhinoscleromatis
Gas from glucose	+	D	—
Acid from lactose	+	D	—
MR	—	+	+
VP	+	—	—
Citrate	+	D	—
Urease	+	D	—
Malonate	+	—	+
Lysine	+	D	—

- Urinary infection
- Abscesses and wound infections
- Meningitis
- Septicemia

Laboratory Diagnosis

It is done by culture and biochemical tests.

Other Pathogenic Species of Klebsiella

K. ozaenae—causes ozaena, foul smelling discharge from the nose. *K. rhinoscleromatis*—causes rhinoscleroma, chronic granulomatous hypertrophy of nose. *K. oxytoca* rarely isolated from human specimens.

Treatment

Carbapenems as imipenems and meropenems are recommended. Strain causing **KPC**—*Klebsiella pneumoniae* carbapenemase was isolated from hospitalized patients in New Delhi, for this drug resistance strains **(NDM-beta-lactamases)**, tigecycline, colistin should be reserved. **KPC** is extended spectrum beta-lactamase (ELBL) type enzyme that causes resistance to third and fourth generation cephalosporins. The resistance is plasmid mediated.

NDM was first described in a strain of *Klebsiella* in a Sweden patient who had travelled to India. The strains may show resistance to many antibiotics thus limiting treatment options (resistance to aminoglycosides, fluoroquinolones). Such patients are often placed on maximum infection control precautions to prevent spread to other patients.

Differences between *E. coli* and *Klebsiella* are given in Table 32.4.

TABLE 32.4: Differences between *E. coli* and *Klebsiella*

Property	E. coli	Klebsiella
Capsule	Absent	Present
Motility	Motile	Non-motile
Colonies on MacConkey's medium	Pink flat colonies	Pink mucoid colonies
IMViC reactions	++— –	– —++

PROTEEAE

Tribe Proteeae consists of 3 genera: *Proteus, Morganella and Providencia.*

All the members of tribe Proteeae give **PPA test positive**: They have ability to deaminate amino acid phenylalanine to phenyl pyruvic acid. This property is tested by growing on PPA medium and next day adding few drops of ferric chloride, slant becomes green (Table 32.5).

PROTEUS

They are normal intestinal commensals and opportunistic pathogens. They may be present in nature as saprophytes in sewage, soil, decomposing animal matter.

The medically important species of proteus are:
- *Proteus mirabilis*
- *Proteus vulgaris*
- *Proteus myxofaciens*
- *Proteus peeneri*

Of these all, the infections in humans are produced by first two species.

Morphology

Gram-negative non-capsulated, pleomorphic, motile rods.

Cultural Characteristics

They grow on routine media: Characteristic **'fishy' or 'seminal'** odor is present.

Swarming on solid media: The growth spreads on surface of plate in waves, a filmy layer in concentric circles; shown by *Proteus vulgaris* and *P. mirabilis*.

MacConkey's medium: There is no swarming (it is inhibited by bile salts) and non-lactose fermenting (colorless) colonies are produced.

CLED medium (cysteine lactose electrolyte deficient medium): On this medium, swarming is inhibited.

Methods of Inhibiting Swarming

- Increased concentration of agar (6%)

TABLE 32.5: Biochemical tests of Proteeae

	Pr. mirabilis	Pr. vulgaris	Morg. morganii	Prov. alcalifaciens	Pro. stuartii	Pro. rettgeri
Urease	+	+	+	—	+/—	+
Ornithine decarboxylase	+	—	+	—	—	—
Indole	—	+	+	+	+	+
Adonitol fermentation	—	—	—	+	+/—	+/—
Trehalose fermentation	+	+/–	+/–	+/–	+	—

- Incorporation in medium
  - Chloral hydrate (1:500)
  - Sodium azide (1:500)
  - Alcohol (5–6%)
  - Sulphonamide
  - Surface active agents
  - Boric acid

Biochemical Tests

- Phenylalanine deaminase is produced converting phenylalanine to phenyl pyruvic acid.
- Degrade tyrosine.
- Indole is negative in *Proteus mirabilis* and it is positive in *Proteus vulgaris.*
- MR positive, VP negative.
- Lactose, dulcitol, malonate not fermented.
- Rapid urease production is positive except in some species of *Providencia.*

Antigens

It possess somatic 'O' and flagellar 'H' antigens—so named because of production of misty growth on agar by flagellated strains (H—Hauch—mist) and absence of mist in non-flagellated strains (O—Ohne Hauch—without mist).

Certain non-motile strains of *Proteus (OX2, OX19,* and *OXK)* agglutinated by sera from typhus fever patients which is the basis of heterophile **agglutination**—Weil-Felix test for diagnosis of Rickettsial infections.

Diene's Phenomenon

It can be used as one of the typing method for *Proteus* for demonstration similarity of two different strains of proteus.

When two different strains of *Proteus* (e.g. two strains isolated from two different patients in ward) are inoculated on solid medium as nutrient agar or blood agar (these media should not contain substances that will inhibit swarming) at two different points, if these two strains as identical, swarming caused by both will coalesce and no clear demarcation can be made (Fig. 32.6). On the other hand, if these two strains are not identical, the point where their swarming meet each other, there is clear cut demarcation produced. In this method, if two strains are identical, it means both are originated from a common source.

Diseases Caused by Proteus

They are urinary tract infections, nosocomial infections (wound infection, burn infections, and septicemia).

The speciality of urinary tract infection caused by proteus is that due to the production of enzyme urease which breaks down urea into ammonia that makes pH alkaline and may cause **tubular damage**. The alkalinity leads to formation of **phosphate stones**. (Uric acid stones will be formed in acidic urine.)

MORGANELLA MORGANII

It doesn't swarm, but motile, the biochemical reactions are indole positive, MR-positive, VP, citrate negative, urease positive, PPA positive and no H_2S is produced hence TSI shows K/A reaction. Infections produced by it are urinary, nosocomial wound infections and pneumonia.

PROVIDENCIA

It has following species:
- *Providencia alkalifaciens*
- *Providencia rettgeri*
- *Providencia stuartii*
- *Providencia rustigianii*

Infections

They include nosocomial infections as UTI; blood, burns and wound infections.

Swarming of Proteus

Types of swarming: Continuous and discontinuous swarming.

Continuous swarming: Swarming in which uniform film of growth is formed.

Discontinuous swarming: In which series of concentric circles or waves-like pattern is seen (Fig. 32.6).

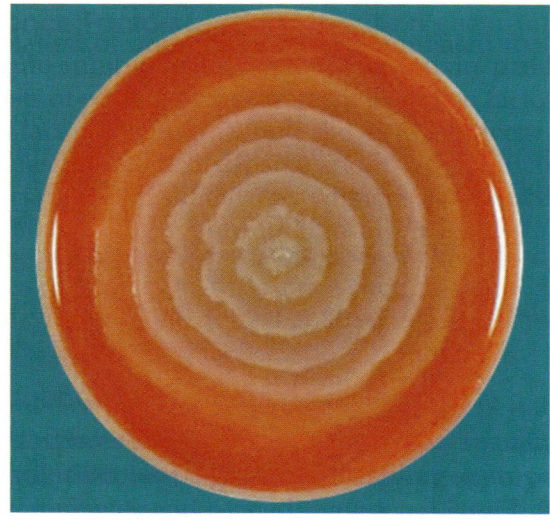

Fig. 32.6: Swarming of proteins on BA

Stimuli for swarming or possible causes of swarming are:

- Positive chemotactic movement in search of nutrients.
- Negative chemotactic response to metabolic products which are accumulated in the medium due to their growth and multiplication.
- Swarm cells originate under conditions of rapid growth, in which due to depletion of nutrients, flagellar synthesis becomes uncontrolled which leads to deficiency of substances necessary for growth.

Process of swarming: When *Proteus* is cultured on medium, after 2–4 hours, short forms having few flagella are stimulated and result in production of 'swarm cells' which are mutiflagellate forms having multiple nuclei and length 2–4 microns. These swarm cells emerge from the edge of colony in groups, swarm short distance on slime produced, and return back. As swarming progresses, more and more cells are converted into mutiflagellate forms, which come out, travel the distance, and come back.

In **discontinuous swarming**, after few hours forward movement stops, cells revert back to short forms with few flagella. These short forms grow and multiply until swarm cells are produced. The cycles of swarming and consolidation (stage during which swarm cells revert back) are repeated which gives alternate concentric rings of growth.

CITROBACTER

It forms normal flora of human intestine.

These are Gram-negative motile bacilli. They are non-lactose fermenter (or late lactose fermenter). *C. frundii* gives typical reactions, *C. koseri* (formerly known as *C. diversus*) and *C. amalonacticus* do not form H_2S. It produces urinary tract infection, infections of gall-bladder, meninges and middle ear.

Some strains of *C. frundi* which have 'Vi' antigenic sharing with salmonella were previously classified as 'Bethesda–Ballerup' group.

ENTEROBACTER

- They are motile, lactose fermenting bacilli.
- IMViC reactions are –, –, +, +
- Two important species, i.e. *E. cloacae* and *E. aerogenes* are differentiated by biochemical tests.

	E. cloacae	*E. aerogenes*
Gas from glycerol	—	+
Aesculin hydrolysis	—	+
Lysine decarboxylase	—	+
Argine dihydrolase	+	—

- Other species include *E. sakazaki*, *E. taylore*, and *E. gergoviae*.
- *Normal habitat*: Enterobacter is found in sewage, soil, water and also in human and animal feces.
- Infections produced are urinary tract infection, sepsis, wound infection.

SERRATIA

It has been associated with nosocomial infections. Multiple drug resistant strains are common. It produces characteristic red pigment, pink or magenta, non-diffusable pigment called as prodigiosin. The only species *S. marcescens* (*Bacillus prodigious*) is of medical importance. It is a saprophyte and may grow in the container of sputum (**pseudohemoptysis**) will confuse with true hemoptysis.

33

Salmonella

History

- Willium Jenner in 1850 first differentiated the terms typhus fever and typhoid fever.
- Typhoid bacillus is first observed by Eberth (1880) in mesenteric lymph nodes and spleen of a patient suffering from the disease.
- Graffy isolated the typhoid bacillus (1884) from spleen of patient. The name **Eberthella Graffky** bacillus or **Eberthella typhi** was given to this organism.

Classification

The members of the genus *Salmonella* were classified based on antigenic structure, epidemiology, biochemical tests and host range. The studies of **DNA: DNA hybridization** have grouped into **7 evolutionary groups.** Currently the genus *Salmonella* is divided into **two species** each having multiple subspecies and **serotypes.** The two species are **S. enterica and S. bongori** (formerly subspecies V). The species **enterica contains five subspecies,** i.e. **salmae, arizonae, diarizonae, houttenae,** and **indica.** Most of the human infections are caused by subspecies *enterica*, named and written as *Salmonella enterica subspecies enterica*. Rarely infections may be caused by subspecies *arizonae, diarizonae;* other species cause infections in cold-blooded animals. The widely accepted nomenclature is *S. entrica subspecies*

enterica serotype typhimurium which can be shortened as *S. typhimurium*. But as per as clinical microbiology laboratory is concerned, old classification is followed (Table 33.1). Salmonellae are classified by Kaufmann and White-Scheme into 67 serogroups based on antigenic structure.

Diseases Caused

- *Enteric fever or typhoid fever*: S. typhi, S. paratyphi A, S. paratyphi B
- *Food poisoning*: S. typhimurium, S. enteritidis
- *Septicemia*: S. cholerasuis, S. paratyphi C

Entric fever group: Most of the cases are caused by *Salmonella typhi* followed by *Salmonella paratyphi A*, and *Salmonella paratyphi B*.

Other less common causes of typhoid fever or enteric fever include:
- *Salmonella paratyphi C*
- *Salmonella enteritidis*
- *Salmonella typhimurium*
- *Salmonella dublin*
- *Salmonella bairley*
- *Salmonella panama*
- *Salmonella sendai*
- *Salmonella saintpaul*

TABLE 33.1: Old classification of salmonellae based on biochemical tests

Property	Subgenera of Salmonella			
	I	II	III	IV
Lactose	—	—	+	—
Dulcitol	+	+	—	—
Malonate	—	+	+	—
d Tartrate	+	—	–	–
Salicin	—	—	—	+
KCN	—	—	—	+

SALMONELLA TYPHI

Morphology

- They are Gram-negative rods, with parallel sides, rounded ends.
- *Size*: 1–3 μm × 0.5 μm.
- Bacteria are motile with peritrichate flagella (*Salmonella gallinarum pullorum* is non-motile).
- They are non-capsulated, non-sporing.

Cultural Characteristics

- They are aerobes, facultative anaerobes.
- Optimum pH 6–8, optimum temperature 37°C (15–40°C).
- It has simple growth requirements, it grows on ordinary media as nutrient agar.
- *Nutrient agar*: Colonies are large, 2–3 mm, grayish white circular, low convex, smooth, translucent. The degree of opacity varies with the strain.
- *Liquid media*: In peptone water or nutrient broth, it produces uniform turbidity. On prolonged incubation, a thin pellicle may be formed as pili may be present.

Enrichment Media

These media are used for stool samples. These media are incubated for 6–8 hours to inhibit the growth of commensals present in stool sample and then, from this medium subculture can be performed on selective medium.

a. *Selenite 'F' broth*: It is a good enrichment medium for *Salmonella* but some species, as **S. paratyphi A**, inhibited in this medium.

b. *Tetrathionate broth* is another enrichment medium used for culturing *Salmonella* from feces.

Differential Medium

- *MacConkey's medium*: Non-lactose-fermenting (NLF) colonies are produced. Which are pale colorless, smooth, shiny and translucent (Fig. 33.1).

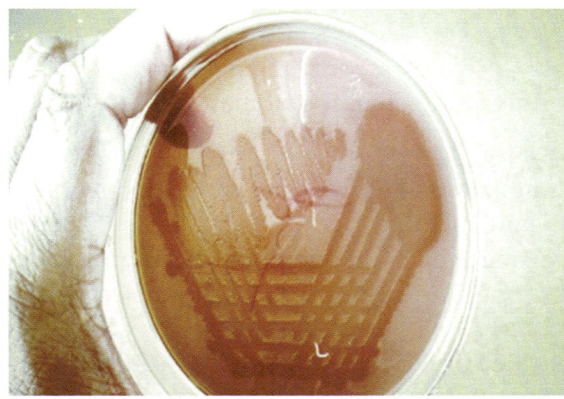

Fig. 33.1: Non-lactose fermenting colonies on MAC

- *Brilliant green MacConkeys agar*: On this medium pale green translucent colonies are produced.

Selective Media

- *DCA (deoxycholate citrate agar)*: This medium has same contents like MacConkey's medium but salt concentration is more and extra bile salts are added to make a selective medium. This medium is inhibitory to *Shigella* hence DCA is mostly preferred as a selective medium. Non-lactose-fermenting colorless colonies are produced on this medium.

- *Wilson and Blair bismuth sulphite agar*: Colonies are **green with or without black center** indicating production of H$_2$S. Crowded colonies may take up dye from the medium and appear green or pale brown. Large discrete colonies have black center and clear edge. *Salmonella* may produce H$_2$S, hence there is metallic sheen surrounding the colonies.

- *XLD (xylose lysine deoxycholate medium)*: This medium has the advantage that it can distinguish *Salmonella* and *Shigella*. Colonies of *Salmonella* and *Shigella* are red (alkaline with phenol red) because *Shigella* do not ferment xylose, lactose, sucrose in the medium within 24 hours and because *Salmonella* neutralize the acid they form with limited amount of xylose by decarboxylation of lysine.

  Most *Salmonella* **species** produce H$_2$S which react with ferric ammonium citrate in the medium to produce **black centers in their red colonies** (Fig. 33.2).

- *Salmonella–Shigella* agar is also selective medium used for isolating *Salmonella* from stool sample.

Hektoen-enteric agar: It is a selective medium for *Salmonella* and *Shigella*. It contains bile salts, lactose,

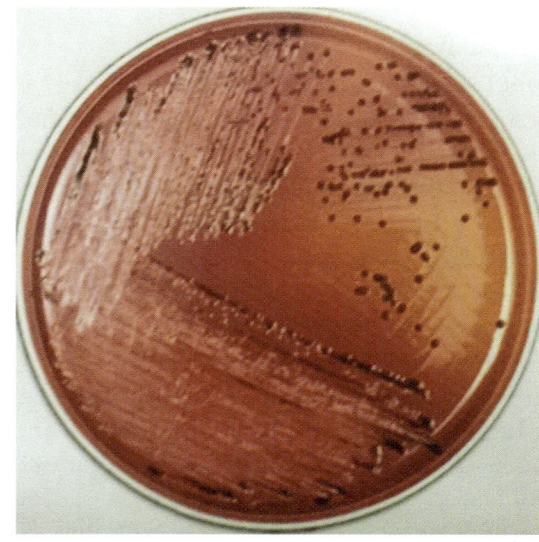

Fig. 33.2: XLD showing pink colonies with black center suggestive of *Salmonella typhi*

sucrose, sodium thiosulphate, ferric ammonium citrate, acid fuschin and thymol blue. Sodium thiosulphate is source of sulphur while H_2S is detected by ferric ammonium citrate. Colonies of *Salmonella* are **bluish green with black centers.** High salt concentration in the medium inhibits Gram-positive bacteria and many coliforms.

Biochemical Reactions

- They ferment glucose, mannitol, and maltose and produce acid with gas (*S. typhi* is anaerogenic).
- Indole is negative, MR positive, VP negative, citrate positive (*S. typhi* does not grow in Simmon's citrate medium-requires tryptophan) except *S. paratyphi A*. *S. typhi* gives kosers citrate test positive.
- H_2S is produced (except *S. paratyphi A*, *S. cholerasuis*), urease is negative.
- IMViC is – + – +
- *Salmonella* decarboxylase lysine, ornithine and arginine but *S. typhi* is exceptional in lacking ornithine decarboxylase and paratyphi lack lysine decarboxylase.
- TSI show K/A with H_2S (anaerogenic) in *S. typhi* and K/A with gas without H_2S in *Salmonella paratyphi* A and *Cholera suis*.

Resistance

Bacteria are killed by boiling of water, chlorination of water and pasteurization of milk. They may retain viability in cultures for years by preventing drying.

Antigenic Structure

It has flagellar '**H**', somatic '**O**', and surface '**Vi**' antigen.

Flagella 'H' Antigen

- It is heat labile.
- Protein in nature.
- Alcohol susceptible, formalin resistant.
- When motile species are treated with formalin the labile protein 'H' antigens of flagella are preserved which are used for agglutination reaction.
- When it is mixed with its antiserum on a slide, it forms loose, large, fluffy clumps.
- Numerous peritrichous flagella explain the nature of clumps.
- It is stronger immunogenic so that antibody formed against this antigen following infection appears early and high titer. Hence significant titer of antibody against 'H' antigen is more that of 'O' antibody in widal test.
- This antigen may occur in either of two phases, hence when an organism is tested for agglutination; it should be tested with both sets of flagellar antigens.

(Usually this is done at Central Research Centre, Kasauli.)

- Identification of antigenic structure of 'H' antigens helps in serotyping of *Salmonella*.

Somatic 'O' Antigen

- It is heat-stable phospholipid-protein-polysaccharide complex, which is the integral part of cell wall (endotoxin).
- It is less immunogenic as compared to 'H' antigen hence antibodies against it following infection occur late and titers are low.
- It forms chalky granular, compact clumps.
- Agglutination takes place slowly at high temperature (50°–55°C).
- 'O' antigen is not a single factor, it is made up of many factors hence it may crossreact with other species.
- Identification of 'O' antigen is used for grouping of *Salmonella*.
- Treatment with trichloracetic acid extracts this antigen from bacteria. This was first shown by Boivin hence 'O' antigen is also called as **Boivin antigen.**

Vi Antigen

- Almost all recently isolated strains of *Salmonella typhi* have Vi antigen as a covering layer outside their cell wall.
- It is surface polysaccharide.
- Heat labile, resistant to alcohol and phenol.
- It causes trouble while performing agglutination from suspected colonies of *S. typhi* with its group specific antigen 'O' antisera. It renders organisms non-agglutinable with 'O' antiserum.
- Vi antigens can be removed by heating a suspension for 1 hour at 100°C. The suspension is without Vi and it forms visible agglutination with 'O' antisera.
- Similar Vi antigens have been found in some strains of *Paratyphi C*, Dublin, and *Citrobacter frundi*.
- Freshly isolated strains of *S. typhi* rich in 'Vi' antigen produce more opaque colonies.

Importance of Vi

1. It inhibits phagocytosis, resists complement activation and bacterial lysis.
2. Persistence of Vi antigen indicates carrier state.
3. It is poorly immunogenic, only low titers are produced following infection.
4. Detection of 'Vi' antibody is not helpful for diagnosis of typhoid fever hence 'Vi' is not included in Widal test.

5. Total absence of 'Vi' antibodies indicates poor prognosis in a proved case of typhoid fever. The antibody disappears in early convalescence. Its persistence indicates carrier stage.
6. 'Vi' antibodies are detected by coagglutination test. Titer more than 10 are considered significant. For this test, **Bhatnagar Strain** is used to prepare 'Vi' antigen.
7. 'Vi' antigen affords a method of **epidemiological typing** of *S. typhi* as phage typing is done by using **'Vi' bacteriophages.**

Fimbrial Antigen

- Only some isolates have fimbria. Hence, it is not important in diagnosis.
- Fimbrial antigens is nonspecific, it crossreacts with other becteria.
- Antigens used for widal test should be free from fimbria.

Antigenic Variations seen in S. typhi

1. **H-O variation:** It is seen when grown on 1:800 phenol agar.
2. **Phase variation:** Flagellar antigens occur in either phase I or II, generally any one phase predominates.
3. **V-W variation:** 'V' form agglutinates only with 'Vi' antisera, 'W' form only with 'O' antiserum (V-has Vi, W-does not have Vi)
4. **S-R variation:** It indicates loss of antigen and loss of virulence, prevented by culturing on Dorset's medium in cold; or by lyophilization.
5. **Variations in O antigen:** It may be caused by lysogenic phages.

Phase Variation

- Salmonella flagellar 'H' antigens occur in either of two phases. In phase I, antigens are either specific for the species or shared by only few species while **antigens in phase II** are widely shared hence called **nonspecific** or **group-specific phase.**
- Some strains possess both the phases, while *S. typhi* occurs in phase I only.
- A culture in phase I will be converted into phase II by growing oraginisms in presence of antiserum against phase I antigens. Craigie's tube is used for this conversion (Fig. 33.3).

H-O Variation (Phenotypic Variation)

When organism is grown on phenol agar, they loose flagella, i.e. 'H' form. This is a phenotypic change and reversible because if it is grown again on agar without phenol, flagella develop on bacterial cells.

Use of Craigies tube to obtain cells with many flagella (Fig. 33.3):

Craigie's tube consists of soft agar (0.2%) in first tube in which there is small tube which is opened at both the ends. The second tube slightly projects above the surface of agar.

The strain of *Salmonella* is inoculated in the inner tube and incubated. The highly flagellated strains are motile and they will travel the semisolid medium and will appear in outer tube. Multiflagellated forms will be obtained from growth on the surface of outer tube.

(For preparation of 'O' antigen of *Salmonella* for Widal test, a stable non-motile mutant *S. typhi* 901 is used).

V-W Variations (Phenotypic Variation)

'V' form is with presence of Vi antigen on the surface of cell of *Salmonella* while when it is lost either by heating or with the action of chemicals, organisms occur in 'W' phase.

S-R Variations

Due to mutation, smooth to rough variation occurs with change in the colony morphology from smooth to rough and it is associated with loss of 'O' antigens and virulence.

Variations in 'O' Antigens

It may be induced by lysogenic conversion, for example, *S. anatum* is converted into *S. newington* by one bacterio-phage.

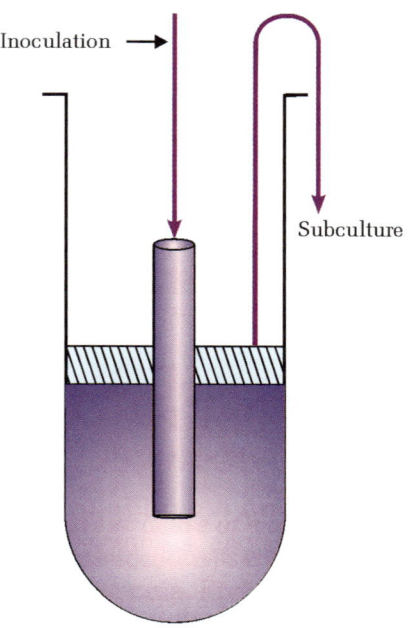

Fig. 33.3: Craigie's tube

Kaufmann–White Classification

This classification is based on antigenic structures of *Salmonella* species.

Grouping of Salmonella

Salmonella are **grouped on the basis of common, distinctive 'O' antigen.** For example *Salmonella paratyphi* **'B'** has antigenic structure of 'O' antigen as **1, 4, 12** while *S. chester* has **4, 5, 12** pattern of **'O'** antigen. *S. typhimurium* has pattern as **1, 4, 5, 12. As factor '4' is shared by all the three species,** they are grouped together in group **'B' or group with factor '4'.** Similarly *Salmonella* in group 'D' share common '9' or 'O' antigen factor.

Most of the clinical isolates of *Salmonella* species fall into group **A–G** (Flowchart 33.1).

Serotyping is based on identification of antigenic pattern of flagellar 'H' antigens.

The most important aspect of this classification is that it gives species status to serotype, e.g. if we identify serogroup and serotype as *S. typhi* based on common 'O' – factor 9 and 'H' antigen, we call the serotype *Salmonella typhi* as separate species. Table 33.2 gives the antigens used for serogrouping and serotyping of *Salmonella*.

Pathogenesis (Flowchart 33.2)

Mode of infection: Ingestion, source of infection is patient or carrier, incubation period 7–14 days. ID50 = $10^3 – 10^6$ bacilli. Infective dose is $10^3 – 10^6$; this variability reflects the ability of this organism to resist the acidic pH of stomach.

Flowchart 33.1: Identification of *Salmonella* serogroup and serotype

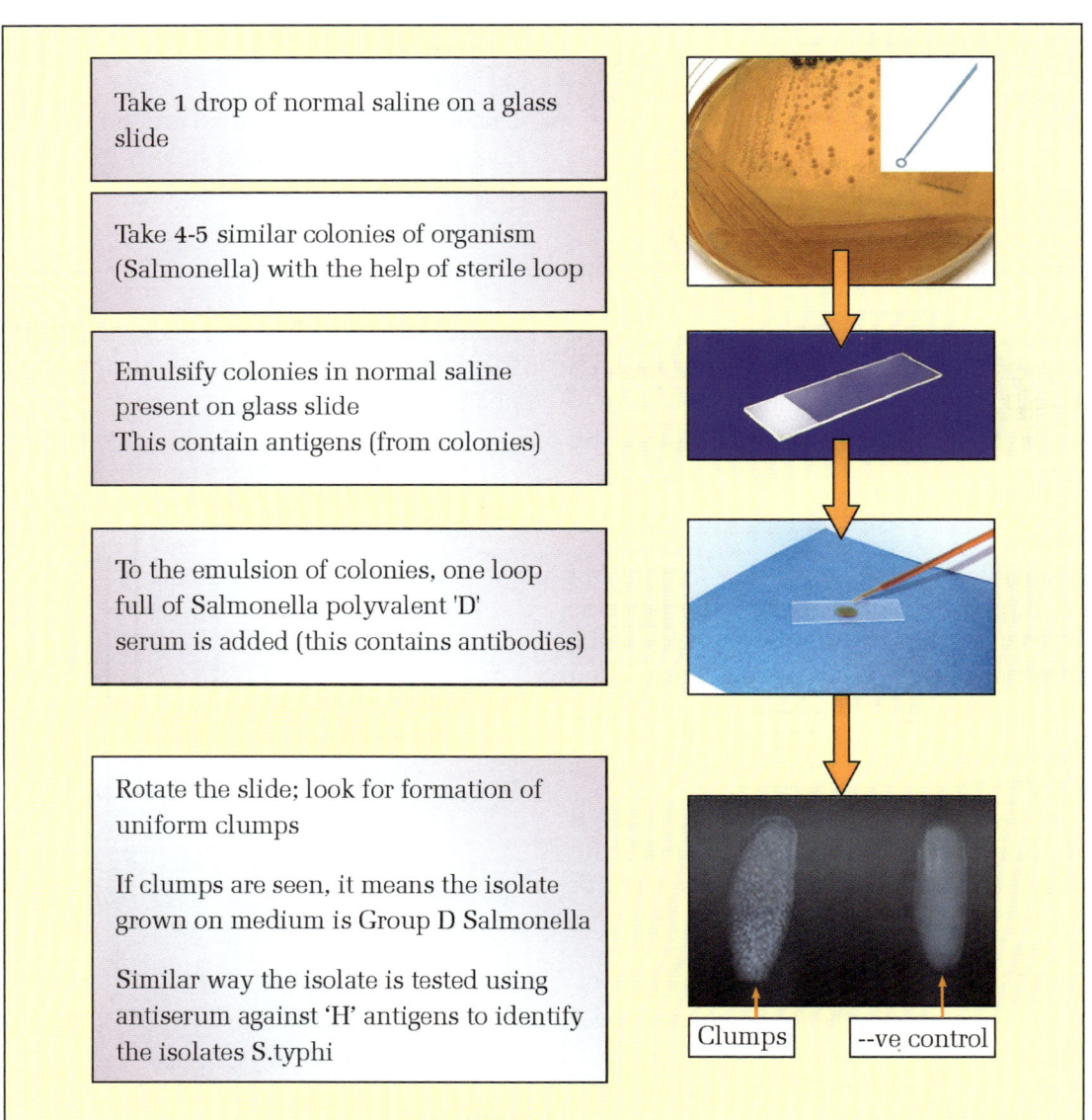

Take 1 drop of normal saline on a glass slide

Take 4-5 similar colonies of organism (Salmonella) with the help of sterile loop

Emulsify colonies in normal saline present on glass slide
This contain antigens (from colonies)

To the emulsion of colonies, one loop full of Salmonella polyvalent 'D' serum is added (this contains antibodies)

Rotate the slide; look for formation of uniform clumps

If clumps are seen, it means the isolate grown on medium is Group D Salmonella

Similar way the isolate is tested using antiserum against 'H' antigens to identify the isolates S.typhi

Clumps   --ve control

TABLE 33.2: Kauffmann–White scheme—examples

Serogroup	Serotype	O	H-phase I	H-phase II
2-A	S. paratyphi A	1, 2, 12	a	—
4-B	S. paratyphi B	1, 4, 5, 12	b	1, 2
	S. typhimurium	1, 4, 5, 12	i	1, 2
	S. chester	4, 5, 12	e, h	e, n, x
7-C1	S. paratyphi C	6, 7(vi)	c	1, 5
	S. choleraesuis	6, 7	c	1, 5
8-C2	S. muenchen	6, 8	d	1, 2
9-D	S. typhi	9, 12, (vi)	d	—
	S. enteritidis	1, 9, 12	g, m	—
	S. gallinarum	1, 9, 12	—	—
10-E1	S. anatum	3, 10	e, h	1, 6

Conditions that increase or decrease the susceptibility are:

- Conditions that decrease acidic pH—achlorhydric disease, antacids ingestion
- Conditions that break the integrity of mucosa
  - Inflammatory bowel disease
  - History of surgery
- Conditions that decrease the normal flora—by antibiotics

Pathogenicity (Flowchart 33.2)

- Various defense mechanisms of innate immunity which try to resist *Salmonella* are—bile salts, lysozyme, complement, cationic antimicrobial substances.
- The organism invades mucosa. Travel of organism is through 'M' cells which are phagocytic microfolds present in Peyer's patches.
- The organism induces formation of membrane muffles in epithelial cells. These muffles surround the bacteria within large vesicles. The process is called 'bacteria-mediated endocytosis'. The bacterial proteins mediate alteration in actin cytoskeleton which is required for uptake.
- The organisms lie within vesicles. They are resistant to liposomal contents and cryptins which are bactericidal peptides made by epithelial cells.
- The vesicles containing bacteria ultimately travel through basement membrane where they release organisms in lamina propria.
- Organisms are phagocytosed by macrophages so that they are protected from antibodies, complement and polymorphs.
- Bacteria are able to resist killing by macrophages, on the other hand they multiply inside the cells. This changes regulatory system of macrophages.

Flowchart 33.2: Pathogenesis of *Salmonella typhi*

- Environmental signals within macrophages trigger alteration of regulatory system of phagocytized bacteria.
- Bacteria get disseminated through infected macrophages and reach tissues having cells of reticuloendothelial system. Infection of liver, spleen, lymph nodes and bone marrow takes place. Secretions of macrophages under the influence of cytokines are responsible for signs and symptoms of the disease.
- Bacteria enter mesenteric nodes, and through thoracic duct, enter bloodstream. **First bacteremia** occurs which is of short duration, bacteria go the other organs as gallbladder, liver, spleen, bone marrow, lymph nodes, lungs, kidneys, where further multiplication occurs.
- **Second bacteremia** coincides with onset of clinical feature, i.e. high grade fever, headache.
- Multiplication of bacteria in gall bladder takes place as bacteria grow in bile. From gall bladder, bacteria are released in the intestine and infects Peyer's patches and other lymphoid tissue. Inflammation of intestinal mucosa is followed by necrosis of cells, and there is sloughing of mucosa producing ulcers. Ulcers may perforate and produce complications as hemorrhages. Lesions may heal in 3–4 weeks.

Clinical Features of Enteric (Typhoid) Fever

- Incubation period is 7 to 14 days, it varies with the dose of infection.
- Clinical presentation varies from undifferentiated pyrexia **(ambulant typhoid)** or severe fever.
- Gradual onset, anorexia, malaise, coated tongue, abdominal discomfort
- Step ladder fever
- Bradycardia (relative bradycardia)
- Soft palpable spleen, hepatomegaly
- 'Rose spots' – fade on pressure

Complications

- Intestinal perforation, hemorrhage
- Circulatory collapse, venous thrombosis, hemolytic anemia
- Bronchitis, bronchopneumonia
- Psychoses, deafness, meningitis
- Cholecystitis
- Abscess, arthritis, nephritis, peripheral neuritis
- Osteomyelitis

Epidemiology—Typhoid Fever (Enteric Fever)

Enteric fever is a global public health problem. Almost 80% of the cases and deaths are in Asia and the rest occur mostly in Africa and Latin America. It is estimated that there are 22 million new cases of enteric fever annually, with 200,000 deaths. Regions with the highest incidence of enteric fever (>100 cases per 100,000 persons per year) are South Central Asia and Southeast Asia. In India, the incidence of enteric fever is 9.8 cases per 1,000 person-years. *Salmonella enterica serovar typhi* and *paratyphi A* are the predominant types of etiological agents responsible for enteric fever in India, particularly during summer.

Due to safe water supply and environmental sanitation, typhoid fever in developed countries is controlled. Paratyphi-A is prevalent in India and Asian countries, Eastern Europe and South America. Paratyphi-B is common in Western Europe, Britain and North America while paratyphoid-C is seen in Eastern Europe and Guyana.

Source of infection: Cases and carriers act as source of infection.

Carriers may be convalescent carriers who shed bacteria in feces for 3 weeks to 3 months after clinical recovery.

Temporary carriers shed bacteria for 3 months to one year while **chronic carriers** shed bacteria for more than one year. Carriers may be fecal carrier or urinary carrier. Urinary carrier is associated with calculi or schistosomiasis.

If food handler becomes carriers, it is dangerous. One such example is of cook Mary Mallon (referred as typhoid Merry) contracted disease over 15 years with at least 7 outbreaks affecting 200 persons.

Laboratory Diagnosis (Fig.33.4)

a. *Isolation of bacteria, i.e. culture from these specimens*:
   - Blood culture
   - Urine culture
   - Stool culture
   - Bone marrow culture
   - Duodenal aspirate
   - Bile culture

b. *Demonstration of antibody*:
   - Widal test
   - CIE, ELISA, IHA

c. *Demonstration of antigen* by staphylococcal coagglutination test.

d. *Other tests*:
   - WBC count
   - Diazo test of urine

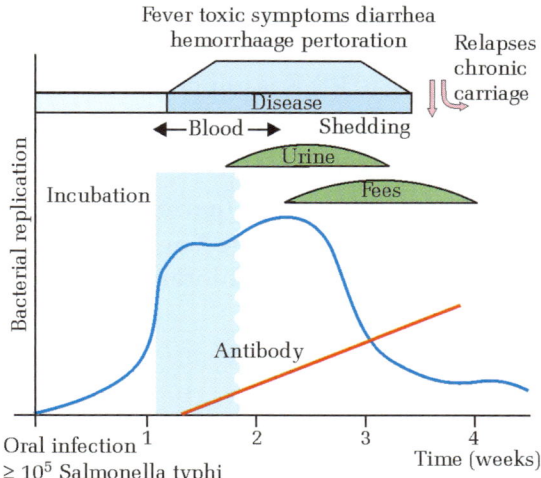

Fig. 33.4: Laboratory diagnosis of typhoid fever

Tests used for diagnosis and stage of infection and when they are used:

Blood culture	1st week
Antibodies (Widal test)	2nd week
Stool culture	3rd week
Urine culture	4th week

Blood Culture

Typhoid fever is septicemic illness. Blood culture is positive in 1st week of infection, also in 2nd, 3rd, weeks of infections. The positivity of blood culture is 90% in first week of fever, 75% cases in second week and 60% in 3rd week of intection and 25% thereafter till subsidence of fever.

Blood culture is the gold standard method of diagnosis of infection. It becomes rapidly negative after effective treatment.

Procedure of blood cuture: Under aseptic precautions 5–10 mL of blood is collected by venepuncture and directly inoculated in 50–100 mL blood culture media. The large volume dilutes the inhibitory substances present in blood. The blood culture media are then incubated at 37°C for 48 hours. After that, subculture is done on solid media, i.e. blood agar and MacConkey's medium. (As blood is normally sterile and it doesn't have commensal flora, selective media are not inoculated from blood culture bottles.)

Blood culture media
- Glucose broth and taurocholate broth
- Tryptic soy broth
- Brain heart infusion broth

Biphasic medium (Tryptic soy agar and tryptic soy broth). Blood is collected in this medium and initially the bottle is incubated in erect position for 48 hours. For subculture, only thing one need to do is tilt the medium so that broth flows over slant portion and automatically get inoculated. Colonies are observed on slant after overnight incubation in tilted position.

There are **advantages** of this biphasic medium. As both solid and liquid media are present in the same medium, **manipulations are avoided** which reduces the chances of contamination, also biphasic medium **minimizes the material.**

Clot Culture

5–10 mL of blood is collected in a sterile bottle. Blood is allowed to clot. To the bottle, sterile glass beads are added to break the clot.

Advantages of clot culture
- Serum becomes available for detection of antibodies in patients serum by Widal test. Even if the test is performed in 1st week of infection, as serum is available, we can determine the basic titer which can be compared with the repeat test.
- In the clot, organisms get trapped hence isolation rate from clot culture is more than blood culture.
- Duodenal aspirate is also recommended in the first week of infection especially if both blood culture and bone marrow cultures are negative.

Feces Culture

It is positive throughout course of disease and even in convalesence. Repeat sampling which increase the isolation rate is possible as this sample is easy to obtain. Use of enrichment (Selenite F) and selective media (Wilson-Blair or Salmonella-Shigella agar)are helpful in diagnosis.

Urine Culture
- It is positive in second and third week of disease. It is used for the for detection of carriers.
- Urine is centrifuged and deposit is used for culture.

Other Materials for Culture
- Bone marrow
- Bile or duodenal aspiration (for detection of carriers)
- Rose spots
- Pus
- CSF
- Sputum

Processing of Blood Cultures
- Blood culture bottles are incubated for 48 hours in incubator at 37°C and then subcultured on solid

media, blood agar and MacConkey's medium (nutrient agar may be added as agglutination of colonies is done from those grown on nutrient agar).

- Next day look for colony morphology, nonlactose fermenting colonies from MacConkey's medium are processed for biochemical test and antibiotic susceptibility testing.

Other semiautomated and automated blood culture systems are also in use.

Processing of Stool Culture

Microscopy: Look for pus cell and organism in Gram's stain, perform motility.

Enrichment of stool sample is done in **selenite broth or tetrathionate broth** which is incubated for 6–8 hours and plated on one of the selective media as SS agar, DCA, XLD. *S. typhi* will produce pink colonies with central blackening due to production of H_2S on XLD medium. (On MacConkey's medium—non-lactose fermenting colorless colonies are produced. Colourless colonies are produced on DCA.)

Identification of Cultures

Biochemical tests

- Catalase positive and oxidase negative, motile Gram-negative bacilli means it is member of family Enterobacteriaceae.
- Identification of the genus is done by IMViC tests, and decarboxylase test.
- Further identification is done by **agglutination test** which identifies the antigens of the isolate grown as colonies on solid media (Flowchart 33.1).

Agglutination

The colony which is identified as *Salmonella* is selected. The colony is emulsified in sterile saline, to the emulsion, group specific polyvalent antiserum, i.e. **group D antiserum** is added. The slide is gently rotated, if clumps are seen, it means test is positive and the organism is group 'D' *Salmonella*. Further identification of species as *Salmonella typhi* is done by agglutination with antiserum against flagellar antigen. (This agglutination test is based on **Kauffmann-White classification**).

Other antisera used for identification of other species are factor 2, factor 4 antisera which identify organisms as group A and group B which contains the species **S. paratyphi A** and **S. paratyphi B,** respectively. Final identification of these species is done by testing agglutination with antisera against flagella in both the phases.

For identification of unusual serotype, help of the National Salmonella Reference Centre at Central Research Institute (CRI) Kasauli may be taken.

The reference center for salmonellae of animal origin is located at the Indian Veterinary Institute, Izatnagar.

Antibiotic sensitivity testing (antibiogram)

The isolate of *S. typhi* is tested against cefotaxime, cefuroxime, ceroperazone, chloramphenicol, cipro-floxacin, nalidixic acid.

DETECTION OF ANTIBODIES

Widal Test

- It measures antibody to 'H' and 'O' antigens of *S. typhi*, 'H' antigens of *S. paratyphi A* and *S. paratyphi B*.
- Dreyer's conical bottom tube used for 'H' agglutination.
- Felix round bottom tube used for 'O' agglutination.

Method for Widal Test

Serial dilutions of patients sera (1; 25, 1; 50; 1; 100, 1; 200) are taken in glass tubes and equal volume of these dilutions taken, i.e. **0.5 mL** in each test tube.

$$\downarrow$$

Add equal volumes of 'H', 'O' AH and BH antigens

$$\downarrow$$

Incubated in water bath (37°C) overnight

$$\downarrow$$

Agglutination titres read

Interpretation of Widal Test

Before interpretation of Widal test, following **history** is taken which is relevant in interpretation of this test.

- *History of vaccination*: If there is history of recent vaccination, test will be positive with all antigens, i.e. *S. typhi* 'H' antigen, *S. typhi* 'O' antigen, *S. paratyphi A* 'H' antigen. If vaccine was taken by patient long back, due to immunological memory, the test may appear **false positive.**
- *History of duration of fever*: This is important as Widal test is positive only in **second week of fever**. If the test is performed earlier, it may give false negative results.
- History of any **other illness** to rule out anamnestic responses.
- History of previous Widal test done and its titer. If the test was also performed earlier we can compare the titers of the two tests. **Demonstration of rise in titers, fourfold** in the second test as compared to previous test is significant finding in favor of diagnosis of enteric fever. Antibodies appear only by end of first week.

- *Significant titers*: O1:100, H1:200.
- Antibodies may be present due to prior disease, inapparent infection or immunization.
- Anamnestic response may be seen during unrelated fever.
- Fimbria-free bacterial suspensions should be used as antigens.
- Early antibiotic treatment will show poor antibody response.
- If titer is more than the endemic titer test will be considered as significant.

Diagnosis of carriers is done by:
- Stool culture
- Bile culture
- Urine culture
- Vi antibody detection by tube agglutination test (significant titres 1:10), ELISA, CIE, RIA, IHA
- Sewer swab technique used to trace carriers.

Detection of Antigen

This test is done in only **first week** of infection, as antibodies appear in second week and the test becomes negative. Antigen is detected by coaglutination test, ELISA.

Newer Serological Tests

There is a need for a quick and reliable diagnostic test for typhoid fever as an alternative to the Widal test. Recent advances include:
- **IDL Tubex® test** can detect IgM antibodies from patients within a few minutes.
- **Typhidot®**, takes three hours to perform. It was developed in Malaysia for the detection of specific IgM and IgG antibodies against a 50 kD antigen of *S. typhi*.
- A newer version of the test, Typhidot-M®, was recently developed to detect specific IgM antibodies only. The dipstick test, developed in the Netherlands, is based on the binding of *S. typhi*-specific IgM antibodies in samples to *S. typhi* lipopolysaccharide (LPS) antigen and the staining of bound antibodies by an anti-human IgM antibody conjugated to colloidal dye particles.
- *IgM dipstick test*: The typhoid IgM dipstick assay is designed for the serodiagnosis of typhoid fever through the detection of *S. typhi*-specific IgM antibodies in serum or whole blood samples.

Phage typing is used to trace source of an epidemic and for epidemiological purposes.

National Phage Typing Centre is at Maulana Azad Medical College, New Delhi. Bacteriophage acting on Vi antigen (Vi phage II) made specific for a particular strain by serial cultures through that strain. Ninety seven Vi phage types of *S.typhi* are recognized. Phage **types A and E1 are most common in India.**

Other typing methods are biotyping, antibiogram, bacteriocin production.

SALMONELLA GASTROENTERITIS

Nontyphoidal Salmonellosis

- Common species are **S. typhimurim** and **S. enteritidis.**
- Some infections may be caused by other species as *S. heidenberg, S. cholera suis, S. dublin.*
- It is **zoonotic disease** hence animals act as source of infection.
- *Mode of transmission*: Ingestion of contaminated food products as eggs, poultry, dairy products.
- As they are more resistant to environmental conditions, they can cause outbreaks.
- They may be multiple drugs resistant. The practice of feeding cattle food along with antibiotic has led to drug resistance and its transfer to human beings.

Clinical Features

- **Gastroenteritis** after 6–48 hours of incubation period which presents as watery diarrhea, nausea, vomiting and cramps in abdomen.
- **Septicemia** with metastatic lesions.
- Endocarditis
- Arteritis
- *Abscesses*: Hepatic abscess, splenic abscess, cholecystitis, lung abscess, brain abscess.
- Urinary tract infection especially in patient with sickle cell disease. Pyelonephritis with cystitis occurs, if renal stones are present.
- Osteomyelitis
- *Genital infections*: Testicular abscess, ovarian abscess.
- Reiter's disease is reactive arthritis, seen in patients with HLA-B27.

Treatment

- Gastroenteritis is treated conservatively with fluid and electrolytes.
- Ciprofloxacin is given for severe gastroenteritis.
- Systemic infections are treated with ceftriaxone.

Drug resistance: Strains resistant to ampicillin, chloramphenicol, streptomycin, sulphonamides and tetracyclines are found. Also due to increased use of ciprofloxacin and ceftriaxone for treatment of MDR, strains of organisms have led to resistance to ceftriaxone by production of Amcβ lactamases and ciprofloxacin due to point mutation of gene of DNA gyrase.

Laboratory Diagnosis

- Isolation of *Salmonella* from feces
- Isolation from article of food

Control of *Salmonella* food poisoning is done by prevention of food contamination.

Treatment is symptomatic in uncomplicated, non-invasive salmonellosis. Antibiotics should be used for serious invasive cases.

Septicemia: *Cholera-suis* causes septicemic disease with focal suppurative lesions like osteomyelitis, deep abscess, endocarditis, pneumonia and meningitis.

Gastroenteritis may or may not be present. Case fatality is up to 25%.

Carriers in Salmonella

Carrier is a person shedding the organisms without clinical disease.

- Convalescent carrier is a patient recovered from the disease and shedding organisms in feces.
- Temporary carriers shed organisms for 6 months.
- Chronic carriers shed organisms for more than 6 months.
- Carriers harbor bacilli in gallbladder and kidney. Based on these carriers may be urinary carriers or fecal carriers.
- Carriers in *S. typhi* are **diagnosed by bile culture, urine cultures, detection of Vi antibodies by staphylococcal coagglutination test**.
- Food handlers who are carriers are an important source of infection (e.g. typhoid Mary transmitted many epidemics).

S. paratyphi-B can infect dogs or cows; animals can be a source of infection.

Typhoid Vaccines

- *Heat-killed vaccine*: It is inactivated by phenol. It is whole cell vaccine which may be monovalent or bivalent or trivalent (TAB). It is given by subcutaneous route and immunity lasts for short period of 3 years, after which boosters are necessary.
- **Ty21a vaccine (typhoral/vaccine):** It is live vaccine prepared from stable mutant of *S. typhi* lacking UDP-galactose-4-epimerase. (GalE mutant). The vaccine strain multiplies for sometime, produces immune response and self destructs after 4–5 divisions. Vaccine is available in lyophilized form as enteric-coated capsules. Vaccine is given before food on days—1, 3, 5 and 1 or 7. No antibiotics are given during this period. It gives protection for 3 years after which boosters are recommonded. The vaccine is recommended to travellers.
- *Typhim-Vi (ViCPS)*: It is purified Vi antigen which can be given subcutaneously or intramuscularly. *S. typhi* Ty2 strain is used for vaccination. Single dose containing 25 µg of antigen is given IM or sub-cutanously. Vaccine is given only after 2 years of age. Vaccine gives protection for 2 years. The vaccine is recommended to travellers.
- *Vi–rEPA*: The Vi polysaccharide is conjugated with nontoxic recombinant protein similar to *Pseudomonas* exotoxin A.

Treatment

Ampicillin, and cotrimoxazole were the effective drugs but because of **drug resistance,** extended cephalo-sporins and fluoroquinolones as ciprofloxacin are suitable. For most of infections, the drugs of choice are ciprofloxacin and ceftriaxone.

NARST (nalidixic acid resistant *Salmonella typhi*) will not respond to ciprofloxacin or norfloxacin. The resistance is due to point mutation in **DNAgyrase gyr A and B**. Ceftriaxone, and azithromycin are antibiotics used against NARST. (Amc – beta-lactamases are also detected in *S. typhi*.)

MDR

Multiple drug resistance is transferred through 'R'. plasmids such as MDR strains were given along with animal feeds. MDR strains are then transferred from animal to human beings.

Treatment for carriers inludes ampicillin or cipro-floxacin with or without cholecystectomy.

TABLE 33.3: Biochemical reactions of *S. typhi, S. paratyphi*, A, B, C

	G	M	L	S	Indole	Citrate	MR	VP	H2S	X	D-tartarate	Mucate
S. typhi	A	A	—	—	—	—	+	—	+	d	A	d
S. paratyphi A	AG	AG	—	—	–	—	+	—	—	—	—	—
S. paratyphi B	AG	AG	—	–	—	+	+	—	+	AG	—	AG
S. paratyphi C	AG	AG	–	–	—	+	+	—	+	AG	AG	—

G = glucose, M = mannitol, L = lactose, X = xylose, A = acid, AG = acid and gas, d = variable

34

Shigella
(Common Cause of Bacillary Dysentery)

DYSENTERY

Shigellae cause in human a disabling disease known as **bacillary dysentery (Gr. dysenteron, sick gut).** Passage of loose motions along with blood and mucus in stool sample and patient has pain in abdomen and tenesmus.

It differs from diarrhea:
- In diarrhea, there is no blood and mucus in stool sample.
- Pus cells are scanty or absent in diarrhea which are present in dysentery.
- Also tenesmus is absent in diarrhea which is there in dysentery.
- Usually, those organisms which **infect large intestine** and cause disease due to invasion are responsible for **presence of mucus and pus cell** in stool sample while those **infect small intestine** produce diarrhea due to production of exotoxin and not by invasion. Hence there is **watery diarrhea**.

Organisms causing dysentery:

Bacteria
- *Shigella*
- *EIEC*
- *Vibrio parahaemolyticus*
- *Campylobacter*
- *Yersenia entrocolitica*

Parasites
- *Entamoeba histolytica*
- *Balantidium coli*
- *Trichuris trichuria*
- *Few Schistosomes*

SHIGELLA

Shigella is named after 'Shiga' who isolated first member of the genus.

Morphology

- They are short Gram-negative bacilli.
- *Size*: 0.6 μm × 2–4 μm.
- **Non-motile**, non-sporing, non-capsulated.
- Fimbriae may be present (only in *Shigella flexneri* some strains other than 6).

Cultural Characteristics

- Aerobes and facultative anaerobes.
- Temperature range 10–40°C (optimum 37°C), optimum pH 7.4.
- It grows on ordinary media, showing small (2 mm), circular, convex, smooth, translucent, grayish colonies.
- It produces NLF pale colonies on MacConkey agar except *Shigella sonnei* which is late lactose fermenter (Fig. 34.1).

Selective Media

- *XLD agar*: Red-colored colonies are produced by *Shigella*, it is the best medium for *Shigella* (Fig. 34.2).

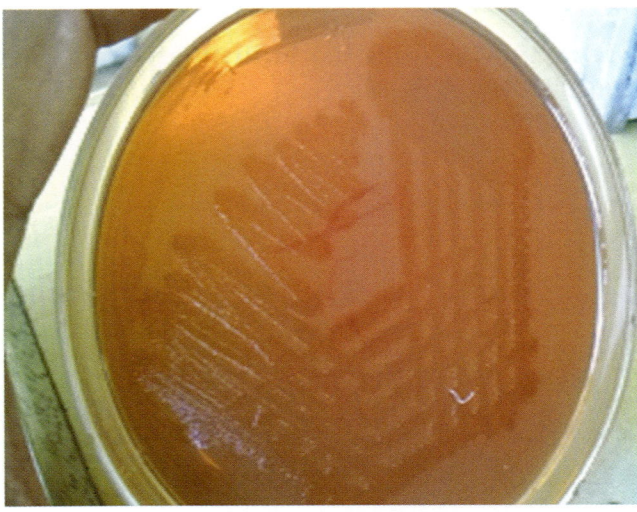

Fig. 34.1: MacConkey's agar showing NLF colonies

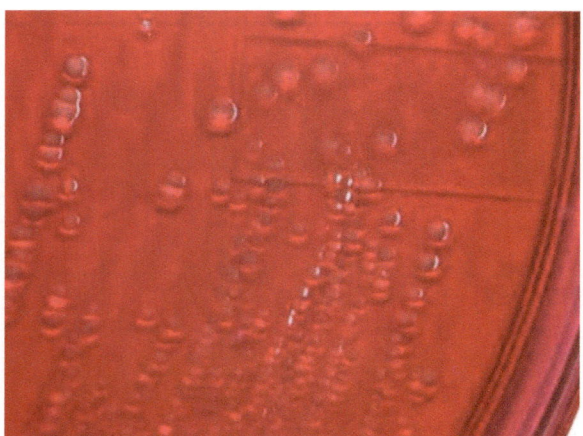

Fig. 34.2: XLD medium shaving red colories

- *Salmonella Shigella agar*: This medium contains high concentration of bile salts, lactose, neutral red as indicator and one more indicator for H$_2$S; pale colorless colonies are produced.
- *DCA*: Non-lactose fermenting colorless colonies are produced by *Shigella* on DCA. (*Shigella sonnei* is late lactose fermenter and may produce pink colonies after 24 hours of incubation. Colonies are more translucent than *Salmonella*.)
- *Hekton-enteric (HE) agar*: It is a selective medium, colonies of Shigella appear green and the colour fades towards periphery.

Liquid Media

Peptone water, and *glucose broth*: They produce uniform turbidity, piliated strains form pellicle.

Enrichment Media

- **Selenite F** (sodium selenite F' inhibits normal flora of gut, F-stands for feces) enrich *Shigella sonnei* and *Shigella flexneri* serotype 6, but inhibitory to other shigellae.
- **Tetrathionate broth** and **brilliant green** broth are unsuitable for *Shigella*.

- **Gram-negative broth** (inhibits Gram-positive bacilli and comparatively less inhibitory to other Gram-negative bacilli) is used.

Resistance

It is killed at 56°C in 1 hour and by 1% phenol in 30 minutes. It remains live for 1–6 months in ice. It dies rapidly on drying. It dies in few hours in faeces. *Sh. sonnei* is more resistant than other species.

Antigenic Structure

It is simple, compared to complicated structure of *Salmonella*, there is considerable antigenic sharing between Shigellae and *E. coli*. Fimbrial antigens may be present. *Shigella* has major antigens and large number of minor somatic 'O' antigens. Identification must be made by combination of antigenic and biochemical properties.

Biochemical Tests (Table 34.1)

- Catalase positive **except** *shigella flexneri* type 1
- Oxidase negative.
- Reduce nitrates to nitrites.
- IMViC: v+– – (variable, positive, negative, negative).
- Indole: *Shigella flexneri* serotype 6, *Shigella dysenteriae* serotype 1 and *Shigella sonnei* are always indole negative. Strains of other serotypes differ.
- Glucose is fermented with acid and without gas except Manchester, New castle biotypes of *S. flexneri* and some strains of *S. boydi* 14 and 15.
- *Decarboxylase test*: Members of A, B, C fail to decaroxylase lysine, ornithine.
- H$_2$S negative.
- PPA negative.
- Mannitol fermented by all except *Shigella dysenteriae*, this test helps to classify shigella.
- Lactose is not fermented (*S. sonnei* ferments it late).

TABLE 34.1: Biochemical tests of Shigella species

Subgroup	Fermentation of				Indole	Lysine decarboxylase	Ornithine decarboxylase	Serotype
	L	M	S	D				
Sh. dysenteriae	–	–	–	–	d	–	–	15
Sh. flexneri	–	A	–	–	d	–	–	6 + 2 varients
Sh. boydii	–	A	–	d	d	–	–	19
Sh. sonnei	A #	A	A #	–	–	–	+	1

A = Acid, d = variable, # = Late lactose fermenter, L = Lactose, M = Mannitol, S = Sucrose, D = Dulcitol

Classification of Shigella

Four species (subgroups) based on biochemical and serological characteristics are:

- *Sh. dysenteriae*
- *Sh. flexneri*
- *Sh. boydii*
- *Sh. sonnei*

Serotypes and biotypes distinguished within the species. Colicin typing is done for *Sh. sonnei*.

Shigella Dysenteriae—Subgroup A

Bacteria in this subgroup show following characteristics:

- Mannitol fermentation negative.
- This group consists of 15 serotypes.
- Type 1 (**Sh. shigae**) is always catalase negative, indole negative.
- *Sh. dysenteriae* type 1 forms a toxin—Shiga toxin.
- *Sh. dysenteriae* type 2 (previously called *S. schmitzi*) forms indole.
- Types 3–7 form Large-Sachs group.

Shigella Flexneri—Subgroup B

- Classified into 6 serotypes.

- There are several subtypes (1a, 1b, 2a, 2b, 3a, 3b, 3c, 4a, 4b, 5a, 5b). In addition, two antigenic 'variants' called 'X' and 'Y' are present which lack type-specific antigens.
- Serotype 6 is always indole negative, occurs in 3 biotypes of which Manchester and Newcastle biotypes produce gas from glucose (while *Shigella boydii* doesn't).
- *Sh. flexneri* type 2a produces enterotoxin ET-1; ET-2 is more widespread.

Shigella Boydii—Subgroup C

- It resemble *Sh. flexneri* biochemically but not antigenically.
- Nineteen serotypes identified.
- It is least frequently isolated from cases of dysentery.

Shigella Sonnei—Subgroup D

- It is indole negative, ferments lactose and sucrose late.
- Antigenically homogeneous, may occur in 2 phases (phase I and phase II).
- It causes mildest form of bacillary dysentery.

Flowchart 34.1: Pathogenic mechanisms of *Shigella*

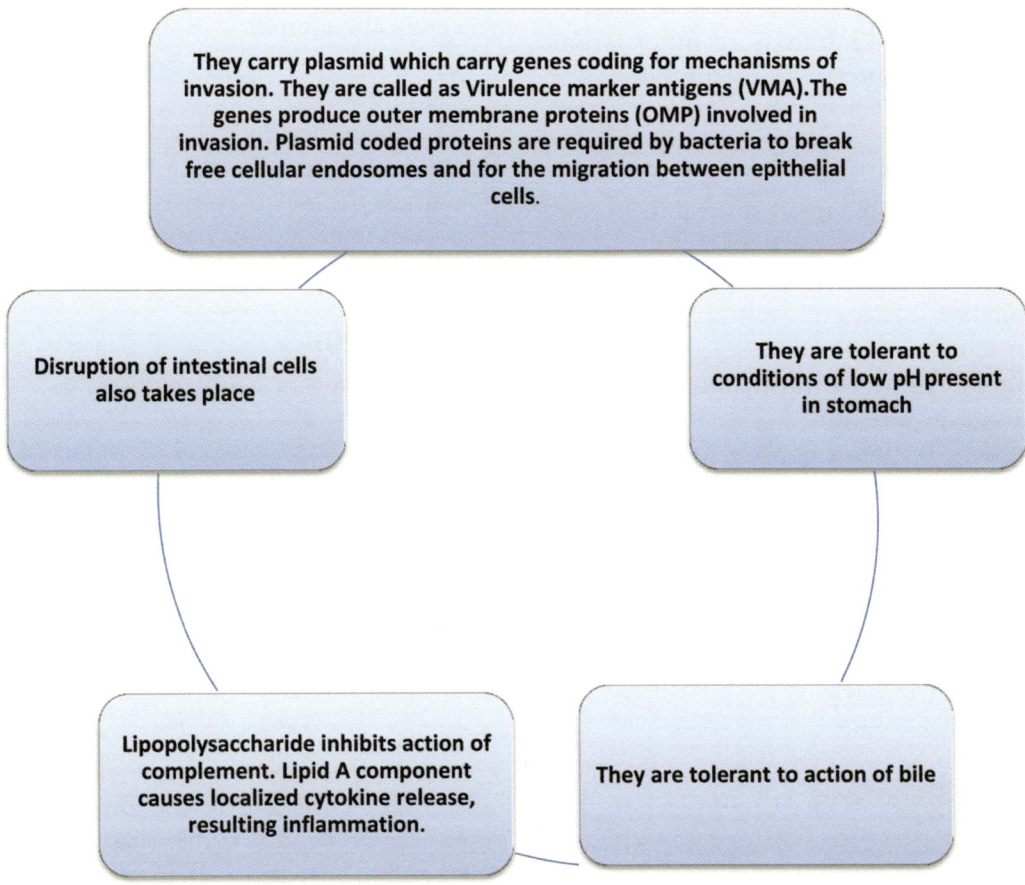

They carry plasmid which carry genes coding for mechanisms of invasion. They are called as Virulence marker antigens (VMA). The genes produce outer membrane proteins (OMP) involved in invasion. Plasmid coded proteins are required by bacteria to break free cellular endosomes and for the migration between epithelial cells.

Disruption of intestinal cells also takes place

They are tolerant to conditions of low pH present in stomach

Lipopolysaccharide inhibits action of complement. Lipid A component causes localized cytokine release, resulting inflammation.

They are tolerant to action of bile

Pathogenicity of Shigellosis

Infection by ingestion, infective dose low, 10–100 bacilli

↓

Bacilli multiply in epithelial cells of large intestinal villi

↓

Spread laterally to adjacent cells and penetrate into lamina propria

↓

Inflammatory reaction, capillary thrombosis occurs

↓

Slough off

↓

Transverse superficial ulcers are formed

Enterotoxins

Shigella enterotoxin (ShET-1 and ShET-2)

ShET-1 is found in *S. flexnei* 2a and it is similar to cholera toxin.

ShET-2 is present in all *S. flexneri* isolates.

Shiga toxin which is a cytotoxin produced by *S. dysenteriae* type 1. It is similar to verotoxin of EHEC. It inhibits protein synthesis by inhibiting 60s ribosome. It causes local vascular damage in intestine and internal organs as kidney and brain.

Endotoxin: It is similar to endotoxin of other Gram-negative bacilli. It causes intestinal inflammation and ulceration.

Virulence Marker Antigen (VMA)

- Outer membrane proteins are responsible for cell penetration and invasive property of bacillus.
- They are coded for by large **plasmids (VMA—virulence marker antigens which are outer membrane proteins).**
- Invasive property is more important for patho-genesis than toxin production.
- Invasive property is demonstrated by ability to penetrate cultured HeLa or Hep-2 cells or by Congo red binding test, or by detection of VMA by **ELISA.**

Fermentation of:		
Biotype	Glucose	Mannitol
Boyd 88	Acid	Acid
Manchester	Acid and gas	Acid and gas
Newcastle	A or A and gas	—

Clinical Features of Shigellosis

It presents as transient fever, watery diarrhea or dysentery or it may be asymptomatic.

Incubation period is 1–7 days, usually 48 hours. There is passage of loose, scanty feces with blood and mucus; abdominal cramps, tenesmus; fever and vomiting may be present.

The whole spectrum of disease ranging from mild disease to severe dysentery is called **Shigellosis.** Severity of illness varies with serotype involved. Infection with serotype *S. dysenteriae* type I is serious in which prostration is marked and young children may have convulsions. *S. flexneri* and *S. boydii* may couse severe illness. Illness due to *S. sonnei* is mild disease with few loose motions and vague abdominal discomfort.

Complications

Disease starts with few loose motions, watery diarrhea, anorexia and vomiting. It is followed by bloody, mucopurulent stools. There is increased tenesmus and abdominal cramps **(dysentery)**. Oedematous hemorr-hagic mucosa along with ulcerations covered with exudates is the common presentation.

- Toxic megacolon, perforation, rectal prolapse are the surgical complications.
- Metabolic disturbances include hypoglycemia, hyponanatremia and dehydration.
- *Toxic encephalopathy (Ekiri syndrome)*: Its manifes-tations are altered sensorial, seizures, delirium, and cerebral oedema.
- Bacteremia is rare, may lead to septicemia, meningitis.
- Keratoconjunctivitis.
- **Reactive arthritis**: People with **HLA-B27** infected with *S. flexneri* may develop this syndrome, which is characterized by ocular inflammation, urethritis and reactive arthritis.

Epidemiology

Shigellosis is associated with wars, lack of sanitation and poverty.

Human beings, cases or carriers, are the only source of infection.

Modes of Transmission-(6F)

- Fomites
- Fingers
- Food
- Flies
- Feces

Feces contaminating food is the commonest mode of spread. Direct infection through fomites; water, contaminated food or drink, mechanical vectors, e.g. flies cause infection. It may occur in young male homosexuals as part of the gay bowel syndrome. In India, *Sh. sonnei*, followed by *Sh. dysenteriae* are the predominant species. Recently, *Sh. dysenteriae type 1* has emerged important cause of dysentery.

Entry, spread, multiplication

- Shigella is somewhat resistant to acidic environment during stationary phase of their growth and multiplication.
- Organisms resist acids but they are less capable of invading cells. When they rich intestine they again grow. At this point, their property to resist acids is repressed and invasive property is also restored.
- Other organisms present in intestine produce anaerobic conditions which are suitable for Shigella to resist acidic conditions.
- Bacteria multiply in the intercellular spaces of intestinal epithelial cells. Invasion involves many genes present on virulence plasmids (VMA or invasion plasmid antigens or IpaB, C, D) and chromosomes.
- Bacteria enter lamina propria. Macrophages engulf bacteria, release IL-1. IL-1 cause inflammation, which invites neutrophils.
- Epithelial cells do not have phagocytic function. The entry of bacteria is mediated by reorganization of actin and cytoskeleton elements similar to those occur in phagocytosis.
- Once bacteria enter epithelial cells, they escape phago-lysosomal vacuoles assisted by bacterial protein which lyses phagosomal membrane. Bacteria enter cytoplasm where they multiply.
- Infected epithelial cell when come in contact with uninfected cell, lysis of cell membrane takes place and cell to cell spread takes place.

Pathogenic mechanisms (Fig. 34.3): Shigella have many pathogenic mechanisms

i. They are tolerant to conditions of low pH of stomach and action of bile.
ii. Plasmid which code for genes responsible for invasiveness are observed in pathogenic strains of Shigella. These genes help bacteria to become free from cellular endosome. These genes are also responsible for spread of bacteria from one cell to other.
iii. LPS prevents action of complement.
iv. Lipid A causes cytokine release leading to inflammation, cellular dysruption so that bacteria enter epithelial cells.
v. Absess breaks down to form ulcer.

Damage: When sufficient number of contagious cells die and slough off, the result is surface erosion in gut wall, the ulcer. The neutrophils that accumulate are shed in feces, where they are detected by microscopy.

The blood and pus containing stools and pain associated with bowel movement (tenesmus) are characteristics of Shigella dysentery.

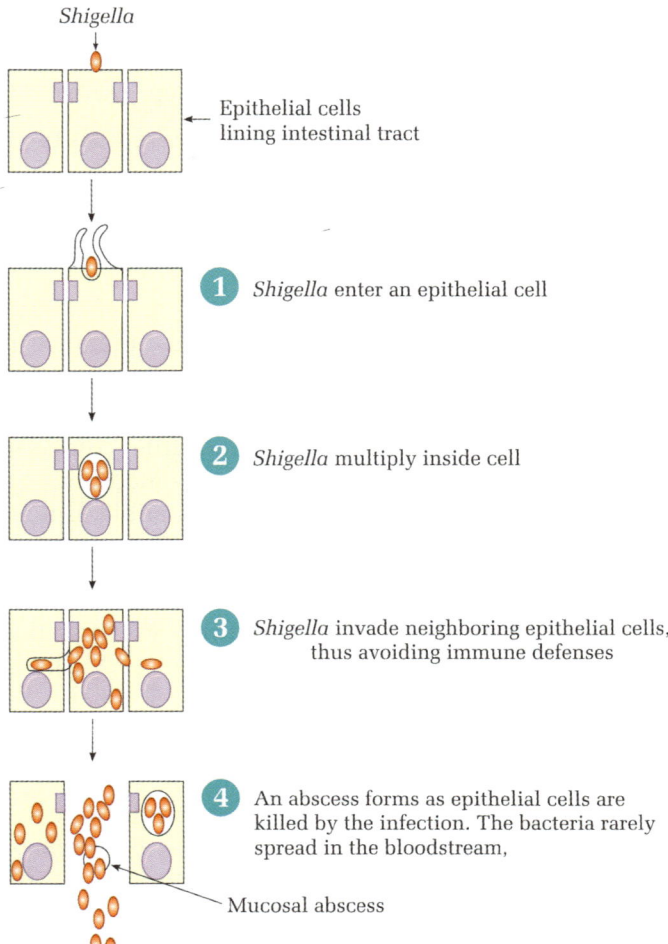

Shigella

Epithelial cells lining intestinal tract

1 *Shigella* enter an epithelial cell

2 *Shigella* multiply inside cell

3 *Shigella* invade neighboring epithelial cells, thus avoiding immune defenses

4 An abscess forms as epithelial cells are killed by the infection. The bacteria rarely spread in the bloodstream,

Mucosal abscess

Fig. 34.3: Pathogenesis of *Shigella*

Despite of invasion, bacteremia is uncommon in *Shigella* except for *Shigella dysentery type*-infection. **Bacteremia** is common in malnourished children in developing countries. ***Shigella dysenteriae* type 1 produces Shiga toxin, which is a cytotoxin** that kills intestinal epithelial cells and endothelial cells. This toxin cleaves mammalian 60S ribosomal subunit; thereby stopping protein synthesis. The action of toxin has two effects. Targeting sodium-absorptive villus cell and decreasing sodium absorption, which leads to excess of fluid in lumen. Second effect is on mucosal endothelial cells which contributes to bloody diarrhea.

It is highly contagious, spread by feco-oral route. Cases and carriers act as source of infection. They first contaminate their hands while cleansing at toilet, then they may contaminate flush handle, door knobs, washbasin taps and other objects when handled by other person, allows transfer of bacteria. Bacilli are also liberated into air when an infective dose is flushed from toilet and after settling down on surface of toilet sit, surrounding survives for some days.

Laboratory Diagnosis of Shigellosis

Diagnosis is done by isolating Shigella from feces. Fresh feces should be cultured (swabs not satisfactory).

Transport medium used is Sachs buffered glycerol saline.

Gross examination: Stool appears blood stained.

Wet mount: It shows pus cells, many RBCs, macrophages.

Gram's stain: Plenty of pus cells and predominance of Gram-negative bacilli will be seen.

Mucus flakes inoculated on **MacConkey, DCA, and XLD** media and hepatoenteric medium—colorless colonies are produced on MacConkey's medium and DCA, while a **pink** colony without central blackening is seen on **XLD** and **green colonies on HE agar.**

Enrichment media: Less inhibitory Gram-negative (GN) broth or nutrient broth are cultured which after 6–8 hours of enrichment subcultured on DCA or XLD.

Processing of colonies: NLF colonies which are catalase positive (*except S. dysenteriae* biotype-1), oxidase negative, nitrates reduced to nitrites, indole test variable depending upon species, MR-positive, citrate-positive, TSI-K/A without H$_2$S and without gas except few biotypes of *S. flexneri* type 6, (New Castle, Manchester and Boyd) non-motile, urease, citrate, H$_2$S and KCN negative.

Slide Agglutination with Polyvalent Antiserum

If the organism is possible *Shigella,* carry out agglutination on bacterial suspension in following order:

- *S. sonnei* (form 1 and 2) serum on one-half of a slide; test suspension without serum on the other half of slide to exclude autoagglutinability in saline. If agglutination positive no further testing is required.
- If negative, test with *S. flexneri* polyvalent antiserum. If positive, test with *S. flexneri* types 1–6, X and Y. If negative, test with *S. boydii* polyvalent antiserum.
- *Shigella dysenteriae* is polyvalent antiserum.

Recent Methods for Diagnosis of Shigella

1. PCR is available targeting gene encoding **invasion plasmid antigen H (ipaH) or VMA.**
2. Gene for shigella enterotoxin 2 can be detected with shET-2PCR.
3. Detection of antibodies against LPS antigen.
4. DNA-array based assay is developed against known serotypes.

Antibiogram: Suphonamide, chloramphenicol, tetracycline, streptomycin, neomycin are recommended.

Treatment and Control

The infection is usually self-limited. Correction of dehydration is important.

Antibiotics should be limited to severe or toxic cases, extremes of age, severely debilitated cases. 'R' plasmid mediated drug resistance was first detected in Shigella. Ciprofloxacin is the antibiotic of choice. Alternate drugs are ceftriaxone, azithromycin and newer generation of quinolones. Treatment is given for 3 days except for *Sh. dysenterae,* it is given for 5 days.

35

Pseudomonas

They are mostly saprophytic, found in water, soil, etc.

They are resistant to common disinfectants and also show resistance to multiple antibiotics. They are predominant organisms causing hospital acquired infections.

The reasons why *Pseudomonas aeruginosa* is emerging as predominant opportunistic pathogen causing hospital-acquired infections are:

I. It has minimum growth requirement. Minimum moisture is sufficient for its growth.
II. Its adaptability.
III. It has many virulence factors.
IV. It is resistant to many disinfectants, hence can grow inside the disinfectants.
V. It is also resistant to many commonly used antibiotics.
VI. More and more patients with decreased immunity, due to age or immunocompromised conditions are admitted in hospitals.

Morphology

- They are Gram-negative bacilli.
- *Size*: 1.5–3 μm × 0.5 μm.
- Actively motile by polar flagellum.
- Bacilli are non-sporing non-capsulated but many strains have a mucoid slime layer.

Mucoid strains have abundance of extracellular polysaccharides composed of alginate polymers. It forms loose capsule which protect bacilli from host defenses. Alginate is different from slime, it is a heterogenous mixture of hexoses produced on prolonged incubation in media with high carbon, low nitrogen.

Cultural Characteristics

- It is an obligate aerobe, can grow anaerobically, if nitrate is available.

- Growth temperature range 6–42°C (optimum—37°C).
- It grows on ordinary media produces large opaque, irregular colonies with a distinctive, musty, mawkish or **earthy smell or grape-like smell (due to production of acetoaminophen),** and **produces diffusible bluish green or greenish yellow pigment**. Pigment may be seen on antibacterial susceptibility testing medium.
- After aerobic incubation on nutrient agar at 37°C for 25 hours, six distinct colony types may be produced.
1. Type I, it is most common, colonies are large, low convex, rough in appearance, often oval with long axis in the line of the inoculum streak, sometimes they are surrounded by a serrated growth.
2. Type II colonies are small, dome-shaped, smooth.
3. Type III is small, rough.
4. Type IV is small, rugose.
5. Type V is mucoid alginate producing, which may even drip into the lid of petri dish.
6. The type VI is drawf, small, mucoid.
   - *Nutrient agar*: Iridescent patches with metallic sheen may be seen. Crystals are seen beneath the patches.
   - *MacConkey's agar*: It forms non-lactose fermenting (NLF) colonies.
   - *Blood agar*: β hemolysis present.
   - *Pseudomonas isolation agar* (Difco) is a selective medium. It contains pigment enhancing component and selective agent, irgasen.
   - *King's medium* is also used for enhancement of pigment.
   - *Broth*: It forms dense turbidity with surface pellicle in liquid medium.
   - *Centrimide agar* is used as selective medium.
     - *Peptone water*: Surface pellicle is seen (due to O$_2$ tension at the surface).

Pigments Produced (Fig.35.1)

They are pyocyanin (bluish green phenazine pigment), pyoverdin (yellowish green), pyomelanin (black), pyorubrin (red). Pyocyanin is soluble in water and chloroform and produced by only *Pseudomonas*, pyoverdin is soluble in water not in chloroform.

Biochemical Reactions

- Glucose utilized oxidatively—forms acid only (it is non-fermenter).
- Nitrates reduced to nitrites and further to gaseous nitrogen.
- Catalase, oxidase, arginine dehydrolase—positive.
- **Indole, MR, VP, H_2S tests are negative.**
- **TSI:** It shows no change.

Resistance

To common antiseptics and disinfectants like quaternary ammonium compounds, chloroxylenol and hexachlorophane. It is sensitive to acids, glutaraldehyde, silver salts and strong phenolic disinfectants.

It shows inert in biochemical reactions.

The **API 20E** can used for biochemical characterization.

Virulence Factors

Alginate, pili, neuraminidase, lipopolysaccharide, phospholipidase, proteases, exotoxin, enterotoxin, elastase, leukocidin, and pyocyanins are virulence factors.

Pathogenicity (Box 34.1)

Pseudomonas commonly causes hospital-acquired infections.
- Infections—wounds, bedsores, infection of eye, burns. Blue pus is produced.
- Urinary tract infections following catheterization.
- Iatrogenic meningitis following lumbar puncture.

> **Box 34.1:** Pathogenesis of *Pseudomonas aeruginosa*
>
> - To cause disease, *P. aeruginosa* must attach to human tissue and get established.
> - It shows two distinct modes of motility, flagella-mediated motility, whereby the organisms swim, and a second system of twitching motility which is due to extension and retraction of organism's polar flagellum.
> - Flagella and pili mediate attachment. This capability is the result of their interactions with the glycolipid asialo GM1 on host cell surface.
> - Flagella also interact with toll-like receptor, TLR5, initiating inflammation.
> - Type IV pili are important for formation of biofilms. Biofilms help in attachment and cells in biofilms avoid cells reorganization by immune cells.
> - Alginate can act as adhesion and it is also important component of biofilm of Pseudomonas.

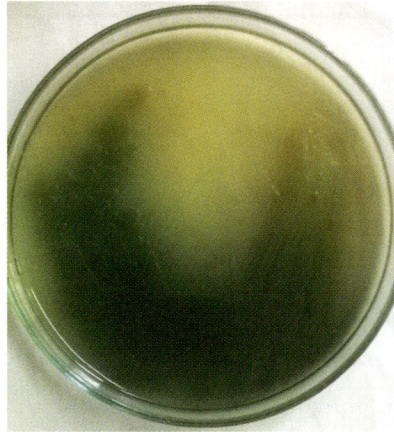

Fig. 35.1: Pigmented Pseudomonas on NA

- Post-tracheostomy pulmonary infections. Ventilation associated pneumonia (VAP)
- Septicemia and endocarditis in debilitated persons.
- Ecthyma gangrenosum and other skin lesions in malignancy.

Green nail syndrome caused by *Pseudomonas* is **paronychia** (inflammation of tissues adjacent to nail with discharge of green pus. Prolonged submersion of hands in water acts as predisposing factor.
- Infection of nail bed following exposure of hands to detergents and water.
- Infantile diarrhea and sepsis.
- Shanghai fever (self-limiting febrile illness like typhoid fever).
- The reasons why *Pseudomonas* is predominant bacterium causing hospital-acquired infections are:
  1. Its adaptability.
  2. It is innately resistant to common disinfectants.
  3. It has many virulence factors.
  4. Number of patients with immunosuppression are increasing.

It is resistant to common antibiotics and antiseptics. Respirators, endoscopes, bedpans, medicines like lotions, ointments, eyedrops, and stocks of distilled water, plants, and flowers may be contaminated with *Pseudomonas* and act as source of infections.

Ear infections in deep sea drivers (swimmer's itch) or it may be recreational as in cases of **whirlpool-associated (Jacuzzi) rash. Malignant otitis externa** may develop which is painful. Pseudomonas is most feared cause of corneal infection following use of contact lenses.

Panophthalmitis following **cataract operations** has been reported in many hospitals across India.

Native valve endocarditis and septicemia may occur in patients compromised by burns, cancer or drug addicts.

TABLE 35.1: Putative virulence factors of *Pseudomonas*

Pili or fimbria	Attachment to epithelial cells
Elastase	Destruction of elastic tissue including that of lamina of blood vessels
Phospholipase C	Breaks lecithin and lipids, causes tissue necrosis, cause hemorrhagic lesion in skin infections and destruction of corneal tissue
Alkaline phosphatase	Tissue breakdown, proteolysis of immunoglobulins and complement
Lipopolysaccharide	Fever, leukopenia, hypotension, shock, adults respiratory distress
Exotoxins A	Inhibition of protein synthesis
Exo-S	Distruction of cellular actin cyto-skeleton
Exo-T	Distruption of cellular actin cyto-skeleton
Exo-U	Acute cytotoxicity
Exo-Y	Increase in intracellular cyclic-AMP

Commonest community-acquired infection is suppurative otitis media.
Other Pseudomonas species, though not common, may cause infections. These are:
- **Fluorescence group:** *P. fluorescence* and *P. putida* which produce pyoverdin pigment.
- Stutzeri group consists of *P. stutzeri, P. mendoma* and CDC group VB-3. *P. stutzeri* produces yellow to brown colonies which may be dry and wrinkle adherent to agar.

Epidemiology of Pseudomonas

It persists and multiplies in moist environments and moist equipment as sinks, drains, flower vases, humidifiers even in distilled water. It may be contaminant in pharmaceutical preparations and may cause ophthalmitis following the faulty chemical sterilization of contact lenses.

Acquisition of this bacterium in hospital is rapid. Burn patients are at risk; it may be present in hospital dust, air suggesting that it may be air-borne infection. Transmission may occur through hands of health care workers or via contaminated instrument. Patients with burn wound and ventilator associated pneumonia may proceed to septicemia.

Eye infections occur following contaminated medicaments, industrialized eye injuries.

Contaminated milk feeds may lead to gastrointestinal infections in newborn and young infants.

Typing Methods for *Pseudomonas aeruginosa*

Being one of the commonest bacterium causing hospital outbreaks, typing method help in investigation of outbreak. By typing methods, isolates from patients and from suspected source are compared.

- *Bacteriocin typing*: *Pseudomonas* produces three types **of bacteriocins—R, F, and S.**
- Indicator strains (known strains maintained in laboratory) are applied on different areas of lawn culture of *Pseudomonas aeruginosa*. Based on growth inhibition of indicator strains by pyocin produced by test bacillus, 105 types are identified.
- *Serotyping*: Based upon structure of 'O' and 'H' antigens, **17 serotypes** are identified.
- *Antibiogram*: Antibiotic susceptibility pattern is simplest and cheap method of typing.
- *Molecular methods*: Pulse filled gel electrophoresis **(PFGE)** is used which has high discriminating power between all isolates of organism.

Laboratory Diagnosis

Ten percent of isolates of pseudomonas are non-pigmented.

Diagnosis is based on culture.
RCR is very sensitive.

Selective media: **Cetrimide agar** is used for isolation from feces or samples with mixed flora. Oxidase test is positive and organism hydrolyses arginine. Repeated isolation is required to confirm diagnosis.

Control

- Prevention of hospital cross-infection requires constant vigilance and strict adherence to asepsis.
- Antibiotic treatment is not always satisfactory.
- Immunotherapy in burn patients with antiserum to *P. aeruginosa* is useful.
- Vaccines are tried in cystic fibrosis patients.

Treatment

- *Penicillins*: Ticarcillin, pipercillin, pipercillin/tazobactum, clavulinic acid.
- *Carbapenems*: Imipenem, meropenem
- *Fluoroquinolones*: Ciprofloxacin, levofloxacin.
- *Aminoglycosides*: Tobramycin, amikacin, gentamicin
- **Polymyxin B**
- **Colistin**
- *Cephalosporins*: Of the cephalosporins, ceftazidime, cefoperazone, and cefipime are active against *Pseudomonas.*

This organism shows high intrinsic resistance to many antibiotics.

Monotherapy with ceftazidime or imipenem is effective in management of hospital-acquired infections. Quinolones; particularly ciprofloxacin is highly active by oral route.

Pseudomonas has drug-resistant plasmids. Some strains produce some β lactamases, carbapenemase and Amc 'C' β lactamases.

STENOTROPHOMONAS MALTOPHILA

- It is saprophyte and opportunistic pathogen.
- It causes wound infection, UTI, and septicemia.
- It can cause many hospital-acquired infections as ventilator associated pneumonia and ecthyma gangrenosum.
- It is oxidase negative. It may produce levander color pigment.
- Acidifies glucose, lactose, sucrose, and maltose.
- Lysine decarboxylase is negative.
- *Treatment*: Drugs of choice are cotrimoxazole, and chloramphenicol. It is resistant to other commonly used antibiotics as aminoglycosides, cephalosporins, imipenem and quinolone.

BURKHOLDERIA CEPACIA

Burkholderia cepacia with other **9 genospecies** make **B. cepacia complex**. They are environmental organisms which may grow in water, soil, plants, animals, and decaying vegetable materials. In hospitals, they have been isolated from a variety of environmental sources from which they can be transmitted to patients. **Patients with cystic fibrosis and chronic granulomatous disease are particularly susceptible to infection with this organism.** It is likely that the organism may be transmitted from one cystic fibrosis patient to other by close contact. Although a small number of patients with cystic fibrosis become infected, the association makes major concern for patients.

A diagnosis of this bacterium in patient with cystic fibrosis alters the life of patient as the patient may not be allowed to form association with other patients. Also the patient may be refused for lung transplant.

It grows on most of the culture media, medium containing colistin is used as a selective medium for growing *B. cepacia*. Colonies slowly appear after 3–4 days.

It is plant pathogen causing **onion rot.** Cepacia (Latin for onion) is an opportunistic environmental pathogen. It causes fatal narcotizing pneumonia, urinary tract infection, respiratory tract infection, wound infections, peritonitis, endocarditis and septicemia.

In healthy individuals, *B. cepacia* causes foot infection **(trench foot or jungle foot)** in troops training in swamy environment. Outbreaks have been reported which are linked to exposure to pressure monitoring devices, **contaminated povidone iodine solutions** and contaminated parental fluids.

Like *Pseudomonas*, it grows in disinfectants and it can use penicillin-G as sole source of carbon for its growth. It is oxidase positive, acidifies mannitol, sorbitol, sucrose, decarboxylases lysine. Many strains from patients with cystic fibrosis are multiple drug resistant. Cotrimoxazole is the drug of choice.

BURKHOLDERIA MALLEI (GLANDERS DISEASE)

- It is Gram-negative, non-motile bacillus with irregular staining and beaded appearance.
- It grows on ordinary media, colonies are initially translucent becoming opaque later. On potato, it produces characteristic honey-like growth.
- It doesn't grow on MacConkey medium.
- Natural disease in equines occurs in two forms.
  1. **Glanders** which is respiratory disease with nodules.
  2. **Farcy** which is infection of skin, lymphatics.
- Human infection is occupational disease. Infection begins as ulcer of skin and mucosa followed by lymphangitis and sepsis. Inhalation of organisms may produce primary pneumonia. Acute disease presents with fever, nasal discharge, and severe prostration with high mortality or subcutaneous infections.
- Guinea pigs are susceptible. Intraperitoneal injection of small amounts of pure cultures cause 'Strauss reaction', testicular swelling in 2–3 days due to invasion of tunica vaginalis.

BURKHOLDERIA PSEUDOMALLEI (MELIDIOSIS)

It is also known as **Whitmore's bacillus.**

- It is Gram-negative, motile bacillus, gives safety pin appearance due to bipolar staining with methylene blue stain (Fig. 35.2).
- It is obligatory aerobe. Colonies on BA, MC are rough, corrugated. On **Ashdown's** medium which is a selective medium, wrinkled, purple-colored colonies are produced.
- It is soil saprophyte, cause infection in rodents and accidentally in humans. It is causative agent of **melidiosis.**
- Human infections occur commonly through skin abrasions or inhalation.

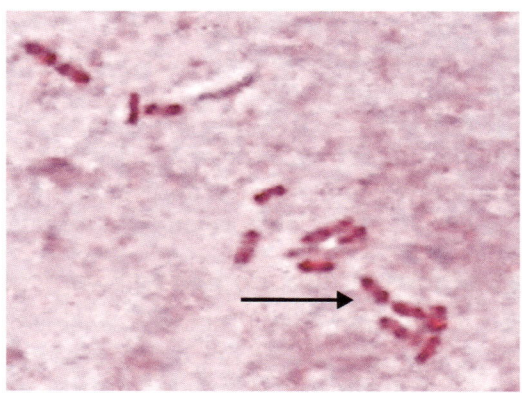

Fig. 35.2: Bipolar staining

Melioidiosis

Different presentations are:
- *Acute septicemia*:
  - Acute pulmonary infection (this is most common manifestation)
  - Mild bronchitis to extensive necrotizing pneumonia, it may resemble TB, chest X-ray shows upper lobe infiltrate.
- *Acute localized skin disease*: Ulceration, abscess formation, lymphangitis, lymphadenitis may occur
- Suppurative parotitis
- *Chronic form*: Liver abscess, splenic abscess, septic arthritis, osteomyelitis, genitourinary infection or involvement of CNS are clinical presentations.

Diagnosis

- *Microscopy*: Gram's stain—Gram-negative bacilli are seen. Methylene blue stain shows bipolar safety pin appearance.
- Culture is done on BA.
- Organisms from culture can be identified by latex agglutination test or by direct immunofluorescence test.
- *Serology*: ELISA, Indirect hemagglutination detect antibodies.
- Identification of **19.5 kDa** may be used for rapid diagnosis.

Treatment

Ceftazidime is the treatment of choice; other options are cotrimoxazole, tetracycline, amoxycillin clavulanate, cefotaxime.

Originally, the disease was restricted to South East Asia, but became important in USA military forces returning from Vietnam war. The disease may occur after a considerable time after exposure (hence term **Vietnam bomb**).

ACINETOBACTER

It is Gram-negative coccobacillus, non-motile, biochemically inert, does not ferment sugar. It is saprophytic and it may be found on skin. It causes hospital-acquired infections. It grows on ordinary media. On MacConkey's medium, it produces pale colonies which are identified by morphology, biochemicals (oxidase negative, IMViC are +).

Classification

Various DNA homology groups called '**genospecies**' exist as shown by DNA hybridization studies. Clinical isolates are called as *Acinetobacter calcoaceticus-baumanii* complex. This complex is further subdivided into *A. baumanii* (for *A. anitratus*), *A. lwoffii* and hemolytic strains as *A. hemolyticus*.

A. baumanii gives glucose oxidation positive and non-hemolytic, *A. lwoffii* is glucose negative non-hemolytic while *A. haemolyticus* is hemolytic.
- *A. baumanii*: It forms pinkish colonies on MacConkey's medium. It forms acid in 10% but not in 1% lactose.
- *A. lwoffii*: It forms pale color colonies on MacConkey's medium.
- Various hospital-acquired infections are produced by *Acinetobacter* which are urinary tract infection, wound infection, burn infection and ventilator-associated pneumonia.

MORAXELLA (BRANHAMELLA CATARRHALIS)

- They were classified as *B. catarrhalis*, again as *Moraxella catarrhalis* which form commensal flora of upper respiratory tract but become pathogenic causing respiratory tract infections, sinusitis, otitis media (third commonest cause), tracheobronchitis and pneumonia (pulmonary disease in elderly patients especially with COPD.
- They are Gram-negative cocci arranged in pairs.
- Sputum is collected for diagnosis of lower respiratory disease which is inoculated on nutrient agar.
- It is differentiated from meningococci by growth on simple medium as nutrient agar at 18–42°C. It doesn't produce pigment.
- It does not ferment sugars.
- PCR is sensitive method for diagnosis.
- *Treatment*: This organism is beta-lactamase producer hence resistant to penicillin, but penicillin combined with clavulanic acid is useful.

MORAXELLA LACUNATA

- Short Gram-negative bacillus arranged in pairs, shows sluggish motility.
- It is aerobic bacterium with simple growth requirements (NA can be used for culture).
- Catalase, oxidase positive and H_2S negative, no fermentation of sugars.
- It was first reported as cause of angular conjunctivitis (by Morax and Axenfeld) also known as **Morax-Axenfeld bacillus**.

KINGELLA KINGAE

- Gram-negative coccobacilli, non-motile, oxidase positive.
- Though it is usually oral commensal, it may cause endocarditis, infections of bones and joints.

36

Vibrio

HISTORY

- The bacillus was observed by Pacini (1854).
- Koch isolated the bacterium from cholera patient in Egypt (1883).

Family Vibrionaceae consists of genera: *Vibrio, Aeromonas* and *Plesiomonas*.

Morphology of *Vibrio cholerae*

- They are Gram-negative, short, curved, bacilli (coma-shaped; Fig. 36.1). Closely arranged two or more bacilli give spiral or (s) shaped forms.
- 1.5 µ × 0.2–0.4 µ in size.
- Non-sporing, non-capsulated.
- Gram-stained smear shows "fish-in-stream" appearance in stained films of mucous flakes from acute cases.
- 'Darting' type of motility is because of single polar flagellum and its coma shape. The wavelength of flagellum is 1.6–2 µ.
- Motility is also called 'shooting star motility'.
- Darting motility gives "swarm of gnats" appearance.
- The name 'Vibrio' is given to this bacterium due to its vibratory motility. (Vibrare = to vibrate).

- Motility is inhibited by addition of specific antiserum and this test is used to give provisional report, so that treatment is started early.
- Speed of the bacillus is 200 µm/sec.

Cultural Characteristics

- It is aerobic bacillus.
- Optimum temperature is 37°C (16–40°C).
- Optimum pH 8.2 (6.4–9.6).
- 0.5–1% NaCl required for optimal growth.
- It grows well on ordinary media.
- Colony morphology on nutrient agar (which is simple solid medium): Colonies are moist, translucent, round, 1–2 mm with **bluish tinge in transmitted light** (bluish tinge is due to action of enzyme **luciferase**).
- Colonies on BA are initially surrounded by a zone of greening which afterwards becomes clear, this is called hemodigestion (Fig. 36.2).
- Hemodigestion is seen on BA (digestion of blood agar surrounding the colonies some authors describe it as pseudohemolysis instead of hemodigestion). It differs from beta hemolysis, as zone of lysis is large

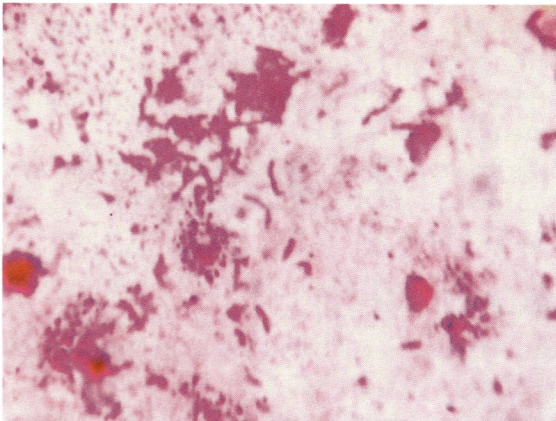

Fig. 36.1: Coma-shaped vibrios

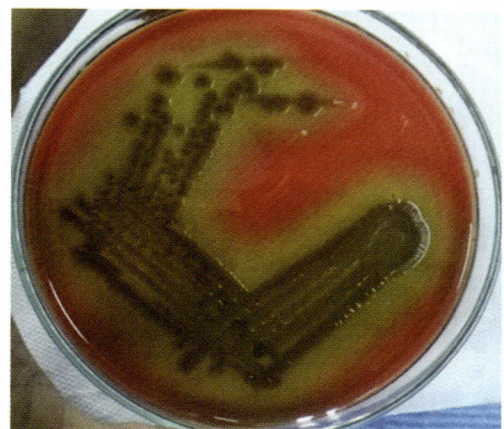

Fig. 36.2: Hemodigestion on BA

and hemolyisis is due to other metabolic products other than hemolysin.

- The medium surrounding main inoculums becomes greenish without change in the medium surrounding isolated colonies.
- *Vibrio* is late lactose fermenter on MacConkey agar.
- Fine **surface pellicle** is formed in peptone water.

Transport or Holding Media for Vibrio

- Venkatraman-Ramakrishnan (VR) medium (pH 8.6–8.8): 20 gm of crude sea salt and 5 gm peptone are dissolved in 1 litre of distilled water.
- Cary-Blair medium (pH 8.4). It is a semisolid medium hence prevents the spillage of stool sample during transportation. It contains buffered solution of NaCl, $CaCl_2$, disodium phosphate and Na-thioglycolate.

Enrichment Media

- Alkaline peptone water (APW)—pH 8.6
- Monsur's taurocholate tellurite peptone water—pH 9.2
- Autoclaved sea water.

Plating Media: Selective Media

- ***Alkaline bile salt agar (BSA) (pH 8.2):*** Colonies have similar apperance to those on nutrient agar.
- ***Monsur's gelatin taurocholate trypticase tellurite agar (GTTA):*** Colonies have greyish black center surrounded by turbid halo due to gelatin liquefaction.
- ***Thiosulphate citrate bile-salt sucrose (TCBS) agar:*** Yellow colonies due to fermentation of sucrose are formed on this medium (Fig. 36.3).

Biochemical Reactions (Table 36.1)

- Catalase positive.
- Oxidase positive.
- TSI medium shows A/A reaction without gas and without H_2S.
- ***Sensitivity to substance O129:*** *Vibrio cholerae* is sensitive to this chemical while similar genera like

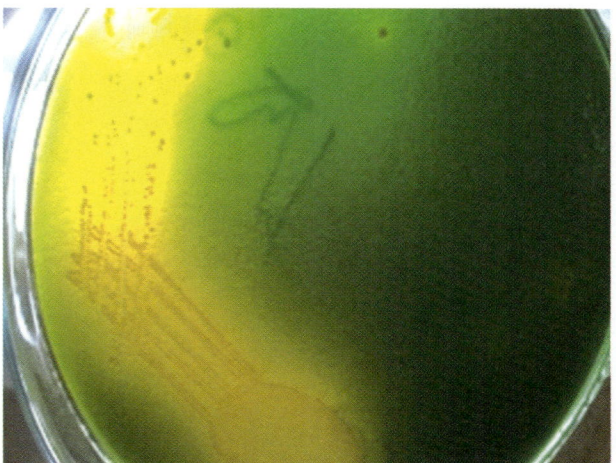

Fig. 36.3: TCBS with yellow colonies

Aeromonas, Plesiomonas are resistant; hence 0129 (IOEG) identification disk can be placed on plated medium and zone of clearing is observed.

- Ferments glucose, mannitol, mannose, maltose, sucrose producing acid, no gas.
- It is late lactose fermenter.
- It is indole positive, MR negative, urease negative.
- **Cholera red reaction** is positive due to production of nitroso-indole. This bacterium is indole positive and reduces nitrates to nitrites. This reaction is tested by addition of few drops of concentrated H_2SO_4 to 24 hours incubated culture of *Vibrio cholerae* in peptone water, a reddish color develops due to formation of nitroso-indole.
- **String test is positive** with 0.5% sodium deoxycholate. On a glass slide, a loopful of growth of organism is mixed with few drops of 0.5% sodium deoxycholate. The suspension loses its turbidity and loop dipped in the suspension is drawn slowly away from the suspension. It forms a thread (Fig. 36.4).
- The string produced by *Vibrio cholerae* lasts longer than 60 seconds, those formed by other *vibrio species* fade after 40–60 seconds.
- Stringing occurs because bile lyses the bacterium and releases DNA.

TABLE 36.1: Differentiation of vibrios from allied genera

Genus	Oxidation-fermentation test		Utilization of amino acids			String test
	Oxidative	Fermentative	Lysine	Arginine	Ornithine	
Vibrio	+	+ 1	+	—	+	+
Aeromonas	+	+2	—	+	—	Variable
Pseudomonas	+	—	V	V	V	—
Plesiomonas	+	+	+	+	+	—

1 = no gas produced, 2 = gas may or may not be produced

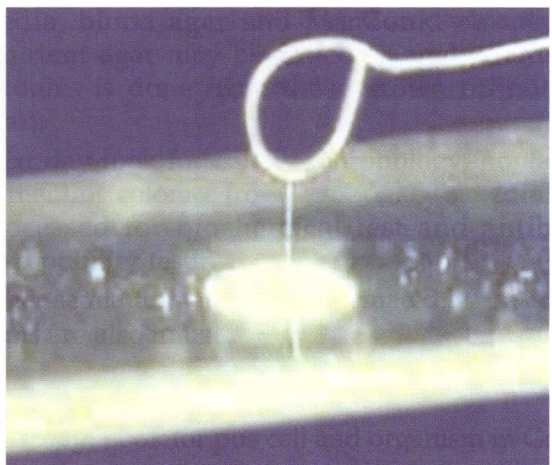

Fig. 36.4: String test

- **Salt tolerance test:** Organism is inoculated in various tubes of peptone water with gradded concentrations of salts (NaCl). *Vibrio cholerae* tolerates maximum up to 6% NaCl.
- Decarboxylation of lysine and ornithine is positive while orginine is negative.

Resistance of Vibrio

Vibrios are susceptible to heat, drying and acids. They are destroyed at 55°C in 15 minutes. El Tor survives longer than classical strains. They survive for months in sterile sea water, do not survive in grossly contaminated water. They survive for days in night soil and on fruits kept at room temperature, and for >2 weeks in the refrigerator. Organisms are susceptible to common disinfectants. Presence of bacteriophages in water or environment as seen in water of river Ganga kills the bacteria (Flowchart 36.1).

Classification of Vibrio

Heiberg classification is based on fermentation of mannose, sucrose, arabinose (Table 36.2).

Gardner and Venkatraman Classification (Flowchart 36.2)

Cholera vibrio and biochemically similar vibrios possessing a common 'H' antigen were classified as Group 'A', rest of the vibrios in group 'B'.

Flowchart 36.1: Vibrio in environment

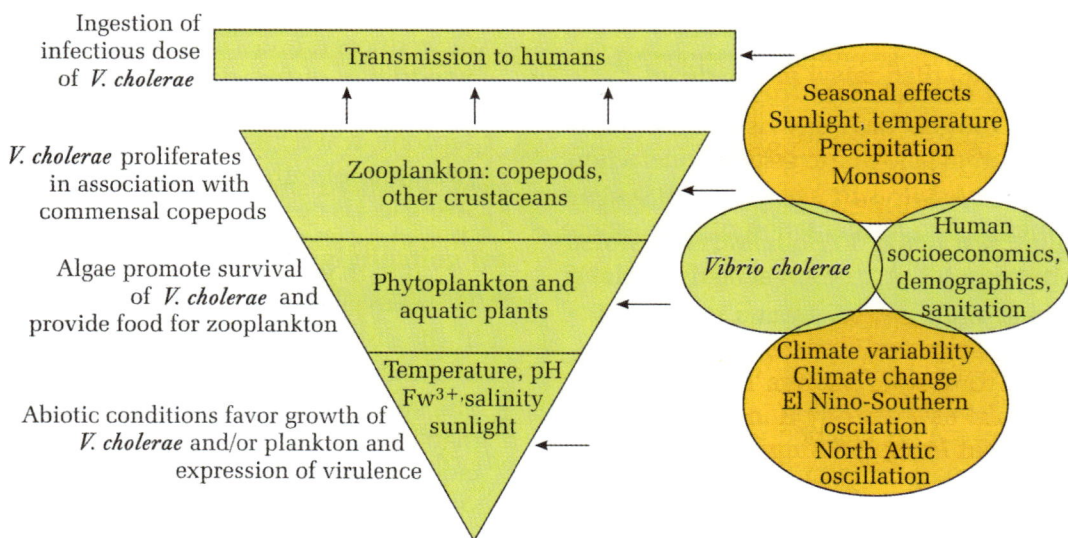

Group	Fermentation of mannose	Sucrose	Arabinose
I	A	A	—
II	—	A	—
III	A	A	A
IV	—	A	A
V	A	—	—
VI	—	—	—
VII	A	—	A
VIII	—	—	A

TABLE 36.2: Heiberg grouping of Vibrios

Flowchart 36.2: Gardner and Venkatraman classification

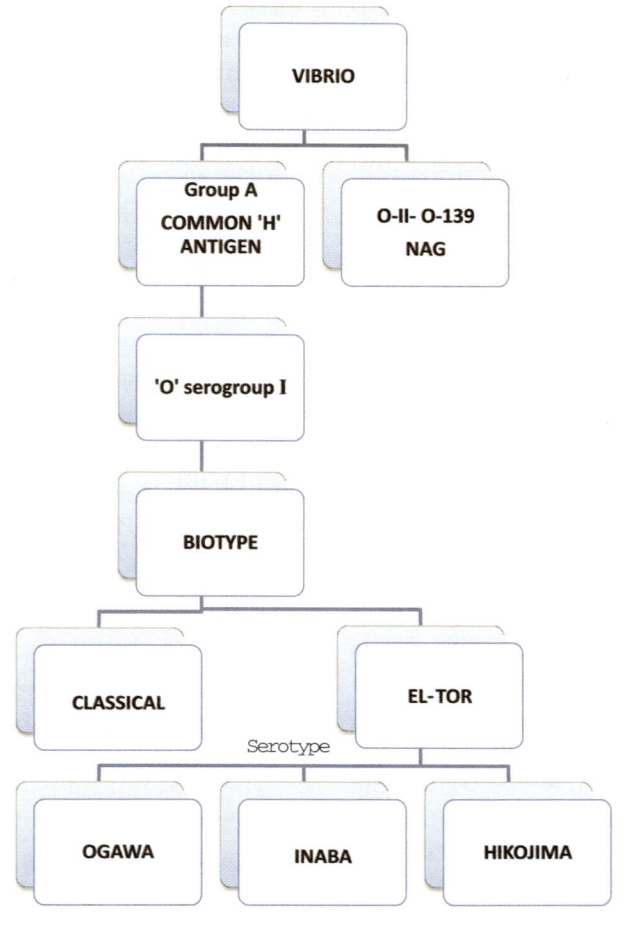

Classification is based on major somatic antigen (O antigen). Isolates from group-A are classified into six serogroups (or serovars—I–VI). Most of the strains of *Vibrio cholerae* causing epidemic belong to serogroup O1.

Other Vibrio isolates, producing no agglutination with anti-O1 antiserum, were called as non O1 vibrios or non-agglutinable vibrios **(NAG)**. They were considered as non-pathogenic vibrios, i.e. non-cholera vibrio (NCV).

Based on minor antigens, the cholera vibrios are classified into three serotypes, i.e. ogawa, inaba and hikojima. Ogawa and inaba strains form agglutination with their specific antisera while hikojima strains form agglutination with both ogawa or inaba antisera.

Non-O1 vibrios may sometimes cause diseases similar to cholera. Though they were called as non-agglutinating vibrios, as they do not agglutinate with O1 antiserum, they agglutinate with their specific antiserum; hence the term NAG is not proper. The NCV are now up to serovar O-139. (There are at least 206 O-groups.)

There are some variants which do not fix exactly into both El-Tor or classical biotypes, which are known as **El-Tor varients.**

Cholera

Under natural conditions, *V. cholerae* is pathogenic only to humans. Infective dose is 10^{10} or more in a person with normal gastric pH. When vehicle is food, as few as 10^2–10^4 organisms may cause the disease because of buffering capacity of food. Any medication or condition that decreases stomach acidity makes a person susceptible to infection. Cholera is not a invasive disease. The bacteria remain attach to microvilli of brush border of epithelial cells. They multiply and liberate toxin.

Formula of WHO Oral rehydration solution (ORS)

Constituent	Amount (g)
Sodium chloride	2.6
Potassium chloride	1.5
Trisodium chloride	2.9
Glucose	13.5
Dissolve in one lit. of water	

O-139 has similar action. It produces O-139 LPS and an immunologically related 'O' antigen. These factors increase the virulence and cause bacteremic illness seen in infection with O-139.

Pathogenicity

Vibrios enter orally through contaminated water or food

They cross protective layer of mucus in small intestine by motility, protease, hemagglutinin (protease and hemagglutinin break mucin and fibronectin of mucosa)

Adhere to epithelial cells by special fimbriae **(TCP)** – toxin coregulated pilus

Combined action of CTx, TCP, and other virulence factors is regulated by **Tox R** genes products called **master switch (Tox R protein)**

Produce cholera toxin

Activation of adenylate cyclase and intracellular **accumulation of cAMP** which **inhibits the absorption** of sodium and **activates excretory chloride** transport in the lumen of the intestine, the high chloride content in intestine increases high osmolality. To balance this **large excretion of water** which tries to overcome absorptive capacity of lumen occurs.

Watery diarrhea

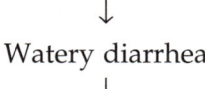

Cholera toxin is a complex of 6 subunits—a single copy of 'A' subunit and 5 copies of 'B' subunits. 'A2' links 'A1' to 'B 'subunits, B binds to GM1 ganglioside, 'A1' causes ADP ribosylation of 'G' protein which leads to stimulation of adenylyl cyclase and increased production of cAMP occur. **Cholera toxin** – causes **secretion** of water, chloride, bicarbonate, and it **inhibits reabsorption also.**

Detection of CT (Cholera Toxin)

- Fluid accumulation in rabbit ileal loop.
- Elongation of Chinese hamster ovary (CHO) cells.
- Increased capillary permeability (permeability factor-PF—"skin-blueing test" positive).
- Changes in adrenal tumor (Y) cells and Vero cells.
- ELISA, IF

CT is antigenic and can be toxoided.

Clinical Features of Cholera

Incubation period: 24 hours – 5 days. There is sudden onset of nausea, profuse watery diarrhea, copious vomiting, and **rice-water stools.** The stool contains few mucus flakes, epithelial cells and a large number of vibrios. It has fishy odor. There is increase in thirst, postural hypotension, weakness, tachycardia and decreased skin turgor. It is painless, effortless diarrhoea. Electrolyte rich diarrhea occurs as much as **20–30 litres/day**. Renal failure occurs due to acute tubular necrosis. Renal failure and fluid loss results in sunken eyes, oliguria, weak or absent pulse, somnalescence and coma. Diminution of extracellular fluid volume leads to hemoconcentration, hypokalemia, acidosis, anuria, and shock.

Vibriocidal IgA antibodies (coprobodies) (serum titre >20) have been associated with protection against colonization and disease.

Complications include cramps, renal failure, and pulmonary edema, cardiac arrhythmias, paralytic ileus, renal failure.

Epidemiology

Cholera has smoldered in an endemic fashion on the Indian subcontinent for centuries. There are references to deaths due to dehydrating diarrhea dating back to Hippocrates and Sanskrit writings.

Epidemic cholera was described in 1563 by Garcia del Huerto, a Portuguese physician at Goa, India.

The mode of transmission of cholera by water was proven in 1849 by John Snow, a London physician.

In 1883, Robert Koch successfully isolated the cholera vibrio from the intestinal discharges of cholera patients and proved conclusively that it was the agent of the disease.

The first long-distance spread of cholera to Europe and the America began in 1817, such that by the early 20th century, six waves of cholera had spread across the world in devastating epidemic fashion. Since then, until the 1960s, the disease contracted, remaining present only in southern Asia.

In 1961, the "**El-Tor**" biotype (distinguished from classic biotypes by the production of hemolysins) reemerged and produced a major epidemic in the Philippines to initiate a **seventh global pandemic.** Since then, this biotype has spread across Asia, the Middle East, Africa, and parts of Europe.

The 7th pandemic started from Sulawesi (celebes), Indonesia. The El-Tor was first isolated by Gotsclich at the El-Tor quarantine station in Egypt.

There are several characteristics of the El-Tor strain that confer upon it a high degree of "epidemic virulence" allowing it to spread across the world as previous strains have done. First, the ratio of cases to carriers is much less than in cholera due to classic biotypes (1:30–100 for El-Tor *vs* 1:2–4 for "classic" biotypes). Second, the duration of carriage after infection is longer for the El-Tor strain than the classic strains. Third, the El-Tor strain survives for longer periods in the extraintestinal environment.

The 7th pandemic was the only pandemic which originated outside India, it produced much milder cholera but was associated with high carrier rate. It was much hardier than classical and survived much longer in the environment.

Between 1969 and 1974, El-Tor vibrio replaced the classic strains in the heartland of endemic cholera, the Gangas River Delta of India. El-Tor broke out explosively in Peru in 1991 (after an absence of cholera there for 100 years), and spread rapidly in Central and South America, with recurrent epidemics in 1992 and 1993.

In 1982, in Bangladesh, a classic biotype resurfaced with a new capacity to produce more severe illness, and it rapidly replaced the El-Tor strain which was thought to be well-entrenched. This classic strain has not yet produced a major outbreak in any other country.

In December 1992, a large epidemic of cholera began in Bangladesh, and large numbers of people have been involved. The organism has been characterized as *cholerae* **O139 "Bengal"**. It is derived genetically from the El-Tor pandemic strain but it has changed its antigenic structure such that there is no existing immunity and all ages, even in endemic areas, are susceptible. It is capsulated, more invasive, caused many cases of bacteremia and extraintestinal manifestations. It has district IPS. The epidemic has continued to spread and *V. cholerae* **O139** has affected at least 11 countries in southern Asia.

Cholera is notifiable disease; any case should be notified to the public health authority. Approximately 2–3 lakh cases are reported worldwide. Recent outbreaks are reported from Zimbabwe (2009) and Haiti (2010).

Seasonal pattern of transmission has observed. It is common in rainfall flooding. Poor sanitation, poverty, overcrowding and malnutrition are predisposing factors for infection. Persons with low immunity, malnutrition, and persons with a particular blood group (group 'O') are at increased risk of severe disease.

Humans are the only reservoirs of the disease and patients or carriers act as source of infection. Cholera is maintained during epidemics by carriers and sub-clinical cases. In the intraepidemic period, it is maintained in sea water, crustaceans and planktons.

Carriers in Cholera

- *Incubatory carriers*: Due to short incubation period, these carriers shed bacilli 1–2 days before clinical disease.
- Convalescent carriers are patients recovering or recovered from disease and shed bacilli in feces for 2–3 weeks.
- Contact or healthy carriers get inection from cases, shed bacilli for 10 days.
- Chronic carriers shed bacilli for longer period.

Apart from cholera toxin, other virulence factors which help in pathogenesis of *Vibrio* are:

- Motility of Vibrio and proteolytic enzymes produced by it as mucinase help to penetrate mucus.
- Toxin coregulated pilus is special fimbria helps in adhesion to intestinal epithelial cells.
- CTX-gene for cholera toxin encoded by bacteriophage.
- ToxR gene regulates expression of CT, TCP and other virulence factors.
- Zona occludens toxin use breaks tight junctions between epithelial cells.
- Accessory colonization factors also help in colonization and adhesion.

Carriers may be incubatory (1–5 days), convalescent (2–3 weeks); healthy, occur after subclinical infection (<10 days) or chronic infection (months to years).

Laboratory Diagnosis of Cholera

Samples Collected

- **Stool** is collected by inserting sterile rubber catheter and allowing the sample to run through the tube into container (Fig. 36.5).

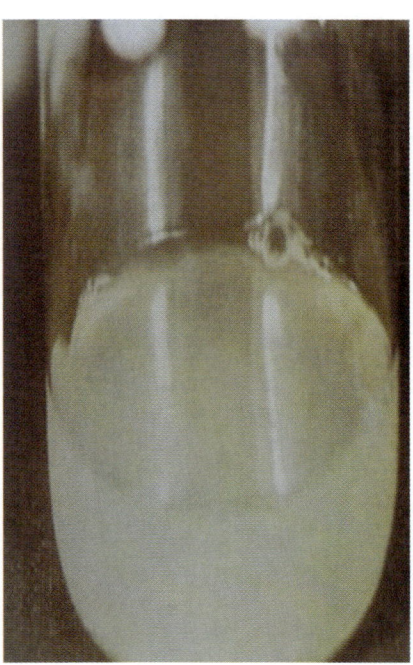

Fig. 36.5: Rice watery stools

- *Rectal swabs:* These are suitable for detection of carriers, or patient's recovering from the disease. Cotton swab is inserted and held for a few seconds in rectum and then transported in transport medium.
- Stool samples may be collected on strip of filter paper which is transferred in plastic container. It is used especially when transport medium is not available.

Sample is transported in transport medium; if any delay, it is preserved in refrigerator.

If transport period is longer (few hours), transport sample in enrichment media (e.g. **APW**).

If there is delay in transportation, transport media Venkatraman-Ramakrishna medium or Cary Blair medium or autoclaved sea water are used.

Cary Blair medium has advantages:

1. As this medium is semisolid, spillage is avoided during the transport of stool sample.
2. As Cary Blair medium acts as transport medium for other enteric pathogens as *Salmonella, Shigella, Campylobacter*, and if clinical diagnosis is not clear, it can be used as transport medium whatever the pathogen.

Rapid tests

In areas with limited to no laboratory testing, the **Crystal VC → dipstick rapid test** can provide an early warning to public health officials that an outbreak of cholera is occurring.

Although removing access to an implicated water source is often not as simple as when **Dr. John Snow famously ordered the** handle removed from the Broad Street pump. Recently, WHO prequalified the WC/rBS vaccine for purchase by UN agencies, and has suggested that it may have a role to play in protecting populations at high risk for epidemic cholera. A second vaccine, marketed as ShanChol and manufactured by **Shantha Biotec, India,** is pending WHO prequalification.

ELISA CT is highly immunogenic for humans and laboratory animals. As a result, many immunologic techniques have been developed for detecting CT. The discovery the GM1 ganglioside is the natural receptor for CT and LT and its subsequent purification led to the development of **ganglioside-capture** enzyme-linked immunosorbent assay **(GM1-ELISA),** culture supernatants are added to microtiter plate wells coated with GM1 ganglioside. Toxin bound to the GM1 receptors is then detected by adding antiserum to CT, followed by enzyme-conjugated antiglobulin antibody.

Coagglutination

The test reagent is relatively inexpensive to prepare but requires a specific anti-CT (cholera toxin) (or anti-LT) antibody.

The **latex agglutination** test uses specific anti-CT or anti-LT bound to latex particles.

DNA Probes used for detection of toxin is sensitive method.

Direct Microscopy

Microscopy: Demonstration of 'darting motility' can be done preferably by dark ground microscope, but if it is not available, motility can also be seen by light microscope by hanging drop method.

Simple Tests

Inhibition of motility:

- Addition of **specific antiserum** to stool sample inhibits the motility of *Vibrio cholerae.*
- *Distilled water inhibition test:* Motility of *Vibrio* is inhibited by addition of distilled water. This test is simple and cheap but must be interpreted with using control, i.e. one preparation without adding distilled water.
  - *Direct immunofluorescence:* This is used on stool sample for rapid diagnosis of cholera bacillus.
  - **Gram-stained** smear shows **coma**-shaped Gram-negative bacilli, pus cells are scanty or absent.
  - Sample is plated on to selective media (**TCBS**) as well as non-selective media (**MacConkey medium**), enriched media as **blood agar and blood agar with identification disk O-129.**
  - **Identification of *V. cholerae* colonies is done by blood agar—hemodigestion is seen.**
- *MacConkey's medium:* Pale **non-lactose-fermenting** colonies are produced.
- *TCBS:* **Yellow colonies** due to sucrose fermentation are produced.
- *BA with O-129:* Presence of zone of inhibition around the disk will be present.
- **Catalase positive, oxidase positive.**
- Urease—negative
- **Cholera red test**—positive
- **String test**—positive
- *Decarboxylase tests:* Lysine and ornithine decarboxylase tests positive

L	G	M	S	Indole	MR	VP	Citrate	TSI
Negative	Positive	Positive	Positive	Positive	Negative	Negative by classical biotypes and positive by El-Tor	Negative	A/A

Biochemical tests done for identification and for differentiation of classical and El-Tor biotypes (Table 36.3).

Chick RBCs Agglutination

A loopful of the colony is emulsified in saline drop on a glass slide to which a drop of 2.5% chick RBCs suspension is added. Clumping of RBCs means the test is positive. El-Tor biotypes give this test positive while classical biotypes give the test negative.

Sensitivity to Polymyxin B

Polymyxin disk containing 50 units is placed on antibiotic susceptibility plate. All strains of classical Vibrio are sensitive while El-Tor strains are resistant.

Sensitivity to Cholera Phage IV

All strains of classical cholera vibrio are lysed by Mukherhee's group IV phage with routine test dilution while El-Tor strains are not lysed.

Modified CAMP Test for the Identification of Vibrio cholerae Biotype El-Tor

It is similar to CAMP test used for group B streptococci. A single straight line streaking of *S. aureus* (beta lysine producing) is done on blood agar. The Vibrio species to be tested is inoculated perpendicular to streak of *S. aureus*. The test is positive with El-Tor biotype and negative with classical biotype of *V. cholerae*. However, O139 strains also give strong positive reaction while non-O1and non-O139 vibrios give a weak positive reaction.

Serotyping: Suggestive colonies agglutinated with polyvalent O1 antiserum and then with specific Ogawa or Inaba antisera.

Serological tests: Complement based vibriocidal antibody test, and antitoxin assay are used. The tests are useful in epidemiological purpose.

Phage typing: The isolates of *Vibrio cholerae* may be sent to National Institute of Cholera and Enteric Disease

(NICED) at Kolkata. It is also an international reference center for cholera.

Diagnosis of Carriers

- More than one cycle of enrichment may be required while doing stool culture.
- Repeated examination is done due to intermittent shedding of *Vibrio cholerae*.
- Collection of stools after purgative and bile after duodenal intubation can be helpful.

Examination of Water Samples for Vibrio

- Enrichment is done with alkaline peptone water
- *Sewer-swab technique*: Filtration through millipore membrane filter.
- Sewage to be diluted in saline filtered through gauze and then treated as for water. **Filter is placed on double strength MacConkey's medium.**

Prophylaxis of Cholera

Types of Oral Vaccines

- Killed oral whole cell vaccine with or without 'B' subunit of cholera toxin.
- Live oral vaccines with classical, El-Tor and O-139 strains, with toxin genes deleted.

Newer Vaccines

Dukoral: It was developed in Sweden. It is whole cell killed vaccine, conjugated with B subunit of cholera toxin.

Two doses are given orally one week apart. One more dose is given for children between 2 and 5 years. It is not adviced below 2 years. It gives 85% protection for 6 months and 50% in 3 years.

Shanchol and moRCVAX: These are closely related bivalent vaccines (oral vaccines).

Treatment of Cholera

Replacement of fluids and electrolytes is the most important aspect in the management of patients. Antibiotic therapy is only of secondary importance. Tetracycline, chloramphenicol, ciprofloxacin, 3rd generation cephalosporins are commonly used. Multiple drug-resistant strains becoming increasingly common.

Prevention

- Use of safe water for drinking purpose.
- Proper fecal disposal by sanitary methods.
- Food sanitation.
- Investigation and control of outbreak.

TABLE 36.3: Differentiation of classical and El-Tor biotypes		
Properties	Classical	El-Tor
Hemolysis of sheep RBCs	Negative	Positive
Agglutination of chick RBCs	Negative	Positive
Voges-Proskauer test	Negative	Positive
Polymixin B sensitivity (50 IU/disc)	Sensitive	Resistant
Susceptibility El-Tor phage 5	Negative	Positive
Susceptibility to Mukherjee Group IV phage	Positive	Negative

- Notification—locally and nationally
- Health education.
- Tetracycline is used for chemoprophylaxis of household contacts.

HALOPHILIC VIBRIOS

Vibrios which require high concentration of salts for their growth and will not grow in absence of salts are called as halophilic vibrios (Table 36.4).

- *V. parahaemolyticus*
- *V. alginolyticus*
- *V. vulnificus*

They are found in sea water and marine life. They can tolerate up to 10% salt concentrations.

V. PARAHAEMOLYTICUS

- It was first isolated from cases of food poisoning due to sea fish in Japan.
- It is found in coastal areas, in fish, crabs, oysters, etc.
- It differs from *V. cholerae* in being **capsulated**, showing **bipolar staining** and pleomorphism.
- They have peritrichous flagella when grown in solid media and polar flagella when grown in liquid media.
- These bacteria can tolerate up to 8% salt concentration.
- They produce **green**-colored colonies on **TCBS agar** (sucrose not utilized).

TABLE 36.4: Characteristics of *V. parahaemolyticus* and *V. alginolyticus*

	V. parahaemolyticus	*V. alginolyticus*
Indole	+	+
VP	—	+
Nitrate	+	+
Urease	—/+	—
Sucrose fermentation	—	+
Swarming	+	—
10% NaCl	—	+

Kanagawa Phenomenon

When grown on Wagatsuma agar (special high salt blood agar); the organisms from environmental sources nearly always give non-hemolytic colonies whereas those from human patients always give hemolytic colonies. Hence this is used as a laboratory test to determine pathogenicity.

It causes food poisoning. It causes invasion of intestinal epithelial cells leading to diarrhea, accompanied by fever, vomiting and abdominal pain, this is of moderate degree and recovery is seen in 1–3 days.

V. AGINOLYTICUS

- It has a higher salt tolerance.
- It utilizes sucrose.
- It is seen in sea fish.
- It causes infection of the eyes, ears and wounds.

V. VULNIFICUS

- It is VP negative, utilizes lactose, tolerates salt concentration of <8%.
- It causes wound infections.
- In immunocompromised hosts like in patients of liver transplants, it causes penetration of gut mucosa, though no gastrointestinal manifestations are seen, bloodstream is invaded leading to septicemia and high mortality.

V. MIMICUS

- It mimics *V. cholerae* in biochemical features.
- It doesn't utilize sucrose.
- It can tolerate 0.5–1% salt.
- It is found in sea food like oysters.
- The disease is self-limiting.
- Clinical features are similar to those caused by *V. parahaemolyticus*.

37

Campylobacter and Haemophilus

CAMPYLOBACTER

Morphology

- It is Gram-negative curved rod (Fig. 37.1). It shows 'S' shaped or multispiral forms (S or gull wing shape).
- Size is 0.2–0.5 µm × 0.5–5 µm
- It is motile by polar flagella at one or both ends.

Characteristics

- It is microaerophilic, requires 5% O_2 with added 10% CO_2. Simplest way to produce micro-aerophilic atmosphere is to keep plates in anaerobic jar without catalyst and to produce gas with gas pack system or by gas exchange.
- Thermophilic, grows at 42°C.
- Oxidase is strongly positive.
- Carbohydrates are not utilized.

Medically important species are:
1. **Causing diarrhoeal diseases:**
   - *C. jejuni*
   - *C. coli*
   - *C. lari*

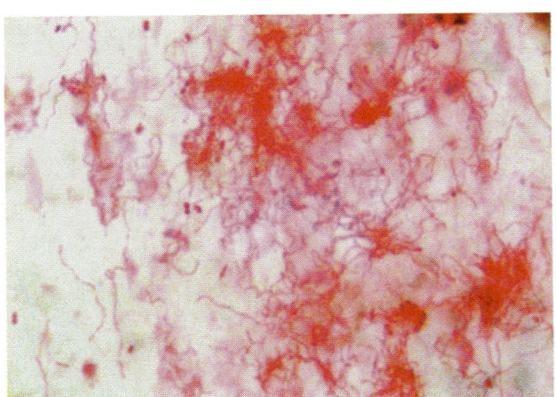

Fig. 37.1: Gram-stained smear showing Gram-negative spirals of Campylobacter (X1000)

2. **Causing extraintestinal infections:**
   - *C. fetus*

3. **Causing abscess:**
   - *C. sputorum*
   - *C. concisus*

C. JEJUNI

It is a zoonotic infection. It gained prominence for the first time in the 1970s causing human diarrheal disease affecting children and adults.

It is transmitted by consuming raw milk. It can cause both diarrheal and systemic illness. (It is the most common diarrheal pathogen in developed countries compared to *Salmonella, Shigella* in developing nations.) It is endemic in developing countries, where children are affected, the older age groups being immune due to sub-clinical infections. It is normal intestinal flora in domestic animals and birds, shed in faces. It is found in surface water. After infection, it is localized in jejunum or ileum. It rarely infects the lower intestine.

C. jejuni is susceptible to gastric acid and infective dose is 10⁴. Organisms multiply in small intestine, invade epithelium, produce inflammation (presence of RBCs and pus cells in stool), occasionally invade bloodstream.

Localized tissue invasion and toxic activity cause enteritis.

Clinical Features

It produces highly invasive disease involving lymph nodes and causing bacteremia. It presents clinically with fever, abdominal pain and watery diarrhea. It usually causes a self-limiting disease but in few cases, the severity is more.

C. jejuni produces diarrhea by three different mechanisms:

a. Production of toxin, like cholera toxin, causing watery diarrhea.
b. Penetration of gut epithelium, like *Shigella,* leading to bloody diarrhea.
c. Penetration of mucosa like *Salmonella.* Organisms proliferate lamina propria and mesenteric lymph nodes.

If patient is HLA-B27 positive, reactive arthritis may occcur. The bacterium also acts as triggering factor in development of Guillain-Barre syndrome.

Laboratory Diagnosis

Microscopy

- Look for **RBCs** and **leukocytes.**
- Look for **darting** or **tumbling** motility. Phase contrast or dark field microscopy can be used for demonstration of motility.
- Gram-stained smear shows presence of pus cells and Gram-negative spiral bacilli.

Culture

- Feces or rectal swabs are transported in **Cary Blair medium.**
- Samples are inoculated on **Skirrow's, Butzler's, Campy BAP medium.** These are incubated at 42°C in an atmosphere of 5% O_2, 10% CO_2 and 85% N_2 (Can also grow at 37°C, but the higher temperature is believed to inhibit the fecal flora).
- Colonies are seen after 48 hours, which are non-hemolytic, grey, confirmed by Gram's staining, motility, oxidase catalase and nitrate reduction tests.

Treatment

It includes fluid and electrolyte replacement and antibiotic—erythromycin is drug of choice.

C. COLI

It is found in healthy pigs. It can be differentiated from *C. jejuni* by hippurate hydrolysis test. It can cause diarrheal disease.

C. LARIDIS

It can be differentiated from *C. jejuni,* as it is resistant to nalidixic acid. It may cause diarrhea.

C. FETUS

This bacterium is first seen in a case of infectious abortion in cattle. It may cause extraintestial disease.

HAEMOPHILUS INFLUENZAE

- Pfeiffer observed that small Gram-negative bacillus is constantly present from influenza pandemics, it was called as 'influenza bacillus' (Pfeiffer's bacillus).
- Later it was proved that influenza is caused by virus, the relationship between viral pandemic and influenza bacillus was disapproved.
- The bacterium is later on renamed as *Haemophilus influenzae* (Fig. 37.2).

Morphology

Gram-negative bacilli showing pleomorphism, bacillary or filamentous forms are seen in CSF. Coccobacillary forms seen in sputum.

- *Size*: 1–2μ × 0.3–0.5μ
- They are non-motile, non-sporing
- Often capsulated
- Stain with Loeffler's methylene blue or dilute carbol fuschin.

Culture (Table 37.1)

- These bacteria are fastidious.
- These bacteria are capnophilic and require 5–10% CO_2 for their growth.
- Optimum temperature is 35–37°C.
- Bacteria require 'X' and 'V' factor for growth.
- **X factor:** It is heat-stable iron porphyrin hematin present in blood, necessary for synthesis of enzymes catalase, peroxidase, cytochrome oxidase which are important in aerobic respiration.
- **'V' factor:** It is heat labile, coenzyme nicotinamide adenine dinucleotide (NAD) or NAD phosphate which is hydrogen acceptor. It is produced by fungi, *Staphylococcus aureus* in large amount. It is present in RBCs. It shows satellitism when grown on a plate streaked with hemolytic *S. aureus* at the center.

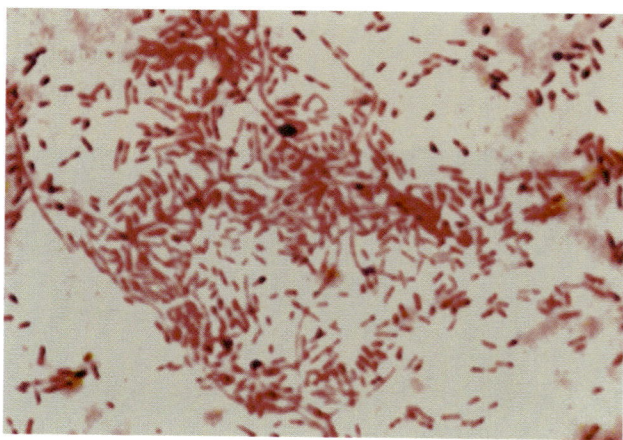

Fig. 37.2: Gram-stained smear of Haemophilus (X1000)

TABLE 37.1: Growth characteristics of *Haemophilus* species

Species	Growth requirements			Hemolysis on horse blood agar
	X	V	CO₂	
H. influenzae	+	+	–ve	–ve
H. aegyptius	+	+	–ve	–ve
H. ducreyi	+	–ve	V	V
H. parainfluenzae	–ve	+	–ve	–ve
H. haemolyticus	+	+	–ve	+
H. parahaemolyticus	–	+	–ve	+
H. aphrophilus	+	–ve	+	–
H. paraphrophilus	–	+	+	–

- **Chocolate agar with isovitalex** is good enriched medium.
- **Chocolate** agar with penicillin and bacitracin is also used for isolation of bacteria from samples as sputum.
- The differential medium of **Robert** contains bacitracin, sucrose and phenol red to differentiate *H. parainfluenzae* which ferments sucrose and form yellow colonies while *H. influenzae* forms **non-fermenting colorless colonies.**
- *Colony characteristics*: Capsulated strain produces large colonies which are translucent and show **iridescence**, non-capsulated strains produce small transparent colonies.
- For isolation of *H. influenzae* from sputum sample, addition of **bacitracin** (10 IU/mL) makes the medium **selective**.
- Special media used for growth are: Filde's agar, Levinthal's agar.
- Tests for factor X and V can be done by several ways:
  - Filter paper disks containing factor 'V' can be placed on medium and growth around the disk is observed.
  - Strip containing 'X' factor can be placed parallel with one containing 'V' factor on agar deficient in these factors. Growth will be seen in the area between two strips.

> If subcultured on transparent medium as levinthal agar, colonies of capsulated strains of *H. influenzae* show iridescence, if a beam of light is directed from the side through the underside of the colonies. It is thought to be due to optical properties of capsular layers, and it shows different shades of colors with the angle of observation.

Satellitism (Fig. 37.3)

It shows **dependency** of *H. influenzae* on **'V'** for their growth.

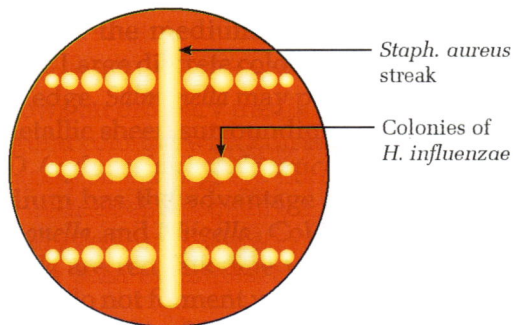

Staph. aureus streak

Colonies of H. influenzae

Fig. 37.3: Satellitism

A plate of blood agar is inoculated with the sample containing *H. influenzae* and a streak of beta hemolytic *Staphylococcus aureus* is made across the initial streaking. *Staphylococcus aureus* which is beta hemolytic releases factor X from RBCs and staphylococci themselves supply factor 'V'.

Biochemical Tests

- Glucose and xylose are fermented.
- Catalase positive, oxidase positive and nitrates are reduced to nitrites.

Resistance

This bacterium is inactivated by refrigeration (0–4°C) and heating at 55°C for 30 minutes. Hence CSF should not be refrigerated.

Three Major Antigens

- *Capsular polysaccharide*: It is classified into types **a–f;** (Hi 'b' is most relevant in clinical infections). Antibody against it gives protection. Type 'b' capsular polysaccharide contain polyribosyl ribitol phosphate **(PRP)**, hence it is used in the vaccine (PRP vaccines and PRP-conjugate vaccines). As **Hib vaccine** is widely given, other serotypes 'c' and 'f' are increasingly reported causing infections along with non-capsulated strains.

- Outer membrane protein
- Lipo-oligosaccharide (LOS)

Typing Methods

- Serotyping is based on capsular antigen, 'a' to 'f'. Serotyping is done by various methods as agglutination, coagglutination, ELISA, CIE, Quellung reaction.
- Biotyping is based on indole test, urease test and ornithine decarboxylase test. 6 biotypes I to VI are known, most infections are produced by types I, II, III.
- *Phage typing*: Four types, i.e. HP1, HP3, S2 and N3 identified.

Variation: Colonies of *H. influenzae* show a smooth to rough (S-R) variation with loss of capsule and virulence. Genetic transformation has been demonstrated in this bacterium.

Pathogenesis of *H. influenzae*

It is strictly human pathogen. Non-capsulated strains may colonise nasopharynx and oropharynx in mostly all children within few months after birth.

Virulence Factors

- **Capsule** resists phagocytosis. Capsule is the most important virulence factor. On the basis of capsule, the bacterium is divided into 6 capsular types **'a' to 'f'**. Most of the strains which cause invasive infections belong to **capsular type 'b'.**
- **Lipid 'A'**: It probably induces meningeal inflammation.
- **IgA protease** breaks down IgA on mucosal surfaces, helps bacteria in adhesion.
- **Pili** help in adhesion

Mode of infection is by respiratory route. Bacilli adhere to mucosa by pili and other factors. Viral infection facilitates infection. The presence of anti-capsular antibodies, complement, phagocytes try to limit infection. In absence of anti-PRP antibodies, bacterial multiplication occurs. Bacteremia spreads the organisms to various sites including meninges. Non-capsulated strains spread locally after colonization and cause sinusitis, otitis media, bronchitis, and pneumonia.

Clinical Presentation

Invasive Disease

It is usually seen in children; mostly capsular Type 'b' causes invasive disease.

- Meningitis (common in age group 2 months to 2 years, mortality is high in untreated children—90%).
- Laryngoepiglottitis (croup): There is obstructive edema, common in 3 to 18 months of life.
- Bacteremia
- Pneumonia
- Arthritis (septic arthritis in children, involves large joints)
- Endocarditis and pericarditis
- Brain abscess

Noninvasive Diseases

Usually it is seen in adults, secondary infections caused by non-capsulated strains.

- Otitis media
- Sinusitis
- Exacerbation of COPD
- Chronic bronchitis and bronchiectasis

Epidemiology

Non-capsulated strains are present in nasopharynx or throat in 25–80% of healthy people; capsulated strains (50% type b) are present in 5–10%. Most of the invasive infections are caused by capsular serotype-b. Outbreaks occur in close communities. The mortality rate associated with meningitis is around 5%. Neurological sequelae as intellectual impairment, seizures, hearing loss is seen in 10–20% of survivors.

Laboratory Diagnosis of *H. influenzae*

Meningitis

Diagnosis is done by CSF Gram's stain, culture and antigen detection by latex agglutination or counter-immunoelectrophoresis. In croup or pneumonia—sputum is collected, it should be homogenized before culture.

Sample collection: CSF is collected under aseptic precautions by lumbar puncture.

Transport: Transport CSF immediately to laboratory or keep in incubator, or at room temperature but **never refrigerate** the sample as it hampers the viability of bacilli.

CSF examination: It shows increased pus cells, 4000–5000 WBCs/mL, with predominance of neutrophils. It shows decreased CSF glucose and increased CSF proteins.

Gram-stained smear shows pus cells with Gram-negative cocobacilli. It may show pleomorphism. (Long bacillary forms, short bacilli, coccobacilli; Gram-negative bacilli may be capsulated.)

Culture

- CSF is cultured on blood agar with central streak of *Staphylococcus aureus*
- Chocolate agar with disks of factors X and V may also used.

- Incubate the plates at 37°C with 5–10% CO_2 in candle jar and 60% humidity (by placing a guage piece soaked in water in candle jar).
- After 24–48 hours of incubation, 1–2 mm smooth, opaque colonies will be observed.
- On clear solid medium, smooth transparent, glistening colonies are produced after several days. The organism has ability to mutate which is rough nonvirulent form produced on subculture. The smooth colonies are called as **'honey droplet'** colonies.
  - Capsule can be detected by Quellung test.
  - **Biochemical tests:** It is catalase positive, oxidase positive.

Antigen detection: Hib capsular antigen in CSF is detected by Latex agglutination test or ELISA or coagglutination test or CIEP. The test has the advantage that it is rapid but disadvantage that it detects only common capsular type.

Treatment and Prevention

Drugs of choice: Cefotaxime or ceftazidime; amoxyclav or clarithromycin also effective. Carriage of non-capsulated strains in URT of young children is common. Rifampicin is used for chemoprophylaxis of susceptible contacts.

Conjugate vaccines available are PRP-OMPC (polysaccharide linked to outer membrane protein complex), the outer membrane complex of *Neisseria meningitidis* serogroup B, and PRP-T uses tetanus toxoid, in HbOC, mutant diphtheria acts as a carrier protein.

Some strains of *H. influenzae* are resistant to ampicillin through penicillin binding protein 3. It is beta-lactamase negative ampicillin resistance **(BLNAR)**.

HAEMOPHILUS AEGYPTIUS

- It is also called as **Koch-Weeks bacillus.**
- It causes **'pink-eye'** conjunctivitis.
- It is causative agent of **Brazilian purpuric** fever in infants and young children.
- It differs for *H. influenzae* being more fastidious, not fermenting xylose.

HAEMOPHILUS DUCREYI (Causes STD)

- It causes chancroid or **"soft sore"** which is painful, non-indurated, irregular ulcer which bleeds easily. Inguinal lymph nodes are enlarged and become painful.
- **'School of fish'** or **'railroad track'** appearance is seen in **Gram's stain.** The bacterium shows **bipolar staining.**

- Material is collected from ulcer base by scraping and cultured on media after Gram's staining. It grows on **chocolate agar** with **isovitalex** fetal calf serum and vancomycin which acts as selective agent. It requires factor 'X' and not 'V'.
- Chorioallantoic membrane of chick embryo is also used for cultivation.
- Growth is identified by agglutination with anti-serum.
- A multiplex PCR is developed for simultaneous detection of *H. durcei, T. pallidum* and herpes simplex virus in genital specimens.

Treatment: Single dose of azithromycin is used for treatment. Other drugs are ciprofloxacin, ceftriaxone, and erythromycin.

HAEMOPHILUS PARAINFLUENZAE

- It requires only 'V' and not 'X' factor.
- It forms larger colonies than *H. influenzae* which are yellow and opaque, ferments sucrose.
- It is commensal in URT : It causes subacute bacterial endocarditis, urethritis, and pharyngitis.

HAEMOPHILUS APHROPHILUS

It may present as commensal in mouth and throat. On chocolate agar, it forms yellowish large colonies, and requires factor 'X' not 'V'. It requires high concentration of CO_2. It may rarely cause subacute endocarditis, brain abscess, pneumonia, and sinusitis.

HACEK GROUP OF ORGANISMS

- These are fastidious, slow-growing bacteria.
- They form normal mouth resident flora.
- It can cause infections; especially endocarditis. Other infections include otitis media, pneumonia, conjunctivitis, septic arthritis, wound infection, brain abscess, and periodontal infections.
- Blood culture takes 7–30 days to be positive.

The organisms in this group are *Haemophilus parainfluenzae, H. aphrophilus, H. paraphrophilus, Actinobacillus actinomycetemcomitans, Cardiobacter hominis, Eikenella corrodens,* and *Kingella kingae.*

Haemophilus species are responsible for 1% of causes of infective endocarditis. Majority are caused by *H. aprophilus* (following dental disease and sinusitis, otitis), followed by *H. parainfluenzae.*

Actinobacillus actinomycetemcomitans may cause periodontitis and infective endocarditis in patients with prosthetic heart disease.

It forms normal oral flora. The species name contains word 'Actinomycete' and part of word 'concomitiant' (means at the same time). It is facultative anaerobe, grows under CO_2 and humid conditions. Colonies adhere to agar and have 'star-like' structure at the center.

CARDIOBACTER HOMINIS

- Gram-negative, pleomorphic rods
- Form normal flora of mouth
- Rarely causes endocarditis
- Pleomorphic rods 'rossetes'
- Grows on BA, chocolate agar and pit the agar
- No growth on MacConkey agar
- It may cause meningitis.

EIKENELLA CORRODENS

- It is Gram-negative coccobacillary form. It may form normal flora of mouth.
- On blood agar and chocolate agar, small spreading yellowish colonies are produced. No growth on MacConkey agar. Colonies may be bleach-like odor. Rapid identification kits are available.
- It shows twitching or jerky motility by contraction of fimbria.
- Oxidase +ve, asaccharolytic
- It has the ability to corrode the agar during growth, hence the name.
- It causes cellulitis following human bites, clenched fist injuries, endocarditis in drug addicts, respiratory infections as pneumonia, empyema.

KINGELLA KINGAE

It is Gram-negative coccobacillary form and may rarely cause endocarditis.

- Infections produced in young patients include wound infection, bacteremia, endocarditis, and osteomyelitis.
- BA, CA used for culture, better growth is seen under 5–10% CO_2.
- Can grow on gonococcal selective medium.
- Oxidase +ve, glucose utilizers.
- Out of *K. kingae* and *K. detrificans,* later one is nitrate positive.
- Growth around penicillin disk is used for staining. It becomes rod-shaped (differentiates from gonococci).

Laboratory Diagnosis

- *Blood culture*: Subcultures are done on chocolate agar with vitamins.
- Plates are incubated with 5–10% CO_2 for 24–48 hours, blood culture bottles are incubated further if no growth occurs, up to at least 14 days after which subcultures are done on chocolate agar.
- Detection is done in one week by BACTEC.
- PCR is highly sensitive method.

Treatment

Ceftriaxone is the drug of choice, ampicillin along with gentamicin can be used.

38

Bordetella

BORDETELLA PERTUSSIS

Bordet and Gengou identified the bacterium from sputum of patient suffering from disease, pertussis—means intense cough.

The genus *Bordetella* also includes following species— *Bordetella parapertussis* which causes mild disease, *Bordetella avium* causes respiratory disease in birds and *Bordetella bronchiseptica* (originally isolated from dogs).

Morphology

- They are small 0.5 µ, ovoid, capsulated (tend to loose capsule on repeated subculture); non-sporing Gram-negative coccobacilli. **Capsule doesn't give Quellung reaction**.
- **Bipolar metachromatic granules** are seen on staining with toludine blue.
- If Gram-stained smear is prepared from colony on culture, bacteria tend to occur in clumps and there will be space in between, giving **thumb print** appearance.

Cultural Characteristics (Table 38.1)

- It is strictly aerobic and growth takes place in presence of 5–10% CO_2.
- Optimum temperature is 35°C, longer incubation (at least 5 days) with enhanced humidity required (a bowl of water should be placed on the floor of incubator).
- Bordet-Gengou glycerine potato blood agar (blood neutralizes the inhibitors).
- Charcoal blood agar (charcoal also adsorbs inhibitors).
- Charcoal blood agar with cephalexin is selective medium.
- Colonies appearance on Bordet-Gengou medium is dome-shaped, shining giving **'bisected pearl'** or **'mercury drop'** apperance. Confluent growth gives 'aluminium paint' apperance. Charcoal agar supplemented with 10% horse blood and cephalexin.
- **Regan-Lowe (RL)** medium is available as semisolid transport medium as well as solid medium for isolation of organism.

TABLE 38.1 Differentiating features of Bordetella species (note—V = variable)

	B. pertussis	*B. parapertussis*	*B. bronchiseptica*	*B. avium*
Motility	–	–	+	+
Growth on MacConkey	–ve	+ve	+ve	+ve
Growth on Bordet-Gengou	–ve	+	+	+
Medium	3–6	1–2	1	1
Urease	–ve	+ve	+ve	–ve
Nitrate	–ve	–ve	+ve	–ve
Citrate	–ve	v	+ ve	V
Oxidase	+ve	–ve	+ve	+ve
HLT and TCT toxin	+ve	+ve	+ve	+ve
ACT toxin	+ve	+ve	+ve	–ve
PT toxin	+ve	–ve	–ve	–ve

Modulation: It is a reversible change in capsular antigen called as **modulation**. Bacteria occur in any of the 3 modes—X, I, C. Each has special antigen. X, I, C term is derived from color of colonies produced by Bordetella, 'X' for xanthia (yellow), 'C' for cyanic (blue) and 'Z' for intermediate. On Bordet Gengou medium, fresh isolates are in 'X' mode.

- **Lacey's DFP medium** which is Bordet-Gengou medium with diamine fluoride and penicillin is used as **selective medium**.

  It is biochemically inert, oxidase and catalase are positive.

Resistance

Though it is delicate organism, it survies in droplets for 4–5 days. It is easily killed by heat (55°C for half hour) and disinfectant.

Antigens and Virulence Factors

- Antigens are associated with capsule and fimbria.
- *Pertussis toxin (PT)*: It has 3 different actions—lymphocytosis-producing factor, histamine-sensitizing factor, islet-activating protein.
- Marked lymphocytosis seen in patients with *B. pertussis* is due to **lymphocytosis-producing factor (LPF)**.
- Histamine-sensitizing factor increases sensitivity of experimental animal to histamine.
- Islet-activating factor stimulates insulin production by pancreatic cells.
- *Filamentous hemagglutinins (PHA)*: It adheres to cilia of respiratory epithelium and erythrocytes and promotes secondary infection. (It binds to galactoside residues on ciliated cells and CR3 receptors on polymorphs). As the bacterium survives inside leukocytes, it exempts from attack of antibodies.

- *Adenylate cyclase (AC toxin)*: It acts by catalyzing the production of cAMP by various types of cells and help in attachment.
- *Heat-labile toxin*: Its pathogenic role not known.
- *Tracheal cytotoxin*: It causes ciliary damage, inhibits ciliary movements, stimulates release of IL-1, prevents regeneration of cells.
- *Lipopolysaccharide* (endotoxin—heat-stable toxin).
- *Smooth to rough variation*: Fresh isolates (smooth form) after subculture loose surface antigens, become rough (avirulent) forms.
- Reversible change in capsular antigen, bacillus may occur in one of three modes—X, I, C. X refers to xanthic yellow, 'C' for cyanic (blue) and 'I' for intermediate forms.

Pathogenicity (Flowchart 38.1)

The local manifestations of the disease are tracheitis and bronchitis, along with accumulation of mucus, inflammatory cells, bacteria, and epithelial cells. The mucociliary elevator is impaired by damage to ciliary epithelial cells and cough is triggered because cough receptors are sensitized. The intense straining against the closed vocal cords occurs in an effort to expel the mucus and debris in the lower respiratory tract. Deep inspiration and forced expiration make up the 'whoop'.

Infection spreads by droplets and fomites, incubation period is 1 to 2 weeks (Flowchart 38.2).

Clinical Stages

- *Catarrhal*: It is first stage, highly infectious and clinical features are mild cough, corzya, malaise, low grade fever, lacrimation.

Flowchart 38.1: Pathogenicity of *B. pertussis*

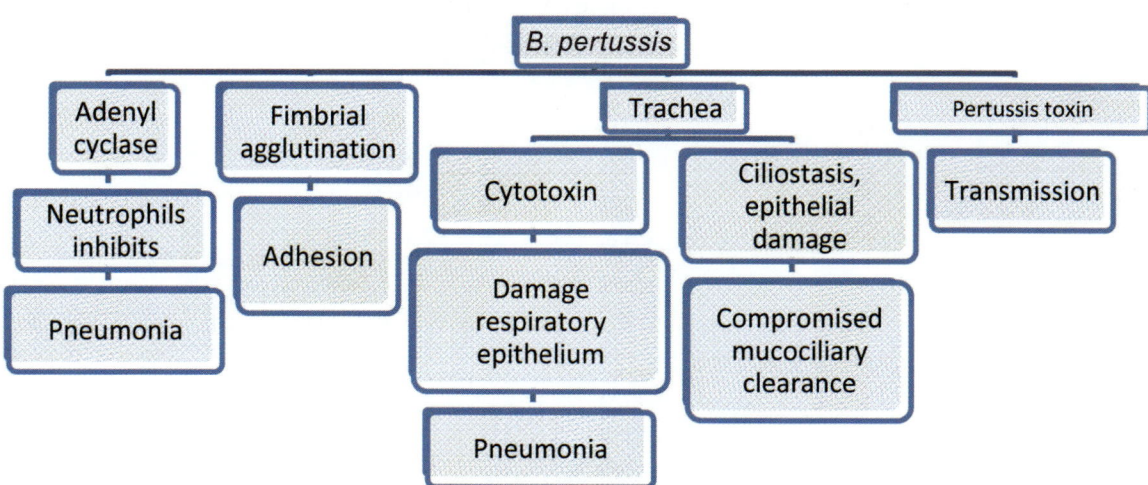

Flowchart 38.2: Mechanisms of damage in pertussis

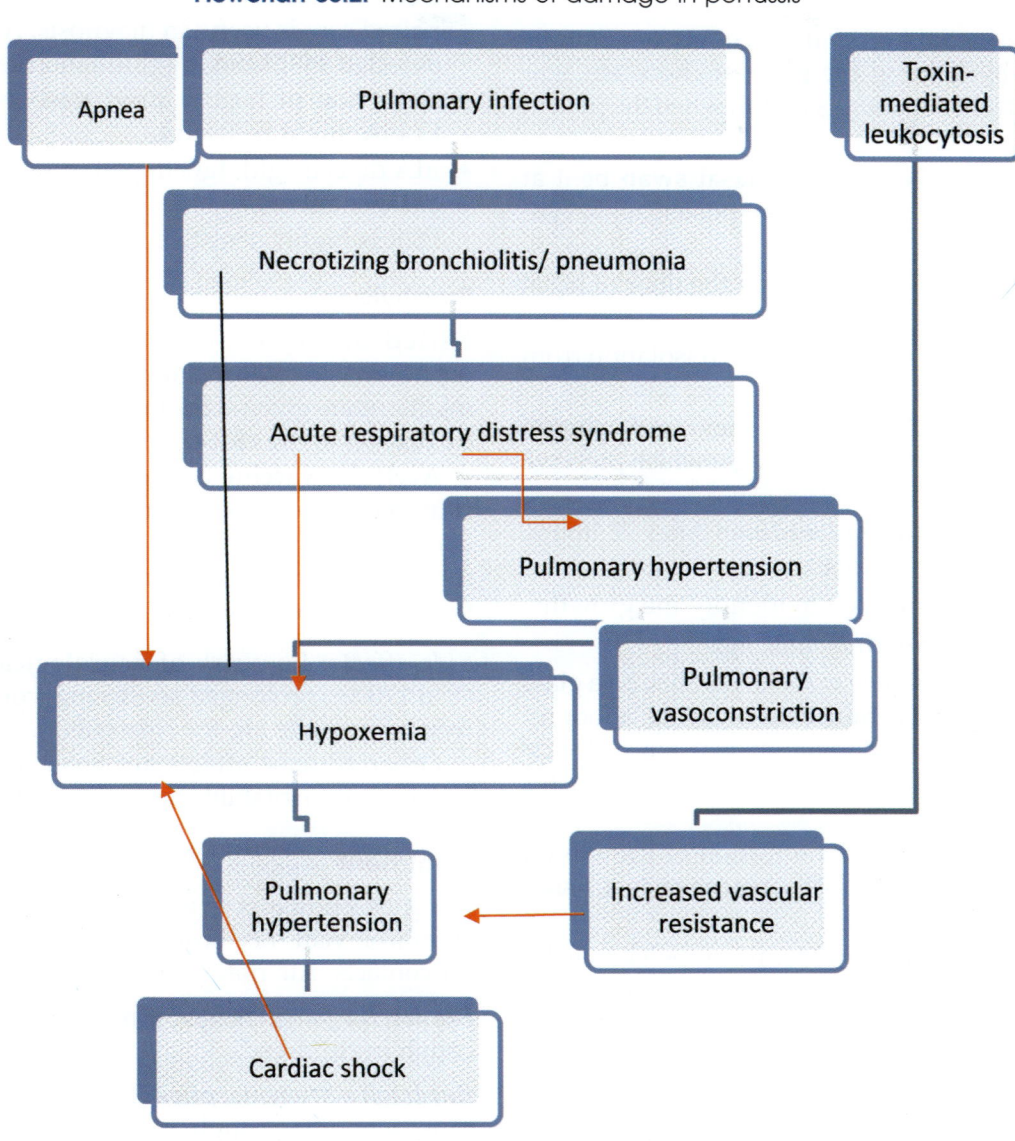

- *Paroxysmal*: Violent spasms of **cough "whooping"**, **cough** becomes more and more spasmodic and there may be vomitings after coughing. It is highly infectious stage.
- **Convalescent phase (2–4 weeks or 1–3 months)**, cough gradually resolves.

Complications

- *Pressure effects*: Subconjunctival hemorrhage, subcutaneous emphysema, pneumothorax, abdominal and inguinal hernia, petechiae on face and abdomen.
- *Respiratory*: Bronchopneumonia, lung collapse, bronchitis, bronchiectasis.
- *Neurological*: Convulsions, coma, paralysis, deafness, mental retardation.
- Bacilli do not invade bloodstream.

Epidemiology

New cases arise from symptomatic patients because cough provides an efficient means of dissemination of bacilli. Long-term carriage is not known. The degree of contact is important: 80–90% of non-immune siblings exposed in household become infected, compared with less than 50% of non-immune child contacts at school.

The disease is more severe and mortality rate highest in first 2 years of life.

Although one attack confers long-lasting immunity, different serotypes may infect everytime. Serotypes 1, 2 and 3 are most prevalent.

B. pertussis causes 95% cases of whooping cough while 5% are caused by *B. parapertussis*. Whooping cough-like clinical picture is also produced by other organisms as adenovirus, *Mycoplasma pneumoniae*. The syndrome is called as '**pseudo-whooping cough'**.

Laboratory Diagnosis

- *Cough plate method of sputum collection*: Sample is collected by holding the plate of chocolate agar 10–15 cm in front of patient's mouth when the patient is coughing.
- *Post-nasal swab*: **Waste's postnasal swab** bent at 40° is used to collect material from posterior pharyngeal wall.
- *Per-nasal swab*: It is passed along the floor of nasal cavity.
- Recent studies have shown improved isolation from suction.
- Transport in 0.25–0.5 mL of casamino acid solution or in Stuart's medium or charcoal agar which preserve viability.
- *Culture on Bordet-Gengou medium*: After 72 hours, colonies are opaque, smooth.
- **Biochemical tests** are used to identify the growth.
- *Identification of growth is done by*:
  1. *Slide agglutination using antisera*. For this, on a glass slide, the colony is emulsified in saline, a loopful of antiserum is added to the suspension and slide is gently rocked for 1 minute and observed for clumping.
  2. Another method for identification of growth on medium is by **immunofluorescence** test using specific antiserum.
  3. Recently immunological identification is done by **rapid immunoblot** method by using monoclonal antibodies.
- **Immunofluorescence** of direct smears of specimens and smears from cultures helps in rapid identification.
- Demonstration of **specific antigens in** nasal secretions is done by **ELISA.**

Detection of Antibodies

- Antibody detection is not much helpful in diagnosis.
- Demonstration of 4-fold rise in titre of antibodies in paired sera is useful in diagnosis. Antibodies can be detected by ELISA, agglutination test.
- Detection of locally produced secretory IgA by ELISA might be useful.
- EIA detects IgM, IgG in paired sera (against PT and FHA antigens).
  PCR is highly sensitive method for diagnosis.

Prophylaxis

Killed alum absorbed vaccine combined with diphtheria toxoid and tetanus toxoid is used. Three injections are given at the interval of 4–6 weeks followed by booster at the end of one year.

Acellular vaccine consists of one or more different components which are chemically or genetically detoxified pertussis, filamentous hemagglutinin, 69 kDa outer membrane antigen, fimbrial 2 and 3 antigens. Vaccination not advised routinely after 7 years of age.

Side effects: Low risk of neurological complications (1 in 17000), prolonged screaming, convulsions, hyporesponsive state are the side effects.

Other adverse effects are fever, tenderness at the injection site, irritability and neurological complications.

Treatment

Drug of choice is erythromycin, azithromycin or clarithromycin. Erythromycin prophylaxis is indicated for contacts. Alternative drug is cotrimoxazole.

Bordetella parpertussis: It may cause mild whooping cough in children.

Bordetella bronchiseptica: It is motile and may rarely cause whooping cough. It can grow on nutrient agar. It is responsible for approximately 0.1% cases of whooping cough.

Bordetella avium: It causes coryza in turkeys. It can grow on nutrient agar. It produces HLT and TCT but does not produce ACT and PT.

39

Brucella

Brucellosis is called Malta fever or undulant fever or Mediterranean fever. Brucellosis is a zoonotic disease affecting goats, buffalos, pigs, other animals (Bruce—isolated organism for the first time, melitiensis—after Melita, the Roman name for Malta).

Different Species

- *Brucella abortus* causes disease in cattle (contagious abortions).
- *Brucella melitensis* causes disease in sheep and goat.
- *Brucella suis* causes disease in pigs.
- *Brucella canis* causes disease in dogs.
- *Brucella pinnipediae* and *cetacea* are newly recog-nized marine mammal species that may also infect humans.

Morphology

They are non-motile, non-capsulated, non-sporing, Gram-negative coccobacilli ($0.5–0.7 \times 0.6–1.5\mu$). They may show bipolar staining.

Cultural Characteristics

- It is strictly aerobic, growth is slow in simple media, it is capnophilic (require 5–10% CO_2), optimum pH—6.6–7.4.
- Optimum temperature is 37°C.
- Growth improved by adition of serum or liver extract to the medium.
- **Media:** Serum dextrose agar, serum potato infusion agar, trypticase soy agar.
- **Biphasic medium** containing tryptic soy agar slant and tryptic soy broth at the bottom of the medium is used for blood culture.
- **Tryptose agar with bacitracin, polymyxin and cycloheximide is a selective medium:** Colonies are small, and low convex, smooth, and transparent.

- **MacConkey's agar:** Non-lactose fermenting colorless colonies are produced.
- In liquid media, it shows uniform turbidity and powdery deposit.

Castaneda's Method of Blood Culture (Fig. 39.1)

It is a biphasic medium having broth as well as solid slant in the same bottle. Usually trypicase soy agar and trypticase soy broth is used.

It is used for blood culture and bone marrow culture.

Under all aseptic measures, 5–10 mL of blood is collected by venipuncture and inoculated in the broth at the bottom of the biphasic medium.

The bottle is incubated for 48 hours in incubator and after that it is tilted, so that broth runs over the agar slant in the same bottle, thus for subculture, just tilt the bottle; while in conventional blood culture, blood is inoculated in broth which after incubation for 48 hours, is subcultured on a solid medium (liquid

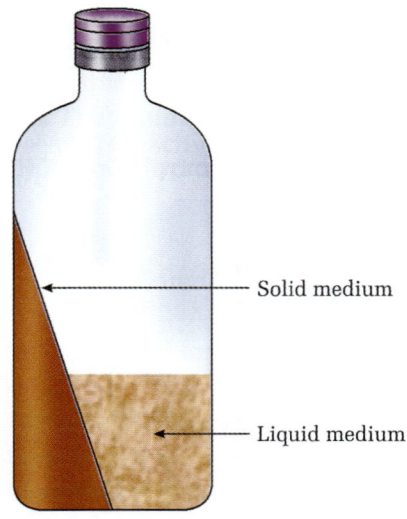

Solid medium

Liquid medium

Fig. 39.1: Castaneda biphasic medium

medium is taken by aspiration with sterile needle and syringe). The colonies are observed on slant portion.

Advantages

- The manupulation is not required in Castaneda's medium.
- There are chances of contamination in routine blood culture bottle while subculturing, which is not there in Castaneda's method.
- Materials are minimized in Castaneda's method.
- The risk of infection in laboratory persons is minimized.
- Growth in embryonated egg: Brucella grows on CAM of chick embryo and growth is indicated by death of egg.

Biochemical Tests

- No carbohydrates are fermented.
- Catalase positive, oxidase positive, urease positive, nitrates reduced to nitrites.
- Indole, MR, VP, citrate negative.

Resistance

They survive 10 days in refrigerated milk, 1 month in ice-cream, 4 months in butter, varied periods in cheese. They are killed at 60°C for 10 minutes. They are killed by pasteurization.

Antigens of Brucella (Table 39.1)

- **Brucella is classified into three species:** B. melitensis, B. abortus, and B. suis.
- **There are two main antigens:** 'A' and 'M', Brucella abortus contains more 'A' antigen, and B. melitensis contains more 'M' antigen.
- They show crossreactions with Vibrio cholerae, E. coli O:116, O:157, Salmonella, Stenotrophomonas maltophilia, Yersinia enterocolitica and Francisella tularensis.
- Subspecies level identification is done by bacteriophage typing; the reference phage—Tbilisi (Tb) phage is used in typing.

Species

Species identification is done by CO_2 requirement, H_2S production, sensitivity to dyes, agglutination by

TABLE 39.1: Differentiation of Brucella species

Species	Biotype	Lysis by bacteriophage RTD	Lysis by bacteriophage RTD × 10⁴	CO₂ requirement	H₂S	Growth on dye media — Basic fuchsin 1.50000 (1:25000)	Growth on dye media — Basic fuchsin (50000)	Thionin	Agglutination by Mono specific sera (A)	Mono specific sera (M)	Anti-rough serum
B. melitensis	1	–	–	–	–	+	–	+	–	+	–
	2	–	–	–	–	+	–	+	+	–	–
	3	–	–	–	–	+	–	+	+	+	–
B. abortus	1	+	+	+/–	+	+	–	–	+	–	–
	2	+	+	+	+	–	–	–	+	–	–
	3	+	+	+/–	+	+	+	+	+	–	–
	4	+	+	+/–	+	+	–	–	–	+	–
	5	+	+	–	–	+	–	+	–	+	–
	6	+	+	–	+/–	+	–	+	+	–	–
	9	+	+	+/–	+	+	–	+	–	+	–
B. suis	1	–	+	–	+	–	+	+	+	–	–
	2	–	+	–	–	–	–	+	+	–	–
	3	–	+	–	+	+	+	+	–	–	–
	4	–	+	–	–	+	+	+	+	+	–
B. neotomae		–	+	–	+	–	–	+	–	–	–
B. ovis		–	–	+	–	+	+	+	–	–	+
B. canis		–	–	–	–	+	+	–	–	–	+

monospecific antisera, phage lysis and metabolic tests. *Br. melitensis*, *Br. abortus* and *Br. suis* infect goats or sheep, cattle and swine, respectively. Further classification is based on biotyping.

Biotypes

   i. *Br. abortus*—7 biotypes (1–9, number 7, 8 are deleted)

   ii. *Br. melitensis*—3 biotypes

   iii. *Br. suis*—5 biotypes

   Br. suis strains which produce H_2S are called as **'American strains'** while those not producing H_2S are called **Danish strains.**

Phage Typing

The Tbilisi (Tb) reference phage is used for phage typing. *B. abortus* is lysed by Tb phage at 1 RTD and 1000 RTD while *B. suis* is lysed at 1000 RTD and *B. melitensis* is not lysed at all.

Pathogenicity

All major species are pathogenic, of which most pathogenic is *B. melitensis* followed by *B. abortus*, *B. canis* and *B. suis*. The pathogenicity in human brucellosis is attributed due to factors like LPS, adenine and guanine monophosphate, virB, 24 kDa protein, and urease enzyme. Brucellae may enter the host via ingestion or inhalation, or through conjunctiva or skin abrasions. The brucellae colonize in different organs with predilection for lymphoreticular system.

Modes of Transmission

- Direct contact with animal tissue as in farmers.
- Ingestion of contaminated milk.
- Inhalation of aerosolized organisms.
- Infection in laboratory person by inhalation or accidental injury.

   It mainly affects reticuloendothelial system. Organisms spread from the site of infection to local lymph nodes where they multiply and enter bloodstream and cause disseminated disease.

Three types of infection are seen:

1. *Latent infection*: No clinical disease, only serological evidence may be present (antibodies positive in serum).
2. *Acute or subacute brucellosis*: It is called as undulant fever, presents with musculoskeletal pain, asthmatic attacks, sweating at night, exhaustion, anorexia, constipation, irritability and chills.
3. *Chronic brucellosis*: It presents as sweating, lassitude, joint pains, nervousness.

Complications

- Epididymo-orchitis
- Hydrocele
- Urinary tract infection
- Pyonephrosis
- Infertility
- Meningitis
- Meningoencephalitis
- Peripheral neuritis
- Facial palsy
- Hemiplegia
- Endocarditis
- Cutaneous or mucous membrane lesions
- Chronic liver disease
- Splenic abscess
- Acute cholecystitis
  - Pneumonia
  - Bronchitis
  - Hematologic complications
  - Severe anemia

Epidemiology

Brucellae are animal pathogens transmitted to humans by accidental contact with infected animal faces, urine, milk or tissues. The common sources of infection are unpasteurized milk, milk products, cheese and occupational contact (e.g. farmers, veterinarians, and slaughterhouse workers). Occasionally, airborne route is important.

Laboratory Diagnosis

Culture

- *Blood culture*: TSB culture kept for 6–8 weeks. **Castaneda method** is recommended.
- **Bone marrow culture.**
- **Other samples** which can be cultured are lymph node, CSF, urine, abscesses, occasionally sputum, breast milk, vaginal discharge and semen.

Identification is done by:

- Preparing smears from colonies, it shows Gram-negative coccobacilli.
- Oxidase test, ability to use glutamic acid, ornithine, lysine, ribose, production of H_2S are used for identifications.
- **Agglutination** with specific antisera is done for which colonies are emulsified in saline and antiserum added followed by mixing, clumping occurs.

Antibodies Detection

- Standard **agglutination test** (SAT): It is a tube agglutination test for detection of antibodies.

- Detects mainly IgM; **titer 1:160 is significant**. Due to presence of blocking antibodies, Coomb's serum should be used for detection of antibodies by agglutination.
- **Modified test:** Serum is first treated with 2-mercaptoethanol and then agglutination performed, it detects IgG. IgM is sensitive to it, while IgG is resistant. It differentiates acute from chronic brucellosis. This test is superior to routine agglutination test for determinig the response to treatment.

Other tests for antibodies detection are (Table 39.2):
- **Complement fixation test** is more useful in chronic cases (detects IgG as well as IgM)
- IgG or IgM specific **ELISA** can be done.

ELISA yields higher sensitivity and specificity.
- **Lateral flow** is used for antibodies detection.
- **Latex agglutination** is also used for antibody detection.
- **Indirect immunofluorescence** test is sensitive test.
- **PCR is done with primers specific for OMP2, OMP25, rrs-rrl genes.**
- Delayed type of hyposensitivity to brucellin antigen is not helpful in diagnosis.

Diagnosis of Brucellosis in Animals

It is done by microscopy (Gram's and direct immunofluorescence test), rapid plate agglutination test, **milk ring test** and **rose Bengal card test.**

Modified ZN staining method (Brucella differential stain)

Brucella abortus in tissues and exudates is stained by modified Z-N stain. Dilute carbol fuschin (1 in 10) is added to smear without heating for 15 minutes, decolorization is done with 0.5% acetic acid for 15 seconds and after washing the slide, counterstaining is done for 1 minute with methylene blue.

Rose Bengal card test: It is a rapid slide agglutination test with a buffered stained antigen. Though it is widely used as screening test in animals, it also gives good results with human brucellosis.

Rapid plate agglutination test is developed for antibodies detection.

Test to detect antibodies in milk is milk ring test. The sample of milk is mixed with a drop of brucella antigen stained with hematoxylin and incubated at 70°C in water bath for 40–50 minutes. If antibodies are produced against brucella in milk, bacilli are agglutinated and rise with cream to form a blue ring at the top, the remaining milk is unstained.
- *Whey agglutination test*: It is another test useful in detection of antibodies in milk.

Treatment

Gold standard treatment is doxycycline plus streptomycin while rifampicin plus doxycycline is alternative treatment. Cotrimoxazole is given in children and pregnant women. Patients with neurological diseases are treated with combination of doxycycline, streptomycin and ceftriaxone.

The treatment recommended by the World Health Organization for acute brucellosis in adults is rifampicin 600 to 900 mg and doxycycline 100 mg twice daily for a minimum of six weeks.

Prophylaxis

- Persons handling animals should use protective clothing and gloves.
- Pasteurization of milk should be done.
- Cattle should be immunized with live-attenuated *Br. abortus* strain 19 vaccine while goats and sheep should be immunized with *Br. melitensis* **Rev.1 vaccine.**
- *Br. abortus* **strain 19-BA** (more attenuated strain 19) is used for human immunization in USSR. Slaughter the unimmunized infected animals.

TABLE 39.2: Results of serological tests in diagnosis of brucellosis in various clinical types

Type of brucellosis	Agglutination test	Mercaptoethanol	CFT	ELISA
Acute	+	+/–	+	+
Chronic	+/–	+	+	+
Past infection	(—)	—	—	(—)

40

Mycobacterium Tuberculosis

Mycobacteria are "fungus-like bacteria", as they may show branching. They are slender, acid-fast, aerobic bacteria which cause one of the dreadful infections of lungs. Hansen first discovered *M. leprae*. Koch first isolated tubercle bacillus and satisfied Koch's postulates.

Morphology

- Acid-fast bacilli (Fig. 40.1): Acid-fast nature of the organism is due to presence of mycolic acid (unsaponifiable wax) in the cell wall.
- It is straight or slightly curved rod.
- Size: 3 × 0.3 μ, even long bacillary forms may be seen.
- Arrangement: Single, in pairs or as small clumps.
- **Beaded or barred** forms can be seen in which fragmented appearance is present.
- Non-acid-fast rods and granules may be present in culture which are called Much's granules as he suggested that these are non-acid forms of bacilli.

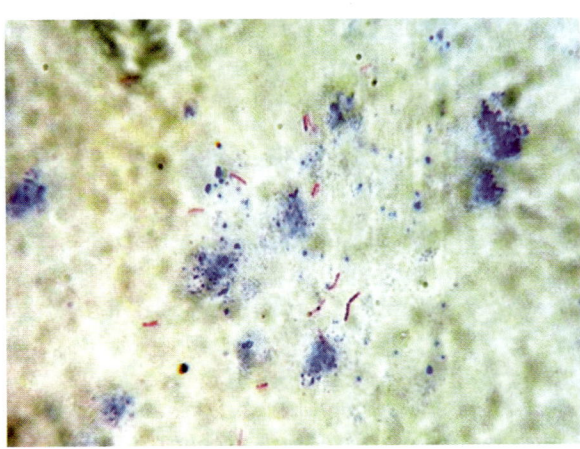

Fig. 40.1: AFB

Cultural Characteristics

They are aerobic, slow growing (due to mycolic acids on cell wall, nutrients cannot reach inside easily, hence slow growth and generation time is more). Generation time is 14–20 hours. The colonies appear in 2–8 weeks.

- Optimum temperature 37°C (25–40°C), pH—6.4–7.0.
- Organism is highly susceptible to fatty acids and other toxic substances produced in the media, which are neutralized by albumin or charcoal.
- Lowenstein-Jensen (LJ) medium is commonly used for isolation.

Other Media used for Cultivation of MTB

- **Solid**: Petragnani, Dorset egg, Tarshi's (blood), Loeffler (serum), Pawlowsky (potato).
- **Liquid**: Dubos, Middlebrook, Sula and Sauton's, Proskauer and Beck's.
- In liquid media, growth starts from the bottom and creeps up the side and forms a pellicle.
- Diffuse growth is seen in liquid media by addition of Tween 80.

Liquid media are used in automated methods; also they are used for preparation of antigen sensitivity tests. Virulent strains tend to form **serpentine cords** in liquid medium.

M. Tuberculosis (MTB) (Flowchart 40.1)

- Luxuriant growth (eugonic) is produced by MTB on L-J medium as compared to *M. bovis*.
- It produces dry, rough, irregular raised colonies with wrinkled surface.
- Colonies become buff-colored on further incubation.
- The **colony** is not easily emulsified, it is tenacious **(rough, buff, tough)**.

Flowchart 40.1 Role of mycolic acid in MTB pathogenesis of TB

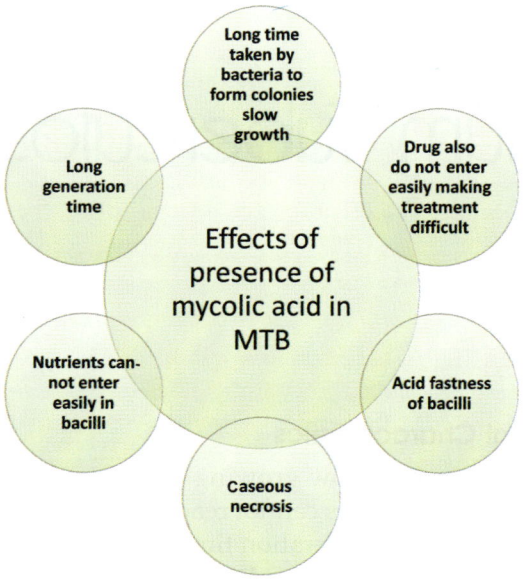

- MTB (0.5% improves the growth) grows on medium with glycerol.
- MTB also **doesn't grow** in medium containing **P-nitrobenzoic acid (500 mg/µl).**

M. bovis

- Sparse growth (dysgonic) on L-J medium (Fig. 40.2).
- Colonies are flat, smooth, moist.
- It produces white colonies.
- Colony breaks easily when touched.
- *M. bovis* grows better in conditions of reduced O_2 tension on soft agar media containing tween 80.

M. tuberculosis grows on the surface, while *M. bovis* forms a band of growth a few millimeters belew surface (Table 40.1).

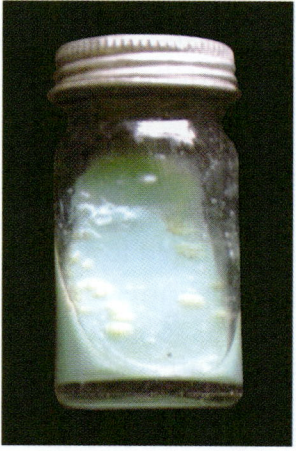

Fig. 40.2: L-J medium with growth of *M. tuberculosis*

TABLE 40.1: Differences between human and bovine tubercle bacilli

Mycobacterium tuberculosis	*Mycobacterium bovis*
Mode of infection mostly by inhalation of droplets	Mode of infection is by ingestion of milk or other animal products
Primary infection usually occurs in lungs	Infection of intestine
It grows luxuriously on L-J medium (eugonic)	Grows sparsly (dysgonic)
Growth in L-J medium with glycerol is present	No growth
Strictly aerobic	Initially microaerophilic
Dry, rough, irregular colonies on L-J medium	Flat, smooth, moist colonies are produced on L-J medium
Colonies are not easily emulsifiable	Colonies can be easily emulsifiable
Niacin test positive	Niacin test negative
Nitrate test is positive	Nitrate test negative
Vaccine strain is not derived from *M. tuberculosis*	Vaccine strain is derived from bovine TB bacilli
Comparatively low pathogenic to experimental animals	It is more pathogenic for experimental animals

Resistance

- Heating at 60°C for 15–20 minutes kill the bacilli.
- It survives longer in sputum (20–30 hours).
- Survival in droplet nuclei is 8–10 days.
- Cultures can be stored up to 2 years at 20°C.
- MTB is sensitive to formaldehyde, glutaraldehyde, tincture iodine and 80% ethanol.

Biochemical Reactions

- Niacin test differentiates human (+ve) and bovine strains.
- Aryl sulphatase test positive only with atypical mycobacteria.
- Neutral red test positive for virulent strains of tubercle bacilli.
- Tubercle bacilli give catalase weak positive, peroxidase positive.
- Atypical mycobacteria: Catalase strong positive, peroxidase negative.
- If *M. tuberculosis* looses catalase, peroxidase activity, resistance to INH may be predicted.

  Nitrate reduction test is positive with *M. tuberculosis*.

Niacin Test

M. tuberculosis doesn't produce enzyme which converts niacin to niacin ribonucleotide and accumulates niacin in the culture medium. When 10% cynogen bromide and 4% aniline in 96% ethanol are added to bacterial suspension, a canary yellow color shows a positive reaction. *M. tuberculosis* gives the test positive while *M. bovis* is negative. Other niacin positive bacteria are *M. simiae* and *M. cheloni*.

Arylsulphatase Test

Arylsulphatase is an enzyme produced by some atypical mycobacteria. The organisms are grown in a medium containing 0.001 M tripotassium phenophthalein disulphate. If the enzyme is produced, it liberates free phenophthalein from tripotassium phenophthalein disulphate. This can be detected by adding 2N NaOH dropwise to culture medium. If the test is positive, pink color develops.

Neutral Red Test

Virulent strains of tubercle bacilli can bind neutral red in alkaline buffer solution. Positive results are present with *M. tuberculosis*, *M. bovis*, *M. avium* and *M. ulcerans*.

Catalase Peroxidase Test

A mixture of equal volumes of 30% H_2O_2 and 0.2% catechol in distilled water is prepared to this 5 mL test culture and left for few minutes. Effervesce are produced, if test is positive. Brown discoloration means positive peroxidase test. *M. tuberculosis* and *M. bovis* are peroxidase positive and weak catalase positive while most of the atypical mycobacteria are strong catalase positive.

Amidase Test

Ability of an organism to break three amides, i.e. acetamide, benzamide, carbamide, nicotinamide and pyrizinamide is used in this test. A 0.00165 M solution of amide is incubated with the bacillary suspension at 37°C and to this 0.1 mL of $MnSO_4$, $4H_2O$, 1 mL of phenol solution and 0.5 mL of hychlorite solutions are added. The tubes are placed in boiling waterbath for 20 minutes. Blue color develops in positive test. *M. tuberculosis* splits nicotinamide and pyrazinamide.

Nitrate Reduction Test

Nitrate test positive bacteria reduce nitrate to nitrite by an enzyme nitroreductase. This test is positive with *M. tuberculosis* and negative with *M. bovis*. *M. kansasii*, *M. fortuitum* and *M. chelonei* may give this test positive. Part of colony is emulsified in a buffer solution containing nitrate and incubated at 37°C for 2 hours. Then sulphanilamide and n-naphthyl-ethylene diamine dihydrochloride solutions are added. Development of pink or red color indicates a positive test.

Susceptibility to Pyrizinamide

M. tuberculosis is sensitive to 50 µg/mL pyrazinamide while other mycobacteria including *M. bovis* are resistant.

Susceptibility to Thiophen-2-Carboxylic Acid Hydrazide

M. bovis is sensitive to 10 µg/mL of TCH. *M. tuberculosis* is not inhibited by this chemical. Some South Indian strains give positive results.

Tween 80 Hydrolysis

Enzyme lipase produced by some mycobacteria splits Tween 80 into oleic acid and polyoxyethylated sorbitol which modifies optical properties of test solution from yellow to pink. Pink color indicates hydrolysis of Tween 80. *M. tuberculosis* shows variable results. *M. kansasii* is positive while *M. bovis*, *M. africanum*, *M. avium* complex are negative.

Antigenic Structure

1. *Cell wall antigens*: The cell wall consists of lipids, proteins and polysaccharides. Lipids carry 60% of cell wall weight. Lipids of cell wall particularly mycolic acids are responsible for acid fastness of bacilli. Cell wall is made of four distinct layers.

a. Peptidoglycan is the innermost layer which gives shape and rigidity to cells.

b. Arabinogalactan lies external to peptidoglycan layer.

c. Mycolic acid layer is the principle constituent of cell wall.

d. Mycosides (phenolic glycolipids) form the outermost layer.

The cell wall antigens include arabinomanan, arabinogalactan and lipoarabinomanan.

2. *Cytoplasmic antigens*: These antigens are used for typing of mycobacteria. These antigens include antigen 5, antigen 6, antigen 14, antigen 19, antigen 32, antigen 38 and antigen 60. Antigen 60 is lipopolysaccharide while rest are proteins.

Typing

Antigenic Properties

- Group specificity is due to polysaccharide antigen.
- Type specificity is due to protein antigens.
  - There is some degree of relationship between MTB and atypical mycobacteria, also between *M. tuberculosis* and *M. leprae*.

– *M. tuberculosis* strains are antigenically homogeneous.

– Bacteriophage typing: There are four phage types, **type I common in India and worldwide.** The types are A,B,C and intermediate type-I.

– **Bacteriophage type 33D** isolated from environmental Mycobacterium, lyses all strains of *M. tuberculosis* but not BCG. This test is used to check vaccines.

– Bacitracin typing: Two types are seen.

– **Molecular typing** by DNA fingerprinting, RFLP, most strains contain a chromosomal insertion sequence **(IS6110),** the fingerprinting of it is used for epidemiological typing. **Spoligotyping:** It is based on typing the direct repeat locus **(DR).**

Entire genomic sequencing has been done for *M. tuberculosis and M. bovis.*

There is evidence that members of the *M. tuberculosis* complex (tubercle bacilli) mentioned above, developed from a common progenitor by successive loss of short chromosomal segments known as **'Regions of difference'—RD).**

M. canetti and some strains of South India are closest to progenitor strain.

M. bovis is developed from *M. tuberculosis.*

There are certain strains highly virulent in each species, e.g. *M. tuberculosis* and one family, **Beijing or W/Beijing family** spreading fast and have high virulence and easily develop drug resistance.

Virulence

- Virulent strains of *M. tuberculosis* form microscopic **serpentine cord** in which mycobacteria are arranged in parallel chains. **A cord factor** has been extracted from bacteria by treatment with ether. It inhibits migration of WBCs, causes chronic granuloma.

- **Lipoarabinomannan:** It facilitates the survival of bacilli within macrophages.

- **Kat G:** It encodes for catalase, an enzyme protective in oxidative stress.

- **Rpov:** It is **the main sigma factor** facilitating transcription of several genes.

- **Erp gene:** Encodes protein for multiplication.

- Virulence is also associated with cell wall lipids.

- Region of difference -1: It encodes for **early secretory antigen-6 (ESAT-6), culture filtrate protein-10.**

- Leu D, Pan CD and isocitrate lyase gene (icl 1).

- **Sigma factors: sigC, sigH genes.**

- **Varients of human *M. tuberculosis:* African varient** shows properties intermediate between human and bovine type; the **Asian strain shows** low virulence for guinea pigs (originally isolated from South India).

MYCOBACTERIUM TUBERCULOSIS COMPLEX

Mycobacterium tuberculosis refers to a group of genetically very closely related variants of what is strictly speaking is single species (Table 40.2).

Host range: Natural infection occurs in humans, dogs, and other primates. *M. bovis* is more pathogenic for animals.

Mode of infection: (1) Direct inhalation of aerosolized bacteria in droplet nuclei. (2) Sometimes infection can occur by ingestion (milk) or (3) Inoculation (rare). Virulence depends on ability to survive in macrophages and multiply. Only 1/10 of infected persons develops active tuberculosis. Cell-mediated immunity plays a major role.

Pathogenesis of Tuberculosis (Flowchart 40.2)

- TB bacilli: Enter by inhalation (Fig. 40.3).
- Source of infection is a open case of pulmonary tuberculosis.
- They are taken by pulmonary or alveolar macrophages.
- Invasion of macrophages may result partly due to the association of C2a with bacterial cell wall followed by C3b, opsonization of bacteria and recognization by macrophages.
- Macrophages are unable to kill, bacteria proliferate inside macrophages.
- Macrophages secrete IL-1.
- It stimulates TH cells.
- TH cells produce IL2 which activates macrophages.

TABLE 40.2: Tuberculosis complex

M. tuberculosis	The predominant cause of human tuberculosis
M. bovis	Causes tuberculosis in cattle
M. africanum	It appears to be intermediate between human type and bovine type. It causes human tuberculosis and it is mainly found in Africa. Type I is more common in West Africa and has many features similar to *M. bovis,* type II is seen in East Africa and it closely relates with human *M. tuberculosis*
M. caprae	It is isolated from goats, causes few cases of TB in veterinary surgeons
M. pinnipedi	Uncommon pathogen of seals and rarely causes infection in a occupationally involved person having contact with seals
M. microti	It is rarely encountered pathogen of voles but attenuated in humans
M. canetti	It is very rare and genetically primitive form

Flowchart 40.2: Pathogenesis of primary tuberculosis

Airborne droplet nuclei enter alveoli, multiplication of MTB starts.

Site of primary infection is usually middle zone (airflow is greatest)

Bacteria taken by alveolar macrophages which may clear bacilli. But for most of the time bacilli multiply inside the macrophage, destroying macrophages. The bacilli can multiply both extracellularly and intracellularly

Lymphocytes and monocytes are invited at the site of infection. Monocytes get converted into macrophages which engulf bacilli release from damaged cells.

Infected macrophages are carried by lymphatics to regional lymph nodes.

Some patients develop area of lung inflammation along with enlarged hilar lymph nodes draining the infected area of lung. This is called Ghon's complex

In non immune persons, the organisms may spread hematogenously throughout the body

During the dissemination, the bacteria localized in certain tissues, including lymph nodes, vertebral bodies, meninges and most importantly upper part of lungs.

Until the effective cell-mediated response develops, the bacilli proliferate at the sites of infections.

Primary infection can have various outcomes. CMI and delayed hypersensitivity develop in 3-8 weeks .

In most of the patients, the immune response does not control the infections and progressive pulmonary disease develops

The manifestations occur in very young , the elderly and patients with AIDS.

Pneumonia worsens, tuberculous meningitis may develop

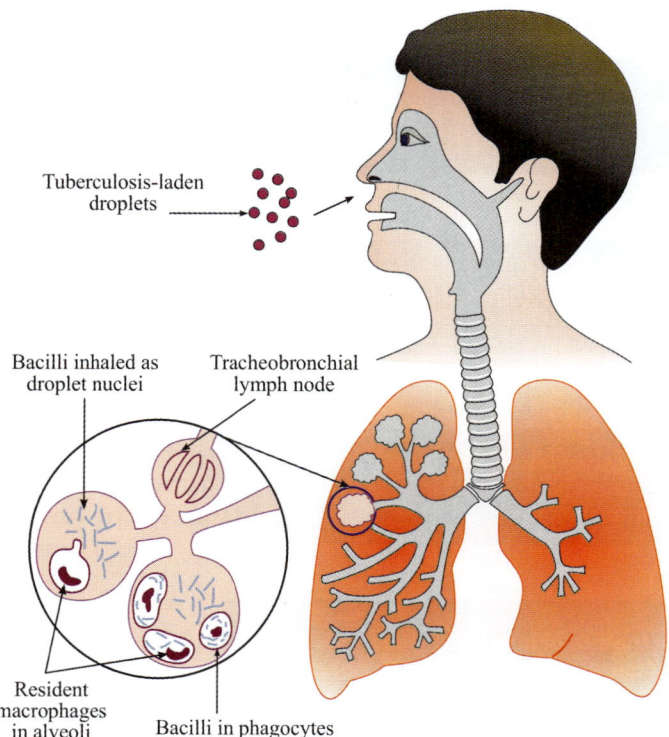

Tuberculosis-laden droplets

Bacilli inhaled as droplet nuclei

Tracheobronchial lymph node

Resident macrophages in alveoli

Bacilli in phagocytes

Fig. 40.3: Mode of infection

- In presence of cytokines and in an attempt to kill bacilli, macrophages undergo proliferation and are converted into epitheloid cells and giant cells, activated macrophages kill bacilli.

- Lipids present on bacilli cause central necrosis which is caseous necrosis, surrounded by lymphocytes, macrophages, fibroblasts, and fibrin is laid down in an attempt to seal the lesion.

- The balance between bactericidal activity of macrophage and number and virulence of bacteria determines the outcome of infection.

- If central necrotic material is connected to bronchus, material is coughed out which may contain live tubercle bacilli, infective to others, and **cavity formation occurs**.

- **Outcome:** CD4 cell is key cell in immune response. There are two types of CD4 cells—TH_1 and TH_2 secreting $INF\gamma$, IL-1, IL-2, $TNF\alpha$ and other cytokines. TH_1 dependent cytokines activate macrophages resulting in protection and limiting the infection while TH_2 induces delayed hypersensitivity and tissue destruction.

- **Role of genetic factor:** The human gene called **natural resistance associated macrophage protein-1 (NRAMP-1)** may have role in determining the susceptibility of person to tuberculosis.

Pathology

Avascular granuloma called '**tubercle**' has central zone of **Langerhans giant cells** with or without caseation surrounded by peripheral zone of lymphocytes and fibroblasts. It is an example of **type IV hypersensitivity**.

Exudative lesion: Acute inflammatory reaction, bacilli more virulent, host response more DTH in nature and there is accumulation of inflammatory cells and edema formation.

Productive type: Predominantly cellular, more associated with protective immunity than DTH.

Classification

Primary Tuberculosis (Pulmonary TB)

In endemic countries, it occurs in young children. Bacilli taken by macrophages, proliferate, form a subpleural focus of pneumonia called **Ghons focus**. Areas involved are upper part of lower lobe or lower part of upper lobe. The Ghon focus along with involved hilar lymph nodes form—**primary complex.** Usually, it heals spontaneously—a few bacilli may remain latent. It can cause miliary, meningeal or other disseminated TB. Lesion is small. Cavity formation is rare with primary infection. Local spread is uncommon in primary infection.

Post-primary Tuberculosis

It is seen in adults. The lesion is in upper lobe of lungs. It is due to reactivation of latent focus. Cavity formation occurs. Expectoration of bacteria-laden sputum acts as a source of infection for others. Lesion is larger. Lymph node involvement is uncommon. Local spread is common. In immunocompromised patients, dissemination to other organs may occur.

Extrapulmonary Tuberculosis (EPTB)

It due to dissemination of bacilli to various organs, Normally, it counts 20–40% cases of TB but much more common in HIV seropositive patients.

- *Tuberculous lymphadenitis:* 30% cases of EPTB are due to this type of TB. Commenest sites affected are cervical lymph node, supraclavicular lymph nodes. It is painless swelling without warmness and discoloration (cold abscess).
- *Pleural effusion:* It is responsible for 20% of EPTB cases.
- **Upper respiratory tract** involves larynx, pharynx and epiglottis.

Genitourinary TB

- Renal TB
- *Genital TB:* Females—MTB infects fallopian tubes, endometrial which may lead to infertility. Males—epididymitis is common.

- ***Skeletal TB*:** It is common in weight-bearing joints—Pott's spine, hip, knees are common sites. As the disease advances, there is collapse of vertical bodies with formation of kyphosis, and paravertebral abscess.
- ***Tuberculous meningitis*:** It is common in children. The presentation may be meningitis or tuberculoma formation.
- ***Pericarditis*:** It results from either by direct spread or by hematogenous method.
- ***Intestinal TB*:** Ileum and cecum are commonest sites affected. Modes of infection are ingestion of sputum, hematogenous spread or ingestion of contaminated milk with *M. bovis*.

Skin Lesions

- ***Scrofulaceum*:** It results from direct extension from underlying lymphadenitis.
- ***Lupus vulgaris*:** Nodules develop on face.
- ***Miliary tuberculosis or disseminated TB*:** It develops by hematogenous dissemination of bacilli and results in formation of small, yellowish granulomatous lesions **similar to millet** seeds in various organs.

HIV AND TB

HIV reactivates TB infection, makes disease more serious, and renders treatment ineffective.

TB hastens the progress of HIV infection to active disease.

Emergence and spread of MDR TB, XDR-extensively drug resistant bacilli and XXDR are reported which are difficult to treat.

The theme for World TB Day 2014 is "Reach the 3 Million". One-third of the estimated 9 million people falling ill with TB each year do not get the care they need. Moreover, traditional diagnostic tests can take more than 2 months to get results. But the situation is beginning to change. New technologies can rapidly diagnose TB and drug-resistant TB in as little as two hours. The EXPAND-TB multi-partner project to enable effective and sustained access, and use of recommended new TB diagnostic technologies in 27 low- and middle-income countries. These countries together carry 40% of the estimated global MDR-TB burden. Over 30% of the MDR-TB cases detected globally in 2012 were from EXPAND-TB countries. 90% of India's detected MDR-TB cases were through EXPAND-TB supported services. Use of these tests requires strengthened laboratory services. By the end of 2013, 92 laboratories were fully operational. From 2009 to 2013, the number of MDR-TB cases diagnosed in the 27 countries tripled, with 36 000 diagnosed in 2013 alone.

Epidemiology

- ***Incidence*:** 2.2 million new TB cases annually—176 cases per 100,000 population.
- ***Prevalence*:** 2.8 million cases—230 cases are seen per 100,000 population.
- ***Deaths*:** About 270,000 deaths occur each year—22 deaths per 100,000 population.
- Approximately 5% of TB patients estimated to be HIV +ve.

DR-TB (drug resistant-TB) 2.2% in new cases and 15% in previously treated cases. India is the highest TB burden country in the world, accounting for about 23.3% of the global prevalence. India has contributed to approximately 25.5% of the total global new cases detection during the year 2012 as per WHO Global Report 2013. In the year 2010, 3.5% of MDR cases in India have XDR.

Laboratory Diagnosis of Pulmonary TB Samples

- Sputum—early morning sample
- Laryngeal swabs
- Bronchial washings, BAL
- Gastric lavage in small children

Under **Revised National Tuberculosis Control Programme (RNTCP),** two sputum samples are recommended, i.e. early morning and one spot sample (Table 40.3).

Microscopy

- It is performed on direct or concentrated samples. Smears are stained by Ziehl-Neelsen technique.
- At least 10,000 bacilli per mL of sputum should be present to be detectable in direct smears.
- **Fluorescent microscopy: Auramine phenol or auramine-rhodamine dyes** are used for staining the smears. Smears are seen under high power. As smears are screened at high power in fluorescent microscope; **screening is rapid** which is helpful, if sample load is high.
  - Previously saprophytic bacilli were differentiated by the property that they are only acid-fast, not alcohol-fast. This concept is changed, it is proved

TABLE 40.3: Reporting as per RNTCP guidelines

	Result	Grading	No. of fields
>10/field	+	3+	20
1–10/field	+	2+	50
10–99/100 fields	+	1+	100
1–9/100 fields	+	Scanty	100
No. of AFBs in 100 fields	–		1000 fields

Flowchart 40.3: Pathogenesis of tubercle

Antigens of MTB processed by APCs activated by bacterial components and presented to antigen specific T lymphocytes which undergo clonal proliferation

↓

Activated T cells produce cytokines
INFγ with calcitrol activate macrophages and lead them to forms granuloma around foci of infections

↓

Activated macrophages become epithelioid cells which morphologicaly resemble epithelial cells

↓

Some of the epithelioid cells become giant cells.
Center of granuloma contains mixture of necrotic tissue, dead macrophages, cheese like- caseation

that alcohol fastness cannot be further used for differentiation and what alcohol does is just clearing of the smear.

Kinyoun's modification of acid-fast stain: In this modification of AFB staining, no heating is required (**cold method**). More concentrated phenol is added to smear for longer period.

Concentration Methods

Petroff's method: It is simple method and most commonly used for concentration of sputum sample. It has three important steps.

1. *Homogenization*: Sputum is mixed with equal volumes of 4% NaOH at 37°C with shaking for 20 minutes.
2. *Concentration by centrifugation*: Sputum is centrifuged at 3000 rpm for 20 minutes.
3. *Neutralization*: As alkali is added in the first step. It should be neutralized, for this, add few drops of N/10 HCl.

Advantages of Petroff's method: Reagents are easily available, organisms are not killed during concentration procedure hence, suitable for microscopy as well as culture.

NALC combined with 2% NaOH: This method is considered better than Petroff's method. N-acetyl-cysteine liquefies the sputum, NaOH kills the bacteria

and the sample is then neutralized with buffer and concentrated by centrifugation. **Most of the automated systems use this method**.

Concentration techniques are classified as follows:
A. *Concentration techniques for microscopy alone (culture not possible as bacteria are killed)*:
- Treatment with antiformin
- Treatment with sodium carbonate or sodium hypochlorite
- Use of detergents (tergitol)
- Floatation methods using hydrocarbons
- Autoclave

B. *Microscopy and culture (bacteria survive the concentration method, hence culture possible on the concentrated specimens)*:
- Petroff's method (sputum + 4% NaOH)
- Sputum + NaOH + cetrimonium bromide (no centrifugation or neutralization)
- Treatment with dilute acids
- Treatment with N-acetyl-cysteine with NaOH
- Treatment with pancreatin, desogen, zephiran, cetrimide
- Flocculation methods

Culture of Specimen

- It is very sensitive: It detects 10–100 bacilli per mL of sputum.
- L-J medium is widely used.
- Culture examined at 4 days (rapid growers) and twice a week thereafter.
- Negative report is given only after 8–12 weeks of incubation.
  Growth tested by ZN staining. Confirmation is done by biochemical tests.

Identification is done by following characteristics:
- Rough, buff, tough colonies on L-J medium, no pigment production.
- No growth on L-J medium with P-nitrobenzoic acid (PNB).
- Weak catalase positive.
- Niacin positive.
- Nitrate reduction—positive.
- Resistance to TCH.

Other Methods for Diagnosis

1. *BACTEC 460*: Radiolebeled C14 in palmitic acid is used as substrate in the **7H12** medium.When MTB grows, it utilizes the substrate for their growth and CO_2 is released. The 'C' in CO_2 is radiolabeled which is detected by radiometric method.

2. *MGIT*: The growth detection is based upon **AFB metabolism, O$_2$** utilization and subsequent O$_2$ quenching fluorescent dye in the medium.

   BACTEC 9000MB: It is an automated method and uses fluorescent quenching method.

3. *Nucleic acid methods to identify isolate*:
   - *PCR*: Most of the molecular methods based upon **rRNA, 16S rRNA, 16S rDNA**
   - **LCR, RFLP, IS fingerprinting**
   - **Line probe assay (line immunoassay)**
   - **Gene expert** detects the **multidrug resistance within short time**
   - *DNA chips, DNA microarrays*: It has been used to simultaneous identification of mycobacterial species and to detect mutation of gene which causes rifampicin resistance. It determinates specific nucleotide sequences, **diversity of rpoB** and **16S rRNA genes** help in speciation.
   - **Fluorescent in situ hybridization**

4. *Chromatographic analysis*: Analysis of mycobacterial mycolic acids be done by **gas liquid chromatography.**

5. *Mass spectrometry*: It has high sensitivity.

6. *Animal inoculation* in guinea pigs, now rarely used for the diagnosis.

7. *Quantiferon TB assays*: It is also called **interferon gamma release assay** because these tests detect release of INFγ from persons who have been exposed to *Mycobacterium tuberculosis*. It is an ELISA based test. Based on antigens, there are three types of generations.

   1st generation responds to 1-tuberculoprotein, PPD, 2nd generation test responds to 2 proteins, i.e. **ESAT6** (early secretory antigen target 6) and **CFP-10** (culture filtrate protein-10). These proteins secreted by both *M. tuberculosis* and *M. bovis* hence the test is positive with both bacilli. The nontubercle bacilli do not secrete both proteins except *M. kansasi, M. szulgai* and *M. marimum,* therefore, they may give the test negative. The 3rd generation responds to three tubercular proteins, ESAT-6, CFP-10 and TB7.7. These assays are **comparable with tuberculin** test in **evaluating latent infection,** particulary in those with BCG vaccine.

Animal Inoculation

Animal inoculation is performed in two healthy; tuberculin negative guinea pigs. Specimen is inoculated intramuscularly into the thighs. The animals are weighed prior to test and thereafter weekly. If the animal develops infection, tuberculin test becomes positive and there is progressive loss of weight. Animal is killed after six weeks. Autopsy is performed which shows following findings:

1. Caseous lesion at the site of inoculation.
2. Enlargement of caseous inguinal lymph nodes with spread to other lymph nodes as lumbar, mediastinal, and cervical lymph nodes.
3. Tubercles may be seen in spleen, lungs, liver and peritoneum.
4. Kidneys remain unaffected.

Acid-fast bacilli are demonstrated in the lesions. Sometimes the organisms produce only enlarged lymph nodes only and animals may have to observed for 12 weeks. *M. tuberculosis* is highly pathogenic to guinea pigs and hamsters and nonpathogenic for rabbits, while *M. bovis* is less pathogenic for rabbits and highly pathogenic for guinea pigs. Catalase negative and INH resistant strains and most of Asian strains isolated from South India show low virulence for guinea pigs. Animal inoculation method nowadays is rarely used for the diagnosis of tuberculosis.

Antitubercular Sensitivity Tests (Flowchart 40.4)

- *Absolute concentration method*: A standard inoculum of bacterium is cultured on media containing graded concentrations and medium without drug. The lowest concentration of drug which inhibits the growth is minimum inhibitory cocentration (MIC).
- *Resistance ratio method*: Two sets of media, one with test and one with standard strain (H37RV), (RV = rough virulent) are used.

  Bottles of L-J medium containing doubling concentrations of drugs are inoculated with a test strain and a known sensitive strain (H37Rv). Culture media are incubated at 37°C and observed for growth after 3 weeks. The medium with the lowest concentration of drug showing no more than 20 colonies is taken as minimum inhibitory concentration (MIC). The result is expressed as resistance ratio.

Interpretation

Resistance ratio of 1 or 2 = sensitive strain

Resistance ratio of 4 = doubtfully resistant strain, test should be repeated.

Resistance ratio of 8 = Unequivocally resistant stains

- **Proportion method** determines average sensitivity of strain. Standard inoculum of bacterium is cultured on one L-J medium with drug and one L-J medium without medium and colonies are counted. When more than 1% of mycobacteria grow in presence of drug, it is considered as resistant strain.

Flowchart 40.4: Identification of mycobacteria

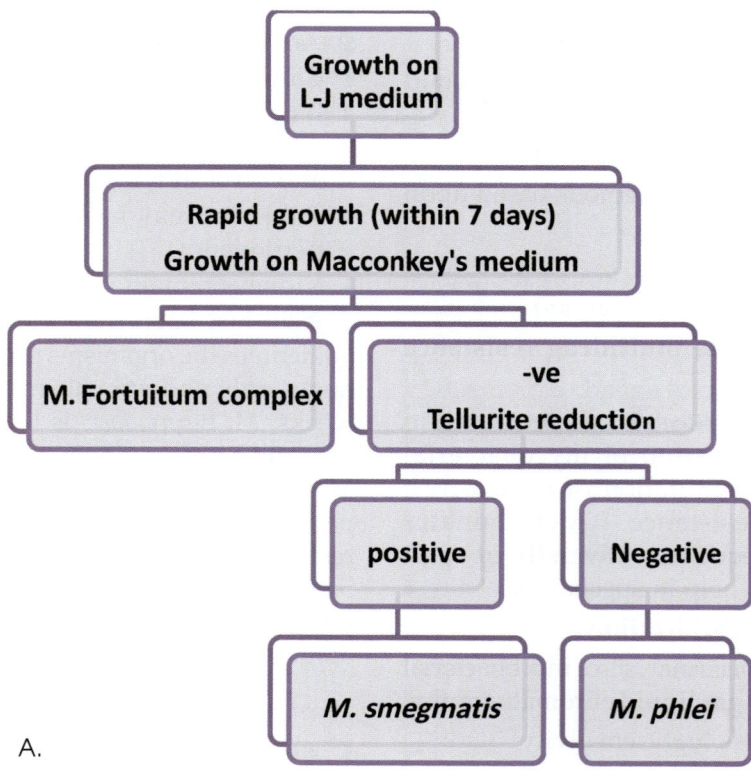

A.

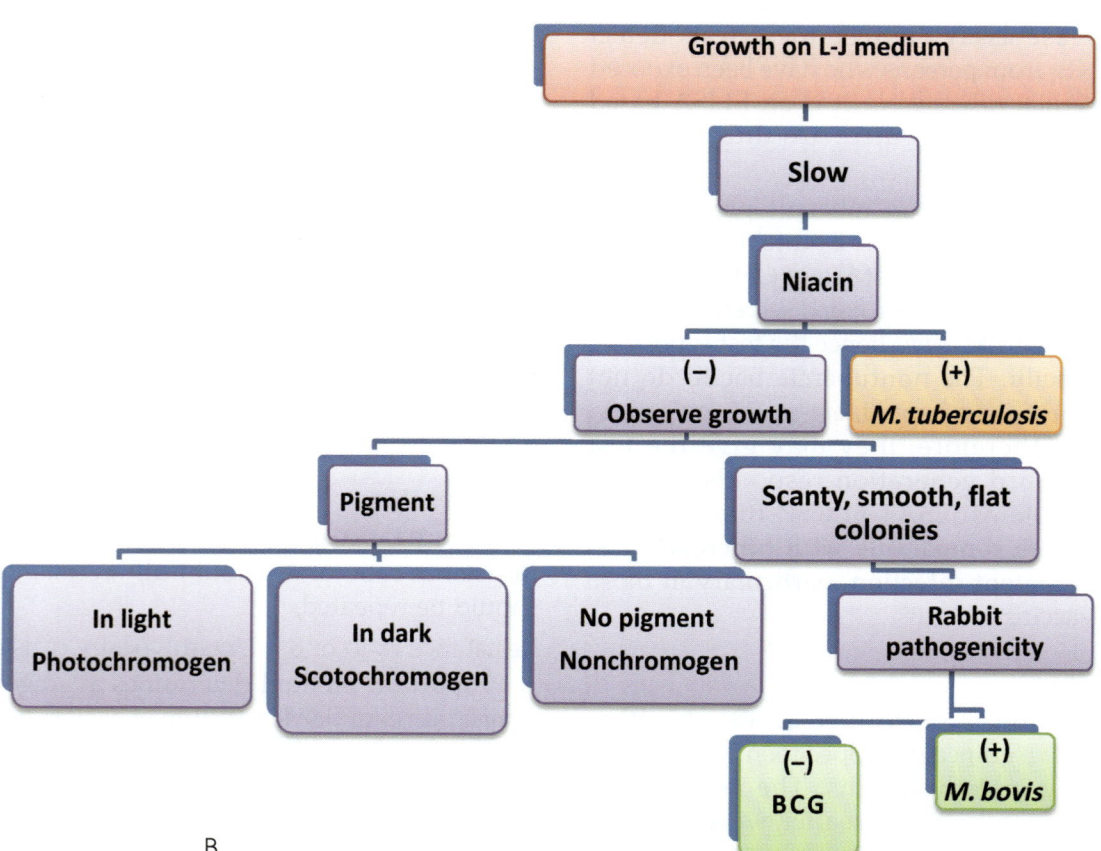

B.

- **Molecular methods—PCR to detect resistance genes.** The most common mechanisms of drug resistance are:
  - INH—catalase-peroxide gene (Kat G) or inh A gene (encodes an enzyme that functions in mycolic acid synthesis)
  - Rifampin—rpoB gene (alteration in B subunit of RNA polymerase)
  - PZA—pnc A gene
  - ETB—embB gene
  - Streptomycin: Mutation I gene coding ribosomal S12 protein (rpst/rpsL) and 16S RNA gene(rrs)
  - Fluoroquinolones: Mutation in DNA gyrase gene gyrA
  - Another method for drug susceptibility is radiometric broth method.

Diagnosis of Extrapulmonary Tuberculosis

Specimens

These depend upon the site of infection: urine, CSF, joint fluid, biopsy material, other body fluid, and blood. Problem in diagnosis is that bacilli are present in very few in numbers in the specimen.

- *CSF*: It develops cob web clot on standing. Examination may be useful. PCR, DNA probes can be used for diagnosis.
- *Bone marrow, liver biopsy* from cases of miliary tuberculosis (from patients with HIV-TB co-infection) are processed for culture. Pus from abscess may be used for microscopic examination.
- *Pleural effusions, other body fluids* may be collected in citrated bulb to prevent protein coagulation. Culture can be performed from sample directly or after concentration.
- *Urine*: It is used for the diagnosis of renal tuberculosis. It is advisable to collect 5–6 whole morning samples, centrifuge each at 3000 rpm for 30 minutes and sediment is used for culture.

Koch Phenomenon

Patient infected with *M. tuberculosis* develops CMI and allergy (delayed hypersensitivity). **Koch phenomenon** is combination of immunity and hypersensitivity. Subcutaneous infection of virulent bacilli in guinea pig produces a nodule in 10–14 days, it breaks down to form ulcer till animal dies. If bacilli are given to a guinea pig already infected with TB 4–6 weeks prior, indurted lesion appears in 1–2 days, ulcer is formed which gets healed. This is called Koch phenomenon. It is a combination of hypersensitivity and immunity.

Mantoux Test (Tuberculin Test)

0.1 mL of PPD injected intradermally on flexor aspect of forearm

- *Positive*: At 24–48 hours, induration of 10 mm or more seen
- *Negative*: Induration of 5 mm or less

Interpretation of Mantoux test:

- *Positive*: Infection with TB (recent or past) or BCG immunization.
- It indicates hypersensitivity to tuberculoprotein.
- *Negative*: It means the patient never had contact with tubercle bacillus.

Old tuberculin is concentrated filtrate of broth in which TB bacilli have grown for 6 weeks.

PPD is partially purified protein antigen contains in additional to reactive tuberculin protein, a varity of other constituents of bacilli and of growth medium.

1 Tuberculin unit (TU) = 0.01 mL of OT (original tuberculin) or 0.00002 mg of PPD-S.

TU is defined as the activity contained in a specified weight of **Sieberrt's PPD Lot No. 49608 in buffer.** First strength tuberculin has 1 TU, intermediate strength has 5TU and second strength has 250TU. A large amount of tuberculin injected in hypersensitive host may give severe reaction, flare up inflammation and necrosis at the site of injection, therefore, **in surveys 5TU in 0.1 mL is used to begin** with.

CDC cut off points: CDC has set off three cut off points defining a positive test result, depending upon the sensitivity, specificity of the test and prevalence of the disease.

Patients at higher risk of developing TB (AIDS patient) 5 mm or longer induration is considered positive, larger than 10 mm is considered positive for persons with increased probability of recent infection. It may include health care workers, IV drug users. For persons at low risk of infection 15 mm or larger induration is considered as positive.

False negative may be due to miliary TB, measles, malignancy, sarcoidosis, malnutrition, immunosuppressive therapy or impaired CMI, inactive PPD, improper injection, and AIDS.

Tuberculin test becomes positive after 4–6 weeks after infection; after BCG the test becomes positive and it may last for 3–7 years.

Peoples who were PPD positive years ago and are healthy, may fail to give test positive, retesting with PPD after 2 weeks, the test will be positive because of booster effect of PPD.

Other methods of tuberculin test are:

Heaf test: It is done by multiple puncture method, may be useful in screening but results are not satisfactory.

Tine test: Disposable prongs carrying dried PPD can be used for testing of an individual.

Uses of Mantoux test:
- Select population for vaccination.
- To diagnose active infection in infants.
- Positive test is considered as an indicator of successful immunization.
- To find out prevalence of disease in community.

Montoux test in AIDS: As CMI is decreased in AIDS patients, the test may be interpreted wrongly. In AIDS patients, hypersensitivity to *Candida albicans* is last to go, thus CMI is accessed by using skin test with *Candida albicans*. If skin test is positive with Candida and Montoux test negative, it is considered negative.

Prophylaxis of TB

BCG (Bacillus Chalmette-Guerin): Strain of *M. bovis* attenuated by 239 serial subcultures on glycerine bile potato medium over 13 years is used. BCG causes self-limited infection. It gives delayed hypersensitivity and immunity (up to 10–15 years). It is given to newborns, intradermal on the deltoid muscle, immediately after birth.

Contraindications
- Infants with active HIV disease
- Babies born to mothers with AFB positive sputum (BCG given after prophylactic chemotherapy)

Complications of BCG
- ***Local:*** Abscess, ulcer, keloid, lupus vulgaris, confluent lesions
- ***Regional complications:*** Enlargement of lymph nodes, suppuration of lymph nodes.
- ***Generalized complications:*** Fever, mediastinal adenitis, erythema nodosum, rarely meningitis
- ***BCGitis:*** Very rarely, non-fatal meningitis, progressive tuberculosis and disseminated BCG infections are reported in people with low immunity.

Chemoprophylaxis
- Isoniazid 5 mg/kg given daily for 10–12 months.
- It is given to babies of mothers with active TB.
- It is also given to children living with patients of active TB cases.

Treatment

The antitubercular drugs include bactericidal agents such as rifampicin (R), isoniazid (I), pyrazinamide (Z), streptomycin while bacteriostatic drugs are ethambutol (E), ethionamide, thiacetazone, para-aminosalicilic acid (PAS) and cycloserine. Short course regimen of 6–7 months is used. Four drugs (HRZE) are given three times a week during initial intensive phase of 2 months, followed by continuing phase of two drugs (HR) three times a week for 4–5 months.

In MDR-TB cases, treatment is given with second line drugs under DOTS plus. There are 5 categories (I–V) of patients under RNTCP, from newly diagnosed cases to MDR and XDR cases. MDR cases are in category IV while XDR cases are in category V.

Multi-drug resistant TB: It is resistance to rifampicin and isoniazid, with or without resistance to one or more other drugs. Concomitant HIV infections are more dangerous.

Drugs used are quinolones, aminoglycosides, macrolides, PAS, ethambutol, thiacetazone, cycloserine, capreomycin.

DOTS (Directly observed therapy under supervision)— ensures patient compliance.

Revised National Tuberculosis Control Programme (RNTCP): It is a national program started in India in 1993. The important components of this program are direct observation treatment (DOTS) which is a short-term chemo-therapy based on the results of AFB in sputum samples. The protocols for diagnosis and treatment for pulmonary and extrapulmonary treatment are standardized (Flowchart 40.5).

With emergence of drug resistance in TB, **DOTS plus** is incorporated in RNTCP which include second line of drugs for TB (Table 40.4).

Though initially only microscopy was started in the programme, genetic method, **Gene expert** is also started to **find out multiple drug resistant TB.**

TABLE 40.4: Standard RNTCP-DOTS plus regime

Intensive phase (6–9 months)	Continuation phase (for 18 months)
Kanamycin	Ofloxacin or levofloxacin
Ofloxacin or levofloxacin	Ethionamide
Ethionamide	Cycloserine
Cycloserine	Ethambutol
Pyrizinamide	
Ethambutol	

Flowchart 40.5: RNTCP guidelines for diagnosis of pulmonary tuberculosis

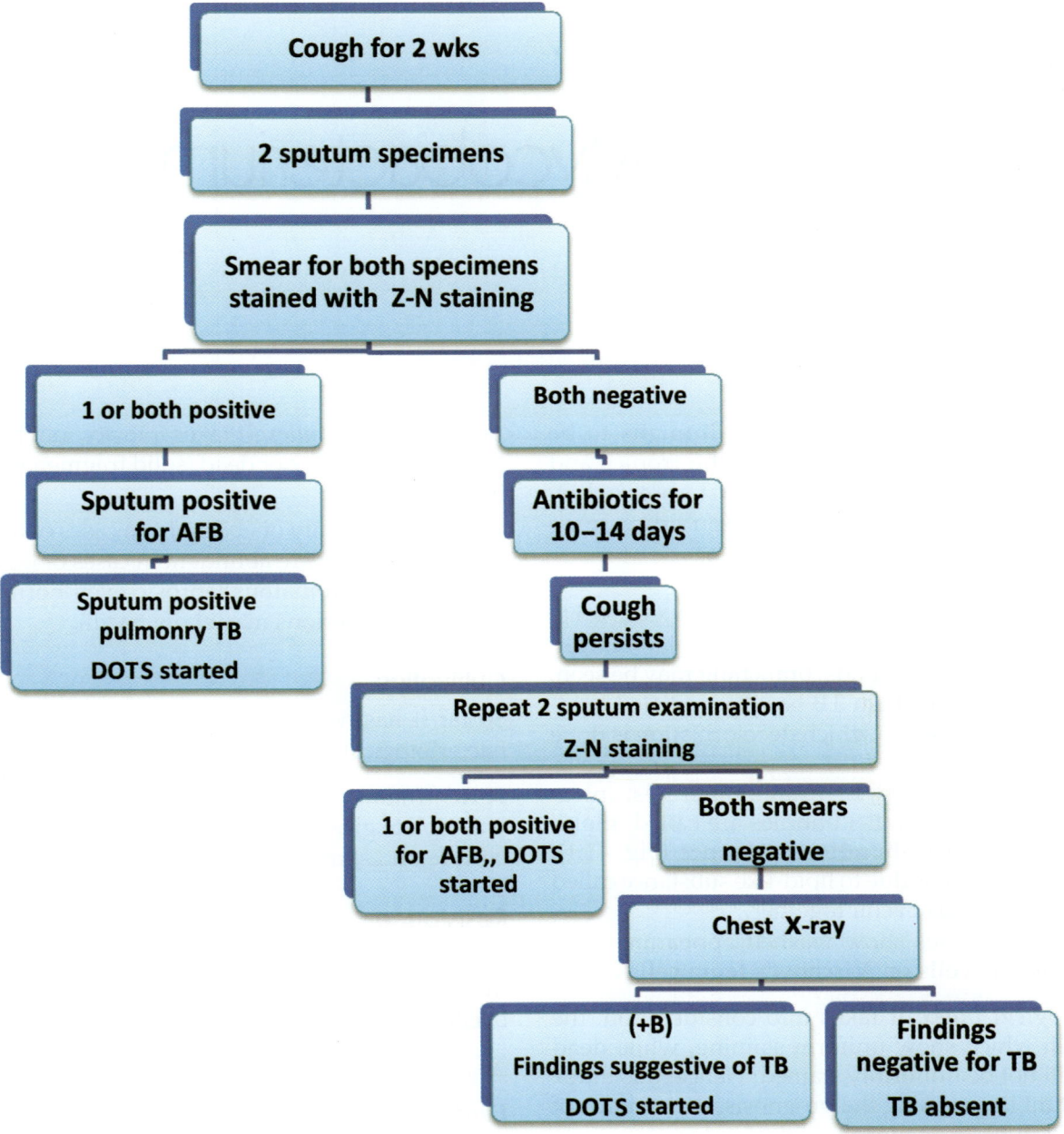

XDR-extensively drug resistant tuberculosis: These strains of *M. tuberculosis* are resistant to INH, rifampicin, any quinolone and also resistant to one of the injectable second line aminoglycosides, i.e. amikacin, capreomycin, kanamycin. Such resistant strains are recognized globally.

DOTS-Plus Programme (2010)

Six drugs are given in intensive phase for 6–9 months.

Four drugs are given for 18 months in continuation phase.

41

Mycobacterium Leprae

It is the first bacterial pathogen of humans to be described. It probably originated in the tropics and spread to rest of the world. It was first observed by Hansen (1868). It causes leprosy (Hansen's disease).

Morphology

- It is straight or slightly curved rod 1–8 µm × 0.2–0.5 µ.
- Variations of morphology such as polar bodies, clubbed forms, lateral buds, branching may be seen.
- Being less acid-fast than TB bacilli, **modified acid-fast staining** is used in which decolorization is done with **5% H$_2$SO$_4$.**
- **Arrangement**—singly or in agglomerates, intra-cellular bacilli in parallel bundles are called **'globi' which gives 'cigar'-bundle** appearance (Fig. 41.1). Bundle formation is due to lipid-like substance called **'glia'** which binds bacilli together.
- Infected histocytes show washed appearance and called **'foamy'cells** or **'Virchow's lepra cells'.**

Morphological index: It takes into consideration, the live bacilli which show uniform staining, while dead bacilli will not be uniformly stained. Hence, this index is important in accessing the prognosis. (Percentage of live bacilli in tissue is morphological index.)

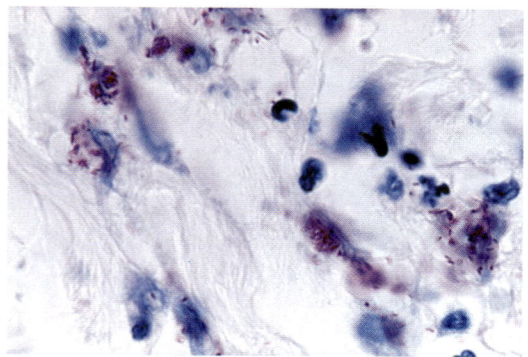

Fig. 41.1: Macrophages studded with globi of acid-fast Lepra bacilli

Bacteriological index: It takes into account all acid-fast bacilli, whether live or dead (solid fragmented granular bacilli).

Bacilli are scanty or absent from cases of tuberculoid leprosy and they are abundant in cases of lepromatous leprosy. In lepromatous leprosy, even normal skin in between two lesions may show bacilli.

Cultivation

So far it has not been possible to culture it either in bacteriological media or in tissue culture.

ICRC (Indian Cancer Research Institute) bacillus: It was isolate grown on human fetal spinal ganglion cell culture on L-J medium. (It was not Lepra bacillus.)

Resistance

Bacilli remain viable in environment for 9–16 days and in moist soil for 46 days. Direct sunlight may kill the bacilli in 2 hours.

Animal Inoculation

Footpad of mice: It forms granuloma in 6 months, infection resembles human tuberculoid leprosy.

Mice: Use of mice has the advantage that it is easily available but yield of bacilli per gram of tissue is low (10^6 bacilli/gm of tissue).

Nine banded Armadillos have adavantages that the lesion resembles with lepromatous leprosy, yield of bacilli is more (10^{10} bacilli/gm of tissue in 6–8 months) but disadvantages are that they are not available in India; they do not multiply in captivity and do not survive easily at high temperature.

Other animals which can be used in experimental infection include chimpanzee, monkey, Indian pangolin, golden hamsters, chipmunks.

Classification (Flowchart 41.1 and Table 41.1)

Leprosy is classified into four forms.

Madrid Classification

1. **Lepromatous** is multi-bacillary form highly infective, deficient CMI, exaggerated humoral response, auto-antibodies are present, lepromin test negative.
2. **Tuberculoid** is paucibacillary form, macular anesthetic patches, neural involvement are seen. CMI is good, lepromin test positive, prognosis is good.
3. **Borderline forms (dimorphic) have lesions of both forms.**
4. **Indeterminate leprosy.** In early stages of leprosy, a small macule may form which is not sufficiently developed to be classified into one of the recognized clinical forms described. This is called indeterminate. It may persists for several years or heal completely. Rarely it may progress to one of the clinical forms. (Generation time—12 to 13 days).

Ridley-Jopling Classification

The clinical forms of leprosy and progress is dependent on CMI of the patient. Leprosy is classified into following types:

- Tuberculiod tuberculoid (TT)
- Borderline tuberculoid (BT)
- Borderline bodreline (BB)
- Borderline lepromatous (BL)
- Lepromatous lepromatous (LL)
  TT, BT, BB, BL, LL, of these polar forms are TT and BT.

Flowchart 41.1: Characteristics of tuberculoid and lepromatous leprosy

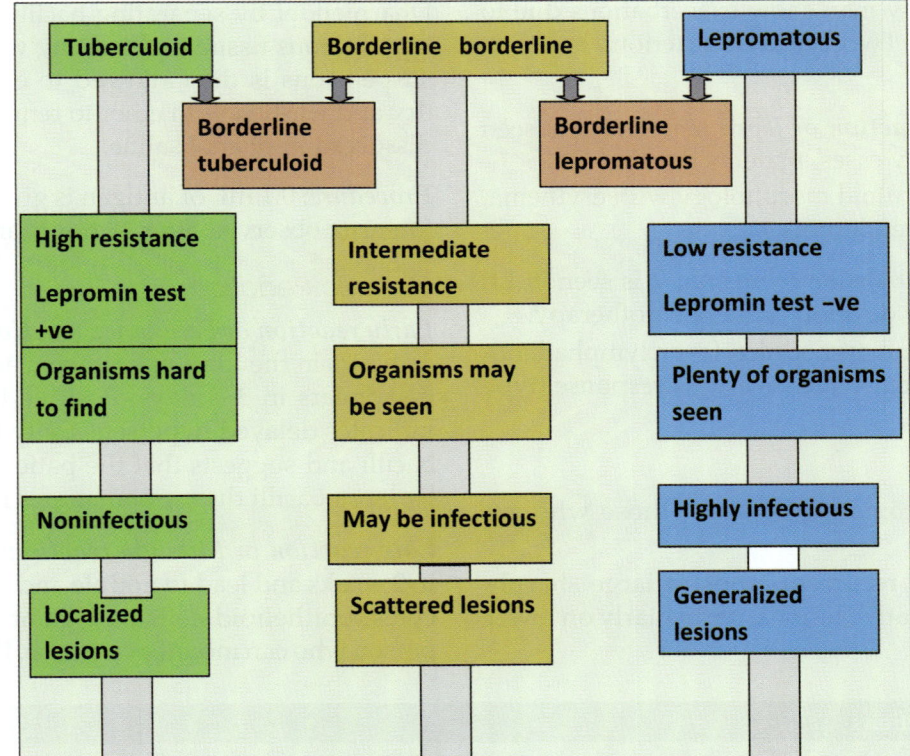

Leprosy group	Skin lesions—macules, papules, nodules	Nerve damage resulting in loss of sensation or weakness of muscles
Paucibacillary	1-5 lesions hypopigmented or erythematous Assymetrically distributed Definite loss of sensations	Only one nerve trunk
Multibacillary	More than 5 lesions Distribution more symmetrical Loss of sensation	Many nerve trunks

TABLE 41.1: Clinical classification of leprosy

Different antigens of lepra bacilli: Lipoarabinomannan (LAM), phenolic glycoproteins (PGL-1).

Leprosy is exclusively human disease. Classification as lepromatous, tuberculoid, dimorphous and indeterminate is based on host resistance.

It is **chronic granulomatous disease affecting skin, peripheral nerves, and nasal mucosa.** Superficial granulomatous lesions in the form of nodules **(lepromata)** having vaculated cells are seen in lepromatous leprosy. Nodules ulcerete, secondary infection occurs. There is mutilation and distortion. Mucosa of nose, mouth, respiratory tract are involved along with reticuloendothelial (RE) system (eyes, testes, kidneys and bones). Tuberculoid type has few macules but nerve involvement is early leading to deformaities of hand and foot.

Lepra Reactions

Patients with leprosy may show exacerbations due to immune reactions. Two types of reactions are seen (Box 41.1).

Type 1. *Reversal reaction or lepra reaction*: It is seen in borderline leprosy cases, patients develop CMI.

BL, shift to tuberculoid morphology with erythema, swelling, pain and tenderness.

Type 2. *Erythema nodosum leprosum*: It is seen in LL or BL types, usually develops after chemotherapy.

Inflamed subcutaneous nodules, fever, lymphadenopathy, arthralgia occur which is arthus response (type III hypersensitivity).

Lucios phenomenon

1. It is seen in lepromatous leprosy, those who are untreated.
2. Patients develop recurrent crops of large sharply demarcated ulcerative lesions, particularly on lower extrimity.

3. It is due to parisitism of endothelial cell, proliferation and thrombus formation which leads to ischemic necrosis.

Lepromin Test

It is an example of type IV hypersensitivity. The test was first described by Mitsuda in 1919.

Antigen: Initially crude antigens obtained from human lepromatous tissue was used as antigen. This is Mitsuda test. This standard Mitsuda antigen contains 4×10^7 bacilli per mL with self-life 2 years.

Standard antigen is replaced by the antigen prepared from armadillo-derived bacilli (lepromin A) then by human derived bacilli (lepromin-H).

Dharmender's antigen: This antigen contains more bacillary component and very less tissue component. This antigen was first prepared by Indian scientist Dharmender by separating bacilli from finely ground lepromatous tissue and treating with chloroform. The suspensions is then allowed to evaporate to make it dry and washed with ether to remove lipids. Finally, it dissolved in phenol saline.

Procedure: 0.1 mL of antigen is given intradermally on forearm; observed after 48 hours and then regularly.

Biphasic Reaction

Early reaction or Fernandez reaction: It is seen in 24 to 48 hours in the form of erythema and induration. This disappears in 3–4 days. Positive Fernandez reaction indicates delayed hypersensitivity to antigens of lepra bacilli and suggests that the patient has been infected by lepra bacilli during sometimes in the past.

Late reaction or Mitsuda reaction: It develops after 1 to 2 weeks and lead to nodule and ulceration (lymphocytes, epithelioid cells and giant cells). It identifies person who can mount a response. It is more important.

BOX 41.1: Lepra reactions	
Type I **downgrde or reversal reaction**	Type II reaction
It occurs in first 6 months	**Erythema nodosum leprosum**
Occurs in patients with borderline BT, BB, BL	Rare in first 6 months
There are classical signs of inflammation within previously involved macules, papules, plaques	Occur in patients with **BL or LL**
It is two types:	It is **Arthus** reaction (type III hypersensitivity)
	It occurs after starting therapy.
Downgrade reaction, before starting treatment, lesions become more lepromatous histopathologically / Reversal reaction after initiation of antileprosy therapy, lesions become more tuberculoid histopathologically	Crops of painful erythematous papules develop, many also develop symptoms of neuritis, lymphadenitis, orchitis, glomerulonephritis.
Treatment: Steroids	*Treatment*: Antipyretics, glucocorticosteroids, clofazimine, thalidomide

Uses of Lepromin Test

- To classify the lesions. Lepromin test is positive in tuberculoid leprosy and negative in lepromatous leprosy.
- To assess the prognosis.
- *To assess the resistance*: Those showing positive reactions have CMI and are capable of responding to infection. Such individuals are allowed to work in Leprosaria (where leprosy patients are isolated).
- To verify the identity of candidate lepra bacilli.

Epidemiology

Once leprosy was thought to be restricted to humans. It is reported in chimpanzees and sooty mangaby monkeys in Africa. It was thought that leprosy was transmitted by close skin to skin contact but now it appears more likely that bacilli are disseminated from nasal secretion of patients with lepromatous leprosy. The main route of transmission is the nasal mucosa. Less commonly, transmission can occur by skin erosions. Other transmission routes, such as blood, vertical transmission, breast milk, and insect bites, are also possible.

It is assumed that infected individuals, even those who did not develop the disease, may have a transitional period of nasal release of bacilli. The presence of specific DNA sequences *M. leprae* in swabs or nasal biopsies and seropositivity for specific bacillus antigens in healthy individuals living in endemic areas suggest that carrier plays a role in the transmission of leprosy.

- Official figures from 103 countries from 5 WHO regions show the global registered prevalence of leprosy to be 180 618 at the end of 2013; during the same year, 215 656 new cases were reported.
- Pockets of high endemicity still remain in some areas of many countries—Angola, Bangladesh, Brazil, People's Republic of China, Democratic Republic of Congo, and Ethiopia.
- A dramatic decrease has been achieved in the global disease burden: from 5.2 million in 1985 to 805 000 in 1995, 753 000 at the end of 1999 and 180 618 cases at the end of 2013.
- Leprosy has been eliminated from countries where the disease was considered a public health problem in 1985. Multi-drug therapy (MDT) has been the key factor against leprosy since its inception in 1981 and by 2005, the prevalence in India was less than 1/10000. This was a landmark achievement in the history of leprosy in India. By the end of 2010, the prevalence had come down to 0.69/10000. Cases of leprosy are not uniformly distributed but tend to cluster in certain localities, villages or talukas. Hence, while the country as a whole has eliminated leprosy, two states, Bihar and Chhattisgarh are yet to achieve elimination (with a prevalence rate of 1.12 and 1.94, respectively).

Laboratory Diagnosis

Bacteriological diagnosis is done in lepromatous leprosy, which is difficult in tuberculoid cases (Table 41.2).

TABLE 41.2: Differences between tuberculoid and lepromatous leprosy

	Tuberculoid leprosy	Lepromatous leprosy
CMI	Present	Absent
Organisms in tissue	Scanty or absent	Plenty
Infectivity	Noninfective	Highly infective
Lepromin test	Positive	Negative
Skin lesions distribution	Asymmetrical	Symmetrical distribution
	One or two hypopigmented plaques	Lesions are more in mumber
	Lesions are confined, in skin and peripheral nerves	Multiple skin nodules and raised plaques
		All organ systems except lungs and CNS may be involved
Granuloma formation	Present	Absent
	The predominance of CD4 cells, IL2, IFNγ, IL-12	CD8 cells, IL-4, 5, 10
Autoantibodies	Absent	Plenty
Antibodies to PGL-1	Less commom	More commomn
Lesions	Few	Plenty
Antibodies to lepra bacilli	Absent or present	Present
Prognosis	Good	Bad
Nerve involvement	Early, nerve involvement is due to external compression by external pressure of granulomma	Late, nerve involvement is due to direct involvement of nerves
Type II lepra reaction	Negative	Positive
Lesions	Macular, dry, scaly	Nodular lesions

Lepromatous Leprosy (Fig. 41.2)

Skin clippings from various sites are taken. Sites on body where lesions are most prominent such as nodules, thick patches and areas of infiltration are selected. If patches are present, material from edges is taken. Usually 5–6 different sites are selected which include ear lobule, buttocks, forehead, chin and chicks. The sites are **nasal mucosa, skin lesions and ear lobules (5–6 different areas)**. The selected portion of skin is cleaned with spirit. Skin is pinched up and raised using thumb and index finger of left hand. This will minimize bleeding when cut is made. With scalpel blade, an incision, 5 mm long and 3 mm deep, is taken on pinched skin. If blood comes out it is wiped out. Scalpel blade is turned at right angle to incision. Bottom and sides of slit are scraped with blade many times in same direction and tissue fluid and pulp is collected on blade. Material is spread on glass side.

Nasal scrapings: A blunt scalpel is used to scrape septum to get piece of mucosa which is teased to form smear.

Smears are stained with modified Z-N staining using 5% H_2SO_4 as decolorizing agent.

Grading of smears

1–10 bacilli/100 fields	= 1+
1–10 bacilli/10 fields	= 2+
1–10 bacilli per field	= 3+
10–100 bacilli per field	= 4+
100–1000 bacilli per field	= 5+
>1000 bacilli/clumps/globi	= 6+ in every field

Bacteriological index: Total number of pluses scored divided by number of smears observed (minimum of 4 skin lesions, a nasal swab and both ear lobes).

Morphological index: It is the percentage of uniformly stained bacilli or solid fragmented granular bacilli **(SFGB)** out of the total number of bacilli counted.

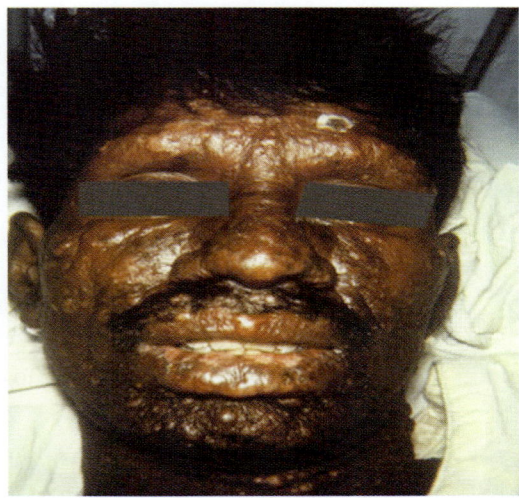

Fig. 41.2: Lepromatous leprosy

Tuberculoid Leprosy

Laboratory diagnosis in tuberculoid leprosy is made by **biopsy** specimens which show granuloma formation and bacteria in the lesions are scanty or absent.

Molecular diagnosis: **PCR** that encodes **65** and **18 Kda proteins** of *M. leprae* used to identify bacilli in specimens and used to assess prognosis. Delection limit of PCR is as low as one bacillus.

Antibody detection

- *FLA-ABS (fluorescent leprosy antibody absorption test)*: It is used for identification of subclinical cases. It detects antibodies irrespective of duration and stage of disease. It claims to be 92% sensitive and 100% specific.
- *ELISA*: It detects IgM to PGL-1 (phenolic glyco lipid-1) antigen found in 95% patients with untreated LL patients. Its titer decreases with treatment. The test shows low sensitivity (60%) in TT patients.

Treatment

Paucibacillary (I, TT, BT)
- Dapsone—100 mg. Daily × 6 months
- Rifampicin—600 mg. Once a month for 6 months

Multibacillary (BB, BL, LL)
- Dapsone—100 mg. Daily × 6 months
- Rifampicin—600 mg. Once a month
- Clofazimine—50 mg. Daily × 2 years/till smears are negative (Ethionamide/prothionamide may be added as a substitute.)

Prophylaxis

There is antigenic relationship with MTB.
- BCG vaccine was observed to induce lepromin positivity, hence was suggested by Fernandez.
- Field trials with different vaccines (BCG + killed lepra bacilli, ICRC bacillus) are going on but no conclusive results so far.
- Possible second generation vaccines, either natural or recombinant form of 18, 31, 65 and 70 kDa proteins.

The national institutes for leprosy are:
- National JALMA. Institute of Leprosy and Other Mycobacterial Diseases, Agra.
- CLTRI (Central Leprosy Training and Research Institute), Chengalpattu, Tamil Nadu.

Mycobacterium Lepraemurium

It, is causative agent of rat leprosy. DNA studies show that *M. leprae* and *M. lepraemurium* are not related species. The disease in rat exist in two forms—glandular (lymph nodes involved) and mucocutaneous type.

42

Atypical Mycobacteria/ Anonymous/Unclassified/ Paratubercle/Tuberculoid/MOTT
(Mycobacteria other than Tubercle Bacilli)

Mycobacteria other than human and bovine TB bacilli which may cause infection in humans are called atypical mycobacteria. They are also called environmental (saprophytic) mycobacteria as they are present in environment. Other names are paratubercle bacilli or MOTT—Mycobacteria other than human and bovine TB bacilli (Table 42.1).

These bacteria cause infections in developed countries where human infections are not common. In India; MTB is common even in AIDS patients.

Based on pigment production, rate of growth, they are classified by Runyon into four types.

RUNYON CLASSIFICATION

These bacteria cause infections in developed countries where human infections are not common. In India; MTB is common even in AIDS patients.

Group I (photochromogens) produce pigment in light on LJ medium. Group II (scotochromogens) produce pigment in dark. The Group III (non-chromogens) do not produce any pigment. Group IV are rapid growers.

TABLE 42.1: Diseases and associated atypical mycobacteria

Primary infection-tuberculosis like	M. kansasii, M. avium intracellulare, M. simiae
Lymphadenopathy	M. scrofulaceum, M. avium intracellularae, M. kansasii
Chronic ulcers	M. marinum
Skin abscess	M. fortuitum, M. chelonei
Burulis ulcer	M. ulcerans
Swimming pool granuloma	M. marinum
Surgical wound infection	M. chelonei

Group I. Photochromogens

They produce pigment in light.

M. kansasii

- It is photochromogen which requires complex media. It causes pulmonary disease especially in immuno-deficient person.
- Though it has been isolated from tap water, the exact source of infection is not known.
- It is the second common cause of pulmonary disease caused by MOTT.
- It forms loose serpentine cords as compared to cord formed by MTB.
- Morphology is characteristic. They are long, broad, **banded forms** (stain smears appear as **cross-bars**).
- It produces yellow orange pigment.
- Tween 80 hydrolysis test and nitrate tests are negative.
- It can be identified by using **antisera** by **latex agglutination test.**
- **DNA probe** is sensitive method for its identification.

M. marinum

- These are long rods with **cross-bands.**
- Optimum temperature for growth is 30°C, poor growth or no growth.
- **Tween 80 test is positive, urease test positive**.
- **Nitrate test is negative**.
- It can be identified by latex agglutination test.
- **DNA probe** can also be used for its identification.
- It causes skin lesion. It is called as 'swimming pool granuloma' or 'fish tank granuloma'.
- Tendonitis
- Tender nodules may appear which are distributed along the lymphatics.

- It gives nitrate test negative which along with poor growth at 35°C differentiates it from *M. kansasii.*
- Natural pathogen of cold blooded animals (fish, amphibians).
- Papule forms due to injury, breaks to form indolent ulcer on prominent surfaces, as—elbows, knees, ankles, nose, fingers and toes.
- It is distributed in temperate areas; may cause epidemics due to common source, i.e. swimming tank (**swimming tank granuloma**).
- Bacilli are very few in lesions; the lesions are self-limiting which undergo spontaneous healing.

M. simiae

- Originally it was isolated from monkeys.
- It causes pulmonary lesions.
- It is niacin positive.

M. asiaticum

It may occasionally cause pulmonary disease.

M. genavense

- It grows slowly.
- It may occasionally cause pulmonary lesions in advanced AIDS patients.

Group II. Scotochromogens

They produce pigments (yellow, orange, red) even if cultures are incubated in dark. If medium is exposed to light, the intensity of color increases.

M. scrofulacum

- It is scotochromosome, found in water, and patients with chronic lung disease. It causes **cervical lymphadenopathy** in children (**scrofula**).
- It is nitrate and tween 80 tests negative.

M. gordonae

- It is found in tap water and it is a contaminant of clinical specimen.
- It is called as 'tap water scotochromogen'.
- It is a rare cause of disease. Its pathogenic potential is doubtful.
- Tween 80 test positive, nitrate test negative.

M. szulagi

It is photochromogen at 25°C and scotochromogen at 37°C. It may occasionally cause pulmonary disease.

M. celatum

It is rare cause of pulmonary disease.

Group III. Nonphotochromogens

They do not produce any pigment. They include following organisms:

M. Avium-intercellulare Complex (MAC)

M. intercellulare and it along with a related species *M. avium*, form a complex called '**MAC—*Mycobacterium avium intercellulare complex*'.

- This causes pulmonary infection in AIDS patient, lymphadenopathy, or disseminated disease.
- *M. avium* is called **Battery bacillus** as it was isolated from patient in Battery State Hospital, Georgia.
- The organism grows optimally at 41°C and form smooth colonies.
- The infection is seen in AIDS patients with CD4 counts below 200 cell/μL.
- Pulmonary disease is described in middle-aged ladies without chronic pulmonary disease, hence the name **Lady Windermer disease**.
- The differentiation between two species can be done by **DNA probe** or high performance gas liquid chromatography (**HPLC**).
- Organisms are low catalase positive; Tween 80 hydrolysis, nitrate reduction and urease tests are negative.
- They reduce potassium tellurite to metallic tellurium.

M. xenopi

- It is found in hospital water supply, caused nosocomial outbreaks.
- It may be a commensal but may cause disease in AIDS patient.
- Originally it was isolated from toads.
- Though it is nonphotochromogenic, it may produce yellow colonies.
- Colonies have '**bird-nest' appearance** (stick-like filaments probe from colonies).
- Optimum temperature for the growth is 42°C.
- Nitrate, tween 80 and urease—all are negative.

M. ulcerans

- It is present in water.
- It causes a condition known as '**Buruli's ulcer'**
- This name is derived from Buruli district of Uganda where a large outbreak took place.
- Lesions are in the form of painless ulcers, small nodules which become necrotic.
- It may cause osteomyelitis.
- An exotoxin is produced by it which may be responsible for the disease.

- It has narrow temperature requirement (31°C to 34°C).
- It is slow grower; colonies appear in 4–8 weeks.

M. malmoense

- It causes pulmonary disease.
- Occasionally, it may cause lymphadenopathy.

M. paratuberculosis

- It is known as **Johne's** bacillus.
- It is pathogen of cattle.
- It is associated with pathogenesis of **Crohn's disease**. But its role is uncertain. **Others:** Other very rarely found mycobacteria are *M. shinoides, M. terrae*, and *M. gastri.*

Group IV. Rapid Growers

Organisms producing rapid growth (within 7 days) at 37°C or 25°C, are included in this group thus it is heterogeneous collection of mycobacteria. *M. phlei* is chromogenic rapid grower.

M. fortuitum and M. chelonae

- They are present in soil. Injury acts as predisposing factor. They produce **chronic abscess** as **injection abscesses.**
- They **do not produce any pigment.**

M. fortuitum

- Optimum temperature for growth *of M. fortuitum* is 28°C, grows best at 37°C.
- They are refractory to treatment hence if *M. fortuitum* produces pulmonary disease; it is difficult to treat the condition.

- It **grows on MacConkey agar without crystal violet.**
- Nitrate test is positive.
- It is more resistant to drugs hence differentiation is required.
- It's nitrate test positive.
- It takes iron from medium.

M. abscesses: It causes pulmonary disease.

Salt tolerance test is used for differentiation between *M. fortuitum* and *M. chelonae.*

M. chelonae and *M. abscesses* are nitrate negative, differentiation of *M. cheloni* and *M. abscesses* is done by 5% salt tolerance test. *M. chelonae* shows no growth in medium with 5% sodium chloride. *M. abscesses* grows in present 5% sodium chloride while *M. chelonae* does not.

M. smegmatis: It may cause soft tissue infections.

M. genevense, M. confluentis, and *M. intermedium* show common features as poor growth in liquid media. They are isolated from blood of AIDS patients.

M. vaccae is rapid grower and acts as good immunomodulatory.

SKIN PATHOGEN (Table 42.2)

- They are exclusively skin pathogens (multiply optimally at skin temperature) which produce skin ulcers and granulomatous skin disease, without systemic invasion and there is no lymphadenopathy.
- According to Runyon classification, *M. ulcerans* belongs to group III while *M. marinum* comes from group I.

TABLE 42.2: Differences between skin pathogens, i.e. *M. marinum* and *M. ulcerans*

Character	M. ulcerans	M. marinum
Geographic distribution	Tropics	Temperate zone
Clinical course	Chronic progressive ulcer	Self-limiting ulcer
Bacilli in lesions	Abundant	Scanty
Rate of growth	Slower, 4–8 weeks	Faster, 1–2 weeks
Growth temperature	25°C no growth 37°C no growth Best temperature is 30–33°C	Growth is seen at 25 and 37°C
Bacilli in cord	Cords are present	No cord formation
Pigment in light	No	Yes
Lesion in foot pad of mice	Edema, rarely ulcers are seen on legs and arms A toxin is produced by this bacillus which causes inflammation and necrosis in guinea pig	Purulent ulcer
Mode of infection	Infection follows minute trauma	Infections occur from infected swimming pools or fish tanks
Site of lesions	Sites of infection are legs and arms	Elbows, knees, ankles, nose, fingers

- *M. ulcerans* **(Buruli ulcer):** The name Buruli ulcer is derived from Buruli district of Uganda where large epidemic occurred. The bacterium grows slowly at 34°C but not at all at 37°C in primary culture.
- Sampling is done from edge of ulcer in the initial phase of the disease.
- It produces toxins which produce inflammation and necrosis in injected guinea pigs.

Ecology

- Environmental bacteria are present in soil, water, and air.
- There are no secondary cases as person to person transmission is absent.
- They may cause weak sensitivity with Mantoux test and also affect immune response with BCG in their locality due to cross-antigen with MTB.
- Common laboratory contaminants.
- *M. avium, M. kansasii,* and *M. xenopi* present in water may cause confusion in diagnosis of TB caused by MTB (false positives).

The summary of diseases caused by various MOTTs is given in Table 42.3.

TABLE 42.3: Differences between typical and atypical mycobacteria

Typical MTB	Atypical MOTT
Souce of infection is an open case	Source is in the environment
Secondary cases do occur	No secondary cases
May be sensitive to primary line of treatment	Usually resistant to primary line of drugs
Obligate pathogen	Opportunistic pathogen
Slow growth	Some are rapid growers
Niacin positive	Negative
Arylsulfatase negative	Positive
Pathogenic to guinea pigs	Nonpathogenic
Weak catalase positive	Strong catalase positive

Treatment

- MOTTs are resistant to first line of therapy; but pulmonary lesions caused by MAI complex or **'MAIK' complex** (MAI with *M. kansasii* added) may be treated with INH, rifampicin, ethambutol in combination with quinolones, clofazimine, and rifabutin.

43

Spirochetes

These are elongated, motile, flexible bacteria twisted spirally along the long axis (Speira—coiled, chaite—hair).

Endoflagella are polar flagella wound along the helical protoplasmic cylinder; situated between outer membrane and cell wall, it gives motility to the spirochetes.

Spirochetes (Fig. 43.1) are aerobic, anaerobic or facultative, some are non-cultivable. Reproduction occurs by transverse fission.

CLASSIFICATION

a. *Spirochetaceae family:* Genera *Spirochaeta, Treponema, Borrelia, Cristispira* are included in this family.
b. *Leptospiraceae:* It contains genus *Leprospira.*

Medically important spirochetes are *Treponema, Borrelia,* and *Leptospira* (Fig. 43.2).

Treponemas are further classified based on pathogenicity
a. Venereal syphilis—*T. pallidum*
b. Non-venereal treponematoses
   • *T. pallidum*—endemic syphilis
   • *T. pertenue*—yaws
   • *T. carateum*—pinta

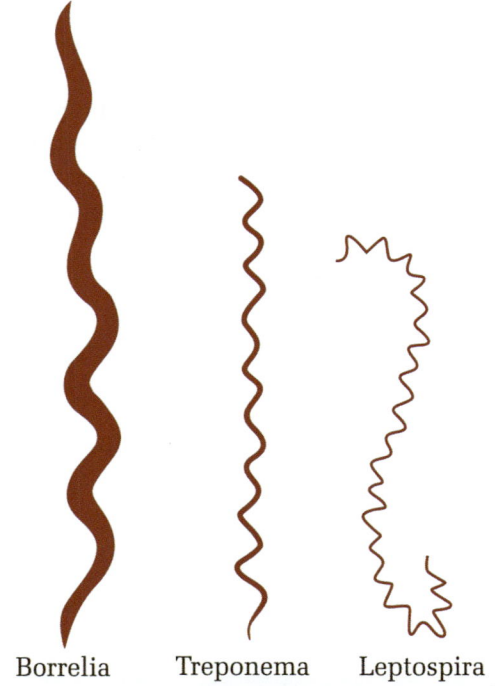

| Borrelia | Treponema | Leptospira |

Fig. 43.2

Treponema (Trepos—to turn, nema—thread).

TREPONEMA PALLIDUM

Treponema pallidum (pallidum = pale staining).

Morphology
• Size: 4–14 µ long × 0.1–0.2 µ wide.
• These are flexible bacteria, twisted along the long axis.
• About 10 regular spirals, at intervals of 1µ are present.
• It is actively motile. It shows following types of motility:
   – Backward-forward movement
   – Flexion of whole body

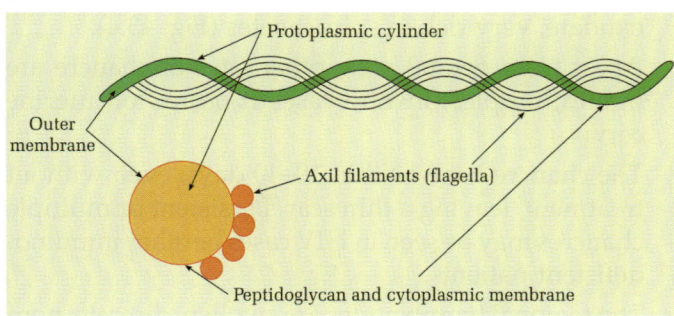

Fig. 43.1: Structure of *Spirochaete*

- Corkscrew motility
  Motility is due to presence of endoflagella.

Methods of Demonstration of T. pallidum (Fig. 43.3)

- They are seen by negative staining with India ink and **dark ground** or phase contrast microscopy.
- **Giemsa:** Bacteria stain light rose red.
- **Silver impregnation methods: Fontana's** method is used for films, **Levaditi's** for tissue, bacilli appear dark brownish against yellowish brown background.

Cultural Characteristics

- They do not grow in artificial culture media.
- *Nichol's* **strain** is virulent strain of *T. pallidum* maintained by serial passage in rabbits; which was isolated from a case of general paralysis of insane in 1912.
- **Reiter's strain:** *T. phagedenis* (non-pathogenic) is used for group specific tests; it grows well in thioglycollate medium with serum.
- *T. refringens* (Noguchi strain) is nonpathogenic strain.

Resistance of Treponema

It is very delicate, readily inactivated by drying and heat, killed in 1–3 days at 0–4°C. It is inactivated by distilled water, oxygen, soap, bismuth, mercurials, arsenicals, common antiseptic agents and antibiotics.

Antigenic Structure

By serological tests, three types of antibodies are identified. These antibodies react with three types of antigens.

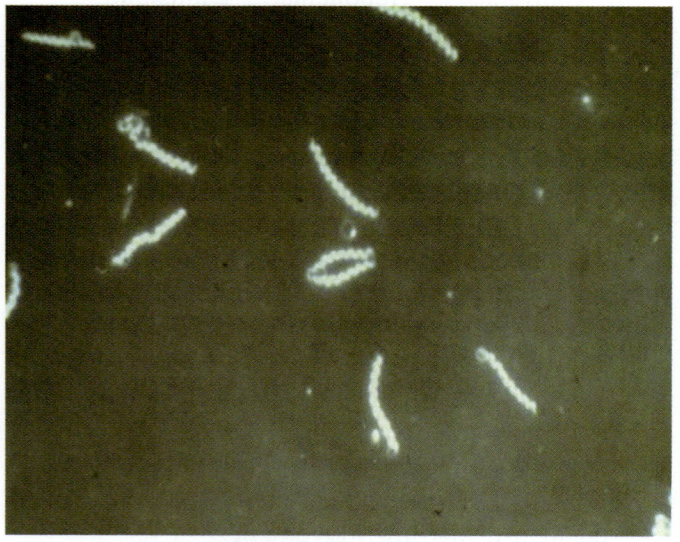

Fig. 43.3: DGM showing *T. pallidum*

Three types of antigens:

1. *Reagin antigen*: Hapten extracted from beef heart is used as antigen to detect antibodies against this antigen. The antigen is cardiolipin, chemically diphosphatidyl glycerol. This antigen is used in **non-specific tests**, also called standard tests for syphilis (**STS**).

2. *Group antigen*: It is found in *T. pallidum* and non-pathogenic strains, e.g. *Reiter's* strain.

3. *Species specific antigen*: **It is polysaccharide** in nature; antibodies seen only in sera of patients with pathogenic *T. pallidum* infection.

Venereal Syphilis

Transmission: It occurs by sexual or by transplacental route.

It is inactivated by heating and drying (41–42°C) hence fomites don't play a role. As it is killed at the refrigeration temperature, transfusion syphilis doesn't occur.

Pathogenicity: The name syphilis is derived from a poem written by Fracastorius of Verona describing the legend of a shepherd named Syphilus who had been stuck with the disease. It a sexually transmitted disease. It is rarely transmitted in doctor, nurse and laboratory workers nonvenereally.

The infectivity is maxium during first two years of disease—primary, secondary and early latent stages. Infective dose: 60 organisms infect 50% of volunteers.

Clinical incubation: 10–90 days.

Primary Syphilis Lesion

It is characterized by (ulcer) chancre and lymphadenopathy.

- There is papule on the genital area, that ulcerates, forms classical chancre of primary syphilis, called **hard chancre**. It is a **painless**, relatively avascular, indurated and a circumscribed lesion. There is thick exudate, very rich in spirochaetes (Fig. 43.4).

  Apart from genital area, other sites of chancre are mouth, nipples, in rare cases it occurs on uterine cervix.

  The chancre heals within 10–40 days, even without treatment, leaving a thin scar. Persistent or multiple chancres may be seen in HIV cases or other immunodeficient patients.

- The regional lymph nodes are swollen, discrete, non-tender and rubbery.

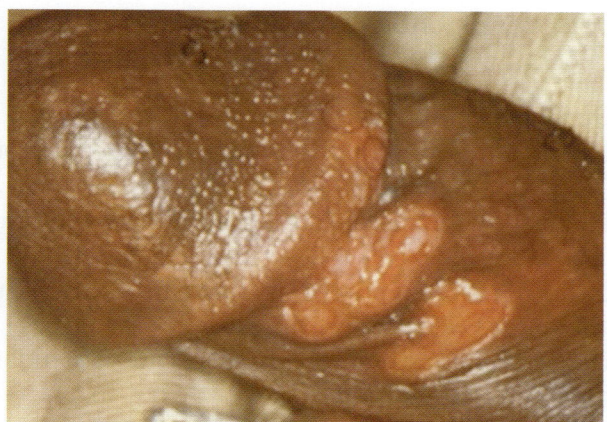

Fig. 43.4: Primary chancre

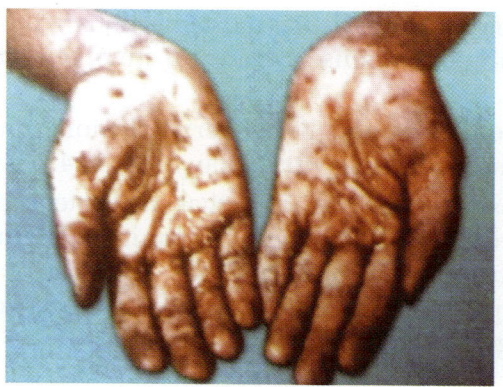

Fig. 43.5: Skin lesions of secondary syphilis

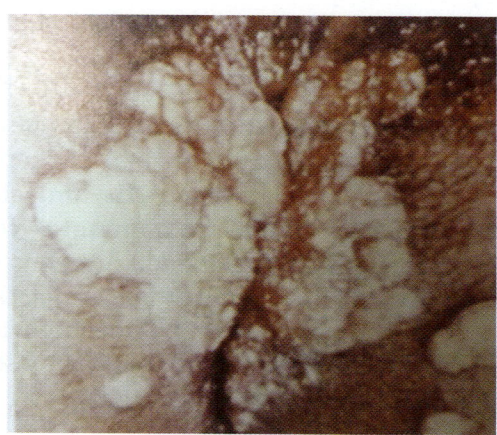

Fig. 43.6: Condyloma

The spirochetes spread from the site of entry into bloodstream, even prior to appearance of chancre. Hence, the patient may be infectious during the late incubation period.

Secondary Syphilis

3–6 weeks after ulcer heals, the lesions of secondary syphilis develop. It results from spread of infection. Treponemes replicate in lymph nodes, skin, joints, muscles, and mucosae.

The lesions of secondary syphilis are roseolar or papular skin rashes (Fig. 43.5), **condylomata** at muco-cutaneous junctions (Fig. 43.6), mucous patches in

Flowchart 43.1: The natural history of untreated syphilis

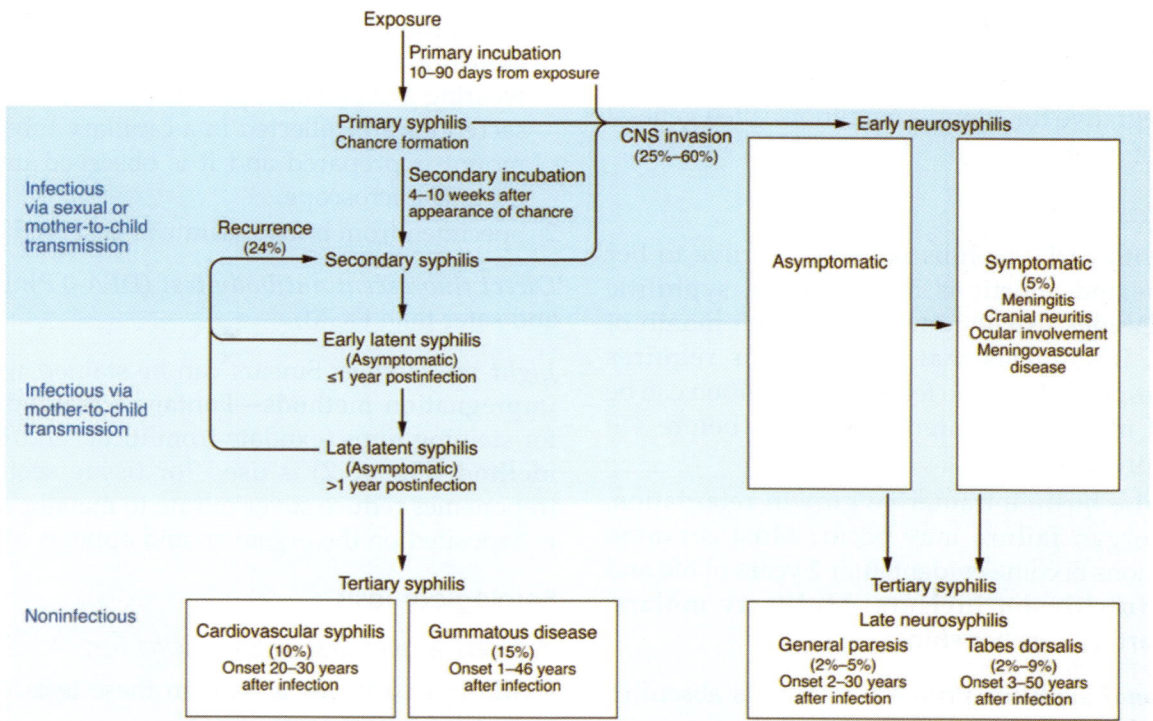

oropharynx. The patient is most infectious in this stage; ophthalmic, osseous, meningeal involvement may occur.

Depending upon the severity, lesions undergo spontaneous healing which may occur in 4–5 years.

It has been demonstrated that the bacteria contain hundredfold fewer **membrane spaning proteins** than outer membrane protein of GNBs. They play a role in handling host defences. Also they **coat plasma proteins** helping them to escape host defences.

Latent Syphilis

It is the period of quiescence for several years, the disease can only be diagnosed by serological tests.

Tertiary Syphilis

The hallmark of this stage is destruction of tissue caused by host responses against treponemal antigens. The change is in the form of **vasculitis and chronic inflammation.** Soft masses or **gammatas** contain inflammatory cells and treponemal antigens which destroy bones and soft tissues. Cardiovascular lesions-aneurysms, chronic granulomata and meningovascular lesions develop; which may represent manifestations of delayed hypersensitivity.

Quaternary or Late Tertiary Syphilis

Tabes dorsalis: Involvement of dorsal column of spinal cord results in loss of sensation of position, resulting ataxic gait.

General paralysis of insane: Generalised involvement of brain leads to impaired motor functions as well as higher integrative functions, a condition called general paralysis of insane.

Congenital Syphilis

Woman with early syphilis is more infective to her fetus, repeated abortions may occur in syphilitic patients. Lesions usually develop after 4th month of gestation. It suggests that pathogenesis requires immune response from the fetus. The condition can be treated, if mother is treated adequately before 4th month of pregnancy.

Premature birth, intrauterine growth retardation, multiple organ failure may occur. Most common manifestations become evident after 2 years of life and include **Hutchinson incisors, Mulberry molars,** deafness, arthritis, **saber shins.**

Occupational syphilis: Primary chancre is absent or extragenital, usually on fingers.

Laboratory Diagnosis of Syphilis

Direct Microscopy

- **Dark ground microscope**
- **Light microscope** to observe stained preparations (silver impregnation)
- **Fluorescent microscope:** Direct immunofluorescence is used
- **Immunohistochemistry** on formalin fixed tissue sections gives definitive diagnosis
- **Detection of antibodies by** nonspecific or standard tests (STS)
- **Specific antibodies tests**
- **Newer specific antibody tests:** Lateral flow assay
- **PCR**
- **Western blot**

Specimens collected include:
- Exudate from chancre
- Lymph node aspiration
- Blood for the serological test

Microscopy

It is useful in:
- Primary syphilis
- Secondary syphilis
- Congenital syphilis with superficial lesions

Dark ground microscope: **Sensitivity of DGM:** 10^4 treponemes/mL are required to be detected by DGM.
1. *Specimen from ulcer*: Wet films are examined under dark ground or phase contrast microscopy. Serum exuding from base of lesion is collected. With wearing gloves, slight pressure is given at base. The secretions are collected in a capillary tube or direct mount is prepared and it is observed under dark ground microscope.
2. Specimen from bubo aspirate is observed by DGM.

Direct fluorescent antibody test (DFA-TP): It is better and safer than DGM.

Light microscope: Smears can be stained with **silver impregnation methods—Fontana's method** is useful for staining films (exudate from ulcer) and **Levaditi's method** (Fig. 43.7) is used for tissue sections. The treponemes reduce silver nitrate to metallic silver that is deposited on the organism and appears black.

Serological Tests

A. Nonspecific Test or Standard Tests for Syphilis

Cardiolipin antigen is used in these tests. These are also called **reagin tests.**

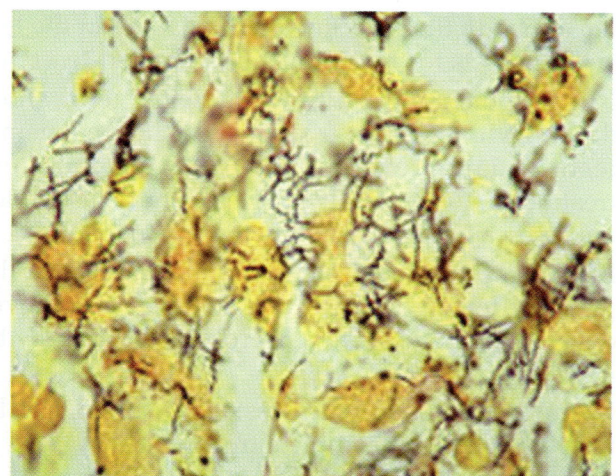

Fig. 43.7: Levaditi stain showing *Treponema pallidum*

Cardiolipin is purified extract of beef heart with lecithin and cholesterol added. (Lecithin increases the avidity of antigen antibody complexes, while cholesterol increases the surface area for the reaction.)

Wasserman's complement fixation test is no longer in use.

Kahn test is a tube flocculation test.

VDRL: **Slide flocculation** test (Venereal Diseases Research Laboratory Test, the laboratory is in New York). Test requires inactivated serum; results are seen under low power lens of microscope. If negative, reported as non-reactive, while when positive, reported as reactive. Titer more than 1:8 are significant.

Rapid plasma reagin test (RPR): Antigen is coated on fine carbon particles; so reaction is easily visible to naked eye, but this test is not suitable for testing CSF.

Advantages of RPR: Test can be performed on serum as well as plasma, results can be read with naked eye, rapid , simple, prior heating of serum is not required.

Advantage of reagin tests: As these tests become negative 6–18 months after treatment, they are used to access the prognosis.

Other modifications of VDRL include:
• Toluidine red unheated serum reagin test (TRUST).
• Automated reagin test (ART)
• Unheated serum reagin test (UST)
• VDRL-ELISA

Disadvantage of reagin tests or STS or nonspecific tests is biological false positive reactions.

Biological false positive (BFP) reactions: Positive reactions with cardiolipin tests, negative with specific treponemal tests, in absence of present or past infection, no technical error.

These BFP reactions may occur in about one percent of normal sera. BFP antibody is usually of IgM type, while reagin antibody in syphilis is mainly IgG.

Acute BFP <6 months: It is seen in following conditions: Acute infections, injury, inflammation, *HIV*, malaria, *Mycoplasma pneumoniae* and parenteral drug use.

Chronic BFP >6 months: Relapsing fever, hepatitis, tropical eosinophilia, aging, SLE, RA are the conditions which give chronic BFP reactions.

Other causes are cardiovascular disease, tuberculosis, leprosy, other STDs, multiple blood transfusions, lyme disease, endemic treponemiasis, and age.

B. Group Specific Tests

Non-pathogenic strain (Reiter's strain) proteins are used as antigens, e.g. Reiter protein complement fixation test, ELISA.

C. Specific T. pallidum Tests

Strain used is virulent *Nichol's* strain as antigen.

Treponema pallidum immobilization (TPI): It is the most specific but complex test as Treponemes should be maintained. Live suspension of Nichol's strain is incubated with patient's serum in presence of complement. If 50% of organisms are immobilized, the test is considered positive.

Fluorescent treponemal antibody (FTA) test: Indirect immunofluorescent test: Smear of Nichol's strain on slide is used as antigen. The patient's serum is added to the slide, which is washed to remove unattached antibodies, the smears are observed under microscope.

FTA-ABS: Test serum preabsorbed with sonicate of Reiter's treponemes so that nonspecific antibodies in the serum are removed by washing then indirect fluorescent treponemal antibody test is performed. It is a standard reference test.

FTA-ABS 200: Patient's serum is first diluted as 1: 200, then it is preabsorbed with sonicate of Retier's strain and the serum then used for FTA. The test has good sensitivity 80%,100%, 95% in primary, secondary and tertiary syphilis.

Treponema pallidum hemagglutination (TPHA): Antigen used—tanned erythrocytes coated with sonicate of treponema; it is mixed with patients serum, if positive, clumpings of RBCs seen. It is simple, more economical than FTA-ABS, standard kits available; it is standard confirmatory test.

TPPA test: *Trponema pallidum* particulate agglutination test.

This test has replaced TPHA, instead of RBCs, the **gelatin** particles are coated with *T. pallidum subspecies pallidum* antigen. There is no separate absorption test, hence simple to set up and requires less preparation time. Serum is diluted in microtiter plate, sensitized gelatin particles are added to 1:40 dilution making it final 1:80. Antibodies react and form a matt of agglutination particles.

Enzyme Immune Assay

Capita syphilis-M test and Trep Check M test based of antihuman antibody to capture IgM antibody in patients serum followed by use of purified *T. pallidum* antigen to detect IgM anti-*T. pallidum* antibody in patient's serum. IgM ELISA is most powerful in diagnosis of congenital syphilis.

Western blot test (WB): EIA format is used in the WB test which has more sensitivity and specificity than IgM ELISA for diagnosis of congenital syphilis.

Rapid Test

Lateral flow assay: Results of this test are available in 30 minutes.

PCR: It can be performed on whole blood and tissue from lesions.

Advantages of PCR are:

- It is especially useful in suspected **neurosyphilis** (serum is reactive, history of syphilis present with abnormal findings in CSF).
- Diagnosis of congenital syphilis on amniotic fluid.
- It also helps to distinguish various strains of *T. pallidum subspecies pallidum*.

Interpretation of Serological Tests

- Reagin antibodies appear in the serum only four weeks after acquiring the infection; hence tests for these antibodies may sometimes be non-reactive in primary stage of the diseases. Diagnosis of early primary syphilis can be done either by repeating a VDRL test after 1–2 weeks, if the same was initially negative or by performing a FTA-ABS test.
- With primary chancre, tests for reagin antibody are reactive only in 70% of cases. Thereafter, antibody levels increase and become maximum in the secondary stage, when all standard tests for syphilis are invariably reactive. During the next several years,

the antibody titres decline gradually and in the late syphilis, tests for reagin may become non-reactive.

- Non-treponemal tests become negative or show decline with effective treatment, while treponemal tests usually remain positive after complete treatment. VDRL test or RPR test is more useful for the assessment of cure following treatment.
- If adequate treatment is given immediately after the primary lesion appears, the patients may never develop antibodies and all serological tests may be negative.
- In late syphilis, serological tests may continue to be reactive even after complete treatment.
- In congenital syphilis, it is necessary to distinguish between maternal antibodies passively transferred across the placenta and the antibodies produced as a result of active fetal infection. In the former, repeat tests will show an decrease in titer, whereas in the latter titre will rise. Demonstration of IgM antibody in the newborn is indicative of active infection, as IgM does not normally cross the placenta. Hence, IgM FTA-ABS confirms the diagnosis of congenital infection.

Choice of Serological Tests

- VDRL and RPR tests are used for screening or for diagnostic purposes of large number of sera.
- These tests are also used for quantitative measurement of regain titre for assessment of clinical activity.
- Treponemal tests (TPHA or FTA-ABS) are used to confirm the diagnosis with a positive reagin test.

Some Facts of Serological Tests

- The test of choice for serologal diagnosis in a clinic setting is VDRL or RPR.
- Most sensitive test in primary syphilis is TP-PA.
- First test to positive is FTA-ABS.
- Tests for monitering therapy are VDRL and RPR.
- Tests for confirmation of diagnosis: TPHA, FTA-ABS, and TP-PA.
- Measurement of IgM in neonate or congenital syphilis: 19S IgM FTA-ABS or Capita 'M' test.

Nonveneral Treponematosis

Diseases vary in different clinical conditions, regions. Transmission occurs by body contact.

a. **Endemic syphilis:** It is caused by *T. pallidum subspecies endemicum*. It was also reported from India. Different names were given to disease in different skin lesions, progresing to gummata. The involvement of CVS, CNS not seen.

b. *Yaws*: Different names of this disease are 'pian', 'frambesia', 'parangi'. With penicillin it was almost irradicated but it reappeared. In India, the disease was seen in Andra Pradesh, Madhya Pradesh, Orrisa. Primary lesion is called **'mother jaw'**.

It starts as extragenital papule which enlarges and ultimately breaks down to form ulcerative granuloma. As in syphilis, clinical course involves secondary and tertiary manifestations except CVS and CNS involvement. Mode of infection is by direct contact. Diagnosis and treatment is similar to syphilis.

c. *Pinta*: It is characterized by extragenital papule which without ulceration develops into psoriaform lesion. Hypopigmented or hyperpigmented secondary skin lesion also seen. The condition is caused by *T. carateum*.

Treatment

a. *Early syphilis*: Primary, secondary and latent infection of two years or less is included in this category. Benzathine penicillin 2.4 lacs units are given intramuscularly as a single dose after sensitivity testing. Alternatively doxycycline 100 mg twice a day is given orally for 15 days.

b. *Late syphilis*: Infection more than 2 years is included in late syphilis. Benzathine penicillin 2.4 lacs units given intramuscularly, once in a week for three weeks. In certain patients, treatment with penicillin may lead to Jarisch-Herxheimer reaction. The reaction is either due to liberation of toxic products from massive destruction of treponemes or due to hypersensitivity reaction. It is a systemic response with fever, chills, myalgia and hypotension.

BORRELIA

1. *B. recurrentis* (Fig. 43.8), *B. duttoni* cause relapsing fever.
2. *B. burgdorferi* causes Lyme disease.
3. *B. vincenti* causes Vincent's angina.

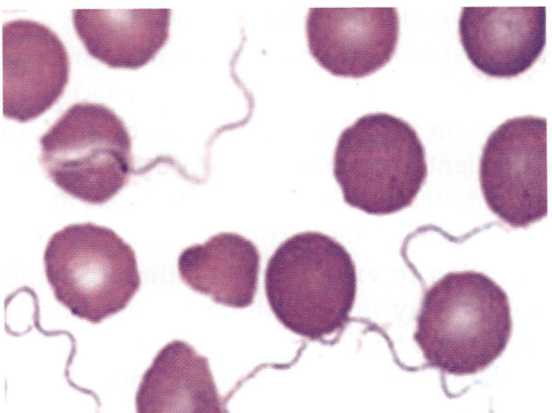

Fig. 43.8: Borrelia recurrentis in blood smear

Morphology

- Size: 8–20 × 0.2–0.4 µ.
- 5–10 loose coils at 2µ intervals are seen.
- Ends of bacterium are pointed.
- They are Gram-negative, stained better by Giemsa staining.
- Spirals are wide open, coarse, irregular.
- They are motile with endoflagella.

Cultural Characterisitics

- It is micro-aerophilic, difficult to cultivate.
- It grows on CAM of hen's egg.
- It can be grown by intraperitoneal inoculation in rats and mice.

Relapsing fever: It is either louse-borne or tick-borne.

Incubation period is 2 to 10 days. Fever of sudden onset occurs which subsides in 3–5 days followed by afebrile period for 4–10 days, and then fever relapses. DNA rearrangements in linear plasmids present in bacteria are reponsible for antigen variations. Recovery from disease is associated with development of immunity against all antigenic variants. **Relapses** are due to antigenic variations. Borrelia are present in blood during febrile periods. Disease subsides after 3–10 relapses.

Epidemic or louse-borne RF: **Vector is louse.** It is exclusive human disease. It is comparatively more severe disease (jaundice and hemorrhage), relapse less common. There is no transovarial transmission in lice. The mode of transmission is not by bite, but because rubbing into abraded skin.

Endemic or louse-borne RF: **Vector is soft tick.** It is an accidental human disease with less severe clinical disease. Transovarian transmission in vector is present, relapse more common. It is transmitted by bite or discharges of ticks.

The places as caves or other dwelling of infected ticks are common sites of infection, hence it is called 'place' diseases.

Examination of blood during febrile periods is only useful as bacteria rarely appear during afebrile period.

Laboratory Diagnosis

- **Sample examined** is blood collected by veni-puncture.
- **Microscopy:** Wet films are observed under dark ground or phase contrast microscope. Bacteria show lashing movement.
- Giemsa, Leishman are used to stain blood smears. Dilute carbol fuschin can be used for staining bacilli.

- **Animal inoculation:** After intraperitoneal inoculation in white mice, organisms multiply and detected in the peripheral blood examination.
- **Serology:** It gives false positive tests for syphilis; serum may show agglutinins to Proteus OXK.
- **GlpQ test:** It is immunoblot test that detects glycerophosphodiester phosphodiesterase (GlpQ) antigen.

Treatment

Antibiotics used for treatment are tetracycline, chloramphenicol, penicillin, and erythromycin.

BORRELIA VINCENTI

- Size: 5–20 × 0.2–0.6 μ wide.
- 3–8 coils of variable size are present.
- It is Gram-negative, stained with diluted carbol fuschin (1 in 10).

Pathogenicity

It is normal mouth commensal. In presence of predisposing factors as malnutrition, viral infection, it causes gingivostomatitis or oropharyngitis (Vincent's angina or pharyngitis) associated *Fusobacterium spp.* The association is called as **fusospirochaetosis** (Fig. 43.9).

Laboratory Diagnosis

Stained smears of exudates from lesions show the spirochete and spindle-shaped fusobacteria. Anaerobic culture will grow the organisms.

Treatment

Penicillin, and metronidazole are used for the treatment.

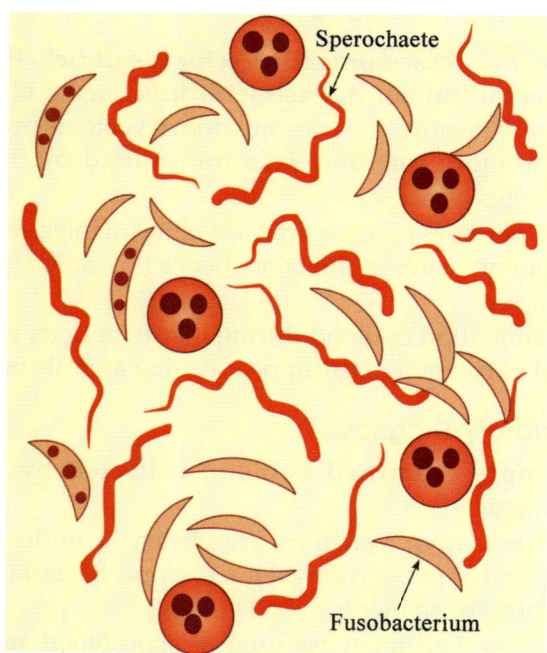

Fig. 43.9: Fusospirochaetoses

LEPTOSPIRA

Several species of Leptospira are saprophytic, many are parasitic in rodents. They are delicate spirochetes with close spirals and they have hooked ends. They cannot be seen under light microscope as they are very thin. (Leptos means fine or thin.)

Infection in natural host is usually asymptomatic.

Genus Leptospira has 2 species:
- I. *L. interrogans* (pathogenic)
- II. *L. biflexa* (saprophytic): These leptospirae are found in surface waters.

Morphology

- Size: 6–20 × 0.1μ thick.
- It has pointed ends which are hooked (umbrella handles).
- Numerous closely placed coils are seen.
- Two type of motility: Translation (forward backward movement) and rotational along long axis are present.
- It is seen under dark ground or phase contrast microscope as actively motile bacteria.
- It is stained best by silver impregnation.

Culture of Leptospira

- They are aerobic, microaerophilic.
- Temperature: 25–30°C
- pH: 7.2–7.4
- Generation time is 12–16 hours in media while it is 4–8 hours in experimental animals.
- They are cultivated in media enriched with rabbit serum.
- Liquid and semi-solid are Korthof's, Stuart's, Fletcher's.
- Semi-synthetic medium is EMJH (Ellinghausen-McCullough-Johnson-Harris) medium.
- As leptospirae are microaerophilic, their growth occurs few millimeters below the surface.
- **Cultivation in chick embryo:** Leptospira grow on chorioallantoic membrane of chick embryo. They are demonstrated in allantoic blood vessels in 4–5 days by dark ground microscope.
- **Cultivation in experimental animal:** Samples are inoculated by intraperitoneal route into guinea pigs. After 15 minutes, the blood is withdrawn from the animal. As leptospirae invade bloodstream more rapidly, the blood withdrawn is free from contaminants.

Resistance

Heating at 60°C for 10 seconds or 50°C for 10 minutes kill leptospirae. They are acid labile, destroyed by sodium hypochlorite. The factors which influence their survival in sewage are pH, salinity, temperature and amount of pollution.

Antigens

Genus-specific antigens are common to all members of the genus. Classification into serogroups and serovars based on **surface antigens.** Previously agglutination reactions were used to find out serotypes or serovars. With the availability of molecular methods, **RFLP and DNA probes** are used for identification of types.

Classification

They are classified into two species, each contains several serogroups and serovars. The pathogenic leptospirae belong to the species *L. interrogan* and non-pathogenic leptospirae belong to serogroup *L. biflexa.*

Another classification is based on DNA—DNA hybridization studies. There is high degree of heterogenicity within the two species of traditional classification. The phylogenetic analysis based on 16S rRNA gene sequencing indicates **that there are three clades of Leptospires, pathogenic, saprophytic, and some uncertain pathogenicity**. The 19 species (13 pathogenic and 6 saprophytic) do not correspond to the traditional classification. Also some serovars in traditional classification occur into multiple species in DNA classification.

Under the new classification, the species are further divided into 24 serogroups and 250 serovars based *upon surface polysaccharide.*

L. interrogans serogroup Icterohaemorrhagiae has 22 serovars, e.g. Icterohemorrhagiae, Pomona, Canicola, Grippotyphosa, Australis, Autumnalis, Hebdomadis, and Grippotyphosa. The serogroup Interrogan contain serovars as Icterohaemorrhagae, Smithi, Copenhageni.

L. biflexa: It contains saprophytic leptospirae found in environment, water sources. Approximately there are 22 serogroups and 200 serotypes.

Pathogenicity

It is a **zoonosis;** humans infected when water contaminated with urine of carrier animals **enter body through cuts or abrasions or intact mucosa.**

Incubation period: 10 days (2–24 days).

Disease ranges from mild **undifferentiated pyrexia to Weil's (disease) syndrome** (severe disease with hepatorenal damage, which can be fatal).

Clinical Features (Table 43.1)

Fever with rigors, vomiting, headache, conjunctival suffusion, calf pain, purpuric hemorrhages is the common clinical feature. Albuminuria, and jaundice seen in 10–20% of infected persons. Urine examination shows albuminuria.

Aseptic meningitis or abdominal symptoms may predominate in some cases.

Late Sequelae in Leptospirosis

Late sequelae include chronic fatigue and other symptoms are headache, paralysis, mood swings and depression. In some cases, uveitis and iridocyclitis may be a late presentation of leptospirosis. Ocular symptoms are probably attributable to the persistence of leptospires in the eyes, where they are sheltered from the patient's immune response.

Apart from eye involvement, the pathogenesis of alleged late or persistant symptoms is unknown. The existence of persistant or chronic infections has not been confirmed and "scars" caused during the acute disease have not been demonstrated.

Laboratory Diagnosis

Collection of Specimens

Organisms can be isolated from **blood, CSF, peritoneal dialysate** during first 10 days of illness. Speimens should be collected before antibiotics are started. Leptospirae persist in kidneys, hence they can be demonstrated in urine and can be cultured in later stage of the disease. **Citrated or EDTA** containing tubes are used for **PCR.**

Examination of blood: 1st week

Examination of urine: 2nd week

DGM: From 2nd to 4th–6th week.

Microscope

- Leptospira can be detected by DGM in blood, urine, CSF, dialysate fluid: 10^4 organisms per mL are required to be detected by DGM.
- Organisms in tissues are visualized by silver staining.
- **Immunohistochemical** method is performed at reference laboratory.
- **Direct immunofluorescence** can be used for detection of leptospira in samples.

Culture Methods

Specimens for culture in 1st week of infections are blood, CSF (in case of meningitis), and dialysis fluid.

TABLE 43.1: Diseases caused by Leptospira species

Leptospira serogroup	Source of infection	Human disease	Distribution
Autumnalis	?	Peritibial fever—fever, rash over tibia	USA, Japan
Bovis	Cattle	Fever, prostration	USA, Australia
Canicola	Dog urine	Infectious jaundice Influenza-like illness, aseptic meningitis	Worldwide
Grippotyphosa	Rodents, water	Marsh fever Fever, aseptic meningitis	UK, USA, Africa
Hebdomadis	Rats, mice	7 day fever, jaundice	Japan, Europe
Icterohaemorrhagae	Rat urine, water	Weil's disease Jaundice, hemorrhages, aseptic meningitis	Worldwide
Mitis	Swine	Swineherd's disease Aseptic meningitis	Australia
Pomona	Swine, cattle	Swineherd disease	Australia, Europe, USA
Pyrogens	Pig	Febrile illness	SE Asia, Europe, USA
Bataviae	Rat	Fever	SE Asia, Africa, Europe
Hardjo	Cattle	Dairy farm fever	UK, USA, New Zealend

Urine culture is possible in 2nd week of infection.

- *Blood culture*: Leptospiremia occurs in the first stage of disease, i.e. in **first week of illness**. Hence blood cultures should be collected as early as possible. One or two drops of blood inoculated in 5 tubes containing 5–10 mL of semisolid EMJH medium. After 1–2 weeks, the leptospirae produce a diffuse zone of growth near top of the test tube and later a ring of growth at the level in the tube appears corresponding to the level of optimum oxygen tension for the organism.
- *CSF culture*: Other samples which can be cultured in first week are CSF and dialysis fluid. The quantity of CSF used for culture in EMJH medium is 0.5 mL.
- *Urine culture*: Urine culture is positive in second week. Urine should be processed immediately by neutralization of pH by sodium bicarbonate followed by centrifugation.

Cultures in EMJH medium are incubated at 28–30°C and examined weekly by DGM till 13 weeks. Growth occurs as descrete band just below the surface of the medium known as **Dinger's ring**. Culture that shows growth of other bacteria should be passed through membrane filters before taken for DGM.

Identification of Leptospira

It is done by MAT method or by molecular method. **PCR, and RFLP are used.**

Serological Tests

Antibodies in serum appear at end of 1st week, increase till 4th week.

Genus Specific Tests

Antigen used is *L. biflexa Patoc 1* strain. Tests are:
- Complement fixation
- Indirect immunofluorescence
- ELISA (IgM, IgG)
- IgM specific dipstick

Type Specific Tests

It identifies serovars.

- **Microscopic agglutination test (MAT)** which is more specific, done in reference laboratories.

Antibodies are detected in 5–7 days after onset of symptoms.

MAT: Patient's sera are treated with live suspension of leptospira serovars. After incubation, the mixture is observed under microscope for the formation of agglutination and titers can be detected. The range of antigens used should include serovars representative of all serogroups. The test is read by DGM. The end point is the highest dilution in which 50% of the leptospira agglutinated, the end point is determined by presence of approximate 50% free leptospira compared to control suspension.

Determination of rise in titers is important. If the patient presents with early course of disease or if date of onset not known then interval of 10–15 days is sufficient. If symptoms typical of leptospirosis are present the gap between two serum samples should be 3–5 days.

Titer of **200** is a probable case (**CDC),** in endemic areas titers as high as 800 are seen.

Formalized antigens are used in MAT to overcome difficulty with live bacteria.

Rapid Tests for Detection of Antibodies

- IGM dipstick
- ELISA
- Latex agglutination
- Lateral flow assay
- Complement-fixation test (CFT)
- Counterimmunoelectrophoresis (CIE)
- Dipstick tests: LEPTO Dip-S-Tick
- Dried latex agglutination test (LeptoTek Dri-Dot)
- Indirect fluorescent antibody test (IFAT)
- Indirect hemagglutination test (IHA)
- Patoc-slide agglutination test (PSAT)
- Sensitized erythrocyte lysis test (SEL)

WHO criteria: **Faine's criterion** is WHO approved guidelines for diagnosis based on clinical, epidemiological and laboratory findings.

Inoculation into guinea pigs: **Centrifuged deposit** is neutralized with alkaline solution and injected.

Diagnosis in animals can be done by culturing pieces of kidneys.

Examination of water for pathogenic leptospirae: Young guinea pig is shaved and some area of skin scarified. Guinea pig immersed in water. Infection of scarified area develops.

Leptospirosis

The disease was first described by Larrey in 1812 among Napoleon's troops at the siege of Cairo, and was initially believed to be related to the plague.

Adolph Weil (1886) published his historic paper describing the most severe form of human infection that was later known as Weil's disease.

Noguchi (1918) proposed the name leptospira (thin spirals) following microscopic observations.

Outbreaks of **'Andaman hemorrhagic fever'** were first reported in 1988, and identified as leptospirosis in 1993.

The principal strains are *Leptospira interrogans serovars, icterohaemorrhagiae, automnalis, pyrogenes, grippotyphosa, canicola, australis, javanica, sejroe, louisiana* and *pomona*

- *Serovars, automnalis* and *icterohaemorrhagiae* have been reported from the mainland.
- A single infection by serovar, *javanica* was reported in Madras in 1996—the latter had previously been found only in bandicoots (Bandikota bengalensis).
- *Leptospira interrogans serovar valbuzzi* has been identified as a cause of hemorrhagic pneumonia in the Andaman islands.
- *Leptospira interrogans sensu stricto* is the predominant infecting species in the Andaman islands.

The disease is endemic in Kerala, Tamil Nadu, Gujarat, Andaman, Karnataka, Maharashtra. It has also been reported from Andhra Pradesh, Orissa, West Bengal, Uttar Pradesh, Delhi and Puducherry.

Clinical Features

Leptospirosis can manifest in many ways. The various syndromes of presentation are as follows.

- Acute febrile illness
- Weil's syndrome characterized by jaundice, renal failure and myocarditis with cardiac arrhythmias
- Pulmonary hemorrhage with respiratory failure
- Meningitis
- Meningoencephalitis

The incubation period is 7–14 days, but ranges from 2–21 days.

The incidence rate ranges from 0.1–1/100,000 per year in temperate climates to 10–100/100,000 in tropical countries. The number of districts in Maharashtra reporting leptospirosis has expanded from two in 1998 to ten districts in 2005. The important districts are Mumbai, Thane, Kolhapur, Sangli and Sindhudurg which are affected by leptospirosis. The serovars isolated were L. *icterohaemorrhagiae* (rats), *L. canicola* (canines) and *L. australis* (cattle).

Serovar Specific Tests

Microscopic agglutination test (MAT): MAT is the gold standard test for diagnosis of leptospirosis because of its unsurpassed diagnostic specificity. The main advantage is that serovars can be identified which is of epidemiological importance. The difficulties in utilizing MAT are due to the following factors.

The antibody titers rise and peak only in 2nd or 3rd week, making it a less sensitive test. A fourfold rise in titer or seroconversion is the most definitive criteria for diagnosis of leptospirosis. Therefore, a second sample is mandatory, which is difficult to obtain. In such circumstances, a single high titer in MAT can be taken as diagnostic criteria. As MAT titres peak and persist for a long time (5–10 years), they would interfere with current diagnosis. Therefore, many workers use different criteria. A titre of 1:100 is taken as significant criteria, but there is controversy on the single diagnostic titre as it depends on endemicity. In non-endemic areas, 1/100 titre is taken as the diagnostic criteria. It is preferable to do rapid tests along with single high titres. Positive rapid tests with high titres suggest current infection while negative rapid tests are probably due to past infection. In Andaman, a titre of 1/200 is taken as diagnostic titre.

Treatment

Severe cases of leptospirosis should be treated with high doses of intravenous penicillin. Less severe cases can be treated with oral antibiotics such as amoxycillin, ampicillin, doxycycline or erythromycin. Third-generation cephalosporins, such as ceftriaxone and cefotaxime, and quinolone antibiotics also appear to be effective. Jarisch-Herxheimer reactions may occur after penicillin treatment.

India National Leptospirosis Reference Centre: Regional Medical Research Centre: Indian Council of Medical Research, Andaman and Nicobar Islands.

44

Actinomycetes

These are mold-like bacteria described first in the lesion of 'lumpy jaw' (actinomycosis) in cattle.

CHARACTERISTICS OF ACTINOMYCETES

- They are true bacteria having superficial resemblance to fungi.
- They are forms between bacteria and fungi.
- Actinomyces in tissues appear as sulfur granules, 0.3–1 µm, white to yellow.
- They are Gram-positive filaments with Gram-negative club ends.
- Clubs surround the granule-like 'ray of petals', hence called ray fungus. The name Actinomyces refer to ray-like organism in the granule of lesions.
- Characteristic similar to fungi is network of branching filaments.
- Characteristic similar to bacteria: Thin bacteria (0.6–1 µ), cell wall has muramic acid, susceptible to antibiotics, they have prokaryotic nuclei.
- They are closely related to mycobacteria.
- Important genera include *Actinomyces*, *Nocardia*, *Streptomyces* and *Actinomadura*.
- They cause actinomycosis or mycetoma called **'actinomycotic mycetoma'**
- Thermophilic Actinomyces as Micropolyspora and Thermoactinomyces may cause allergic pneumonitis (farmer's lung and baggassosis).

Species

A. israelii (commonest), *A. viscosus*, *A. odontolyticus*, *A. meyeri*.

Actinomyces cause chronic granulomatous infections accompanied by other bacteria, which enhance pathogenic effect. They are *Bifidobacterium dentium*, *Actinobacillus actinomycetemcomitans*, *Eikenella corrodens*, *Haemophilus aphrophilus*, *Bacteroides*, fusobacteria, staphylococci and anaerobic streptococci.

Infections: They have low virulence. Predisposing factors include surgery, trauma.

ACTINOMYCOSIS

Clinical Features

There are indurated painless swellings with multiple discharging sinuses which discharge **sulfur granules.**

Sulfur granules are 0.25–2 µm in size, white to yellowish. Granules are microcolonies which consist of Gram-positive filaments surrounded by zone of swollen club-shaped structures giving 'sunray' apperance (Fig. 44.1). These clubs appear Gram-negative, probably they are antigen–antibody complexes.

Common Sites Involved

1. **Cervicofacial (cheek and submaxillary regions)**
   - Jaw is often involved.
   - Infection is endogenous in origin.
   - Dental carries acts as predisposing factor. Infection takes place after tooth extraction or other dental procedures. Men are affected more frequently.
   - Infection is common in rural agricultural workers.

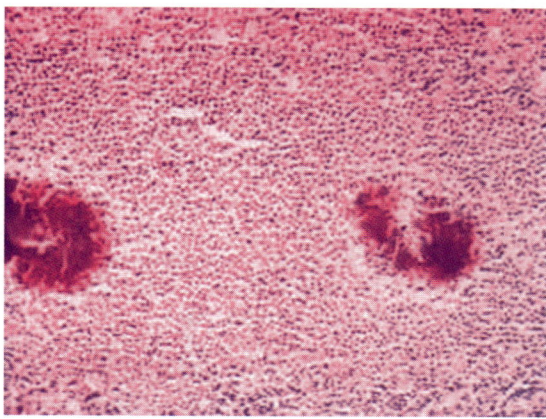

Fig. 44.1: H and E section showing sunray appearance

2. Thoracic (lung, pleura, pericardium and spread outward to chest wall).

- Infection occurs as a result aspiration from oral actinomyces from mouth.
- There may be multiple sinuses formed in chest wall. Ribs and spine may be erroded.

3. Abdominal (around cecum, neighboring tissues and abdominal wall. Infection may spread to liver via the portal vein).

4. Pelvic (with use of IUCD).

5. CNS

6. Gingivitis, periodontitis with sublingual plaques leading to root surface carries.

Most of the infections are endogenous except pelvic disease which is exogenous infection associated with use of intrauterine contraceptive devices (Flowchart 44.1).

Laboratory diagnosis

Specimens: Pus, discharge, tissue biopsy, sputum, granules are collected for diagnosis.

Gross examination: Take pus in a test tube with sterile saline; sulfur granules are seen.

Flowchart 44.1: Clinical types of actinomycosis

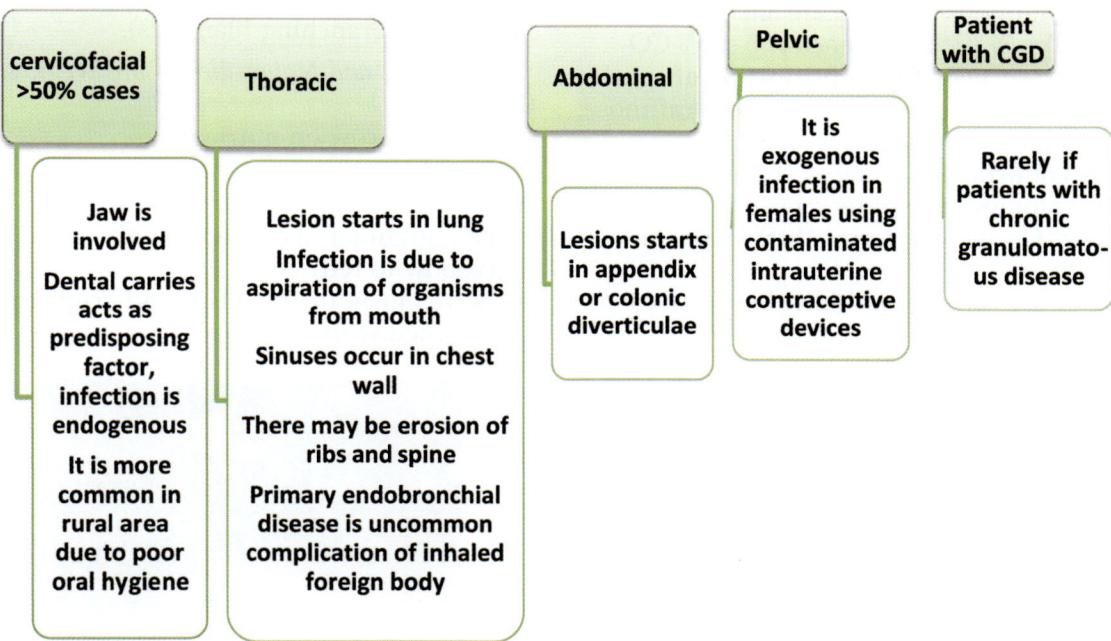

Flowchart 44.2: Comparison of actinomycotic and eumycotic granuloma

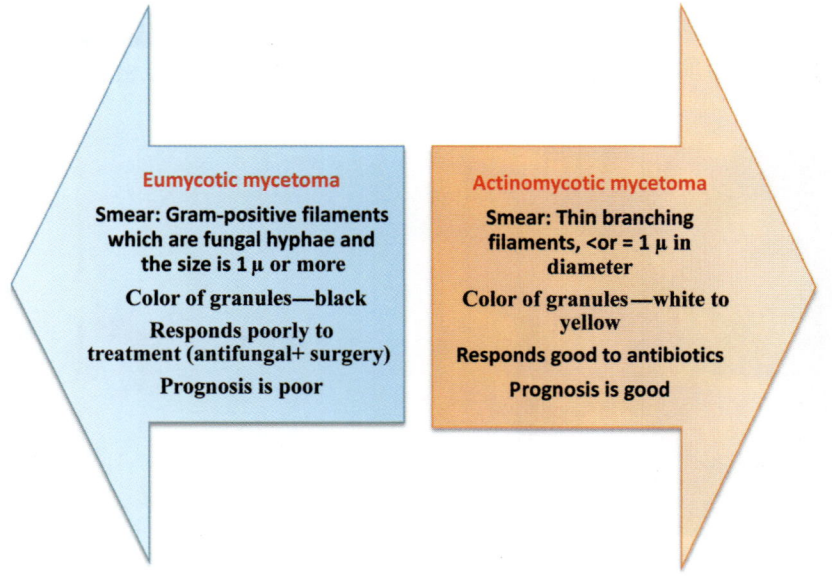

Microscopy

- In a sterile test tube containing sterile saline, granules are mixed. Granules settle at bottom which are withdrawn with capillary tube.
- Crush the granules between slides and prepare smears. Gram stain shows Gram-positive filaments and clubs (Fig. 44.2).
- Direct immunofluorescence detects antigen in specimens.
- **Biopsy** (H and E): It shows filaments surrounded by pus cells and chronic inflammatory cells.
- **Culture:** Granules are washed with saline—crushed with glass rod, inoculated in thioglycollate broth, brain heart infusion agar (BHIA), BA.
- Incubation conditions required are anaerobic, 24–48 hours to weeks, 37°C, in presence of 5–10% CO_2.
- **Biochemical tests used for identification of species are** acid from glucose, mannitol, starch, raffinose, xylose; catalase –ve, NO_3 +ve or –ve.
- Isolates are confirmed by fluorescent antisera.

A. israelii colonies are spidery resembling **molar teeth,** irregular (Fig. 44.3). It forms **fluffy balls** in thioglycollate broth.

A. bovis produces general turbidity in thioglycollate broth.

Treatment

Penicillin, tetracyclines are given for several months supplemented with surgery.

Metronidazole, trimethoprim, penicillinase resistant penicillins have no action against actinomyces.

NOCARDIA

Nocardia is named after 'Nocard' who described bovine disease. It is an environmental or soil saprophyte.

Species: *N. asteroides* (star-shaped colonies), *N. brasiliensis, N. madurae, N. caviae.*

Morphology (Figs 44.4 and 44.5)

Strict aerobic, Gram-positive bacteria and form mycelium (branching filaments).

N. asteroides and N. brasiliensis are **weak acid-fast** (1% H_2SO_4).

- Readily grow on nutrient agar.
- Broad temperature range.
- Slow growing (5–14 days).
- Dry, granular, wrinkled colonies with pigmentation (yellow to red).
- Better growth in BHIA and trypticase soy agar enriched with blood.

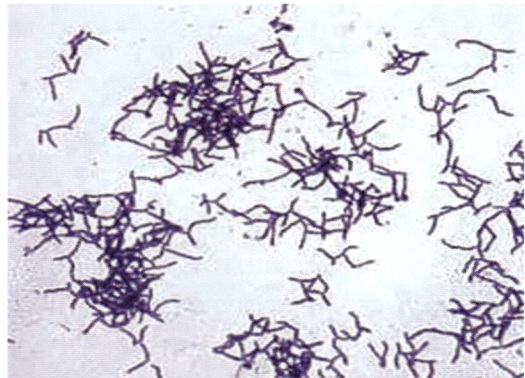

Fig. 44.2: Gram-positive branching filaments suggestive of actinomycosis

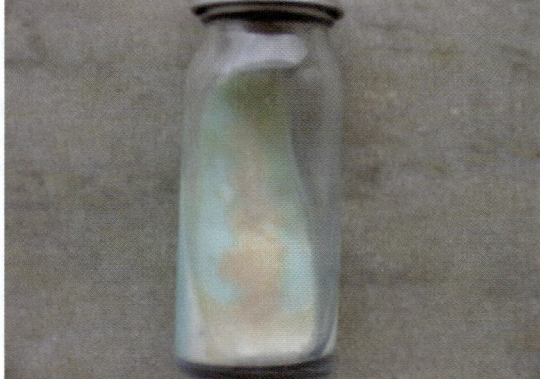

Fig. 44.4: Growth of *Nocardia* on LJ medium

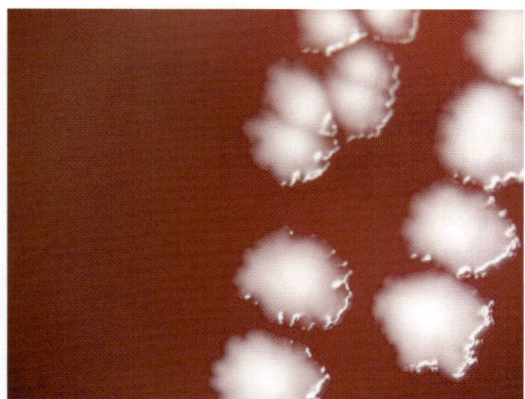

Fig. 44.3: Molar tooth-like colony of *A. israelii*

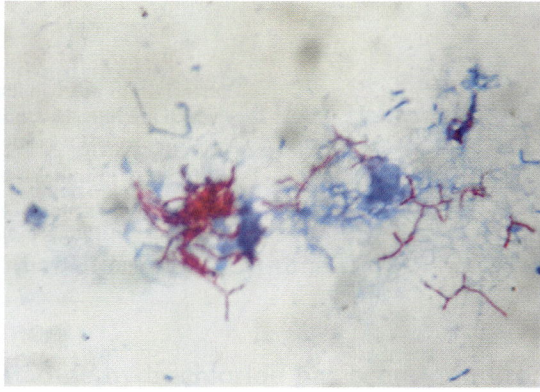

Fig. 44.5: Acid-fast filaments (1% H_2SO_4) of *Nocardia asteroides*

TABLE 44.1: Differences between Actinomyces and Nocardia

	Actinomyces spp.	Nocardia
O$_2$ requirement	Facultative anaerobe	Strict aerobe
Temp. range	Grow at 35–37°C	Wide range
Habitat	Oral commensals	Environmental saprophytes
Acid fastness	Non-acid-fast	Weak acid-fast
Mode of infection	Endogenous	Exogenous

Pathogenicity

Systemic nocardiosis may occur in immunocompromised patients. Pulmonary nocardiosis is also one of the common infections produced by *Nocardia*. These bacteria may produce mycetoma, cutaneous lesion or mucocutaneous lesions.

Differences between Actinomyces and Nocardia are given in Table 44.1.

STREPTOMYCES SOMALIENSIS

It causes mycetoma in Somalia, Sudan. Microscopically filamentous forms with chlamydospores are seen. Colonies translucent to opaque. Dry chalky colonies are produced on BA, Sabourad's dextrose agar (SDA).

Treatment

Sulphonamide is the drug of choice. Sulphadiazine is used for CNS infections. Nocardia are also sensitive to carbapenems as imipenem and cilastatin, cefotaxime or ceftriaxone. Cotrimoxazole is better than sulphadiazine.

ACTINOMADURA

- It is most frequent cause of actinomycetoma.
- Important species are *A. madurae* and *A. pellettieri*.
- White to yellow granules are produced except *A. pellettieri* produces red granules.
- Amikacin and imipenem are effective against Actinomadura.

TROPHERYMA WHIPPLEI

- Whipple's disease is multi-system disease. Patient presents with diarrhea, malabsorption with fever, arthalgia, lymphadenopathy. Mainly intestine is affected.
- The organism is present in environment as a saprophyte.
- Diagnosis is done by histopathological examination (PAS staining) of duodenal biopsy, electron microscopy and by PCR.
- Ceftriaxone (IV route) should be given for 2 weeks followed by cotrimoxazole for 1 year.

45

Rickettsia

- The rickettsiae (*Rickettsia* and *Orient species*) and anaplasmas (*Anaplasma, Neorickettsia,* and *Ehrlichia*) of medical importance are obligatory intracellular bacteria transmitted by arthropods.
- Rickettsia species, *Orientia tsutsugamushi, Ehrlichia species* and *Anaplasma species* are evolved from a common ancestor.

MORPHOLOGY

- They are small (0.3–0.5 μm) Gram-negative bacilli.
- Non-motile, non-capsulated.
- Do not stain well with Gram stain (purple) but they can be seen under light microscope by staining with Giemsa, Gimenez, and Macchiavello (red).
- They have trilaminar cytoplasmic membrane and cell wall.

- Generation time is 8–10 hours.
- Pathogen parasitizes endothelium cells.
- They lack genes for many essential enzymes, hence they depend on host cells for their nutrition.
- The genus *Rickettsia* is divided into two groups based on lipopolysaccharide.
- The immunodominent protein, outer membrane protein omp-B occurs in all *Rickettsia* species.

Initially they were thought to be viruses but they show following characteristics similar to bacteria.
- They have cell wall similar to Gram-negative bacteria.
- They contain both DNA and RNA; they have enzymes for Kreb's cycle and ribosomes for protein synthesis.
- They multiply by binary fission.
- Susceptible to antibiotics.

TABLE 45.1: Features of rickettsiaceae

Group	Species	Disease	Vector	Reservoir	Distribution
Typhus	R. prowazekii	Epidemic typhus	Louse	Human beings	Worldwide
		Brill-Zinsser disease	Louse	Human beings	America, Europe, Australia
	R. typhi	Endemic typhus	Rat flea	Rat	Worldwide
Spotted fever group	R. rickettsii	Rocky Mountain spotted fever	Tick	Rabbit, dog, small rodents	North America
	R. sibirica	Siberian tick typhus	Tick	Wild animals, cattle	Russia, Mongolia
	R. conorii	Fever Boutonneuse	Tick	Rodents	Mediterranean
		South African tick typhus		Rodents, dogs	South Africa
		Kenyan tick typhus	Tick	? Rodents	Kenya
		Indian tick typhus		? Rodents	India
	R. australis	Queensland tick typhus	Tick	Rodents	N. Australia
	R. japonica	Oriental spotted fever	Tick	?	Japan
	R. akari	Rickettsial pox	Gamsid mite	Mouse	USA, Russia
Scrub typhus	O. tsutsugamushi	Scrub typhus	Trombiculid mite	Small rodents, birds	East Asia, Pacific Islands, Australia

CULTURE

They do not grow in cell free cultures. The following methods are used for their culture.

- Yolk sac of 5–6 days old chick embryo.
- They multiply in membrane surrounding the yolk sac. This method is widely used for preparations of antigens and vaccines.
- They grow in continuous cell lines (HeLa, HeP2, and Detroit-6) but growth is not satisfactory.
- Animal inoculation: Guinea pig, mice are used.

Susceptibility

They are rapidly killed by heating at 56°C and also at room temperature. Na-hypochloride (1%), 5% H_2O_2, 70% ethanol are able to kill them.

Antigens

1. Group specific soluble antigen is present on the surface of all organisms.
2. Species specific antigen is present on cell wall.

An alkali stable polysaccharide found in some *Rickettisa* and in some nonmotile strains of *Proteus* (OX-19, OX-2, and OX-K) which form the basis of Weil-Felix test.

New or emerging rickettsioses have been described in last few decades, including tick-borne lymphadenopathy (TIBOLA) and *Dermacentor*-borne-necrosis eschar-lymphadenopathy (DEBONEL) related to *Rickettsia slovaca* infection, as well as lymphangitis-associated rickettsiosis attributed to *Rickettsia sibirica* infection.

1. Typhus Fever Group

A. Epidemic Typhus

- Transmission is by lice feeding on blood of patient, shed in feces, enter through abrasions.
- *R. prowazekii*, the agent of classical epidemic typhus, transmitted by the human body (clothing) louse, *Pediculus humanus* (but not by head lice) from active human cases or from healthy carriers or subclinical cases, so-called Brill-Zinsser disease.
- The infectious agent in the feces of the body louse is usually inoculated by scratching of the site of the louse bite, but in epidemics, in closed communities an aerosol of dried louse feces may be inhaled.
- Burundi outbreak (1995), which started in a prison at N'Gozi and spread to the malnourished inhabitants of refugee camps in the central highlands (over 1500 m), causing over 50 000 cases with a mortality of 2.6%.

- The genome of the organism has recently been sequenced, providing new evidence of an evolutionary relationship between rickettsiae and intracellular mitochondria in general.

Pathophysiology

- After proliferation at the site of the louse bite, the organism spreads hematogenously.
- *Rickettsia prowazekii*, like other most rickettsia, produces vasculitis by infecting the endothelial cells of capillaries, smaller arteries and veins resulting in fibrin and platelet deposition causing occlusion of blood vessel. The pathology is similar to that described for the spotted fever group of rickettsial diseases.
- Typhus group rickettsiae extensively multiply and accumulate intracellularly until they burst the endothelial cell and disseminate into the bloodstream.
- The angiitis is most marked in the skin, heart, nervous system, skeletal muscle and kidneys. If local thrombosis is extensive, it can cause gangrene of skin and distal part of extremities.
- Incubation period is 7 to 12 days.
- Headache, chills, fever and myalgia are common symptoms. The fever worsens quickly and become unremitting and remains high until death or if untreated, resolution by crisis toward the end of the second week.
- The conjunctivae are suffused and face congested. There may be epistaxis, dry cough, delirium and splenomegaly.
- The typhus rash appears on the second to fourth day of fever, starts in axillary folds and upper part of trunk and spreads centrifugally to limbs. It consists of small irregular pink macules which rapidly darken to a mulberry or purple color and rarely become frank petechial. There is no eschar.
- Meningoencephalitis may occur in 50% with meningism, tinnitus, hyperacusis followed by deafness, dysphagia, dysphoria, agitated delirium and coma. Survivors may suffer transverse myelitis, hemiparesis, peripheral neuropathy with hyperesthesia and prolonged psychiatric disturbances.
- The petient becomes stuporous and delirious in the second week of infection. The name typhus comes from the cloudy state of consciousness in the disease (from typhos, meaning cloud or smoke).
- In population at risk of epidemic typhus fever, nutrition and general immunity to infection are inadequate and illness is often severe with overall mortality rate up to 20% and >50% in the weak and aged. **Delirium (Typhus = cloud).**

B. Recrudescent Typhus or Brill-Zinsser Disease

It is due to reactivation and is a mild sporadic illness. Transmission is by lice feeding on blood of patient, bacteria shed in feces cause abrasions.

C. Endemic Typhus (Murine Typhus)

- Causative agent: *R. typhi*.
- Vector is rat flea and reservoirs are rats.
- Transmission by bite of flea.
- *Xenopsylla cheopis* typically infects man in markets, grain stores, garbage depots. It is often a mild illness, but can become more aggressive in refugee camps.
- After an incubation period of 1 to 2 weeks, there is an abrupt onset of illness and the initial presentation is often nonspecific. Fever, severe headache, chills, myalgia, and nausea and vomiting are most common.
- Hepatomegaly and splenomegaly (10%) may be present.
- Neurological signs and symptoms include confusion, stupor, seizures and localizing sign such as ataxia.
- The rash is macular or maculopapular and petechiae are noted in some patients. These lesions are most often distributed on trunk and involvement of extremities is not infrequent.
- The clinical course of murine typhus is usually uncomplicated. However, some patients may develop central nervous system abnormalities, renal insufficiency, hepatic insufficiency, respiratory failure and hematemesis requiring intensive care.

2. Spotted Fever Group

- The "spotted fever" group of rickettsiae, which contains a large number of species transmitted from rodents, dogs, and wild animals by ticks.
- *R. rickettsii*: It causes Rocky Mountain spotted fever, so-called because of the area of its discovery, but now mainly occurring in the eastern Atlantic states of USA, especially in trekkers and hunters exposed to wild animal ticks.
- Rocky Mountain spotted fever resembles epidemic typhus with rash and petechiae on body, palms, soles, and buccal mucosa.
- *Rickettsia rickettsii* is transmitted transstadially (stage to stage) and transovarially in tick and thus maintains infection in nature. The tick transmits the disease to human during a prolonged period of feeding that may last for 1–2 weeks.
- The bite is painless and usually unnoticed. Rickettsiae are injected from salivary glands of attached tick after 6–10 hours of feeding on human. Human may be infected by exposure to infected tick hemolymph while removing tick from person or animal especially if tick is crushed between fingers.
- The laboratory-acquired infection by aerosols or parenteral inoculation of rickettsiae has been reported.
- *R. conorii*, the cause of tick typhus in the Mediterranean area and in India, which is transmitted by the brown dog tick *Rhipicephalus sanguineus*.
- *R. akari*, rickettsial pox: Vector is mite; it is a mild disease with vesicles. Infection acquired from domestic mouse.
- *R. africae*, which is found in the African veld, is transmitted in game park areas by ticks living on cattle, hippo, and rhino.
- *R. japonica*, *R. australis*, and a variety of other similar organisms, which are widely distributed in Asia and Australia and infect man through various species of animal ticks.
- *R. tsutsugamushi*, recently renamed as a new genus with only one species, **Orientia tsutsugamushi**, the agent of **scrub typhus,** acquired from the bite of larval trombiculid mites (mitelarre-chiggers) living on the waist high Imperata grass growing in previously cleared jungle around villages and in plantations.
- The area of risk includes South East Asia, the Indian subcontinent, Sri Lanka, and other Indian Ocean islands, Papua New Guinea, and North Queensland.
- Fever, headache, rash, characteristic escher at site of bite are clinical presentations.

3. Trench Fever

- It is caused by *Rochalimaea quintana*.
- The name of the genus is given after da Rocha Lima, an early investigator of riskettsial diseases. The species name **'quintana' means fifth, referring to 'five-day fever', a synonym for the disease.**
- It is transmitted by body louse which shows poor growth in yolk sac.
- It is the only species which grows on bacteriological media (blood agar).

4. Q Fever

- It is caused by *Coxiella burnettii*, transmitted by ixodid ticks.
- Human transmission is by ingestion, inhalation from domestic livestock as cattle, sheep, goat, dogs, pigs, camels, mules, and fowls.

- Rickettsiae shed in milk, wool, hides, and conception products. It is occupational disease presents as pneumonia, hepatitis, and endocarditis.
- Q fever was so named by Derrick in 1937 as 'query fever' caused by *Coxiella burnetii* and occurs worldwide. It is a very small rickettsia-like organism which is a zoonosis of rodents, rabbits and birds that is particularly resistant to heating and drying.
- It is transmitted to domestic goats and cattle by ticks and to human by direct infection through milk, placental products and dried feces in dust. Workers who handle livestock (e.g. cattle, sheep, goats), especially at the time of slaughter or parturition, are at an increased risk of infection.
- It causes an intracytoplasmic infection in which organism multiplies, especially in splenic histiocytes and Kupffer cells of the liver.

Clinical Manifestations

- Incubation period ranges from 2–6 weeks.
- Acute Q fever has an abrupt onset, with fever, intractable headache, chills, myalgia, cough, and chest pain. Characteristically, rash is absent.
- Chronic Q fever infection is less common. It may present as endocarditis, chronic or relapsing multifocal osteomyelitis, chronic hepatitis, chronic vascular infection, pericarditis, or myocarditis.
- Humans contract the disease by inhaling contaminated aerosols when they come in contact with infected animals or materials contaminated by them.
- The acute illness may subside spontaneously and complicating endocarditis may occur after a few months in 10% patients. Pneumonitis occurs in more than half of patients. Hepatosplenomegaly is a common finding; it usually is accompanied with elevation of liver enzymes.
- Chronic Q fever infection must be excluded in patients with multifocal osteomyelitis, especially if a history of exposure to farm animals is noted.
- **Complications** include chronic Q fever, endocarditis, myocarditis, meningoencephalitis, glomerulonephritis, and syndrome of inappropriate antidiuretic hormone (SIADH).

EHRLICHIA

Human Monocytic Ehrlichiosis

Ehrlichia replicate in **cytoplasmic vacuoles** and form **'inclusion'** called as **'Morla cells'**.

Clinical incubation period is 1–2 weeks. Clinical feature are fever, headache, myelgia, athralgia, cough, pharyngitis, other manifestations are diarrhea, vomiting, altered sensorium. A petechial macular or maculopapular rash appears in some patients.

Cytopenia seen in early stage of disease gives clue in diagnosis. Mild to moderate leukemia, thrombocytopenia seen in 60–90% patients. Mortality is due to renal failure, metabolic acidosis, DIC, myocardial dysfunction or encephalitis.

Human Granulocytic Ehrlichiosis

It has short incubation period (7–10 days). The disease is similar to monocytic form but it is mild. Infection is seen in immunocompromised patients.

Indirect immunofluorescence test is used for detection of antibodies. Human granulomatis type of disease is diagnosed by Giemsa-stained peripheral blood smear.

Doxycycline reduces the duration of illness and mortality.

TIBOLA AND DEBONEL

- New or reemerging rickettsioses include tick-borne lymphadenopathy (TIBOLA) and *Dermacentor*-borne-necrosis-escher-lymphadenopathy (DEBONEL) related to *Rickettsia slovaca* infection, as well as lymphangitis-associated rickettsiosis attributed to *Rickettsia sibirica* infection.
- Patients may develop persistent asthenia and alopecia at the site of the eschar.
- The first proven case of *R. slovaca* infection was reported only in 1997 in France and is called tick-borne lymphadenopathy (TIBOLA). In Spain, the same condition is called *Dermacentor*-borne-necrosis-erythema lymphadenopathy.
- The tick (*Dermacentor* spp.) bite is commonly located on the scalp region with a characteristic local reaction (eschar) which can be surrounded by a circular

TABLE 45.2: Newer Rickettsia

Species	Disease	Transmission	Geographical distribution
E. chaffeensis	Monocytic ehrlichiosis	Tick bite	North and South America, Asia
A. phagocytophilum	Granulomatic ehrlichiosis	Tick bite	USA, Eurassia
E. ewingii	Ehrlichiosis ewingii	Tick bite	USA
N. sennetsu	Sennetsu ehrlichiosis	Fluke-infested fish	Japan, Southeast Asia

erythema. The other main symptoms are enlarged and sometimes painful lymph nodes in the region of the tick bite, characteristically in the occipital region and/or behind the sternocleidomastoidal muscle.

- The most frequent general symptoms are low-grade fever, fatigue, dizziness, headache, sweat, myalgia, arthralgia, and loss of appetite. Without treatment, the symptoms are seen to persist for as long as 18 months.

Doxycycline treatment can shorten the illness.

Laboratory Diagnosis of Rickettsial Fevers

Diagnosis is done by culture and serology (antibody detection).

Being a hazardous pathogen, biosafety level 3 is used.

Isolation

Animal inoculation: Mice and guinea pig are used for isolation of rickettsia.

Samples collected are blood (in skimmed milk) or other suitable sample as sputum in Q fever. The animals are observed daily, temperature is recorded.

Neil-Mooser (tunica) reaction: In Rocky Mountain spotted fever, guinea pig develops fever, scrotal necrosis and it may die.

R. typhi, R. conori, R. akari develop **tunica reaction.** Fusion of layers of testes occur, hence testes cannot be pushed back into abdomen.

R. prowazekii and *C. burnetii* develop only fever.

R. tsutsugamushi multiplies in mice and develops ascites.

Xenodiagnosis

Ro. quintana doesn't grow on mice or guinea pig. Xenodiagnosis is done. Healthy lice are allowed to feed on patients and organisms are detected in gut of lice.

Weil-Felix Reaction

Weil-Felix test is used for the diagnosis of rickettsial fevers. It is a tube agglutination test. It is called as **hetrophile agglutination** as proteus antigens are used for the detection of rickettsial diseases.

Flowchart 45.1: Pathogenicity of *Rickettsia*

Rickettsia enter by bite of vector or through feces

↓

Disseminate through blood and attached to endothelial cells by ompA, ompB or other surface protein

↓

Encountering endothelial cells, they attach to cell membrane and induce the cells to engulf them——induced phagocytosis

↓

Bacilli rapidly escape from phagosome into cytoplasm by lysis of cell lysis of phagosomal membrane by their phospholipase

↓

In cytoplasm, they multiply and spread to other endothelial cell through long cellular of cell membrane. Eventually destroy host endothelial cells

Damage may be due to phospholipase, protease, or by free radicals induced membrane lipid peroxidation

↓

Endothelial damage is responsible for clinical presentation

↓

Host defences: clearance of bacteria by cytotoxic T cells and their products

Flowchart 45.2: Mechanism of endothelial damage

Leakage of RBCs from damaged area of endothelial cells causes hemorrhagic spots

Dilatation of blood vessels produce pink rash

Pinpoint hemorrhages of blood vessels of brain, liver, lungs, heart lead to encephalitis, pneumonitis, cardiac arrhythmia, vomiting, and abdominal pain

Effects of endothelial damage

The reasons why *Proteus* antigens are used and not their known antigens are used for detection of antibodies against Ricketssia are:

- There is a sharing antigen between (carbohydrate antigen) rickettsiae and *Proteus* strains OX19, OX 2, OX K.; thus though *Proteus* and *Ricketssia* are different bacteria, they have some antigenic similarity called hetereophilia (Phila means loving, hetero means two different).
- Another reason is Proteus antigens can be prepared easily and safe as compared to rickettsial own antigens as this organism is dangerous to handle and may cause fatal infection in laboratory person.

Reactions

- Test is positive with OX19 and OX2 in epidemic typhus, endemic typhus and tick-borne spotted fever.
- The test is negative or weakly positive in Brill-Zinsser disease. In spotted fever, both OX19 and OX2 are agglutinated.
- Scrub typhus gives positive reaction with OX K antigens.

The antibody titer rises during acute stage of disease, reaches peak titer up to 1:1000 or 1:5000 by second week and then starts declining.

Agglutination pattern with

	OX19	OX2	OXK
Epidemic typhus	+++	+	—
Brill-Zinsser disease	Usually negative or weak positive		—
Endemic typhus	+++	+ or –	—
Tick-borne spotted fever	++	++	–
Scrub typhus	–	–	+++

Disadvantage

- The test is false positive in UTI or other Proteus infections, typhoid fever, liver disease.
- It is not possible to differentiate between epidemic and endemic diseases.
- Antibodies to spotted fever group can be demonstrated by direct immunofluorescence.
- Immunohistology: This technique uses either fluorescence labeled or enzyme labeled antibodies. Idientification of antigen is possible in tissue.
- These tests have 70% sensitivity and they are used in Rockey Mountain spotted fever group. PCR is also 70% sensitive.

Other tests developed to detect antibodies are:

- ELISA
- CFT
- Latex agglutination
- Indirect immunofluorescence.
- Immune peroxidase
- Western blot.

Immunoprophylaxis

- No effective vaccine is available to protect rickettsial fevers.
- The Weigl's strain vaccine used previously contained killed contents of lice infected with *R. prowazekii*.
- **Formalized mouse brain vaccine** was obtained by **Castaneda**
- **Cox** developed inactivated **yolk sac** vaccine.
- A live-attenuated vaccine using **'E strain'** was found to be effective but the disadvantage is that it may produce mild disease in vaccinated persons.

Treatment

Tetracycline, doxycyclines are effective provided the treatment is started early. Sulphonamides enhance the disease and they are contraindicated.

Additional Points

Rickettsial infection has been one of the great scourges of mankind, occurring in devastating epidemics during times of war and famine. Napoleon's retreat from Moscow was forced by rickettsial disease breaking out among his troops. Lenin is said to have remarked, in reference to rickettsial disease rampant during Russian revolution that "either socialism will defeat the louse or the louse will defeat the socialism". Rickettsial disease in **India** has been documented from Jammu and Kashmir, Himachal Pradesh, Uttaranchal, Rajasthan, Assam, West Bengal, Maharashtra, Kerala and Tamil Nadu. **There is a high magnitude of scrub typhus, spotted fever and Indian tick typhus caused by *R. conorii*.** An extensive study on tick-borne rickettsiosis in **Pune district of Maharashtra** revealed that Indian tick typhus exists as **zoonosis**.

Pathology: These organisms after entering human body multiply, locally and enter the bloodstream. Then they invade target cells, which are vascular endothelium, reticulo-endothelial cells and in case of ehrlichiosis and anaplasmosis, blood cells. Once inside host cells, organisms multiply and accumulate in large numbers before lysing the cell (in case of typhus group) or they escape from cell, damaging its membrane and causing influx of water (in case of spotted fever group). Unlike rickettsiae in the spotted fever group, which can survive and replicate for several days after the death of their host cells rickettsiae of the typhus group die rapidly after killing their host cells. Vasculitis is the basic pathogenic mechanism. **Vasculitis is responsible for skin rash, microvascular leakage, edema, tissue hypoperfusion and end-organ ischemic injury. Formation of thrombi can lead to tissue infarction and hemorrhagic necrosis.** Inflammation and vascular leakage leads to interstitial pneumonitis, noncardiogenic pulmonary edema, cerebral edema and meningoencephalitis. Infection of endothelial cells also induces procoagulant activity that promotes coagulation factor consumption, platelet adhesion and leukocyte emigration and may result in clinical syndrome similar to disseminated intravascular coagulation (early signs and symptoms of these infections are nonspecific and mimic benign viral illnesses, making diagnosis more difficult). Symptomatology may vary from mild to severe. Unless there is a high index of suspicion, it is likely to be missed as the clinical presentation may mimic other common infections in the tropics. Incubation period of various rickettsial infections varies between 2 and 21 days. Clinical manifestations of rickettsial infections are detailed herein.

Fever: Fever of undetermined origin is the most frequent presentation of disease. Fever is usually abrupt onset, high grade, sometimes with chills, occasionally with morning remissions and associated with headache and myalgia. Diagnosis of rickettsial disease should always be considered in patients with acute febrile illness accompanied with headache and myalgia, particularly in endemic areas with history of tick exposure or contact with dogs.

Headache and myalgia: Severe frontal headache and generalized myalgia especially in muscles of the lumbar region, thigh and calf is seen in variable proportion of cases. Headache is noted less frequently in young children than in adults, but when it occurs, it is often intractable to therapy.

Rash: Though rash is considered as hallmark of rickettsial disease, it is neither seen at presentation nor in all the patients. Thus it should be remembered that spotted fevers could be spotless too! Rash usually becomes apparent after 3–5 days of onset of symptoms. Initially, rash is in the form of pink, blanching, discrete macules which subsequently becomes maculopapular, petechial or hemorrhagic. Sometimes palpable purpura (typical of vasculitis) is seen. Occasionally, petechiae enlarge to ecchymosis and gangrenous patches may develop. Rarely gangrene of digits, earlobes, scrotum, nose or limbs may occur secondary to vasculitis and thrombosis. Distribution of rash is initially near ankles, lower legs and wrists. Thereafter, rash spreads centripetally to involve whole body. The rash of typhus group rickettsioses is quite atypical, initially appearing on trunk, spreading centrifugally and usually sparing palms Eschar, a black necrotic area, resembles the skin burn of cigarette butt. A necrotic eschar usually associated with regional lymphadenopathy. Gastrointestinal symptoms including nausea, vomiting, abdominal pain and diarrhea are seen with varying frequency. Constipation is seen particularly in epidemic typhus. Respiratory symptoms include cough and distress are sometimes seen. Following are the life-threatening manifestations of rickettsial infections.

(1) *Respiratory*: Interstitial pneumonitis and noncardiogenic pulmonary edema secondary to pulmonary microvascular leakage. (2) *Neurological*: Meningoencephalitic syndrome is known to occur with rickettsial infections. (3) *Renal*: Acute renal failure is associated with bad prognosis and can be a presenting feature of rickettsial disease. (4) Disseminated intravascular coagulation like syndrome, hepatic failure, gangrene and myocarditis.

GENUS BARTONELLA

Human pathogenic species are *B. bacilliformis, B. quintana and B. henselae.*

B. bacilliformis (Oroya fever): It presents with fever, anemia due RBCs invasion. **Verruga** is a late sequelae in survivors or in those with asymptomatic disease. Daniel Carrion inoculated himself with material from verruga and developed Oroya fever due to which he died, Oroya fever is also known as **Carrion's disease.**

Bartonella henselae: It is febrile illness with lymphadenopathy following cat scratch hence called **cat-scratch disease.** It also causes other conditions. In bacillary angiomatosis, vascular nodules and tumors develop on skin, mucosa while bacillary peliosis involves spleen and liver.

The causative agent can be demonstrated in lymph node biopsy section stained with **Warthin-Starry stain.**

Bacillary angiomatosis may also be caused by *R. quintana* or *R. afipia.*

46

Chlamydia

CHARACTERISTICS

- They are obligate intracellular parasites.
- They are filterable and fail to grow on cell free media, hence considered to be viruses.
- Based on the diseases produced, they were initially called as psittacosis-lymphogranuloma-trachoma (PLT) viruses.
- They lack enzymes of electron transport chain and require ATP (hence called **energy parasites)** and nutrient resources from host cell.
- They have trophism for columnar and transitional epithelial cells lining mucosae.
- They produce basophilic inclusion bodies hence called **'basophilic viruses'.**
- They possess both DNA and RNA.
- As Sir Samuel Bedson studied extensively on psittacosis, the name Bedsonia was also proposed to this group. However, they are officially classified as bacteria belonging to genus Chlamydia, in the family Chlamydiaceae.
- They have cell wall and ribosomes.
- They replicate by binary fission without an eclipse phase.
- They are susceptible to antibiotics.

- They are intracellular parasites of humans, birds, and animals.
- They are Gram-negative small bacteria which are nonmotile.

Family Chlamydiaceae consists of two genera—Chlamydia and Chlamydophila. The genus Chlamydia has one species—C. trachomatis and genus *Chlamydophila* has three species—*C. psittaci, C. pneumoniae* and *C. pecorum*.

C. TRACHOMATIS

Morphology

Two forms (Table 46.1)

1. *Elementary body*: Extracellular form, also it is the infective form (200–300 nm). It is spherical particle with rigid cell wall, (similar to the cell wall of Gram-negative bacilli) and nucleoid.

2. *Reticulate body*: Intracellular and growing, multiplying form, inside the body large number of elementary bodies (EB) produced called inclusion bodies. (500–1000 nm). Its cell wall is fragile and pliable, leading to pleomorphism.

TABLE 46.1: Differences detween elementary body and reticulate body

Characteristic	Elementary body	Reticulate body
Size	0.2–0.3 μ (200–300 nm)	1 μ (500–1000 nm)
Morphology	Electron dense core rigid spore like	Fragile, pleomorphic
Infectivity	Infectious	Noninfectious
RNA:DNA ratio	1:1	3:1
Metabolic activity	Inactive	Active
Replication	Absent	Present, by binary fission
Trypsin digestion	Resistant	Sensitive
Growth	No	Yes
Projections	Few	More

Inclusion bodies surround the nucleus like a 'shield'. Inclusion body is demonstrated by Giemsa stain, Lugol's iodine stain, Macchiavello and Giminez stain.

Growth Cycle of Chlamydia (Fig. 46.1)

- Infection is started with attachment of elementary body to epithelial cell, followed by endocytosis.
- Inside the host cell, the elementary body (EB) lies in endosome, thus remains separated from rest cytoplasm by endosomal membrane.
- By 6–8 hours, EB undergoes transformation to a large reticular body (RB).
- Division begins by binary fission, by 40 hours the development of Chlamydia microcolony (containing many elementary bodies) within host cell is formed and it is called inclusion body.
- Inclusion body contains 500–1000 elementary bodies ready to come out, the mature inclusion exocytosed in 72–96 hours. EB released which can infect other cells.

Cultivation

Yolk Sac Inoculation

They grow in yolk sac of chick embryo. They infect the endothelial cells. Specimen is pretreated with streptomycin, polymyxin B and then inoculated into yolk sac. Growth is detected by demonstration of inclusion bodies by Giemsa, Giemnez, Macchiavello stains.

Tissue Cultures

This is the method of choice. Cell cultures used are McCoy cell, mouse fibroblasts, monkey kidney cell cultures, HeLa, HeP2. Cell cultures are pretreated with metabolic inhibitor, cycloheximide. Growth in cell cultures is detected by demonstration of inclusions by Iodine staining (Fig. 46.2), Giemsa and Giemnez. Direct immunofluorescence is used for rapid detection.

Animal Inoculation

Mice are used as experimental animals, they are inoculated with intranasal, intraperitoneal and intracerebral routes. The animal dies in 10 days. Elementary bodies can be seen in smears from lungs, spleen, brain, peritoneal exudate.

Antigenic Properties: Three Major Antigens

- *Heat-stable genus-specific antigen*: It is stable polysaccharide, responds to CFT.
- *Species-specific protein antigen*: It is present on envelope of all strains of a species. Based on this antigen, chlamydiae are classified into different species.
- *Serotype-specific antigen* is present on major outer membrane (MOMP). Intraspecies typing helps to classify into many serotypes.

Resistance to Physical and Chemical Agents

- They are inactivated at 56°C within few minutes.
- At 37°C, infectivity is lost in few hours.
- At 4°C they remain viable for several days.
- They are killed by ether, formalin, phenol.

Ocular Infections (Table 46.2)

Chlamydia causing eye infections are known as **TRIC (trachoma inclusion conjunctivitis)** agent. Two types of eye infections occur.

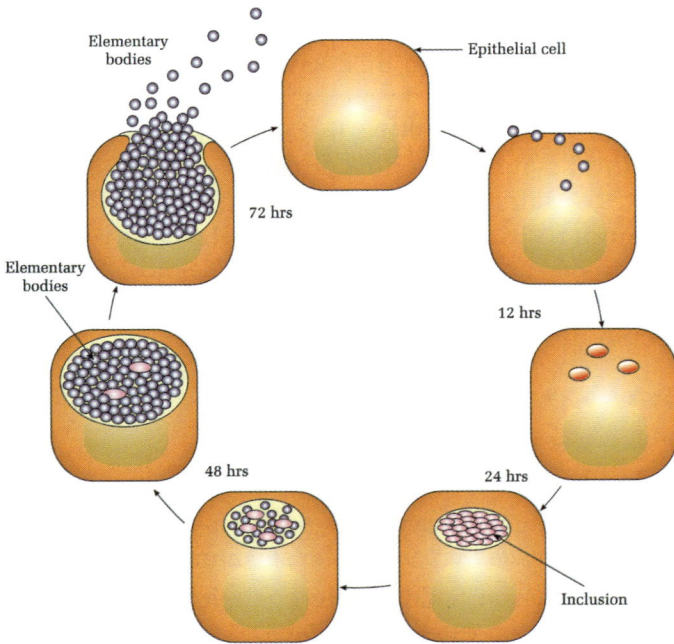

Fig. 46.1: Life cycle of Chlamydia

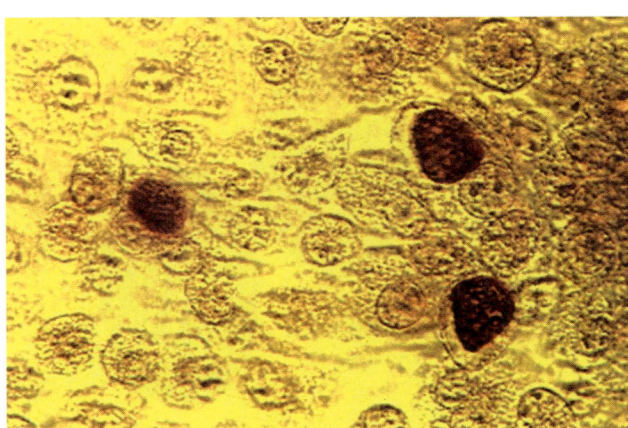

Fig. 46.2: Iodine staing showing chlamydia inclusions

TABLE 46.2: Chlamydia infections

Species	Serotype	Disease
Chlamydia trachomatis	A, B, Ba, C	Endemic blinding trachoma
Chlamydia trachomatis	D, E, F, G, H, I, J, K	Inclusion conjunctivitis
		Genital Chlamydia
		Infant pneumonia
Chlamydia trachomatis	L1, L2, L3	Lymphogranuloma venereum (LGV)
Chlamydophila psittaci	Many serotypes	Psittacosis
Chlamydophila pneumoniae	Formerly called TWAR strain	Acute respiratory disease

Trachoma

- It is a major preventable cause of blindness.
- It is caused by *Chlamydia trachomatis* serotypes A, B, Ba, C.
- It is exclusive human infection transmitted from eye to eye by fingers, fomites or through flies.
- Incubation period is 7–14 days.
- It is chronic keratoconjunctivitis, characterized by follicles, papillary hyperplasia, pannus formation and cicatrization.

Trachoma dubium (suspicion), protrachoma (conjunctivial lesion before follicle formation) are different stages followed by established trachoma.

Laboratory Diagnosis

- Scraping is taken from the lesion which shows inclusion bodies surrounding the nucleus like as a shield (Fig. 46.3).
- The inclusions can be demonstrated by Giemsa stain.
- Other simple method is staining with Lugol's iodine.
- *Inclusion bodies*: Halberstaedter-Prowazek or HP bodies demonstrated in conjunctival scraping.
- **Direct immunofluorescence (IF) can be used for the detection of antigen.**
- **ELISA can also be used for antigen detection.**
- **Culture** can be done in HeLa or HEp-2 cells and inclusions can be demonstrated in cell culture or by IF test.

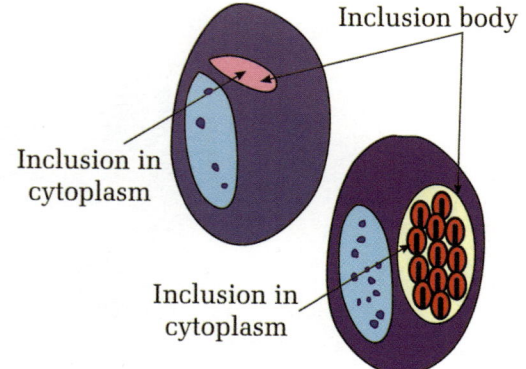

Fig. 46.3: Inclusion body of *Chlamydia* (surrounding nucleus like a shield)

- Other methods used for the diagnosis are PCR, LCR.

Inclusion Conjunctivitis

It is caused by *Chlamydia trachomatis* serotypes D-K. It is also called as paratrachoma. It spreads from genital secretions to eye by hand contact or by bathing in contaminated swimming tanks **(swimming pool conjunctivities)**. The disease is common in sexually active individuals.

Ophthalmia Neonaturum

It is called blenorrhea. It is the neonatal infection; infection takes place while passing through infected birth canal. Infection apperars 5–12 days after birth.

Infant pneumonia: Usually infants between 4 and 16 weeks of age are affected. Patients present with cough, sneezing with minimum fever and toxicity. High titers of IgM antibodies are present in sera.

Genital Infections (Flowchart 46.1)

Nongonococcal Urethritis

Serotypes D-K cause this condition. It is a sexually transmitted disease. In males, it causes epididymitis, proctitis, conjunctivitis. In female, it causes acute urethral syndrome, mucopurulent cervicitis, endometritis, salphingitis, pelvic inflammatory disease, conjunctivitis, perihepatitis **(Fitz-Hugh-Curtis syndrome)** and **Reiter's syndrome**. Diagnosis is based on isolation of organisms, detection of antigen by ELISA, IF.

Lymphogranuloma Venereum (LGV)

- It is a sexually transmitted disease.
- Incubation period is 3–5 days to 5 weeks.
- The condition is caused by serovars—L1, L2, and L3 of *Chlamydia trachomatis*. Most common L2.
- *Primary lesion*: Small painless papulovesicular lesion is present on external genitalia.
- Secondary stage develops after 2 weeks.

Flowchart 46.1: Chlamydia genital infections

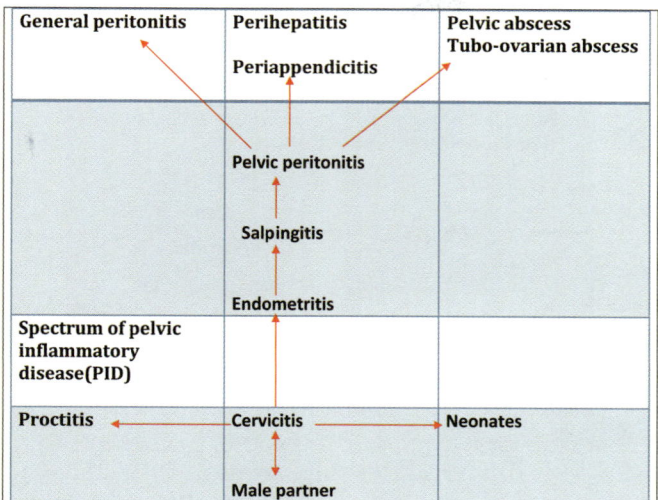

- It causes suppurative inguinal adenitis (Bubo), which may breakdown forming discharging sinuses. Intrapelvic and paracortical lymph nodes are involved in females.
- Joints, eyes and meninges are affected in few cases.
- *Tertiary stage*: Late sequelae in women are rectal stricture and elephantiasis of vulva **(esthiomene).**
- There may be involvement of joints, eyes, meninges.

Laboratory Diagnosis

- Smears from material aspirated from the bubos may show elementary bodies **(Miyagawa's granulo-corpuscles).**
- Patients develop antibodies with titres of 1:64 or more in CF test and 1:52 or more in micro-IF (immune fluorescence test)
- Detection of antigen by direct immunofluorescence increases sensitivity.
- Molecular methods are DNA probes and PCR.

Respiratory Infections

Pneumonia

It is caused by *Chlamydophila pneumoniae* strains originally known as TWAR strains (TW-18, AR-39), now designated as *Chlamydia pneumoniae*. The strain was called as TWAR as they were isolated from acute respiratory disease in adults in Taiwan (TWAR from Taiwan Acute Respiratory). Incubation period is 1–3 weeks. Clinical presentation includes pharyngitis, sinusitis, bronchitis, pneumonia. Diagnosis is based on detection of antigen by IF or ELISA, antibody detection by CFT, ELISA and by PCR.

Psittacosis

It is a disease of birds of parrots family caused by *Chlamydophila psittaci*. It is shed in nasal discharge and feces of birds. Infections are transmitted to humans by dusts or aerosols. It is an occupational disease seen in poultry workers and clinical spectrum varies from mild influenza-like symptoms to pneumonia, endocarditis, meningoencephalitis, pericarditis, myocarditis, and arthritis. Diagnosis is done by isolation, detection of antigen, and detection of antibodies. **Ornithosis** is disease of other birds, it is now merged with psittacosis.

Inclusion bodies produced in **Psittacosis** are known as **'Levinthal Coles-Lillie'** bodies.

Lines of evidence suggesting that *C. trachomatis* is associated with atherosclerotic coronary artery disease and cerebrovascular disease consists of seroepidemiological studies, detection of organisms in atherosclerotic tissue, cell culture studies, animals models, trial of prevention using antibiotics. Possible link is still controversial.

Laboratory Diagnosis of Chlamydial Infections
(Flowchart 46.2)

Specimens collected are corneal scrapings, bubo aspirate, genital secretions, and sputum based upon the infection.

Transport specimens in SPG or SPS medium.

TABLE 46.3: Differences between different Chlamydia species

Properties	Chalmydia trachomatis	Chlamydophila pneumoniae	Chlamydophila psittaci
Inclusion morphology	Round vacuolar	Round, dense	Large variable shape, dense
Glycogen in inclusison	Yes	No	No
Morphology of elementary body	Round	Pear-shaped or round	Round
Susceptibility to sulphonamides	Yes	No	No
Plasmid	Yes	No	Yes
Natural host	Humans	Humans	Birds
Mode of transmission	Person to person Mother to infant	Airborne, person to person	Airborne bird excreta to humans

Flowchart 46.2: Laboratory diagnosis of *Chlamydia*

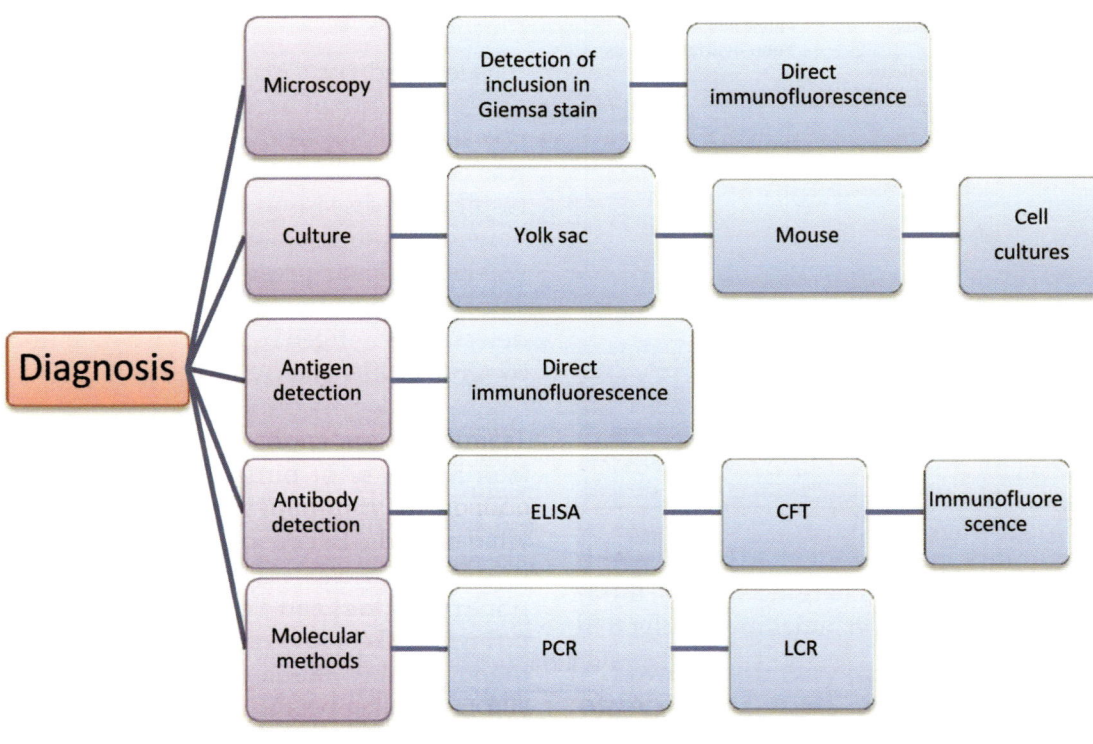

Microscopy

Inclusion bodies which are stained as **basophilic** with Giemsa stain, iodine staining is also used as inclusion contains glycogen. It is mainly important in diagnosis of neonatal conjunctivitis. (HP bodies in trachoma).

Direct immunofluorescent staining (DF) is used for the direct detection of Chlamydia in specimens and in growth in tissue cultures.

Demonstration of Chlamydia antigens
- Commonly used method is Micro-IF (titre-1:8)
- ELISA

Isolation of Chlamydia

- Cell cultures preferred one are HeLa, HEp-2. McCoy cell lines which are treated with substances as metabolic inhibitors which inhibit metabolism of host cell so that the host's machinary is used by organisms for their growth.
- Cell cultures can be treated with DEAE dextran, which increases the contact between organisms and cell culture is increased.
- Growth of Chlamydia is detected by staining inclusions and direct immunofluorescence test.

Growth in Embryonated Eggs

Samples are inoculated in embryonated eggs (grow in yolk sack of 6–8 days old embryo): Group specific antigen is detected by CFT and inclusion body can be demonstrated.

Experimental animals: Mice were used, nowadays this is not done.
- ***Antibodies detection*** (group specific): CF tests (1:64), ELISA tests for IgG and IgM antibodies are common tests. Fourfold rise in titers for both tests is diagnostic.
- **DNA probe is molecular method.**
- **Amplification techniques used in diagnosis are PCR, ligase chain reaction.**
- ***Demonstration of hypersensitivity by skin testing (Frei's test):*** 0.1 mL of antigen derived from yolk sac material is inoculated intradermally on the forearm. Same amount of noninfected material is inoculated on other arm which acts as control. In 2–5 days, induration 7 mm or more is formed indicating positive test.

Treatment

Doxycycline and erythromycin (for pregenet women) are drugs of choice.

TABLE 46.4: Differences between Chlamydia and viruses

	Chlamydia	*Viruses*
Cellular organization	Present	Absent
Binary fission	Present	Absent
Both DNA and RNA	Present	Either DNA or RNA
Ribosomes	Present	Absent
Sensitivity to antimicrobials	Present	Absent

NEW VARIANT OF CHLAMYDIA TRACHOMATIS

A new variant *Chlamydia trachomatis* (nvCT) strain has been recently isolated in Sweden (2006)62, which has a 377 bps deletion in a portion of the plasmid that is the target area for some of the nucleic amplification tests (NAATs). Consequently, these tests often give false negative results when presented with this strain. Therefore, it is important to select primers for NAAT carefully particularly those targeting the endogenous plasmids. The symptoms and treatment of this strain do not differ from those for normal chlamydiae. So far, this strain has been found in Sweden and Norway. The clinicians and microbiologists should remain vigilant for suspicious negative results as well as unexplained fall in positive results. However, other commercially available NAAT systems that use a different sequence (Gene Probe Aptima Combo AC 2, Probe Tech, BD, etc.) accurately detect this agent.

Prevention

WHO has started SAFE program to prevent trachoma.

S – Surgery for deformed eyelids

A – Periodic azithromycin therapy

F – Face washing and hygeine

E – Environmental improvement as building latrines, decreasing number of flies

Treatment

Tetracycline is used for genital infections except in pregnant women in which azithromycin is used. Topical tetracycline or erythromycin is used for neonatal infections.

LGV: Sulphonamides and tetracycline are used for the treatment of LGV.

47

Mycoplasma

Initially, this organism was isolated from a case of bovine pleuropneumonia, later on many isolates were found in human, animal and environmental sources; they were called **pleuropneumonia-like organisms—PPLO.** The term **Mycoplasma was replaced (Myco-fungus-like form)** which describe their morphology. *Mycoplasma pneumoniae* was also called **Eaton's agent** as it was first isolated by Monroe Eaton.

General Characteristics

- These are bacteria devoid of cell wall, highly pleomorphic.
- They are resistant to penicillin and other antibiotics which act on cell wall.
- They have no fixed shape or size.
- Cell bound by membrane containing sterols.
- They can pass through filters.
- They multiply by binary fission.
- They have the ability to synthesize purines and pyrimidines.

Morphology

- It is the smallest free living organism.
- They are pleomorphic, occur as granules or filaments, coccoid, disc-like, ring forms.
- Size varies, smallest mycoplasma is 125–250 nm in size.
- Growth on solid media consists of protoplasmic masses of indefinite shape, these are structures of size 50–300 nm.
- Morphology appears different with different methods of demonstrations, e.g. dark field microscopy, Giemsa-stained smear from solid and liquid media.
- No flagella, spores, fimbria but motile with **apical knob-like structure** which is responsible for its gliding motility.

- They can cause hemadsorption.
- They are Gram-negative but better stained by Giemsa stain.

Cultural Characteristics

- They are facultative anaerobes.
- They grow at incubation temperature of 22–41°C (optimum—35–37°C).
- They are cultivated in solid or liquid media.
  - Media for cultivation are enriched with 20% horse or human serum and yeast extract. High concentration of serum is required to provide cholesterols.
  - **Medium with penicillin and thallium acetate is used as selective medium**
  - PPLO broth is liquid medium for it (heart infusion peptone broth with 2% agar, yeast extract, horse serum). For enrichment, 30% human ascitic fluid or animal serum is added (serum provides cholesterol)
- Most species are hemolytic due to production of hydrogen peroxide.
- They grow in 2–6 days, producing small colonies (10–600 μ).
- Colony is typically biphasic—"fried egg appearance"—colonies are round with granular surface, and dark center typically burried in agar. Colonies of *M. hominis* are typically "fried egg" like while those of *M. pneumoniae* are smaller and lack typical appearance. Rapidly growing colonies of mycoplasma can be detected by hand lens (Fig. 47.1).
- Colony studied by **Dienes method:** Agar block containing colony is cut and taken on a slide, a cover slip is placed on the block and alcoholic solution of methyl blue, azure is added. With help of lens, colony is studied.

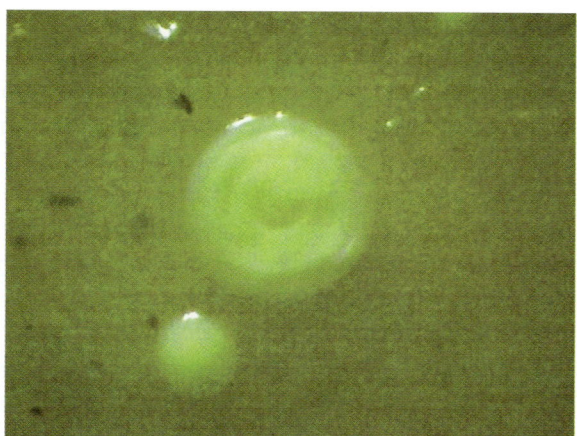

Fig. 47.1: Colony of *Mycoplasma*

Resistance

Lipolytic and surface active agents are effective. They don't have cell wall hence antimicrobials acting on cell wall are not effective. They are sensitive to tetracycline. Sensitivity to methylene blue (0.002%) is used as test for identification of *M. pneumoniae*.

Biochemical Reactions

- They can utilize glucose or arginine as sole source of carbon. Unique feature is requirement of cholesterol and related sterols by most mycoplasmas.
- They are chemoorganotrophs, the metabolism is mainly fermentative.
- Urea is not hydrolysed except by *Ureaplasma*.

Pathogenicity (Flowchart 47.1)

Transmission is by droplet secretions. It causes two types of infections: respiratory tract infections and genital infections.

Respiratory tract infection: Incubation period—1–3 weeks.

Clinical presentation: Pneumonia produced is called **'primary atpical pneumonia'.** It is also known as **walking pneumonia.** Fever, malaise, headache, sore throat, cough are common symptoms. Consolidation of lungs may occur and cough with blood-tinged sputum (primary atypical pneumonia) may be produced (*Mycoplasma pneumoniae*).

Complications: Rashes, meningitis, otitis, encephalitis, hemolytic anemia, myocarditis, pericarditis, cerebellar ataxia, transverse myelitis, GB syndrome, peripheral neuropathy, arthralgia, and coagulopathies are complications of the infection.

Genital infections: It is a common cause of **non-gonococcal urethritis**.

Classification

Pathogenic

- **Respiratory**: *Mycoplasma pneumoniae*
- **Genital**: *M.hominis, M. genitalium, Ureaplasma urealyticum*

Flowchart 47.1: Pathogenic mechanisms of *Mycoplasma*

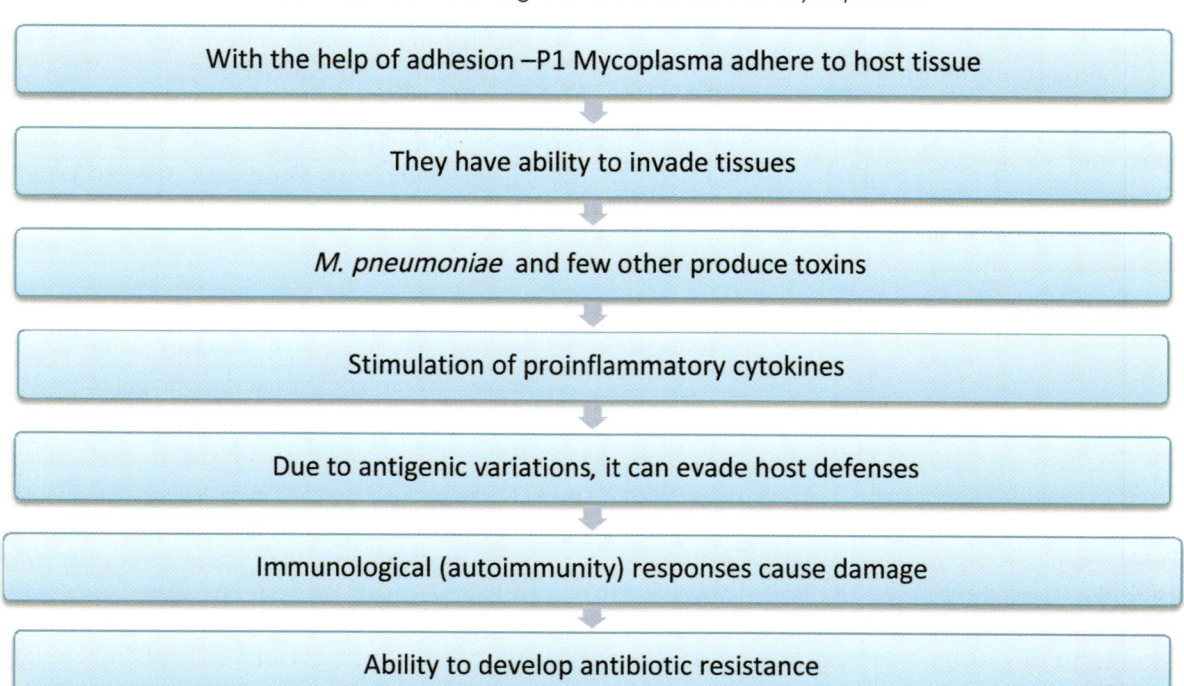

With the help of adhesion –P1 Mycoplasma adhere to host tissue

↓

They have ability to invade tissues

↓

M. pneumoniae and few other produce toxins

↓

Stimulation of proinflammatory cytokines

↓

Due to antigenic variations, it can evade host defenses

↓

Immunological (autoimmunity) responses cause damage

↓

Ability to develop antibiotic resistance

Nonpathogenic

Respiratory
* *M. orale*
* *M. buccale*
* *M. salivarium*
* *M. faucium*

Genital
* *M. fermentans*
* *M. primatum*
* *M. penetrans*

M. fermentans is found in oropharynx and gut. Recenty few strains discoved from AIDS patient known as **'AIDS Associated Mycoplasma'**.

Laboratory Diagnosis

1. Isolation of Mycoplasma

Specimens: Throat swabs and respiratory secretions are collected for diagnosis.

* Isolation is done into **Mycoplasma medium** containing glucose and phenol red. The color change indicates growth.
* Growth on solid medium: It is identified by hemolysis; colonies adsorb RBCs of guinea pigs.

2. Serological Methods

a. *Specific tests for antibody detection are*:
  * Immunofluorescence
  * Metabolic inhibition
  * Complement fixation
  * Indirect hemagglutination
  * RIP
  * Western blot

b. *Nonspecific tests*: The heterophile tests used for the diagnosis are:
  * *Streptococcus MG test*: Serial dilutions of patients' serum are mixed with heat killed suspension of *Streptococcus MG,* incubated at 37°C overnight and looked for clumping, titer **1:20** is significant.
  * *Cold agglutination test*: Titer of **1:32** or more is suggestive. The test is based on the principle that antibodies produced in *Mycoplasma* react with human **'O' antigens** at low temperature.

3. Molecular Methods

DNA probe, PCR.

Treatment

Tetracyline and erythromycin are drugs of choice.

UREAPLASMA UREALYTICUM

It is isolated from urogenital tract. It hydrolyses urea. Genital infections are caused by *M. hominis* and *U. urealyticum*. They are transmitted by sexual contact and may cause urethritis, balanoposthitis, Reiter's syndrome in men and salpingitis, PID, cervicitis, vaginitis, infertility, abortion, postpartum fever in women.

Treatment

Teracycline and erythromycin are used for treatment. Also newer macrolides and quinolones are effective.

TABLE 47.1: Mycoplasma and L forms of bacteria	
L forms	*Mycoplasma*
Resemble parent bacillius antigenically	Stable form
DNA homology with parent cell	
Don't initiate the disease	Initiate the disease
Absence of sterols	Sterols are present

48

Helicobacter Pylori

Morphology

Gram-negative spiral bacteria, motile by lophotrichous flagella.

Size: $3\mu \times 0.5$–0.9μ.

Cultural Characteristics

It is microaerophilic. Media used for cultivation are chocolate agar, Skirrow's medium, Butzler's medium, CampyBAP medium.

- It grows in an atmosphere of 5% O_2, 10% CO_2 and 85% N_2.
- High humidity and 5–10% CO_2 are required for the growth.
- The optimum temperature for growth is 37°C.
- It produces circular, convex and translucent colonies.

Biochemical Reactions

It is inactive in most of the tests but produces urease, catalase and oxidase. Urease produced by it is 100 times more powerful than that produced by *Pr. vulgaris.* It gives Cristensen's urease test positive in a few minutes.

H. pylori is resistant to nalidixic acid and sensitive to cephalothin. This property is used in identification of *Helicobacter sp.*

Virulence Factors

- *Protease*: It is very powerful, almost **100 times more powerful than *Proteus*** which is vital for its survival in stomach. Amidase and arginase contribute in production of ammonia.

  Ure-1 protein regulates passage of urea across cell membrane.

Adhesions: Majority of bacteria remain within mucus but some of them may adhere to mucosal surfaces with lipoprotein or blood group antigen binding proteins.

- *Cag PaI genes*: Cytotoxin is associated with gene, encodes a secretion system through which a specific protein Cag A, is translocated into epithelial cells. This interferes with host cells signaling, causing proliferation and cytoskeletal changes, produces a proinflammatory cytokine response. **It is highly immunogenic and patients with peptic ulcer disease or gastric adenocarcinoma have antibodies to CagA.**
- *Vac A*: Vacuolating cytotoxin is common in peptic disease. It induces formation of vacuoles in the cytoplasm of epithelial cells.
- *Bab A*: An adhesin and is associated with increased gastric inflammation.

Pathogenicity (Flowchart 48.1)

Organism is acquired in childhood, human transmission is through feco-oral route, and source of infection is human gastric mucus.

Most infected persons do not develop disease, it is noninvasive, the organism lives in gastric mucus. Gastric antrum is the commonest site of infection. More than 80% of duodenal ulcers and more than 60% of gastric ulcers are related with *H. pylori* infection.

Antral colonization causes depletion of stomatin producing 'D' cells which cause decreased production of stomatostatin. This leads to loss of inhibition of gastric release which causes hypergastrinemia.

Lesion: It is associated with duodenal ulcers, B cell lymphoma, and atrophic gastritis.

Other: Pernicious anemia, autoimmune gastritis, iron deficiency (role of *H. pylori* in these conditions is uncertain).

Flowchart 48.1: Pathogenesis of *H. pylori*

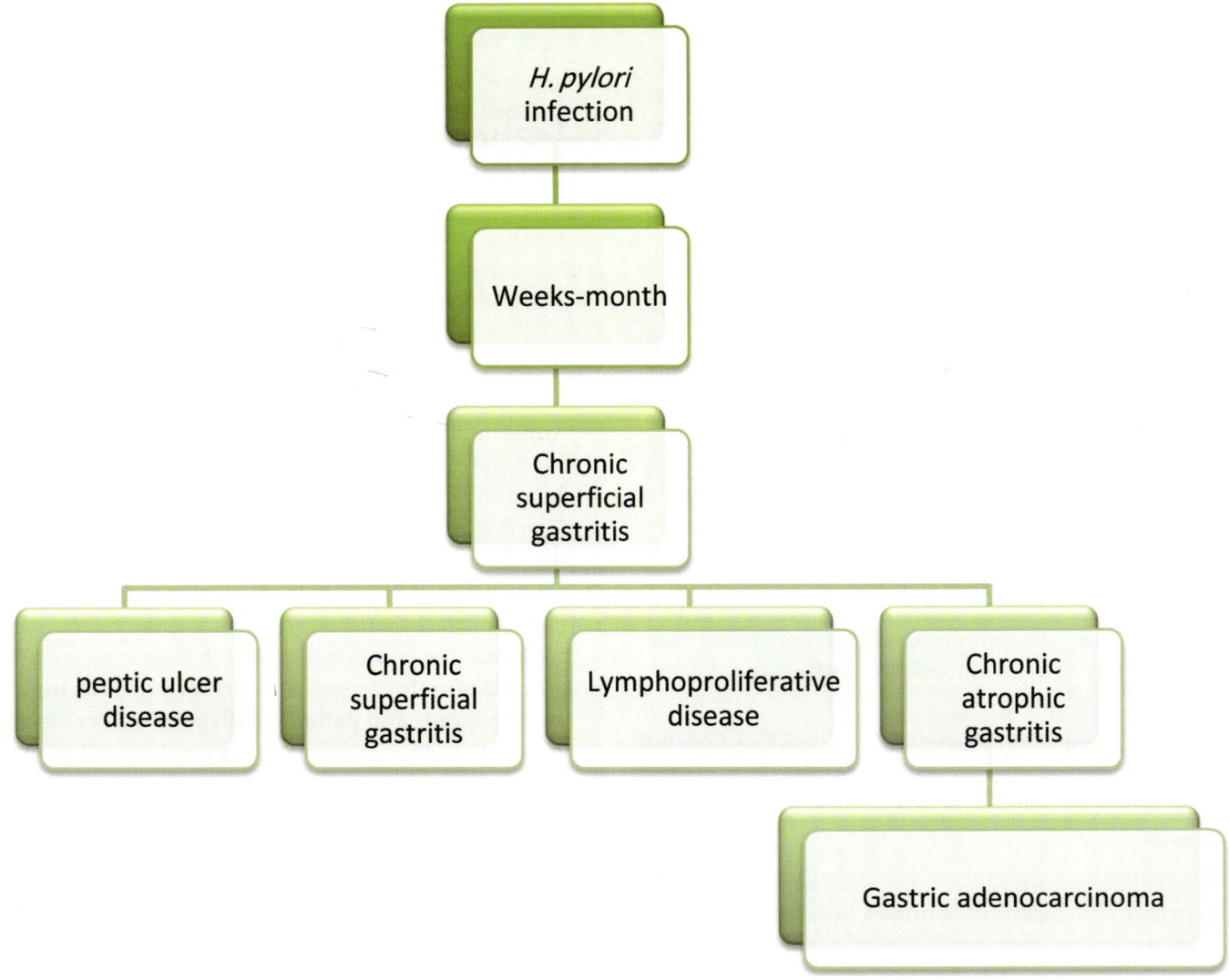

Laboratory Diagnosis (Flowchart 48.2)

Invasive Tests

- Endoscopic biopsy gives **rapid urease** test positive.
- The biopsy material is placed in urea broth with indicator and incubated at 37°C. If tissue contains *H. pylori*, change of pH occurs within few minutes to 2 hours due to ammonia production.
- Histopathology section stained with Giemsa stain or silver stain shows spiral bacilli.
- Culture is most specific but less sensitive.

Noninvasive Tests

- **C13 or C14 urea breath test**. It is most accurate test, useful for prognosis also. In chronic infections, it remains positive.

- Urea labeled isotope of carbon (C_{13} or C_{14}) is given orally to the patient. If patient's stomach has *H. pylori*, urea is converted into ammonia and CO_2. The lebeled CO_2 appears in breath which can be measured.
- **Stool antigen test**: This test is less accurate.
- Detection of antibody by ELISA or Immunoblot is less useful.
- PCR is highly sensitive.

Treatment

A combination of bismuth subsalicylate, tetracycline (or amoxycillin) and metronidazole are given for two weeks. Another alternative is omeprazole and clarithromycin.

Flowchart 48.2: Tests for diagnosis of *H. pylori*

Noninvasive tests

Serology: ELISA or IA are used to screen patients with dyspepsia

They are less helful for screening children and unreliable to exclude infection in elderly patients

Urea breath test: It detects bacterial urease activity in stomach by measuring output of CO_2 resulting from spliting of C13 or C14 labelled isotope into CO_2 and ammonia

It is highly sensitive and specific test.

The test cannot be used during or after antibiotics.

Fecal antigen test

Tests using monoclonal antibodies are more accurate

Polymerase chain reaction

It is helpful for detection of *H. pylori* in gastric juice, feces, water supplies, dental plaque

Invasive tests

Sample collection

Endoscopic mucosal biopsy from gastric antrum within 5 cm of pylorus, and also from body of stomach (patient should not have received antibiotic 1 month prior)

Biopsy—urease test

It is simple, bedside procedure, biopsy is kept in urea broth with phenol red as indicator, formation of amonia give alkalnity and color change in 2–72 hours

Histopathology and culture

It helps to grade biopsy. Bacteria are seen smear-stained with Giemsa

Fluorescent based molecular probes are able to detect bacteria and virulence factors

Culture is useful for testing antibiotic sensitvity and for typing of bacteria

49

Yersinia

HISTORY

- Alexandre Yersin discovered plague bacillus.
- The genus name Francisella was given after Franscis for his studies on tularemia.

Gram-negative bacilli, primary pathogens of rodents are grouped in Pasteurella. There are three genera:

a. Yesinia—*Y. pestis* causes plague, *Y. enterocolitica* causes enteric and systemic disease, *Y. pseudotuberculosis* is a rodent pathogen.

b. *Pasteurella multocida* causes hemorrhagic septicemia.

c. *Francisella tularensis* causes tularemia.

The organism belongs to family Enterobacteriaceae.

YERSINIA PESTIS

Morphology

- Short, plump, ovoid Gram-negative bacteria, 1.5 µm × 0.7 µm.
- **Bipolar staining (safty pin appearance)** is seen on Giemsa or methylene blue staining (Fig. 49.1).

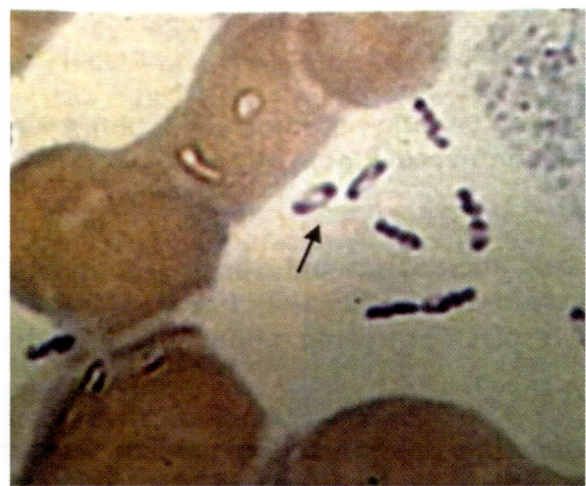

Fig. 49.1: Smear showing bipolar staining (*Y. pestis*)

- **Wayson's stain** is special stain used for *Y. pestis*. (Bipolar staining is done to condensation of protoplasm at two ends of bacilli.)
- Smear prepared from NA with 3% NaCl shows pleomorphism. Various forms as cocci-like, ghosts, 'club shaped', yeast-like cells, elongated bacillia are seen.
- Involution forms may be seen.
- Bacterium is surrounded by slime layer.
- It is non-motile, non-sporing.
- **Direct immunofluorescence** is used to demonstrate bacteria in specimens.

Cultural Characteristics

- Aerobic and facultative anaerobic.
- It grows over wide range of pH (5–9.6) and optimum temperature is 27°C (range 2–45°C) (envelope develops at 37°C).
- It grows on ordinary media, on nutrient agar, small delicate transparent disc-like colonies are formed.
- **Dark brown** colonies produced on blood agar due to absorption of hemin pigment (Fig. 49.2). Bacteria store hemin pigment in outer membrane.
- **NLF** colonies are produced on MacConkey agar. Like other *Yersinia*, it grows on this medium but colonies disappear due to autolysis.
- **CIN agar** (cefsulodin, irgasan, novobiocin) is a selective medium. Typical dark red 'bull's eye' appearing colonies are produced in 24 hours.
- **Stalactite growth** is seen in ghee broth (Fig. 49.3): If a drop of oil is allowed to float on the surface of inoculated medium in a flask, characteristic growth develops, consisting stalactites hanging down from oil drop.

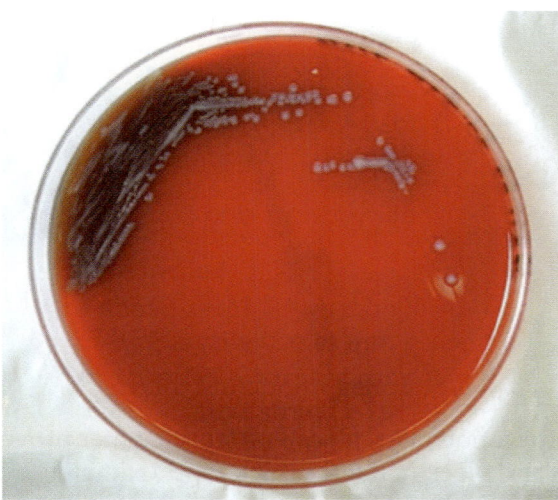

Fig. 49.2: BA with growth of *Y. pestis*

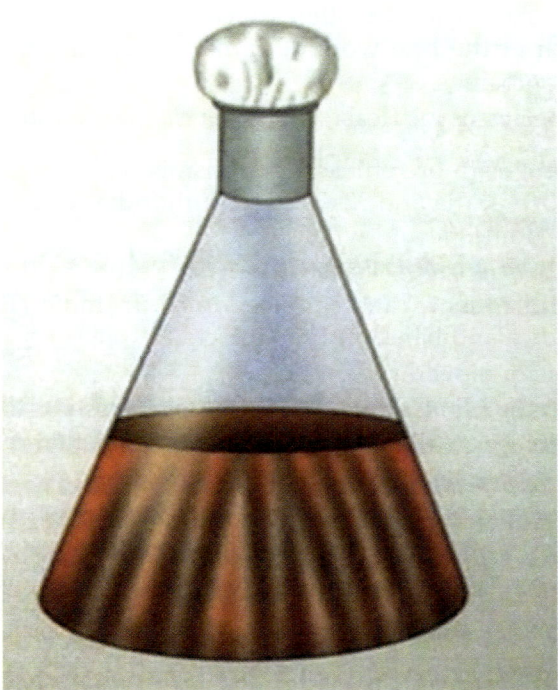

Fig. 49.3: Stalactite growth of *Yesinia pestis* in ghee broth

TABLE 49.1: Virulence factors of plague bacillus

Virulence factor	Mechanism of action
V-W antigen	Yield requirement of Ca for growth at 37°C
Plasmid Ppcp-1	Codes for plasminogen activating protease that has temperature dependent coagulase activity. It causes dissemination of organisms from flea bite
Capsular protein	Antiphagocytic
Phospholipidase-D	It is responsible for survival of organisms in gut of rat flea

TABLE 49.2: Biotypes of *Yersinia pestis*

Varity	Glycerol fermentation	Nitrate reduction
Y. pestis var orientalis	—	+
Y. pestis var antiqua	+	+
Y. pestis var medievalis	+	—

Biochemical Reactions of *Y. pestis*

- It ferments glucose, maltose, and mannitol.
- Indole positive, MR positive, VP negative, citrate negative.
- Oxidase negative, urease negative, catalase positive.
- It is classified into three physiological varieties based on glycerol fermentation and nitrate reduction.

Resistance

The organisms are easily destroyed by disinfectants. It can survive longer in deep burrows.

Antigens, Toxins and Virulence Factors (Table 49.1)

- **HL** protein envelope antigen (Fraction I) inhibits phagocytosis. It is encoded by plasmid. It is best formed, if cultures are incubated at 37°C.
- 'V 'and 'W' antigens are coded by plasmid, inhibit phagocytosis and intracellular killing of organisms.
- Bacteriocin, coagulase, fibrinolysins are produced by virulent strain.
- *Toxins*:
  - *Protein toxin*: It is murine toxin, its role in human infection is not known.
  - *Endotoxin*: It is lipopolysaccharide similar to other Gram-negative bacilli.
- Surface component absorbs hemin and basic aromatic dyes.
- Virulence is associated with ability for purine synthesis.

PLAGUE (Fig. 49.4)

Incubation period is 2–5 days.

1. *Bubonic* (Bubo means enlarged lymph node in grain): It is transmitted by bite of rat flea (Fig. 49.5), commonly inguinal lymph node is involved. Organisms enter bloodstream, cause septicemia, hemorrhages in skin, mucosa leading to disseminated intravascular coagulation (DIC) and gangrene of skin, penis, and fingers. Fatality: 30–90%.
2. *Pneumonic*: It spreads by droplet infection, hemorrhagic pneumonia occurs which leads to bloody mucoid sputum and cyanosis. This is highly infectious.

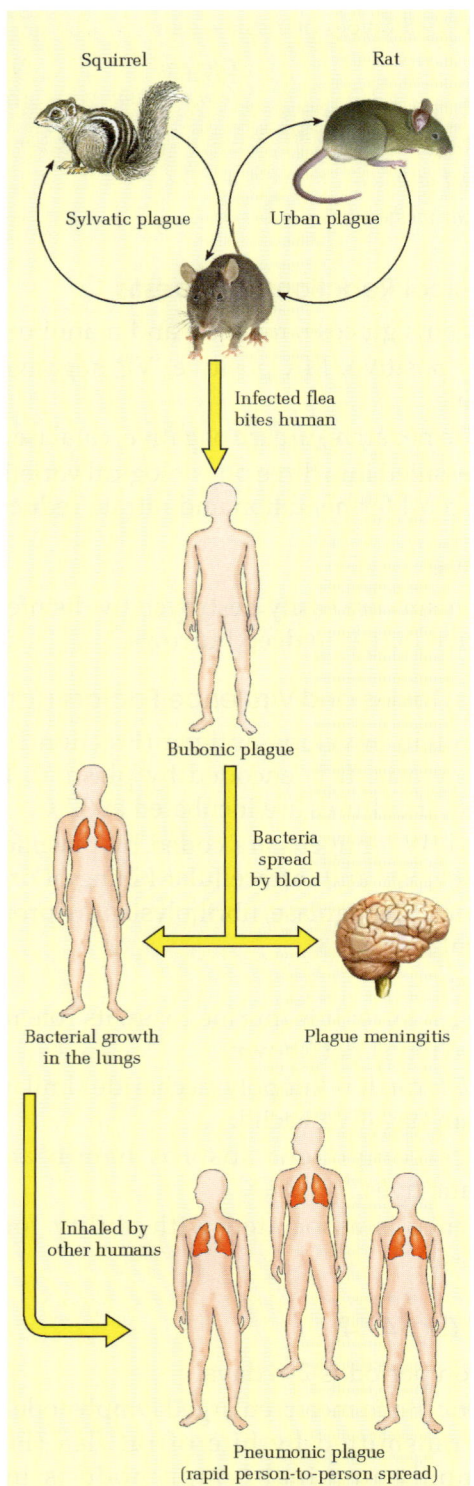

Fig. 49.4: Modes of infection of plague

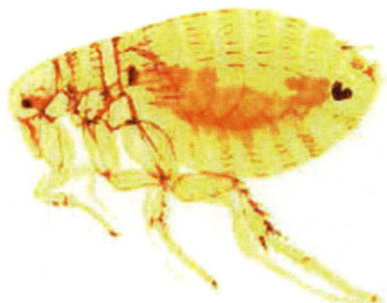

Fig. 49.5: Rat fleas

Cycle in Rat Flea

Multiplication takes place in stomach, enter proventriculus and block it. Rat flea sucks approximately 0.5 mL of blood (5000–50,000) bacillia which are enough to infect flea. The extrinsic incubation period is the time from entry of bacilli till blocking the proventriculus.

Blocked flea bites other rodents, but it regurgitates bacilli at the bite wound. It may leave rat and bite human beings.

Species of rat fleas: *Xenopsylla cheopis, X. astia.*

X. cheopsis (more efficient in transmission) is common in North India and *X. astia* in South India. Two cycles exist, domestic and wild.

1. *Sylvatic (wild) cycle of plague*: Reservoir (foci) is **wild** rodent (rabbits, mice, dogs). In India, Tatera indica and bandicoot are infected.
   Vector is wild rodent flea.
2. *Urban (domestic) cycle of plague*: Reservoirs are domestic (urban) black rat. Vector is oriental rat flea (*Xenopsylla cheopis*).
3. *Human cycle of plague*: Bubonic plague is acquired from contact with either sylvatic or urban reservoirs or arthropod vector bite and further transmitted in human population by spread of pneumonic plague.

Bubonic plague presents with swollen and painful **axillary** (arm pit) and **inguinal** (groin) lymphadenopathy **(bubos)**.

Transmitted from **mammalian reservoirs by flea (arthropod) bite** or contact with contaminated animal tissues.

Plague epidemics usually occur in cool, humid seasons which favour multiplication of fleas. '**Flea index'** is mean number of fleas per rat.

Epidemiology

Cases of human plague have been known from time immemorial. Although it is difficult on the basis of the information that has survived from the distant past to distinguish plague from other acute communicable diseases, from what is known plague is an ancient

3. *Septicemic plague*: It is terminal event in bubonic or pneumonic plague.

Massive involvement of blood vessels takes place. There may be hemorrhages in skin and mucosa (hence called '**black death'**).

disease which originated in the cradle of human civilization in Central Asia. The first plague epidemic on record was the outbreak among the Philistines in 1320 BC, described in the Bible (I Samuel, V and VI) as characterized by the appearance of "emerods in their secret parts".

In the last two millennia, plague has become widespread, affecting a large number of countries on most continents during several pandemics. The first certain pandemic, known as Justinian's plague, was recorded in the sixth century AD. Between 542 and 546 AD epidemics in Asia, Africa and Europe claimed nearly 10,000000 victims. The second plague pandemic is the well known "Black Death" of the fourteenth century (1347–1350). It was the cause of some 50,000000 deaths, half of them in Asia and Africa and the other half in Europe, where a quarter of the population succumbed. This pandemic was the beginning of a number of outbreaks of plague which ravaged Europe and Africa in subsequent centuries. The third pandemic began in Canton and Hong Kong in 1894 and spread rapidly throughout the world, carried by rats aboard the swifter steamships that replaced slow-moving sailing vessels in merchant fleets. Within 10 years (1894-1903), plague entered 77 ports on five continents: Asia, Europe, Africa, North America, South America and Australia. Plague spread widely in India where it caused nearly 13000000 deaths and claimed many victims in a number of other countries. Early in the pandemic, important discoveries enabled plague prevention and control to be placed on a scientific basis. In 1894, the causal agent was discovered. It was also established that rats contract plague and that the rat flea *Xenopsylla cheopis* is the common vector.

In India, large plague outbreaks occurred during the first half of the 20th century. The last laboratory confirmed human cases were reported in 1966 from Karnataka state. Since then, several suspected outbreaks have occurred, in the historic plague-endemic areas of south India and Himachal province in north India. In August-October 1994, human plague was reported in India for the first time in 30 years. During this outbreak, 876 cases 54 of which were fatal characterized as presumptive plague. Most cases (596) were reported from Maharashtra state: 151, in Gujarat state, 68 in Delhi, 50 cases in Karnataka, 10 in Uttar Pradesh, and 12 cases in Madhya Pradesh. Fifty-two of the 54 fatal cases occurred in Gujarat, 1 in Delhi and 1 in Karnataka. Although the exact circumstances are unknown, factors contributing to the re-emergence of plague in India have been identified by the National Technical Advisory Committee on Plague constituted by the Government of India. Beed district (Maharashtra State) has had sylvatic plague in the past. Ecological changes created by the earthquake in September 1993 disturbed the equilibrium density of domestic rodents (*R. rattus*) and

their fleas (*X. cheopis*), generating large energy supplies for domestic rodents in the form of stored food grains, this resulted in a gradual growth of *R. rattus* population in the subsequent 10-month period. On 5 August 1994 in Mamla village in the Beed district, rat-fall was reported, followed by reports of flea nuisance. Three weeks later, suspected cases of bubonic plague were notified, followed by reports from other villages in Beed and other districts. The resurgence of plague in Surat, Gujarat state, was related to a record high rainfall during the September monsoon. While cleaning up local residents have become infected after contact with dead animals. Shortly after the flood the Ganapati festival brought huge crowds of people together in the city which would facilitate the spread of acute respiratory illness.

In 2002, plague was reported from Simla.

Diagnosis of Plague in Humans

Specimens: Bubo aspirate, sputum, blood culture, impression from spleen are the specimens collected.

Microscopy

- Bipolar staining with safety pin appearance is seen.
- Wayson's stain is special stain used.
- Direct immunofluorescnce detects F1 antigen in specimens.

Culture

- *BA*: Brown colonies are produced due to hemadsorption.
- *MacConkey's medium*: Pale nonlactose fermenting colonies are seen.
- *Ghee broth*: Stalactite growth is seen.

Suspected case: Compatible clinical presentation; and consistent epidemiological features: exposure to infected animals or humans, and/or evidences of flea bites, and/or residence in or travel to a known endemic focus within the previous 10 days.

Presumptive case: Definition of suspected case plus: Putative new or re-emerging focus: at least two of the following tests positive:
- *Microscopy*: Material from bubo, blood or sputum contains Gram-negative coccobacilli, bipolar after Wayson or Giemsa staining;
- F1 antigen detected in bubo aspirate, blood or sputum;
- A single anti-F1 serology without evidence of previous *Y. pestis* infection or immunization; and
- PCR detection of *Y. pestis* in bubo aspirate, blood or sputum.

Confirmed case: Strain isolation from a clinical sample identified as *Y. pestis* by phage lysis of cultures at 20–25°C and 37°C or a fourfold rise in the anti-F1 antibody titer in paired serum samples.

In pneumonic plague, sputum is collected.

In septicemic plague, blood culture is done.

Serological tests
- Antibody to **F1** antigen detected by IgG and IgM **ELISA.**
- Antibodies to F1 antigen are also detected by **passive hemagglutination or CFT.**

PCR: It is rapid and sensitive method for diagnosis of plague in clinical specimens and flea.

Diagnosis of Plague in Rats
- Smears from bubo from carcasses of dead rats stained with Gram's stain, Giemsa stain which shows Gram-negative bacilli with bipolar staining.
- Fluorescent antibody technique is used for direct detection of antigen.
- Bacilli demonstrated in spleen smears, heart blood and bone marrow.
- In badly putrefied carcasses, demonstrations of 'F1' antigen is done by direct immunofluorescence (titer 1:128).

Prophylaxis of Plague
- Control of fleas and rodents.
- Killed vaccine (whole culture antigen): It has 2 doses, given subcutaneously at 1–3 months interval. Booster is given after 6 months. Vaccine is effective against bubonic but not pneumonic plague. It gives protection for less than 6 months. This vaccine is prepared in Haffkine Institute, Mumbai.
- Live-attenuated vaccine based on strain EV76 has side effects but still used in Soviet Union.
- Chemoprophylaxis of exposed persons: Tetracycline orally for at least 5 days are given. Other alternative is cotrimoxazole.
- Other tests are IgG, IgM ELISA and rapid dipstick assays using F1 antigen.

Treatment
Streptomycin is the drug of choice for bubonic and septicemic plague. Early treatment is necessary to reduce mortality. Combinations of streptomycin with tetracycline is also effective.

YERSINIA PSEUDOTUBERCULOSIS
- It is Gram-negative bacillus with bipolar staining.
- It is motile at 22°C (non-motile at 37°C), non-capsulated.
- On blood agar, it forms non-hemolytic colonies.
- On MacConkey's medium, it grows poorly.
- It ferments rhamnose, melibiose, it is urease positive, indole negative.
- On basis of somatic and flagellar antigens, it is divided into 6 serogroups and 9 serotypes. Most of the infections are caused by serotype 1.
- Infection in animals takes place by alimentary route.
- It produces multiple nodules in lungs, liver, spleen in animals.
- Man is infected by ingestion of contaminated food. It rarely presents as typhoid-like illness. Autoimmune condition is due to deposition of immune complexes in joint and other site occurs. Few strains of *Y. pseudotuberculosis* express super antigen, which cause autoscarlet type of fever in Russia, similarly in Japan which has been linked pathogenesis of idiopathic acute systemic vasculitis in childhood known as '**Kawasaki disease**'.
- Diagnosis is done by microscopy and culture. Antibodies are detected by tube agglutination test.

YERSINIA ENTEROCOLITICA

Morphology
It is small Gram-negative rod, motile at 22°C. It grows at wide range of temperatures (up to 44°C), aerobically and anaerobically.

On blood agar, it produces small translucent colonies and on MacConkey's medium it forms pinpoint non-lactose fermenting colonies. **Schiemann CIN medium** is used as a selective medium.

It is Indole and VP positive. It is reactive at 28 rather than 37°C. It differs from pseudotuberculosis in its

TABLE 49.3: Differences between Yersinia and Pasteurella

	Y. pestis	*Y. pseudotuberculosis*	*Y. enterocolitica*	*P. multocida*
Motility at 22°C	—	+	+	—
Growth on MacConkey medium	+	+	+	—
Acid from sucrose	+	—	+	+
Acid from maltose	—	+	+	—
Indole	+	—	+	+
Oxidase	—	+	—	+
Urease	—	+	+	—
Ornithine decarboxylase	—	—	+	+

ability to ferment sucrose, sorbitol, cellibiose but not salicin. Ornithine decarboxylase test is positive.

Antigenicity: More than 60 'O' and more 20 'H' antigens are identified; most of human infections are due to O3, O8, and O9.

It withstands freezing and survives in dampsoil, pasteurization destroys them, somewhat resistant to chlorine. It is susceptible to sulphadiazine, streptomycin, tetracycline and chloramphenicol, but not penicillin.

Diagnosis is based on culture of blood, lymph node or tissues. Antibodies are detected by aggultination and ELISA. PCR is sensitive method.

Virulence Factors for *Y. enterocolitica*

Invasion protein (Inv) helps in adhesion to M cells of gastric mucosa.

- Yersinia adhesion—'A' binds to extracellular proteins as collagen and fibronectin, thus contributing to the pathogenicity.
- *Y. pseudotuberculosis* produces super antigen which binds to T cells in a non-specific manner leading to cytokine release.
- Post-infective phenomenon—reactive arthritis— especially patients with HLA-B27 are prone for this condition.
- Erythema nodosum.
- Graves' disease

Y. enterocolitica contains an antigen similar to thyroid stimulating binding site but its pathogenic role in Graves' disease is not established.

Toxin Production

Pathogenic serotypes produce heat-stable enterotoxin, but toxin is not produced above temperature 30°C, hence it is unlikely that it is associated with the disease. However, toxin may be produced by organisms present in contaminated food kept at room temperature. This may be responsible for occurrence of few cases in which no organism is isolated.

Pathogenesis

It adheres and penetrates terminal ileum, invades intestinal mucosa, multiplies in lymphoid tissue. Incubation period is 7 days.

Infective dose is unknown. Children more than 4 years and adults 20–34 years are susceptible for infection.

Sources

The bacteria have been isolated from various animals. Human infection occurs probably by ingestion or contact. Family and short outbreaks suggest that person to person transmission occurs.

Clinical Lesions

- *Enterocolitis*: Abdominal pain (confused with appendicitis), headache, fever, diarrhea, nausea, vomiting (children—watery, mucoid diarrhea) are clinical features.
- Inflammatory terminal ileitis is seen in children.
- People with HLA-B27 are more susceptible for infection.
- Transfusion-related septicemia
- Mesenteric lymphadenitis
- Erythema nodosum, polyarthritis, Reiter's syndrome, bacteremia and meningitis.

Diagnosis is made by culture. Incubation of tubes of broth is done at 37°C and 22°C for demonstration of motility at 22°C.

PASTEURELLA MULTOCIDA

It is Gram-negative bacillus, non-motile, indole and oxidase positive. Human infection may occur by animal bite or trauma. Different strains from different animals cause septicemia in animals.

P. aviseptica is chicken cholera bacillus used by Pasteur for development of first attenuated bacterial vaccine. Human infection may occur in the form of wound infection, cellulitis, abscess. Human infections can be treated with penicillin, and tetracycline.

GENUS FRANCISELLA

F. tularensis

It is Gram-negative bacillus, non-motile, capsulated and size is approximately 0.3–0.7 × .02 µ.

It may show bipolar staining; stains best with diluted carbol fuschin. Smears from postmortem material may require gentle heating for the penetration of the stains. It may be pleomorphic with bacillary or filamentous forms in cultures.

Growth Characteristics

It is strictly aerobic bacillus. Fresh isolates are fastidious. It grows well in blood agar containing 2.5% glucose, 0.1% cysteine. Optimum temperature is 37°C. Minute droplet-like colonies develop in 72 hours. Casein hydrolysate is used as liquid medium.

Biochemical Tests

It forms acid from glucose and maltose. Indole and urease are negative.

Modes of Infections

- Handling of infected animals and organisms may enter through minor cuts in skin or mucosa
- Animal bites
- Bite of blood sucking insects
- Ingestion of contaminated food and water
- Inhalation of aerosols

The disease is called **'rabbit fever'** as it is common in rabbits handless. But, it may occur while handling other animals.

Laboratory Diagnosis

It is done by isolating and identifying the bacteria from clinical material obtained from local lesions. As this organism is biohazardours, processing of specimens and cultures are carried out in biosafety cabinets.

- Glucose-glycine cysteine blood agar is used for culture which is incubated for 7 days.
- Identification can be done by direct immuno-fluorescence.

Antibodies detection is done by tube agglutination test, CFT, Coomb's test, ELISA and latex agglutination.

Treatment

Streptomycin and gentamicin are antibiotics of choice. Tetracycline is used for chemoprophylaxis.

TULAREMIA

The genus name is given in honor of Francis who extensively studied the disease. The disease originally described from Tulare country, California. Infection may be transmitted by direct contact with rodents or through tick bites. It can also be transmitted by ingestion of contaminated water or meat or by inhalation of aerosols.

Oropharyngeal Tularemia

Membranous pharyngitis with cervical lymphadenopathy in Norvey may be caused by consumption of water (with animal's excreta of lemmings). Hence, it is also known as **'Lemming' fever.**

50

Other Bacteria

LEGIONELLA PNEUMOPHILA

The name Legionaire's disease is given to illness which occurred in members of American Legion who attended a convention in Philadelphia in 1976. All the members suffered from hemorrhagic pneumonitis, fever, cough, chest pain. The causative agent is then called as *Legionella pneumophila.* Aerosols of water from building's air conditional system was the source of outbreak.

Morphology

- It is thin, non-capsulated, Gram-negative bacillus of size 2–5 μ × 0.1–0.3 μ.
- It is motile with polar or subpolar flagellum.
- It is stained better by silver impregnation methods. Immunoperoxidase and immunofluorescence.

Cultural Characteristics

- It is fastidious, requires complex media, **BCYE** (buffered charcoal yeast extract) agar with L-cysteine and antibiotics.
- It grows under 5% CO_2, temperature 35°C, and pH 6.9.
- Colonies grow in 3–6 days.
- Colonies are 1–2 mm in diameter, circular, grey, low convex with irregular edge. When colonies are examined under microsope, "cut glass" apperance is seen.

Biochemical Reactions

It is catalase positive, oxidase is variable. It hydrolyses hippurate, starch and gelatin.

Sensitivity

It is killed by 1% formalin, 2% gluteraldehyde, 70% ethyl alcohol and chlorine (5 ppm) in one minute.

Serogrouping: It is divided into more than 14 serogroups.

Epidemiology

Bacteria are widely distributed in natural water sources. They grow inside free-living amebae and protozoa, and in man-made aquatic environments. Infection takes place by inhalation of aerosols, air condtions and shower heads. The risk factors are smoking, alcohol, advanced age, illness, hospitalization, and immunodeficiency.

Pathogenesis of Legionella

Through aerosols, bacteria enter in the alveoli and multiply in macrophages and monocytes. Hematogenous, lymphatic or contiguous spread occurs. Cellular immunity is responsible for recovery. The **serogroup-1(SG-1)** causes most human infections, while **serogroup 6 causes hospital-acquired infections.** A virulence factor 'M' associated protein **(Mip protein)** is important which prevents fusion of phagosome with lysosome evading defence of phagocytic cells.

Legionnaires' Disease

It presents as fever, dry cough, dyspnea, chest pain, diarrhea and encephalopathy, if untreated.

Legionnaires' disease is an interstitial pneumonia. Incubation period is 2–10 days.

- Extrapulmonary complications result from spread of bacteria from lung through blood which may result in myocarditis, pericarditis, prosthetic valve endocarditis, peritonitis and pyelonephritis.
- Other infections include sinusitis and soft tissue infections

Pontiac Fever

Milder, "influenza-like" illness; fever, chills, myalgia, headache are the symptoms.

Laboratory Diagnosis of Legionella

- Samples collected are sputum, bronchial aspirate, lung biopsy, serum for antibody detection.
- *Microscopy*: Direct fluorescent antibody test is sensitive method.
- *Culture*: BCYE (buffered charcol yeast extract) agar medium is used for cultivation and growth detected by immunofluorescence staining.
- **MALDI-TOF** is used for rapid identification.
- Antigen detection in urine is done by **latex agglutination or ELISA.**
- Antibody detection in serum is done by ELISA, indirect immunofluorescence.

Treatment

Macrolides, ciprofloxacin, tetracycline, azithromycin and quinolones are the drugs of choice.

Prevention

Legionellae from water can be irradicated by chlorination of water (5 ppm of chlorine in one minute) or by heating (60°C).

BORRELIA BURGDORFERI

- It causes Lyme's disease (Flowchart 50.1)—first observed in Lyme, Connecticut, USA.
- It is transmitted by bite (regurgitation of gut contents) of Ixodid ticks; natural hosts are rodents, deer, other mammals.
- *Groups*: B. burgdorferi, B. garinii and B. afzelii.

Morphology

It is a spiral organism, 20–30 μ long and 0.2–0.3 μ wide, radially stained by silver impregnation method.

Clinical Features

Incubation period is 3–30 days.
- **Localized infection** presents as expanding annular skin lesion (**erythema migrans**).
- **Disseminated infection** presents with fever, myalgia, arthralgia, and lymphadenopathy and there may be meningeal or cardiac involvement.
- **Persistent infection** occurs after months or years. Chronic arthritis, neuropathy, encephalopathy, acrodermatitis, 3rd degree heart block are the complications.

Neurological abnormalities are observed in a small percentage of patients in the form of meningitis, encephalitis and lymphocytic meningoradiculitis (cases from Asia, and Asia). The syndrome is known as **Bannwarth's syndrome.**

Laboratory Diagnosis

- Isolation is done from skin lesions, CSF, blood or from ticks.
- Media used are **modified Kelly's (BSK) medium**; culture will be positive after 2 weeks or more.
- Serology: Immunofluorescence is used for screening,
- Immunoblotting is used for confirmation.
- False positive FTA-ABS results may be seen.

Treatment

Tetracycline, penicillin, newer macrolides, cephalosporine are used for treatment. For skin lesion, joints and 1st, 2nd degree heart block, doxycline is the drug of choice, followed by ampicillin, cefuroxime. For CNS infections, ceftriaxone is used.

LISTERIA MONOCYTOGENES

- It is a Gram-positive bacillus (coccoid).
- It is motile by peritrichous flagella, showing **tumbling motility**, it is **motile when grown at 27°C** while non-motile when grown at 37°C.
- It is aerobic or microaerophilic, grows better in presence of 5–10% CO_2.
- On blood agar, beta hemolysis is produced.
- It ferments glucose and salicin, catalase is positive. Oxidase, indole urease are negative, MR and VP positive.
- CAMP test (+ve).

Virulence Factors

- Internalin helps the bacterium to evade from phagocytic killing.
- Listerolysin causes disruption of phagolysosome membrane.
- Phospholipases help in cell to cell spread by dissolving cell membrane.
- Inoculation in rabbits causes marked monocytosis (hence the name monocytogenes). Monocytosis is also seen in human beings.
- Instillation of culture filtrate of the bacillus into the eyes of rabbits causes keratoconjunctivitis. This is called **Anton test.**

Pathogenicity (Table 50.1)

The organism is saprophytic in soil, water, sewage, plants. It acts as opportunistic pathogen in immunocompromised host. Gastrointestinal is mostly mode of infection in neonates and adults. Milk, raw vegetables, cheese, and unpasteurized milk act as vehicles of transmission. Other modes of infection are contact with infected animals; inhalation of contaminated dust. Infection in newborn may be due to transplacental

Flowchart 50.1: Pathogenesis of Lyme disease

```
                    Bite of Ixodes tick
                    infected with
                    B. burgdorferi
                    ┌──────────┴──────────┐
            Organisms                    Dissemination
            multiply in                  of organisms in
            skin                         blood
                │                              │
            Erythema                           │
            migrans                            │
                │                              │
            Secondary                    Meningitis
            annular skin                 Carditis
            lesions                      Musculoskeletal pain
                │                        Eye abnormalities
            Residual bacteria in
            protected places
            ┌──────┴──────┐
    Acrodermatitis      Intermittent
    chronica            or chronic
    atrophicans         arthritis
                            │
                    Chronic encephalopathy
                    Polyneuropathy
                    or leucoencephalopathy
                            │
                    Chronic cardiomyopathy
```

TABLE 50.1: Infections caused by *Listeria monocytogens*

Pregnancy associated	*Neonatal*		*Infections due immunosuppression*
Transplacental infections result in abortions Intrauterine growth retardation Premature labor Chorioretinitis	Early onset: Clinical features in 1st week of life—granulomatous infantisepticum disseminated disease in liver, spleen, adrenal glands, lungs, respiratory distress	Late onset: After 1st week of life— nosocomial infection— meningitis	Sepsis, meningitis Endocarditis Peritonitis Osteomyelitis Cholecystitis Visceral abscess Acute diarrheal disease

transmission. After entering in GIT, the bacterium multiplies in hepatic and splenic macrophages destroying them. Serotypes 1/2a, 1/2b and 4b are responsible for most of the infections.

Laboratory Diagnosis

Laboratory diagnosis is based on isolation of bacteria from various clinical specimens as cord blood, lochia, meconium, CSF, cervical and vaginal secretions. Isolation is increased by cold enrichment.

- *Cold enrichment*: Materials are stored in tryptose phosphate broth or thioglycolate broth at 4°C and subcultures are done weekly for 1–6 months.
- Rapid detection is possible by DNA probe, PCR and FISH.

Treatment

Ampicillin, penicillin, tetracycline, and erythromycin are effective against it.

ERYSIPELOTHRIX RHUSIOPATHIAE

- It is a slender Gram-positive bacillus, non-motile, non-sporing, tendency to form filaments.
- It is microaerophilic, grows on ordinary media, blood agar with rabbit blood is used for primary isolation. Black colonies are produced on BPT.
- It is a natural disease of animals. Human infection occurs on hands or fingers of those handling animals, fish or animal products. It is called 'seal finger or whale finger' disease.
- Lesions are red, edematous, with involvement of joints and lymph nodes.

Treatment

Penicillin, ampicillin (drug of choice) and erythromycin are useful against this bacterium.

ALCALIGENES FAECALIS

Gram-negative, non-sporing, strict aerobic, non-fermenter, motile by peritrichous flagella, oxidase positive. It is a saprophyte and may cause urinary infections, fever, infantile gastroenteritis and suppurative lesions.

CHROMOBACTERIUM VIOLACEUM

Gram-negative, motile bacillus which produces violet pigment. It is oxidase negative. It is saprophyte and may cause skin infection or multiple abscesses.

- Colonies have cyanide color due to production of hydrogen cyanide.
- Pigment may cause confusion in oxidase test, hence the test is performed on culture grown on anaerobic conditions so that pigment production is inhibited.

FLAVOBACTERIUM MENINGOSEPTICUM

Gram-negative, non-motile bacillus which produces yellow pigment. It is oxidase positive and causes outbreaks of neonatal meningitis.

KLEBSIELLA GRANULOMATIS (CALMATOBACTERIUM GRANULOMATIS, DONOVANIA GRANULOMATIS)

Donovan first described this bacterium in smear from ulcer. It is sexually transmitted disease. It causes ulcerative lesions in genital area. The beefy red ulcer formed in the disease bleeds easily on touching. Due to autoinoculation, **multiple ulcers occur**. This bacterium is stained better with Giemsa stain (Fig. 50.1). They are Gram-negative, coccobacilli (1–2 μ) or pleomorphic, capsulated bacilli which show **bipolar staining with safety pin appearance**. Egg yolk medium and Levinthal medium are used for its culture. It responds to tetracycline, gentamicin, and chloramphenicol.

RAT BITE FEVER

This condition is caused by two different bacilli, i.e. *Streptobacillus moniliformis* and *Spirillum minus*. **Fever, rash and arthralgia are the common signs and symptoms following rat bite.**

STREPTOBACILLUS MONILIFORMIS

Gram-negative, non-motile non-capsulated bacilli (5 × 0.1–0.5μ). Bacilli form chains which appear as filaments with club-shaped swellings (monniform) giving string of bead's appearance. Enriched media are used for cultivation. It grows well on Loffler's serum slope.

Catalase, oxidase, indole and urease tests are negative, ferment glucose.

Fever develops 2–10 days after exposure; other manifestations are headache, myalgia, petechial rash, and arthritis. The clinical presentation is also called as **erythema artriticum epidemic** or **Haverhill fever**. The

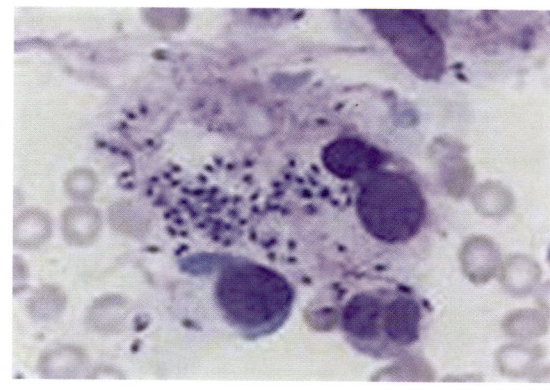

Fig. 50.1: Giemsa stain showing *K. granulomatis*

mode of infection is probably through consumption of bacilli in milk or water contaminated by rats.

Laboratory Diagnosis

It consists of isolation of bacteria from blood or other fluid or antibodies detection by CFT, indirect fluorescence and ELISA.

SPIRILLUM MINUS (Fig. 50.2)

(Carter was first to identify it from India in a rat. Japanese worker called it **sodoku**).

It is short, Gram-negative bacillus better stained with Giemsa staining or demonstrated by dark ground microscope. It is actively motile; size is 3–5 × 0.2–0.5 μ with 2–3 regular spirals. This bacterium cannot be cultivated. It has incubation period of 1–3 weeks, deaths may be due to endocarditis. Diagnosis consists of microscopic demonstration of bacilli in blood or exudate, or inoculation in experimental animal.

Treatment: The bacillus is sensitive to penicillin, tetracycline, and streptomycin.

GARDNERELLA VAGINALIS

It causes bacterial vaginosis. **Bacterial vaginosis** is characterized by:
- Increased vaginal pH >4.5.
- Foul smelling discharge (rotten fish with KOH).
- Presence of **clue cells**, which are vaginal epithelial cells studded with Gram-negative coccobacilli on their surface.
- Other anaerobes as *Mobilincus, peptostreptococci* are associated with *G. vaginalis.*
- **Nugent scoring** on Gram-stained smear from vaginal swab is done for microscopic diagnosis and it is based on presence or absence of bacteria morphologically resembling *Lactobacilli*, Gram-negative coccobacilli and presence of clue cells.

Amsel Criteria

Bacterial vaginosis is diagnosed, if any 3 or 4 findings are present:
1. Profuse thin, homogenous vaginal discharge uniformly seen over vaginal wall.
2. pH of vaginal discharge more than 4.5.
3. If few drops of 10% solution of KOH is added to vaginal discharge, intense fishy odor is produced **(Amide test).**
4. *Clue cells* (Fig. 50.3): These are vaginal epithelial cells studded with Gram-negative coccobacilli, which have granular appearance and indistinct borders. These cells can be observed in wet mount or in Gram-stained smear.
   - *Morphology*: Gram-negative pleomorphic rod. They are non-motile.
   - *Culture*: It is difficult to culture; sample is inoculated on blood agar or chocolate agar in anaerobic jar. Minute colonies appear after 48 hours of incubation.
   - Identification is done by smear, aerotolerance test.
   - Immunofluorescence is also used for demonstration of clue cell.
   - Presence of pili helps in adhesion to vaginal epithelial cells.
   - *Treatment*: Metronidazole is the drug of choice.

AEROMONAS AND PLESIOMONAS

These bacteria belong to the family Vibrionaceae and may cause diarrhea.

Both genera are Gram-negative, oxidase positive, motile (*darting motility*) with the help of **polar flagellum.** They are differentiated by **decarboxylase tests** and sensitivity to chemical substance O129 (available on disc) from vibrios.

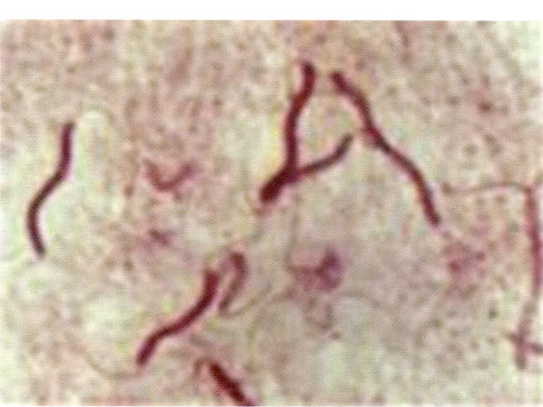

Fig. 50.2: Spirillum

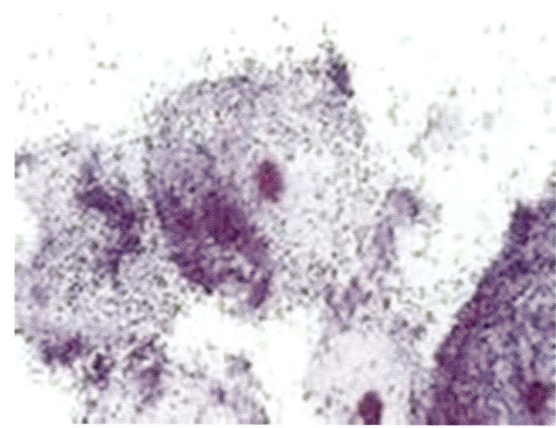

Fig. 50.3: Clue cell

AEROMONAS

The important species of aeromonas are isolated from human beings *A. hydophila, A. caviae,* and *A. veronii biovar sorbia.* All these are grouped in *A. hydrophila group.*

- These bacteria are associated with fresh water, salty water, may be found in meat and sea foods.
- Diseases caused by aeromonas are divided into two—**intestinal (diarrhea) and extraintestinal.**
- *Diarrhea:* Role of aeromonas is not firmly established but their presence has been associated with diarrhea.
- The **extraintestinal manifestations** are wound infections, bacteremia, osteomyelitis and pneumonia.
- *A. hydrophila* was isolated from frog with '**red leg disease**'.
- Aeromonas produces beta hemolysis on blood agar.
- **Ampicillin blood agar** is used as selective medium for aeromonas as it is resistant to ampicillin.
- *CIN agar:* Colonies with '**bull's eye' appearance** are produced. Colonies have red center surrounded by clear edge.

PLESIOMONAS SHIGELLOIDES

- This species **may agglutinate antisera** produced against **Shigella,** hence the name.
- They are found in water, soil, animals (shellfish, lizard, dog, and cat).
- The intestinal manifestation is diarrhea while extra-intestinal manifestations are bacteremia, wound infection and meningitis.

DIFFERENTIATION FROM VIBRIOS

- **String test** of *Vibrio cholera* lasts for 60 seconds while others may give weak reaction.
- Vibrio is **resistant to chemical-O-129** (disk is placed on plated medium) at both concentrations of O-129 (150 and 10 µg). Plesiomonas sensitive to both concentrations while Aeromonas is resistant to O-129.
- *Decarboxylase test*: Plesiomonas give all; arginine, lysine and ornithine decaroxylase tests positive. Aeromona gives arginine test positive.

CAPNOCYTOPHAGA

Gram-negative fusiform bacilli which form normal oral flora and may rarely cause systemic disease in patient with immunosuppression.

51

Introduction to Virology

Viruses are the smallest infectious particles that separate living from non-living organisms. Viruses can be crystallized like chemicals; infectious nucleic acid could infect host cells and yield complete progeny.

TABLE 51.1: Differences between viruses and other organisms

Viruses	Other unicellular microbes
No cellular organization	Present
DNA or RNA—never both	Contain both DNA and RNA
Obligate intracellular parasites, do not grow on cell free media	They can grow on cell free media
Reproduced by a complex process	Reproduced by binary fission
Rely on host synthetic machinery	Do not rely on host cells
They also lack enzymes necessary for their synthesis of proteins and nucleic acids	They have their own enzymes
Viruses can be crystallized like chemicals	Cannot be crystallized
Ribosomes are absent	Ribosomes are present

Properties of Viruses

- Viruses are the smallest infectious particles.
- There is no cellular organization.
- They have either DNA or RNA, never both.
- They are obligate intracellular parasites.
- Viruses rely on host synthetic machinery.
- They are dependent on host cells for energy.
- Viruses reproduce by a complex process.
- Viruses can be crystallized like chemicals, infectious nucleic acid.
- Viruses could infect host cells and yield complete progeny.
- They are too small to be seen under microscope, require electron microscope.
- They also lack enzymes necessary for their synthesis of proteins and nucleic acids.

- They are filterable through filters which hold bacteria.
- They do not respond to antibiotics.
- Their size is measured in nanometer.

Structure of Virus (Fig. 51.1)

- Central nucleic acid, either DNA or RNA is called core of virus.
- Core is surrounded by a protein covering or shell called **capsid**, the smallest unit of it is called capsomere. Core and capsid together form **nucleo-capsid.**
- *Functions of capsid*:
  - Protection of nucleic acid.
  - Adsorption to host cell surface thus helps in attachment, which starts infectious process of virus.
  - Transfer of nucleic acid from one host cell to another.
- Outermost covering is called **envelope** which is made up of glycoproteins. The proteins of envelope are virus-coded while lipids come from the cell membrane of infected host cell.

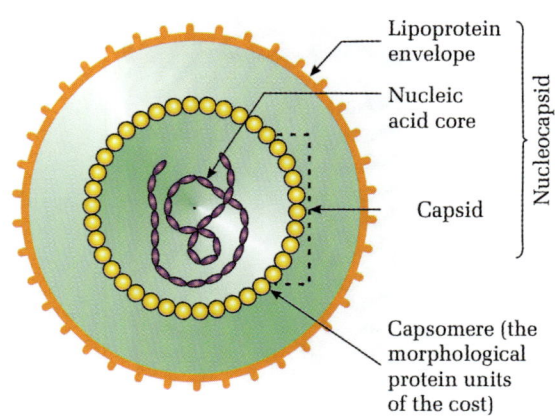

Fig. 51.1: Structure of virus

- Peplomere is the smallest protein unit of envelope. These may be seen as projecting spines on surface.
- The whole extracellular infectious virus particle is called **virion.**

Size: Size variable from 20 to 300 nm, largest, e.g. *Poxvirus—300 nm,* smallest, e.g. *Parvovirus—20 nm.*

Capsid

Symmetry of capsid

a. *Icosahedral or cubical symmetry:* In this type of symmetry, there are 12 vertices or corners and 20 sides or facets forming a polygon. Each facet is equilateral triangle. Pentons are present at vertices and hexons make facets. **Examples** of viruses having icosahedral symmetry are *herpes virus, papovavirus, parvovirus, adenovirus, HBV* which are DNA viruses while *picornavirus* and *reovirus, togaviridae, HIV, calcivirus,* are RNA viruses which show icosahedral symmetry (Fig. 51.2).

b. *Helical symmetry:* Capsomeres surround the nucleic acid core forming spiral-like pattern (Fig. 51.3).

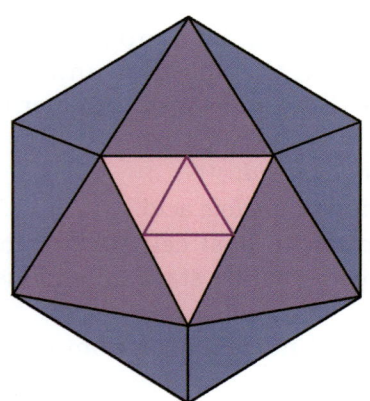

Fig. 51.2: Icosahedral symmetry

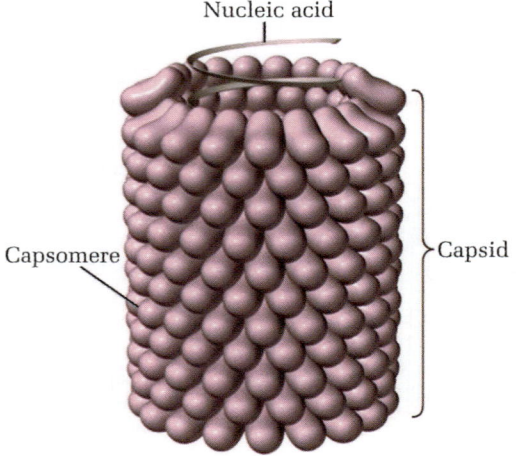

Fig. 51.3: Helical symmetry

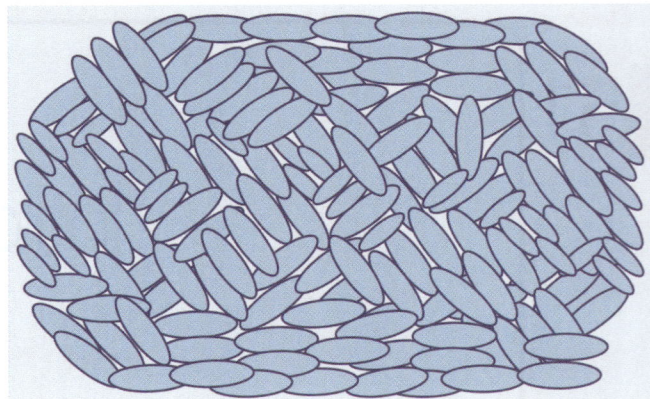

Fig. 51.4: Complex symmetry of vaccinia virus

Viruses showing this type of symmetry are *tobacco mosaic virus, arboviruses, rhabdoviruses, myxoviruses, corona virus, arena virus,* Bunyaviridae

c. *Complex symmetry:* Some viruses do not show typical pattern as above and have complex symmetry. *Poxviruses,* Filoviridae show complex symmetry (Fig. 51.4).

Envelope

It is lipoprotein in nature, it may or may not be present, and it may have projecting spikes of protein subunits on the surface called peplomers.

Importance of viral envelope: It confers chemical, antigenic and biological properties. For example, surface peplomers of *HIV* give two important antigens, i.e. gp 120 and gp 40. Enveloped viruses are more susceptible to lipid solvents. These are examples of chemical property given by envelope. Surface molecules help in attachment to host cells, hence if antibodies are produced against envelope; it causes neutralization by specific antibodies.

Methods of Estimating Size of Virus

Electron microscopy: It is the most common method to visualize viruses in tissue extracts and ultrathin sections of infected cells.

Rate of sedimentation in ultracentrifuge: In utracentrifuge, forces more than 100000 times gravity may be used to drive the particles down to bottom of tube. Viral particles will settle down at a rate proportionate to their size. This relationship between size, shape and sedimentation rate gives the idea of viral particles.

Passing through membrane filters of different sizes: The viral preparation is passed through a series of membranes of known pore size, the approximate size of virus is determined based upon the membranes which allowed the viruses to pass and membrane which held the viruses. The size of viruses is calculated by the average pore diameter multiplied by 0.64.

Comparative measurements: While observing the preparation under EM, by comparing the size of viruses with other objects, the size of viruses is measured. The following are the examples of objects which are compared: *Staphylococcus* has diameter of 1000 nm. *Bacteriophages* vary in sizes between 10 and 100 nm. Protein molecules range between 5 (serum alumin) and 7 nm (gloulin) (Fig. 51.5).

Shape of Viruses

- Bullet shaped, e.g. *Rabies virus*
- Filamentous, e.g. *Ebola virus*
- Brick-shaped, e.g. *Pox virus*
- Rod-shaped, e.g. *Tobacco mosaic virus*
- Complex morphology, e.g. *Bacteriophage*.

Chemical Properties of Viruses

- Viruses contain only one type of nucleic acid: Single or double-stranded. Nucleic acid can be extracted by treatment with detergents or phenol.
- Capsid is protein which confers antigenic specificity.
- Lipid is present on envelope.
- Some viruses contain carbohydrate.
- Viruses have enzymes, e.g. neuraminidase, reverse transcriptase.

Resistance of Viruses

- Usually they are heat-labile, inactivated by heating at 66°C for 30 minutes.
- Viruses are stable at low temperature (lyophilization for prolonged storage).
- All viruses are susceptible to alkali, but varied susceptibility to acids.
- Viruses are more resistant than bacteria to chemical disinfectants.
- 50% glycerol-saline is a preservative for many viruses, e.g. *rabies, vaccinia*.

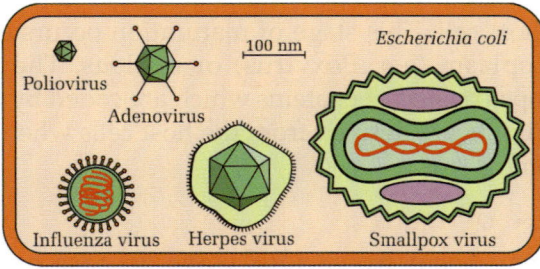

Fig. 51.5: Comparison of sizes of viruses

- Most effective virucidal agents are the oxidizing agents as gluteraldehyde, formaldehyde, H_2O_2 and BPL.
- Lipid solvents are active against enveloped viruses.

Origin of Viruses

Two theories of evolution of viruses are postulated. Viruses may have DNA or RNA of host cells that probably became independent for replication and evolved. Another theory suggests that viruses may be degenerated forms of intracellular parasites.

Viral Hemagglutination

It is originally observed in Influenza virus. It is due to hemagglutinin spikes on surface of viruses.

RBCs are taken in ELISA microtitre plate. Serial dilutions of viral suspensions are performed which are obtained from viruses grown from allantoic cavity or amniotic cavity and they are added to RBCs in ELISA plate. After incubation for 37°C or 4°C, the highest dilution showing carpet formation, i.e. hemagglutination is noted. Negative test shows just settled RBCs forming compact button.

Applications

Detection and assay of influenza virus and other viruses having hemagglutinin on their surface is done by this test. Hemagglutination in some viruses is specific to RBCs of specific animals. Also some viruses react with specific RBCs at specific temperatures; these properties are used for the identification of such viruses.

When viruses grown in different routes in chick embryo amniotic cavity or allantoic cavity, the growth of viruses is detected by **hemagglutination (HA)**.

Similarly growth of hemagglutinating (HA) viruses in cell cultures is determined by hemadsorption and antibody in serum is detected by **hemadsorption inhibition (HAI)**.

Hemagglutination inhibition test (for antibody): If patient is infected with virus having heagglutinin on their surface, the patients will produce antibodies which will inhibit hemagglutination, e.g. patient having infection with Influenza viruses will produce antibodies against hemagglutinins, if viruses are grown in cell cultures and if RBCs are added to cell cultures, in presence of such antibodies, the antibodies will inhibit the hemagglutination. Hemagglutination and elution are used to **purify and concentrate** viruses. Elution: It is caused by neuraminidase (receptor-destroying enzyme). It is reversal of hemagglutination.

Types of Viral Infections

- **Clinical or overt** or apparent infections—can be acute, subacute or chronic
- **Subclinical** or inapparent infections
- **Latent infections,** e.g. *Herpes simplex* and *Herpes zoster*
- **Persistent tolerant infection**, e.g. lymphocytic choriomeningitis in mice
- **Slow viruses**, e.g. scrapie, kuru, *HIV* infection

Viral of Multiplication

Steps involved in multiplication include adsorption, penetration, uncoating, biosynthesis, maturation, release.

Viruses do not have enzymes and synthetic machinery; hence they are dependent on host cells. They also dependent for energy on host cell. The host cell also gives precursors required for the synthesis of viral nucleic acids and early proteins. The genetic information is present in viral nucleic acid.

Attachment or Adhesion

- This is the first step to initiate the viral multiplication. Viruses come in contact with the host cells by random collision and it is reversible process.
- For attachment to host cells, viruses use their surface receptors. For example, enveloped viruses utilize surface spikes and in case of RNA viruses, exposed capsid proteins take part in attachment.
- Suitable ionic condition, pH and temperature should be available for virus attachment. If they find suitable complementary sites on host cells, they adhere. Viruses have adapted to attach a variety of receptors.
- Some viruses carry specialized receptors for attachment to particular tissues. For other viruses, attachment is initiated by ubiquitous components of cell membranes. Some viruses may use multiple receptors also.
- Specific receptors on virus surface which are meant for attachment may determine the tropism for particular tissues, e.g. HIV has surface gp 120 which binds to CD4 receptors of host cell and then enter it. Other example is presence of hemagglutinins on the surface of influenza virus which attach to epithelial cells of respiratory system. Approximately 10^4–10^5 virus binding sites are present on any cell.

Penetration

- It depends upon the type of viruses. Enveloped viruses use different strategies for penetration.
- Influenza viruses bind to cell surface receptors which aggregate at distinct sites on plasma membrane **(clathrin-coated pits)**. Virions are endocytosed in clathrin-coated vesicles and are delivered to endosomes.

- In contrast, most paramyxoviruses **fuse directly** with the plasma membrane with use of fusion proteins.
- Some **non-enveloped** viruses, such as *Adenoviruses*, undergo **receptor-mediated endocytosis** and appear in the cytoplasm within endocytic vesicles **(viropexis).**
- Some non-enveloped viruses probably **cross the plasma membrane directly** and enter in the cytoplasm in absence of vesicle formation.
- In *HIV*, surface **gp40 fuses** with the host cell membrane and facilitates the entry.

Uncoating

The physical separation of viral nucleic acid from other viral structures is called accounting. Free nucleic acid or nucleocapsid may occur. The ability of infectivity is lost at this stage. Lysosomal enzymes help in separation of viral nucleic acids and capsid which are released in host cell.

- *Biosynthesis*: In initial stages of synthesis, viral nucleic proteins, capsid proteins and enzymes are produced which are necessary for next steps in which synthesis of other viral structures are involved. As viruses depend upon host cells for synthetic machinery as well as energy, the host cell processes should be halted and diverted for the production of virus products. Proteins required for this purpose are synthesized.
- In case of RNA viruses, biosynthesis of viral nucleic acids takes place in cytoplasm of host cells while that of DNA viruses it takes place in the nucleus. But in some viruses, it may occur partially in cytoplasm and partially in nucleus.
- Viral mRNA carries the genetic information; **transcription occurs** followed by translation which produces early or structural proteins necessary for viral synthesis of viral components. **Translation** is followed by replication which forms many virus particles.

Maturation

Important events which occur in stage include assembly of viral proteins, viral nucleic acid is surrounded by capsid. Envelope is glycoprotein in nature; of which proteins are produced by virus and lipid is obtained from host cell. This stage of maturation occurs either in cytoplasm (e.g. Poxvirus) or nucleus. The viral envelope consists of proteins which are coded by them while lipids are derived from the host cells when they are coming out.

Release of Virions

- It may occur by various ways, in case of **non-enveloped viruses,** they come out by **cell lysis.**

Enveloped viruses are usually released by **budding**. Some viruses are capable of inducing **apoptosis.**

- HIVs come out by lysis of cell membrane. Some viruses accumulate inside host cells, degeneration of host cells occur and viral particles are released.

Types of RNA Virus and Transcription

Positive Sense RNA Viruses

- Positive sense viral RNA can be immediately translated by host ribosomes into proteins.
- Negative sense RNA viruses cannot be translated immediately; negative strand is first transcribed into positive strand RNA by viral RNA dependent RNA polymerase then translation occurs.

Retroviruses: RNA is first converted into DNA by reverse transcriptase, the DNA is then transcribed into mRNA, and then translation occurs.

Positive strand RNA viruses are *Picornaviridae, Togaviridae, Coronaviridae, Calciviridae, Flaviviridae.*

RNA viruses with negative strand RNA are *Rhabdoviridae, Orthomyxoviridae, Paramyxoviridae, Bunyaviridae, Filoviridae,* and *Aerenaviridae.*

Smallest virus (also smallest DNA virus)	*Parvovirus*
Largest virus (also largest DNA virus)	*Poxvirus*
Smallest RNA virus	*Picornaviridae*
Largest RNA virus	*Paramyxoviridae*

DNA Viruses

Poxviridae family: Large, brick shaped or ovoid viruses (300 × 240 × 100 nm). Core has single linear double-stranded DNA. Multiplication and maturation takes place in the cytoplasm. Family is further divided into genera.

Herpesviridae: Medium-sized DNA viruses with linear double-stranded DNA. The icosahedral nucleocapsid have 162 capsomeres. Lipid envelope is present.

Adenoviridae family: Medium-sized viruses with icosahedral symmetry. They are nonenveloped viruses with 252 capsomeres.

Papovaviridae: Small (40–55 nm), non-enveloped, double stranded DNA viruses with 72 capsomeres. The family has two genera: Papillomavirus and polyomavirus.

Parvoviridae family: Small (18–26 nm), enveloped viruses with single stranded DNA.

Hepadnaviridae family: The name comes from hepa = liver, dna for DNA core. It includes HBV. The virus is 42 nm in size and it is enveloped.

RNA Viruses

Picornaviridae: Small (20–30 nm), non-enveloped, single-stranded viruses with icosahedral symmetry. Three gerera are included:

1. Enterovirus including polio, coxsackie, echo viruses and related viruses.
2. Rhinovirus includes human, bovine, equine rhinoviruses.
3. Hepatovirus which includes Hepatitis A virus.

Orthomyxoviridae: Medium-sized (80–120 nm), spherical or elongated, enveloped viruses which carry hemagglutinin and neuraminidase peplomers. Genome is single-stranded RNA fragmented into 8 pieces. The family contains only one genome, influenza virus.

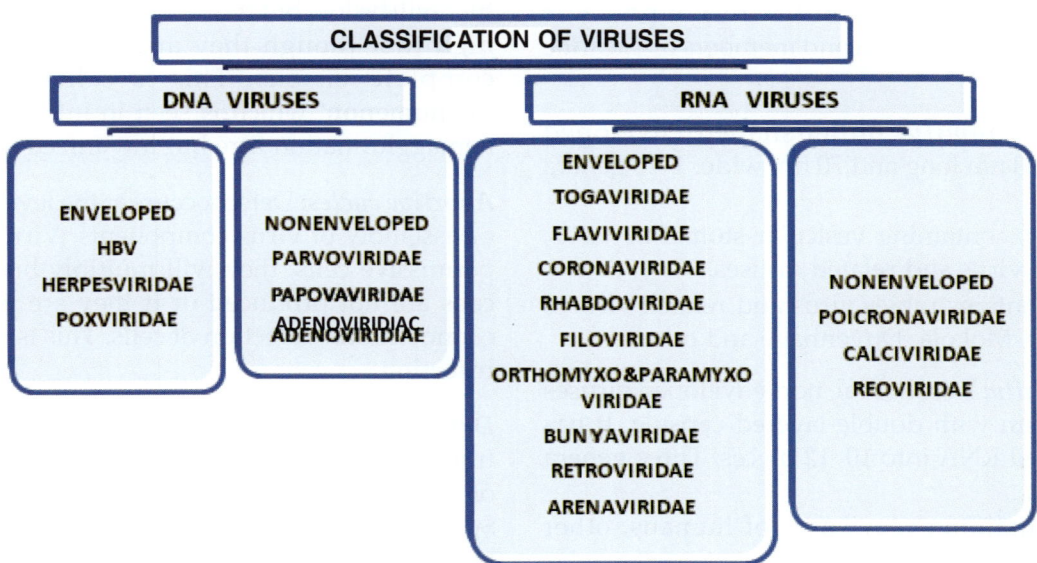

***Paramyxoviridae family*:** Pleomorphic viruses with single-stranded linear RNA. Envelope is present. This family has three 3 genera:

- *Paramyxovirus*: It consists of Newcastle disease virus, mumps virus and parainfluenza viruses of humans, other mammals and birds.
- *Morbillivirus* contains measles, canine distemper, rinderpest and related viruses.
- *Pneumovirus* contains respiratory syncitial virus of humans and related viruses.

***Togaviridae family*:** Single-stranded enveloped viruses. These are spherical viruses with 40–70 nm in size. Most members multiply in arthropods as well as in vertebrates. Three genera are included:

- *Alpha virus*, consisting of viruses previously classified as group A arboviruses.
- *Rubivirus* consists of rubella virus.
- *Pestivirus*, consisting of mucosal disease virus, hog cholera virus and related viruses.

***Flaviviridae*:** Previously grouped under Togaviridae, as group B arboviruses, have been classified as separate family because of difference in their molecular structure and replication strategy.

***Bunyaviridae*:** Spherical, enveloped viruses of size 90–100 nm. All are arthropod-borne viruses. It includes four genera—bunya virus, hantavirus, nairovirus, phlebovirus, and ukuvirus.

***Arenaviridae family*:** Spherical or pleomorphic viruses of 50–300 nm in size, contain electron dense ribosome like particles giving a sandy appearance **(arena means sand in Latin).** These are rodent parasites but rarely cause human infections leading to severe hemorrhagic illness. This family has only one genus—Arenavirus. Species included in this family are lymphocytic choriomeningitis virus, Lassa and members of Tacaribe complex.

***Rhabdoviridae family*:** Bullet-shaped enveloped viruses, 130–300 nm long and 70 nm wide. Two genera are included:

- *Vesiculovirus*, containing vesicular stomatitis virus, Chandipura virus and related viruses.
- *Lyssavirus* contains rabies virus and related viruses as Lagos bat, Mokola, Duvenhage and others.

***Reoviridae family*:** Icosahedral, non-enveloped viruses of size 60–80 nm with double-layered capsule. It has double-stranded RNA into 10–12 pieces. Three genera are included:

- *Reovirus* containing reoviruses of humans, other mammals and birds.
- *Orbivirus* containing several arboviruses as blue tongue virus, Afican horse sickness virus and Colorado tick fever virus.
- *Rotavirus* includes human rotavirus, calf diarrhea virus and related viruses.

***Coronaviridae family*:** Pleomorphic enveloped viruses of size 100 nm. They have club-shaped peplomers projecting as a fringe from surface resembling the solar corona, hence the name. This family includes only one genus, Coronavirus. Members include human corona viruses causing upper respiratory illness, SARS avian infectious bronchitis virus, calf neonatal diarrhea virus, murine hepatitis virus.

Retroviridae family (re = reverse, tr = transcriptase): These are RNA tumor viruses and related viruses. Viruses are icosahedral, about 100 nm in size with lipoprotein envelope. RNA dependent DNA polymerase (reverse transcriptase) is present in the viruses. Three subfamilies are included:

- Oncovirinae, the RNA tumor viruses group.
- Spumivirinae, the foamy viruses group.
- Lentivirinae (lenti = slow), visna and maedi viruses of sheep.

***Calciviridae family*:** Spherical viruses (35–39 nm) with 32 cup-shaped depressions arranged in symmetry.

***Filoviridae*:** Long filamentous, enveloped viruses (80 nm diameter and up to 14000 nm long) with helical nucleocapsid and ss RNA genome. It contains Marburg and Ebola viruses.

***Abnormal replicative cycles*:** If influenza viruses are cultivated in amniotic cavity, viruses multiply inside but because of defective assembly of viruses, the virus titer will be low but the hemagglutinins produced show high titer though they are not assembled to form complete virions. This is called **'Von-Magnus phenomenon'** which is seen in influenza virus (high hemagglutination titre but low infectivity).

***Abortive cycles*:** Defect occurs at the level of maturation or assembly of virus components. Viruses infect non-permissive cells, they will multiply but the daughter cells are not produced or if they are produced, they cannot initiate infection of cells. This is called **abortive infection.**

***Defective viruses*:** These viruses lack one or more functional genes. Deletion mutants may lack portion of genome. These genes are necessary for replication. Spontaneous deletion mutant may affect replication of viruses. They are called defective interference particles.

They have capsid but require help of homologous virus for replication. Another type of defective virus is when a defective virus requires the help of other unrelated virus but replication competent virus. Examples are *Adenoassociated virus* and *Hepatitis D* virus which require help of *Adenovirus* and *HBV*, respectively.

Pseudovirion: It is a defective particle containing host cell DNA, as during viral replication, capsid encloses host genetic material. They may appear as normal viruses under electron microscope but will not replicate.

The **transforming retroviruses** are **defective viruses** as a portion of viral genome deleted and replaced with a piece of DNA of host cell. This gene produces transforming protein.

Examples of viruses with segmented genome

- ***Orthomyxoviridae:*** *Influenza virus*—8 segments (single strand)
- ***Bunyaviridae:*** 3 segments (single strand)
- ***Reoviridae:*** *Rotavirus, Reovirus*—10–12 segments (double-stranded RNA viruses)
- ***Arenaviridae:*** 2 segments (single-stranded RNA virus).

Cultivation of Viruses (Figs 51.6 and 51.7)

As viruses are obligatory intracellular organisms, they do not grow in cell-free media. They are dependent on host for biosynthetic machinery and also for energy. The different methods of viral cultivation are animal inoculation, growth in embryonated eggs and use of tissue cultures.

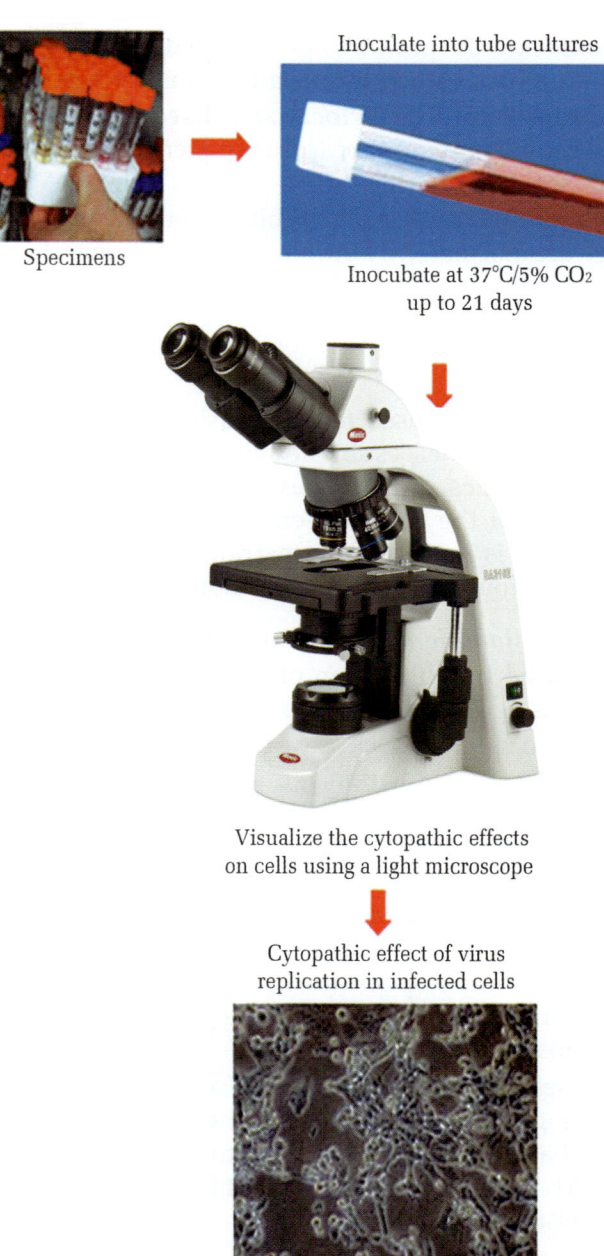

Specimens

Inoculate into tube cultures

Inocubate at $37°C/5\%$ CO_2 up to 21 days

Visualize the cytopathic effects on cells using a light microscope

Cytopathic effect of virus replication in infected cells

Fig. 51.7: Viral cultivation

Animal Inoculation

These methods are of importance in special viruses such as arboviruses and coxackie viruses which do not grow in embryonated eggs. Animals are used for studying the efficacy of vaccines and drugs.

Most common animals used are **suckling mice**. Arboviruses and coxsackie viruses are grown in suckling mice. Only suckling animals are susceptible to arboviruses and not the adult once. In case of *Coxsackie viruses,* it is possible to differntiate between types 'A' or 'B' based upon the lesions produced. The mode of inoculation is intraperitoneal or intracerebral.

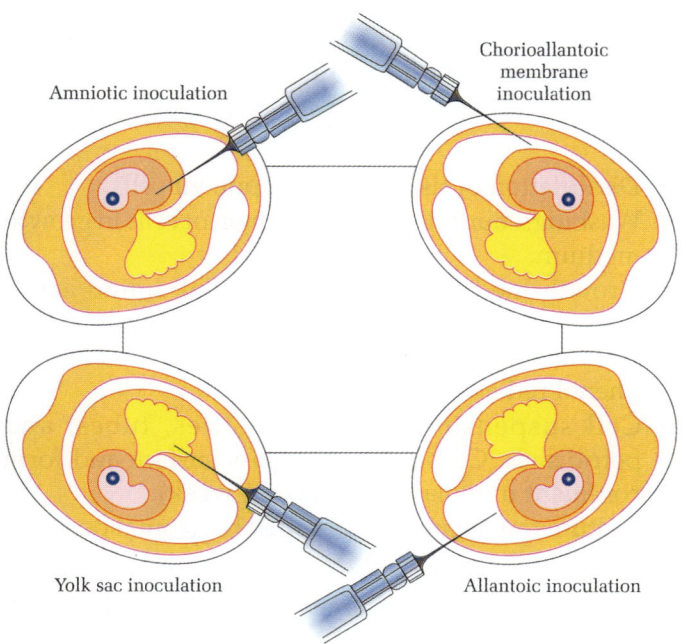

Amniotic inoculation

Chorioallantoic membrane inoculation

Yolk sac inoculation

Allantoic inoculation

Fig. 51.6: Virology laboratory methods

Coxsackie 'A' produces **generalized myositis**, and flaccid paralysis leading to death within a week.

Group 'B' produces **localized disease** with focal myositis, hepatitis, myocarditis, pancreatitis, spastic paralysis.

Other animals used are rabbits, monkeys, hamsters which are inoculated by intraperitoneal, intranasal, and subcutaneous routes. The growth in animals is indicated by the lesions, disease, or death.

Embryonated Eggs

These are mainly used for **diagnosis of** infections as influenza virus, herpes simplex viruses and for production of **vaccine**s. Advantages of using embryonated eggs are that they are cost-effective, easily obtained, harvesting is easy to demonstrate various viruses. Following routes are used (Fig. 51.6):

1. *Chorioallantoic membrane (CAM)*:
- It is used for cultivation of poxviruses and herpes viruses.
- It is also used for pock asay. Each pock is one colony produced by one virion.
  - The morphology of pocks is helpful to differentiate between *Herpes simplex 1* and 2. *HSV* 1 produces smaller, white shiny pocks; they are non-necrotic.
  - *Vaccinia* pocks are large, irregular, necrotic and some of them are hemorrhagic.
  - Inhibition of pock formation may be used for demonstration of antibodies produced against those viruses.
- Viruses are also differentiated by 'ceiling temperature'. Ceiling temperature is the highest temperature of incubation of embrionated egg to produce pocks on CAM. This property is used to differentiate between *Variola* and *Vaccinia*.

2. *Allantoic cavity (sac)*: It is used for cultivation of influenza viruses for the diagnosis as well as for vaccine preparation. This route is also used for rabies viruses and yellow fever viruses for the production of vaccines. After harvesting, the growth of viruses is demonstrated by hemagglutination. After few passages, only viruses grow in allantoic cavity. Except type C, influenza viruses grow well in allantoic cavity.

3. *Amniotic cavity (sac)*: It is used for primary isolation of influenza viruses. Viruses grow well in this route producing high yield, hence for production of influenza viral vaccines, this route is preferred. The *Mumps*, *Newcastle* disease viruses are also cultivated by this route.

4. *Yolk sac*: It is used for rabies viruses and for *Chlamydia* and *Rickettsia*.

Chick embryo vaccines in routine use
- *Influenza*
- *Yellow fever* (17 D strain)
- *Rabies* (Flury strain)

Tissue Culture

They are of three types—organ cultures, explant cultures and cell cultures. The cell cultures are further classified into primary, secondary and continuous cultures. The primary and secondary cell cultures are suitable for cultivation of viruses for preparation of vaccines, the continuous cell lines are not used for vaccines preparation as they may harbor tumor virus. They are used for cultivation of viruses for diagnosis and also for the production of some viral vaccines. It is suitable to use.

1. Organ Cultures

Small bits of organs are maintained in growth medium, preserving their original architecture and function. It is used for cultivation of virus which has affinity for certain organs. For example, Tracheal ring is used for *Coronavirus*.

2. Explant Cultures

They are fragments of minced tissue, grown as explants, embedded in plasma clots. For example, adenoid tissue explants culture. It is used for *Adenovirus*.

3. Cell Cultures

A. *Primary cell cultures*: The origin of primary cell culture is normal cells which are freshly taken from tissue. They are capable of only 5–10 divisions. Tissues dissociated into component cells by the action of proteolytic enzymes like trypsin or mechanical shaking. Cells are washed, counted and suspended in growth medium.

Steps
- Dissociation of tissue into component cells.
- Washing, counting, and suspension of cells in growth medium.
- Growth medium contains essential amino acids, vitamins, salts, glucose, buffer system, calf serum, antibiotics (to prevent bacterial contamination) and phenol red as indicator.
- Cell suspension is put in bottles, tubes, and petridishes. Cells adhere to glass surface and form confluent monolayer (in about 1 week).
- Cultures are incubated in sloped horizontal position.

Contents of medium for cell culture: These are Eagle's minimum essential medium base, hank's balanced salt solution, L-amino acids, vitamins, glucose, antibiotics, growth medium (10% serum), phenol red as indicator.

Primary cell cultures: Primary cell cultures are preferably used for production of vaccines as there is no possibility of cell culture harboring oncogenic virus. They may be used for growth of viruses for diagnosis. They are derived from normal cells. For example, rhesus monkey kidney cell culture, human amnion cell, chick embryo fibroblast culture. Also embryo fibroblast cell culture is used for cultivation of fastidious viruses as *Cytomegaloviruses*. Primary cultures have **short life** and they are costly to maintain.

B. Diploid cell strains: These are of **single cell type**; the original **diploid chromosome** is maintained for up to **50 cell divisions**. Examples are **WI38,** which is human embryonic lung cell strain. **HI-8** are rhesus monkey embryo cell cultures. **Human diploid cell cultures** are used for preparation of vaccines and for cultivation of fastidious viruses. WI-38 used for preparation of rabies vaccines. WI-38 is human embryonic lung cell line used for isolation of *HSV, CMV,* and *VZV.*

C. Continuous cell lines: These are derived from **cancer cells,** therefore, capable of indefinite growth. Their chromosome is **haploid**. They are subcultured regularly to maintain, and even stored at low temperature.

The list of continuous cell lines and their origin is given below:

- *HeLa*: Human carcinoma of cervix cell line
- *HEp-2*: Human epithelioma of larynx cell line: good for respiratory syncitial virus
- *Vero*: Vervet monkey kidney cell line
- *KB*: Human carcinoma of nasopharynx
- *McCoy's*: Human synovial carcinoma cell line
- *BHK21*: Baby hamster kidney cell culture

Continuous cell lines are used for primary isolation of viruses from clinical specimens. The advantages of continuous cell lines are they can be easily obtained, cheaper and easy to handle. Disadvantages are they do not support growth of few viruses and some oncogenic viruses may be present in these cultures, hence they are not good for preparation of viral vaccines.

Detection of Virus Growth in Cell Culture
(Figs 51.8 and 51.9)

1. **Cytopathic effects**
   - *Entero virus (poliovirus)*: It causes crenation of cells, degeneration of sheet.
   - *Measles*: Causes syncytium formation.
   - *Herpes* leads to focal degeneration.
   - *Adenovirus* forms large granular clumps (bunch of grapes) and cells become round.
   - *SV 40*: Cytoplasmic vacuolation is seen.
   - *CMV* causes enlargement of cells.
   - *Parainfluenza virus*: Focal rounding and multi-nucleated giant cells appear.
2. **Metabolic inhibition**: Indicator (phenol red) shows color change due to multiplication of viruses and their metabolism (change in pH occurs).
3. **Hemadsorption**: The growth of hemagglutinating viruses as myxoviruses, arbovirus is detected by adding guinea pig RBCs to cell cultures. The RBCs adsorb on cell surfaces which can be detected under inverted microscope, e.g. *influenza*.
4. **Interference**: In the first step, infective material containing suspected noncytopathic virus is added. In the second step, another virus which is known to produce cytopathic effects is added. If the virus which is suspected is grown, it will inhibit the growth of cytopathic virus, thus no cytopathic effects means, suspected virus is grown.
5. **Transformation**: When viruses having oncogenic potential are present in cell cultures they cause various changes as loss of pallisidal arrangement, cells become dark.
6. **Immunofluorescence**: Direct immunofluorescence helps us in early detection, therefore, widely used for diagnostic purposes.
7. DNA probes or PCR are used for eary detection of growth.

Difficulties with cell cultures
   I. Bacterial contamination.
  II. Susceptible to toxic substances.
 III. Someviruses do not grow in cell culture, e.g. *Hepatitis B*, diarrheal viruses, *parvovirus, papillomavirus.*

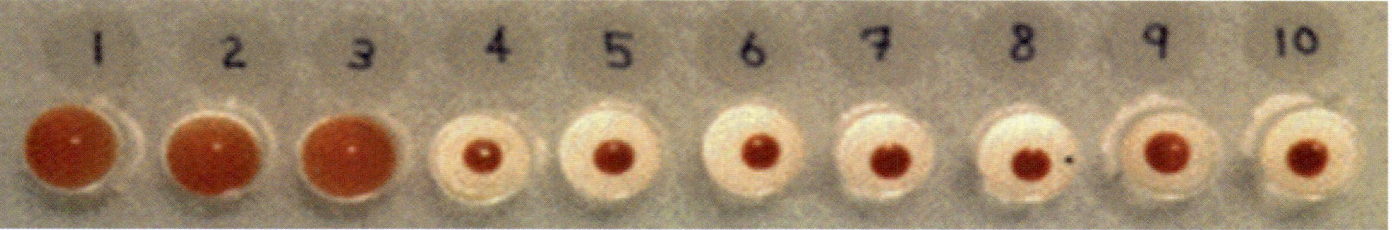

Fig. 51.8: Viral agglutination test

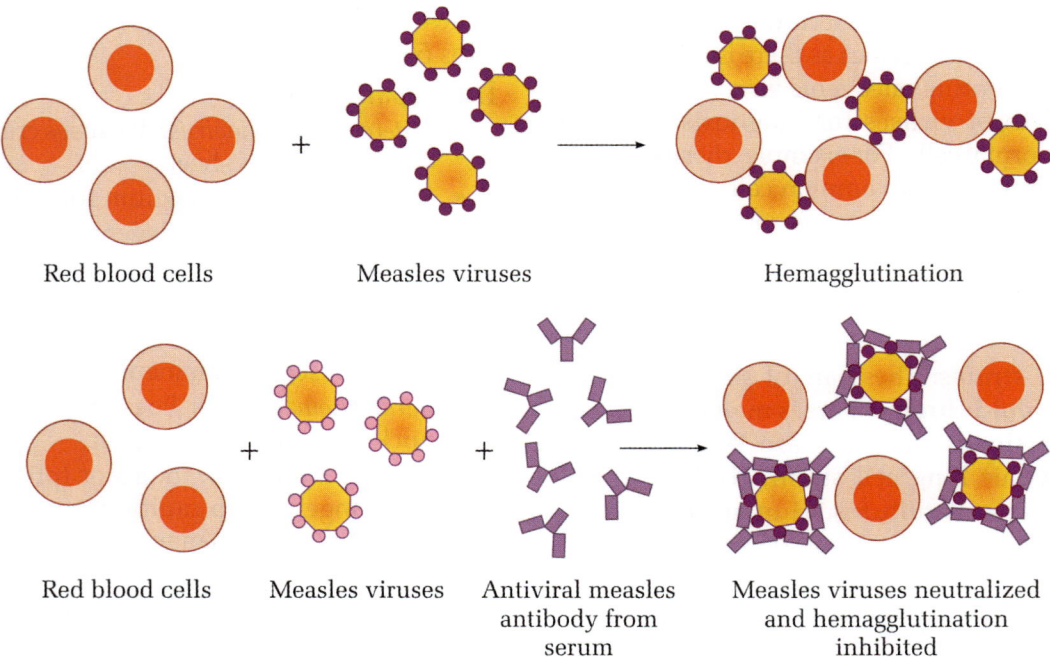

Red blood cells   Measles viruses   Hemagglutination

Red blood cells   Measles viruses   Antiviral measles   Measles viruses neutralized
                                       antibody from   and hemagglutination
                                       serum   inhibited

Fig. 51.9: Hemagglutionation and hemagglutination inhibition

Quantitation of Viruses

Serological tests, as ELISA and RIA after standardization, can be used for quantification of viruses. These tests lack the ability to differentiate infectious particles from non-infectious particles. Though hemagglutination is simple and easy, it is also not possible to quantitate infectious and non-infectious viral particles. Electron microscope can be used to count the particles by comparing with suspension of latex particles of similar size. It has also same disadvantage. Hence, biological tests are used for quantitation.

Assay of Infectivity

Two types of infective assays can be performed: Quantal assay and quantitative assay.

Quantal Assays

The result of this test is either death of animal or plaque or pock formation on CAM of chick membrane. Serial dilution of viral preparations are tested in series of animals or in cell cultures. The reciprocal of highest dilution of viruses which cause effects in 50% of cells or animals is called ID50.

a. *Plaque assay*: It is used for viruses which produce lesions in cell cultures.

   Method: Monolayers of cell cultures are inoculated with viral dilution. The medium containing agar or carboxymethylcellulose is overlayed over cell cultures. After incubation during which viruses repeatedly multiply and kill cells, the cell cultures can be observed under microscope for formation of small area of infection (killing of cells) called 'plaque'. One virus will form its colony and will form one plaque, thus one virus is one colony-forming unit. The number of plaques formed in the cell cultures can be measured.

   Direct immunofluorescence: It determines number of infected cells producing viral antigen.

b. *Pock assay*: Pock producing viruses can be quantified by inoculating virus suspension on CAM of chick embryo and numbers of pocks produced are counted.

Purification of viruses

- High speed centrifugation in density gradients or gradient material as potassium tartrate, sucrose is used for purification of viruses. Viruses migrate to an equilibrium position at a point where the denisity of solution is equal to their buoyant density and form a visible band.

- Viral preparations are concentrated by precipitation with ethanol or polyethylene glycol or ultra-centrifugation and then viruses are separated by column chromatography or density gradient centri-fugation.

Viral Genetics

Properties of viruses as virulence, antigenicity are governed by genes. Knowledge of viral genetics is important to understand host parasite relationships.

Mutation: Mutation in viral genome sequences occurs by deletion, frame shift, base substitution. The frequency of mutation is 10^{-4}–10^{-8}. Most of the mutations are lethal so that they do not survive. A mutant becomes evident only when the mutation confers easily demonstrable property. Mutations may be spontaneous or produced in response to inducers as mutagens.

Conditional lethal mutants: These mutants survive under permissive conditions but not in nonpermisive conditions. They are used in genetic studies and used in vaccine preparation. One such vaccine, e.g. influenza vaccine uses Ts mutants of temperatre sensitive mutant (conditional lethal mutants) of strain of virus which survives at low temperature of upper respiratory tract, but do not survive at high temperature of lower respiratory tract. Hence, they will produce low grade infection of upper respiratory tract giving immunity without producing damage in lower respiratory tract.

Host dependent mutants: Such mutants grow in permissive cells, but in non permissive cells, they produce abortive infection.

Interactions Among Viruses

If two or more viruses infect the cell, the result varies based on either genetic or phenotypic or genotypic interaction of viruses. Genetic interactions results in some progeny viruses which may differ genetically from parent virus. Progeny produced by non-genetic interactions are similar to parent cells. In genetic interaction, the nucleic acid interact while in non-genetic interactions, the genes products are involved.

Intramolecular Recombination

This occurs between two different but closely related viruses simultaneously infecting host cell, two viruses exchange segments of nucleic acids and form a hybrid with genes from both parents. They are genetically stable and replicate producing progeny like itself. This is common in DNA viruses.

Reassortment

Host cell is infected with two viruses with segmented genome. The exchange of genes occurs so that a new progeny virus is produced by genetic re-assortment. The phenomenon also occurs in nature resulting genetic varations in viruses. This may be the way by which pandemic strain of influenza originate in nature.

Reactivation

It is genetic interaction between gene of an active virus with genomes of inactive virus. Both infect a cell at a time. Portion of gene of inactive virus is trapped in active virus genome. The result is formation of progeny viruses with some characteristic of inactive virus. The phenomenon is known as **cross-reactivation or marker rescue**. The phenomenon is used in production of influenza virus vaccine. If new epidemic strain does not grow in embryonated eggs, it is grown along with standard strain inactivated by ultraviolet rays, thus daughter virions with antigenic characteristics of new strain of virus and growth characteristic of standard strain are obtained which are used for preparation of vaccines.

Phenotypic Mixing

Either gene of one virus enters capsid of another virus or capsid of progeny virus contains genetic components of both viruses. If genetic material of one virus is encased in completely heterologus virus, it is called **transcapsidation.** Transcapsidation produces progeny viruses covered with capsid of homologus virus. Phenotypic mixing usually occurs between different members of same family. Phenotypic mixing can occur in non-related viruses, this may happen in case of enveloped viruses in which case two viruses need not be closely related. The nucleocapsid of one virus encased with envelope characteristic of other virus, this phenomenon is called **pseudotype formation**.

Complementation

Host cell is infected with one defective virus and other normal virus, the progeny virus becomes capable of replication under conditions otherwise not suitable for replication of one or both viruses. One virus gives gene products to another allowing the second virus to grow. The genotype of two viruses is not changed. In this process, one virus has complemented second virus by providing the gene product which second virus is lacking. If both viruses are defective in the same gene product, they will not complement for growth any ways.

Interference

Two different viruses infect host cell, one virus prevents multiplication of another virus. Several mechanisms may occur as; one virus may inhibit the ability of another virus to adsorb to cell by blocking cell surface receptor (retroviruses, enteroviruses) or destroying its receptors. One virus may compete with other for some components necessary for replication (e.g. polymerase). The first virus may cause cell to produce an inhibitor.

Viroids

It is a new class of subviral agents. There is apparent absence of an extracellular dormant phase (virion). Their genome is much smaller than viruses. It is free of protein, low molecular weight RNA resistant to heat and organic solvents. They are sensitive to nucleases. There is possibility that causative agents of some diseases may be due to viroids.

Prions

These are proteinaceous infective agents. They may cause chronic degenerative diseases. They do not have nucleic acid, they are resistant to UV rays, heat (90°C for 3 minutes), proteases, nucleases but sensitive to proteases.

The examples of diseases caused by prions are **Kuru** and **Creutzfeldt-Jakob disease.**

52

Host–Rarasite Relationship

Virus host responses differ at community level, individual level and cellular levels.

Viral infections at the level of community: The herd immunity against virus may limit the spread of viruses in community. People in community may have immunity due to exposure or due to vaccination. If immunity is less, viruses may spread causing epidemics or pandemics. Best example is the infection due to new strains of influenza virus, i.e. swine flu virus (*H1N1*). This virus has new antigens completely different from previous circulating influenza virus, hence it spreads rapidly. Herd immunity against viruses can be increased by vaccination. With the global polio irradiation programme, live attenuated vaccines are given. *Pox virus* is the best example of virus disease irradicated with active immunization.

At cellular levels, effect of viruses vary between no damage to cell death.

Viral effects on cells may be:

- Cell death: Polio virus
- *Cytocidal effect*: Viruses lyse cells, e.g. *HIV*
- *Cellular proliferation*: Molluscum contagiosum
- *Malignant transformation*: Oncogenic viruses
- In tissue cultures, viruses produce changes called **cytopathic effects** which are characteristic of the virus. Cell infected with viruses may fuse forming fusion of adjacent cell which is characteristic of *respiratory syncytial virus*. There may be enlargement of cell as seen in infection with *Cytomegalovirus*. Viruses may produce degeneration of cell as in case of *poliovirus*.

Cellular injury may be due to structural or non-structural proteins of viruses which affect metabolism of infected cells. Direct damage may be due intracellular accumulation of viruses. When viruses infect cells, some viral coded antigens appear on the cell which may alter properties of the cells. Certain viruses have ability to cause damage to chromosome of cells. Such viruses infecting the pregnant women may lead to congenital infections, e.g. *CMV*. Histologically, most characteristic feature seen in viral infected cell is formation of inclusion bodies.

Different Routes of Entry of Viruses in Host
(Flowchart 52.1)

1. *Viruses entering through various mucosae*:
   - *Nose and throat*: Viruses entering this route are *influenza, rhinovirus, mumps, measles, rubella, varicella zoster, cytomegalovirus, parainfluenza, Ebstein-Barr virus.*
   - *Gastrointestinal tract*, e.g. *hepatitis A, hepatitis E virus, poliovirus, rotavirus.*
   - *Genital*: HIV, hepatitis B virus, hepatitis C virus, herpes simplex virus, human papilloma virus.

2. *Viruses entering through skin*:
   - Insect bites, e.g. *arboviruses*.
   - Animal bite, e.g. *rabies virus*.
   - Injections, e.g. *HIV, HBV*.

3. *Viruses causing infection by transplacental route*: Viruses cause congenital infections. This transfer is known as vertical transfer. The viruses which cause congenital infections are *rubella, CMV, HIV, HBV, herpes simplex virus, parvo B virus.*

Different Methods of Spread of Viruses (Fig. 52.1)

After entering in human body, viruses may spread locally causing localized infections or viruses may spread causing generalized infections via blood or lymph. The spread of viruses takes place in following ways:

- *Direct cell-to-cell spread*: Viruses spread from one cell to another by forming bridge, e.g. common cold viruses.

Flowchart 52.1: Routes of human infection with different virus

Respiratory	Gastrointestinal	Contact with lesions	Body and body fluids	Insect bites
Airborne small droplets	Enteric adenovirus	Herpes simplex virus		Dengue
Influenza Measles Varicellla-zoster	Hepatitis A virus	Varicella-zoster virus		Westnile virus
Airborne large droplets	Norwalk virus			Chikungunya
	Polio virus and other enteroviruses			Encephalitis viruses
Adenovirus Parainfluenza virus Parvovirus	Rotavirus			Yellow fever virus
Direct contact with respiratory secretion			Hepatitis B viruss	
Respiratory syncytial virus Rhinovirus			Hepatitis C virus Cytomegalovirus Epstein-Barr virus HIV	

- *Spread through macrophages:* After entry of virus in body, viruses may be taken by macrophages in which viruses grow and spread to various parts of body.
- *Lymphatic spread of viruses:* Viruses entering through skin, mucosa may reach lymph nodes and if not cleared, viruses spread along with lymphatics.
- *Some viruses after entry go to lymph nodes,* multiply and enter blood causing primary viremia. With primary viremia, viruses are shed in different organs or cells of reticuloendothelial system where they multiply and spillover in blood causing secondary viremia.

- **Viruses may enter** in different cells in **blood and spread via bloodstrem.**

Cell associated	Viruses
Lymphocytes	HIV, HBV, HCV, measles, mumps, rubella, Epstein-Barr virus
Monocyte–macrophages	HIV, poliovirus, CMV, measles
Neutrophils	Influenza virus
RBC	Parvo B-19
None, free in plasma	Picornaviruses

- *Spread along the nerves:* Neurotrophic viruses, such as *rabies and herpes virus,* may spread along the nerves.

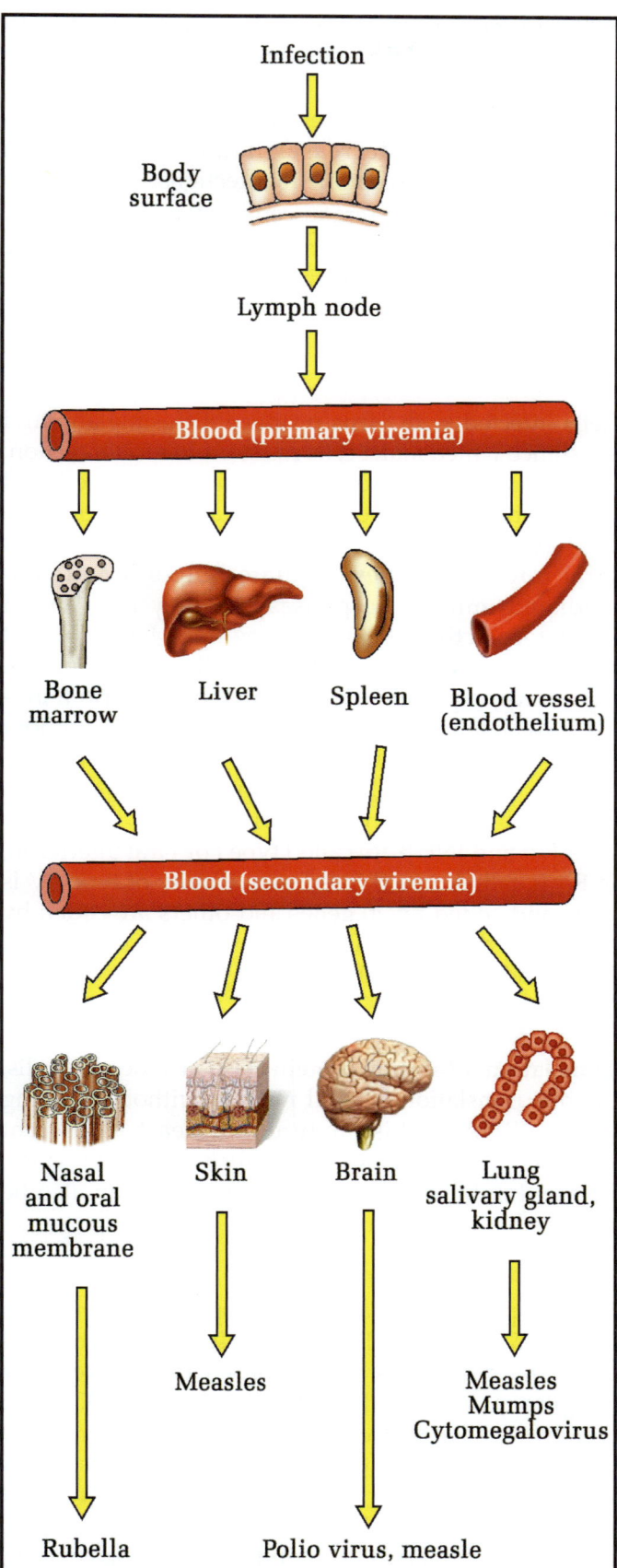

Fig. 52.1: Example of spread of virus to secondary sites

Inclusion Bodies

Definition: Inclusion bodies are structures with definite size, shape, location, staining reaction which can be demonstrated in host cells infected by that virus.

Uses

1. Detection of inclusion body by histopathological examination of specimen and its staining helps in early viral diagnosis.
2. Detection of specific inclusion bodies in cell cultures is one of the cheap and effective methods of detection of viral growth in cell cultures.

Classification of Inclusion Bodies

They are classified on the basis of their location as intracytoplasmic, intranuclear, or both. Intranuclear inclusion bodies are further classified as **Cowdry type A** which are of variable size, and have granular appearance *(herpes simplex viruses, yellow fever virus)* while Cowdry type B are produced by *adenovirus.* These are well demarcated and multiple.

Based on staining properties, they are classified as acidophilic (eosinophilic) and basophilic.

Intracytoplasmic inclusion bodies are produced by *poxviruses, rabies virus.* Intranuclear inclusion bodies are produced by *herpes simplex viruses.* Both intranuclear as well as intracytoplasmic inclusion bodies are produced by *measles.*

Viruses produce eosinophilic inclusion bodies except *adenovirus* which shows basophilic inclusion bodies.

- **Negri** body is eosinophilic inclusion body seen in cells infected with *rabies virus.* It is intracytoplasmic and stained with either Giemsa stain or more specific Seller's method.
- Inclusion bodies in **molluscum contagiosum** are large (20–30 nm) and can be easily seen under light microscopy and stain used on histopathological slide is H and E.
- *Vaccinia* infected cells show small inclusions **(Guarnieri bodies),** while *fowl pox* shows large inclusion bodies (Bollinger bodies). The only bacterium which shows inclusion bodies is *Chlamydia trachomatis* (intracytoplasmic basophilic inclusions which surround the nucleus like a shield).

Pathogenesis of Viral Infections

Viral Immunity

Viruses are good antigens. They stimulate both cellular and humoral immune responses.

Natural infection and multiplication of virus in human body exposes to the whole range of viral antigens.

Individual viruses produce variable immune response, e.g. *smallpox* produces lifelong immunity, *influenza* produces short-lived immunity.

A. Humoral immunity: Factors mediating humoral anti-viral immunity are:

1. *Antibodies*
   - IgG, and IgM give protection in blood and tissue spaces.
   - IgA protect mucosal surfaces. This type of antibody is important in viruses infecting or entering mucosal surfaces, e.g. *poliovirus, influenza virus.* The oral poliovaccine produces local as well as systemic immunity.
   - Antibodies prevent adsorption to cell receptors, e.g. antibodies against hemagglutinin (HA) of influenza prevent entry of virus.
   - Prevention of release of progeny viruses, e.g. antibody against neuraminidase (NA) limits spread of viruses.
   - Antibodies to surface antigens are neutralizing (e.g. anti-hemagglutinin) while to internal antigens, always non-neutralizing.
2. *Complement*: It causes surface damage to enveloped virions and causes cytolysis of virus infected cells.
3. *Harmful effects of antibodies*: Sometimes antibodies increase the infectivity or severity, e.g. increased severity of *RSV* infection in infants due to maternal antibodies. **Antibody in dengue causes immune enhancement. Antibody may cause** complement-mediated injury, e.g. immunothrombocytopenia in viral hemorrhagic fevers.

B. Cell mediated immunity (CMI): Infected cells express viral antigens on surface. As viruses are intracellular, antibodies have no acess inside hence CMI is very important in viruses. Cytotoxic T cells kill virus infected cells.

Some viral infections decrease immunity: Measles, *HIV* decrease CMI, *lymphocytic choriomeningitis,* leukemia viruses decrease humoral immunity.

Non-Immunological Responses (Innate)

Phagocytosis

Macrophages are more important than polymorphs. (Kupffer cells in liver, dendritic cells in skin, etc.).
- Body temperature—fever is a defense mechanism against most viruses.
- *Herpes simplex* is reactivated by fever.
- Hormones, corticosteroids enhance most viral infections, e.g. herpetic keratoconjunctivitis. Patients on steroids may suffer fatal infection due to *varicella zoster* virus.

- Pregnancy increases severity, probably due to suppression of immunity and decreased interferon production.
- *Malnutrition*: In children, it predisposes them to measles which decreases immunity and again making child susceptible to infections.
- *Age*: Extremes of age are susceptible for viral infections.
- Interferon is natural defense mechanism of vertebrate cells against virus infection.

Interferons (Fig. 52.2)

Definition

Cells infected with virus produce diffusible antiviral substance which make cells resistant to viral infection. Interferons are family of host-coded proteins produced that inhibit viral replication. INFs are produced quite early by body. They are the first line of defence against viral infections. They regulate humoral and cell-mediated immune responses and they have broad regulatory activities on cell growth. It has no direct action on virus but it acts on other cells of same species. It produces a protein (translation inhibition protein—TIP) which inhibits translation of viral mRNA without affecting cellular mRNA. Interferons are species-specific. Interferon produced by one virus protects infection by same or related virus.

INF-α and INF-β are called type I or viral interferon, INF-γ is called type II interferon. Family of type 'A' is large and coded by 20 genes and others are coded by one gene. INF-α and INF-β are resistant to low pH. INF-β and INF-γ are glycosylated.

Mode of Action of Interferon

Translation inhibiting protein (TIP) produced by cells, inhibits translation of viral mRNA, without affecting cellular RNA. TIP is mixture of at least 3 different enzymes, protein kinase, oligonucleotide synthatase, RNase. Inhibition of viral transcription may also be responsible (Flowchart 52.2).

Synthesis of INF

They are produced by all vertebral species. Normal cells do not produce INFs. INF-α and INF-β are synthesized by many cell types while INF--γ is produced by lymphocytes, mainly T lymphocytes, NK cells. **Dendritic** cells are also potent INF producers and they can secrete up to **1000 times more** than fibroblast. RNA virus is better inducer. The production is also induced by double-stranded DNA, bacterial endotoxin, synthetic polymers. Potent inducers are togaviruses, Sendai virus, NDV, vesicular stomatitis virus. Avirulent viruses are better inducers than virulent viruses.

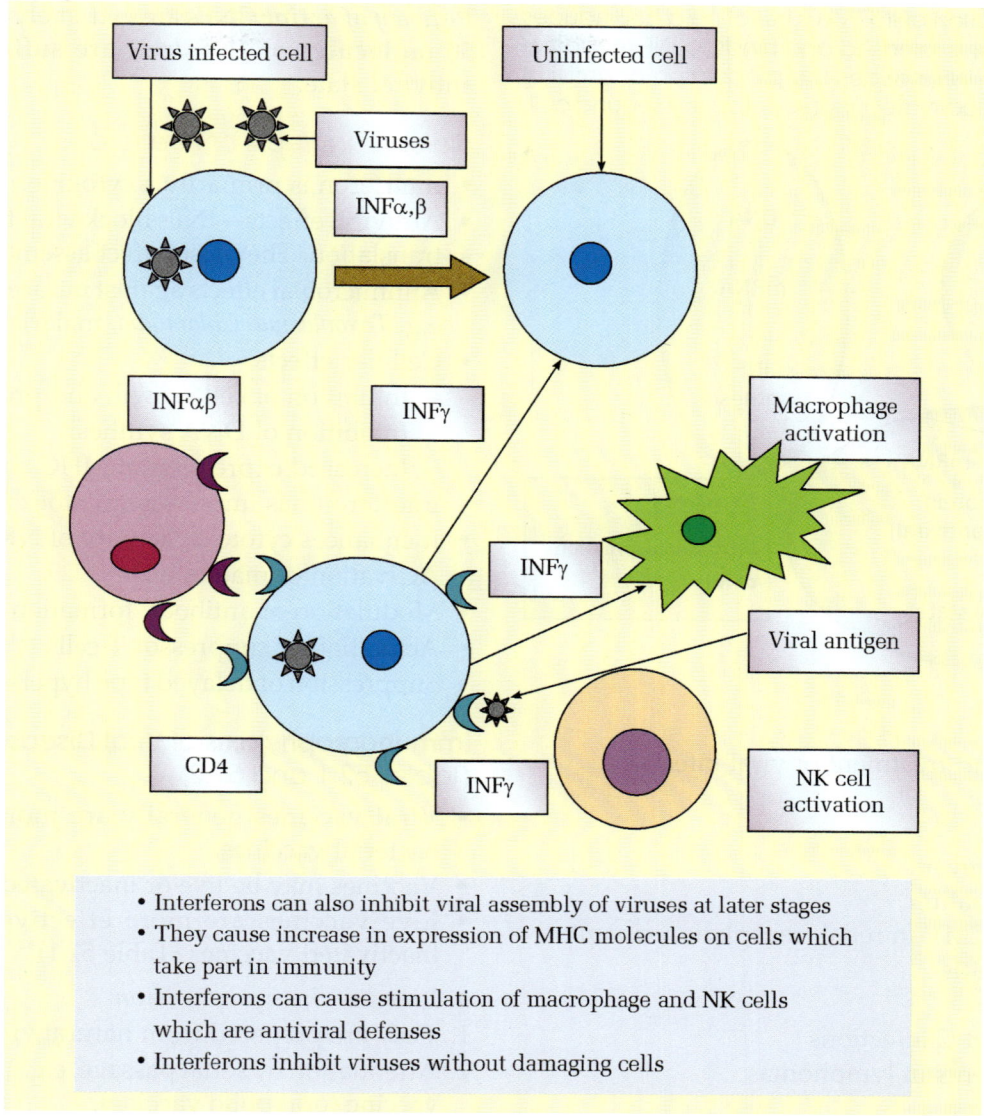

• Interferons can also inhibit viral assembly of viruses at later stages
• They cause increase in expression of MHC molecules on cells which take part in immunity
• Interferons can cause stimulation of macrophage and NK cells which are antiviral defenses
• Interferons inhibit viruses without damaging cells

Fig. 52.2: Role of interferons in viral infection

Production increased by increasing temperature up to 40°C and inhibited by steroids and increasing oxygen tension.

Anticellular Activities of INF

• It inhibits cell growth.
• It has effects on differentiation of cells.
• It increases expression of MHC.
• It enhances natural killer activity.
• INF α-β2 is identical to B cell differential factor.

Specificity of Interferons

• They can only protect cells of same or related species.
• They are not virus specific; INF produced by one virus may offer protection to same or unrelated viruses.
• Viruses vary in their susceptibility to interferon.
• Viruses vary in ability to induce interferon.

Conditions Affecting Interferon Production

• **Stimulating**: Increasing temperature up to 40°C has positive effect on production.
• **Inhibiting**: Steroids, increased oxygen tension inhibit production.

Classification of Interferons

• **Alpha interferon (INF-α)** is produced by leukocytes, it is a nonglycosylated protein, 16 antigenic types. It is usefull as antiviral substance.
• **Beta INF (INF-β)** is produced by fibroblasts and epithelial cells. It is glycoprotein.
• **Gamma INF (INF-γ):** It is produced by T lympho-cytes which is a glycoprotein, immunomodulator, it has less antiviral functions.

Flowchart 51.2: Action of INF: Virus infecting a cell induces production of INF. It is released and binds to INF receptors on other cells. The INF induces the production of antiviral proteins which are activated, if virus enters the second cell.

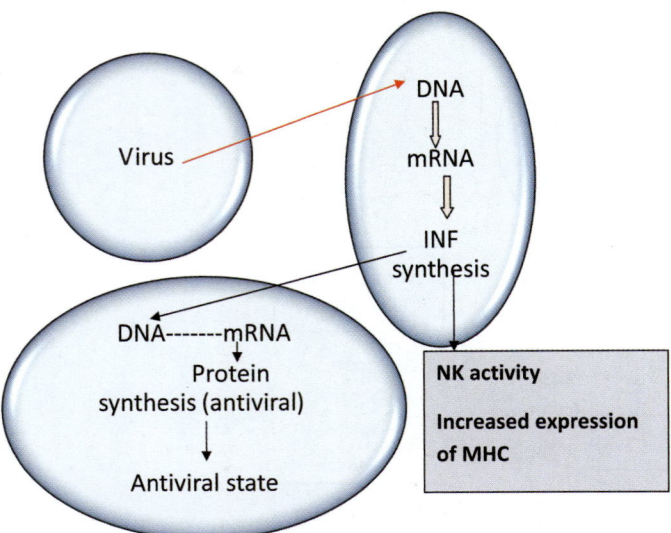

Uses of Interferon

- Prophylaxis and treatment of viral infections
- URTI
- Herpes zoster
- Hemorrhagic fevers
- Herpes encephalitis
- Treatment of CMV in renal transplant recipient
- Herpetic keratitis
- Genital warts
- Hepatitis B and C infections
- Anticancer agents in lymphomas

Side Effects of INF Therapy

- Gastrointestinal side effects
- Nervous system side effects
- Bone marrow suppression

Characteristics

- INFs are inactivated by proteolytic enzymes.
- They resist heating at 56–60° for 30–60 minutes.
- INFs are stable over wide range of pH (2–10).
- Molecular weight—17,000.
- Poorly antigenic.
- They are non-dylasable proteins.
- Assay is based on biological activity, e.g. inhibition of plaque formation.

Production of Human Interferon

INFs are expressed as they can be produced from buffy coat leukocytes from blood banks, with Newcastle Disease Virus or Sendai virus as inducers.

Potency of action: INFs are extremely potent, **less than 50 molecules of INFs/cell** are sufficient to induce antiviral state.

Biological Effects of Interferon

- Interferon is primarily a cytokine.
- Antiviral effects—INFs block viral transcription and translation. They also affect assembly of viruses.
- Antimicrobial effects against intracellular organisms, e.g. *Toxoplasma, Chlamydia*, malaria.
- Cellular effects
  - Inhibition of cell growth and proliferation
  - Inhibition of DNA synthesis
  - Increased expression of MHC antigens
- Interferon has immunoregulatory actions
- It enhances cytotoxic activity of NK, K and T cells
- Activation of macrophage
- Modulation of antibody formation
- Activation of suppressor T cells
- Suppression of delayed type hypersensitivity (DTH).

Immunoprophylaxis of Viral Diseases
(Tables 52.1 and 52.2)

- Viral vaccines generally are more effective than bacterial vaccines.
- Vaccines may be live or inactivated.
- Live vaccines are more effective than killed or inactivated vaccines (Table 52.1).

a. *Live vaccines preparation*
1. They are prepared from natural virus, e.g. *cowpox.*
2. Attenuation by serial passage, e.g. *Yellow fever,* Sabin vaccine (oral polio vaccine).
3. Recombination, e.g. *influenza virus.*

b. *Inactivated vaccines preparation:* Heat, phenol (rabies), formalin (JE, Salk), beta propionolactone (rabies) are used for preparation of vaccines.

c. *Subunit vaccines* have less adverse effects, e.g. *influenza, hepatitis B.* Cloning antigens in bacteria or yeast produce hepatitis B virus vaccine.

Advantages of Live Vaccines

- Single dose sufficient
- Administered by route of natural infection
- Antibodies to whole range of virus antigens are produced
- Induce CMI
- More lasting immunity
- More economical
- Administered conveniently
- They can be given in combination, e.g. MMR

TABLE 52.1: Comparison of live-attenuated vaccine and killed vaccines

Characteristics	Killed	Live vaccines
Number of doses	Multiple	Single
Need for adjuvant	Yes	No
Duration of immunity	Shorter	Longer
Effectiveness of protection (more closely mimics natural infection)	Lower	Greater
Immunoglobulin produced	IgG	IgG, IgA
Mucosal immunity produced	Poor	Yes
CMI	Poor	Yes
Residual viral strain in vaccine	No	Yes
Reversion to virulence	No	Possible
Excretion of vaccine and transmission to non-immune contacts	No	Yes
Interference by other viruses in host	No	Yes

TABLE 52.2: Examples of different vaccines and cell cultures in which they are produced

Vaccine	Type	Cell substrate
Hepatitis A virus	Killed	Human diploid fibroblast
Hepatitis B virus	Subunit HBsAg	Recombinant vaccine in yeast
Influenza A and B	Live intranasal	Embryonated chicken eggs
Influenza A and B	Killed	Embryonated chicken eggs
Measles	Live	Chicken embryo fibroblast
Mumps	Live	Chicken embryo fibroblast
Papilloma	Subunit (l1)	Recombinent DNA
Oral polio	Live	Monkey kidney cells
Killed polio	Killed	Monkey kidney cells
Rota virus	Live	Vero monkey kidney cells
Rubella	Live	Human diploid fibroblast
Varicella	Live	Human diploid fibroblast
Zoster	Live	Human diploid fibroblast
Adenovirus	Live	Human diploid fibroblast
Japanese encephalitis	Killed	Mouse brain
Yellow fever	Live	Embryonated chicken eggs

Disadvantages of Live Vaccines

- Remote risk of reversion to virulence.
- It may be contaminated with other viruses or infectious agents.
- It can spread from vaccines to contacts.
- Dangerous in immunocompromised patients.
- Interference due to pre-existing viruses.
- Heat labile.
- Local and remote complications occur.

Advantages of Killed Vaccines

- Stable
- Safe
- Can be given in combination
- No danger of spread of virus

Treatment of Virus Infections

Drugs which inhibit attachment and penetration: Amantadine inhibits attachment of influenza virus and prevents entry of virus. Rimantadine is derivative of amantadine and has similar effects but less toxic.

Inhibitors of Viral Nucleic Acid Synthesis

Acyclovir: It is a nucleoside analogue active against *herpes simplex* viruses and *varicella zoster*. It inhibits viral coded thymidine kinase. Tropical application is effective in treatment of herpes keratitis, genital herpes.

Ganciclovir is nucleoside analogue of guanosine, it is more active against *cytomegalovirus*. **Vidarabine** is also nucleoside analogue active against *HSV-1*. **Iododeoxyuridine** is nucleoside inhibitor which inhibits replication of viruses. It is given for topical treatment of *HSV*. Another nucleoside inhibitor given for herpes keratoconjunctivitis is trifluorothymidine. **Foscarnet** acts by inhibiting DNA polymerases of herpes viruses and inhibits reverse transcriptase in *HIV*. **Azidothymidine** (AZT, zidovudine) is nucleoside analogue, inhibits DNA synthesis by enzyme reverse transcriptase. It is drug of choice for HIV. **Deoxyinosine** has similar action and used as substitute in patients resistant to AZT. Another substitute for AZT is **dideoxycytidine.**

Ribavirin is nucleoside analogue which inhibits synthesis of guanine. Aerosol form of it is prescribed in respiratory syncytial virus infection and also treatment of influenza B infection.

Diagnosis of Viral Infections

When is specific diagnosis needed?

- Screening of blood donors for *HIV* and *hepatitis B* and *hepatitis C virus*.
- Pregnant women, e.g. *rubella, HIV*.
- Specific therapy, e.g. eye lesions, herpetic encephalitis.
- To find out the etiology of vague syndromes, e.g. aseptic meningitis.
- Epidemics, outbreaks: To perform seroepidemiological studies.
- Discovery of new viral infections, e.g. antigenic variants of influenza, *SARS*.
- Confirming the viral diseases for which specific therapy is available.

Viral Diagnosis (Flowchart 52.3)

Steps in diagnosis include: Samples collection, transport and processing which is done by microscopy, antigen detection, isolation of virus, antibody detection, and molecular methods.

Flowchart 52.3: Viral diagnosis

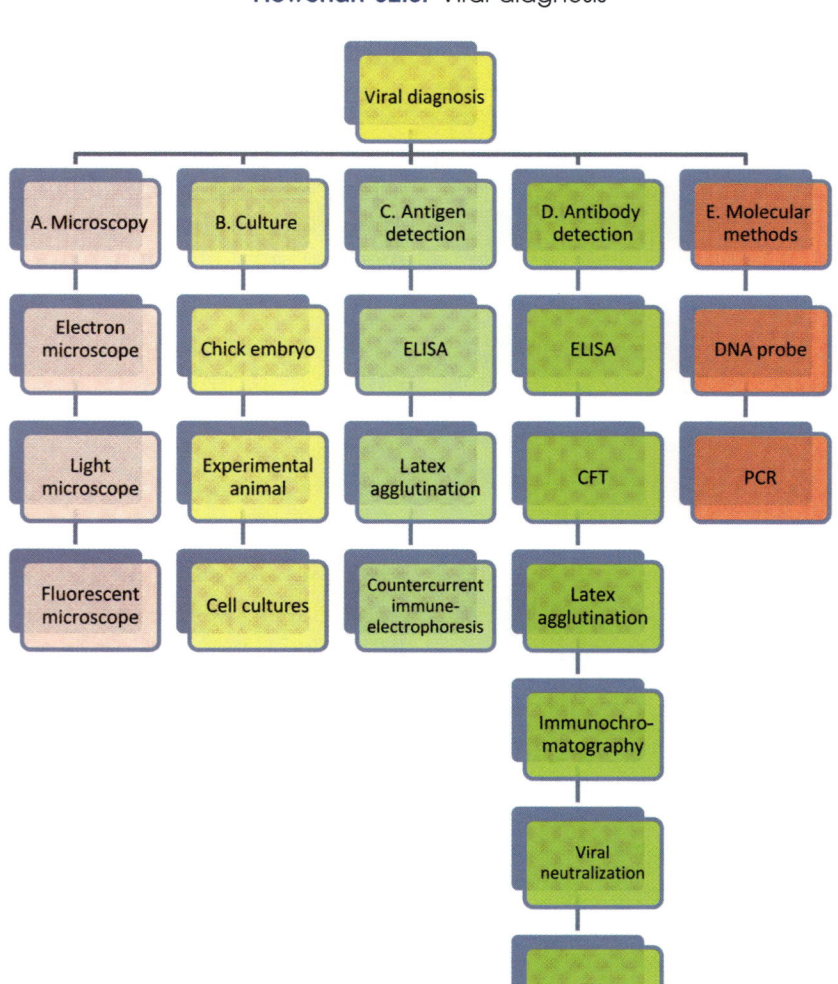

A. Samples Collection

Samples collected depend upon the infections suspected, stage of disease and tests available.

For example, in case of polio, stool samples are collected along with throat swab to confirm the diagnosis by culture, while serum is collected for detection of antibodies.

In hepatitis A infection, during early stage virus is present in stool sample, while in later stage serum collected for antibodies detection.

B. Transport and Storage of Specimens

- Sterile, leak-proof containers are used.
- Minimal interval shoud be there between collection and processing of specimens.
- *Transport media*: Viral transport medium (VTM): If **culture** is to be performed, VTM is used, even if **PCR** is to be performed on specimens other than blood, VTM used, e.g. nasopharyngeal secretions for the diagnosis of *H1N1*.
- Viral infusion broth (VIB)
- Sucrose-phosphate-glutamate (SPG)

Storage temperature

a. 4°C for up to 96 hours
b. 70°C beyond 96 hours
c. Repeated cycles of freezing and thawing to be avoided.

C. Direct Examination

1. Electron
  a. Microscopy
  b. Immune
	It is used to study morphology of virus particles
	Electron microscopy

2. Light microscopy	It is used to study histological appearance Inclusion bodies
3. Antigen detection	Immunofluorescence, ELISA, etc.
4. Viral genome detection	Hybridization with specific nucleic acid probes Polymerase chain reaction (PCR)

i. *Electron microscopy*: 10^6 virus particles per ml required for visualization. Viruses may be detected in the following specimens. (Virus particles are detected and identified on the basis of morphology.)

Feces

- *Rotavirus*
- *Adenovirus*
- *Norwalk-like viruses*
- *Astrovirus*
- *Calcivirus*

Vesicle fluid

- *HSV*
- *VZV*
- *Poxvirus*

Skin scrappings

- *Papillomavirus*
- *Orf*

Biopsy: *Molluscum contagiosum*

Brain biopsy: *Herpes simplex* virus infection

Cell culture: EM is used for detection of viral growth in cell cultures.

Uses of electron microscope for the diagnosis of viral infection based upon the morphology.

ii. *Immune electron microscopy (IEM)*: The sensitivity and specificity of EM may be enhanced by immune electron microscopy. Sample is treated with specific anti-sera before being put up for EM. Viral particles present will be agglutinated and thus aggregated together by the antibody, which are then seen under EM.

Advantage: As viral particles are concentrated in the specimens, sensitivity increases.

Disadvantage: In normal EM, when we observe stool for rota virus, we may detect other viruses present in stool, this is called "**catch all phenomenon**" which is lost in IEM.

iii. *Fluorescent microscopy*: Using monoclonal antibodies viral antigen is detected on cell surface or within cells infected by viruses.

Uses of fluorescent microscope:

- **Use in antimortem diagnosis of rabies:** Skin scrapings from nape of neck are taken on slide or corneal impression smears are taken on glass slide to which rabies antibody coated with a fluorescent dye is attached. The smear is observed under fluorescent microscope.
- Diagnosis of herpes simplex encephalitis on brain biopsy specimen is done.
- Diagnosis of adenovirus infection.
- Diagnosis of orthomyxoviruses and paramyxoviruses.
- Detection of viral growth in cell cultures.

iv. *Light microscopy*: Detection of viral inclusion bodies or cytopathic effects in cell or tissues is done by light miscroscopy.

- Diagnosis of rabies is made by demonstration of Negri bodies in histopathological specimens from brain.
- *Tzank smear*: It is used for the detection of multi-nucleated cell for diagnosis of herpes infection from

vesicular fluid. It is performed by staining material from vesicular scrapings with Giemsa, H and E or Papanicolaou stain or toludine. Multinucleated giant cells are seen with the nuclei having a ground-glass and multifaceted appearance.

- H and E stained smear from kidney biopsy is used for demonstration of owl's eye type of inclusion body in infection with *CMV*.
- Demonstration of syncytial formation is used for diagnosis of parainfluenza viruses.
- Light microscopy is used to observe cytopathic effects in tissue cultures.

v. *Immunologic detection of viral antigens*

a. *Immunofluorescence*: Herpes group viruses, e.g. detection of *HSV*, *VZV*, and *CMV*. Specimens: Vesicular lesions (for *HSV*), BAL (for *CMV* pneumonia), leukocyte fraction from blood (for *CMV* antigenemia)

b. *ELISA*: For example, detection of p24 antigen of *HIV* virus during window period; detection of HBsAg in **serum sample** for *HBV*.

D. Detection of Antibodies

With some assays such as EIA, RIA and neutralization, one can look specifically for IgM or IgG.

Other assays such as CFT and hemagglutination inhibition (HAI), one can only detect total antibody, which comprises mainly IgG.

Newer techniques, such as enzyme immune assays (EIAs), offer better sensitivity, specificity and reproducibility than classical techniques, such as CFT and HAI.

Simple, rapid tests based on immunochromatography are available for detection of antibodies against dengue, *HIV*.

Western Blot is used for detection of HIV specific antibodies which is a confirmatory test for HIV diagnosis.

E. Molecular Techniques

Nucleic acid hybridization: Cloned fragments of DNA or RNA that are complementary to the viral nucleic acid of interest (molecular probe) carrying either an enzyme or a radioactive marker can be directly reacted with a tissue specimen. These techniques can be performed either *in situ* on tissue section or in a test tube. After separating the unreacted nucleic acid from the mixture, the hybridized nucleic acid is quantitated either by measuring radioactivity or the color generated from the enzyme-labeled substrate.

DNA probes are available for the diagnosis *of CMV, papilloma virus, Epstein-Barr virus* in clinical specimens.

DNA probes are also used for detection of viral growth in cell cultures.

Nucleic acid amplification

- **PCR** is used for diagnosis of *HIV* especially in window period and for early infant diagnosis.
- **PCR** available for the diagnosis for *HSV, CMV, HPV, rotavirus, measles virus, HCV*.

Cultivation of viruses

- *Animals*: Suckling mice, rats, monkeys, chimpanzees are used for cultivation.
  Mice: It is used for *coxsackie* and *arbovirus*.
- *Embryonated eggs*: The various routes used are CAM, allantoic cavity, amniotic sac and yolk sac.
  1. CAM: It shows visible pocks, different viruses have different pock morphology. Each infectious virus particle forms a single pock.
  2. Amniotic cavity is used for *influenza and mumps*.
  3. Allantoic cavity is used for *influenza, mumps, newcastle diease virus*.
  4. Yolk sac is used for *herpes simplex virus*.

Tissue culture

Organ culture or explant or cell culture.

Cell culture—three types:

1. *Organ culture*: Small bits of organ, preserving their original architecture and function used, for highly specialized virus of certain organ, e.g. tracheal ring for *coronavirus*.
2. *Explant culture*: Fragments of minced tissue, grown as explants embedded in plasma clots, e.g. adenoid tissue explant cultue for *adenovirus*.
3. *Cell culture*: Tissues dissociated into component cells by the action of proteolytic enzymes like trypsin or mechanical shaking, cells are washed, counted and suspended in growth medium.

Medium for cell culture is Eagle's minimum essential medium (MEM).

a. *Primary cell culture:* Normal cells freshly taken from body and cultured (kidney or lung), these cells are maintained for limited (1 or 2) passages, e.g. primary nonkey, human amnion. They are used for *influenza, parainfluenza*, some *enteroviruses*.

b. *Diploid cell strains:* They retain original diploid chromosome number and karyotype; limited passages possible (<50 to 70), e.g. human diploid fibroblast: *HSV, CMV, VZV, rhinoviruses* can be cultured on them.

c. *Continuous cell lines derived from* cancer cells; continuous passage in vitro is possible, e.g. HeLa, HEp-2 used for *adenovirus, RSV*.

Methods for Detection of Viral Growth

Cytopathic effect: Different cytopathic effects are rounding, swelling, shrinking, granular appearance, glassy appearance, cell fusion causing formation of multinucleated giant cells, cell death, cell rounding or degeneration or/and aggregation.

a. *Influenza virus* causes enlarged granular cells.

b. *Parainfluenza virus* causes focal rounding and multinucleated giant cells.

c. *RSV* and *measles* form syncytial (Fig. 52.3), giant cells or granular rounded cells.

d. *Mumps* virus produces syncytial giant cells.

e. *Adenovirus*: Enlarged, clustered cells produced (bunches or grapes are produced).

f. Inclusion bodies may present in the nucleus or cytoplasm.

Metabolic inhibition: Viruses when growing inside the cell cultures, they inhibit the metabolism of cells.

Hemadsorption: For hemagglutinating viruses (influenza and parainfluenza), viral growth is indicated by adsorption of erythrocyte on to the surface of cell.

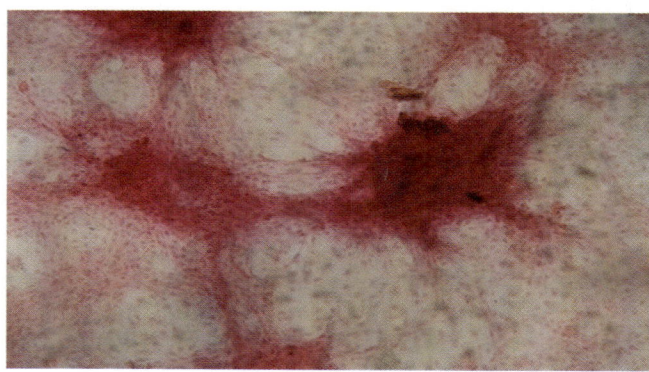

Fig. 52.3: Cytopathic effects of measles (syncytial formation)

Interference: The growth of noncytopathic virus in culture tested by challenge with known cytopathic virus, growth of first will inhibit infection by the second virus by interference.

Transformation: Some viruses transform normal cell into tumor cells leading to formation of tumor cells.

Immunofluorescence: Direct immunofluorescence is used for detection of antigen in tissue cultures. It detects viral growth in cell culture quite early. It is sensitive and specific test.

53

Bacteriophage

Bacteriophages are the viruses which live on bacteria.

Significance of Bacteriophages

- Bacteriophages can be grown easily on bacteria; they act as model to study host parasite relationship at molecular level and cellular level.
- Bacteriophages transfer genetic information from one bacterium to another by a process called *transduction*.
- By transduction, bacteriophages transfer multiple drug resistance amongst bacteria.
- Also by transduction, bacteriophages transfer the property of production of toxin. Hence a bacterium will produce toxin, if it is infected with tox virus. This conversion of non-toxigenic bacteria to toxigenic bacteria is called **lysogenic conversion**.
- The presence of phage genome integrated with bacterial genome gives bacteria some properties by a process called *phage conversion*.
- As bacteriophages live on bacteria, they reduce the burden of bacteria in environment. The water of Ganga is free of vibrios because of presence of vibriophages.
- Bacteriophage typing method is used epidemio-logically to find out source of infection, which helps in investigation of outbreaks.
- Bacteriophage typing is used for differentiation of a bacterial species into subtypes.
- Bacteriophage typing using Mukerjee's phage IV is used for differentiation of classical and El-Tor biotypes of *Vibrio cholerae.*

Morphology

'T' phages are bacteriophages live on *E. coli,* and act as model to study bacteriophage.

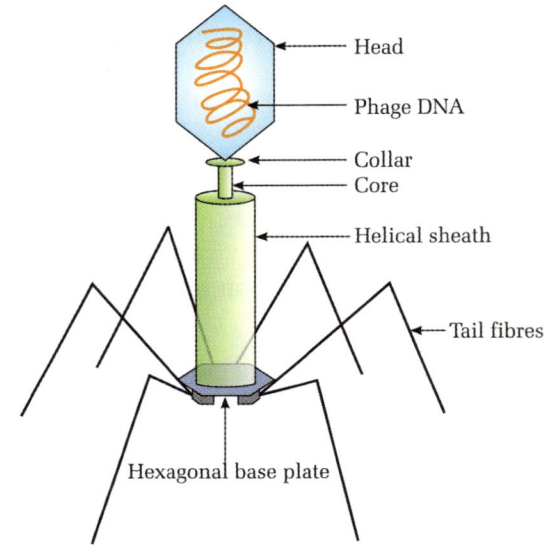

Fig. 53.1: Structure of bacteriophage

- It has head which is hexagonal, with core of double-stranded DNA surrounded by capsid (Fig. 53.1).
- Size is variable, from 28–100 nm.
- Tale which is cylindrical, central portion is hollow called core is surrounded by contractile sheath. The terminal part is base which has hook-like structures called prongs and tale fibers (Fig. 53.1).

Bacteriophage shows two types of life cycles, i.e. **lytic cycle** in which bacteriophages multiply inside the bacterial cell resulting into bacterial cell lysis while in **lysogenic cycle** or temperate cycle, DNA of bacteriophage integrates with host cell genome and replicates with host cell genome.

Lytic Cycle (Fig. 53.2)

Steps of multiplication of bactriophages are adsorption, penetration, biosynthesis, assembly and release.

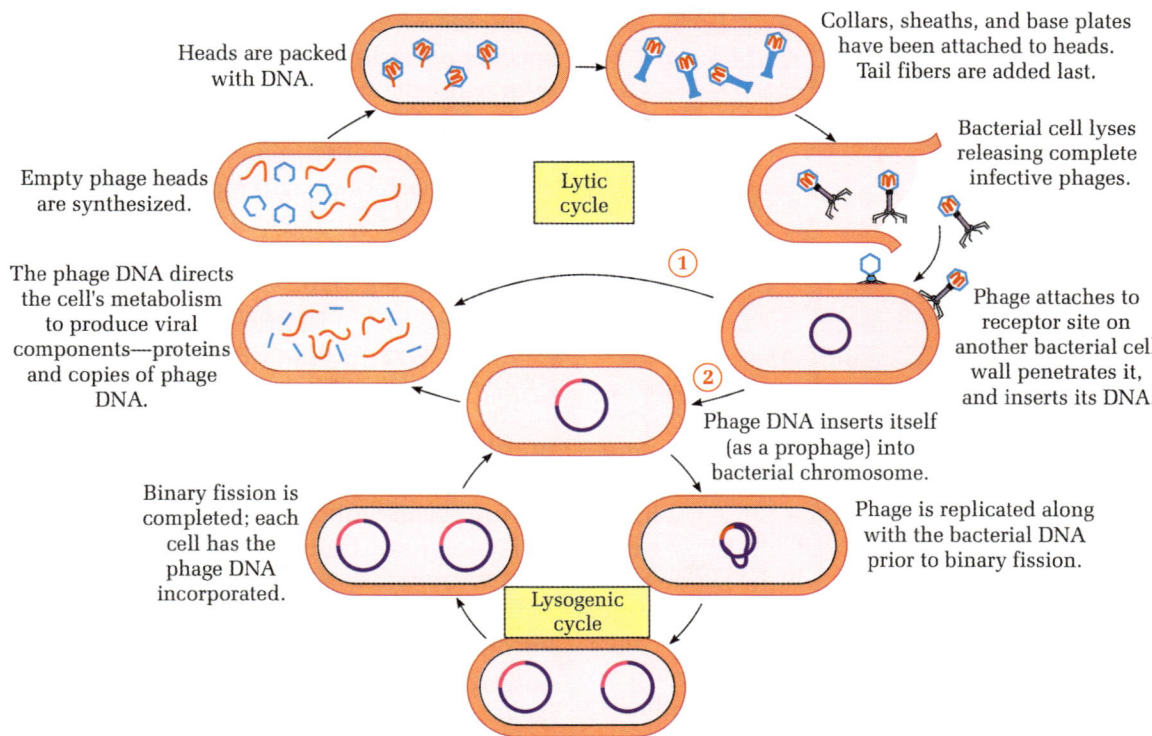

Fig. 53.2: Life cycle of bacteriophage

Adsorption: A bacteriophage attaches to bacterium by tail, it is a specific step. The attachment is brought out by complementary structures present on phage similar to receptors on bacterium (either on cell wall or flagella or pili).

Bacteriophage of one bacterium is specific for that bacterium and does not attach to human cells. Different parts of cell wall or other structures as flagellum, fimbria act as receptors of bacteria for bacteriophage. For example bacteriophages of *Salmonella* are used for typing of *Salmonella* and they attach to Vi antigen present on certain strains of *S. typhi*. In some bacteria, the sites for the attachment are present on flagella or fimbria. If attachement step is bypassed by some means (e.g. injection of phage DNA into cell) infection of other wise non-susceptible bacteria will also occur. The naked bacteriophage DNA can infect the bacterium, a process called **transfection.**

Penetration: The bacteriophage gets firmly attached to cell with the help of basal plate and tail fibers. When contractile sheath contracts and lysozyme present on tail dissolves bacterial cell wall, thus helping the phage to enter cell.

Biosynthesis: After penetration, biosynthesis starts, early proteins are formed, they act as enzymes necessary for biosynthesis of viral proteins called late proteins. Synthesis of head, tail occurs. As bacteriophage is devoid of synthetic machinery, it will use the bacterial machinery. In this time, bacterial DNA or RNA synthesis will not occur.

Maturation: The newly formed DNA is packed into head, tail attaches, thus mature phages become ready to come out.

Release: Phage enzymes act on already weakened cell wall resulting in cell lysis and release of progeny phages.

Eclipse phase: The time between entry of phages nucleic acid and appearance of first intracellular phage particle by maturation is called elipse phase. It is time required from synthesis to maturation.

The nature of cellular receptors for animal viruses is known for only few viruses. Once the adsorption has occurred, the entire virion or substructure containing viral genome and virion polymerases must be translocated across the plasma membrane.

Latent period: It is the interval between infection of bacterium with phage and appearance of first extracellular phage particle.

Like bacterial growth curve, if we plot a graph between numbers of infectious phage particles released against time in minutes after infection of bacterium, one step **growth curve** will be obtained. This has latent period followed by **rise period** in which number of extracellular phages increase (Fig. 53.3).

The average number of new phage particles produced per bacterium is called **burst size.**

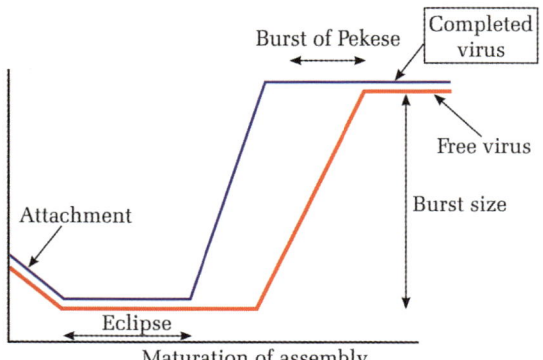

Fig. 53.3: Bacteriophage growth curve

Lysogenic cycle: A special type of bacteriophage enters bacterial cell. Its DNA integrates with host cell nucleus forming prophage (integrated phage DNA) which multiplies synchronously with host DNA. A new characterisric is given by phage DNA which is known as 'lysogenic conversion'. Example, Diphtheria bacterium produces toxin when it is infected with a bacteriophage encoding gene for its toxin production. If the bacterium is made free from that phage (in presence of specific phage antiserum), the bacterium will become nontoxic. When a bacterium is infected with bacteriophage, it resists infection with bacteriophage until the first bacteriophage is cleared. This is called **infection immunity.** It resembles with premunition immunity seen in other infections as malaria or syphilis.

Bacteriophage Typing (Figs 53.4 and 53.5)

This method is used to classify a bacterium below species level. It helps in identification of common source of infection in epidemics. Bacterial strains are identified by type specific phages.

Procedure of Bacteriophage Typing

A lawn culture of bacterium is made. The bacterial colonies are emulsified in saline and spread over a plate by either flooding method or swabbing method.

But before the incubation of bacterial culture plate, specific bacteriophages are applied on the same plate over various areas. The sites where bacteriophages multiply, they will lyse bacteria and form a clear area called 'plaque' after incubation.

Which bacteriophages form plaques are the bacteriophage type of the bacterium; for example, perform a lawn culture of *Staphylococcus aureus* and apply phage types 50, 51, 80, 81, 82 and if the clearing is seen where 50, 51 and 80 are applied and clearing is not seen around where 81 and 82 are applied, the phage type of this strain of *Staphylococcus aureus* is 50, 51, 80.

The lysis is influenced by the dose of virus. Phage preparations should be standardized by titration in which serial dilutions of phage are applied on a lawn culture of susceptible bacterium.

The highest dilution of phage producing confluent lysis is known as **'routine test dose' (RTD).**

Bacteriophage typing of *Staphylococcus aureus* is performed at Maulana Azad Medical College, New Delhi.

Phage typing is used for following bactria: Salmonella *typhi,* Bacillus anthracis, *Classical and El-Tor biotypes of* Vibrio cholerae.

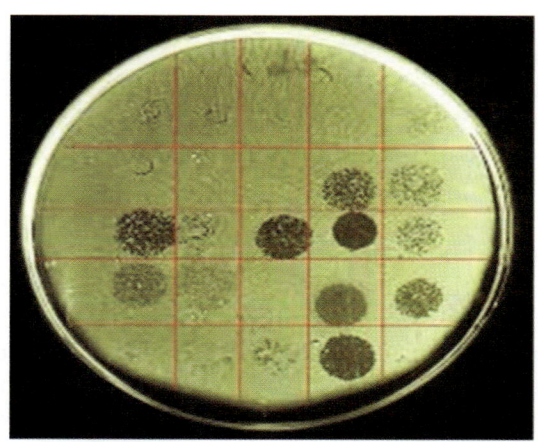

Fig. 53.4: Bacteriophage typing

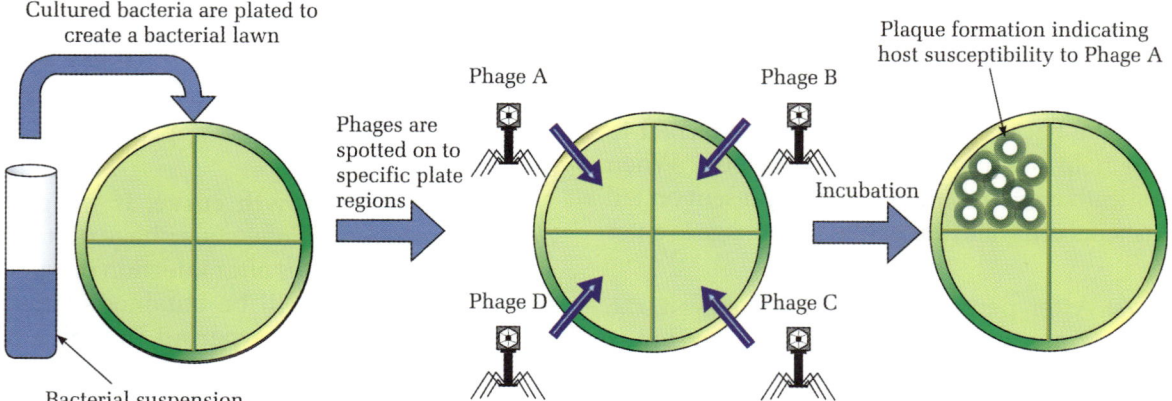

Fig. 53.5: Steps of bacteriophage typing method

54

Adenovirus

They belong to family Adenoviridae, genus Mastadeno-virus. The mastadenoviruses cause infection of mammals. Members of the genus aviadenoviruses cause infection in birds. The name *adenovirus* was given because they were first isolated from adenoids. *Adeno-viruses* are further classified based on hemagglutinating properties and DNA homology.

About **51 serotypes** have been isolated from humans of which only one-third known serotypes cause human infections. Some of the serotypes are used for cancer induction in animals. *Adenoviruses* are also used as vector **for gene therapy**.

Structure (Fig. 54.1)

- These are non-enveloped viruses with a diameter of 70–75 nm.
- The genome is made of linear, double-stranded (ds) DNA with 2 major proteins, 26–45 kbp. It is infectious.
- The capsid is icosahedral, comprised of 252 capsomeres. 240 are hexons; at the vertices are 12 pentons, from which a fiber with a terminal knob projects the virus, morphologically the virus looks like **space vehicle.**
- The penton base carries a substance which has a toxin like action that causes rapid appearance of cytopathic effects and detachment of cells from surface on which they are growing. The fibres are also associated with hemagglutination activity.

Host Range and Cultivation

They are host specific and do not grow in other animals. *Adenoviruses* isolated from humans are classified into groups A to F.

Cell cultures used are **HeLa, HEp-2:** Cells become rounded and aggregate into grape-like clusters. These viruses take several days to grow. The infected cells do not lyse even though they round up.

Resistance

They remain viable at 37°C for 7 days. As they do not have envelope, they are also resistant to bile salts, ethers or other organic solvents.

Antigenic Structure

They have **group specific antigen** present on **hexon protein** and **type specific** antigen is associated **with polypeptide of fibre**. The group specific antigen is detected by ELISA test and type specific antigen is detected by neutralization.

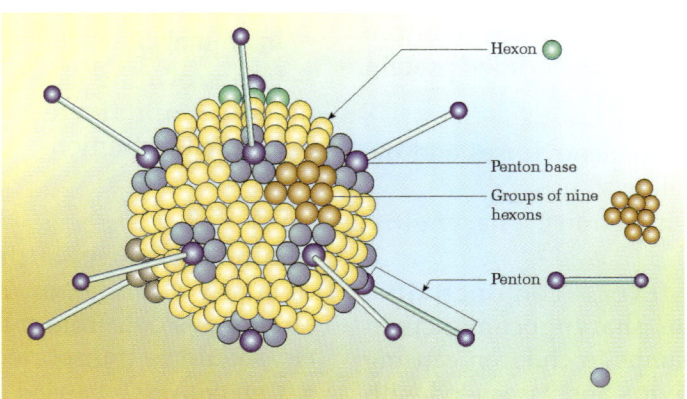

Fig. 54.1: Structure of adenovirus

Classification Scheme of Adenoviruse

Group	Serotype	Hemagglutination		Tumorogenicity in vivo	Transformation of cells
		Group	Result		
A	12, 18, 31	Iv	None	High	+
B	3, 7, 11, 14, 16, 21, 34, 35, 50	I	Monkey	Moderate	+
C	1, 2, 5, 6	III	Rat	Low or none	+
D	8–10, 13, 15, 17, 19, 20, 22–30, 32, 33, 36–3, 942–49, 51	II	Rat	Low or none	+
E	4	III	Rat	Low or none	+
F	40, 41	III	Rat	Low or none	+

Clinical Syndromes

Almost half of adenoviral infections are subclinical. Most infections are self-limited. The subclinical infections produce type-specific immunity. Incubation period is 2–14 days; for gastroenteritis, it is usually 3–10 days.

Transmission: Modes of infection are droplets, feco-oral route (direct and through poorly chlorinated water) and fomites. Adenovirus outbreaks are seasonal. Respiratory diseases mainly occur in late winter through early summer. Pharyngoconjunctival and epidemic keratoconjunctivitis (EKC) infections occur in the summer months, while gastrointestinal disease does not seem to be seasonal.

Pathogenicity

Virus **attaches to mucosal cells** of respiratory tract; gastrointestinal tract by **knob-like structure-fibre**. The host cell receptor is **CAR (coxsackie adenovirus receptor).**

Virus Effects on Host Defence Mechanisms

The small, abundant **VA DNA** affords protection from interferon by preventing activation of an interferon inducible **kinase.** Adenovirus **E3 region proteins inhibit cytolysis** of infected cell by host defences. The **E3 gp 19 kDa protein** blocks movement of MHC class I to cell surface, thus protecting the infected cell from action of cytotoxic (TC) cells. Other **E3-encoded protein blocks** induction of cytolysis by TNF-α.

Various infections caused by adenoviruses and the associated serotypes are as follows:
- Upper respiratory tract infections: Pharyngitis, tonsillitis—1 to 7.
- Pharyngoconjunctival fever, conjunctivitis, pharyngitis—3, 7, 14. The pharyngoconjunctival fever occurs in summer camps in children causing **swimming pool conjunctivitis** and associated with serotypes 3, 7, and 14.

- **Epidemic keratoconjunctivitis** is highly contagious condition caused by serotype 8 (it spread in Australia from Haiwaiian islands). It spreads through shipwards hence called **'shipward'** eye. Fever, conjunctivitis may be followed by keratitis and periauricular lymphadenopathy, other serotypes which may cause this are 19, 37.
- **Acute respiratory distress:** 4, 7, 21.
- Lower respiratory tract infections (LRI): Bronchitis, pneumonia, fever, cough: 3, 7.
- Pneumonia: It is severe in young children and infants—(7) serotype, 3, 7 in adults
- *Pertussis-like syndrome*: Fever, paroxysmal cough, post-tussive vomiting—5.
- Acute follicular or hemorrhagic conjunctivitis: 3, 7.
- Hemorrhagic cystitis: 11, 21
- Gastrointestinal disease—40, 41 cause infantine diarrhea.
- Adenovirus type 12 (Ad 12) has been implicated in development of **celiac disease.** The development of disease appears to depend on protein sequence homology between **Ad 12** an early protein and **A-glidin**, a component of certain grains that activate the disease. It has been suggested that exposure to Ad12 induces antibody response to A-glidin, which predisposes to the disease. (Adenovirus 12 virus was the first DNA containing virus shown to cause cancer in animals.)

Overcrowding causes outbreaks. Out breaks are noted in military recruits, swimming pool users, residential institutions, hospitals, day care centers, etc.

Diagnosis

Clinical specimens, such as swabs (nasopharyngeal, conjunctival, rectal, or other) and washings, corneal scrapings, stool, urine or biopsy and autopsy materials, etc. should be transported in **viral transport medium.**
- Cell culture is carried out in HeLa and human fetal diploid cells.

- Cytopathic effects include swelling and rounding of cells. Cells may become refractile and clustered into irregular clumps.
- Infection of adenovirus detection is made rapid by **shell vial culture**. Viral specimens are centrifuged directly on to tissue culture cells; cultures are incubated 1–2 days and then tested by monoclonal antibodies against group reactive epitope on hexon.
- Viral growth in cell culture is detected by CFT, HA, neutralization.
- Isolation of virus from a pharyngeal specimen is more suggestive of a current clinical infection than from fecal specimen.
- Rapid detection of serotypes 40, 41 is done by **ELISA or immunofluorescence antibody** method.
- Other detection methods in current use include **electron microscopy, polymerase chain** reaction and **nucleic acid probes**.
- Fastidious adenoviruses (enteric viruses) can be detected by **EM, latex agglutination**. With difficulty they can be isolated in a line of human embryomic kidney cells transformed with a fragment of adenovirus 5 DNA.
- Serology is mainly used for epidemiologic studies. The tests for the detection of antibodies include CFT, HAI, RIA, and neutralization.

Prevention

It includes: Handwashing, contact precautions, respiratory precautions in health care settings. Adequate chlorination of swimming pools. Sterilization or disinfection of ophthalmologic equipment and use of single dose vials of ophthalmic medications.

Vaccine: Live, enteric coated, oral vaccine (types 4, 7, and 21) gives some protection against respiratory disease.

Adenoassociated Virus (AAV) or Adenosatellite Virus

As it is genetically defective virus, it multiplies only along with adenovirus, simultaneously. Types 1, 2, 3 are human origin and type 4 is simian. The pathogenic role of this virus is unknown.

55

Poxviruses

Family **Poxviridae** is classified into two subfamilies: *Chordopoxviridae*, which are poxviruses of vertebrates and *Entemopoxviridae* which are poxviruses of insects, do not cause human infection.

There are some **unclassified poxviruses,** i.e. molluscum contagiosum, tanapox, yabamonkey tumor.

The **subfamily Chordopoxviridae** is classified into six groups as given below.

Orthopoxviruses	These viruses tend to cause generalized infections with rash—*variola, vaccinia, cowpox, monkeypox, rabbitpox, buffalo-pox, camelpox, mousepox*
Parapoxviruses	*Orf* (contagious pustular dermatitis), *paravaccinia* (milker's node, bovine stomatitis)
Capripoxviruses	Sheeppox, goatpox, lumpy skin disease
Leporipox	Myxomas, fibromas of leopards
Avipoxviruses	Viruses of birds—*fowl pox, canarapox, pigeonpox, turkeypox*
Suipoxviruses	*Swinepox*

POXVIRUSES

There are largest viruses infecting the vertebrates.

Variola Virus

Variola virus is causative agent of smallpox.

Smallpox is irradicated. The disease occurred in two clinical forms.

Florid form: It caused severe disease which was highly fatal, it was seen in Asia. This type of disease was caused by **variola major.**

Mild form called alastrim: *Variola minor* caused nonfatal disease; it was seen in Latin America.

Vaccinia Virus (Fig. 55.1)

- Originally Jenner used cowpox vaccine for vaccination against smallpox.
- By arm-to-arm passage in humans over several years led to permanent changes in *cowpox virus.*
- *Vaccinia virus* is an artificial virus.
- As *vaccinia virus* is safer to work with, it was studied in great detail.
- It can be used as a vector for recombinant vaccines. Genome of vaccinia can accommodate about 25,000 foreign base pairs.
- It is used for coding antigens of *HBV, HIV*, rabies and neuropeptides.

Differences between Variola and Vaccinia Viruses

Vaccina virus, the agent used for smallpox vaccination, is distinct species.

Restriction endonuclease pattern shows that they are **distinct from** *cowpox virus* which was believed to its ancestor. At some time after its original use as vaccine, the vaccine virus became *vaccinia virus.*

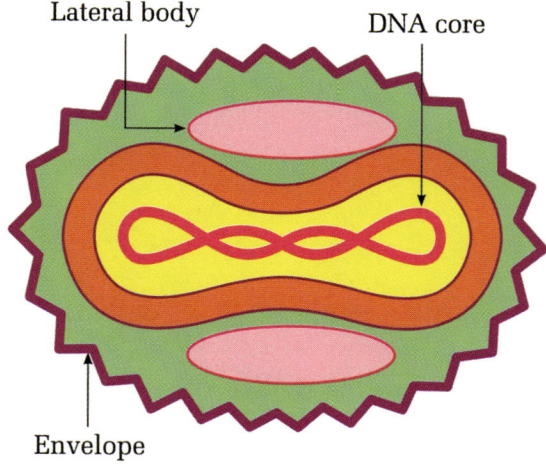

Fig. 55.1: Vaccinia virus

Vaccinia may be the product of genetic recombination, a new species derived from cowpox virus or variola virus by serial passage, or the decedent of new a distinct viral genus.

Variola has narrow host range but *vaccinia* has wide host range that includes rabbits, and mouse, cattle and buffalo. Disease in buffalo is still seen in India. Both viruses grow in CAM of embryonated egg of 10–12 days old, but *variola* produces smaller pocks (Fig. 55.2).

Morphology of Vaccinia Virus

- Size: 300 × 200 × 100 nm in size.
- Virus is brick shaped.
- It has double-layered membrane.
- Virus has biconcave nucleoid containing DNA core.
- There are lens-shaped lateral body on each side of nucleus.
- It produces intracytoplasmic elementary bodies (**Paschen bodies**) in smears from lesions.

Chemical Properties of Poxvirus

- Stable for months at room temperature.
- Stable for years when freeze dried.
- Susceptible to sunlight, UV light and irradiation.
- Inactivated by formalin and oxidizing disinfectants.
- Resistant to 50% glycerol, 1% phenol and ether.

Antigenic structure of poxvirus

- There is a common nucleoprotein antigen for all pox viruses.
- LS antigen (a complex of heat labile and stable antigens).
- Other antigens include agglutinogen and hemagglutinin.

Cultivation and Host Range

Viruses grow on CAM of 11–13-day-old chick embryo. Pocks seen in 48–72 hours. Pocks produced by *variola* are small, shiny, non-necrotic, non-hemorrhagic. *Vaccinia* produce larger pocks which are necrotic and some may produce hemorrhagic pocks.

'Ceiling temperature' is used for identification of viruses. It is the highest temperature of incubation of embryonated eggs which show visible 'pocks'. If the temperature of incubation exceeds ceiling temperature, no growth will be seen. *Vaccinia* virus has the highest ceiling temperature, i.e. 41°C.

Both *variola* and *vaccinia* can be grown in tissue cultures of monkey kidney, HeLa and chick embryo cells. *Vaccinia* viruses are fast growing.

Detection of viral growth in cell culture is done by detecting eosinophilic inclusion bodies (**Guarneri bodies**) in stained preparations.

Animal Inoculation

- *Vaccinia*: Monkeys, calves, sheep and rabbits are infected by scarification.
- *Variola*: Monkeys are used as experimental animals.
- Scarification of rabbit cornea with variola causes keratitis.
- Intranasal instillation of *variola* in monkey causes self-limited attack of smallpox.

Smallpox

- It is exclusively human infection.
- No carriers, patients with clinical disease, patient in early phase (from appearance of buccal mucosal lesions to disappearance of all skin lesions) act as source of infection.
- Infection occurs only in close contacts.

Clinical Features of Smallpox

- Incubation period is 12 days.
- Centrifugal lesions passing through macular, papular, vesicular and pustular stages.
- Lesions heal by scar formation, in 2–4 weeks.
- Exanthems vary in severity.

Laboratory Diagnosis of Smallpox

- Detection of virus antigen.
- Isolation of virus in early phase from blood.
- Isolation in all cases from eruptive lesion.
- Electron microscopy.

Vaccine for Smallpox

Live preparation of vaccinia virus propagated on skin of calves. It is applied by scarification which froms a local pustular lesion, healing takes place by scar formation.

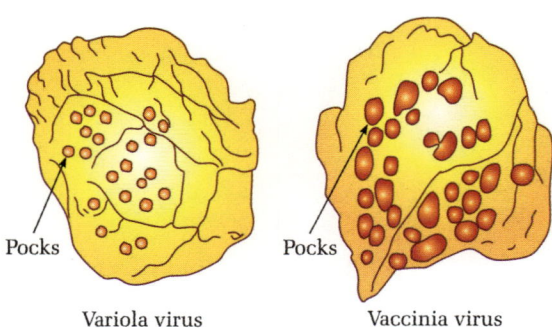

Variola virus   Vaccinia virus

Fig. 55.2: Pocks on CAM

Eradication of Smallpox

Factors contributing to eradication
- Use of freeze-dried vaccine.
- Vaccination by multiple punctures with bifurcated needles which was simple, effective and economical.
- No animal reservoir.
- No human carriers.
- Infection takes place in close contacts.

Global *eradication* of smallpox announced by WHO in May 1980. Last case of *V. major* was found in May 1975 in Assam. While last case of *V. minor* was found in Oct 1977 in Somalia.

Threat of bioterrorism: Last stocks of virus present in CDC Atlanta and Centre for Research on Virology and Biotechnology, Russia. Large stocks of smallpox vaccine are maintained by WHO for rapid development of vaccines in case of emergency.

Monkey Pox

Seen in Central and West Africa. It clinically resembles smallpox. Virus can be distinguished from variola.

Buffalo Pox

Seen in cattle in India. It produces localized lesions on hands of persons in contact with infected animals.

Cowpox

- Lesions are seen in udders and teats of cows.
- Transmitted to humans during milking.
- Lesions are seen on hands and fingers.
- Fever and constitutional symptoms may be present.
- Genetically, distinct from vaccinia.
- It is antigenically related with variola and vaccinia, but can be differentiated by its hemorrhagic pocks and ceiling temperature. Infections are restricted to some geographic areas in UK and Europe.
- The term 'Pseudo-cowpox' is used for paravaccinia virus.

Milker's Node

- Infections are acquired by milking infected cows.
- Small ulcerating nodules develop.
- It resembles *orf virus.*
- It is unrelated to *cowpox.*

Orf Virus

- It causes contagious pustular dermatitis.
- It is a disease of sheep and goats.
- It is transmitted to humans by contact.
- Single papulovesicular lesion with central ulcer appears on hand, forearm or face.

Tanapox

- It is seen in Africa.
- Single pock-like lesion appears in upper part of body.
- Monkeys are the only susceptible animals.

Molluscum Contagiosum

- It is benign epithelial tumor that occurs only in humans.
- *Virus*: The purified virus is oval or brick-shaped and has size about 20×30 nm. Viral genome resembles that of vaccinia. It has G + C content 60%.
- Disease **spreads by direct or indirect contact** (common use of towels, swimming pools).
- **Incubation period** may extend to 6 months.
- Infection is seen in children and young adults, seen as STD in young adults.
- *Lesions*:
  - Pink or pearly white wart-like nodules.
  - Distribution of lesions: Lesions are present on face, arms, back, buttocks.
  - They are rarely found on palms, soles, on mucosal membranes.
- Lesion on moist areas may resemble with that of *herpes simplex* viruses, may become secondary infected and ulcerated.
- Humans are only susceptible host.
- Virus cannot be grown in eggs, tissue or animals.

Laboratory Diagnosis

I. **Histopathology** (Fig. 55.3): The semisolid caseous material can be expressed and used for diagnosis by histopathology (H and E). Sections show large eosinophilic inclusion bodies displacing nucleus to margins. Molluscum bodies composed of virus particles in protein matrix.

II. **Electron microscope** can detect pox-like particles.

III. PCR can detect viral DNA sequences.

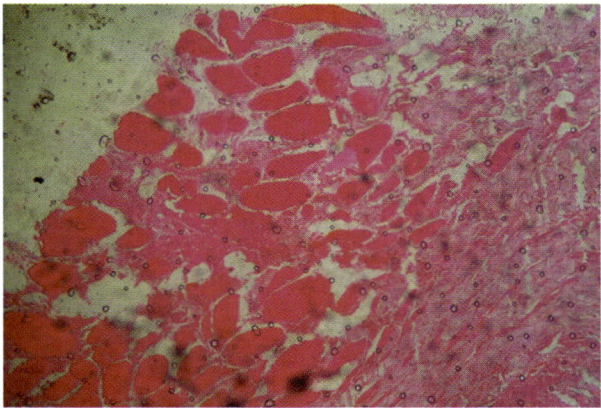

Fig. 55.3: Histopathological staining showing pink molluscum bodies

56

Herpes Viruses

Herpes viruses are leading cause of human viral disease. These viruses have ability to cause overt disease or remain silent for many years and get reactivated. This type of infection is called **latent infection**. Herpes comes from the Latin word *herpes* which, in turn, comes from the Greek word *'herpein'* which means to creep. There are at least 25 viruses in the family **Herpesviridae.**

Viral Structure (Morphology) (Fig. 56.1)

- *Size*: 150–200 nm
- *Core*: Herpes viruses have a core of double-stranded DNA (125–240 kbp).
- *Capsid*: Capsid surrounds core, total 162 capsomeres are present.
- *Symmetry*: Icosahedral
- **Envelope** is made up of glycoproteins (envelope is derived from nuclear membrane of host cell nucleus), it has glycoprotein spikes about 8 nm.

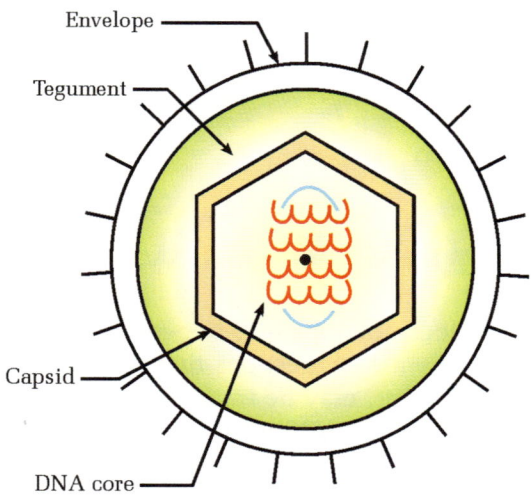

Fig. 56.1: Structure of HSV

- *Tegument*: It is an amorphous substance present between capsid and envelope.
- Replication takes place in nucleus, progeny viruses bud from nuclear membrane.

Replication

Virus fuses with plasma membrane, viral DNA is released from capsid at nuclear pore, transcription of early genes occur, replicate in the nucleus and form intranuclear bodies (**Cowdry type 'A' inclusion bodies**). They are called **Lipseutz bodies.** Several herpes viruses bind to cell surface **glycosaminoglycans, principally heparan** suface. Viral attachment also involves several **coreceptors,** i.e. members of immunoglobulin super-family.

These viruses express many micro-RNAs which are small single-stranded RNAs and they function after transcription to regulate gene expression. It is predicted that these **viral micro-RNAs** are important in regulating entry into or exit from (or both) the latent phase of virus life cycle and may be attractive targets for furture therapy.

Herpes simplex **glycoproteins**: Major glycoproteins are gB–I .Three of the glycoproteins are essential for production of infectious virions, gB, gD are involved in adsorption to and penetration into cells, and gH causes in release of viruses. Some of the glycoproteins have common antigenic determinants shared by HSV1-HSV2 (gD, gB).

Classification of Herpes Viruses

Subfamilies include:

- *Alpha herpesviridae* (Table 56.1): There are fast growing, cytolytic viruses that cause infection of neurons.

TABLE 56.1: Classification of Herpesviridae family

	Alpha herpesviridae	Beta herpesviridae	Gamma herpesviridae
Growth cycle	Fast replicating (12–18 hrs), cytolytic Variable host range Latent infection in sensory ganglion Cytopathic effects develop fast Released from cells	Slowly replicating Narrow host range Latent infection in salivary glands, kidneys, lymphoid tissue Produce cytomegaly. Difficult to grow Associated with cells	Variable Narrow host range Lymphoid tissue —

TABLE 56.2: Properties of different herpes viruses

Official name	Common name	Subfamily	Cytopathy	Site of latency
Human herpes simplex 1	Herpes simplex virus 1	Alpha	Cytolytic	Neurons
Human herpes simplex 2	Herpes simplex virus 2	Alpha	Cytolytic	Neurons
Human herpes simplex 3	Varicella zoster virus	Alpha	Cytolytic	Neurons
Human herpes simplex 4	Epstein-Barr virus	Gamma	Lymphoproliferative	Lymphoid tissue
Human herpes simplex 5	Cytomegalovirus	Beta	Cytomegalic	Secretory glands, kidneys, other organs
Human herpes simplex 6	Human B cell lymphotropic virus	Beta	Lymphoproliferative	Lymphoid tissue
Human herpes simplex 7	RK virus	Beta	Lymphoproliferative	Lymphoid tissue
Human herpes simplex 8		Gamma		

- **Beta herpesviridae** are slow growing, may be cytomegalic, and become latent in salivary glands, kidneys, other lymphoid tissue. **CMV** is classified into *Cytomegalovirus* **genus**. This subfamily also includes genus *Roseolavirus* which has two species, i.e. *HHV6 and HHV7*. (They are similar to gamma herpes viridae as they infect T cells, molecular analysis shows that they are different.)

- *Gamma herpesviridae*: They infect and become latent in lymphoid cells. The genus include *EBV*. It also includes *HHV8*.

Viral Persistance and Latency (Table 56.2)

Viral latency is a part of life cycle of herpes viruses (Fig. 56.2). The processes involved in latency are not understood properly. Some aspects are studied in *EBV*, *herpes simplex*.

Latency in *EBV* requires expression of a complex array of viral gene products. In infected B cell, EBV genes are expressed from widely separated regions of genome. One of these genes, latent infection membrane protein—LMP-1, is present that has receptor for TNF alpha. Some of these genes participate in transformation of B cells in culture. In particular, **latent infection membrane protein-LMP-1** has receptor for **TNF-α**. This interaction prevents TNF-α mediated apoptosis, which ensures cell survival. Cells that express LMP-1 on their surface form tumors in immunodeficient mice.

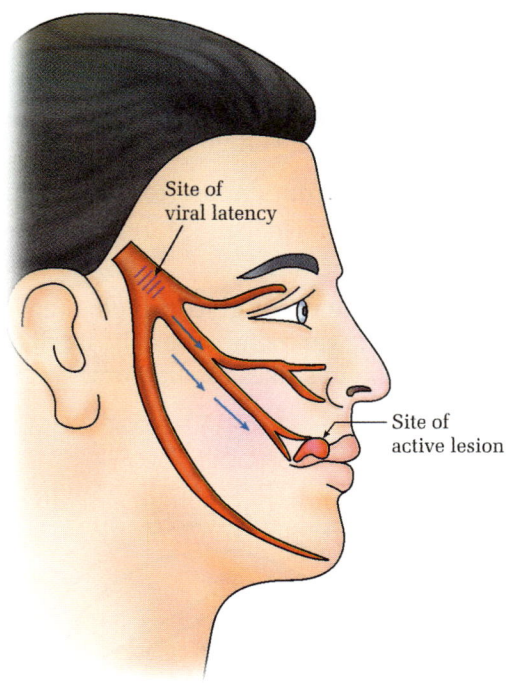

Site of viral latency

Site of active lesion

Fig. 56.2: Latency in HS-VSV-1

Latency does not appear to depend on virus-coded proteins. There are suggestions that **RNA transcripts, in lieu of proteins, may be involved in latency. Such RNA molecules may inhibit the replication pathway**, thus favouring the establishment of latency. Virus-derived mRNA transcripts are found in latently infected neurons.

(Two RNA latency associated transcripts that overlap the immediate early gene products called,**CP-O** are found in large amount in nuclei of latency infected neurons.)

How the infected ganglions are protected from host defences?

- Infected neurons avoid immune recognization and killing by lymphocytes by various mchanisms.
- Part of each infected neuron is protected by blood–brain barrier; most of each axon is sheathed in myelin layers which further protect neurons from immune recognization.
- In addition, **neurons do not routinely express class I or II MHC antigens**.
- Some herpes viruses express **proteins that block production of MHC antigens**.
- Other herpes virus proteins **block the release or activity of cytokines** that would normally aid lymphocytes in clearing virus infected cells.

Reactivation

It is suggested that herpes DNA passes along the nerve axon back to the nerve ending where infection of epithelial cells occur. Not all reactivation will result in a visible lesion; there may be asymptomatic shedding of the virus, only detected by culture.

An increase in CD8 suppressor cell activity is common at the time of recurrences.

Spread of the viruses may be enhanced by some mediators, e.g. prostaglandins, and a temporary decrease in immune effector function, particularly delayed hypersensitivity.

There may be local increase in levels of protaglandins following triggering stimuli of recurrences. Depression of CMI predisposes for herpes recurrences. However, it is achieved, latency is feature of HSV infection. Sometimes it occurs naturally by a variety of stimuli as sunlight, trauma, and stress. The interval between stimulus and apperance of lesions is 2–5 days.

HERPES SIMPLEX VIRUS (HSV-1 AND HSV-2)

The two viruses crossreact serologically but some unique protein exits for each type. HSV growth cycle proceeds rapidly in 8–6 hours. The genome is large (150 kbp) and encodes at least 70 polypeptides. At least 8 glycoproteins are present among viral late genome products. One **(Gd)** is potent inducer of neutralizing antibodies. The **glycoprotein 'G'** is a complement binding protein. Glycoprotein 'G' is type specific and allows discrimination between HSV1 and HSV2 (Table 56.3).

TABLE 56.3: Differentiation between HSV-1 and HSV-2

HSV-1	HSV-2
Small pocks on CAM, replicate poorly in chick embryo fibroblast	Larger pocks, replicate well in chick cell embryo fibroblast
Latency—trigeminal ganglion	Latency—sacral ganglion
Transmission by contact (saliva)	Sexually transmitted
G + C content 67%	69%
Infectivity is not temperature sensitive	Infectivity is more temperature sensitive
Not nurovirulent	More neurovirulent in laboratory animals
Resistance less common	More resistant to antivirals

BOX 56.1: Pathogenesis of HSV

- Typical lesion of herpes virus is vesicle, degeneration of cells lead to ballooning of intraepithelial cells.
- Mononuclear cellular reaction is usual with vesicular fluid becoming cloudy and cellular infiltration in subepithelial tissue.
- The basal layer is intact (as lesion rarely invades subepithelial layers).
- Base of lesion contains multinucleated giant cells, infected nuclei contain eosinophilic inclusions which can demonstrated in Tzank' smear.
- This occur rapidly on mucous membranes and non-keratinized epithelia, on skin the vesicle breaks to form ulcer.
- The ulcer crusts, scab formation takes place followed by healing.
- After resorption or loss of vesicular fluid, the regeneration of epithelium takes place.
- NK cells form early defenses of body, they recognize and destroy viruses.
- Herpes glycoproteins are synthesized during early growth get inserted in host cell membranes, some are secreted into extracellular fluid.
- Cytotoxic cells-(Tc) are important in recovery as they form CMI.
- During replication of viruses at the site of entry, viral particles enter sensory nerve endings which penetrated to parabasal layer of epithelium and transported (probably as nucleocapsid), along axons to neuron in the sensory ganglion by retrograde axonal spread.
- Virus replication in some ganglia causes latent infection.

Pathology

Herpes simplex viruses cause cell lysis and produce inflammation. Lesions produced in skin and mucosa are same, the changes induced in primary and recurrent infections are same but vary in severity.

HSV-1: HSV-1 produces lesions in and around mouth. It is transmitted by direct contact or droplet infection from carriers or patients.

HSV-2: It causes genital herpes. It is sexually transmitted latency occurs in spinal ganglion. Intracerebral infection in rabbits and mice produce encephalitis and corneal scarification produces keratoconjunctivitis in rabbits.

Cultivation

- *Monkey or rabbit kidney or human amnion or HeLa:* Well-defined foci, with heaped up cells, syncytial or giant cell formation occurs on these cell cultures.
- *Chick embryo:* CAM—pocks one formed they are small, non-necrotic.

Pathogenicity

Mode of Infection

Infection occurs by close contact, it may be venereal in genital herpes.

Route of Infection

HSV-1

- Mouth-to-mouth contact (kissing or the use of utensils contaminated with saliva).
- Transfer of infectious virus via any wound or through the eyes.

HSV-2

- It spreads sexually and is found in the anus, rectum and upper alimentary tract as well as the genital area.
- Infant can be infected at birth by a genitally-infected mother or *in utero.*

Course of Disease

Virus enters through skin or mucosa, multiplies locally, enters cutaneous nerve, and goes to ganglion where it remains **latent, HSV-1** becomes latent in **trigeminal ganglion** while **HSV-2** remains latent in **sacral ganglion**. The viruses travel back from nerve to skins and produce vesicles. This happens if the person's immunity is decreased. Stress, exposure to cold or excess heat act as precipitating factors for reactivation of viruses. But reactivation is also observed in some persons with virus specific humoral and cell mediated immunity. Probably immunity decreases severity of the disease by restricting local multiplication of virus. HSV-1 produces lesions above waist and HSV-2 produces lesions below waist. Spontaneously reactivation occurs inspite of HSV specific humoral and cell-mediated immunity in host. The extent to which immune response produced against virus prevents viral multiplication is not fully known but makes recurrence less severe and less extensive. Many recurrences are asymptomatic sheding only viruses in secretions. It is not known why some individuals have reactivations

and others have not though, 80% of human population harbor HSV-1.

Clinical Findings

Infections with herpes simplex viruses may be primary infection which takes in childhood or recurrent infection. Persons with low titer of antibodies usually are primary asymptomatic infection. Symptomatic disease may occur more commonly in small children with involvement of buccal or gingival mucosa. Incubation period is short and the disease last for 2–3 weeks. Primary infection results in latency.

1. *Oropharyngeal disease:* HSV-1 involves buccal and gingival mucosa, frequent in **small childern**, incubation period 2–12 days. Symptoms include fever, **sore throat**, vesicular or ulcerative lesions, **gingivitis or stomatitis** and malaise (Fig. 56.3).

    Primary infection in adults causes tonsillitis and pharyngitis; localized lymphadenopathy occurs.

2. *Recurrent disease:* Clusters of vesicles at border of lips develop, intense pain occurs initially, which reduces in 2–3 days.

3. *Keratoconjunctivitis:* HSV-1 may cause severe keratoconjunctivitis; recurrent lesions are common and produce **dendritic ulcers**, which lead to permanent opacity and blindness. Follicular conjunctivitis with vesicle around mouth is also a common occurrence.

4. *Cutaneous:* Lesions become pustules, break, and heal without scar formation within 8–10 days.
- Fever blisters (herpes febralis) are seen in and around mouth.
- Skin lesions may also occur on cheeks, chin, forehead and buttocks in neonates.
- Localized lesions of abrasion may occur (traumatic herpes).
- Lesions occur on fingers of dentists and hospital person **(herpetic whitlow)**.

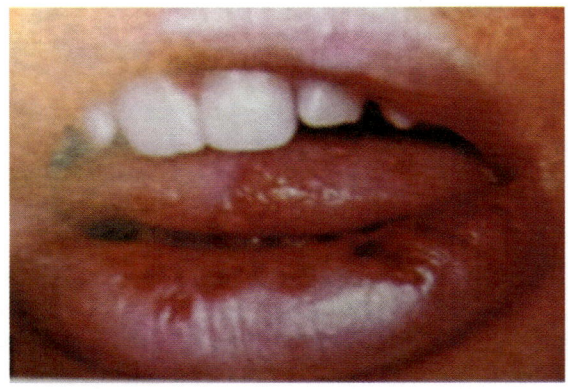

Fig. 56.3: Herpes labialis (vesicular lesions)

- Lesions occur on bodies of wrestlers (**herpes gladiatorum**).
- Cutaneous lesions in **patient with burns and eczema** (eczema **herpeticum**): Cutaneous lesions are painful and life-threatening.

5. *Genital herpes*: Mostly caused by *HSV-2* but *HSV-1* may also cause.
- *Lesions*: Vesicles and ulcers develop on penis, cervix, vulva, vagina, perineum. Lesions are painful and may be associated with fever, malaise, dysuria, inguinal lymphadenopathy.
- **Complications** are aseptic meningitis, extragenital lesions. Recurrent lesions are common and tend to be mild. A limited number of vesicles appear, heal in about 10 days. Virus is shed only for a few days. Whether it is symptomatic or not, a person shedding virus is source of infection to others. Some recurrences are asymptomatic with anogenital shedding lasting for less than 24 hours.
- Because of antigenic crossreactivity between *HSV-1* and *HSV-2*, pre-existing immunity provides some protection against heterotopic virus. An initial HSV-2 infection in a person already immune to HSV-1 tends to be less severe.

6. *Encephalitis*: HSV-1 may cause encephalitis, surviors may have residual deficits. HSV-1 is considered as one of the commonest cause of sporadic encephalitis. About 50% patients have primary infection and 50% have recurrent infection.

7. *Visceral*: It may cause tracheobronchitis, pneumonitis. Hepatitis is an uncommon complication of HSV. Disseminated disease may occur in immunocompromised patients.

8. *Neonatal*: The infection is acquired in uterus or during birth or after birth. Mother is the source of infection. Newborn infant is unable to restrict viral replication and spread. They may develop a severe disease. Most common mode of infection is while passing through infected birth cannel: In such cases, the risk for neonatal infection is 30–40%. Cesarean section is advised in women with genital lesions.

9. *Neonatal herpes* is always symptomatic, diseases produced are:
- Localized lesion on skin, eye and mouth.
- Encephalitis with or without skin lesions.
- Disseminated disease: It may involve many organs including CNS, the cause of death may be viral pneumonia or intravascular coagulopathy. The worst prognosis is in infants with disseminated disease with encephalitis. Many of survivors are left with permanant disease.

10. *Infections in immunocompromised persons*:
- Risk factors are malnutrition, renal disease, cardiac disease, transplant persons, persons with hematological malignancy, AIDS.
- Lesion may involve respiratory tract, intestinal mucosa, and esophagus.
- Malnourished children are prone to fatal disseminated disease. In most of the cases, the disease reflects reactivation of latent HSV infection.

11. *Erythema multiforme*: *Herpes simplex* antigen forms complexes with antibodies which may be circulating in blood or get deposited on skin which can be demonstrated by skin biopsy.

Laboratory Diagnosis

Samples collected are vesicle fluid, corneal scraping in case of conjunctivitis, throat swabs in case pharyngitis, CSF in case of meningitis, brain biopsy in case of encephalitis.

a. *Microscopic examination*: Scrapings from base of ulcers or vesicles are taken on slides.
- **Tzank smear (Fig. 56.4)**: Staining with toludine blue or Giemsa or Papanicolou stain Oshows multinucleated giant cells, with faceted nuclei and ground glass appearance of chromatin material.
- **Giemsa** is used for demonstration of inclusion bodies.
- **Electron microscopy** is used for the demonstration of viral particles in lesions.
- **Direct immunofluorescence** is used for rapid diagnosis of encephalitis (brain biopsy), and other lesions.

b. *Viral isolation*:
- **Eggs**: CAM shows pocks.
- **Experimental animals**: Lesions are produced in mice. HSV-2 produces severe infection of brain.
- **Cell cultures—HeLa**: Growth in cell cultures is detected by:
  - *Cytopathic effects in 2–3 days*: Localized foci, with heaped up cells, syncytial or giant cell formation occur.

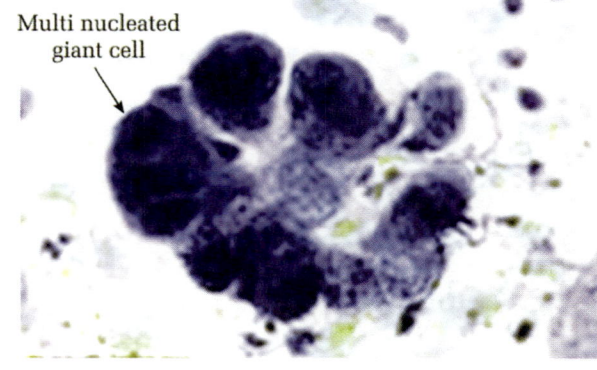

Multi nucleated giant cell

Fig. 56.4: Tzank smear

– *Other methods of detection of viral growth*: Direct immunofluorescence, viral neutralization
– DNA probes
– Typing can be done with monoclonal antibodies or by restriction endonuclease analysis.

c. *Serological test*: ELISA, CFT, RIA, IF, PHA. Serological tests are not helpful in countries like India where large number of normal persons give antibody test positive due to exposure early in life (80–90% of normal individuals are seropositive).
Serological tests are helpful in primary infection only.

d. *PCR*: It is rapid and sensitive method, especially helpful in diagnosis from CSF.
This test has replaced brain biopsy method for diagnosis of **CNS infection.**
Flowchart 56.1 depicts infections produced by herpes simplex virus.

Chemotherapy

There are a variety of nucleoside analog drugs used to treat herpes infections; acyclovir, famciclovir and valacyclovir. These drugs act against the replicating virus (they are incorporated into the DNA as it is copied) and therefore they are ineffective against latent virus. Since once the virus infects, the patient has it for life, the best option is to avoid infection by not coming in contact with the virus. Ocular lesions are treated with topical acyclovir, iododeoxyuridine, trifluorothymidine, vidarabine.

Mother to child transmission: Avoiding vaginal delivery and cesarean section is advised in women with genital lesions.

VARICELLA-ZOSTER VIRUS (ALSO KNOWN AS HERPES ZOSTER VIRUS, HUMAN HERPES VIRUS-3)

Morphology

It is similar to HSV. There is no animal reservoir. Virus propogates in cultures of human embryonic tissue and produce typical inclusion bodies. The same virus causes chickenpox and zoster. Viral isolates from vesicles of chickenpox or zoster patients show no significant genetic variations.

Cultivation

HeLa or human fibroblasts cell cutures:
• *Detection of viral growth*: Viruses form intranuclear inclusion bodies which can be stained by Giemsa stain.
• Cytopathic effects not marked, they are more focal and spread slowly than induced by HSV.
• Infectious virus remains cell associated and serial propagation is more easily accomplished by passage of infected cells than tissue culture fluids.

Entry of viruses take place through respiratory tract or conjunctiva.
• Primary infection in a nonimmune individual (child) causes varicella (chickenpox) while reactivation of latent virus causes zoster.

Flowchart 56.1: Infections produced by herpes simplex viruses

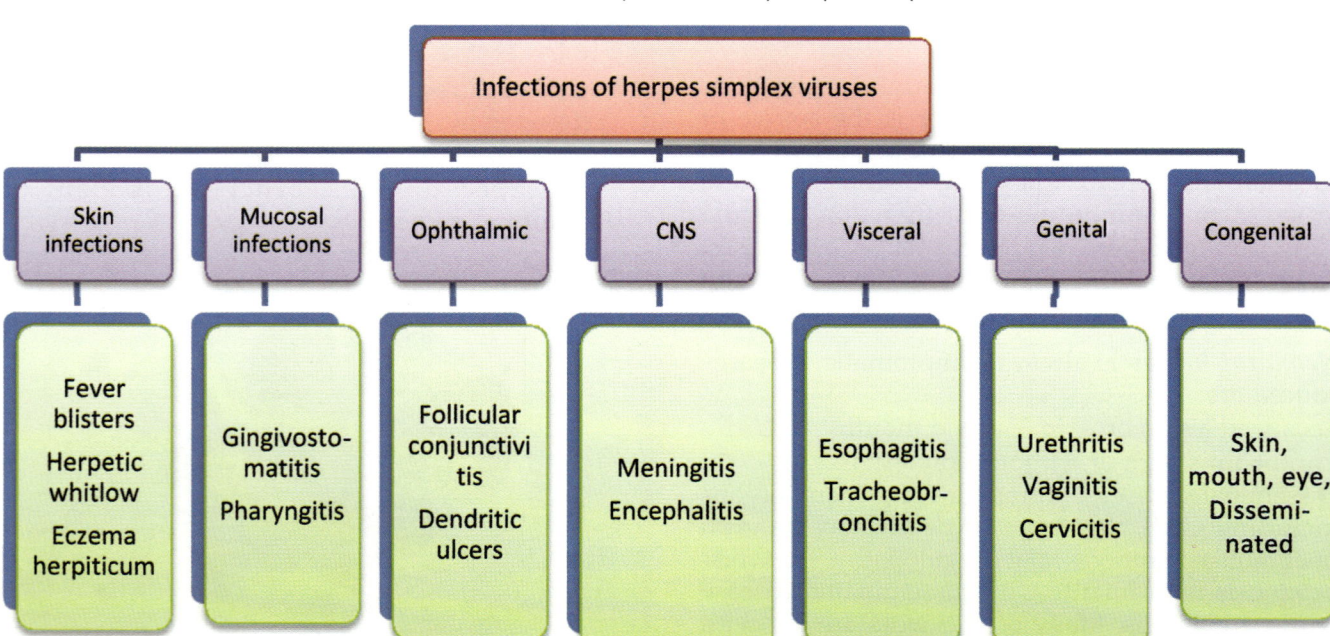

Zoster means **girdle,** the word is derived from the characteristic rash that forms a ring around the thorax in many patients. The structure of varicella virus is very similar to *Herpes simplex virus* although the genome is somewhat smaller.

Chickenpox (Fig. 56.5)

After entry of virus through aerosols or direct contact, viruses multiply initially in lymph nodes. Viruses spill over, enter blood circulation causing primary viremia. Viruses spread and carried to liver and spleen. They multiply in these organs and cause secondary viremia. Infected cells transport the viruses to skin where typical lesions develop. Swelling of epithelial cells, ballooning degeneration and accumulation of tissue fluids result in vesicle formation (Table 56.4).

Viral replication and spread is limited by humoral and cellular responses. Virus-coded protein **ORF61 antagonizes the interferon α pathway.** This contributes to infection.

Prodromal stage: Incubation period 10–21 days, virus multiplies and produces primary viremia which leads to deposition of viruses in various tissues , viruses again enter blood causing secondary viremia (virus travels to the skin, mouth, conjunctiva, respiratory tract, etc.). Malaise and fever are the earliest symptoms.

Maculopapular rash (most pronounced on the face, scalp and trunk and less on the limbs) and fever are main clinical features. The rash is centripetal in distribution. There is vesicle and pustule formation followed by scab formation. Rash is centripetally distributed. Evolution of rash from macule to pustule may be seen at a time as it evolves slowly.

Complications

- Pneumonia can be associated with a varicella infection (about 15% of adult patients) and may be fatal. Varicella pneumonia is rare in children but it is the most common complication in neonates, adults, and immunocompromised patients.

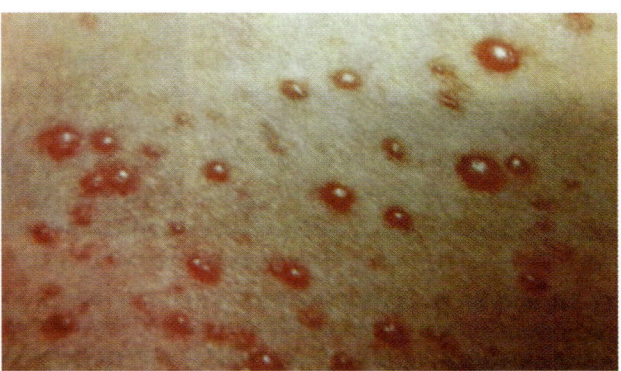

Fig. 56.5: Skin lesions of chickenpox

- *Fulminant encephalitis and cerebellar ataxia*: Though encephalitis is rare but those who survive may be left with permanent sequelae.
- Reye's syndrome, Guillain-Barre syndrome, etc.
- Immunocompromised individuals are at increased risk of complications including those with organ transplantation, malignancy, HIV infection and those receiving steroids. Disseminated intravascular coagulation may occur, that is fatal.
- *Primary infection during pregnancy*: The virus may cause congenital infections called fetal varicella syndrome.

Shingles VZV

Zoster (herpes zoster or varicella zoster): Zoster occurs in patients who had primary infection earlier. Reactivation of latent infection takes place. Immune compromised patients usually suffer from zoster. Aging or compromised conditions may act as precipitating factor. Some cases may be asymptomatic while in others reactivation previous disease takes place. Such cases may be endogenous in origin. Latent virus is carried from primary infection to area of skin supplied by sensory nerve. Latent virus that travels along sensory nerves to area of skin (dermatome) innervated from the affected ganglion. Thoracic nerves are affected. Within few days, crops of vesicles appear on skin supplied by the nerve. The trunk, head, neck are more commonly affected. The ophthalmic division of trigeminal nerve

TABLE 56.4: Differences between smallpox and chickenpox		
	Smallpox	*Chickenpox*
	Fever occurs 2–4 days before rash	If at all occurs, it occurs at the time of rash
Rash	More lesions on face and extremities	More lesions on body
Distribution	Lesions of palms and sole	No lesions on palms and soles
Appearance	Large deep-seated vesicles or pustules in the same stage of development	Small shallow vesicles in various stages of development
Course	Lesions resolve in 14–21 days	Lesions resolve in 7–10 days
Mortality	10–30%	Very uncommon

is involved in 10–15% cases. The most common complication is **post-herpetic neuralgia**—protracted pain which may continue for months. It is common after ophthalmic zoster. Varicella zoster CNS disease most frequently causes meningitis and often presents without rash.

Role of Specific CMI

Varicella and zoster viruses are identical, the two diseases being result of differing host defences. The development of varicella zoster specific cell-mediated immunity is important in recovery from both infections. Apperance of local interferon contributes to recovery.

Evasion of Host Defences

Varicella zoster virus has some mechanisms to evade host defences. It **downregulates major histocompatibility complex class I and II antigen expression and also interferes with a interferon pathway.**

- Virus remains dormant in ganglia.
- It may be reactivated under stress or with immune suppression.
- Recurrence is accompanied by severe radicular pain in discrete areas those innervated by the nerve in which latent infection has occurred.
- Lesions are like in chickenpox and occur in restricted areas (dermatome) that are innervated by a single ganglion.
- Rash unicellular, mostly in dermatome supplied by D3 to L2 and trigeminal nerve (ophthalmic branch).

Complications

- Reactivation can affect the eye via the trigeminal nerve and the brain via the cranial nerve VII and VIII (Bell's palsy and Ramsay-Hunt syndrome)
- Meningoencephalitis
- Lower motor neuron paralysis
- Post-herpetic neuralgia
- Patients with AIDS usually have multidermatomal involvement

Diagnosis (Table 56.4)

Both chickenpox and shingles are diagnosed by their characteristic appearance but a definitive diagnosis can be made by electron microscope, culture of the virus from the lesions (a difficult procedure) followed by detection of specific antigens (ELISA) and **PCR**.

Treatment

Acyclovir (or other nucleoside analogs) can be useful, particularly in preventing dissemination in immuno-suppressed patients. Varicella immunoglobulin can also be used. Only supportive care is used in children who quickly recover, if they mount an adequate cell-mediated response.

Vaccines

- A live-attenuated varicella vaccine **(Oka strain)** is produced against VZV. It leads to antibody production and cell-mediated immunity. Single dose is given in children between 1 and 12 years of age and two doses given 6–10 weeks apart in older children.
- *Zoster vaccine*: Zoster vaccine is more potent (14 times) than varicella vaccine. It is recomonded for those with chronic medical problem and older than 60 years of age.

Passive Protection

Varicella zoster immune globulin (VZIG) from patients of zoster in convalescent phase is used for passive protection of immunocompromised children exposed to infection. The disadvantage is its availability.

EPSTEIN–BARR VIRUS

Morphology

It is similar to HSV but antigenically and genetically different. It grows in human lymphocytes.

Viral capsid antigen (VCA) is of diagnostic importance. It is transmitted through saliva (by kissing, hence called **"kissing disease"**). Persons shed the virus from time to time throughout life. The virus can also be spread by blood transfusion, it enters a latent state in the lymphocyte without undergoining viral replication.

Biology of EBV

- Entry of the virus takes place in the epithelial cells of pharynx through CR2 (or CD21) receptors. Virus multiplies locally in epithelial cells of pharynx and parotid glands. It enters blood circulation and infects B lymphocytes through CR2 (or CD21) receptors.
- Two events may occur—virus remains latent in B cells, get immortalized or transformed acquiring capacity of infinite indefinite growth in vitro. (Other cycle may be lytic cycle.)
- Polyclonal activation of B cells takes place. Mononucleosis represents polyclonal transformation of infected cells.
- Viral antigens appear on infected B cell surface, thus neoantigens appear on infected B cells. T cells get converted into blast cells in response to neoantigens. These T cells are atypical lymphocytes present in peripheral blood (seen in blood smear).

- Intermittent activation of latent EBV leads to clonal proliferation of infected B cells. This is controlled by activated T cells in immunocompetent person. In a person with immunodeficiency, B cell replica is unchecked. It causes lymphoma.
- Genetic and environment factors are considered important in formation of nasopharyngeal carcinoma seen in Chinese men.
- Genetic influence is also evident in X-linked lymph proliferative syndrome (XLP or Dunken' syndrome showing high sensitivity to EBV infection).

Infectious Mononucleosis

- *Symptoms*: Sore throat, malaise, headache, abdominal pain, nausea, vomiting, chills are important symptoms.
- *Signs*: Lymphadenopathy, fever, pharyngitis, splenomegaly, hepatomegaly, periorbital edema, jaundice, and skin rash are the signs of the disease.

Complications include neurological disorders such as meningitis, encephalitis, myelitis and GBS. Secondary infections, autoimmune hemolytic anemia, thrombocytopenia, agranulocytosis, and aplastic anemia are the other complications of the virus.

EBV Induced Tumors (Flowchart 56.2)

Burkitt's lymphoma: This is a tumor of the jaw and face found in children. The tumor cells show evidence of EBV DNA and tumor antigens and patients show a much higher level of anti-EBV antibodies than other members of the population. Tumor cells are monoclonal and show a very characteristic translocation between chromosomes 8 and 14. Persons that are resistant to malaria appear to be susceptible to progression to the lymphoma. This lymphoma is endemic in equatorial Africa but only occurs rarely elsewhere. **Nasopharyngeal**

Flowchart 56.2: Clinical and immunological events in EB virus infections

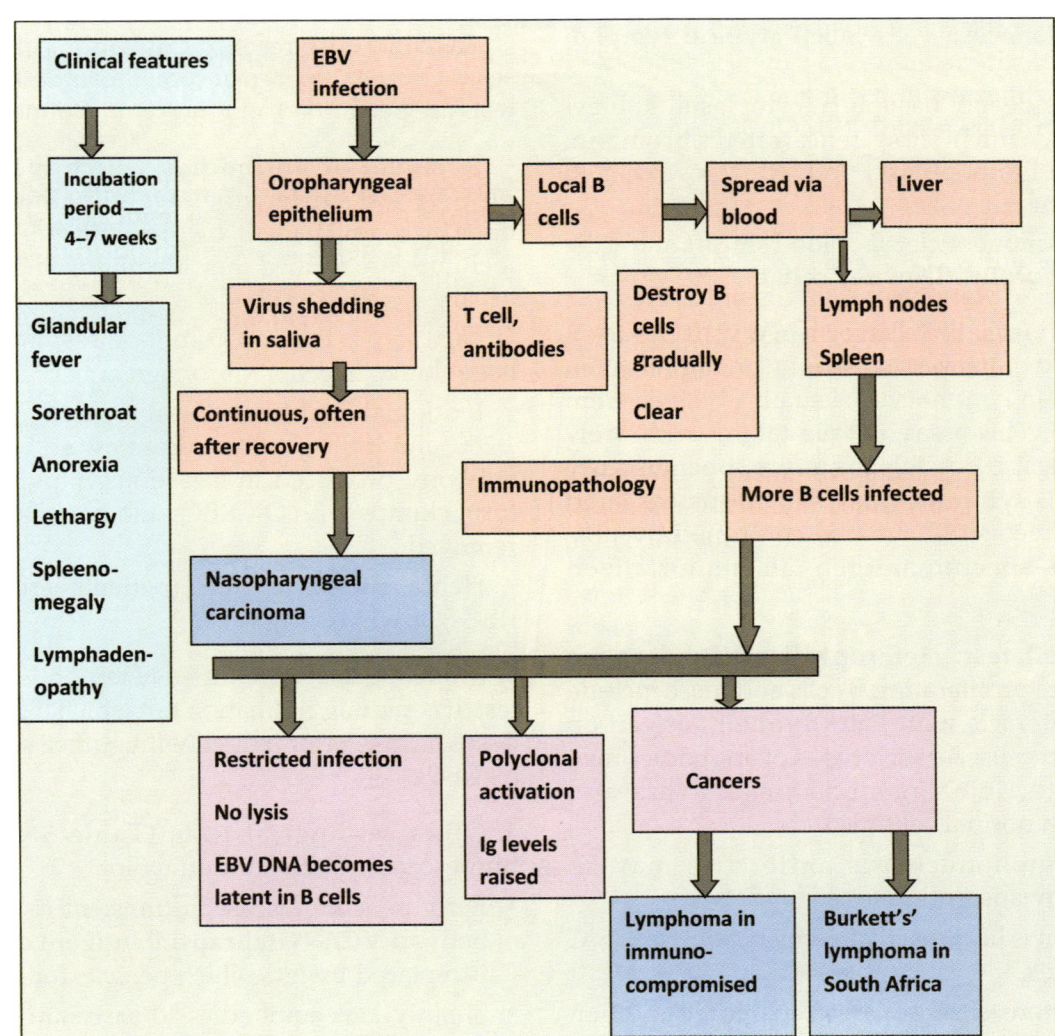

cancer: This disease, which occurs in a number of areas (South China, Alaska, Tunisia, East Africa), is associated with EBV.

Oral Hairy Leukoplakia

This EBV-associated disease results in lesions in the mouth and has increased in frequency recently as it is an opportunistic infection of HIV-infected patients.

Other Diseases

- **Lymphoproliferative diseases.** For example, X-linked lymphoproliferative syndrome (**Dunkun's disease**), is autosomal recessive disorder, children develop fatal lymphoproliferative disorder following infection with EBV.
- **Chronic fatigue syndrome**

Diagnosis

1. Blood examination during early phase shows leukopenia, followed later by leukocytosis with abnormal mononuclear cells called **atypical lymphocytes.**

This cell has deeply basophilic cytoplasm, kidney-shaped nuclei, which show fenestrated chromatin. These cells are **lymphoblasts** derived from T cells in response to virus.

In infectious mononucleosis, blood smears show the **atypical lymphocytes (Downey cells).**

Isolation of virus: EBV can be isolated from saliva, peripheral blood or lymphoid tissue by immortalization of normal human lymphocytes, usually obtained from umbilical cord. This assay is time taking and rarely performed. It is also possible to culture spontaneously transformed B lymphocytes from virus infected patients. Any recovered agent is confirmed by EBV DNA or virus-specific antigens in immortalized lymphocytes.

2. Paul-Bunnell test: Heterophile antibodies are produced by the proliferating B cells and these include an IgM that interacts with **Paul-Bunnell antigen** on sheep red blood cells. As such types of antibodies may also occur after injections of animal's sera and sometimes with normal cells also.

Infectious mononucleosis antibodies may be differentiated by absorption tests.

- Patient serum is heat inactivated by heating for 56°C for 30 minutes.
- Double dilutions of serum are prepared by addition of saline as 1:25, 1:50, and 1:100and 1:200.

- For this, one mL of serum is mixed with 2.4 mL saline to make 1:25 dilution. In the subsequent test tubes, 0.5 mL of normal saline is taken to which 0.5 mL of 1:25 diluted serum is added. It is mixed well and again from this tube 0.5 mL is carried to next tube, so that we get serum dilutions as 1:25, 1:50, and 1:100 and 1:200.
- To these test tubes of dilutions, equal volume of 1% solution of sheep RBCs is added. Thus final dilutions are 1:50, 1:100, 1:200, and 1:400.
- The test is incubated at 37°C for 4 hours. The highest dilution showing clumps is taken as titer. If it is equal to or greater than **1:200**, it is considered significant and the disease will be suspected.

The antigen used in the test is sheep RBC which is heterophile antigen, the test is an example of **heterophile agglutination** test.

As the antibodies may occur sometimes normally or due to injection of foreign sera (Forsman antigen), it is necessary to differentiate the antibodies from false antibodies.

To avoid false reactions due to injection of foreign serum or seen in normal sera, the antibody absorption tests are performed and then Paul-Bunnell test is done.

Removal of antibodies which may give false positive test (differential agglutination test): This is done by mixing patient's serum with guinea pig kidney; if clumps are formed they are removed. Thus one type of false positive antibody is removed.

Next step is to remove antibodies which might have been due to injection of foreign antiserum in patient.

If original Paul-Bunnell test is positive with titer, i.e. 1:200, and if the positive serum mixed with OX RBCs, antibody produced in infectious mononucleosis will form clumps with OX RBCs and by washing it will be removed.

Hence, if test is repeated (patients serum with sheep RBCs), it will be negative.

3. Monospot test is modified heterophile agglutination test. It is slide agglutination test which uses horse RBCs. Test serum is prior treated with guinea pig kidney and ox RBCs.

4. Other serological tests (Table 56.5): Immunofluorescence, ELISA, immunoblot.

- Early in acute disease, a transient rise in IgM antibody to **VCA (viral capsid antigen)** appears which is replaced by IgG which persists for life.
- Slightly later antibodies to **early antigens** develop that persist for several months.

TABLE 56.5: Serological features of EBV associated diseases

| Condition | Heterophile | Anti – VCA antibodies | | Anti-EA | | Anti-EBNA |
		Ig M	Ig G	EA-D	EA-R	
Acute infectious mononucleosis	+	+	++	+	–	–
Convalescence	+/–	–	+	–	+/–	+
Past infection	–	–	+	–	–	+
Reactivation with immunodeficiency	–	–	++	+	+	+/–
Burkitt's lymphoma	–	–	+++	+/–	++	+
Nasopharyngeal carcinoma	–	–	+++	++	+/–	+

(**Note:** VCA–viral capsid antigen, EA–early antigen, EA-D– antibody to early antigen in diffuse pattern in nucleus, EA-R–antibody to early antigen restricted to cytoplasm, EBNA–Epstein-Barr nuclear antigen).

- Several weeks after acute infection; an antibody to **EBNA** and **membrane antigen** appear and persists for life.
- **Antibodies to EB nucleus (anti-EBNA), anti-early antigen (anti-EA)** are useful marker of infection which persists for several months.

5. Molecular methods helps in early detection: No drugs are available to treat *Epstein-Barr* virus. A vaccine is being developed.

CYTOMEGALOVIRUS

These viruses are ubiquitous herpes viruses that are commom cause of human diseases. Previously they were known as **'salivary gland viruses'.** They are agents of most common congenital infections which is a major public health problem.

Morphology

CMV: Size: 150–200 nm (largest among herpes viruses). Virus is strictly host specific. The DNA genome is (240 kbp) larger than HSV. It has the largest genome of all herpes viruses and replicate only in human cells. Only few of viral proteins (200) are characterized. One of the cell surface protein acts as Fc receptor which can nonspecifically bind to immunoglobulin molecule.

Cultivation

CMVs are very host specific, species specific, cell type specific. They replicate only in human fibroblasts and replicate slowly. Very little virus becomes cell free, infection spreads cell to cell. It takes several weeks for the entire cell monolayer to become infected.

There are several families of glycoproteins in CMV, some of which are important antigen targets. **CMV binds to host cell β macroglobulin and can use the class I HLA molecule as additional receptor for cell attachment** and infection. Virions of CMV coated with β macroglobulin are excreted in urine.

Cytopathic effects: CMV produces characteristic cytopathic effects. It forms perinuclear cytoplasmic inclusions **(Owl's eye; Fig. 56.6)** along with typical intranuclear inclusions formed by HSV. Its name is derived from the fact that it can form cell megaly. Some cells such as macrophages and fibroblasts, support a productive infection while a latent infection is set up in several cell types including T lymphocytes and stromal cells of the bone marrow. It is antigenically different from other herpes viruses.

Virus is difficult to grow, human fibroblast cell culture is used for cultivation; it grows very slowly (50 days).

Modes of Spread

- Close contact: It may spread through saliva or other secretions or by sexual contact.
- *In utero* transmission to the fetus in a pregnant woman and to the newborn via lactation is also present.
- In the hospital, the virus can also spread via blood transfusions and transplants.

In developing countries with more crowded conditions, the virus is found in a much higher proportion of the population than in Western countries.

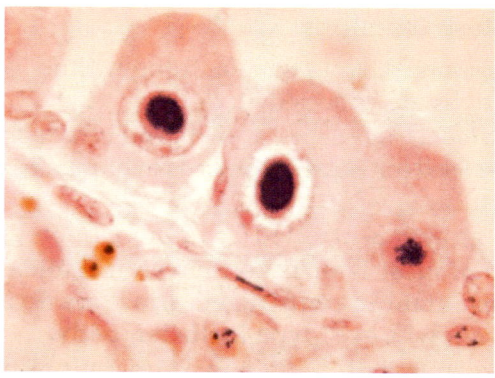

Fig. 56.6: Histopathological section showing owl's eye inclusions

Pathogenesis

No symptoms seen in children and mild disease is seen in adults.

The virus first infects the upper respiratory tract and then local lymphocytes, spleen and lymph nodes, epithelial cells (salivary glands, kidney tubules, testes, epididymis and cervix).

Though infection due to CMV is common, disease is rare and it occurs in two situations, i.e. **congenital disease and disease in immunocompromised patients.**

CMV is the most common viral cause of congenital disease. Abnormalities include microcephaly, rash, brain calcification and hepatosplenomegaly. These may result in hearing loss (bilateral or unilateral) and retardation. Infants may be infected perinatally (mother's genital tract, milk). In either case, the infant remains asymptomatic. Neonates may also receive the virus through infected blood transfusions. In this case, the amount of virus is much higher and symptoms may occur. These usually consist of pneumonia and hepatitis.

Primary infection of older children and adults is usually asymptomatic but occasionally causes "infectious mononucleosis" syndrome, a mild disease, complications are rare, in childern younger than 7 years, hepatomegaly may occur.

Disease in immunosuppressed patients: In patients who have received an organ transplant or have an immunosuppressive disease (e.g. AIDS), cytomegalovirus can be a major problem. Both morbidity and mortality rates are increased with primary and recurrent infections.

- CMV retinitis (15% of all AIDS patients) may lead to progressive blindness. Disseminated disease may occur in AIDS patients; gastroenteritis is common.
- Interstitial pneumonia (it occurs in 10–15% in bone marrow transplant patients).
- Colitis
- Esophagitis
- Encephalitis

Laboratory Diagnosis

- *Specimens*: Urine, saliva, semen, and cervical secretions are collected.
- *Isolation*: Urine, saliva, semen, and other specimens can be used for isolation of virus in human **fibroblast cell culture**.
- Viral growth is detected by immunofluorescence.
- **A simple test is** detection of **cytomegalic cells by Giemsa stain in centrifuged urine or saliva** which shows **"owl's eye" type inclusion body.**
- *Serology*: It is useful in only primary infection and in congenital infection.

- Tests used for antibodies detection are CFT, IF, ELISA. (Detection of IgM)
- Multinucleated cells with characteristic inclusions can be seen in biopsies of many tissues.
- *Direct antigen detection*: Direct immunofluorescence is used for detection of **pp65 and pp67 proteins in** specimens and in leukocytes.
- *Shell vial assay*: Culture and cytopathic effects take 4–6 weeks; early diagnosis is possible with shell vial assay.
- The specimen is added to a vial of cell culture containing a monolayer of cell line, **vial is centrifuged** at low speed and incubated for 24–48 hours, and tissue medium is removed.
- The cells are stained with **fluorescent tagged anti-CMV antibody**, and immunofluorescence is observed under fluorescent microscope.

Treatment

Ganciclovir is used; especially to treat retinitis. Foscarnet is also effective.

A vaccine is being developed but the best way to avoid the virus is to restrict contact between infected children and pregnant women. Also since cytomegalovirus is sexually transmitted, condoms can limit spread.

HUMAN HERPES VIRUS-6

- It is found worldwide and is found in the saliva of the majority of adults (>90%).
- It replicates in B and T lymphocytes, megakaryocytic glioblastoma cell and in the oropharynx.
- It can set up a latent infection in T cells which can later be activated.
- Infected cells are larger than normal with inclusions in both cytoplasm and nucleus.
- Human herpes virus-6 has two forms, HHV-6A and HHV-6B.
- The latter causes exanthema subitum, otherwise known as **roseola infantum (sixth disease)**. This is common disease of young children and symptoms include fever and URTI and lymphadenopathy.
- In adults, primary infection is associated with an infectious mononucleosis syndrome, focal encephalitis and in immunodeficient pneumonia and disseminated disease occur.

HUMAN HERPES VIRUS-7

- This virus binds to the CD4 antigen and replicates in T4 (CD4+) cells and is found in the saliva of the majority of the adult population (>75%).
- Most people acquire the infection in childhood and it remains with them for the rest of their lives.

- It is similar to HHV-6 and may be responsible for some cases of **exanthem subitum.**

HUMAN HERPES VIRUS-8

This was formerly known as **Kaposi's sarcoma associated herpes virus.** It is found in the saliva of many AIDS patients. It infects peripheral blood lymphocytes.

HERPES B

This is a simian virus found in old world monkeys such as macaques but it can be a human pathogen in people who handle monkeys (monkey bites are the route of transmission). In humans, the disease is much more problematic than it is in its natural host. Human cases result in death with serious neurological problems (encephalitis) in many survivors. *In vitro* the virus is sensitive to both acyclovir and ganciclovir.

HERPES SAIMIRI VIRUS

It is a monkey virus which caused fatal infection in a laboratory person bitten by monkey, the B in the name is derived from the initials of the patient. The name of the virus is Cercopithecine herpes virus-1.

57

Picornaviruses

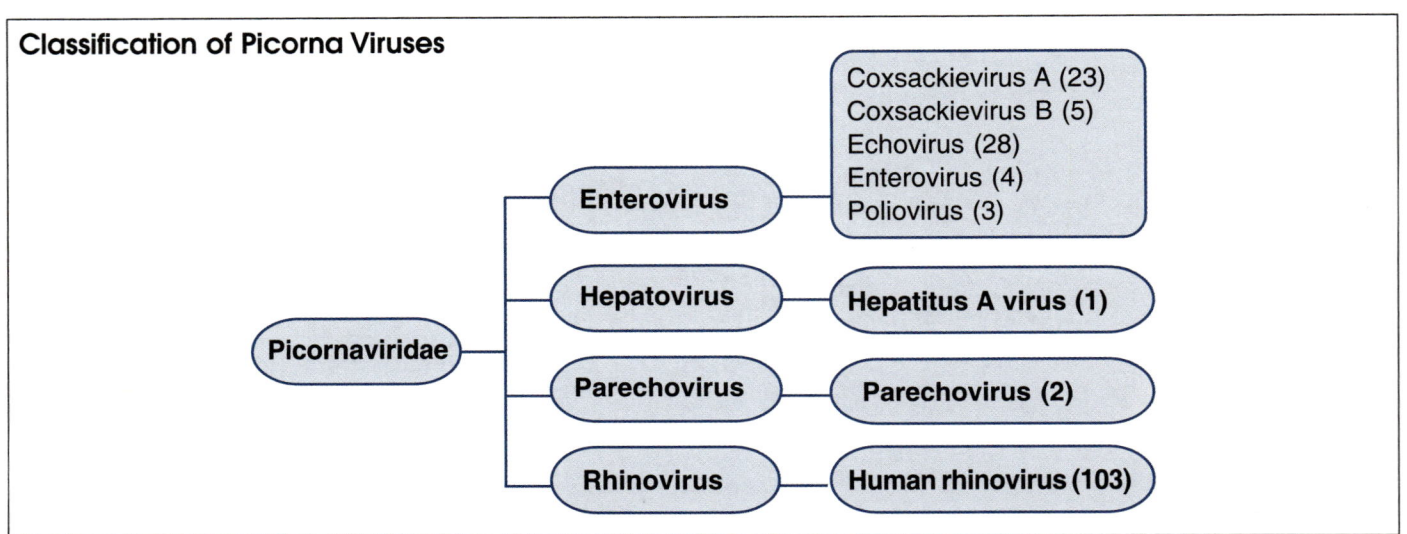

Classification of Picorna Viruses

- Picornaviridae
  - Enterovirus
    - Coxsackievirus A (23)
    - Coxsackievirus B (5)
    - Echovirus (28)
    - Enterovirus (4)
    - Poliovirus (3)
  - Hepatovirus
    - Hepatitus A virus (1)
  - Parechovirus
    - Parechovirus (2)
  - Rhinovirus
    - Human rhinovirus (103)

Pico means small, hence known as small RNA viruses or picornaviruses.

Morphology

- *Size*: 27–30 nm.
- Small positive stranded RNA virus.
- As the genome is positive stranded RNA, it is infectious. It contains genome-linked protein. Virus multiplication occurs in cytoplasm of host cell.
- Viruses do not have a lipid membrane (nonenveloped).
- They have a naked nucleocapsid that is about 30 nm in diameter. Rhinovirus and enterovirus contains capsid shell of 60 subunits, each of four proteins (VP1-VP4) arranged around the genome make single stranded RNA.

Picornavirus Replication (Fig. 57.1)

Replication occurs in host cell cytoplasm. Viruses attach to cells by binding to specific receptors. Binding causes change of virion that leads to release of viral RNA into cell cytoplasm.

A polyprotein is formed by translation of infecting viral RNA which contains coat proteins and proteins required for replication. Polyprotein is broken down into small fragments.

Virus-coded replication proteins including an RNA-dependent RNA polymerase are produced. The infecting viral RNA strand is copied and that strand serves as a template for synthesis of new plus strand. Some new plus strands are recycled as template to amplify the pool of progeny RNA, many plus strands get packaged into virions.

Maturation involves several cleavage events. **Coat precursor protein 'P1'** is cleaved to form aggregates of **VP0, VP3, VP1.** When an adequate concentration is reached, these promotors assemble into pentamers that package plus strand VPg-RNA to form provirions. The **provirions are not infective until a final cleavage changes VP0 to VP4 and VP2.** The mature viruses are released when host cell disintegrates. The multiplication cycle takes place in 5–10 hours.

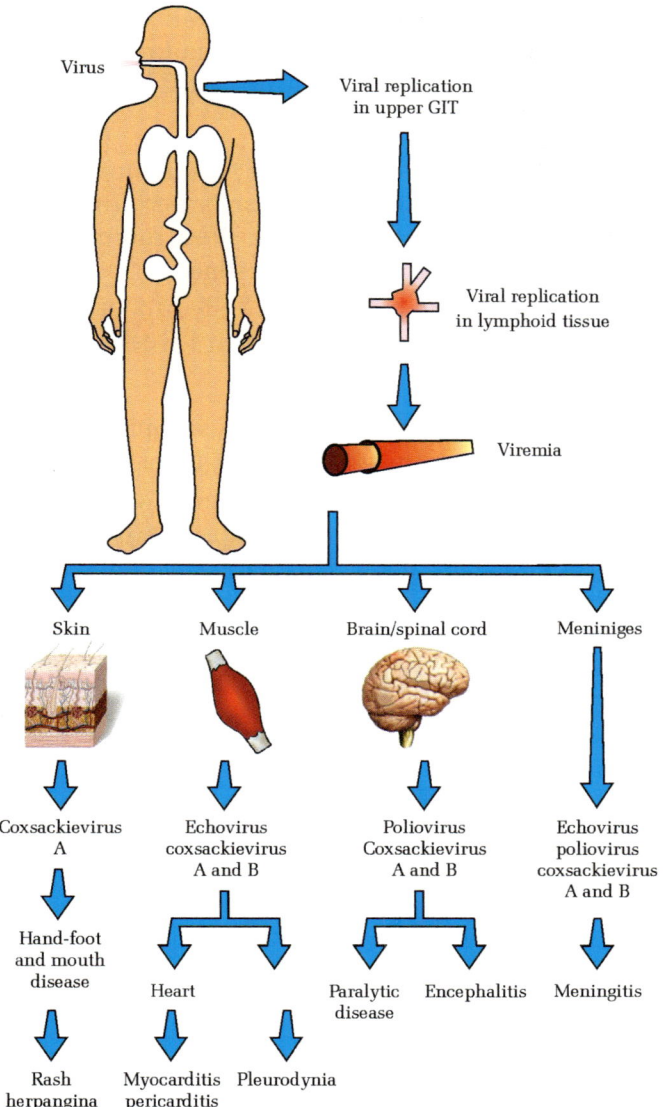

Fig. 57.1: Pathogenicity of picornaviruses

Some Common Properties of Enteroviruses

- They all replicate in the intestinal tract.
- They commonly cause asymptomatic infections which give immunity hence protect against future infection of the virus.
- They can give rise to viremia.
- They occasionally cause infection of central nervous system.
- They are common in children than adults.
- In temperate climate, infections usually occur in the summer and autumn.

There are nine genera within the Picornaviridae.

Genera which infect humans
  i. *Enteroviruses*
 ii. *Rhinoviruses*
iii. *Hepatoviruses*
 iv. *Parechoviruses*

ENTEROVIRUSES

Virus family	Serotypes
Polio	1–3
Coxsackie A	1–22, 24
Coxsackie B	1–6
Echovirus	1–9, 11–27, 29–34
Hepatitis A	*Enterovirus 72*
Other	*Enteroviruses 68–71*

Coxsackievirus and most *rhinoviruses* adhere to ICAM-1, an adhesion glycoprotein expressed on the surfaces of a variety of cells (epithelial, endothelial, fibroblasts).

The expression of these molecules determines tissue tropism.

POLIO VIRUS

The cell surface **glycoCD155,** the **polio virus receptor,** is expressed in spinal cord anterior horn cells, dorsal root ganglia, skeletal muscle, motor neurons and some cells of the lymphoid system (Fig. 57.2).

Morphology

- Spherical particle, 27 nm in diameter.
- Genome is single stranded of positive sense RNA.
- Icosahedral symmetry.
- 60 subunits (each consisting of 4 viral proteins (VP1–VP4), VP1 facing outside carries major antigenic site for combination of type-specific neutralizing antibodies.
- Virus can be crystalized.

Resistance

Virus survives for months at 4°C and year's at –20°C. Heat at 55°C for 30 minutes kill the viruses. Free residual chlorine concentration of 0.3–0.5 ppm and 0.3% formaldehyde kill the viruses. Higher concentration is used to kill viruses in presence of organic matter. Inactivation of viruses is also possible at pH 3. Virus is resistant to chloroform, bile, detergent. Virus survives in feces for a year at 20°C. $MgCl_2$ is used as stabilizer in oral polio vaccine.

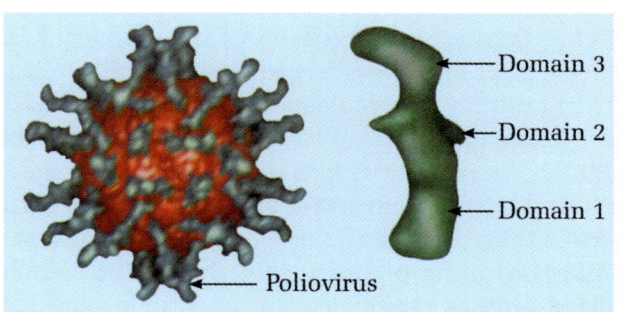

Fig. 57.2: Structure of poliovirus

Antigenic Properties

- By neutralization, three types of polioviruses are identified. Type 1 (epidemic), Type 2 (endemic) Type 3 (epidemic).
  - The **prototype strains** are: Type 1, the Brunhilde, and Mahoney; Type 2, Lansing and MEFI strains; and Type 3, Leon and Saukett strains.
- By CFT, ELISA or precipitation test, two antigens identified—C and D.

C (heated or H antigen): **Coreless or capsid** associated with empty non-infectious virus. It is also called heated antigen. The antigen is less specific, reacts with heterotypic sera. **Anti "C"** does not neutralize virus infectivity.

D–dense (native or N antigen): It is called native or 'N' antigen. The antigen is associated with whole virion. An anti-D antibody is protective and potency of injectable vaccine is measured in 'D' antigen units.

Host range: Humans are natural hosts.
- Experimentally infection is produced in monkeys (intracerebral and intraspinal)—chimpazees and cynomolgus monkeys (orally).
- Established strains grow in rodents and chick embryos (but not fresh isolates).

Cultivation

- Primary monkey kidney cell lines are used (diagnostic and vaccine production).
- *Cytopathic effects:* Infected cells round up and become refractive and pyknotic. Virus forms eosinophilic intranuclear inclusion bodies.
- Plaques develop in infected cell culture layer.

Pathogenesis and Clinical Features (Fig. 57.3)

Mode of Infection

Feco-oral route through ingestion, inhalation or entry through conjunctiva or droplets (respiratory secretions). Virus multiplies in lymphatic tissues and epithelial tissue in alimentary canal (tonsils to Payer's patches). The virus is regularly present in throat and stools before onset of disease. From throat they reach regional lymph nodes—enter bloodstream **(primary viremia)**. Viruses further multiply in reticuloendothelial cells in body and again enter bloodstream causing **secondary viremia**. With the viremia, virus gets disseminated throughout body and infects brain and spinal cord. The cell surface **glycoCD155,** the poliovirus receptor, is expressed on spinal cord anterior horn cells, dorsal root ganglia, skeletal muscle, motor neurons and some cells of the lymphoid system. *Poliovirus* can spread along the axons

of peripheral nerves to CNS where it continues to progress along the fibers of lower motor neurons to involve spinal cord and brain. In CNS, there is degeneration of Nissl bodies.

1. *Asymptomatic infection:* 90–95% individuals do not have symptoms. Virus isolation can be performed from stool or nasopharyngeal secretions. Viral multiplication is limited to oropharynx and intestine.

   Clinical infection occurs in only 5–10% of infected persons. Incubation period 4 days to 4 weeks (average 10 days).

2. *Abortive poliomyelitis:* Primary viremia or **minor illness** (which is transient influenza-like illness).

   Virus multiplies in the epithelial cells of the alimentary canal and the lymphatic tissues (from tonsils to Payer's patches). It spreads to regional lymph nodes, where it multiplies and enter bloodstream causing **minor or primary viremia**. It is characterized by fever,

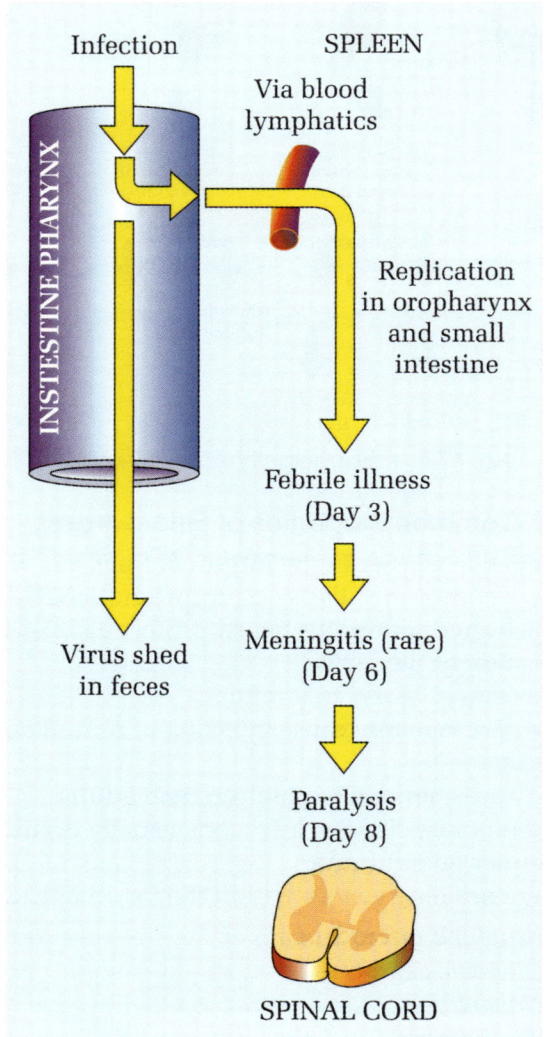

Fig. 57.3: Pathogenesis of poliomyelitis

malaise, headache; sore throat. This is called minor illness.

In many patients, the infection halts at this stage only then, it is called **abortive infection**.

If infection progresses, the minor illness is followed by major illness in 3–4 days.

3. *Nonparalytic poliomyelitis*: After primary viremia, virus goes to reticuloendothelial system where it multiplies and again enters in blood causing **major viremia.**

1–2% of infected patients present with signs and symptoms of aseptic meningitis along with 'influeza like illness'. Fever comes again, with neck stiffness; headache which are the features of **aseptic meningitis. Symptoms make a rapid and complete recovery in less than 10 days.**

Sometimes the disease doesn't progress beyond this stage due to rapid and complete recovery and then it is called **nonparalytic poliomyelitis.**

4. *Paralytic poliomyelitis*: Paralytic poliomyelitis in which patients develop paralysis is very uncommon. **Paralysis** is usually **flaccid** due to destruction of lower motor neurons, along with the invasion of brainstem which can lead to incordination of muscle groups and painful spasms. Paralysis is early in illness, some functions may return in 6 months.

Paralysis may be bulbar, spinal or bulbospinal.

Factors Predisposing to Paralytic Poliomyelitis

- *Violent muscle exercise*: This increases vascularity in the limb or appropriate area of cord and increases access of virus to nerve endings.
- Pregnancy (3rd trimester).
- Immunization of DPT vaccines and irritant substances as heavy metals can result in paralysis of the limb which received inoculation. Paralysis occurs when poliovirus is contracted within 1 month of receiving the inoculation.
- *Tonsillectomy*: It has been associated with reduction in secretory IgA which occurs in pharynx and results reduced neutralization of virus. Virus presents in nasopharynx enters nerve fibers and brain causing bulbar paralysis.

Non-polio enteroviruses (echovirus 4, entero 71) have also been associated with central nervous disease and paralysis; as in polio, paralysis is a rare manifestation of infection.

During the period of viremia, viruses cross the blood–brain barrier and enter spinal cord and brain. It multiplies selectively in neurons and destroy them. The virus shows special affinity for anterior horn cells of spinal cord, dorsal root ganglion, and motor neuron.

Pathologic Changes

- Degeneration of **Nissl** bodies (chromatolysis).
- Degenerative changes of nucleus.
- Lesions are mainly in anterior horn of spinal cord, posterior horn and intermediate columns may be involved.
- When degeneration becomes irreversible, the necrotic cells lyse or are phagocytized by leukocytes or macrophages.

Leisons occur in anterior horns of spinal cord causing **flaccid paralysis.** In paralytic poliomyelitis or spinal paralysis, muscles of one or more limbs are involved. Asymmetrical flaccid paralysis is characteristic finding. It is mostly caused by type 1.

Poliovirus **does not multiply in muscle cells.** The changes that occur in periphery nerves and voluntary muscles are secondary to destruction of nerve cells. Some cells that lost their function may recover completely. Inflammation occurs secondary to attack on nerve cells. In addition to pathogenic changes in nervous tissue, there may be myocarditis, lymphatic hyperplasia, ulcer formation in Payer's patches.

Encephalitis may occur primarily involving the **brainstem** but extending up to the **motor and premotor areas of cerebral cortex.**

Bulbar Poliomyelitis

Cranial nerves are involved, these include 9, 10, 12th. There may be involvement of muscles of **pharynx, vocal cords, respiration**. This condition may turn fatal also.

Post-Poliomyelitis Syndrome

These sequelae develop 20–40 years after infection with poliomyelitis. Weakness and fatigue occurs in those muscles which were early involved.

Progressive post-poliomyelitis muscle atrophy: A recrudescence of paralysis and muscle wasting has been observed in individuals with paralytic polio a decade after. Although progressive muscle atrophy is rare, it is a specific syndrome. **It does not appear to be result of persistant infection but rather due to physiologic and aging changes in paralytic patients already burdened by loss of neuromuscular functions.**

Polio Epidemiology

India has declared polio free since January 2014; the last natural case was detected three years back. Currently polio is endemic in three countries—Pakistan, Afghanistan and Nigeria. In the year 2014, 359 cases reported worldwide, out of which 306 cases reported from Pakistan and 19 cases were reported from nonendemic countries as Somalia, Guinea, Iraq and Cameroon.

Laboratory Diagnosis

Specimen collection: Stools, throat swab, and CSF are the specimens collected for diagnosis.

Microscopy: CSF shows presence of 20–100 cells/mm³. The cells are predominantly lymphocytes.

Direct Demonstration of the Virus

a. **Electron microscope (EM) or immune electron microscope (IEM)**

b. **Isolation of virus is done from:**
   - **Blood** (3–5 days after infection before neutralizing antibodies appear)
   - **Throat swab** (early stage)
   - **Feces:** Viruses are intermittent in feces (**80% in first week, 50% till 3 weeks and 25% till 6 weeks**). Prolonged fecal excretion may occur in immuno-deficient, but no permanant carriers. As viruses are intermitant in feces, repeat samples on next day increase the isolation of viruses.
   - Viral isolation is possible from more than 30 days from stool; during the illness isolation from **throat swab is possible for first few days of illness only.** Isolation from CSF is rare.
   - **CSF** (rare)
   - **Postmortem: Isolation from spinal cord and brain.** Appropriate processing should be done to destroy bacteria (centrifugation, treatment with ether, addition of antibiotics)

Cell cultures used for isolation:
- Primary monkey kidney cell line
- HeLa
- HEp-2
- MRC-5

1. **CPE** appear in 2–3 days. Infected cells round up and become refractive and pyknotic. There is increased cytoplasmic granularity.
2. Viral growth can be identified by neutralization tests with pooled and specific antisera. This also helps in typing of viruses.

   Mere isolation of virus in feces does not constitute diagnosis of poliomyelitis, as symptomless infections are common.

3. *Serodiagnosis*: Antibody rise is detected (in paired sera) by neutralization or CFT (an antibody to 'C' antigen appears first and disappears in few months, whereas anti-D antibodies appear after some weeks, but last for five years).

4. *Molecular diagnosis*: Though PCR is highly sensitive as well as specific; it is done at reference laboratories only.

   Species specific identification on culture can be done by **pan-polio oligonucleotide primers targeted to VP1 coding regions.**

   Sequencing can differentiate between wild viruses and OPV vaccine derived polioviruses (VDPVs).

Shell Vial Culture

Cell vial culture combined with use of monoclonal antibodies for viral detection in cell cultures in absence of cytopathic effects makes the detection of growth in **2–3 days.**

Humoral immunity is produced by circulating and secretory antibodies. IgM is produced within a week lasts for six months. IgG anibody persists for life and secretory IgA antibody in GI tract gives mucosal immunity, prevents intestinal infection and virus shedding. Breast milk containing IgA protects infants from infection.

Cell-mediated immunity is uncertain, as immuno-deficient persons respond normally to infection.

Prophylaxis

Passive immunization by human gammaglobulin is of little value.

Early vaccines: Crude suspensions of spinal cord from infected monkeys, inactivated with formalin (Brodie and Park) or ricinoleate (Kolmer) were tried earlier but found to be ineffective, dangerous, leading to vaccination poliomyelitis.

Salk's Killed Vaccine (1953) (IPV Injectible Polio Vaccine)

It is formalin inactivated preparation of the three types poliovirus grown in monkey kidney tissue culture.

Viral pools of adequate titre are filtered, to remove cell debris and clumps and inactivated with formalin (1:4000) at 37°C for 12–15 days. It is safe and potent (80–90% protection against paralytic poliomyelitis).

Cutter incident (called after manufacturer of the particular vaccine in 1955); 100 cases of paralytic poliomyelitis occurred in those who received vaccines and their contacts following the use of an insufficiently inactivated vaccine. But after this, modifications were done and vaccine became safe.

Killed vaccine is given by injection hence called inactivated or injectable vaccine.

Doses: Three doses given 4–6 weeks apart constitute primary immunization, followed by a booster 6 months later. First dose should be given to babies after 6 months. Booster doses are given every 3–5 years thereafter.

Enhanced potency IPV: It is produced in **human diploid cells**, induces better seroconversion following 2 subcutaneous doses, 4–8 weeks apart. A third dose given 6–12 months later.

Live-attenuated vaccines were developed independently by Koprowsky, Cox and Sabin: Initially all three viruses were used, but now only **Sabin's attenuated strains** are employed **(OPV).**

Criteria Used for Selection of Vaccine Strains

- Vaccine strain should be non-virulent so that it will not multiply in nervous tissue.
- It should be able to set up intestinal infection following feeding and should induce an immune response.
- It should be stable and should not acquire neurovirulence after serial enteric passage.
- It should possess stable genetic characteristics (markers like rct 40, MS and McBride's intratypic antigenic marker) by which they can be differentiated from the wild strains.
- OPV is prepared by growing the attenuated strain in monkey kidney cells. Strict precautions are taken so that the strain should be free from SV40 and B virus. Tests for neurovirulence, genetic stability and potency are carried out.

Vaccine strain can be differentiated from wild strain by different markers as:

- *'d' marker:* Vaccine strain is not able to grow in presence of bicarbonate.
- *rct 40:* Wild strains grow at 40°C, vaccine strain doesn't grow well.
- *MS:* Wild strain grows well in stable line of monkey kidney.

Vaccine is available in monovalent or trivalent form, in pleasantly flavored syrup. $MgCl_2$ or sucrose stabilizes the vaccine against heat inactivation. The vaccine contain Type 1 virus—10 lakh, type 2 virus—2 lakh, type 3 virus—3 lakh TC ID50 per dose (0.5 mL). The liquid vaccine is thermostabilized with $MgCl_2$ which acts only at pH below 7.0. Shelf life of vaccine at 4–8°C is 4 months and at –20°C, 2 years. The vaccine is usually given in trivalent form. It can be given to infants as maternal antibodies have little impact on it. Theoretically, a single dose is sufficient but in practice three doses given at 4–6 weeks apart to make it sure that all three strains multiply in intestine and overcome the interference due to other organisms or within themselves.

Advantage of Live OPV

Ease of administration: The vaccine is given orally and it can be given along with DPT.

Economy: Vaccine is economical hence in mass immunization it is cheaper.

Nature of immunity: This vaccine gives **systemic** as well **as local immunity**, in contrast to killed vaccine which gives only systemic immunity. If killed vaccine is given there is no local mucosal immunity, a wild strain of virus may multiply in intestine hence though the vaccinated person is protected, and there may be dissemination of wild virus.

Thus live virus produces local immunity as well as immunity in community and increases **herd immunity.**

Duration of immunity: Immunity to live vaccine is long lasting while it is short in case of IPV hence boosters are necessary. Natural live immunity is almost lifelong.

Uses in epidemics: Administration of live vaccine, ideally with monovalent vaccine same with that of strains causing epidemic, can lead to halting the epidemic.

Spread of virus in community: The tendency of live vaccine to spread naturally in the community is considered as added advantage. Ideally it is desirable to give OPV simultaneously in whole community at a time, will prevent dissemination of wild virus.

Erradication

Pulse Polio Immunization Programme

Eradication of poliomyelitis
(In 2011 only four countries Afganistan, Pakistan, Nigeria and India remained of Polio free).

OPV was considered as important tool in irradication of polio. But there may be cases of poor response to OPV due to:
- Interference of other enteroviruses.
- Other diarrheal disease may prevent colonization of vaccine strain.
- Neutralization of vaccine strain due to antibodies present in breast milk.
- Some inhibition substances may be present in saliva or intestinal secretions.

In **pulse polio immunization,** all the children below 5 years of age in the area irrespective of their previous

TABLE 57.1: Advantages and disadvantages of live vaccine and killed vaccine

Vaccine	Advantantages	Disadvantages
Live vaccine	Effective Lifelong immunity Gives local immunity Gives herd immunity Ease of administration No need for booster doses Cheap Useful in epidemics	Risk of vaccine-related poliomyelitis Not safe for immunocompromised individuals Unstable, hence cold chain has to be maintained
Killed vaccine	Effective Stable Safe in immunodeficient persons No risk of vaccine related disease	Does not produce local secretory antibody Boosters needed for long immunity Costly Not useful in epidemics

vaccine status are given two extra doses on the same days, usually in the winter. Vaccinated children may shed vaccinated strain in feces; hence if there is a chlid which is not vaccinated and comes in contact with vaccinated child, he will get infection with vaccinated strain. Thus herd immunity is increased.

Advantages and disadvantages of live vaccine and killed vaccine are given in Table 57.1.

The additional doses in pulse polio programme are given in winter season because:
- The efficiency of cold chain is maintained well in winter season.
- This is the season of low transmission of poliomyelitis.
- The government gets time to plan the budget.

With 'pulse polio immunization' polio has been eradicated from India. No case has been reported since 11-02-2014.

Vaccine Derived Poliovirus (VDPV)

On rare occasions, if a population is seriously under-immunized, an excreted vaccine-virus can continue to circulate for an extended period of time. The longer it is allowed to survive, the more genetic changes it undergoes. In very rare instances, the vaccine-virus can genetically changed into a form that can paralyse. This is known as a circulating **vaccine-derived poliovirus (VDPV). Most VDPV isolate belong to sabin type 2.**

It takes a long time for a VDPV to occur. Generally, the strain will have been allowed to circulate in an under immunized population for a period of at least 12 months. Circulating VDPVs occur when routine or supplementary immunization activities (SIAs) are poorly conducted and a population is left susceptible to poliovirus, whether from vaccine-derived or wild poliovirus. **Hence, the problem is not with the vaccine itself, but low vaccination coverage.** If a population is fully immunized, they will be protected against both vaccine-derived and wild polioviruses.

COXSACKIEVIRUS

These viruses were isolated from the village of coxsackie in New York.

Classification

Coxsackie A and B, (by neutralization). 'A' is classified into 24 serotypes and group 'B' into 6 serotypes. coxsakie A-23 is same as ECHO9 and coxsakie A-24 is same as ECHO 34.

These viruses have the ability to infect suckling but not adult mice. Pathological changes produced in suckling mice are:

Type A: It causes **generalized myositis** and flaccid paralysis leading to death within a week.

Type B: It causes patchy **focal myositis,** spastic paralysis, necrosis of the brown fat and often pancreatitis, hepatitis, myocarditis and encephalitis.

Coxsackie (A-7, 20, 21, 24 and B-1, 3, 5, 6) agglutinate human or monkey erythrocytes. Viruses grow well in suckling mice (subcutaneous or intraperitoneal routes). Suckling hamsters can be infected experimentally.

Cultivation

All coxsackie B viruses grow well in monkey kidney tissue cultures, while in **group A, 7 and 9 grow well.** Type 'A' 21 grows in **HeLa cells.**

Clinical Features

- *Herpangina (vesicular pharyngitis):* It is seen in chidren with group-A. There is severe pharyngitis with vesicles on posterior half of palate, pharynx, tonsils or tongue. It is a self-limiting illness.
- *Aseptic meningitis* (Most groups 'A' and all group 'B'): Most commonly the condition is caused by **A7** and **A9.** The disease may sometimes progress to mild muscle wekness suggestive of paralytic poliomyelitis (infantile paralysis).

- *Hand-foot-and-mouth disease (HFMD) (A-16, 9; B 1–3 and enterovirus 71).* It is characterized by oral and pharyngeal ulcerations and vesicular rash on palms and soles that may spread to arms and legs. The vesicles heal without crusting.
- Minor respiratory infections resembling **common cold** (A 10, 21, 24 and B3) (Flowchart 57.1).
- **Epidemic pleurodynia or Bornholm disease** (first described on the Danish island of Bornholm). **Stabing pain in the chest and abdomen is caused by all group B viruses.**
- **Myocarditis and pericarditis** in the newborns are associated with high fatality caused by **group B viruses.**
- *Juvenile diabetes (B4):*
  1. Orchitis
  2. **Transplacental and neonatal transmission (B virus)** leading to hepatitis, meningoencephalitis and adrenocortical involvement.
  3. Post-viral fatigue syndrome (B virus).

Laboratory Diagnosis

- **Virus isolation** is done from the lesions or from feces by inoculation into suckling mice. Identification is done by studying the histopathology in infected mice and by neutralization tests. Serodiagnosis is not practicable (due to several antigenic types).

- **Real-time PCR is higly sensitive method for diagnosis.**

ECHOVIRUSES

As initially they could not be associated with any particular disease, they were called then **'orphans'** (enteric cytopathogenic human orphan—ECHO viruses). Total **34 serotypes** are identified by neutralization test (10, 28 removed from group). Most of human infections are asymptomatic. **Fever, rash, aseptic meningitis** are the manifestations of illness caused by these viruses. Aseptic meningitis is predominantly produced by types **4, 6, 9, 16, 20, 28,** and **30.** Other infections include respiratory illness (types 1, 11, 19, 20, 22) and gastroenteritis (type 18). **Laboratory diagnosis** is done by **isolation of viruses from feces, throat, or CSF; specimens are inoculated in primary monkey kidney tissue cultures.** Viruses are identified by hemagglutination and neutralization.

New enteroviruses
- *Enterovirus 68* causes pneumonia.
- *Enterovirus 70* causes acute hemorrhagic conjunctivitis.
- *Enterovirus 71* causes meningitis.
- *Enterovirus 72* is hepatitis A virus.

Flowchart 57.1: Pathogenesis of common cold

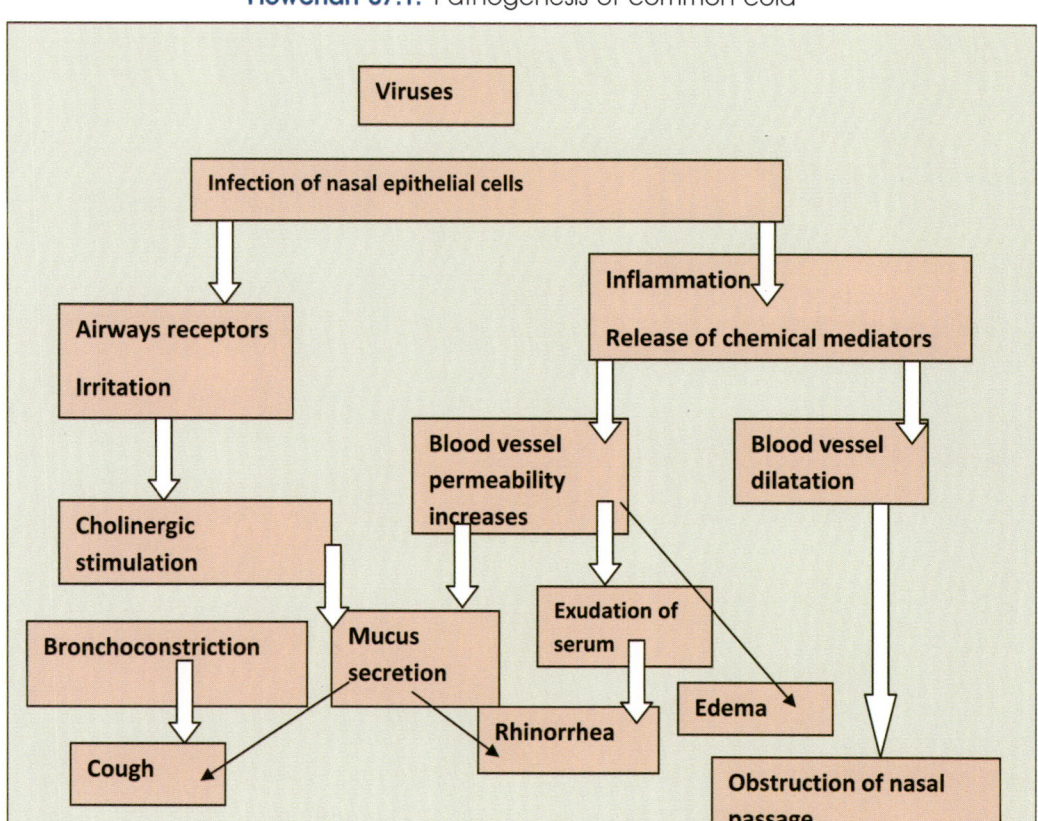

RHINOVIRUSES

Viruses isolated from cases of common cold are called rhinoviruses; rhino refers to nose, which is infected mostly. There are more than 150 serotypes of this virus. They are divided into major and minor receptors groups.

Viruses with major group use cellular adhesion molecule-1 **(ICAM-1) as receptor**, minor group use receptors of the **members of low density lipoproteins family (LDLR).**

Morphologically, they resemble other picornaviruses. They are more heat stable, acid labile. These viruses can grow in human or monkey cells. They are fastidious viruses which require oxygen, low pH, and low temperature.

In the year 2009, genomes of all known rhinoviruses were sequenced.

There are three groups of rhinoviruses. 'H' strains grow in human cells, 'O' could grow in nasal and tracheal ciliated cells, 'M' grows well in human and monkey cells. Droplets or contact, as hands shaking spreads the virus. The viruses may be associated with other viruses causing common cold as *RSV, coxsackie, coronavirus, echoviruses, adenoviruses, influenza and parainfluenza viruses*. There is no special treatment for the condition and laboratory diagnosis is seldom done.

PARECHOVIRUS GROUP

They contain 14 types, 1 and 2 originally classified as echoviruses 22 and 23. **The capsid of these viruses contains 3 proteins because the VPO precursor protein does not break up.** These viruses are acquired in early childhood, replicate in respiratory and gastrointestinal tract and may cause **mild respiratory** disease or **mild gastrointestinal illness,** rarely they cause neonatal sepsis and meningitis.

Foot and Mouth Disease (Apthovirus of Cattle)

This is a **highly contagious disease in cattle and sheep. Infected animals become poor producers of milk.** There are 7 types of viruses. All infected animals are slaughtered and their carcasses destroyed to control the infections. The infection may be transmitted in human beings and infections are characterized by fever, salivation, and vesicles formation on oropharynx, skin of palms, soles, fingers and toes.

58

Orthomyxoviruses

MYXOVIRUSES

Myxoviruses are RNA viruses, adsorb to mucoprotein receptors on RBCs causing hemagglutination (myxa means mucus, affinity to mucins).

Family: Orthomyxoviridae.

Genus: *Influenza viruses*—3 serotypes based on ribonucleoprotein 'RNP' antigen: *Influenza A, Influenza B, Influenza C.*

INFLUENZA VIRUS (Fig. 58.1)

Morphology

- It is spherical virus.
- *Size*: 80–120 nm, long filamentous forms may be seen.
- **Genome** is negative sense single-stranded RNA. Filamentous, RNA is segmented in **eight pieces**. Genetic assortments may occur.
- Hence it is **antigenically unstable**.

Influenza "C" virus contains **7 segments** of RNA lacking a neuraminidase gene. Most of the segments code for a single protein.

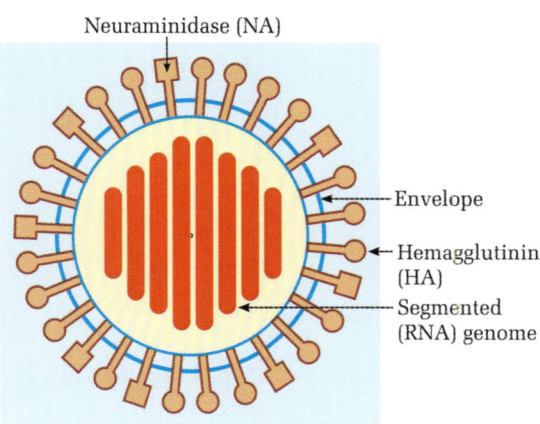

Neuraminidase (NA)

Envelope
Hemagglutinin (HA)
Segmented (RNA) genome

Fig. 58.1: Influenza virus

Sizes and protein coding are assigned to segments. The complete nucleotide sequences are known for influenza viruses. The first 12–13 nucleotides at each of genome segment are conserved among all 8 segments, these sequences are important for transcription.

Structural proteins: Influenza virus contains **9 different structural proteins**. The nucleoprotein (NP) associates with the viral RNA to form ribonucleoprotein (**RNP**) structure, 9 nm diameter and forms **nucleocapsid**. **Capsid** has helical symmetry. The 3 large proteins are (**PB1, PB2, PA**) bound to viral RNP and responsible for viral transcription and replication.

Envelope: Inner membrane protein forms shell beneath envelope (or **matrix protein**) composed of two parts 'M1' and 'M2'. The matrix protein 'M1' is a major component of virion and it is important in morphogenesis.

M1 is enclosed in host plasma membrane-derived lipid bilayer envelope. M2 projects through envelope.

Envelope glycoproteins: Two types of spikes are present, i.e. hemagglutinin (**H**) and neuraminidase (**N**).

Antigens

Internal antigens are type specific.

Ribonucleoprotein: It is the basis of classification into types A, B, C. This protein is found free in infected tissue. Antibody develops after infection only.

Matrix protein: V or viral surface antigens: It contains two antigens: Hemagglutinin (HA) and neuraminidase (NA).

Hemagglutinin (HA): There are 15 types of 'H' antigens, H1–H15. HA binds to receptors present on epithelial cells. As this helps in adhesion to epithelial cells, antibodies produced against HA causes viral neutralization.

Neuraminidase (NA): It is of 9 types, N1–N9. It plays role in release of virus from infected cell. Antibody against 'NA' is not neutralizing antibody. But it prevents spread of viruses to other cells.

Neuraminidase (NA) is receptor destroying enzyme (RDE), it causes reversal of hemagglutination.

Entry of virus takes place by receptor-mediated endocytosis. Fusion of cell membrane with viral envelope takes place, which is mediated by 'HA'.Viral nucleocapsids enter cell cytoplasm. 'M1', 'M2' cause stabilization of lipid envelope and important in viral assembly. 'P'-polymerase proteins are essential for transcription and synthesis of viral RNA. Two nonstructural proteins function as **INF antagonist** and post-transcriptional regulator (**NS1**) and nuclear export factor (**NS2, or NEP**).

Hemagglutination (HA): It is responsible for adsorption and crosslinking of RBC mucoprotein receptors. It is used as a method for detection and titration of virus.

Hemagglutination inhibition (HAI): It used for detection and titration of antibody to virus.

Elution: It is reversal of hemagglutination.

Hemagglutination and elution are used for purifying and concentrating influenza viruses.

Antigenic Variation (Tables 58.1 and 58.2)

RNP, 'M' and two of 'internal proteins' are stable antigens, variations occur in 'H 'and 'N'.

The antigenic differences of the stable antigens are used for classification of virus into three types—A, B, C. The antigenic varitions in 'HA' and 'NA' used for subtyping the virus. Only 'A 'has designated subtypes. So far there are 9 subtypes of 'NA' and 15 subtypes of 'HA' in many combinations have been recovered from human, animal, bird influenza viruses. **Four HA (H1-H3, H5) and 2 NA (N1, N2)** subtypes recovered from humans.

Function of HA: It binds viral particles to susceptible cells.

Function of NA: It is sialidase enzyme which removes sialic acid from glycoconjugates. It facilitates release of viral particles fom infected cells during budding process and helps to prevent self-aggregation of viruses by removing sialic acid residues from viral glycoproteins.

As this virus has segmented genome, antigenically it is not stable. There are two main types of antigenic changes.

Antigenic Drift (Table 58.3)

* It is gradual, sequential change in antigenic structure occurring regularly at frequent intervals.
* The change is due to mutation and selection.
* It accounts for periodical epidemics.
* The new antigen though different from previous, is related to it. Hence, in population, the antibodies produced against the previous virus are present which give some protection against new virus.

Antigenic Shift (Table 58.3)

* It is abrupt, discontinuous variation in antigenic structure.
* The newly formed virus may be completely different; hence people may not have antibodies against it.

TABLE 58.1: Types and subtype of influenza virus

Orthomyxoviridae	Virus	H1N1 (A1)
	Influenza virus A	Human, Hsw N1, H2N2 (A2), H3N2 (A3, Hong Kong)
	Influenza virus B	B (human)
	Influenza virus C	C (human)

TABLE 58.2: Comparision of influenza A, B, C

	A	*B*	*C*
Severity of illness	+++	++	+
Animal reservoir	Yes	No	No
Spread in humans	Pandemic	Epidemic	Sporadic
Antigenic changes	Shift, drift	Drift	Drift
No. of RNA segments	8	8	7
No. of surface glycoproteins	2	2	1
	Some strains agglutinate only guinea pig RBCs on initial isolation	It agglutinates both guinea pig and fowl RBCs	Type C agglutinate only fowl RBCs at 4°C

TABLE 58.3: Differences between antigenic shift and drift

Shift	Drift
Abrupt drastic change	Gradual sequential change
Discontinuous variation	Change occurs frequently at regular intervals
Results in novel virus which is totally antigenically different from previous one	New antigen is related to previous antigen
Antibodies to predecessor strains do not neutralize it	Influenced by antibodies to predecessor strains
It is due to genetic reassortment	It is due to mutation and selection
It may cause epidemics and pandemics	It causes epidemics
People are not protected against new strain	People are protected against new virus at least some extent

- It is because of **genetic reassortment**.
- Antibodies to previous strains do not neutralize it.
- It spreads rapidly over large geographic areas. It accounts for major epidemics and pandemics because there is no antibody in community aginst this totally different virus.

Virus Variability

- Viruses replicate via virally encoded RNA dependent RNA polymerase.
- These enzymes lack a proofreading (error correction) function.
- It leads to formation of large number of mutants especially in influenza 'A'.
- Viruses carrying mutations do not provide a disadvantage in replication; hence evolve rapidly, a feature called genetic drift.
- Genetic recombination between diverse influenza 'A' types occurs when more than one serotype infects a single host creating new combinations of viral gene segments (reassortment) and altering the replicating and virulence properties of progeny virus.
- The combination of genetic drift and genetic reassortment provide mechanisms to generate genetic diversity among influenza type 'A' viruses. The genetic assortment mainly occurs in type 'A' (B and C may show some limited genetic assortment).
- The genetic mechanisms also generate adaptive flexibility; hence the virus becomes capable of infecting different host.

Shifts

The pandemics are associated with antigenic shifts. 'HA' or 'NA' or both changed.

It results from acquisition of new RNA segment 4 and/or 6 either due to genetic reassortments or infection of human with animal virus.

Host Range

Influenza 'A' virus has wide host range and infects human, pig, horse, seal, whale, bird, chicken, and duck.

Influenza 'B' virus and Influenza 'C' virus: Only humans are the host, hence there is no question of genetic reassortment.

Growth in chick embryo: Virus grows well in the amniotic cavity of chick embryo. After adaption, virus also grows in allantoic cavity. Type 'C' does not grow in allantoic cavity. Viral growth is detected by detection of hemagglutinins in amniotic cavity and allantoic cavity.

Cultivation in Cell Cultures

Viruses grow in primary monkey kidney cell cultures. It does not produce cytopathic effects. The viral growth in cell cultures is detected by hemadsorption or demonstration of HA in culture fluid.

Pathogenesis

- Virus transmission occurs via aerosols generated via coughing, sneezing, hand to hand contact and by fomites. Small aerosols less than 10 microns are more efficient in transmission than large droplets.
- Virus enters through mucosa of respiratory tract. With the help of surface spikes, virus attaches to respiratory epithelial cells.
- Viscosity of respiratory secretion is reduced by neuraminidase, H binds to cell receptors. Virus causes destruction and desquamation of ciliated cells, hence mucosa becomes susceptible to secondary bacterial infections.
- Initially columnar epithelial cells are involved afterwards alveolar cells, mucous glands and pulmonary macrophages are infected.
- Virus replicates in 4–6 hours and infectious virions released, cause infection of adjacent cells. Thus infection spreads in respiratory tract in few hours.
- Upper and lower respiratory tract is affected. Due to lysis of cells, there is release of destructive enzymes from epithelial cells.
- Basal layer of respiratory tract remains intact. Local symptoms are due to edema and infiltration of mononuclear cells. Release of cytokines occurs which may cause systemic manifestations.
- There is influx of macrophages and lymphocytes at the sites of infection. Cytokines, released from macrophage, cause fever, muscular pain, fatigue, vasodilatation, stiffness of nose, and rhinorrhea. The irritation caused by debris and host responses lead

to production of mucus. Humoral immunity plays important role in recovery from infection.

Superinfection with other bacteria and fungi occurs. Release **of interleukin-1** from macrophages causes fever, while **INF-α** porbably causes diffuse muscular pains, fatigue. Inflammation, edema and vasodilation result in stiffness, and rhinorrhea. In tracheobronchial tree, the irritation caused by debris and host responses stimulates mucus production. Humoral immunity plays important role in curing the infection.

The pathogenesis of **systemic symptoms** may be related to **TNF-α, INF-α, IL-6** in respiratory scretions and blood. **Antibodies >40 (HA) have been** associated with **protection** from infection. **Secretory antibodies IgA>4 are associated with protection.**

T cell responses include: Tc, NK directed against conserved regions of internal proteins (NP, M) and surface proteins (H, N).

Original antigenic sin: When a previously infected person gets a repeated infection with a different antigenic variant of influenza, antibodies are produced against both the serotypes, but predominant response would be against the original strain. This phenomenon is called "original antigenic sin".

Clinical Features

Incubation period is 1–3 days. Disease varies mild coryza to fatal pneumonia.

Fever, chills, headaches, dry cough, muscular ache, malaise, anorexia, are common symptoms while abdominal pain and vomitings occur in infection with type B.

Complications

- Pneumonia
- Congestive cardiac failure
- Myocarditis
- Encephalitis

- Type B: Reye's syndrome, degeneration in kidney, liver, brain
- Type B sometimes present with gastrointestinal symptoms.

Complications occur in following groups:
- Old age
- Chronic cardiac and pulmonary disorders
- Diabetes
- Renal dysfunction
- Immunosuppression
- Pregnancy—2nd and 3rd trimesters
- Hemoglobinopathies
- Acute laryngotracheobronchitis (croup) in age <1 year

Influenza C virus: Mild coryza causes sporadic upper respiratory tract (URT) illness, it is rarely associated with severe LRT illness.

Immunity to influenza: Antibody to 'HA' is protective while antibody to 'NA' decreases severity. Serum antibody persists for years, secretory antibody persists for months.

Epidemiology (Fig. 58.2)

Factors responsible for epidemics and pademics are immunity to viruses and antigenic variations, i.e. antigenic drift and shift.

Pandemic of Influenza 'A Virus (Table 58.4)

1918-19	**"Spanish flu"**	(H1N1)
1957-58	**"Asian flu"**	(H2N2)
1968-69	**" Hong Kong flu"**	(H3N2)

1977 Redflue (HN) Re-emergence of previous strains occurred in Russia and China.

Antigenic variations occurred in influenza viruses.

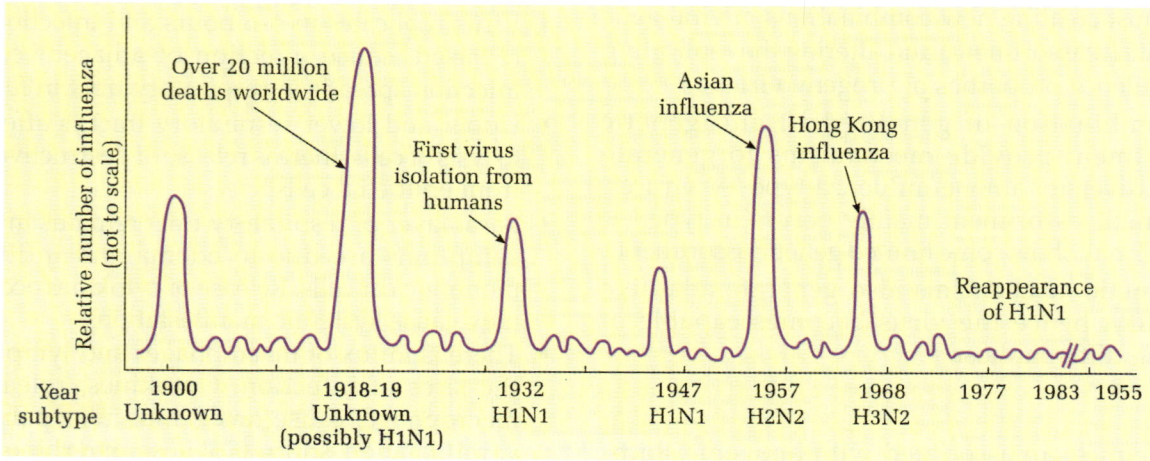

Fig. 58.2: Epidemiology of influenza virus

TABLE 58.4: Different subtypes of influenza viruses causing outbreaks

Year	Subtypes	Type of variation
1918	H1N1	Unknown
1918-57	H1N1	Antigenic drift
1957	H2N2	Antigenic shift
1957-68	H2N2	Antigenic drift
1968	H3N2	
1968-90	H3N2	Antigenic drift
1976-89	H1N1	Reappearance of viruses from 1918, 1950. Prevalence of influenza A virus subtypes

Genetic Reassortment (Fig. 58.3)

The genome of influenza virus is segmented; the reassortment may occur if a host is infected with viruses of two different strains at a time. This causes emergence of novel strain of virus. Pigs act as mixing vessel where virulent genes of fowl mix with genome of influenza virus, producing a novel virus.

Designation of Influenza Virus

Influenza virus type 'A' can be classified into **subtypes** based on surface antigens (Table 58.1). Complete designation of virus may include type, place of origin, series number, year of isolation, antigenic subtypes of 'HA' and 'NA' in parenthesis. For example, *influenzaA /Singapore/1/57/ (H2N2)*.

Laboratory Diagnosis

Virus can be demonstrated in clinical specimen by 'immune electron microscopy'. For this, large number of viruses ($>10^5$–10^6 per mL) should be present in clinical specimens.

1. Demonstration of **viral antigen** on nasopharyngeal cells by **immunofluorescence.**
2. Detection of viral RNA **by RT-PCR.**
3. Isolation of viruses
   a. **Throat garglings** are collected in buffered salt solution.
   b. **Transport** in viral transport medium **(VTM)**.
   c. **Embryonated eggs:** 12–13 days old eggs are used. Inoculation is done in **amniotic and allantoic cavity**: Eggs are incubated at 35°C for 3 days. Fluids harvested from cavities and tested for hemagglutination with guinea pig and fowl RBCs.
   d. **Cell cultures: Primary monkey kidney cell cultures** or continuous cell cultures are used for cultivation. **Identification of growth is done by IF or hemadsorption**.
4. Serological tests to detect antibodies are:
   I. *CFT*: Detects antibodies against RNP
   II. *HAI*: Hemagglutination inhibition tests

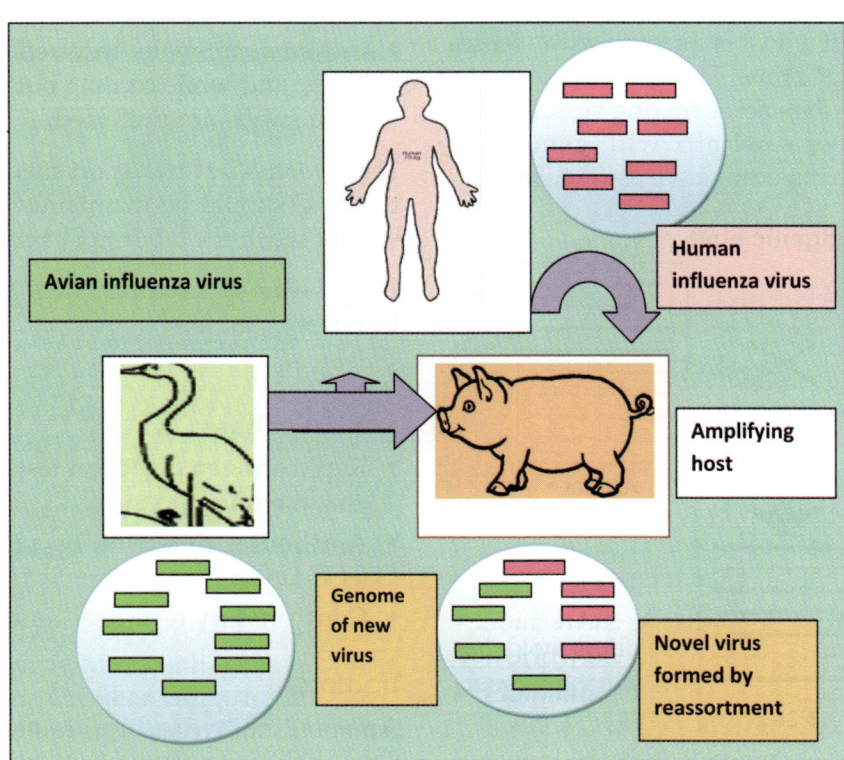

Fig. 58.3: Genetic reassortment in influenza virus

III. ELISA

IV. Immunochromatography.

V. Latex agglutination tests.

5. Genetic methods for differentiation of type of virus:

    a. *RT-PCR (reverse transcriptase PCR)* is preferred for the diagnosis of influenza. The results are available in 1 day, the assay is sensitive and specific. Multiplex technologies have been developed that allow the rapid detection of multiple pathogens in a single test.

    b. Hybridization

    c. Microarray analysis

    d. Restriction analysis.

Bird Flu Virus H5N1—Avian Influenza Virus

First described in Hong Kong in 1997,18 patients infected and 9 deaths occurred. After that more than 240 cases reported with 140 deaths due to poultry outbreaks. Most deaths occurred in Vietnam, and Indonesia. There is no evidence to show human-to-human transmission of H5N1.

These strains are more virulent as they have PBIF$_2$ protein that targets host mitochondria producing apoptosis.

Genetic Assortment

The genome of influenza virus is segmented; the assortment may occur if a host is infected with viruses of two different strains at a time. This causes emergence of novel strain of virus. Pigs act as mixing vessel where virulent genes of water fowl mix with genome of influenza virus, producing a novel virus (Fig. 58.4).

Antigenic shift

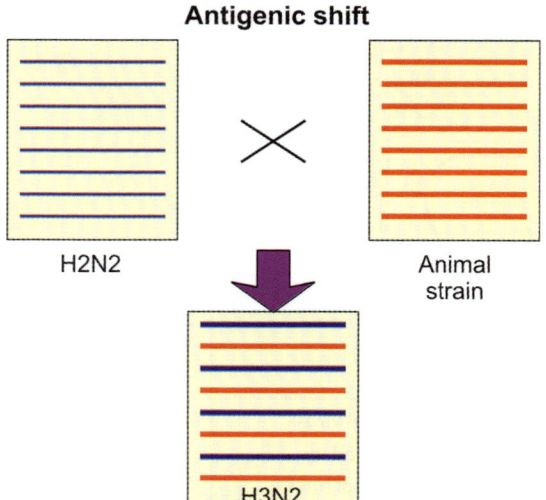

Fig. 58.4: Diagrammatic presentation of genetic reassortment between two viruses producing novel virus

Swine Flu

Swine influenza or swine flu is caused by **H1N1.**

It causes highly contagious acute respiratory disease caused by new strains of influenza formed by genetic assortment. It is reassortment of human influenza A virus, subtype H1N1, including one strain endemic in humans, one endemic in birds and two endemic in swine. This novel strain started producing outbreaks in 2009.

Pigs acted as mixing vessel as human strains and bird strains can infect pigs simultaneously, which combined to produce novel virus. The mode of spread was through droplets expelled by coughing, sneezing; fomites also helped to spread the infections.

Sialic Acid Receptors

These are found on host cell surface which are specific for HA antigens of influenza virus.

- α 2–6 receptors are specific for human influenza strains.
- α 2–3 receptors are specific for avian influenza strains.

Both the receptors are found on the respiratory epithelial cells of pigs. Hence, pigs can be infected with human as well as avian influenza viruses.

Laboratory Diagnosis

Specimens: Nasal swab, nasal washing, sputum, bronchoalveolar lavage, tracheal aspirate, and blood are the samples collected.

Nasal swabs: Swabs inserted in nostrils, left for 10 seconds, and while coming out rotated in nasal cavity. Dacron swabs are preferred.

Transport: **Viral transport medium** is used, temperature 4°C should be maintained in cold chain. Sample should reach the laboratory within 48 hours.

Processing of samples: It is processed in **class III biosafety** cabinets.

Tests Performed

- **Viral culture**
- **Rapid antigen detection tests:** Immunofluorescence, enzyme immunoassay
- **Antibodies detection** by viral neutralization test, CFT, LA
- **Confirmatory test:** Real-time PCR.

Treatment

Amantadine hydrochloride has been found to be of some help in treatment of influenza. It reduced the duration of illness.

TABLE 58.5: Differences between orthomyxoviruses and paramyxoviruses

Characteristics	Orthomyxoviruses	Paramyxoviruses
Size	80–120 nm	100–300 nm
Shape	Spherical	Pleomorphic
Genome	Segmented—8 pieces of RNA	Single, linear
Genetic stability	Unstable	Stable
Genetic reassortment	Yes	No
Hemolysin	Absent	Present
Site of synthesis of ribonucleoprotein	Nucleus	Cytoplasm
DNA dependent RNA synthesis	Required for multiplication of virus	Not required

- Amantadine and rimantasine reduce average duration of illness and cause symptomatic improvement.

- Eseltamivir is new drug whick blocks neuraminidase. It is useful in chemoprophylaxis and treatment.

Earliest vaccine was virus attenuated by **repeated egg passage,** it was given by intranasal instillation. Another vaccine was use of **temperature sensitive mutants** which are able to grow at lower temperature of nasopharyngeal mucosa but not in lungs at 37°C. Third vaccine was **recombinant vaccine** obtained by recombination between ts mutants of known strains and new antigenic variant.

Chemoprophylaxis: Type A—amantadine, rimantadine, for types B and A—zanamivir, oseltamivir are used.

Treatment

A/H₁/N₁/2009 flu: Neuraminidase inhibitors are used for treatment. Oseltamivir (Tamiflu) tablet is given (75 mg) twice a day for 5 days. Zanamivir is available in inhalation form.

General measures for prevention of Swine flu are:
- Stay at home, if you are sick.
- Avoid contact with infected person.
- Contain sneezes and coughs.
- Use N95 respirator in health care settings.
- Washing of hands.

59

Paramyxoviruses

General Characteristics

- Spherical shape (100–300 nm), it may be pleomorphic.
- Giant forms of size 800 nm, may be seen.
- Helical nucleocapsid (18 nm) (larger than orthomyxoviruses) is present.
- Linear single-stranded RNA.
- Fusion protein is responsible for syncytium formation.
- Genome is not fragmented.
- There is no genetic reassortment, do not undergo genetic changes, genetically stable.
- Nucleocapsid is surrounded by **lipid envelope having matrix protein at base.**
- Lipid envelope carries two types of spikes, **hemagglutinin** (has neuraminidase activity also) and **F—fusion protein** which causes fusion of viral envelope with host cell membrane. It is also responsible for syncitia formation.

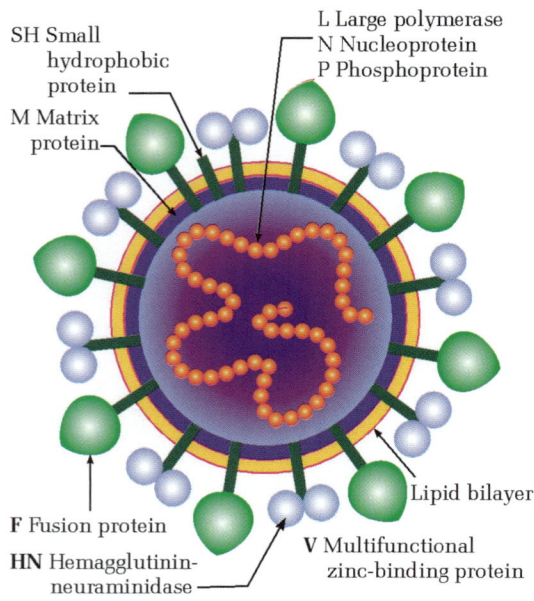

Fig. 59.1: Parainfluenza virus

Classification

There are two subfamilies, i.e Paramyxoviridae and Pneumovirinae. Paramyxoviridae include 4 genera, i.e. *Respirovirus, Rubulavirus, Morbillivirus, Henipavirus*. The Pneumovirinae include two genera, i.e. *Pneumovirus, Metapneumo virus*. The genus *Respirovirus* contains 2 human parainfluenza viruses and the genus *Rubulavirus* contains two other parainfluenza viruses as well as *mumps*. *Sendai virus* of mice which was the first parainfluenza virus isolated and it is now recognized as a common infection in mouse colonies, is a subtype of human type 1 virus. *Simian parainfluenza virus 5 (PIV5)*, a common contaminant of primary monkey kidney cells, is the same as *canine parainfluenza virus type 2; shiping fever virus of cattle* and sheep is a subtype of type 3. *Newcastle disease virus,* the prototype of avian parainfluenza virus of genus *Avulavirus*, is also related to the human viruses.

PARAMYXOVIRUSES

This family includes respiratory parainfluenza viruses (Fig. 59.1), respiratory syncytial viruses which cause acute respiratory tract infections and measles, mumps which cause childhood fevers with rash.

Properties of Paramyxoviruses (Table 59.1)

- Viruses are spherical in shape.
- *Size*: Large, size varies from 100–300 nm. Some of the filamentous forms are large and giants up to 800 nm.
- **Nucleocapsid** is **helical,** diameter is 18 nm.
- *Envelope*: Lipid envelope has matrix protein at its base and two types of glycoprotein spikes.
- *Glycoprotein spikes*: Longer spike is **H** and it has neuraminidase **(NA)** activity also, hence called **'HN' protein.** Short spike is **'F'-fusion protein**, responsible for fusion of viral envelope with plasma membrane of host cells. Cell to cell fusion, syncytia formation and giant cell formation are also associated with F protein.

TABLE 59.1: Properties of paramyxoviridae

	Respirovirus Parainfluenza 1, 3	Rubulavirus Mumps, Parainfluenza 2, 4b, 4a	Morbillivirus Measles	Pneumovirus respiratory synsytial virus
Diameter of nucleocapsid	18	18	18	13
Fusion protein	+	+	+	+
Hemolysin	+	+	+	−
Hemagglutination or hemadsorption	+	+	+	−
Neuraminidase	+	+	−	−
Intracellular inclusions in cytoplasm-C or nucleus –N	C	C	N, C	C
Antigenic types	4	1	1	1
Antigenic relationship	Mumps	Parainfluenza	—	—-

- Apart from NA and F proteins, there is non-glycosylated third protein 'M' which forms the inner layer of envelope, maintaining its structure and integrity.
- *Viral genome*: Single, linear stranded RNA (15000 nucleotides); genome is unsegmented, hence the genome is stable.
- *Proteins*: 6 structural proteins are present.
- *Replication*: It takes place in cytoplasm of host cells, particles bud from plasma membrane.

Cultivation

Primary monkey kidney cell culture: Cytopathic effects produced are **syncytial formation** and acidophilic intracytoplasmic inclusion bodies. Hemadsorption and immunofluorescence are used for identification of growth in cell cultures.

PARAINFLUENZA VIRUSES

Types

1. *Parainfluenza virus-1 includes Sendai virus and human adsorption virus-1.*
2. *Parainfluenza type-2 includes croup associated virus* (CAV).
3. *Parainfluenza type-3*: Causes respiratory disease in animals, bronchitis, and pneumonia (*shipping fever in cattle*).
4. *Parainfluenza type-4 causes* mild respiratory infections in children, sore throat, hoarseness of voice.

Parainfluenza viruses cause repiratory illness in all ages.

Pathogenesis and Pathology

Viruses are transmitted by direct person-to-person contact or by large droplet aerosols. Replication is restricted to respiratory tract. Viremia is uncommon.

Infection may be mild involving nose and throat causing **common cold. Occasionally, types 1 and 2 may cause laryngotracheobronchitis 'croup',** which is characterized by respiratory obstruction due to swelling of larynx and related structures. The infection may spread deeper to trachea, bronchi causing bronchitis or pneumonia or both, especially with type 3.

More than 50% of infections with parainfluenzae types 1–3 result in febrile illness. About 25% primary type 1 infection produce bronchitis, but only 2–3% develop croup.

Presence of host cells proteases able to cleave and activate the fusion protein enabling virus to replicate well and disseminate throughout respiratory tract. **Primary infection tends to be severe and occurs below 5 years of age. It has been suggested that rapid and abundant production of virus specific IgE antibodies causes histamine release in trachea causing croup symptoms.** Parainfluenza type 4 doesn't cause serious disease.

Newcastle disease virus is an **avian parainfluenza virus.** In humans, it may produce **conjunctivitis.**

Laboratory Diagnosis

- Virus is **isolated** from samples like throat swab, nasal swab, nasal washings.
- **Direct identification of viral antigens** in specimens is done by ELISA or direct immunofluorescence (DIF).
- Isolation is done in human and **monkey kidney cell lines** and viral growth is detected by **hemadsorption** (with guinea pig RBCs) and by **IF.**
- *Serology*: Paired sera used for antibodies detection by ELISA, CFT, HI.
- *Treatment*: **Ribavirin** shows beneficial results when delivered by small particle aerosols.

RSV (GENUS—PNEUMOVIRUS)

As it causes cell fusion and form **multinucleated syncytia,** it is called respiratory syncytial virus.

- *Shape*: Pleomophic
- *Size*: 150–300 nm
- Envelope has 2 glycoproteins, **'G'-protein** for attachment, **'F' protein for fusion.**
- **No hemagglutinin** activity.

Infections transmitted by close contact, through contaminated fingers; fomites may transmit the infections. Respiratory tract is involved. Most infections are symptomatic.

Respiratory infections present as febrile rhinorrhea, cough, sneezing, lower respiratory tract infection as tracheobronchitis or pneumonia. About 1% babies develop into severe disease which may require hospitalization. About one-third children with RSV respiratory disease develop into middle ear infections.

Laboratory Diagnosis

- *Specimens*: Nasopharyngeal swabs or nasal washing
- Direct antigen detection in specimens is possible with direct immunofluorescence test.
- Cultivation: Cultivation is done in HeLa, HEp-2 cell lines; virus causes syncytial formation in 10 days.
- Viral growth is also detected by immunofluorescence.

MEASLES (Fig. 59.2)

It is an acute highly contagious infection affecting children. The study of epidemic (1864) in Faroe Island by Danish medical student named Peter Panum helped to understand many aspects of the infection.

Morphology

- Spherical or pleomorphic
- 120–250 nm in size

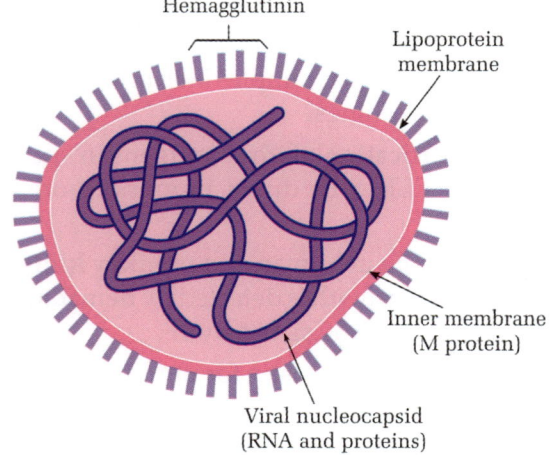

Hemagglutinin

Lipoprotein membrane

Inner membrane (M protein)

Viral nucleocapsid (RNA and proteins)

Fig. 59.2: Measles virus

- Tightly coiled helical nucleocapsid
- Envelope has hemagglutinin spikes
- Envelope has also 'F'—fusin proteins

Cultivation

Human or monkey kidney cell culture or human amnion cell cultures (these are preferred for primary isolation) or HeLa, HEp-2 (viruses grow in these cell lines after adaption) are used for cultivation.

Cytopathic effects are **multinucleate syncytial formation and both intranuclear as well as intra-cytoplasmic inclusion bodies are produced** which are **eosinophilic.** Multinucleate giant cells, called **Warthin–Finkeldey** cells, are produced in lymphoid tissues of patients.

Mode of Infection

Humans are natural hosts. Respiratory secretions and aerosols created by coughing and sneezing transmit the infections. The virus multiples locally, the infection then spreads to regional lymph nodes where further multiplication occurs. **Primary viremia** disseminates the virus, which then multiplies in cells of reticulo-endothelial cells. With the **secondary viremia,** the viruses enter in epithelial cells, skin, respiratory tract, conjunctiva where further multiplication of viruses takes place.

Measles can replicate in certain lymphocytes, which helps in dissemination of infection throughout the body. Multinucleated giant cells are seen in lymph nodes, tonsils, appendix. All these events last for 9–11 days. Onset of illness is abrupt with fever, cough, coryza, conjunctivitis (Flowchart 59.1).

Clinical Features

Prodromal illness: It clinically presents as fever, malaise, cough, nasal discharge and conjunctival infection.

Rash: Rash is red maculopapular, appears on forehead, spread downwards, lead to desquamation. The rash develops as a result of interaction of immune T cells with virus infected cells in small blood vessels.

Koplik spots: Koplik spots are small **bluish white ulcers on buccal mucosa, oppositive lower molar and contain giant cell, viral antigens, viral nucleocapsids and inclusions.** Rarely they appear on conjunctiva and intestinal cells. Though Koplik spots are patho-gnomonic of the disease, they may be missed as they develop a day or 2 days before the skin rash. During prodromal illness, viruses are present in tears, nasal

Flowchart 59.1: Pathogenesis of measles

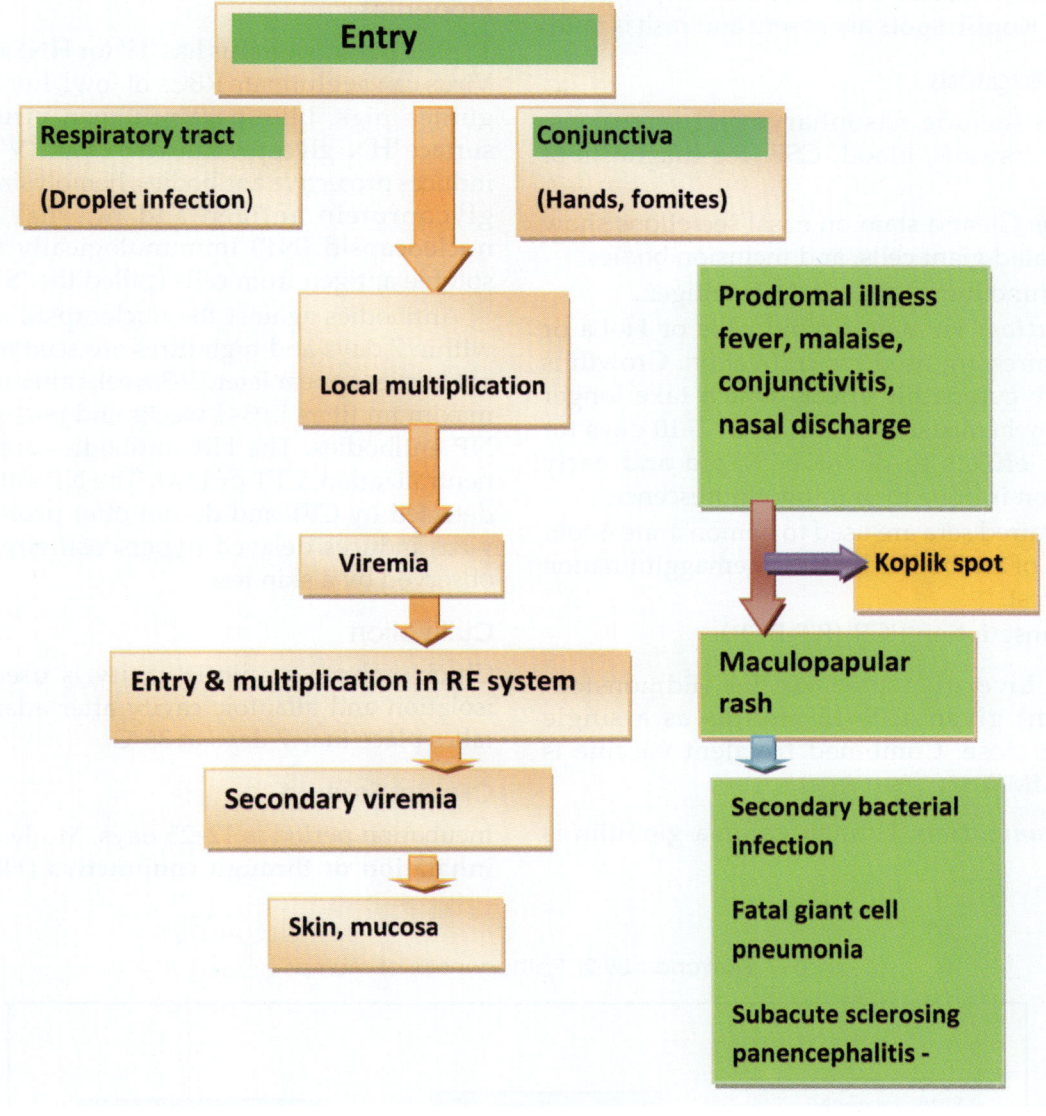

secretions, throats secretions, urine, blood. Antibodies appear with appearance of rash. Viremia disappears. Fever falls.

Complications

- **Secondary bacterial infections** involving beta hemolytic streptococci are common. Pulmonary complications may occur in few cases.

- **Pneumonia (giant cell pneumonia)** in immuno-compromised patients, is due to unchecked viral replication. Extensive cell fusion occurs in lung tissues. It is a fatal condition.

- **Meningoencephalitis:** It develops in 1 in 1000 infected cases. There is second bout of fever with convulsions and pleocytosis in CSF. Survivers may show some signs of permanent damage.

- **Subacute sclerosing panencephalitis (SSPE):** It is a rare late complication of measles. It develops 1 year after infection and it is caused by viruses that remain in the body after acute infection. Large number of measles antigens are present within inclusion bodies in infected brain cells but no viral particles mature. It happens probably due to failure of patient's immune system to clear viruses. By expression of fewer viral antigens on surface, cells may avoide attack of humoral or cell-mediated immune responses. Patients show very high titres of antibodies in CSF and in serum and defective measles virus in brain cells.

- Suppression of delayed hypersensitivity (Montaux) occurs.

- Underlying TB worsens.

- Premature labor, spontaneous abortion.

- Thrombocytopenia, purpura, hemorrhages may occur.

- Modified measles occurs in infants with residual maternal antibodies. The incubation period is prolonged, **Koplik spots** are absent and rash is mild.

Laboratory Diagnosis

- **Specimens** include nasopharyngeal secretions, conjunctival swabs, blood, CSF (for diagnosis of SSPE).
- *Microscopy*: Giemsa stain on nasal secretions show multinucleated giant cells, and inclusion bodies.
- Direct immunofluorescence detects antigen.
- *Virus isolation*: Human diploid cells or HeLa or HEp-2 cultures are used for cultivation. Growth is detected by cytopathic effects which take longer period or by hemadsorption. It takes 7–10 days for cytopathic effects to develop. Rapid and early identification is done by immunofluorescence.
- *Serology*: Paired sera are used to demonstrate 4-fold rise in titre of antibodies by CFT, hemagglutination inhibition test.
- Reverse transcription PCR **(RT-PCR).**

Prophylaxis: Live-attenuated vaccine (Edmonston-Zagreb strain) given at 9–15 months as a single subcutaneous dose. Combined trivalent vaccine is prepared as MMR.

Passive immunization: Human gamma globulin is given.

MUMPS

Properties

Typical paramyxovirus has **'H' (or HN) and 'F' antigen**. Virus can agglutinate RBCs of fowl, human beings and guinea pigs. Like parainfluenza virus, it contains surface 'HN' glycoprotein, also called **'V'** antigen which induces protective antibodies, hemolysin, cell fusion (F) glycoprotein antigen and internal RNA-protein nucleocapsid **(NP)** immunologically identical with soluble antigen from cells (called the **'S' antigen**).

Antibodies against the nuclocapsid antigen appear within 7 days and high titres are seen in 2 weeks. HN antibodies appear later, 2–3 weeks after infection, attain maximum titers in 3–4 weeks and persists longer than NP antibodies. The HN antibodies are measured by neutralization, CFT or HAI. The NP antibodies can be detected by CFT and do not offer protection. Mumps virus induces delayed hypersensitivity which can be observed by a skin test.

Cultivation

Chick embryo amniotic cavity is used for primary isolation and allantoic cavity after adaption. Growth takes place in 6–7 days at 35°C.

Clinical Feature

Incubation period is 12–25 days. **Mode of infection is inhalation or through conjunctiva** (Flowchart 59.2).

Flowchart 59.2: Pathogenesis of mumps

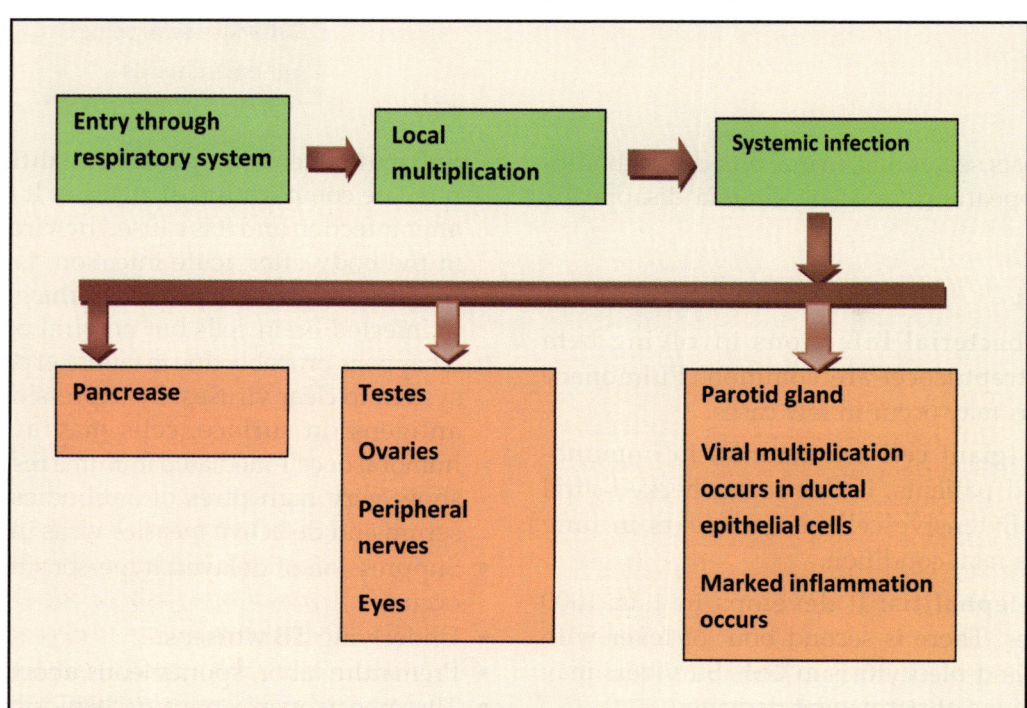

After initial multiplication in respiratory tract and cervical lymph nodes, **viruses enter bloodstream and enter 2nd time in repiratory system.**

Unilateral or sometimes bilateral nonsuppurative **parotid swelling**, fever, tenderness are presenting symptions, resolution may occur in 7 days.

Complications

- *Epididymo-orchitis*: Testes become swollen, painful, there may be unilateral or bilateral involvement, testicular atrophy may lead to sterility.
- **CNS complications are aseptic meningitis, meningoencephalitis.** Virus can be isolated from early stage of meningitis.
- Pancreatitis
- Oophoritis
- Nephritis
- Arthritis
- Myocarditis
- Thyroiditis

Laboratory Diagnosis

Specimens: Respiratory secretions, saliva, urine, and CSF are collected for viral culture and blood for antibodies detection and antigen detection.

- **Direct antigen test in clinical** specimens is done by direct immunofluorescence **(DIF).**
- *Virus isolation*: Saliva (4–5 days), urine (up to two weeks), CSF (7–8 days after onset of illness) are cultured in **chick embryo or in cell cultures.**
- *Chick embryo*: 6–8 days old embryos are used for culture by amniotic route. After incubation for 5–6 days; amniotic fluid is taken and **tested for hemagglutination.**
- *Cell culture*: Monkey kidney, human amnion, HeLa cell lines are used.
- Viruses grow in 1–2 weeks, growth is detected by immunofluorescence (1–2 days), hemadsorption (if RBCs are added to cell cultures containing viruses, RBCs get adsorbed as viral antigen (HA) is expressed on the surface of cell culture which attach to RBCs).
- *Serology*: Paired sera collected and tested by CFT, HAI, and IgM-ELISA. Detection of antibodies against 'S' antigen is used for detection of early infection.
- ELISA is useful as it can be designed to detect mumps specific IgM antibodies. These antibodies are uniformly present in infected persons and do not last more than 60 days. Hence, demonstration of mumps specific IgM antibody in serum strongly suggests recent infection. Another advantage of the test is that crossreaction with parainfluenzae does not occur.
- PCR (RT-PCR) is highly sensitive.

Prophylaxis

- *Live virus vaccine*: Jeryl-Lynn strain, attenuated by egg passage and grown in chick embryo fibroblast is used for prophylaxis.
- Vaccine is given intradermally only after one year of age.
- Vaccine is contraindicated in pregnancy, immuno-suppression.
- Subcutaneous dose either monovalent or given as MMR.
- Protection lasts for 10 years.

NIPAH AND HENDRA VIRUSES

These zoonotic viruses are associated with outbreaks in **fruitbats.**

Nipah virus caused severe encephalitis in **Malaysia** in 1998, 1999 with high mortality (>30%), suvivers had neurologic deficit. It appeared that infections were caused by direct viral **transmission from pigs to humans.** Some patients may develop late onset encephalitis months to several years after initial infection.

HENDRAVIRUS

It is equine virus which caused many deaths of horses in Australia. An equine virus outbreak in 2008 resulted 2 cases in humans. One case was fatal.

Fruitbat (flying foxes) are natural host for both, Nipah and Hendra viruses. The emergence of these new viruses is due to ecological changes including land use and animal husbandary practices.

HUMAN METAPNEUMOVIRUS

It is respiratory pathogen first described in 2001. It was detected using a molecular approach on clinical samples from children with respiratory illness in which no known respiratory viruses were isolated. Human metapneumovirus is able to cause respiratory illness varying from mild upper respiratory tract infection to lower respiratory tract infection, in all ages.

Virus is restricted to respiratory tract. Mostly children are affected, infections resemble with RSV. The specimens for diagnosis are nasopharyngeal aspirate or secretion and RT-PCR is the test of choice used for diagnosis.

RINDERPEST

It is most severe disease of cattle caused by rinderpest virus, a relative of measles virus. In year 2010, it is irradicated after successful global efforts launched in 1994. This is the first animal disease irradicated world-wide. The success was due to vaccination programs and long-term monitoring of cattle and wildlife.

60

Arboviruses

- **Arboviruses (arthopod-borne viruses)** are viruses of vertebrates transmitted biologically by hematophagous insect vectors (Table 60.1).
- Viruses are worldwide in distribution but more common in tropical than temperate zones.
- They multiply in blood sucking insects and are transmitted by bite to vertebrate host.
- Insect viruses and viruses of vertebrates that are sometimes **mechanically transmitted** by insects are **not** in this category.

- Most of them cause silent infection in rodents and wild animals, about 100 of them cause human disease.
- They have been placed into toga, flavi, bunya, and reo and rhabdoviruses.
- Arboviruses have wide host range.
- Their ability to mutiply in arthopods is special character.
- Most important vectors are mosquitoes, ticks.
- Flowchart 60.1 and Table 60.2 depicts taxonomy of arboviruses.

TABLE 60.1: Characteristic properties of arboviruses

Property	Alphavirus	Flavivirus	Bunyavirus	Rhabdovirus	Reovirus
Symmetry	Cubic	Cubic	Helical	Bullet shaped	Cubic
Size	60–65 nm	40–50 nm	90–100 nm	170 × 70 nm	60–80 nm
No. of serotypes	29	29	251	50	74
Nucleic acid	+ssRNA	+ssRNA	–ssRNA	–ss RNA	Ds RNA
No. of molecules	1	1	3	1	10–12

Flowchart 60.1: Taxonomy of arboviruses

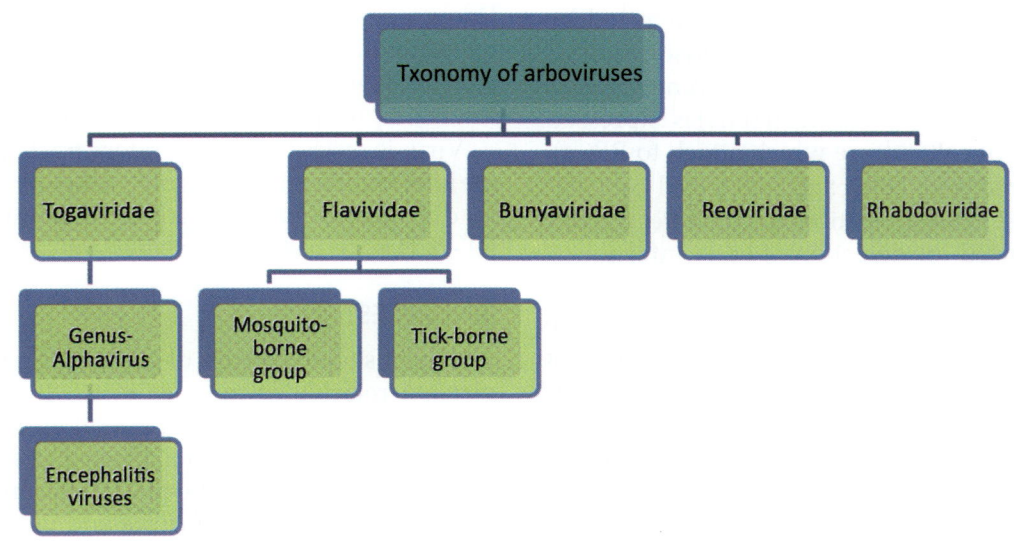

a.

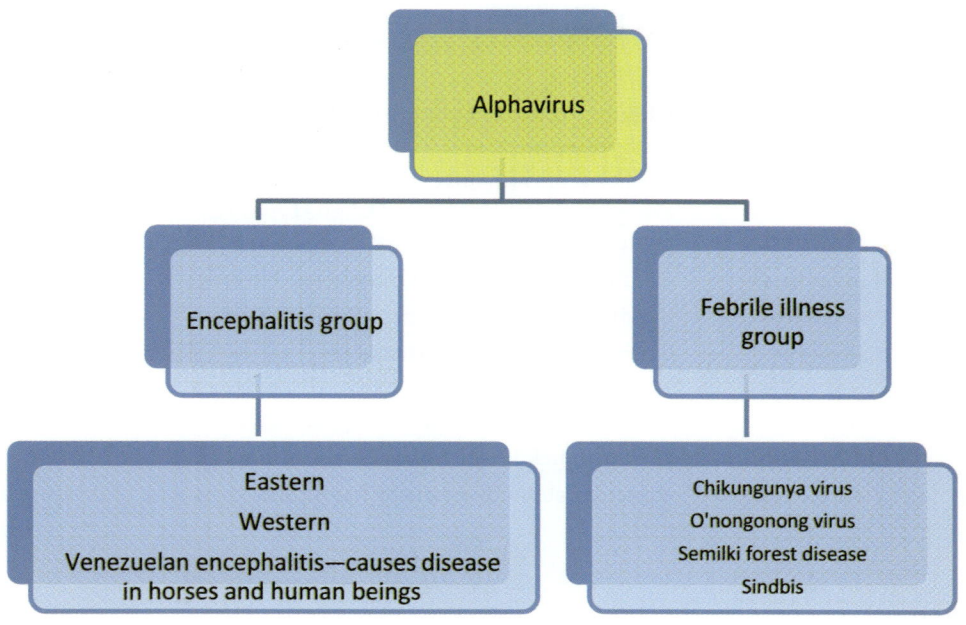

b.

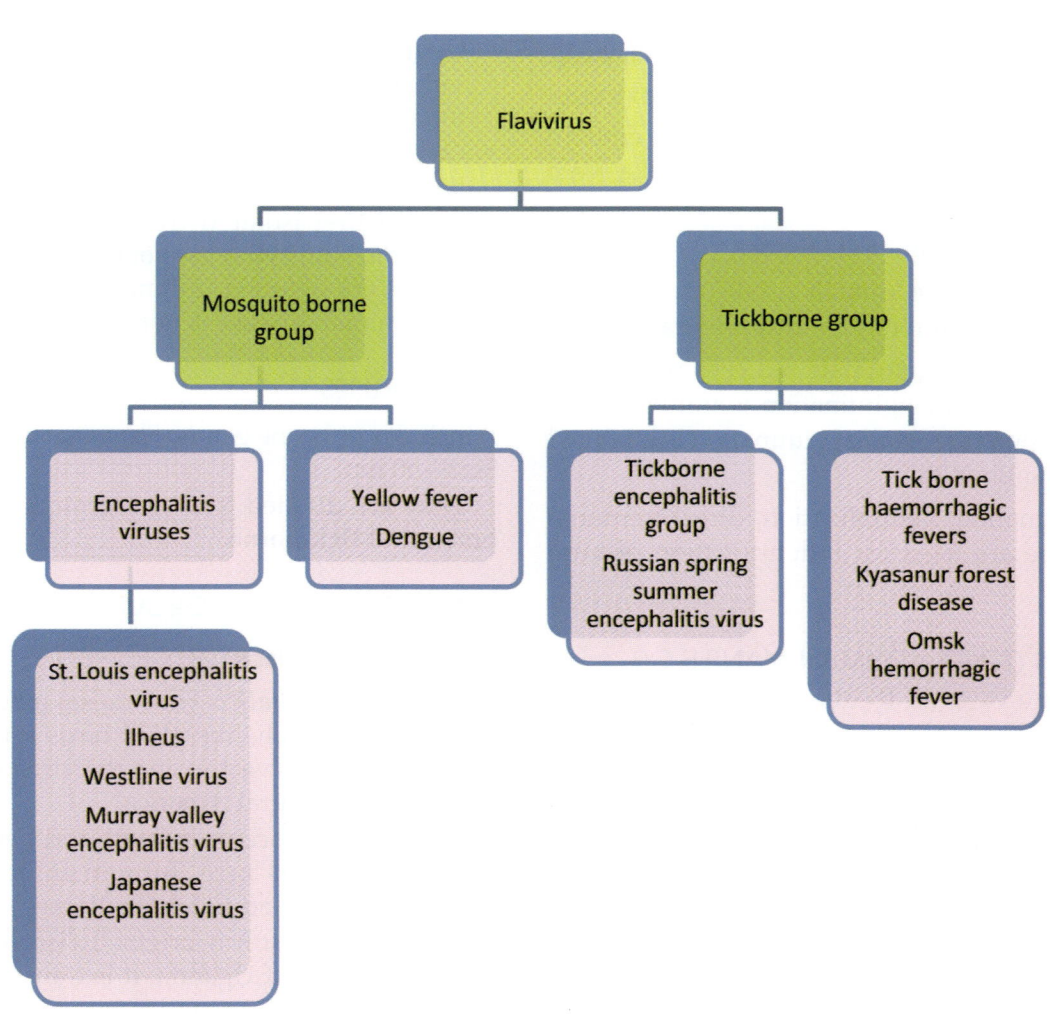

c.

TABLE 60.2: Taxonomy of some important viruses

Family	Genus	Important species
Togaviridae	Alphavirus	Chikungunya, O'nyong-nyong, Mayaro, Semliki Forest, Sindbis, Ross River, Eastern, Western and Venezuelan equine encephalitis viruses
Flaviviridae	Flavivirus	Japanese encephalitis, Murray valley encephalitis, West Nile, Ilheus, St.Louis encephalitis, Yellow fever, Dengue types 1,2,3, Russian Sring Summer encephalitis complex, Looping ill, Powassan, Kyasanur Forest disease, Omsk hemorrhagic fever
Bunyaviridae	Bunyavirus	California encephalitis, Oropouche, Turlock
	Phlebovirus	Sandfly fever viruses, Rift valley fever virus
	Nairovirus	Crimean Congo hemorrhagic fever viruses, Nairobi sheep disease virus, Ganjam virus
	Hantavirus	Hantan, Seoul, Puumala, Prospect Hill, Sin Nombre viruses
Reoviridae	Orbivirus	Colorado tick fever, African horse sickness
Blue tongue viruses Rhabdoviridae	Vesiculovirus	Vesicular stomatitis virus, Chandipura virus

Methods of Isolation

All arbovirus infections are viremic, blood collected during acute viremic phase are positive.

- They can be grown on chorioallantoic cavity or in yolk sac of chick embryo. Primary cell cultures, as chick embryo fibroblasts or continuous cell lines as Vero or HeLa, are used for cultivation of arboviruses.
- Tissue cultures of primary cells like chick embryo fibroblasts or continuous cell lines like HeLa, vero cells are used for cultivation.
- Culture is also done in insect tissues.
- Suckling mice are the animals used for cultivation and route of inoculation is by intracerebral.
- Most arboviruses agglutinate red cells of gosse or day old chicks; hemagglutination is influenced by pH and temperature. Hemagglutination is inhibited by specific antibodies.
- Hemagglutination, neutralization, direct immuno-fluorescence are used for indentification of viral growth.

TOGAVIRUSES (TOGA—ROMAN MANTLE OR CLOA—REFERS TO ENVELOPE)

Enveloped, spherical viruses with single strand of RNA, virus multiplies in host cytoplasm and is released by budding through host cell membrane. Within the family, the genus Alphavirus included.

Alphaviruses

Thirteen species infect human beings, all are mosquito-borne, and they produce epidemics in America and dengue-like fever in tropics.

Encephalitis Viruses

- Eastern, Venezuelan equine encephalitis viruses: Western seaboard of USA.
- *Western equine viruses* widely distributed in USA.
- Venezuelan equine encephalitis—distributed in Central and South America, usually may cause influenza-like infections, culex and anophelines are the vectors, and wild birds are the reservoirs.
- *Onyong–nyong virus:* First isolated from Uganda, it is confined to Africa, transmitted by Anopheline.
- *Semliki* first isolated from anopheline vectors in Uganda, human disease not known and in India anti-bodies are detected in human sera, but association with human disease is not known.

FLAVIVIRUSES

It includes only one genus, *Flavivirus* (flavus—yellow): Size—40 nm.

They are divided into **two groups,** i.e. **mosquito-borne and tick-borne.**

1. MOSQUITO-BORNE GROUP

Encephalitis Viruses

- *St. Louis encephalitis virus* causes mild febrile illness to severe encephalitis. Wild birds act as reservoirs, culex tarsalis is vector, and the virus is prevalent in North and Central America.
- *Ilheus virus:* It occurs in South and Central America, encephalitis is rare, human infections largely subclinical or lead to febrile illness.
- *West Nile virus:* It is originally isolated from West Nile province of Uganda. It is transmitted by culex mosquito. In India, virus has been isolated from culex

and from a patient with fever. Its role as pathogen is confirmed following its culture from brains of fatal cases from Karnataka.

- *Murray valley encephalitis*: Culex is the vector. It has cycle in birds and moisquitoes occasionally produce epidemics.

Arboviruses prevalent in India
- *Chikungunya virus*
- *Dengue virus*
- *Japanese encephalitis virus*
- *Kyassanur forest disease*
- *Chandipura virus*
- *West Nile virus*
- *Ganjam virus*

Japanese Encephalitis Virus (Fig. 60.1)

The disease first recognized in Japan and was named as Japanese B encephalitis (type A was already prevalent in Japan).

It has abrupt onset with fever, headache, vomitings, 1 to 6 days after patients develop signs of encephalitis, i.e. neck rigidity, convulsions, and altered sensorium, coma. The neutrophil counts increase, CSF has normal or raised sugar, raised proteins. Mortality rate is 50%.

In India, it was first seen in 1955, the virus was isolated from Culexvishnui complex from Vellore.

JE cases reported all parts of India. When infected mosquitoes rich high density human infection occurs.

The high cattle pig ratio in the country is limiting human infection.

A formalin inactivated mouse brain vaccine using **Nakayama strain** has been developed in Japan and to small scale in India. Preventive measures include mosquito control, locating piggeries away from human dwellings.

A live-attenuated vaccine JE strain SA14-14-2 is developed by growing the virus in baby hamster kidney cells. It has 2 doses schedule given 1 year apart.

Yellow Fever

Geographic distrubition: It is confined to Central and South America and Africa, **not seen in India**. It is likely that any virus introduced have been kept in check due to prevalence in local mosquitoes with dengue virus. Another reason could be yellow fever is seen in West Africa. In India, mosquitoes are common in eastern part, so that any virus entering by sea may not have suitable vector.

Government of India has laid down strict guidelines for vigilance and quarantine of travelers in international airports.

Clinical features are acute onset fever, chills, headache, nausea, vomiting, relative bradycardia, jaundice, albuminuria and hemorrhagic manifestations, death may be due to hepatic or renal failure. Virus has sylvatic cycle and urban cycle. Human cycle is between humans and *Aedes aegypti* mosquito in which humans act as source of infection. The sylvatic cycle takes between wild monkeys and forest mosquitoes.

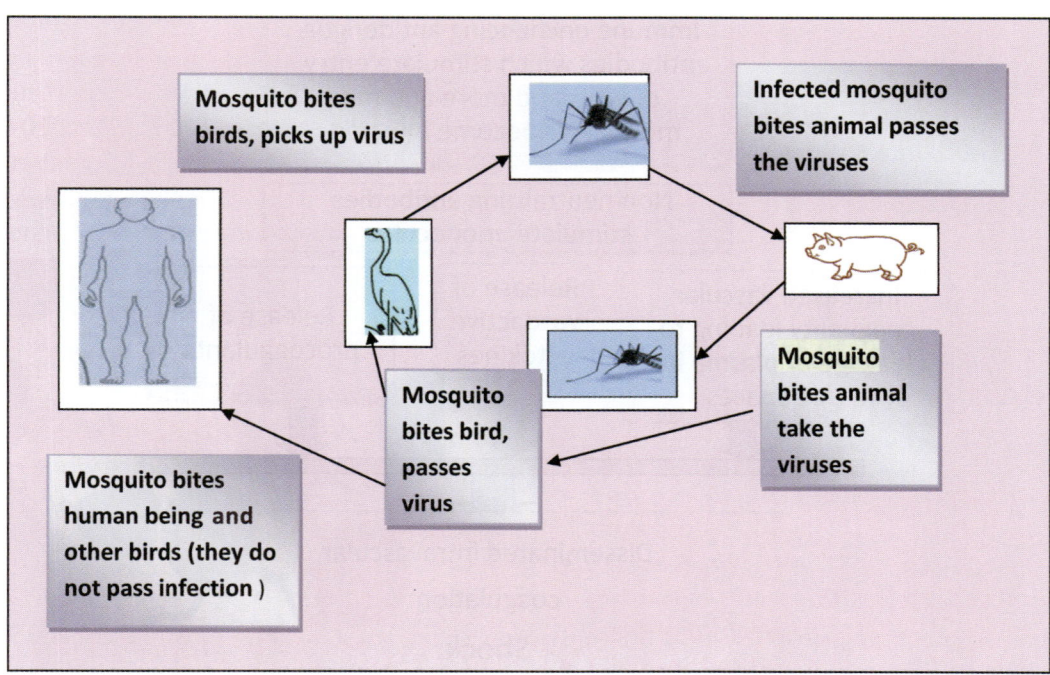

Fig. 60.1: Japanese encephalitis virus—life cycle

Control Dakar vaccine was used previously which was infected mouse brain vaccine. Vaccination with it was stopped as it was encephalitogenic. The **17D vaccine** was developed by passaging the 'Asibi' strain is safe, and effectively given by subcutaneous route. The vaccine is manufactured by Central Research Institute Kasauli. It is mandatory for travel to and from endemic area (valid after 10th day of vaccination till next 10 years).

Dengue Virus (Flowcharts 60.2 and 60.3)

An **arbovirus** (arthropod-borne virus) belongs to family **Togaviridae**, genus **Flavivirus**, composed of **single-stranded RNA.**

There are 4 **serotypes (DEN-1, 2, 3, 4)**. Each serotype provides specific immunity, and short-term cross-immunity. All serotypes can cause severe and fatal disease.

Genetic variation within serotypes: Some genetic variants within each serotype appear to be more virulent or have greater epidemic potential. It transmitted by mosquito *Aedes aegpti*.

Incubation period is 2 to 7 days.

Dengue virus infects peripheral blood mononuclear cells. Dengue viruses cause dengue and dengue hemorrhagic fever and shock.

Pathogenicity: Antibodies developed cause **immune enhancement**.

Clinical Features

They are sudden onset, high fever (>100° F), which is typically biphasic (saddle back) headache, myalgia, pain in back **(break-bone fever)** retro-orbital pain, lymphadenopathies (cervical or occipital), maculo-papular rash. Other associated elements may include upper or lower respiratory involvement, pharyngitis, vomiting and diarrhea.

Hemorrhagic manifestations occur in dengue hemorrhagic fever and dengue shock syndrome.

Two types of immune responses: Primary and secondary.

Flowchart 60.2: Pathogenesis of dengue shock

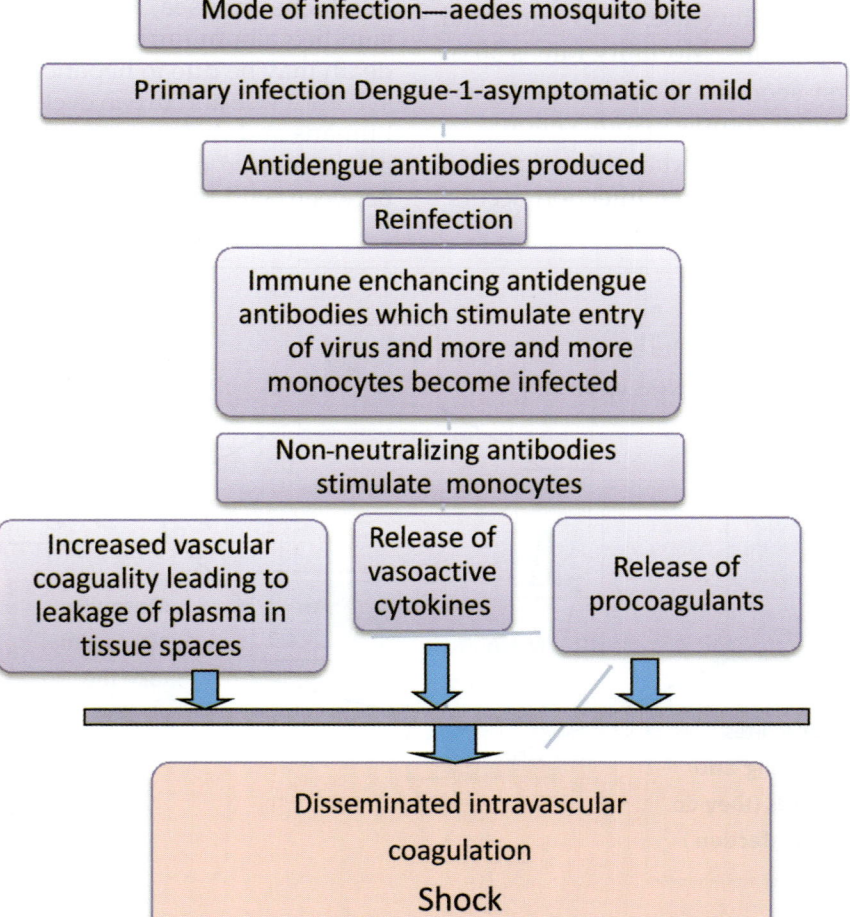

Flowchart 60.3: Pathogenesis of dengue

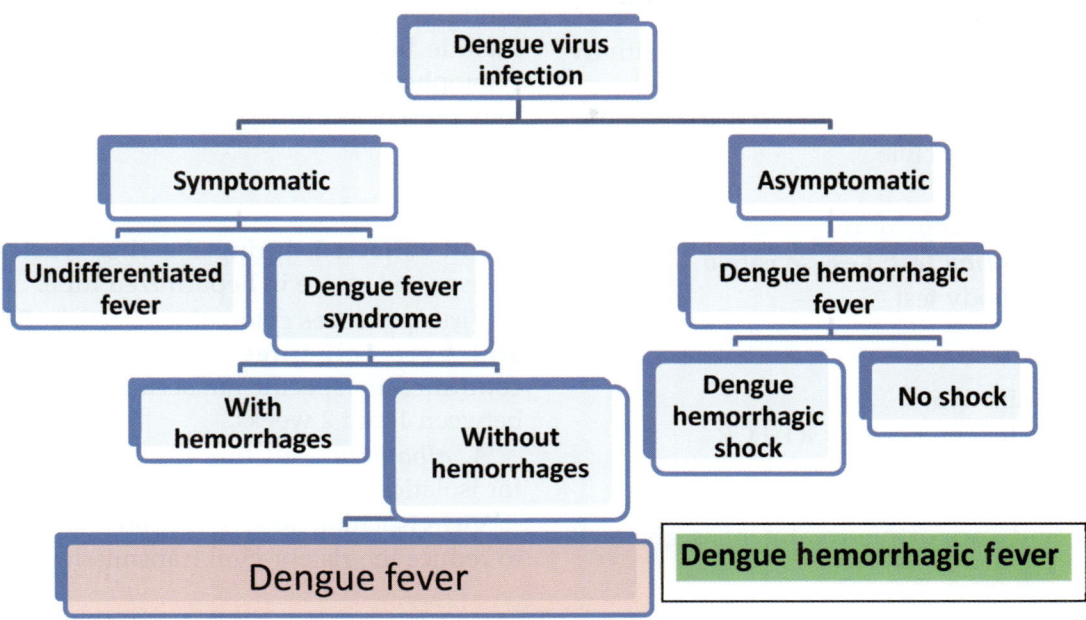

Kinetics of Dengue Virus Replication and Host Response

Primary response: This type of response occurs in persons never previously infected with flavivirus nor immunized with flavivirus vaccine (yellow fever, Japanese encephalitis, etc.). The dominant immunoglobulin isotype is IgM (anti-dengue IgM detected by MAC ELISA) (capture ELISA). About 80% cases had detectable IgM antibody by day 5 of illness and 99% by day 10. IgM peak level by 2 weeks and then declined over 2 to 3 months.

Secondary response (anamnestic response): It is seen in persons with immunity due to previous flavivirus infection or immunization. It is seen in most cases of DHF. Dominant immunoglobulin isotype is IgG (high level) and IgM fraction is lower. Both IgG and IgM anti-dengue antibodies neutralize dengue virus.

Antibody response against dengue consists of production of neutralizing and non-neutralizing antibodies. The neutralizing antibodies are protective in nature; they are produced infective serotype as well as other serotypes. These antibodies give long protection against infective serotype while protection against others is short-lived. Non-neutralizing antibodies are produced against other serotypes. Such antibodies produced against first serotype can bind to second serotype, but instead of protection it inhibits bystander B cell activation against second serotype. **This antibody dependent enhancement is responsible for the severity of secondary dengue infection.**

Laboratory Diagnosis

Clinical laboratory tests are CBC, WBC, platelets, hematocrit, albumin, liver function tests, urine (check for microscopic hematuria).

Viral Culture

Virus culture is the definitive diagnosis but not done routinely. (PCR is used in India for definitive diagnosis.)

Isolation is done by:

1. Inoculation of mosquito, mammalian cell line; other cell lines are Vero, LLC-MK$_2$. Mosquito cell lines are C6/36, AP-61.
2. Intracranial inoculation of suckling mice.

   Detection of viral growth is done by immunofluorescence, cytopathic effect, and plaque formation.

Antigen detection in fixed tissues: Antigen can be detected in peripheral blood leukocytes and in autopsy cases from liver, and lung.

Detection of NS1 antigen is done in early stage of disease before antibodies are developed (from day 1 to 18th day).

Immunoperoxidase test may be done for tissue:
- *Antibody detection*: Conclusive diagnosis of acute infection can be made only when rising levels of anti-dengue antibodies are detected in paired sera.
- In primary infection, IgM appears after 5 days of fever and disappears in 3 months. IgG is detected in low titer from 14th to 21th day, then it gradually increases. In secondary infection, IgM is significantly low while IgG titres rise rapidly.

- *Ig capture (MAC)-ELISA:* Sensitivity 72%; specificity 98%.
- *Duo ELISA (for both IgM and IgG) test:* Sensitivity 95%; specificity 94%.
- *Hemagglutination inhibition test (HI test)* is simple, sensitive and reproducible.
- Neutralization tests
- *Dot-blot immunoassay:* More specific and sensitive
- *Complement fixation test:* Less sensitive
- Fluorescent antibody test

Detection of RNA

   i. *In situ* hybridization
  ii. Detection of dengue RNA by RT-PCR

Treatment

Symptomatic and supportive treatment is given. It consists of:

- Replacement of plasma loss.
- Correction of electrolyte and metabolic distrubances.
- Platelet transfusion, if required.

Prevention: No licensed vaccine is available. The live-attenuated tetravalent vaccine based on chimeric yellow fever-dengue virus (Sanofi Pasteur) is undertrial.

Chikungunya Virus

Family: Togaviridae, Genus: *Alphavirus*
- Lipid-enveloped; 50–70 nm in size
- ++RNA strand.
- Structural proteins: 2 glycoproteins—E1 and E2, inserted in lipid membrane.
  - I. E1 helps in attachment to cell surface, generates neutralizing antibody.
  - II. E2 has hemagglutinin activity.

Chikungunya is a relatively rare form of mosquito-transmitted viral fever associated with acute epidemic polyarthralgia. It spreads by mosquito bites from *Aedes* spp. The arthropod vectors acquire the virus by sucking blood during this period. The virus then spreads to the targeted organs and immune system starts functioning at this stage leading to the activation of both humoral and cellular immunity.

Chikungunya virus has three genotypes—West African, East African and Asian.

Most of the current strains of *Chikungunya* virus circulating in India are believed to be of **East or Central African genotype.** The common **reservoirs** for *chikungunya* virus are **monkeys** and other vertebrates.

Fever typically lasts for two days and then comes down abruptly. Fever may reappear: **"saddle back fever".** A petechial or maculopapular rash usually involves limbs and trunk. Arthralgia or arthritis affects multiple joints (debilitating). The symptoms could also include headache, conjunctival injection, and slight photophobia. Ocular inflammation from chikungunya may present as iridocyclitis, and have retinal lesions as well.

Virus Isolation

Blood collected during the **first week** of illness is transported on ice in heparinized tube.

Virus produces cytopathic effects **in BHK-21, HeLa and Vero cell lines**. The cytopathic effects are confirmed by specific antiserum and results can take between 1 and 2 weeks.

A. albopictus **cell line has** been used successfully for isolation of virus.

Virus isolation must be carried in **BSL-3 laboratories** to reduce the risk of viral transmission.

Serological Diagnosis

Tests
1. Neutralization test
2. Hemagglutination inhibition test
3. Plaque reduction (neutralization test)
4. IgM capture ELISA
5. Rapid immunochromatography or lateral flow assay.

Serologic diagnosis made by demonstration of fourfold increase in antibody in acute and convalescent sera (14 days apart) or demonstrating IgM antibodies specific for virus. Crossreactions are reduced by plaque reduction neutralization test.

RT-PCR: Recently, reverse transcriptase, RT-PCR for diagnosing virus is developed using nested primer pairs amplifying specific components of three structural gene regions—capsid (C), envelope E-2 and part of envelope E1. Specimen for PCR is heparinized whole blood. PCR results for E1 and C genome either singly or together constitute a positive result for *chikungunya virus.*

Epidemiology

Chikungunya was first reported from Tanzania in 1952, afterwards it produced outbreaks in African and Southeast Asian countries. In India from 1963-1973, several outbreaks were reported (Kolkata, Chennai, Maharashtra). In 2005, it re-emerged in Reunion Island of Indian Ocean. Mutated virus caused the re-emergence and there was change of vector from *A. aegypti* to *A. albopictus* and the mutated strain was 100 times more infective to new vector than previous one. Presently the disease is endemic in Karnataka, Andhra Pradesh, and West Bengal.

2. TICK-BORNE GROUP

The viruses produce two clinical syndrome, i.e. encephalitis and hemorrhagic fevers.

Tick-borne encephalitis viruses: **Russian spring summer encephalitis** complex causes serious disease and paralytic sequelae. Infection is transmitted by Ixoid ticks. A formalin-derived vaccine is effective in the prevention of disease.

Tick-Borne Hemorrhagic Fevers

- *Kyasanur forest disease (KFD)*: This hemorrhagic fever was found in villagers in the forest area in Karnataka. NIV (National Institute of Virology, Pune) identified it as a new virus and the named it as KFD.
- *Clinical features*: Clinical features are fever, headache, conjunctivitis, bodyache, hemorrhages into skin and mucosae. Forest birds and small mammals are probably reservoirs of the disease and mode of infection is by bite of ticks, monkeys being amplifier host.
- *Omsk hemorrhagic fever*: It is seen in Russia and Romalia.

BUNYAVIRIDAE

These are single-stranded RNA viruses, size is 100 nm.

1. *Genus—Bunyavirus*: It causes meningitis, encephalitis and disease is seen in America.

California encephalitis virus complex: There are many antigenically related viruses, the important are:
- La Crosse virus accounts for majority of cases transmitted by *Aedes triseriatus.*
- California encephalitis virus.
- Jamestown Canyon encephalitis virus.

Oropouche virus: It presents with rash and meningitis. It is transmitted by *Culicoides paraensis.*

2. *Genus—Phleboviruses*:
  I. *Phlebotomus* or **sandfly fever** or 3 day fever is a nonfatal infection. The virus has been isolated from patients and sandflies from India.
  II. **Right valley fever** common in sheep and domestic animals in Africa. It causes mild infection in human beings.

3. *Genus—Nairovirus*: It is named after the type species Nairobi sheep disease virus. Main pathogens to human beings are from the group **Crimean congo hemorrhagic fever.** The disease is endemic in eastern Europe, central Asia and many parts of Africa. Cattle, sheep, and goat act as reservoir of the disease and it is transmitted by **Haemaphysalis** and **Hyalomma** ticks. During acute phase of the disease, the blood of the patient is highly infectious and infection may be transmitted by direct contact.

Ganjam virus is isolated from ticks collected from sheeps and goats in Orissa. The viruses have also been isolated from human souces.

REOVIRIDAE

It contains genus *Orbivirus. Colarado tick fever* virus, causes self-limiting disease. It caused extensive disease in horses and mules in India. Some mosquito viruses, like Palyam, Kasba, Vellore viruses, belong to orbiviruses. They are not isolated from India.

RHABDOVIRIDAE

Chandipura **virus** was isolated from blood of patient during epidemic of dengue-chikungunya in Nagpur. The virus multiplies in sandflies and Aedes mosquitoes. The role in human disease is not established.

VESICULAR STOMATITIS VIRUS

It is responsible for oral mucosal ulcers, vesicle in cattle, horses and pigs. Human infection is transmitted by *Lutzomyia shannoni*. It is of medical importance as it has been used for oncolytic therapy.

UNGROUPED ARBOVIRUSES

- *Wanori virus*: It was isolated from ticks in India and fom brain of young girl who died after 2 days of fever.
- *Bhanja virus*: It is isolated from Haemophysalis ticks from goats in Orrisa. Human infection is not reported.

RODENT BORNE VIRUSES

Robovirus, some of them are similar to rhabdovirus.

GENUS HANTAVIRUS

It causes **hemorrhagic fever with renal syndrome (HFRS).** The disease occurs in two forms, a **mild disease epidemic nephritis and serous epidemic hemorrhagic fever.** The genus has following species.
- *Hantaan virus:* Infection HFRS in Far East, North Asia, Russia.
- *Soul virus:* It is milder form of disease, probably worldwise.
- *Pummals virus:* It is nephropathic virus common in Europe.
- *Prospect Hill virus:* It is isolated from voles in America, human disease is not known.

Hantavirus: Rodents are reservoirs (field mice, *Rattus rattus* and *R norvegicus*). Viremia is seen in rodents, viruses are shed in urine, feces and saliva. Transmission is by droplet infections. Demonstration of antibodies by ELISA test is used for the diagnosis.

A new syndrome **'Hantavirus respiratory syndrome'** was identified from USA. The clinical features include fever, myalgia, gastrointestinal symptoms, pulmonary edema, hypotension, hypoxia and death. The disease caused by a new virus **Sinnombre virus.** It was associated with mice and rodents. Infection occurs by inhalation and no arthropod is involved in the disease.

In India alone, Japanese encephalitis (JE) and acute encephalitis syndrome (AES), claimed nearly 1,000 lives in 2012. In Oct 2012, Government of India launched a plan to tackle JE problem.

Main target states: Uttar Pradesh, West Bengal, Tamil Nadu, Bihar and Assam.

If untreated, it can result into coma, paralysis, mental retardation or death. fatality rate can be as high as 60%. Flavivirus reproduces in pigs but doesn't infect them. So, pigs are amplifying hosts (also water birds).

Mosquitoes belonging to the *Culex tritaeniorhynchus* and *Culex vishnui* groups—they usually breed in flooded rice fields.

These Culex mosquitoes are normally zoophilic, i.e. they prefer to take blood meals from animals rather than from humans.

These mosquitoes usually prefer to drink the blood of such pigs. But when the population of such mosquitoes increases exponentially (during rainy season, around August), human biting rate increases.

Man is the dead end host, i.e. JE is not transmitted from one infected person to other.

Existing vaccine against JE is a mouse brain derived killed purified vaccine. Although it confers protective immunity, three doses are needed. Studies at NIV have been directed using all the major approaches of vaccine development.

The institute has conducted vaccine trials with inactivated mouse brain derived JE vaccine prepared at Kasauli. The results indicated that three dose regimen is required for vaccination against JE. Studies on **chick embryo derived killed vaccine** for JE have shown that it induces better protection in mice as compared to that of Biken vaccine.

Attempts to use **temperature sensitive (Ts)** mutants have also been carried out.

Immunostimulating complexes (ISCOMs) offer an alternative to produce particles with defined composition. JE ISCOMs prepared from monomers of Egp JE virus have shown nearly tenfold increase in immunogenicity as compared to the monomeric Egp.

Efforts are also going on to develop a DNA vaccine for JE.

Ganjam: RNA virus. (Family—Bunyaviridae).

Ganjam virus was isolated from a tick species Haemaphysalis intermediate collected from sick goats (suffering from lumbar paralysis) as well as from healthy goats, in Orissa state. Later, another agent identical to the prototype strain of Ganjam virus was isolated from the mosquito *Cx. vishnui*. A virus isolated from acute phase serum of a 12-year-old European boy suffering from febrile illness in India was found to be serologically identical to Ganjam virus. The disease was characterized by fever of 2–3 days duration, headache, listlessness, nausea and vomiting. A laboratory infection with Ganjam virus is also on record wherein a 30-year-old technician suffered from fever, backache, joint pains and headache. Neutralizing antibodies to Ganjam virus were detected in animal and human sera collected from Arunachal Pradesh, Tamil Nadu, Orissa, Gujarat, Karnataka and Kashmir states.

Rift Valley Fever (RVF) (Family—Bunyaviridae)

RVF is an important arthropod-borne zoonotic viral disease primarily causing epizootics and high mortality in domestic animals particularly sheep and goats. The disease is known to be prevalent in the countries of African continent and Middle East.

It has not been known to occur in India until 1990 when a serological survey of sheep and goats conducted in Jodhpur, Bikaner and Barmer districts of Rajasthan state showed the presence of HI antibodies as well as RVF virus specific IgG antibodies.

Subsequently, in August – September 1994 an epizootic of febrile illness in sheep with abortions was reported from Veerapuram, Tamil Nadu, resulting in 80% morbidity and 22% mortality. Based on clinical findings, histopathological and electron microscopic studies a presumptive diagnosis of RVF-like illness was made. Although no virus could be isolated from autopsy specimens of sheep, HI antibodies to RVF virus antigen as well as anti-RVF IgG were detected in the convalescent sheep sera. Results of the post-epizootic sero-survey of sheep, goat and humans also revealed the presence of HI and anti-RVF IgG antibodies in the survey sera.

61

Rhabdoviridae

Rhabdoviruses belong to **two genera—Vesiculovirus containing vesicular stomatitis virus** and **Lyssavirus** containing rabies virus.

Order: Mononegavirales

Family: Rhabdoviridae

Genus: *Lyssavirus* (Lyssa—rage, synonym to rabies).

RABIES VIRUS (Fig. 61.1)

Morphology

- It is a bullet-shaped virus.
- Size approximately 180 nm long and 75 nm wide.
- Nucleocapsid shows helical symmetry.
- It is single-stranded, linear RNA, negative sense virus.
- One end of the virus is rounded and other is concave or planar.
- Envelope has knob-like spikes composed of **glycoprotein G** (it is absent on planer end).
- Below the envelope, there is membrane or matrix protein 'M'.
- Enzymes present in nucleocapsid is **RNA dependent RNA transcriptase.**

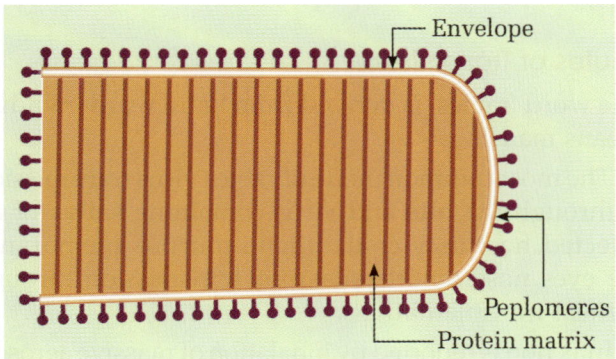

Fig. 61.1: Rabies virus

Antigens

"G" protein (on surface spike): Extraction of outer envelope releases a glycoprotein-G. It is important in virulence and from it purified "G" protein subunit vaccine may be prepared. A substitution of amino acid position 333 of glycoprotein results in loss of virulence indicating essential role of glycoprotein in pathogenesis. The "G" protein can induce **neutralizing antibodies** and antibodies are more **serotype specific**. 'G' protein also induces hemagglutination-inhibiting antibodies. It also produces cylotoxic 'Tc' response. Glycoprotein helps the virus adhesion to acetylcholine receptors of nervous systems. This antibody is **species specific**. The antibodies develop following infection and vaccination. Chemical analysis shows that variations in this protein are associated with the virulence of viruses.

Nucleocapsid protein (N) or nucleoprotein has complement fixing activity (antibody not protective). It provides the **group antigen** of the genus. The antigen may have role in cell-mediated immunity.

Antibodies produced against nucleocapsid protein antigens are used in direct immunofluorescence for diagnosis of rabies.

Other antigens are phosphoprotein **(P)**, matrix protein **(M)**, and polymerase **(L)**. The **matrix or membrane protein (M)** lies between core and outer lipoprotein envelope.

Viral Multiplication

- Virus attaches to cells via glycoprotein receptors. In neural tissue, virus attachment occurs at neuromuscular junctions via acetylcholine receptors. However, this may account for localization of and spreading of virus in nervous tissue, there must be other receptors since host cell range is broad.
- Entry of virus occurs by endocytosis.

TABLE 61.1: Differences between street virus and fixed virus

Characteristics	Street virus	Fixed virus
Susceptibility to laboratory animals	Following inoculation by any route it can cause fatal encephalitis in experimental animals	This virus is infective to experimental animal by intracerebral route only
Incubation period in experimental animal	Long , variable incubation period Usually 21–60 days in dogs	Short and fixed incubation period of 6–7 days (virus multiplies rapidly)
Demonstration of Negri bodies (Fig. 61.2) in brains of animals dying due to rabies	Yes	Negri bodies are usually not demonstrated in the brain of animals dying of fixed virus infection
	It is not used for vaccine production	It is used for vaccine production

- Transcription of 5 messenger RNA is catalyzed by viral RNA polymerase.
- The corresponding viral proteins are: N, the nucleoprotein; 'L' and 'NS', together forming the polymerase; 'M', the internal membrane protein; and 'G', the protein which is glycosylated and inserted into viral envelope.
- Viral RNA is replicated on a positive strand template by a viral polymerase. Only negative strands are enclosed in new virions. The 'M' protein appears to be important in packaging RNA and 'N' protein and linking to the envelope.
- Virions are formed by budding in associated with endoplasmic reticulum of the cell.
- The **virus affects the cell protein synthesis and the cell will die, but before this, it is possible to detect viral antigens by immunofluorescence or immune precipitation tests.** Accumulation of viral inclusions is also shown by histopathology.

Antigenically there is **only one serotype** of rabies virus. There are many strain differences between viruses isolated from different animals and from different geographic areas. The **strains** can be distinguished by **epitopes** in **nucleoprotein** and **glycoprotein**. There are at least **7 antigenic variants found** in animals and bats.

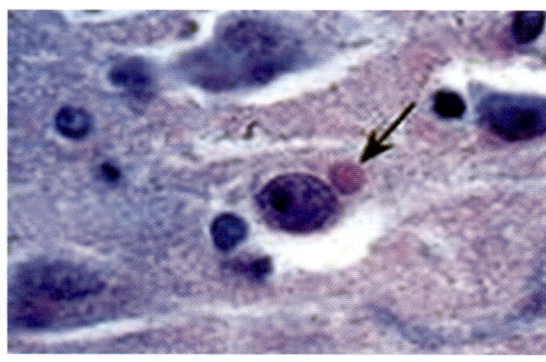

Fig. 61.2: Negri body

Host Range and Cultivation

Animals: All animals are susceptible to rabies; cattles, foxes, and cats are highly susceptible. Humans and dogs are intermediate susceptible and fowls, skunks, and opossums are relatively resistant.

Mice are used as experimental animals for cultivation and infection can be produced by any route. Intracerebral inoculation produces encephalitis and death in 5–30 days.

Street virus: The virus isolated from natural human and animal case is called **street virus** (Table 61.1).

Fixed virus: After serial intracerebral passages in rabbits, the virus undergoes changes and it is called **fixed virus** (Table 61.1).

Reservoirs: Terrestrial mammals, including raccoons, skunks, foxes, insectivorous bats and most importantly dogs are the reservoirs.

Chick embryo: Virus grows in yolk sac of chick embryo. This method is used for isolation of virus for vaccine preparation as well as for diagnosis.

Tissue cultures: Primary and continuous cell lines as chick embryo fibroblast, human diploid cell culture, vero cell culture, chick embryo cell culture are used for diagnosis and vaccine preparation.

Routes of Transmission

The word 'rabies' is derived from Latin word 'rabidus' means mad.

The most common mode of rabies virus transmission is through the **bite** and virus-containing **saliva** of an infected host may contaminate mucous membranes (i.e. eyes, nose, mouth) or aerosol transmission, through corneal transplantations.

Infection is reported by inhalation of massive aerosols generated in bat caves and in laboratory workers.

TABLE 61.2: Clinical features of rabies virus infection

Phase	Duration	Features
Exposure		Bite, it may unrecognized
Incubation period	3–4 weeks–3–4 months mostly 1–2 days or 1–7 years in some cases	—
Prodrome	1–2 days – 1 week	Fever, headache, anorexia, nausea, vomiting, malaise, lethargy, focal pain, paraesthesia, anxiety, agitation, depression
Acute phase—neurologic (encephalitic) phase	1–2 days – <1 week	Confusion, delirium, hallucination, hydrophobia, pharyngeal spasms, aerophobia, hyperventilation, hypoxia
Coma, death	Several weeks to 1 week	Apnea, respiratory arrest, hypo/hyperthermia, hypotension, pituitary dysfunction, cardiac arrhythmia, cardiac arrest

Pathogenicity (Fig. 61.3)

- Bitten by rabid animal, rabies virus enters through infected saliva, virus is deposited in wound caused by bite.
- Virus multiplies in muscles and connective tissues or nerve endings at bite site for 48–72 hours.
- It enters nerve endings, travels in axoplasm towards spinal cord and brain.
- It spreads centripetally from axons to neuronal bodies, infection progresses upwards in the spinal cord through synapses of neurons (3 mm/hour).
- It reaches brain. It multiplies there and causes encephalitis. The virus then travels centrifugally along the nerves to various parts of body including salivary glands, where it multiplies and shed in saliva.
- Encephalitis causes irritability. Virus may multiply in each and every tissue.
- It is present in cornea and facial skin as these sites are near to CNS. The virus may also be present in milk and urine.

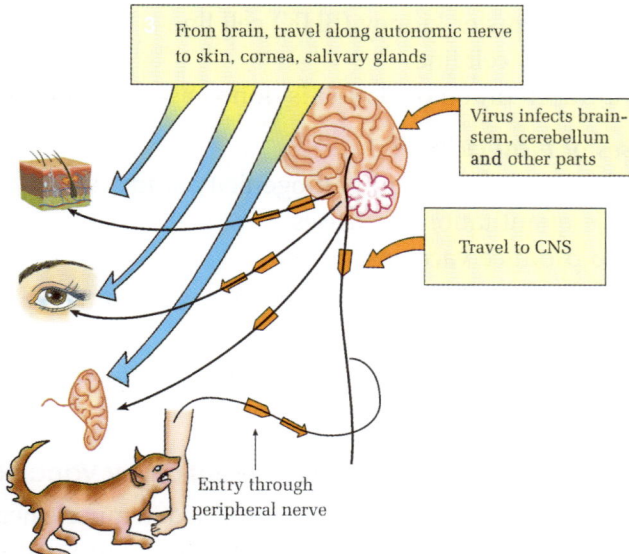

Fig. 61.3: Pathogenesis of rabies

- Virus spreads through nerves to the spinal cord and brain (50% of infected develop rabies). Other organs involved in rabies include retina, pancreas, kidney and heart.
- In brain, virus multiplies rapidly and host shows signs of disease.

Factors Determining Susceptibility and Incubation Period

- **Host's age.**
- **Genetic background.**
- **Viral strain involved.**
- **Site of inoculum:** Incubation period is short, if bite occurs on head or face, lower mortality if bite occurs in legs. (This determines the distance required for the virus to travel from its point of entry to CNS.)
- **Size of inoculum.**

Incubation period: It varies usually 1–3 months (it may be 7 days to year). It depends upon the site of bite.

Rabies in Dogs

- Incubation period is 3–6 weeks.
- *Prodromal stage:* Dog is alert, restless, licking at bite site, snapping imaginary objects.
- *Furious rabies:* It is more common, dog runs amok, bites without provocation. There may be dropping of jaw, dribbling of saliva and convulsions.
- *Dumb rabies:* Dog remains quite and it may not bite without provocation. It is unable to feed.

Clinical Stages

Rabies in Humans (Table 61.2)

Prodromal symptoms and signs: Initial symptoms are fever, fatigue, malaise, headache, and anorexia. Also neurotic pain or paresthesia is present at the site of bite. Other clinical findings are anxiety, depression, nervousness, insomnia, excessive libido or premature ejaculation. Prodromal stage lasts for 2–4 days.

Acute neurological stage: Altered, bizarre behavior, seizures. Patient may be hyperactive and gets stimulated by external stimuli. Even sight of water or noise causes dread of water. Though there is intense thrust, patient is unable to drink water, on the other hand drinking causes painful spasm of larynx, pharynx and chocking. This is called **hydrophobia.**

Generalized convulsions follow and death is due to respiratory failure.

Pathology

Features of encephalitis and myelitis are present. Perivascular infiltration takes place with lymphocytes, polymorphonuclear leukocytes, and plasma cells throughout the CNS. Babes nodules consist of glial cells. Cytoplasmic eosinophilic inclusion bodies **(Negri bodies)** are seen in **neuronal** cells, especially **pyramidal cells of the hippocampus and Purkinje cells of the cerebellum.**

Laboaratory Diagnosis

Antemortem

- Several tests are necessary, no single test is sufficient.
- *Samples*: The samples collected include saliva, serum, spinal fluid, and skin biopsies of hair follicles from the nape of the neck.
- Saliva can be tested by **virus isolation** or reverse transcription followed by polymerase chain reaction **(RT-PCR).**
- Serum and spinal fluid are tested for **antibodies** to rabies virus.
- Skin biopsy and corneal impression smears are examined for rabies antigen by direct immuno-fluorescence (DIF).

Postmortem

- Histopathological examination of brain tissues should be performed.
- *Experimental animal*: Intracerebral inoculation in mice is done with specimens as CSF, saliva and urine.
- Immunofluorescence study is done on impression smear of cut section of brain and salivary glands.
- The nature of rabies disease dictates that laboratory tests be standardized, rapid, sensitive, specific, economical, and reliable.
- *Antigen detection*: Direct fluorescent antibody (DFA) test is done on animals suspected of having rabies.
  - **DFA test is** primarily directed against the nucleoprotein **(antigen)** of the virus.
  Negri bodies **(Fig. 61.2):** In 1903, Dr Adelchi Negri reported the identification of etiologic agent of rabies, the Negri body.

- These are round or oval inclusions within the **cytoplasm of nerve** cells of animals infected with rabies.
- **Size is up to 27 µm.** They are found most frequently in the **pyramidal cells** and the **Purkinje cells of the cerebellum.** Also found in the cells of the medulla and various other ganglia, intracytoplasmic, round or oval, purplish pink structures with characteristic basophilic inner granules. Demonstration of a Negri body is done in **brain tissue and stained by seller's technique.**

Newer Methods for Diagnosis

1. *Direct rapid immunohistochemical test*: The test uses biotinylated antirabies virus nucleocapsid monoclonal antibodies. The advantage of the test is the rapidity of test.
2. *DFA*: 5–6 mm diameter biopsy taken from shaved area just within hairline (biopsy contains minimum 10 hair follicles and it is full thickness biopsy so as to contain nerves at the end of follicles is taken).
3. *Fluorescent focus inhibition test or FAVN— fluorescent antibody-neutralization test* measures the ability of test serum or CSF to neutralize known standards of virus dose.
4. *FFDFA*: Formalin fixed tissue is not suitable for DF. Hence **formalin fixed direct immunofluorescence** test is used. It is a modification of DFA, proteinase 'k' digestion used to dissociate chemical bonds and expose the virus.
5. *Immunohistochemical (IHC) test*: It is also an alternative test.

Culture can be done on:
- Mouse neuroblastoma cells (MNC)
- Baby hamster kidney (BHK) cell line
- CCL 131 cell line
- Intracerebral inoculation is done in suckling mice

Uses of viral culture:
- Study virulence and pathogenicity study
- For quantitation of viruses
- To produce vaccines
- To check safety of vaccine stocks

Amplification methods:
- Nucleic acid detection
- RT-PCR

Pathophysiology of Rabies Prevention by Vaccine

Presumebly the virus must be amplified in muscle near the site of infection until the concentration of virus in tissue is sufficient to accomplish CNS infection. If vaccine or immunoglobulins are administered promptly, virus replication is depressed and virus can be prevented from entering in CNS. The action of passively transferred antibody is to neutralize some of the inoculated viruses and lower the concentration of virus in the body, providing additional time for vaccine to produce antibody response.

Prophylaxis

There is no treatment for rabies after symptoms of the disease appear.

Pre-exposure prophylaxis: It is protection before an exposure, while post-exposure prophylaxis administered after an exposure.

Pre-exposure Prophylaxis

Indications of pre-exposure prophylaxis: It is indicated in persons in high-risk groups, such as veterinarians, animal handlers, and certain laboratory workers. Three doses of rabies vaccine given on days 0, 7, and 21 or 0, 28, 56. A booster dose is given after 1 year then every 5 years.

Postexposure Prophylaxis

It is given to persons possibly exposed to a rabid animal by animal bites, or mucous membrane contamination with infectious tissue, such as saliva. Administration of rabies PEP is a medical urgency.

Postexposure prophylaxis (PEP) consists of:
- Local treatment.
- Wash the wound thoroughly with soap and water.
- Apply quaternary ammonium compound, tincture iodine or alcohol.
- In severe wound, locally infiltrate antirabic serum.
- Avoid suturing of wound.
- Give tetanus toxoid and antibiotics to prevent sepsis (Refer cell culture vaccines).

Antirabies Vaccines

Neural Vaccines

These are suspensions of nervous tissue of animals, infected with fixed cell virus. The old Pasteur's cord vaccine was prepared by drying out pieces of infected rabbit spinal cord. It was replaced by other brain vaccines.

- *Semple vaccine*: Infected sheep brain with fixed virus, inactivated with phenol at 37°C (5% suspension) (produced by CRI-Kausali) is used.
- *Beta propiolactone (BPL) vaccine*: BPL as inactivating agent. It is more immunogenic, smaller doses are effective. (It is mostly used vaccine in India.)

Infant brain vaccine: A lack of encephalitogenic factor in brain of infant has advantage over vaccines prepared from adult brain, as tissue in newborn is non-myelinated.

Disadvantages of neural vaccines are:
- Poor immunogenic as contain mostly nucleocapsid antigen with small part of glycoprotein 'G' which is protective antigen.
- It may contain infectious agent. (This may not be inactivated.)
- Vaccine may be encephalitogenic and may cause neurological reactions.

Advantage: Vaccines are cheap (widely used in India).

Non-neural Vaccine

- *Egg vaccine*: **Duck egg vaccine** is prepared from fixed virus and inactivated by BPL. It was replaced by a more pure vaccine.
- *Live-attenuated chick embryo vaccine* (Flury strain): Two types of vaccines developed are low egg passage (LEP) and high egg passage (HEP). LEP—low passage vaccine used at 40–50 egg passage level for immunization of dogs. HEP—high egg passage vaccine used at 180 egg passage level for immunization of cattle.
- *Tissue culture vaccine*: For preparation of vaccine, fixed virus is grown on human diploid lung fibroblasts and killed by BPL. This vaccine is highly antigenic and produces good immune response.
- One ml of vaccine is given on deltoid region on day 0, 3, 7, 14, 30 and 90 after exposure. Vaccine is not given on gluteal region because of high fat content of the region which inhibits absorption.
- Other effective vaccines include—**primary cell culture vaccines** grown on chick embryo cell cultures, continuous cell line vaccines grown on **vero cell line.**
- **Purified chick embryo cell vaccine (PCEC), purified vero cell vaccine (PVC).**

Advantage: It is highly antigenic and free from side effect.

Disadvantage: It is costly.
- *Subunit vaccine*: Glycoprotein subunit is cloned and recombinant vaccine prepared.
  - Dosage depends upon degree of risk.

Vaccines used in India are:
- HDC vaccine
- Purified chick embryo vaccine
- Purified vero cell vaccine.

Cell culture vaccines (HDC, PCEC, and PVC) have same doses schedule for children and adults.

Pre-exposure prophylaxis: Three doses given on 0, 7, 21 or 0, 28, 56. A booster is recomonded after one year and then every five years.

Post-exposure prophylaxis: 5 or 6 doses given on 0, 3, 7, 14, 30 and optionally 90.

Vaccine is given in the deltoid and dose is 0.1 ml intradermally or 0.5 mL IM anterolateral aspect of the thigh in children is the site for vaccination. It gives good protection for five years, if exposure occurs during this period one or two doses may be required. A five years full course of immunization is to be given.

Another vaccine schedule is 2-1-1, one dose is given on right arm, one dose on left arm at day and another doses on day 7th and 21.

Neural vaccine: The dosages depend upon degree of risks to the patients who are exposed.

The degree of risk is classified as follows:

Class I risk
- Licks including direct contact with saliva on definitely remembered fresh cuts or abrasions on all parts of body except of head, neck, face, fingers.
- Licks on intact mucosa or conjunctiva.
- Bites or scaratches that have raised epidermis but not blood, on all parts of body except head, neck, face and fingers.
- Consumption of milk (unboiled) or handling flesh of rabied animal.

These exposures have slight risk of transmission of rabies.

Class II risk (moderate risk)
- Licks on definitely remembered fresh cuts or abrasions on fingers.
- All bites or scratches on fingers which are not lacerated, not more than half centimeter and they have not penetrated skin.
- Bites or scratches on all parts of body except head, neck, face, fingers which have drawn blood but excluding bites which have five teeth marks or in which extensive laceration took place.

Class III. Persons who are at great risk
- Licks on definitely remembered fresh cuts or bites or abrasions on face, head, and neck.
- All bites or scratches on fingers which are lacerated, more than half centimeter or have penetrated the skin.

- All bites penetrating the true skin and drawing blood, when there are 5 or more teeth marks.
- All bites on any part of body causing extensive laceration.
- All jakel and wolf bites.
- Any class II patient who has not received treatment within 14 days of exposure.

The immunization schedule recomonded by Pastur institute Coonoor is as follows:

	Semple vaccine	BPL vaccine
Class I	2 mL × 7 days	2 mL × 7 days
Class II	5 mL × 14 days	3 mL × 10 days
Class III	10 mL × 14 days	5 mL × 10 days

Subunit vaccines: The glycoprotein subunit is cloned and recombinent vaccine prepared.

Passive Immunization

Human rabies immunoglobulin (HRIG): Dose is 20 IU/kg body wt. Half is given locally and half IM. Passive immunization should be given before or simulatenously with first dose of vaccine, but not after it. In person taking serum and vaccine, a booster dose of cell culture vaccine may be given on day 90.

Equine rabies immunoglobulin (ERIG): It is produced in horses; may be given after purification, but it is not complete free from risk.

Vaccines Failure

There may be rare instances of development of rabies in vaccinated persons. If person receives local treatment with antiserum along with combined vaccination, the risk is negligible.

Epidemiology

- Rabies is endemic in more than 150 countries. Approximately 55,000 deaths occur due to rabies each year, maximum in rural areas of Asia and Africa. India accounts for 20,000 deaths per year.
- Infected dog is source of infection in 99% of cases. Virus is present in saliva from 3–4 days before onset of symptoms till death of dog.
- There are few countries or places which are rabies free no case of indegenously acquired rabies has occurred in man or animals for 2 years:
  - Australia and Antarctica
  - UK
  - Iceland, Ireland
  - China – Taiwan
  - Japan

– New Zealand
– India—Andaman and Nicobar islands, Lakshadweep.

Two epidemiological cycles recognized. **Urban cycle** transmitted by domestic animals as dogs, cats while **sylvatic cycle** involves wild animals as jackals, wolves, foxes, mongooses, bats, etc.

Primary source in nature—mustelids, viverrids (latency) from whom rabies spreads to wild animals and dogs.

Rabies Related Viruses

The genus Lyssavirus contains rabies-related viruses which are:

• **Lagos bat virus (Lyssavirus serotype-2)**

• **Mokola virus (serotype-3)** which is common in Africa, and virus is recovered from humans
• **Duvenhage virus (serotype-4)**—there is a report from South Africa
• **Rabies-like viruses—European bat Lyssavirus type 1 and 2** (may cause human infection)
• **Australian bat Lyssaviruses** caused fatal infection (human rabies virus).

Progressive Multifocal Leukoencephalopathy

JC virus causes this disease especially in immunocompromised patients. Rarely this disease is complication of treatment of monoclonal antibodies. Demyelination of CNS results from replication and reactivation of viruses.

62 Viral Hepatitis

Viral hepatitis is primary infection by any of the viruses belonging the heterogeneous group, hepatitis viruses which now include A, B, C, D, E, and these viruses, have **tropism for hepatic cells**.

Viruses not included in Viral Hepatitis

Other viruses which primarily infect other system, but in course of disease, if they infect liver, they are not included in viral hepatitis. Such viruses include yellow fever, herpes simplex, lyssa, measles, rubella, varicella zoster, coxsackie and EB viruses.

Old Terminology

- Hepatitis viruses transmitted by feco-oral route were called **infective or infectious hepatitis** (later named as hepatitis 'A' virus).
- Another type of virus transmitted by inoculation or parenteral route (originally observed in persons receiving serum or blood transfusion) was called **serum hepatitis or homologous serum jaundice or transfusion hepatitis** (later called hepatitis B virus).
- Afterward, it was observed that apart from infectious hepatitis virus and serum hepatitis virus, similar syndromes are produced by other viruses and the name '**Non-A, Non-B virus**' was given to this group of viruses. Later on, these viruses were characterized separately and different names are given as the terms used presently.

HEPATITIS A VIRUS

Structure of Virus (Fig. 62.1)

- *Size*: 27 nm
- Non-enveloped
- **RNA virus, single-stranded positive sense virus**
- It is related to enteroviruses, formerly known as **enterovirus 72,** now put in its **own family: Hepatovirus.**

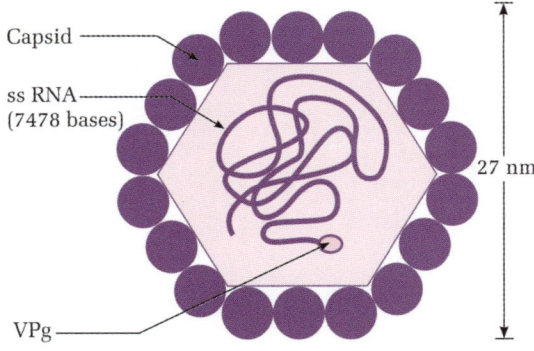

Fig. 62.1: Structure of HAV

The virus has one stable serotype only. Four genotypes exist, but in practice most of them are in **group-1.**

Cultivation

They are difficult to grow in cell culture: Primary marmoset cell cultures are used. Chimpanzees and marmosets are used as experiment animals.

Virus is inactivated by boiling of water for one minute and chlorine 1:4000 ppm for 30 minutes.

Pathogenicity

Source of infection: Cases or carriers act as source of infection to others.

Mode of infection: Infection occurs by contaminated food or water (feco-oral route).

It multiplies in intestinal epithelial cells, reaches liver by dissemination through blood; it is shed in feces during late incubation period and prodromal phase. A short viremia occurs during preicteric phase. Once jaundice is present, by that time virus disappears from feces. Virus persists in nature by continuing subclinical infection.

Clinical Features

Disease varies from mild disease to fulminant hepatitis.

Acute viral hepatitis: Clinical features are flu-like syndrome with fever, headache, anorexia, nausea, abdominal discomfort, and hepatomegaly. The patient has dark urine, pale feces, signs of jaundice and increased levels of AST and ALT. It is usually self-limiting disease which resolves in 2–4 weeks. **Chronic hepatitis or chronic carriers do not occur in HAV. Also it does not produce hepatocellular carcinoma.**

Incubation period: Average 30 days, range 15–50 days.

Complications: They are fulminant hepatitis, cholestasis, hepatitis, relapsing hepatitis.

Chronic sequelae: None.

Laboratory Diagnosis

- *Direct virus detection in stool sample*: This is done during late incubation period and preicteric phase, not thereafter.
- IEM (immune-electron microscope)
- RT-PCR of faces is rapid method for diagnosis and it is highly sensitive.
- **Detection of antigen in feces is done by ELISA test.**

Some patients are IgM negative during acute infection (window period), they are diagnosed by **RT-PCR.**

- **Acute infection** is diagnosed by the detection of **HAV-IgM** in **serum** by **EIA**. **IgM** appears in late incubation period, reaches peak in 2–3 weeks and disappears in 3–4 months.
- **Past infection,** i.e. immunity is determined by the detection of HAV-IgG by EIA. **IgG** appears about same time, peak in 3–4 months and persists longer.
- **Cell culture** is difficult and take up to 4 weeks. It can detect illness earlier than serology but it is rarely performed.

Hepatitis A Prevention

Passive prophylaxis: Immunoglobulin (0.2–0.12 mL/kg) is given intramuscularly, before exposure or early incubation period, can prevent the disease but not infection or disease if occurs, its severity is decreased.

Formalin inactivated vaccine: HAV grown on **HDC** and the vaccine is given intramuscularly (two doses). Protection starts in 4 weeks and lasts for 10–20 years.

Pre-exposure: It is indicated in travelers to intermediate and high HAV endemic regions.

Live-attenuated vaccine: H2 and H-A-I strains of HAV grown in human diploid cell line is developed in China. It is given as single dose subcutaneously.

Post-exposure (within 14 days):
- Household and other intimate contacts
- Selected situations (e.g. day care centers)
- Common source exposure (e.g. food prepared by infected food handler).

HEPATITIS B VIRUS (Fig. 62.2)

Structure (Fig. 62.3)

- Partially double-stranded DNA virus, the +ve strand is not complete. DNA polymerase is associated with positive strand having both actions—DNA dependent DNA polymerase, RNA dependent DNA polymerase. This polymerase can repair the gap in plus strand and makes the genome fully double-stranded (Fig. 62.4).
- The complete negative strand possses 4 genes, i.e. C, P, X, and S.
- Virion is double walled, spherical structure of size 42 nm, originally described as **Dane** particle.
- Nucleocapsid surrounds the core and enzymes. The nucleocapsid also contains a protein, HB core antigen-HBcAg. HBeAg is soluble nucleocapsid protein.

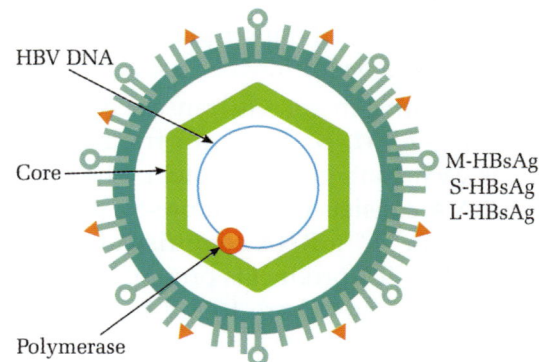

Fig. 62.2: HBV

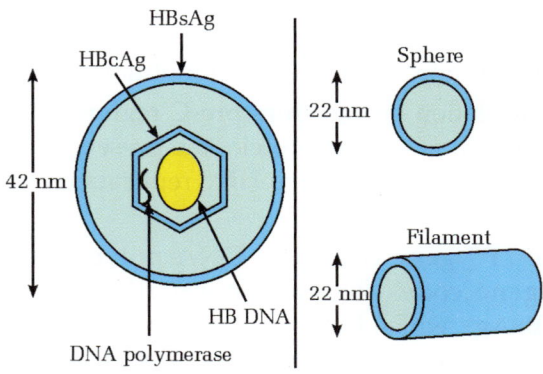

Fig. 62.3: Different particles seen in blood of HBV infected person

Hepatitis B virus genome organization

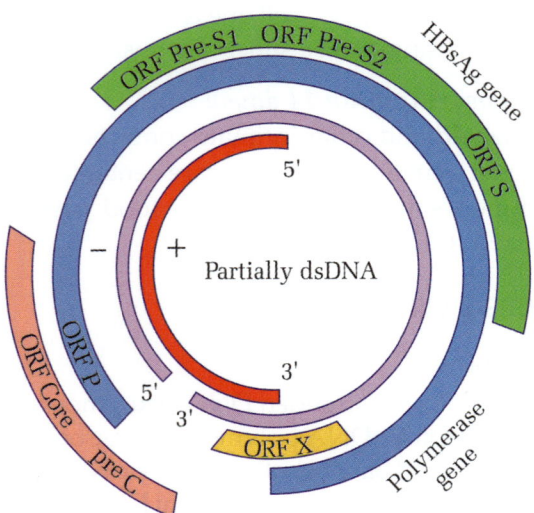

Fig. 62.4: HBV genome

- The envelope consists of HBsAg.
- **HbcAg and HBeAg** are products of "**C**" gene, 'P' codes for **DNA polymerase**, "**X**" gene codes for HBxAg, it acts as activator of transcription and 'S'codes for **HBsAg.**
- There are four overlapping genes coding for the core, surface, polymerase protein and 'X' protein which may act as activator of transcription (4) protein; there is no separate gene for it.
- The surface antigen gene is transcribed to produce **3 mRNAs—L, M, S.** They are translated into 3 proteins each contains "**S**" protein. The product of "**M**" mRNA consists of S and pre-S2 proteins. The **proteins from "L" mRNA comprise of pre-S1, pre-S2 and S.** The "L" product is present only in virion, while the 'M' and 'S' are found in each types of particles seen in patients blood.
- *C-gene:* It has two regions, **C, pre-C**. When "C" region alone is translated, core antigen **HBcAg** is formed. It assembled as nucleocapsid core particle, and it is not secreted, not present in blood, demonstrated in hepatocytes by immunofluorescence.
- If translation begins **from pre-C region, HBeAg is formed**. It is soluble protein, the presence of which in blood indicates active HBV replication and high infectivity.
- The "**P**" gene codes for DNA polymerase. **The 'X'gene** codes for small nonparticulate protein **(HBxAg)**, which has transactivating effects on both viral and some cellular genes. The HBxAg and its antibody are present in patients with severe chronic hepatitis and hepatocellular carcinoma.

By electron microscope, three types of particles can be observed in blood from patient with *hepatitis B virus.* Spherical particles of size 22 nm, filaments or tubular particles of size 22 nm diameter and varying length and double-walled spherical particles of size 42 nm. The former two particles are identical and called hepatitis B surface antigen **(HBsAg)**. The latter particles are complete HBV and called **Dane particles**. The Dane particle is complete HBV.

HBsAg is a complex and contains **group-specific antigens called** 'a' and **type-specific antigens** called '**d**' or '**y**'and '**w**'or '**r**'. Combination of this produces 4 major subtypes: adw, adr, ayw, ayr.

The subspecies show typical geographical distribution. The subtype '**ayw**'is common in Asia, Middle East and India.

Total 8 genotype variants described **(genotypes—A, B, C, D, E, F, G, H)**. Their prevalence varies from place to place. Genotypes 'A 'and 'C' predominate in the US. However, genotypes 'B' and 'D' are also present in the US. Genotype 'F' predominates in South America and Alaska, while 'A', 'D'and 'E' predominate in Africa. Genotype 'D' predominates in Russia and in Asia, genotypes 'B' and 'C' predominate.

Infection with serotype '**C**' is associated with rapid progression.

Diagnostic Importance of HBsAg

This antigen appears in serum during incubation period and during prodrome and acute phase of infection. It is the first serological marker that appears after infection. Its persistence at least 6 months denotes carrier stage and risk of chronic hepatitis. It is not detected in convalescence.

Available data suggests that genotype produces a milder disease, respond better to IFN therapy, and is less likely to develop hepatocellular carcinoma.

Mutants

Few patients may be infected with mutants, two types of mutants observed.

Precore mutants: Patients have severe chronic hepatitis; produce viruses which do **not produce HBeAg.** Initially, it was identified from Mediterranean countries.

Escape mutants: The **mutation** is there in common 'a' **determinant of HBsAg,** preventing them from being neutralized by anti-HBs antibody. These mutant viruses were seen in infants born to mothers with HBeAg and in some liver transplant receivers who had received combined immunization. **If escape mutants occur, vaccinated persons will not respond and will not produce anti-HBs.**

Stability

- Virus is heat stable and remains viable at room temperature for long periods.
- Hypochloride (10,000 ppm available chlorine) or 2% gluteraldehyde for 10 minutes will inactivate virus 1,00,000-fold but HBsAg may not get destroyed by this.

Cultivation of Viruses

It has not yet been possible to propagate the virus in cell culture. Limited production of viruses and proteins can be obtained, if cell lines are infected with viral DNA. The genome of virus has been cloned. Chimpanzee is the susceptible animal which is used as laboratory model.

Replication

Replication of viral nucleic acid starts within hepatocyte nucleus where viral DNA can be either free, extra-chomosomal or integrated at various sites within host chromosomes. However, intergration is not essential for viral replication. To replicate HBV DNA, a full length RNA copy is enclosed in core protein in the hepatocyte nucleus. This is copied to DNA by polymerase, the RNA is destroyed and DNA copied, to form double-stranded DNA as virion matures.

Clinical Features (Flowchart 62.1)

Incubation period varies from 40 days to 6 months. A **prodromal illness** occurs, some patients complain of malaise, anorexia, weakness, and myalgia. Arthralgia may also occur and may be associated with urticarial or maculopapular rash. The rash and arthralgia are due to immunocomplex deposition. Complexes also present in the plasma in cases of fulminant hepatitis B. In an acute case, hepatocellular damage is detectable by biochemical parameters before the onset of jaundice, accompanied by pale stools and dark urine. Carriers are initially symptomless and may remain so. If viral replication continues, some carriers develop the clinical features of chronic hepatitis and cirrhosis, and eventually hepatocellular carcinoma.

Pathogenesis

Acute Disease

- Both B cell and T cell responses are induced by core and surface antigens; damage to hepatocytes could result from action of antibody dependent cytotoxic cell. However, major action causing cell damage is the action of cytotoxic T cells specific for HBcAg in the cell membrane, although NK cells may assist.
- Expression of MHC class I antigen is poor on hepatocytes but can be enhanced, as interferons are produced. This in turn leads to increased antigen recognization and lysis of infected hepatocytes.
- The released HBsAg may induce tolerance; a feature of acute and chronic stages of hepatitis B. This may be due to a specific suppression of lymphocytes or to impairement of function of peripheral blood mononuclear cells due to presence of HBV in these cells.

In asymptomatic carrier, there may be no evidence of damage, despite presence of integrated HBV DNA and HBcAg in liver and HBsAg in the plasma. The lack of production of HBcAg is often detectable in patients with chronic active hepatitis, who usually show evidence of continued viral replication, indicated by presence of HBcAg in the hepatocyte and virus in plasma.

- Autoimmune reaction may also contribute to damage. Superinfection with deltavirus may predispose to progression to cirrhosis.
- It is not clear what determines the progress to carrier stage. The absence or relatively inefficiency of immune system may be responsible.

Persistence of Hepatitis B

- It is indicated by HBsAg present for more than 6 months.
- It occurs in 5–10% of adults, 30% of childhood and 90% of newborn infections.
- It is more common in males.
- It is more likely in immunocompromised individuals.

It has been suggested that **genetic factor** may be important and that an INF response may be one factor.

Hepatocellur Carcinoma (HCC)

Chronic HBV infection is an important factor in this complication. Higher rate of HCC is found where HBV is endemic and infection occurs at very early age. There may be an interval of 30–40 years between primary infection and development of hepatocellular carcinoma (HCC). Integrated DNA can be found in tumor cells, the DNA is extensively rearranged and regions may

Flowchart 62.1: Clinical course of Hepatitis B virus infection

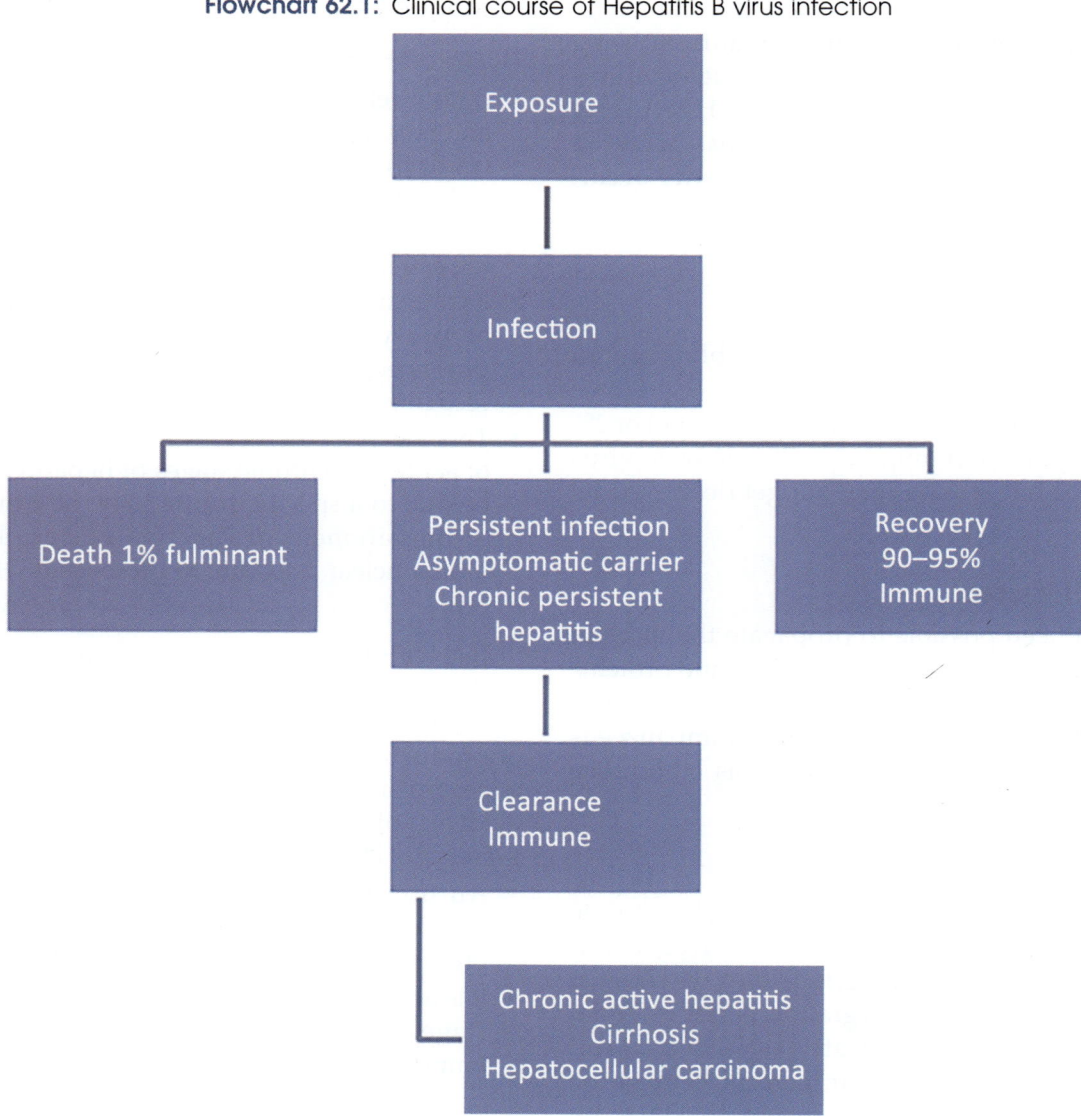

TABLE 62.1: Differences in person presenting as supercarrier versus person presenting as simple carrier		
	Supercarriers	*Simple carrier*
Presence of HBsAg and HBeAg	Both HBsAg and HBeAg are present in high titers	HBsAg is present but HBeAg is not present
Other markers: DNA polymerase and HBV	Both are present in blood along with above mentioned markers	Both are absent
Transaminases levels	They are increased	Not increased
Comparison of transmission between mother as supercarrier with mother as simple carrier % of transmission from mother to fetus	There are more chances of transmission of infection to fetus 60–90%	There are comparatively low chances of transmission of infection to fetus 5–15%

be deleted: The patient is usually negative for HBsAg and other indications of ongoing viral replication. The mechanism of carcinogenesis is not yet clear, although it is associated with cirrhosis. Genetic factor may be necessary.

Carriers in HBV: Two types of carriers are seen in infection with HBV. **Simple carriers** and **supercarriers;** supercarriers pose a threat, as chances of transmission of infection are more if person is exposed to blood of a supercarrier (Table 62.1).

Spectrum of Chronic Hepatitis B Diseases

- *Chronic persistent hepatitis*: It is usually asymptomatic.
- *Chronic active hepatitis*: Symptomatic with exacerbations of hepatitis.
- Cirrhosis of liver.
- Hepatocellular carcinoma.

Concentration of Hepatitis B Virus in Various Body Fluids

- *High*: Blood, serum, wound exudates
- *Moderate*: Semen, vaginal fluid, saliva
- *Low or not*: Urine, feces, sweat, tears, breast milk.

Extrahepatic manifestations of HBV include transient serum sickness-like illness with fever, skin rash, polyarthritis; necrotising vasculitis, glomerulonephritis.

Disease-associated chronic HBV infections include mixed cryoglubulinemia, and glomerulonephritis.

Modes of Transmission

- *Sexual*: Sex workers and homosexuals are particular at risk.
- *Parenteral transmission*: Intravenous drug addicts, health workers are at increased risk. Blood of carriers and patients act as most important source of infection. To prevent this infections, HBsAg testing on donor's blood is mandatory. **(Infective dose is very small as 0.00001 which is smaller than HIV.)**
- Risky procedures are sharing of needles, syringes, other sharp instruments, endoscopes, personal items as razors.
- *Risky practices*: Tattooing, acupuncture, ritual circumcision, ear or nose pricking.
- *Risk with lesions*: Infections by direct contact with open lesions as cuts, scratches, eczema are common, if exposure is there with infected blood or fluids.
- *Perinatal transmission*: Mothers who are HBeAg positive (along with HBsAg) are much more likely to transmit to their offspring than those who are not. Perinatal transmission is the main means of transmission in high prevalence populations. Infections are acquired in the birth canal.

The outcome of infection with HBV varies. In adults, 65–80% of infections are inapperant, with 90–95% of all patients recovering completely. In constrat, 80–90% of infants and young children infected with HBV become chronic carriers.

Fulminant hepatitis occasionally develops during acute viral hepatitis, defined as hepatic encephalopathy within 8 weeks of disease without pre-existing liver disease. It is fatal in 70–90% cases. Fulminant hepatitis is associated with superinfection by other agents including *HDV*. Fulminant disease rarely occurs in *HAV* or *HCV* infection.

About 95% of newborns infected at birth become chronic carriers of virus, often for life. This decreases steadily with time, makes the risk of adults becoming carriers is reduced to 10%.

Epidemiology

Globally chronic hepatitis occurs in about 350 million people. India accounts for second largest burden of infection, next to China. Three epidemiological patterns observed all over the World. **Types I pattern (low endemicity)** where **prevalence is less than 2%.** It is seen in Sri Lanka and Nepal. Type II pattern (intermediate endemicity) is seen in **India,** Bhutan, Indonesia where prevalence is between **2 and 8%. Type 3** pattern with prevalence **more than 8%** is seen in Bangladesh.

The prevalence in India is 3.7%. South Indians have higher carrier rates.

Importance of Vaccination at Birth

Hepatocellular carcinoma is most likely to occur in adults who experienced HBV infection at very early age and become carriers. Therefore, for vaccination to be maximally effective against carrier state, cirrhosis, and hepatoma; it must be carried out during first week of life.

Hepatocellular carcinoma (HCC): 70–90% cases progress to chronic liver disease, 20–50% develop cirrhosis and 5–25% of them develop hepatocellular carcinoma.

Diagnosis (Fig. 62.5)

Batteries of serological tests are used for the diagnosis of acute and chronic hepatitis B infection.

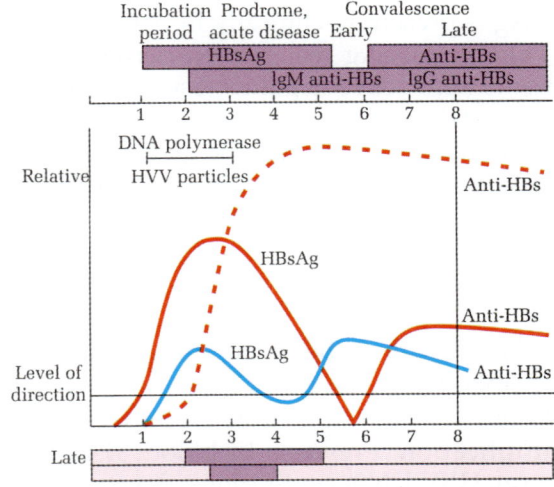

Fig. 62.5: Laboratory diagnosis of HBV

HBsAg

- **HBsAg** is the first marker to appear after infection even before rise in transaminase.
- In typical acute HBV infection, it appears **2–4 weeks before ALT** becomes abnormal and **3–4 weeks** before symptoms of jaundice develop.
- It may last for 6 months or beyond that (chronic carriers).
- **HBsAg** is used as a general marker of infection. Its presence in serum indicates acute or chronic active HBV infection.
- Persistence of HBsAg more than 6 months also increases the risk of chronic hepatitis and development of complication as carcinoma.
- It may disappear during convalescence.
- Presence of HBsAg alone does not indicate that virus is replicating.

When HBsAg is nondetectable, anti-HBs appear and remain for longer period. It is protective antibody.

HBcAg is not detected in serum; it is detected on hepatocytes by immunofluorescence.

Anti-HBc Antibody

- **Anti-HBc antibody appears** in serum a week or 2 after appearance of HBsAg, thus it the first antibody to be detected.
- Anti-HBc of IgM appears when ALT levels begin to rise.
- Anti-HBC initially is of IgM type for 6 months, after it becomes IgG. Anti-HBcAg remains positive lifelong.
- Selective tests for **IgM anti-HBc** differentiate **between recent infection and remote infection**.
- Anti-HBc is marker of prior infection even all other markers become undetectable.
- It has diagnostic value in **window period.**
- Because total anti-HBc is invariably positive when HBsAg is present in clinically ill patients, it is used to validate HbsAg reaction. In perhaps 5–10% of patients with active hepatitis (especially those with fulminant disease) and more frequently during early convalescence, HBsAg may be undetectable in sera.
- Only anti-HBc positive without anti-HBs and HBsAg are patients in window period or HBV infection is resolving.

HBeAg

- HBeAg appears in the blood along with HBsAg or soon after it.
- HBeAg is an indicator of active intrahepatic viral multiplication. Presence in blood of DNA polymerase, HBV DNA, and virions along with HBeAg means high infectivity.

- When HBeAg goes, anti-HBe appears.
- For diagnosis of HBV infection, detection of HBsAg is necessary and presence of anti-HBc IgM indicates recent infection and presence of IgG anti-HBc indicates remote infection.
- The presence of HBV DNA precedes HBsAg by 3–4 weeks. Its presence in high titre (1:100) is evidence of acute infection. The titres decline regardless whether disease resolves or becomes chronic.
- Anti-HBs usually become detectable immediately after disappearance of HBsAg.
- Anti-HBs with or without anti-HBc indicates immunity to reinfection and also indicates adequate vaccination.
- HBeAg indicates active replication of virus and, therefore, infectiveness.
- *Anti-HbeAg*: It means virus no longer replicating. However, the patient can still be positive for HBsAg which is made by integrated HBV.
- *HBV DNA*: It indicates active replication of virus, more accurate than HBeAg especially in cases of escape mutants. It is used mainly for monitoring response to therapy.

Treatment

- Interferon-α—is given for HBeAg positive carriers with chronic active hepatitis. Response rate is 30 to 40%.
- Alpha-interferon 2b (original)
- Alpha-interferon 2a (newer, claims to be more efficacious and efficient)
- Pegylated INF-α
- Lamivudine, a nucleoside analogue reverse transcriptase inhibitor, well tolerated, most patients will respond favorably. However, tendency to relapse on cessation of treatment is seen. Another problem is the rapid emergence of drug resistance.
- *Adefovir*: It is less likely to develop resistance than lamivudine and may be used to treat lamivudine resistance HBV. However, it is more expensive and toxic.
- Entecavir is most powerful antiviral known, similar to adefovir.

Successful response to treatment will result in the disappearance of HBsAg, HBV DNA, and seroconversion to HBeAg.

Vaccination

Highly effective recombinant vaccines are now available. Vaccine can be given to those who are at increased risk of HBV infection such as health care workers. It is also given routinely to neonates as universal vaccination in many countries.

Passive Immunization

Hepatitis B immunoglobulin: HBIG may be used to protect persons who are exposed to hepatitis B. In particular efficient within 48 hours of the incident. It may also be given to neonates who are at increased risk of contracting hepatitis B, i.e. whose mothers are HBsAg and HBeAg positive. It is obtained from human volunteers having high titers of antibodies against HBV.

HBIG must be given as soon as possible after exposure, **preferably within 48 hours;** some protection may be possible after an interval of 1 week. **Second dose** should be given **4 weeks after 1st. Protection** against carrier stage is also provided.

Passive protection is also important to babies born to HBV mother. HBIG should be given at birth but no later than 12 hours after birth. Best protection to babies is achieved by combined immunization. When HBIG not available, the vaccine alone has been reported to protect.

Dose: 300–500 IU should be given soon after the exposure by IM route.

Vaccines

1. **Plasma-derived vaccine**: It is prepared from human volunteers having high titers of antigen (HBsAg). It is killed vaccine prepared by separation of antigen and killed with formaldehyde.

   Disadvantages: It was not totally free from other pathogens and limited availability as it was prepared from human beings. The only advantage is low cost.

2. **Recombinant vaccine**: **It is prepared genetic engineering HBsAg gene, i.e. 'S' gene in yeast**. It contains non-glycosylated particles of HBsAg.
   - Route of vaccination: Intramuscular
   - Sites: Deltoid or anterolateral aspect of thigh
   - Doses: 0, 1, 6 months
   - Seroconversion occurs in 90% of persons.

3. A special vaccine having all components **of HBsAg, (i.e. pre-s, pre-s2 and s) is prepared**. This vaccine produces greater seroconversion, boosters recommended only for those who are at risk.

4. **Recombinant Chinese hamster ovary (CHO) cell vaccine**: This is first vaccine using mammalion cell expression system.

5. **Synthetic peptide vaccine**: It is cheap, safe, but still in experimental stage.

   If a nonimmune person is exposed to HBV, combined immunization is given.

HEPATITIS C VIRUS

- It has linear single-stranded RNA genome, surrounded by capsid.
- *Size*: 50–60 nm
- Enveloped virus, envelope has glycoprotein spikes
- It has:
  a. *Three structural proteins*: Core (c), envelope (E_1 and E_2).
  b. *Nonstructural proteins*: NS_1, NS_2, NS_3, NS_4A, NS_4B, NS_5A and NS_5B.
- Genome resembles that of a flavivirus, positive stranded RNA genome of around 10,000 bases.
- Antigenic diversity: It has **6 genotypes (clades) and 100 subtypes**. Genotypes 1 and 4 have a poorer prognosis and response to interferon therapy. HCV genotype 2 responds best to INF-based therapies. Genotype 3 shows highest rate of clearance and genotype 4 seems to have highest frequency leading to chronic infection after acute infection. Clades differ from each other by 25–35% at nucleotide level while subtypes differ by 15–25%. In Hong Kong, genotype 1 accounts for around 67% of cases and genotype 6 around 25%.
- Genotype 1 is distributed world wide. Genotype 4 is common in Egypt, genotype 5 in South Africa and 6 in Hong Kong. **In India, most prevalent genotypes are 1 and 3.**

Clinical Features

Incubation period: Average 6–7 weeks. Range 2–26 weeks.

Majority of the patients (70–90%) develop chronic hepatitis and many (10–20%) are at risk of progressing to chronic active hepatitis and cirrhosis of liver.

The virus undergoes sequence variation during chronic infection. This complex viral population in a host is called **quasi-species**. The genetic diversity is not very much correlated with virulence but differences exist in response to antiviral therapy depending upon the infecting genotype.

Immunity: No protective antibody response is identified.

The spectrum of chronic hepatitis C infection is essentially the same as chronic hepatitis B infection.

All the manifestations of chronic hepatitis B infection may be seen, with **a lower frequency,** i.e. chronic persistent hepatitis, chronic active hepatitis, cirrhosis, and hepatocellular carcinoma.

Risk factors associated with transmission of HCV:
- Use of commercial immunoglobulin preparations (it caused outbreak in USA in 1994).

- Transfusion or transplant from infected donor
- Injecting drug abuse
- Hemodialysis (years on treatment)
- Accidental injuries with needles or sharps
- Hemophilia patients receiving clotting factors
- Sexual or household exposure to anti-HCV-positive contact
- Multiple sex partners
- *Birth to HCV-infected mother*: The mother to child vertical transmission varies from 3–10%. Mothers with high viral loads or coinfection with HIV more frequently transmit HCV. No risk of transimmion is associated with breastfeading.

Egypt has highest prevalence of HCV **(20%)**. It has been linked with an attempt to treat parasitic disease, schisotsomiasis by therapy that involved **multiple transfusion**.

Laboratory Diagnosis

- *Detection of HCV antibody by ELISA*: It is generally used to diagnose hepatitis C infection. Three successive generations of ELISA are used with different antigens. Even 3rd generation ELISA which contains **NS-5** become positive after 1 month.
- Confirmation is done by **immunoblot method**.
- Antibodies detection is not useful in the acute phase, as it takes at least 4 weeks after infection before antibody appears.
- *HCV-RNA*: Various techniques are available for detection, e.g. **PCR and branched DNA.** It may be used to diagnose HCV infection in the acute phase. It is more sensitive and specific.
- It becomes positive within a few days after infection. However, its main use is in monitoring the response to antiviral therapy.
- *HCV-antigen*: EIA for HCV antigen is available. It is used in the same capacity as HCV-RNA tests but is much easier to carry out.

Prognostic Tests

Genotyping: **Genotypes 1 and 4 have a worse prognosis** overall and respond poorly to interferon therapy. A number of commercial and in-house assays are available.

- *Genotypic methods*: DNA sequencing, PCR-hybridization, e.g. INNO-LIPA.
- **Serotyping** is used particularly, when the patient does not have detectable RNA.
- *Viral load*: Patients with high viral load are thought to have a poorer prognosis. Viral load is also used for monitoring response to IFN therapy. A number of commercial and in-house tests are available.

Treatment

Interferon: It may be considered for patients with chronic active hepatitis. The response rate is around 50%, but 50% of responders will relapse upon withdrawal of treatment.

Ribavirin: There is less experience with ribavirin than interferon. However, recent studies suggest that a combination of interferon and ribavirin is more effective than interferon alone.

Treatment: Combination therapy with INF-α and ribavirin are used for HCV. Newer protease inhibitors developed against HCV are bocevir, telaprevir.

Prevention of Hepatitis C

- Screening of blood, organ, tissue donors
- High-risk behavior modification
- Blood and body fluid precautions.

HEPATITIS D (DELTA) VIRUS

- The delta agent is a **defective virus** which shows similarities with the viroids in plants.
- As it is defective virus, it is dependent on HBV for replication.
- The agent consists of a particle 35 nm in diameter, consisting of the delta antigen surrounded by an outer coat of HBsAg.
- The genome of the virus is very small and consists of a single-stranded RNA.

Clinical Features

- *Coinfection*: *HBV* and *HDV* infect simultaneously; it presents clinically as acute hepatitis B infection varying from mild to severe disease.
- *Super infection*: The patient having already *HBV* infection, leads to more severe and chronic illness.

Laboratory Diagnosis

- **Delta antigen** is expressed mainly on surface of hepatic cells and can be detected on hepatic cells by **immunofluorescence**, it is rarely present in serum.
- **Anti-delta antibody** appears in serum and can be detected by **ELISA.** First IgM appears 2–3 weeks after infection, followed by IgG. In chronic infection, it persists longer.
- Molecular methods are DNA probes and PCR.

No specific vaccine available. Hepatitis B vaccine is effective against it.

HBV screening of donors screens hepatitis D virus and HBsAg.

Modes of Transmission

- Percutaneous exposure
- Injecting drug abuse.
- Per mucosal exposure
- Sex contact

Prevention

HBV-HDV coinfection: Pre- or post-exposure prophylaxis to prevent HBV infection.

HBV-HDV super infection: Education to reduce risk behavior among persons with chronic HBV infection.

HEPATITIS E VIRUS

Different names: **Enterically transmitted hepatitis virus** and as it often occurs in **epidemics,** hence called *E-NANB.*

Source of infection is fecal contamination of drinking water and environment.

Virion:
- Calcivirus-like viruses
- Nonenveloped RNA virus, 32–34 nm in diameter
- +ve stranded RNA genome, 7.6 kb in size.
- Spherical
- Very labile and sensitive
  It has been cultured recently.

Clinical features: Incubation period—2–9 days.

Disease is mild and self-limited, with low **fatality (1%),** fatality is more in pregnancy (20–40%).

Diagnosis: Demonstration of **HEV in bile and stool sample is done by IEM**. It is detectable in early acute phase and during incubation period. **ELISA** tests are available for the detection of IgG and IgM.

Epidemiologic Features

Most outbreaks are associated with fecally contaminated drinking water. Several other large epidemics have occurred in the Indian subcontinent and the USSR, China, Africa and Mexico. In the United States and other nonendemic areas, where outbreaks of hepatitis E have not been documented to occur, a low prevalence of anti-HEV (<2%) has been found in healthy populations. The source of infection for these persons is unknown. Minimal person-to-person transmission is seen.

It was first documented in samples collected during outbreak in **1955** fron **New Delhi** when **290000** samples of icteric hepatitis occurred due to sewage contamination of city's drinking water supply. An epidemic **in Kashmir** in 1978 caused 170 deaths. Pregnant women have high mortality, if infections develop in pregnancy.

Prevention and Control Measures for Travelers to HEV-Endemic Regions

- Avoid drinking water (and beverages with ice) of unknown purity, uncooked shellfish, and uncooked fruit or vegetables not peeled.
- Immunoglobulins prepared from donors in Western countries do not prevent infection. Also efficacy of IG prepared from donor in endemic areas is unknown.
  Table 62.2 shows comparative features of viral hepatitis types.

HEPATITS G VIRUS

Two flavivirus-like isolates were found in serum of young surgeon (GB) with active hepatitis. A similar virus was isolated from another patients. The names **GB viruses A, B, C** were given.

TABLE 62.2: Comparative features of viral hepatitis types

	A	B	C	D	E
Morphology	27 nm, RNA, Picornavirus (Hepatovirus)	42 nm, DNA (Hepadnavirus)	50–60 nm, RNA Flavivirus	35–37 nm, defective RNA Delta virus	32–34 nm, RNA,
Modes of infection	Feco-oral	Percutaneous, vertical, sexual	Percutaneous, vertical, sexual	Percutaneous, vertical, sexual	Feco-oral
Age affected	Children	Any age	Adults	Any age	Young adults
incubation period (days)	12–45	30–180	15–160	30–180	15–60
Onset	Acute	Insidious	Insidious	Insidious	Acute
Illness	Mild	Occasionally severe	Moderate	Occasionally severe	Mild, except in pregnancy
Carrier state	Nil	Common	Present	Nil	Nil
Oncogenicity	Nil	Present	Present	Nil	Nil
Prevalence	Worldwide	Worldwide	Probably worldwide	Mediterranean, North Europe Central, North America	Developing countries India, Asia, Africa, Central America
Prophylaxis	Ig, vaccine	Ig, vaccine	Nil	HBV vaccine	Nil

63

Oncogenic Viruses

Viruses that produce tumors in natural hosts or in experimental animals or which induce malignant transformation of cells in cultures are called *oncogenic viruses*. Oncogenic viruses are responsible for 10–20% of human malignancies.

The association between viruses and malignancy was first described by **Rous (1911)**, who showed that fowl sarcoma, a solid malignant tumor was caused by a virus. He was awarded with **Noble Prize** in 1966.

Transformation

Transformation is the term used for the various changes that are associated with conversion of normal cells into malignant cells by oncogenic viruses. It involves multiple steps. It may be complete or partial as some viruses may only immortalize cell with continuous multiplication. Transformation involves change in cell morphology, loss of property of contact inhibition with formation of microtumors.

All oncogenic RNA viruses belong to family retroviridiae while oncogenic DNA viruses may belong to many families.

Properties of cells transformed by viruses:

Altered cell morphology: Fibroblasts become shorter, parallel orientation is lost.

- Chromosomal aberrations
- Altered cell metabolism
- Increased growth rate, increased organic acids, etc.
- Capacity to induce tumors in susceptible animals

Altered growth characteristics

- Loss of contact inhibition
- Formation of heaped growth (microtumors)
- Divide indefinitely in serial culture
- Capacity to grow in suspension; semisolid agar

Antigenic alterations:

- Appearance of new virus-specified antigen
- Loss of surface antigen
- Cells agglutinate by lectins.

LIST OF ONCOGENIC VIRUSES

RNA Viruses

Retroviruses

- Avian leukosis viruses
- Murine leukosis viruses
- Murine mammary tumor viruses
- Leucosis-sarcoma viruses
- Human T cell leukemia viruses

DNA Viruses

1. Papovaviruses
   - Papillomaviruses of human beings, rabbits and other animals
   - Polyomavirus
   - Simian virus 40
   - BK and JV virus
2. Poxviruses
   - Molluscum contagiosum
   - Yaba virus
   - Shope virus
3. Adenovirus
4. Herpesviruses
   - Marek's disease virus
   - Lucke's frog tumor virus
   - Herpesvirus saimiri, pan, papio, ateles
   - Epstein-Barr virus
   - Herpes simplex viruses types 1 and 2
   - Cytomegalovirus
5. Hepatitis B and C viruses

Oncogenic DNA Viruses (Table 63.1)

Papovaviruses

- *HPV*: Human papillomavirus (HPV) types 16, 18 are associated with carcinoma of cervix uteri. The HeLa cell line has been found to contain HPV-18 DNA.
- *Polyomavirus*: BK and JC viruses can induce tumor in immunodeficient persons which otherwise may cause asymptomatic human infection.
- *Simian virus 40 (SV 40)*: They can transform cultured human species.

Poxvirus

Viruses causing benign tumors are of three groups—rabbit fibroma, molluscum contagiosum and Yaba virus. Similar tumors may be produced in primates including human beings.

Adenovirus

There is no association in human tumors though serotypes 12, 19, 21 may produce sarcoma in experimental animals (newborn rodent).

Herpesvirus

Many viruses of this group have association with natural human and animal cancers.

- *Marek's disease*: It is known as contagious neurolymphomatosis of chickens. Infectious virus particles cannot be isolated from lesions or demonstrated by electron microscope. As vaccine is available, this is first example of malignant condition controlled by vaccine.
- *Luke's tumor of frogs*: This herpesvirus probably causes renal adenocarcinoma of frogs.
- *Herpes saimiri*: When injected into owls, rabbits or monkeys, this virus causes lymphoma or reticular cell sarcoma.
- *Epstein-Barr virus*: This virus is often found in cultured lymphocytes from Burkitt's lymphoma, but in body tumor does not contain virus. However, cell lines obtained from human lymphoma may produce virus in 5–20% cells. Primary infection which takes place in childhood is usually asymptomatic and lymphoma occurs in immunocompromised persons with chronic malaria. EBV-associated lymphomas are reported from transplant recipient. EBV also causes nasopharyngeal carcinoma (China).
- *Herpes simplex virus*: HSV2 infection is proposed to be associated with cancer of uterine cervix and also HSV1 with carcinoma of lip. HSV8 is linked with Kaposi's sarcoma.
- *Cytomegalovirus (CMV)*: It is associated with carcinoma of prostrate and Kaposi's sarcoma.

Hepatitis B virus: It has been associated with hepatocellular carcinoma. Hepatitis C virus is also reported to be associated with this cancer.

Oncogenic RNA Viruses

All oncogenic retroviruses belong to the family retroviridiae. This family also includes other viruses which are not oncogenic. The family retroviridiae is classified into three **subfamilies**:

- *Oncovirinae*: It includes all oncogenic retroviruses.
- *Spumavirinae*: Non-oncogenic 'foamy viruses' (spuma = foam) which cause asymptomatic infections in many animals
- *Lentivirinae*: Viruses causing slow viral infections (lentus means slow) in animals and humans and related immunodeficiency viruses are included in this subfamily.

Based on **host range** (human beings, animals, bird, reptiles), following **groups** exist:

Avian leukosis virus: A group of animals which show some antigenic similarity are included in this group. This group includes avian leukosis animals and sarcoma viruses of fowls (Rous sarcoma virus—RSV).

Mammary tumor virus of mice associated with high incidence of breast cancer.

Leuckosis–sarcoma viruses of other animal: It includes viruses isolated from leukosis and sarcoma in various viruses as monkeys, guinea pigs, hamsters, rats and cats.

TABLE 63.1: Viruses associated with human cancers

Virus family	Virus	Type of malignancy
Papovaviridae	Human papillomaviruses	Cervical, penile cancers
Herpesviridae	EBV	Nasopharyngeal carcinoma, Burkitt's lymphoma
	HSV-2	Cervical carcinoma
Hepadnaviridae	Hepatitis B virus	Hepatocellular carcinoma
Flaviviridae	Hepatits C virus	Hepatocellular carcinoma
Retroviridae	HTLV	Adult T cell leukemia

Human T cell leukemia (lymphotropic) viruses (HTLV): These viruses were isolated (1980) from cell cultures of adult patients with cutaneous T cell lymphoma (**mycosis fungoides**) and leukemia (**Sezwary syndrome**).

HTLV-1 is worldwide distributed but present in endemic areas. It is associated with adult T cell leukemia and a demyelinating disease known as spastic paraparesis. **HTLV-2** is associated with T cells malignancy. HTLV infections spread through infected blood transfusions and other methods in which there is transfer of leukocytes.

Host specificity: Retroviruses exhibit this property due to distribution of their receptors on host cell surface.

They are **ecotropic** (multiplying in cells of naïve species only), **amphotropic** (which multiply in cells of native and foreign species) and **xenotropic** (multiplying only in cells of foreign species but not of native host species).

Viral transmission: It may occur by:
- **Exogenous** retroviruses which spread horizontally.
- **Endogenous** retroviruses are transmitted from parent to offspring as provirus integrates with genome of gem line cells, provirus behaves as cellular genome. Usually these viruses are silent, do not cause disease and cancer formation. Detection is done by nucleic acid hybridization method.

Resistance: Viruses get inactivated at 56°C for 30 minutes, ether and formalin.

Antigens: They possess group specific nucleoprotein antigen (core) and type-specific antigens present on envelope.

Genomic structure: It is simple.

Proviruses have **gag, pol, env genes** in that order from 5′ to 3′ end which are required for replication.
- The **gag gene** codes for group-specific antigen present on nucleocapsid proteins.

- The **pol gene** encodes for RNA dependent DNA polymerase.
- The **env gene** makes envelope glycoproteins.
- **LTRs** (long terminal repeat sequences) regulate control on provirus gene function.
- The **tat** or **tar** gene present in some retroviruses (transregulating viruses) as HIV, HTLV regulates function of viral genes.

Virus transformation
- *Slow transforming viruses*: They possess low oncogenic capacity, generally cause malignancy of blood cells, after a long latent period. The standard retroviruses, as chronic leukemia viruses, belong to this group. They can replicate normally.
- *Acute transforming retroviruses*: They have high oncogenic potential and latent period is short (weeks or months). They can transform cells in culture which slow transforming viruses cannot and they are responsible for different types of malignancies as sarcoma, carcinoma and leukemia.

Acute transforming viruses may be

Replication defective as they carry an additional gene, viral oncogene (**V-onc gene**) which replaces some essential genes required for virus replication. Most acute transforming viruses are of this type so they can replicate only if coinfected with a standard helper retrovirus.

Replication competent as the Rous sarcoma virus carries the oncogenic **src** (pronounced as 'sark'). As it full competent of all genes, they can replicate normally.

Oncogenes (Table 63.2)

Viral oncogenes (V-onc): Genes encode proteins triggering the transformation of normal cells into cancer cells. These genes are not essential for viral replication.

Genes similar to viral oncogenes are found in normal as well as cancer cells.

TABLE 63.2: Some oncogenes* and their chromosomal locations in humans

Viral oncogene	Origin	Natural	Human gene tumor	Chromosomal location
V-src	Chicken	Sarcoma	C-src	20
V-ras	Rat	Sarcoma	C-ras	11
V-myc	Chicken	Leukemia	C-myc	8
V-fes	Cat	Sarcoma	C-fes	15
V-sis	Monkey	Sarcoma	C-sis	22
V-mos	Mouse	Sarcoma	C-mos	8

*Oncoges have given three letter codes based on their origin (animal or tumor), preceded by V- or C- for viral or cellular genes
src = sarcoma of chicken, ras = rat sarcoma, myc = myelomatosis of chicken, fes = feline sarcoma, mos = mouse sarcoma

Cellular oncogene(C-onc) present in cancer cells. **Oncogene** is the term used for genes that are involved in cancer causation. Normal versions of these genes are present in normal cells called **proto-oncogenes**. They are partly responsible for the molecular basis of human cancer. They represent components of pathways responsible for regulating cell proliferation, division, differentiation and maintaining the integrity of genome. Incorrect expression of any component might interrupt that regulation, resulting uncontrolled growth of cells (cancers). Examples are tyrocine-specific protein kinases (src), growth factors mutated growth factor, receptors GTP binding proteins and nuclear transcription factors.

The molecular mechanism responsible for activating a benign proto-oncogene and converting it into cancer gene vary—but all involve genetic damage. The gene may be over expressed, and a dosage effect of overproduced oncogene product may be important in cellular growth changes. These mechanisms might result in constitutive activity, i.e. loss of normal regulation so that gene expressed is at wrong time during cell cycle or in inappropriate tissue types. Mutation might result that alter carefully regulated interactions of proto-oncogene protein or nucleic acids. Insertion of a retroviral promoter adjacent to a cellular oncogen may result in enhanced expression of that gene-promotion—insertion oncogenesis. Expression of cellular gene also may be increased through the action of nearby viral enhancer. Similar genes in normal cells are called as—**proto-oncogenes**—code for proteins involved in regulating cell growth and differentiation.

Transfection: This method is used for the study of oncogenes. Mouse fibroblast cell line (NIH 3T3) has property that they can take up foreign gene (DNA), incorporate in their genome and express transfection. DNA extract of human tumor cells can transform 3T3 cells and such genes (transforming genes) are identical with cellular oncogenes.

GENES REGULATING CELL GROWTH

Proto-oncogenes: Promote growth and proliferations of host cells, essential for life but its overproduction may lead to oncogenesis. They help cells to grow. But when it mutates or there are too many copies of it becomes 'bad' gene that can permanently turned on or activated when it is not supposed to be. When it happens, cell grows out of control, which can lead to cancer. Few cancer syndromes are caused by inherited mutations of proto-oncogenes that cause the oncogenes to turn on (activation). But most cancer causing mutations involving oncogenes are acquired, not inherited.

They generally activate oncogenes by:
- *Chromosomal rearrangements*: Changes in chromosomes that put one gene next to another, which allows one gene to activate the other.
- *Gene duplication*: Having extra copies of a gene which can lead to it making too much of proteins.
- *Anti-oncogenes or tumor suppressor genes*: They control cells growth and proliferation; inactivation may lead to cell transformation.

They are normal genes that slow down cell division, repairing mistakes or tell cells to die. They are negative regulator of cell growth. When they do not work properly, cells can grow out of control, which can lead to cancer. Tumor suppressor genes form complexes with onco-proteins of some DNA viruses which are oncogenic. Inactivation or functional loss of such genes results in tumor formation.
1. The genes identified in normal **retinoblastoma gene (Rb gene)** class, its inactivation causes retinoblastoma.
2. The **p53 gene** is a tumor suppressor gene; the loss of it by chromosomal deletion is associated with some human cancers.

- *Apoptosis–regulatory genes*: They have control on programmed cell death but may occur as proto-oncogenes or tumor suppressor genes or their mutation may be responsible for transformation.
- *DNA repair genes*: Normal host genes which repair any mutations which may occur during cell growth. Failure of DNA repairs may cause persistent mutations.

Events that must occur before oncogenesis:
- **Establishment of long-term persistent infections** which lead to prolonged reaction between virus and host cells.
- *Evasion of host immune response*: Tumor viruses escape host responses as follows:
  - **Restriction of expression of viral genes**, hence immune system may not notice the antigens, e.g. Epstein-Barr virus in B cells.
  - **Viruses infect sites where immune responses cannot reach**, e.g. HPV infecting epidermis.
  - **Mutation of genes**, new virus has altered antigens, hence helps to escape immune responses.
  - Some viruses **infect immune cells** and **cause immunosuppression**.
  - **Host cells susceptibility:** Host cells may be permissive or non-permissive to viruses.
  - Permissive cells support multiplication of viruses.
  - Some cells are permissive to one type of virus but not to another type.

– Oncogenesis may occur in permissive as well as non-permissive cells. Risk is more when virus infects non-permissive cells as for their viruses may undergo some changes making cells immortal, e.g DNA viruses infect to permissive cells, viral particles are released by cell lysis, hence they are not oncogenic to host cells. But if viral cycle is blocked in some way, they grow indefinitely.

– RNA viruses do not cause cell lysis hence may be oncogenic to both, non-permissive and permissive cells.

• **Retention of virus nucleic acid inside host cells** may be important to maintain a stable genetic alteration that occurs in tumor cells.

MECHANISMS OF VIRAL ONCOGENESIS

Virus oncogenesis is slow process (years to decades) having many complex steps. Host factors as immunity and susceptibility decided by genetic factors also contributes to viral oncogenesis. Different mechanisms are used by different viruses but two recurring themes are inhibition of normal growth regulatory processes and stimulation of cell growth.

Series of molecular reactions are involved for progress of normal cells to neoplastic cells. Cells get immortalized which requires repeated entry into cell cycle, which is restricted by cellular retinoblastoma gene protein (Rb); inactivation such suppressor pathway is observed in many cancers. The cellular tumor suppressor protein p53 is disrupted which otherwise involved in programmed cell death.

Transformation of host cells to tumor cells by oncogenic viruses may occur by:

1. *Direct acting oncogenic viruses*: Acute transforming retroviruses of animals have viral oncogenes (*V-onc*), which may cause oncogenesis by directly inserting in host chromosome.

2. *Indirect acting oncogenic viruses*: Most of human oncogenic viruses have transforming genes which get inserted in host genome causing alteration of expression of pre-existing cellular genes(regulate host cell growth) as proto-oncogenes, tumor suppressor genes, DNA repair genes and genes regulating 'apoptosis'.

In case of DNA viruses, viral genome is inserted into cell genome which influences host cells to undergo malignant transformation.

Many molecular mechanisms may be responsible for conversion of benign proto-oncogenes to cancer genes. Overexpression of genes—many genes products may lead to malignant transformation.

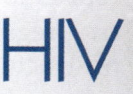

64

HIV

HISTORICAL ASPECT

- First clue of new syndrome came from New York and Los Angelis in 1981. There was an outbreak of rare conditions, i.e. *Pneumocystitis carnii* and Kaposi's sarcoma in homosexuals.
- Luc Montagnier, in 1983 (Pasteur institutie, France) isolated a virus from a West African patient suffering from persistant generalised lymphadenopathy, he gave name lymphadenopathy associated virus (LAV).
- Robert Gallo and his colleagues isolated a retrovirus from a case of AIDS and they gave name as T cell lymphotropic virus III.
- International Committee on viral nomenclature decided the name *HIV* (Fig. 64.1).

First ELISA became available for the detection of antibodies against HIV in 1985.

HIV belongs to **family Retroviridae**, as it has **enzyme reverse transcriptase** which converts RNA to DNA (group Lentivirus).

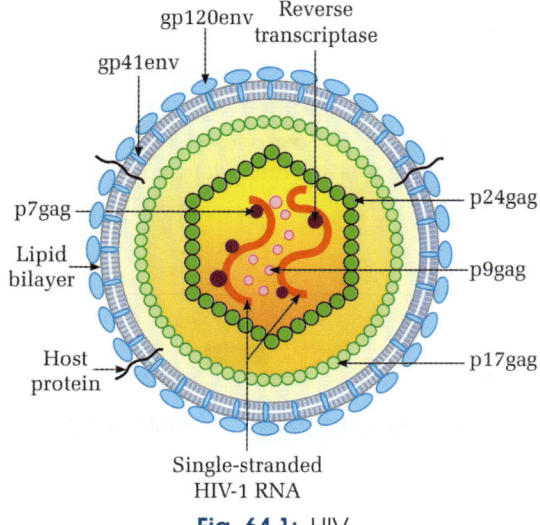

Fig. 64.1: HIV

Morphology

- It is spherical, enveloped virus.
- *Size*: 90–120 nm.
- Nucleocapsid has outer icosahedral shell and cone-shaped core containing ribonucleoproteins.
- Genome is **diploid,** composed of two identical strands of **positive sense RNA.**
- In association of RNA, there is enzyme **reverse transcriptase,** with this enzyme viral RNA is first converted to single-stranded DNA which integrates with host DNA, virus is called **'provirus'.**
- Envelope is made up of lipoprotein, the protein is encoded by virus while lipid is derived from host cell membrane. The **surface spikes (gp$_{120}$)** combine with CD4 receptor of lymphocytes. **Transmembrane pedicle (gp41)** fuses with host cell membrane.

Structural Proteins (Antigens)

- *Gag genes (group associated protein)*: They determine **core and shell of virus.** The precursor protein is p55, which is broken down into **p15, p18, p24. Major core protein is p24.**
  - The p24 antigen can be detected after *HIV* infection when antibody test is negative, late reappearance of this antigen with decrease in its antibody is associated with exacerbation of disease
- The **env (envelope) genes** synthesize **gp120,** forming surface spike and **gp41** forming **transmembrane pedicle.**
- The **pol genes** code for polymerase reverse transcriptase and other enzymes as protease, endonuclease. It is precursor protein which is broken into **p31, p51, p66.**

Nonstructural Genes

- *tat*—transactivating gene enhances expression of viral genes
- *nef*—negative factor gene downregulates viral replication
- *rev*—regulator of virus gene enchances expression of structural proteins.
- *vif*—viral infectivity factor determines the infectivity of viruses
- *Vpu(HIV-1)* and *vpx(HIV-2)* play important role in maturation and release
- *vpr* stimulates promoter region of virus
- *LTR*—long terminal repeats at the ends which has promoter, enhancer and integration signals.

Antigenic Variations in HIV

HIV is highly mutable virus, it shows variations (antigenic variations as well as other properties as growth characteristics, cytopathology) and **variations are due to the error prone nature of the enzyme reverse transcriptase.**

Origin of AIDS

HIV in humans originated from cross species infections by Simian viruses in rural Africa, probably due to direct human contact with infected primate blood. Current evidence is that the primate counterparts of HIV1 and HIV2 were transmitted to humans on multiple (at least 7) different occasions. Sequence evolution analysis placed the introduction of *SIV* cpz into humans that gave rise to *HIV*-1 group 'M' at about 1930, although some estimates push the date back to 1908. Presumably such transmissions occurred repeatedly over the ages, but particular social, economic, and behavioral changes that occurred in the mid-20th century provided circumstances that allowed these virus infection to expand, become well established in humans, and reach epidemic proportions.

Receptors for HIV

CD4 glycoprotein: High affinity receptor and chemokine receptors—CCR5 (new abbreviation R5) and CXCR4 (new abbreviation X4).

Target cells for HIV: T helper cells, cervical cells, astrocytes, CD8+ cells

Megakaryocytes, trophoblastic cells, retinal cells, cardiac myocyte, rectal mucosal cell

Monocyte/macrophage, oligodendroglia and microglia, peripheral blood dendritic cells, follicular dendritic cells, epidermal Langerhan's cells

HIV-1 Genotypes (10. from A-J)

There are **two serotypes of HIV, i.e. HIV1 and HIV2** (Table 64.1). HIV1 (Fig. 64.2) is divided into three groups **(M, N, O).** Group 'M' (major) is responsible for global epidemic. Group 'O' (outliers) seen in West Africa. HIV1 strain related to gorilla. SIV identified in Cameroonian women in 2009 has been proposed as group 'N'. **'M' group** is **worldwide and it has 10 subtypes or clades from A-J.** Subtypes sometimes further split into **sub-subtypes as A1, A2.** Circulating **recombinant forms (CRF)** are derived by recombination between different subtypes. CRF01-AE is recombinant of A and E.

Infected person may have group of closely related subtypes and/or CRF at a given time called **quasispecies.**

Subtype A is seen in West Africa. Subtype B is seen in Europe, America, Japan, and Australia. **Subtype C is most common form worldwide. Asian and African subtypes** (C and E) are more readily transmitted by **heterosexual mode** while **American strains** (subtype B) are mainly transmitted through **blood and homosexual contact.**

TABLE 64.1: Differentiation of HIV1 and HIV2

HIV1	HIV2
	It has 40% genetic identity with HIV1
Vpu	Vpx present
More virulent	Much less virulent than HIV1
Worldwide	Largely confined to restricted areas
Less related to simian immunodeficiency virus	More closely related with simian immunodeficiency virus
Envelope gp41	Envelope antigen gp40

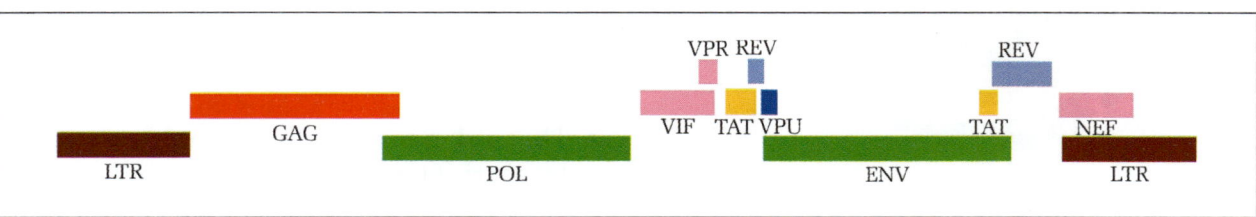

Fig. 64.2: HIV1 genome

Resistance

- It is a thermolabile virus, inactivated by boiling at 100°C in few seconds.
- In dried blood, it may survive for 7 days.
- It is inactivated by—0.5% hypochlorite solution, 2% gluteraldehyde solution; 50% ethanol kills the virus in 10 minutes.

Replication

- Receptor for *HIV* is CD4. After entry, virus infect CD4 cell.
- CD4 cells are mainly T lymphocytes (5–10% of B lymphocytes, 10–20% of monocytes and macrophages, glial cells and microglia of CNS, follicular dendritic cells may be infected).
- The first step of infection is the binding of gp120 to the CD4 receptor.
- Cell fusion occurs as gp 41 of virus fuses with host cell membrane.
- The binding of gp 120 to CD4 cells is not sufficient for the entry of virus. Co-recptors involved are CXCR4 for T cell tropic HIV and CCR5 for macrophages.
- Entry is followed by penetration and uncoating. HIV genome is uncoated and internalised.

- Reverse transcriptase enzyme converts single-stranded RNA to single-stranded DNA and then converts it into double-stranded DNA called **provirus**.
- Double-stranded genome (provirus) integrates with host DNA, with the help of enzyme integrase, causing latent infection.
- From time-to-time, progeny viruses are released by lysis of cells.

It is estimated that **10 billion HIV particles** are produced and destroyed each **day**. The life of virus in plasma is about **6 hours** and **viral cycle takes 2–6 days. Once infected, the half-life of CD4 lymphocytes is about 2–6 days.**

- In an infected person, virus can be isolated from blood, lymphocytes, cell free plasma, semen, cervical secretions, saliva, tears, urine and breast milk.

Pathogenesis (Fig. 64.3)

HIV causes of depletion of CD4 cells, the causes are:
- *HIV* progeny viruses come out of lymphocytes by lysis.
- Uninfected CD4 cells fuse with infected cells and they are also damaged.
- Viral infected cells induce apoptosis.
- Direct *HIV*-mediated cytopathic effects.

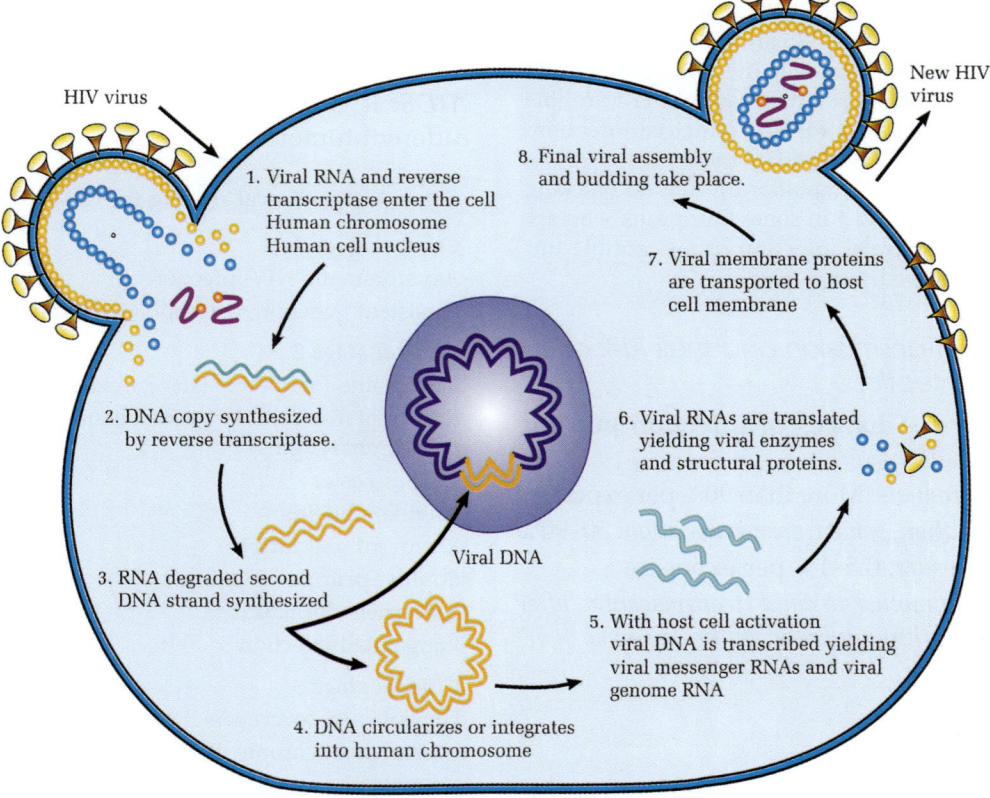

Fig. 64.3: HIV—life cycle

- Autoantibody formed against CD4 cells further damage T lymphocytes (CD4-helper cell).
- Anergy (inappropriate signalling).
- Super antigens (superinfecting organisms).
- Programmed cell death (apoptosis).
- Antibody dependent cellular cytotoxicity (ADCC).
- Natural killer (NK) cells activity.

Due to fall of helper cell, both antibody-mediated immunity and cell-mediated immunity of host decreases leading to immunosuppressive stage. *HIV-specific immune responses are depleted. Cytotoxic CD8 T cells (CTL) activity is decreased.*

HIV trophism: HIV infects CD4 lymphocyte and macrophages with the help of gp120. Entry of virus in the cell is not only mediated by gp120 and gp41 but also with its chemokine receptors. **Macrophage trophic strains (M-trophic) of HIV1** (nonsyncitia inducing strains) use the beta chemokine receptor CCR5 for entry and thus able to replicate in CD4 cells and macrophages. These strains are called **R5 viruses.** The normal legend for this receptor, RANTES, a macrophage inflammatory protein (MIP)-1-beta and MIP-1-alpha are able to suppress HIV1 infection *in vito.* This CCR5 coreceptor is used almost all primary infected HIV1 isolates of viral subtype. T-trophic viruses or SI (syncytial forming) strains replicate in primary CD4 Tcells as well as in macrophages and use alpha-chemokine receptor CXCR4, for entry. These strains are now called **X4 strains.** The alpha chemokine SDF-1, a legend for CXCR4, suppresses replication of T trophic viruses. It does by downregulating the expression of CXCR4 on the surface of the cells. Viruses that use only CCR5 are called R5, those use CXCS4 are called X4 viruses. However, the coreceptor doesn't complete explain the trophism of viruses, as not all R5 are able to use CCR5 on macrophages for a productive infection. Average rate of CD4 decline is 50/mL per year.

Mutation in CCR5 (delta 32 mutation) results in blocking the entry of HIV. It is observed in some Europeans who are either completely resistant to infection or susceptible but progress to AIDS is delayed.

Various Modes of Transmission and their Risk of Transmitting HIV Infection

- *Sexual intercourse:* Chances of infection per one exposure are 0.1–1%
- *Blood and blood products:* More than 90% per exposure
- *Tissue, organ donation, semen, cornea donation:* 50–90%
- *Percutaneous exposure:* 0.5–1% per exposure
- *Transmission from mother to child (transplacental, after birth, during birth, through breast milk):* 15–45%.

Clinical Features

Group I

Acute HIV infection: After 3–6 weeks of infection, some patients present with fever, headache, rash, and lymphadenopathy. Tests for HIV antibodies are negative at onset but may become positive during course of infection, this is called **seroconversion illness.**

In many of the patients infected, **'acute retroviral syndrome'** or seroconversion occurs without any apparent illness.

Group II

Asymptomatic infection or latent infection: All patients pass through stage of symptomless infection, the duration of which varies from patient to patient. Infection continues and presents as persistent generalized lymphadenopathy.

Group III

Persistant generalized lymphadenopathy (PGL): It is presence of enlarged lymph nodes at least 1 cm, at 2 or more different sites, in absence of other causes of lymphadenopathy. This stage is followed by AIDS related complex and then with full blown picture of AIDS. (Some 5% of infected persons remain asymptomatic for 10–15 years; they are called long-term survivors or long-term nonprogressers.)

Group IV

AIDS-related complex: Patients present with constitutional symptoms, and suffer from opportunistic infections as oral candidiasis, TB, herpes zoster.

Group V

AIDS: It is end stage, with different infections and different tumors.

WHO clinical staging for HIV/AIDS in adults

Clinical stage 1
Asymptomatic HIV infection
Persistent generalized lymphadenopathy

Clinical stage 2
Unexplained moderate (10%) weight loss
Recurrent respiratory tract infections (sinusitis, tonsillitis, otitis media, pharyngitis)
Herpes zoster
Angular cheilitis
Recurrent oral ulcers
Popular pruritic eruptions
Seborrheic dermatitis
Fungal nail infection

Clinical stage 3
Unexplained severe weight loss (>10%)
Unexplained chronic diarrhea: >6 months
Unexplained persistent fever: 1 month
Oral candidiasis

Oral hairy leukoplakia

Pulmonary tuberculosis

Severe bacterial infection

Acute necrotizing gingivitis, ulcerative stomatitis, and periodontitis

Unexplained anemia

Clinical stage 4

HIV wasting syndrome (slim disease): Characterized by profound weight loss (>10%), chronic diarrhea (>1 month), prolonged unexplained fever(1 month)

Bacterial opportunistic infections

Recurrent severe bacterial infections

Extrapulmonary tuberculosis

Disseminated non-tubercular mycobacterial infection

Recurrent septicemia (including non-typhoidal salmonellosis)

Viral opportunistic infections

Chronic HSV infection

Progressive multifocal leukoencephalopathy

CMV (retinitis, other organ infection excluding liver, spleen and lymph node)

Fungal opportunistic infections

Pneumocystis jirovecii pneumonia

Esophageal candidiasis

Cryptococcus neoformans-meningitis

Disseminated mycosis (histoplasmosis, coccidioidomycosis)

Parasitic infections

Toxoplasmosis encephalitis

Chronic intestinal cryptosporidiosis

Atypical disseminated leismanial infection

Chronic intestinal cryptosporidiosis (>1 month)

Neoplasma

Kaposi's carcinoma

Invasive cervical cancer

Cervical carcinoma

Lymphoma (cerebral, B cell, and Hodgkin)

Other conditions

HIV encephalopathy

Systemic HIV associated nephropathy or cardiomyopathy

Opportunistic Infections

- *Protozoal*: Toxoplasmosis, cryptosporidiosis, isosporidiosis, generalized strongyloidiasis
- *Fungal*: *Pneumocystis jirovecii,* candidiasis, *cryptococcosis*, histoplasmosis, coccidioidomycosis, aspergillosis
- *Bacterial*: *Mycobacterium avium* complex, *MTB, Salmonella, Campylobacter, Nocardia, Legionella,* multiple or recurrent pyogenic bacterial infection, *Rhodococcus equi*
- *Viral*: CMV, HSV, VZV, and JCV
- *Opportunistic tumors*: Kaposi's sarcoma

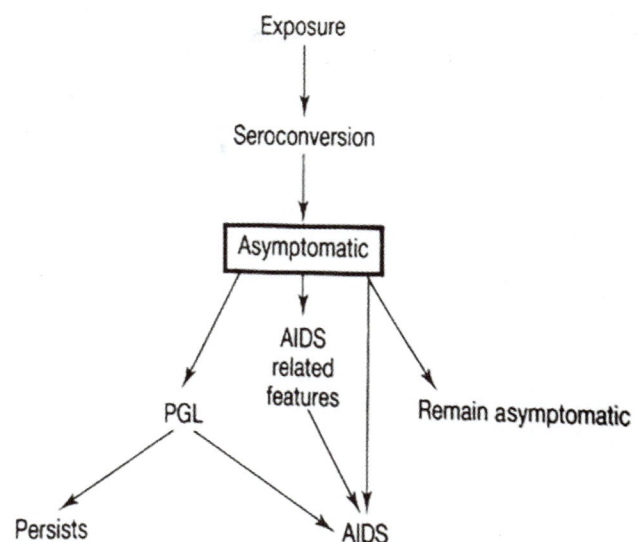

Clinical Course of HIV

Importance of laboratory diagnosis:

a. Prolonged asymptomatic stage

b. Despite treatment, infection invariably fatal

c. No preventive vaccine

d. Implications far beyond physical and mental health of the affected individual

Detection of p24 Antigen by ELISA

If the dose is small, following a needle stick injury, the process may be delayed. **The appearance of viremia, p24 antigenemia followed by IgM response coincides** with acute seroconversion illness. Later p24 disappears from circulation; it remains absent thereafter and reappears in very late stage of disease. However, antibody bound CD4 continues to be demonstrated after dissociation. The **p24 capture ELISA** can be used for this purpose. In this ELISA, antibody to p24 is attached to the solid surface. In first few weeks of infection, and in terminal phase of infection the test is uniformly positive. The test is useful in **window period.**

Viral Isolation

The virus is present in circulation and body fluids, within lymphocytes or cell free. Virus titers are parallel to p24 titers, high soon after infection, low during asymptomatic period and again high towards the end of disease. The virus is present in many parts of body and can be isolated from peripheral lymphocytes. The procedure of viral culture is **co-cultivation** of patient's lymphocytes with uninfected lymphocytes in the presence of interleukin-2. As the risk is high in viral culture, it is done at reference laboratory.

PCR

It is highly sensitive and specific. Two types are used.
- *DNA-PCR*: Peripheral lymphocytes from patient's blood are lysed and provirus DNA is amplified using primers from relatively constant region of *HIV* genome.
- *RT-PCR*: It can be used for diagnosis of infection and monitering the viremia.

Antibody Detection (Table 64.2 and Fig. 64.4)

It is simple test for the diagnosis of HIV infection. The period between the entry of virus in patient till the appearance of antibody in blood is called **window period**. The window varies from 2–8 weeks. If the infection is due to sexual method, antibodies take a longer time to appear in blood. Initially IgM appears and it disappears in 8–10 weeks, while IgG remains positive for longer period.

National HIV Testing Policy

a. No mandatory HIV testing is imposed as a precondition for employment or for providing health care services and facilities.
b. Test is performed after pre-test and post-test counseling
c. Consent should be informed and written
d. General purpose consent not valid

Screening Tests (ELISA/Rapid/Simple Test)

- *ELISA (E)*: It takes 2–3 hours.
- *Rapid (R)*: It gives result few within minutes, e.g. dot blot assays, particle agglutination, HIV spot.
- *Simple (S)*: Test takes half hour—immuno-comb tests
- Line immunoassay

ELISA: Generations of ELISA are one to four, depending upon the antigen used. Third generation is highly sensitive and specific.
- *Generation I*: Viral lysate is used as an antigen.
- *Generation II*: Antigen obtained by recombinant DNA technology.
- *Generation III*: Synthetic peptides are used as antigens.
- *Generation IV*: It detects antigen as well as antibody.

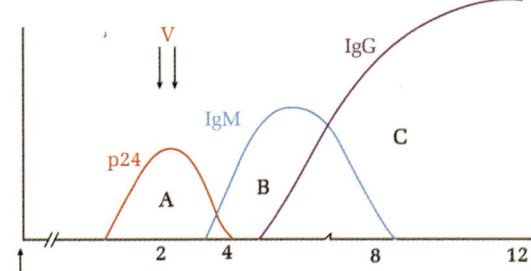

Fig. 64.4: Sequence of appearance of various serological markers after massive infection

Types of ELISA: Indirect, sandwich, competitive and capture ELISA.

Advantages: Large number of samples processed at one time, written record for documentation is available, it is highly sensitive.

Limitations: Technical skill required and equipment are costly.

False negative: Test done in window period, late stage of disease may be false –ve test.

False positive:
- Autoimmune diseases
- Multiple pregnancies
- Hypergammaglobulinemia
- Chronic alcoholics
- Patients with hepatitis
- Recipient of multiple transfusions
- Antibodies to Class II HLA (HLA-DR4)

WHO and UNAIDS recommendations for HIV testing strategies in India: In India the guidelines are given by the organization called NACO (National AIDS Control Organization).

Currently antibody tests used in India are **Coomb AIDS, Tridot and immunochromatography or lateral flow (NACO).**

Other tests for antibodies detection include:
- Line immunoassay
- Radioimmunoprecipitation assay (RIPA)
- Indirect fluorescent antibody test.

TABLE 64.2: Evolution of serological markers during HIV infection				
State of infection	*p24*	*Anti-HIV IgG*	*Anti-HIV-IgM*	*Western blot pattern*
Early infection	Negative	Negative	Negative	Negative
Acute seroconversion illness	Positive to negative	Negative to positive	Positive	Partial p24 and or gp120
Carrier asymptomatic	Negative	Positive	Negative	Full pattern
PGL	Positive	Positive	Negative	Loss of p24 or p55
AIDS	Positive			Absence of p24/p55

Confirmatory Tests or the Supplementary Testing

These are for serum samples which were previously positive with screening test. It has to be done by different systems, using different antigens. If serum is reactive in two different systems, it has to be tested by another method.

Western blot is the confirmative test.

Procedure

- *HIV* proteins are separated by electrophoresis (polyacrylamide electrophoresis).
- The separated products are blotted on strips of nitrocellulose paper.
- The stripes are reacted with patient's sera.
- Their presence is detected by enzyme conjugated antihuman globulin. A suitable substrate is added. Prominent color bands will be produced where specific antibodies attach to different proteins.

Interpretation

A **positive band** with **proteins representing three genes** is conclusive. Positive band with at least two of the following is significant, i.e. **p24, gp41/120, gp41.**

WHO criteria: Presence of at least two envelope bands (out of gp120, gp160 or gp41) with or without gag or pol bands is taken as positive test.

CDC criteria: Presence of any two out of p24, gp120, gp160, gp41 bands is considered as positive test.

Disadvantages

- It is difficult if bands do not occur to satisfy the criteria.
- It may happen in early infection.
- It is a suitable test but interpretation is subjective and it requires expertise.
- The test is costly.
- Intermediate results with Western blot test are possible. In such cases, the test is repeated, later, if no results are seen later, p24 test is done.

In absence of western blot, the policy is to use simple or rapid or EIA in combinations, as recommended by NACO. The various strategies of HIV testing (NACO Guidelines) are as follows:

Strategy I: It is used for donation safety. Single ELISA or rapid or simple test is performed and if it is positive, the blood bag is discarded, similarly the transplants are discarded.

Strategy II: It is used for **surveillance purpose.** If first test is positive, the second test is performed, if second test (based on different system, or different manufacturer or different principle) is also positive, it is considered positive.

Strategy III: This is used for the diagnosis of persons or patients. In this strategy, if the results of two different tests are positive, a third test is performed. If all three tests are positive, it is considered as positive.

It is used for asymptomatic individuals.

Laboratory Diagnosis of HIV

Tests during Window Period

1. p24 antigen estimation
2. HIV specific **DNA PCR**
3. Viral culture

HIV RNA detection (by RT-PCR) detects HIV RNA as early 12th day. p24 antigen is detected in 1–2 weeks (avarage 16th day). Antibody detection is possible by 22nd day with third generation kit.

Indications

1. History of untested blood transfusion
2. History of unprotected or risky sexual exposure
3. Needle stick injury in HCW (contaminated).

Detection of HIV Specific DNA by PCR (Specific Gene Sequence)

- Useful in newborns
- Useful for diagnosis in window period.
- In indeterminate results with E/R/S/WB
- Useful for subtyping of *HIV* and other research

Peripheral blood monocytes from heterologus HIV uninfected donors are stimulated by PHA and after 48–72 hours, the stimulated cells are then cultured along with patient's lymphocytes.

Direct culture method: Peripheral blood mononuclear cells are cultured in-vitro which was stimulated with mitogen-phytohemagglutinin (PHA).

- Detection of viral growth can be done by following method.
- Demonstration of p24 or reverse transcriptase enzymes, syncytia formation or by direct immune fluorescence.

Test for diagnosis in newborn is *HIV* DNA specific PCR on dried blood spot (DBS). Blood is collected by heel prick on DBS card, kept at room temperature and transported to referral laboratory for PCR. It is used for early infant diagnosis.

Monitoring Progress of HIV Disease (Fig. 64.5)

1. *Viral markers:* Plasma **HIV RNA load, p24** antigen
2. *Surrogate markers:* Virus specific markers (antibody to p24 p17, nef, etc.)
3. *Non-specific markers:* Cellular markers—CD4 count
4. *Soluble markers:* Neopterin, beta 2 macroglobulin

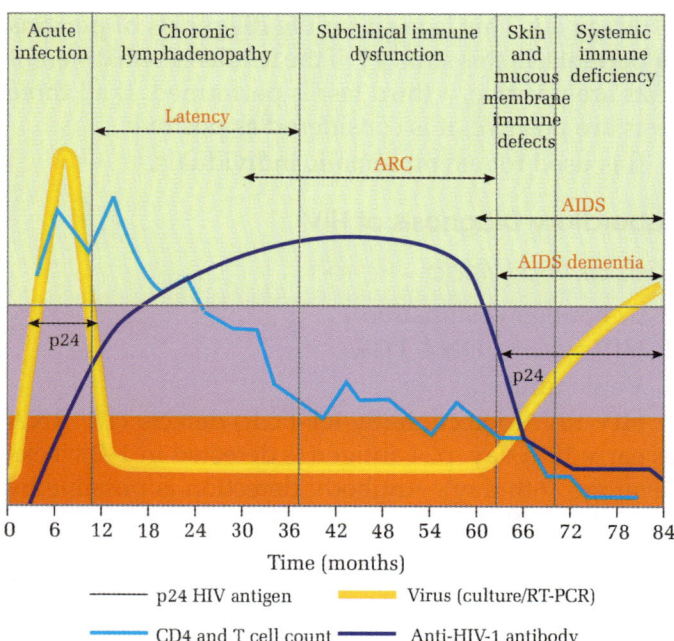

Fig 64.5: Variaus markers of HIV infection

Plasma HIV RNA load: It is best method for monitoring progression and response to ARV therapy (except children). Viral load is **10^2–10^7 HIV RNA copies/mL** in untreated patients. Levels are >10-fold lower in long-term non-progressers than in individuals with progressive disease. **Load >10,000 copies – start ARV therapy.**

Techniques available **for quantification** are:
- Quantitative RNA PCR
- Branched DNA assay
- Nucleic acid sequence based amplification (NASBA)

Epidemiology

HIV/AIDS in India: By year 2011, the adult HIV prevalence is 0.27%. There were 20.8 adults and 1.4 lakh children included in people living with HIV/AIDS, North East states as Nagaland, Mizoram and Manipur are high prevalence states.

Nagaland has higher prevalence rate (0.88%) **than global prevalence (0.8%) in 2012–13.**

Treatment

Antiretroviral treatment (ART) is used to stop progression of disease, increase life, reduce viral loads and reduce HIV transmission.

The indication to start treatment is based on CD4 counts and WHO staging of the disease. For clinical stages I and II start ART if CD4 counts are less than 350 cells/mm³ and for stages III and IV treatment is started with any count. Highly active antiretroviral (HAART) therapy uses combination of at least three drugs. NACO recommends three drugs (2NRTI + 1 NNRTI) in first line therapy. Following regimes are used.

Preferred regime—Lamivudine + AZT + Nevirapin
Alternate regimes are:

Lamivudine + Stavudine + Efavirenz
Lamivudine + Stavudine + Nevirapine

65

Rotavirus, Rubella Virus, Papovaviruses

Viruses causing diarrhea are:

- *Rotavirus*
- *Adenovirus*
- *Calciviruses (norvovirus and sapovirus)*
- *Astroviruses*
- *Norwalk*

HUMAN ROTAVIRUS (Fig. 65.1)

Types A-E plus two tentative species (F and G) based on structural protein-*VP6* are present.

Virion

Icosahedral, 60–80 nm in diameter, double shell virus, contains RNA (double-stranded), structural proteins 9, core contain, several enzymes, it is nonenveloped (transient **pseudo-envelope** is present during rotavirus particle morphogenesis).

Important features: Genetic reasortments occur redially. It is important cause of infantile diarrhea.

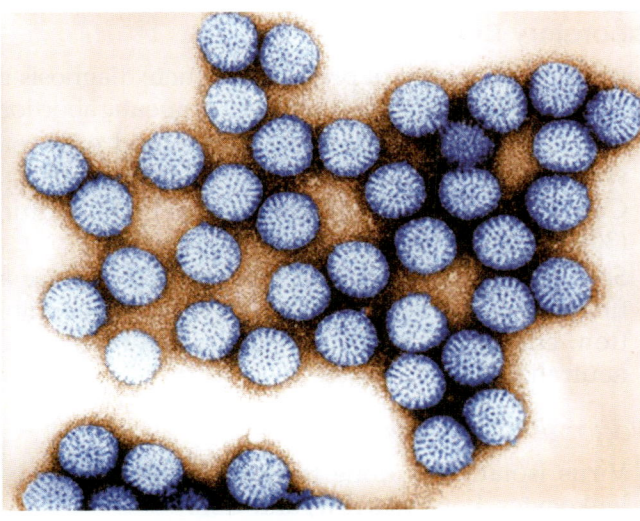

Fig. 65.1: Rotavirus

Pathogenesis (Flowchart 65.1)

It infects cells in the villi of small intestine. Viruses multiply in cytoplasm of enterocytes and damage their transport system. One of the viral encoded proteins, NSP4 is viral **enterotoxin** and induces secretion by signal transduction. Damaged cells may slough off in lumen; large number of viruses appear in stool, viral excretion lasts for 2–12 days in healthy patients, while it is prolonged in malnourished. Diarrhea may be due to impaired Na and glucose absorption as **damaged villi are replaced by nonabsorbing villi.**

Flowchart 65.1: Pathogenesis of rota virus

Ingested viruses infect cells at the tip of vili of small intestine

↓

Virus then infects in large number these cells

↓

Release of viruses in lumen

↓

Infected cells damaged & lost leaving immature cells with decreased absorptive capacity for sugar, water, salts

↓

Fluid accumulation in lumen of intestine leading to diarrhoea and dehydration

Incubation period is 1–3 days. Rota virus is the commonest cause of diarrhea in children and infants. Some outbreaks are reported from China in older children and adults caused by strains known as **'adult diarrhea rotavirus' (ADRV).** Clinical features are fever, pain in abdomen, vomiting and loose motions.

Laboratory Diagnosis

Demonstration of virus in stool is done by EM or ELISA; PCR (most sensitive). Antibodies are detected by ELISA.

Treatment: Supportive treatment given.

Vaccine: Live-attenuated rotavirus vaccine is monovalent. In the year 2006, a **live-attenuated pentavalent** become available. Human bovine virus reassortment rotavirus vaccine has been produced.

Other Agents of Viral Gastroenteritis

Family: Calciviridae
Genus: Nairovirus includes Norwalk viruses
Genus: Sapovirus—sapporo-like viruses

Norwalk is the most important cause of epidemic gastroenteritis in adults.

Sapoviruses cause sporadic cases in infants, children and elderly.

Adenoviruses (type 40, 41) cause diarrhea in infants and young children worldwide.

Astroviruses

- They have star-shaped appearance.
- 28–30 nm in size with positive sense ssRNA genome.
- These viruses cause diarrhea in infants, children and elderly.

Respiratory viruses

SARS coronavirus

Influenza B virus
Togaviridae and picornaviruses cause gastroenteritis in animal and in human beings.

RUBELLA VIRUS

Family: Togaviridae; only member of genus *Rubivirus.*
- It is pleomorphic roughly spherical particle, 50–70 nm in diameter.
- It has single-stranded RNA genome.
- Envelope carrying hemagglutinin peplomers agglutinates goose, pigeon, day-old chick and human RBCs at 4°C.
- Growth in cell lines, e.g. rabbit kidney (RK13), baby hamster kidney (BHK21) cell line and Vero cell lines are used; growth identified by interference.

Clinical Features

- Infection acquired by inhalation.
- Incubation period is 2–3 weeks.
- Generalized rash, first develops on face, spreads to neck, trunk and extremities; spares palms and soles.
- Non-tender enlargement of posterior cervical glands occurs.
- *Complications*: Arthralgia and arthritis; common in women with increasing age.
- It causes chromosomal breakages and inhibits mitosis in infected embryonic cells.
- Viremia occurs in patients with subclinical infection also.

Rubella in Pregnancy

- Fetal damage is related to stage of pregnancy. Infection in early pregnancy may cause death of fetus.
- *First trimester*: Congenital malformations are cardiac defects, cataract, deafness (classical triad).
- *Late pregnancy*: Communication defects, mental retardation; manifest later in life.
- Hepatosplenomegaly, thrombocytopenic purpura, myocarditis and bone lesions are called "**expanded rubella syndrome**".
- Virus present in all excretions of congenitally infected infants.

Postnatal Rubella

- It may occur in neonatal age, childhood or in adults.
- After 1–5 days of prodromal stage, a rash appears in children along with fever and respiratory symptoms.
- *Rash*: It is generalized maculopapular rash which starts from face and spreads to trunk and extremities.
- Occipital or post-auricular lymphadenopathy is seen. Pinhead size petechiae develop on soft palate and uvula called '**Forchheimer spots**.

Laboratory Diagnosis

It is important in case of pregnant women; diagnosis in early pregnancy is an indication for therapeutic abortion.
- *Virus isolation*: It is possible from blood or throat swabs (as early as seventh day before the rash).
- Cultures should be incubated at lower temperature (30–35°C).
- *Serology*: Demonstration of IgM antibody or rise in titer is detected by **ELISA,** hemagglutination inhibition, complement fixation, immunofluorescence, neutralization.

Diagnosis of Congenital Rubella

- Virus isolation is done from urine, throat swabs, leukocytes, bone marrow, and CSF.
- *Serology*: It involves demonstration of IgM antibodies.

Prophylaxis

- Infection confers lasting immunity.
- *Vaccine*: Attenuated RA 27/3 strain grown in human diploid cell culture is used for vaccine preparation.
- It is administered subcutaneously.
- It is given separately or as MMR vaccine (measles, mumps, rubella).
- Contraindications are immunodeficiency, pregnancy.

PAPOVAVIRUSES

It is the term indicating the names of viruses in this group, i.e. human papillomavirus, polyomavirus of monkeys and vacuolating virus of monkeys.

Family: Papovaviridae

Genera

- *Polyomavirus*: It includes simian vacuolating virus (SV-40), and polyomavirus.
- *Papillomavirus*: It includes human papillomavirus and animal papillomavirus.

These are small nonenveloped, DNA viruses with icosahedral symmetry.

PAPILLOMAVIRUSES

Morphology

- Papilloma viruses are former members of family Papovaviridae.
- These viruses have diameter 55 nm.
- *Symmetry*: Icosahedral.
- They contain a large genome (8kbp), which is double-stranded DNA.
- *Proteins*: 2 structural proteins are present.
- Non-enveloped viruses.
- Replicate in nucleus of host cell.

Some of the papillomaviruses infect animals while others infect human beings. These viruses have tropism for squamus epithelium of skin and mucosal membranes.

Pathogenesis

Modes of transmission: HPV infections are transmitted by **direct contact** through minor abrasions, sexually and perinatally.

HPV causes infection of cutaneous and **mucosal sites** which may lead to development of different kinds of **warts**—skin warts, plantar warts, flat warts, anogenital warts, laryngeal papilloma and several cancers of cervix, vagina, vulva, penis, anus and head and neck.

Based upon relative occurrence of viral DNA in certain cancers, **HPV types 16 and 18 are considered to be high cancer risk,** about 15 other subtypes are also considered high risk. Many HPV infections are considered benign.

Integrated copies of viral DNA are present in cervical cancer cells, though it is not integrated in noncancerous cells or premalignant cells. Skin cancers appear to harbor HPV genomes in episomal state.

Viral early proteins E6 and E7 are synthesized **in cancer tissue. These are viral oncoproteins.**

Cervical cancers develop slowly and multiple factors are involved in progression to malignancy. For this, **persistent infection of high-risk HPV is necessary.**

Correlation between Virus Type and Type of Lesion Produced (Table 65.1)

Common warts (verruca vulgaris) usually found on hands and feet of children, mostly associated with types 1, 2, 3, 4.

Condyloma acuminatum or genital wart is due to 6, 11. This may be transmitted venereally and may be occasionally turn malignant.

HPV is **not cultivable virus;** diagnosis can be done by PCR.

A **recombinant vaccine** containing antigens from HPV 6, 11, 16, 18 is prepared which is indicated in adolescent and young adult women. The vaccine is contraindicated in pregnancy.

Types 6, 11 are associated with intraepithelial neoplasia, and type 16, 18 are related to cervical cancers.

HPV type	Clinical lesion	Suspected oncogenic potential
1	Plantar warts	Benign
2, 4, 27, 57	Common skin warts	Benign
3, 10, 28, 49, 60, 76, 78	Cutaneous lesions	Low
5, 8, 9, 12, 17, 20, 20, 36, 47	Epidermodysplasia verruciformis	Mostly benign, some may progress to malignancy
6, 14, 40, 42–44, 54, 61, 70, 72, 81	Anogenital condylomatas, laryngeal papilloma, dysplasia and intraepithelial neoplasia	Low
7	Hand warts of butchers	Low
16, 18, 31, 33, 35, 39, 45, 51–53, 56, 58, 59, 66, 68, 73, 82	High grade dysplasia Carcinomas of genital mucosa Laryngeal and esophageal carcinomas	High correlation between genital and oral carcinomas, especially cervical cancers

TABLE 65.1: Association of different serotypes with different tumors

PARVOVIRUS

- It is small, single-stranded DNA virus, host specific, of all viruses. B19 worldwide. Clinical features are respiratory infection with erythematous maculo-papular rash, arthralgia. Infection starts with erythema of cheeks (**slapped cheek disease**), it spreads to trunk, and limbs. The disease is known as **fifth disease.**
- Aplastic crises occur in children with chronic sickle cell disease.
- In adult females, it causes symmetrical polyarthritis affecting joints of hand and knee.
- In immunodeficient patient, it causes anemia.
- It causes congenital infection, fetus presents with fetus hydrops.
- Modes of transmissions are respiratory route, blood transfusion and congenital.
- Diagnosis is based on demonstration of virus in early infection and by antibody detection.

Virus Hemorrhagic Fevers

Viruses which cause hemorrhages belong to two families, **Arenaviridae and Filoviridae.** These are zoonotic infections, seen in South America, Africa; infections vary from asymptomatic to fatal disease.

Arenaviridae

They are single-stranded RNA viruses. EM shows electron dense granules resembling grains of sands within virus, hence the name **(arena-sand).**

It is spherical, or pleomorphic, 80–300 nm in size.

Lymphocytic choriomeningitis virus causes aseptic meningitis.

Laboratory mice are carriers. Viruses are shed in urine and feces which act as sources of infection.

South American hemorrhagic fever: *Junin* and *Machupo viruses* cause Argentinian and Bolivian hemorrhagic fevers. Rodents are the reservoirs.

Lassa virus: It is highly contagious virus caused many outbreaks in West Africa. Rodents are source of infection but patient-to-patient transmission occurs by droplets as virus is present in throat, saliva, urine and blood.

FILOVIRUSES

Thread-like viruses (filaments thread) with size— 800–1000 nm.

MARBURG

It caused hemorrhagic fever in Margburg (Germeny) and Belgrade (Yugoslavia). African green monkeys were source of infection, person-to-person transmission occurred. The infections are not reported since 1980.

EBOLA VIRUS

Ebola virus and Marburg virus, both cause highly fatal hemorrhagic fever in Africa with 25–90% mortality rate. Both are included in the family Filoviridae.

Ebola virus has produced extensive outbreak in 2014 and it is declared by WHO as public health emergency.

Ebola caused two outbreaks in 1976, one in Sudan and other in Democratic Republic of Congo. The latter outbreak occurred in a village near river Ebola hence the name Ebola virus. There are 4 subtypes or species (Zaire, Sudan, Reston, and Ivory cost).

Morphology: Viruses are pleomorphic, mostly seen as long filamentous threads, average size **805 nm.**

The reservoir hosts for Ebola are not known but infected animals as **fruit bats or primates (apes and monkeys) are suspected as reservoir hosts.**

Transmission: It spreads through **close contact with blood, secretions, organs, or other fluids of infected animals. Human-to-human** transmission occurs via **direct contact** of broken skin or mucosa with the following:
- Blood, secretions, organs or other body fluids
- Infected surfaces and materials, e.g. bedding, clothing, etc.

Clinical manifestations: Incubation period is 2–12 days. The most common clinical features are fever, headache, muscle pain, sore throat. Other symptoms include abdominal pain, vomiting, diarrhea, rash (with bleeding or hemorrhages), and shock leading to death.

Laboratory diagnosis
- Serum antibody (IgM, IgG) against nucleoprotein (NP) and glycoprotein (GP) antigens is detected by ELISA or immunofluorescence test.
- Serum antigens (NP, VP40, and GP) are detected by capture ELISA.
- Molecular methods for detection of viral RNA are RT-PCR and real-time PCR.
- Electron microscopy can be used for detection of viruses.
- Cell culture can be done in vero cell lines.

Treatment: Symptomatic treatment and correction of rehydration are the only options as there is no proven treatment or vaccine against this virus.

Reovirus prototype virus is Respiratory Enteric Human Orphan virus, association with disease is not known.

Orbivirus: The name derived from Orbi means ring in Latin as its innerlayer has ring-shaped capsomeres. Human infection is due to Colorado tick fever.

Bocavirus: It is a new parvovirus which has been isolated from respiratory tract of children presenting with acute respiratory disease.

CORONAVIRUSES

Morphology

- Large (120–160 nm), spherical, RNA virus with helical symmetry.
- Enveloped virus. The envelope has petal- or club-shaped or crown-like peplomers giving appearance of **'solar corona'**.
- **Two groups** exist; **acid labile viruses** (cause common cold-like illness) and **acid-stable viruses** (cause gastroenteritis in human beings and animal).
- It includes two **subfamilies Coronavirinae and Torovirinae**. The Coronavirinae family is classified into **four genera**—alpha corona, beta corona, gamma corona, and delta corona. Most of them infect animals except gamma coronavirinae which infects birds.

Human Coronaviruses

Total six corona viruses causing infections in human beings are known, first two viruses belong to **Alpha-coronavirinae**, and rest belong to **Beta-coronavirinae.**
1. Human coronavirus 229E
2. Human coronavirus NL63 (new haven coronavirus)
3. Human coronavirus OC43
4. Human coronavirus HKUI
5. SARS-CoV(severe acute respiratory syndrome coronavirus)
6. **MERS-CoV(Middle East respiratory syndrome)**

Most coronaviruses produce **mild respiratory disease** except **SARS-CoV** and **MERS-CoV** which are restricted to geographic areas, transmitted from human to human, and produced outbreaks with high mortality.

Mode of transmission: Coughing, sneezing, personal contact as touching mouth, nose, eyes, or shaking hands. SARS-CoV also spreads by droplets and rarely through air.

SARS-CoV

It was first time recognized in **China (November 2002)**. The **WHO physician Dr CarloUrbani** visited Hong Kong died. He infected 12 persons who shared the same hotel and spread the disease to their own countries before themselves died.

Epidemiology: It spread to 30 countries, with 8098 cases and 800 deaths. India was not affected. No case since 2004 has been reported.

Source: Infection probably contracted from animals, including monkeys, raccoon dogs, cats, dogs, rodents and Himalayan palm civets.

Clinical manifestations: Lower respiratory tract infection with muscle pain, headache, sore throat, fever followed by cough, dyspnea and pneumonia was the presentation of SARS.

Laboratory diagnosis

- **Antigen detection** in respiratory secretions by ELISA.
- **Electron microscope** can be performed on stool sample.
- *RNA detection*: **RT-PCR** is useful for respiratory secretions, stools and blood.
- **Isolation** was done in vero cell line.
- **Antibodies detection: ELISA** and **indirect immuno-fluorescence** can be performed on paired sera to demonstrate fourfold rise in antibody titre.

Prevention and treatment: No specific drug or vaccine is available.

Control measures

- Isolation of patients
- Quarantine of exposed person
- Restricted travel to affected area
- Use of barrier precautions
- Frequent handwashing
- Avoid contact with animals

MERS-CoV

- It is severe form with 30% mortality.
- First detected in Saudi Arabia and then affected neighboring countries.
- *Spread*: Infection probably acquired from camels and cats.
- People at risk include—health care providers, close contacts of cases and animals and recent history of travel from Arabian Peninsula within 14 days.

66

Prions and Slow Viral Diseases

SLOW VIRUS DISORDERS

A group of disorders characterized by long incubation period, slow course ending fatally.

The **chacteristics** of slow viral infections are:

a. Long incubation period—months or years.

b. Mostly there is involvement of CNS.

c. Outcome is fatal.

d. Genetic predisposition is seen.

e. There is minimum or no immune response.

Slow viruses are classified into three groups:

Group-A: It is infection of sheep caused by Lentiviruses, e.g. Visna

Group-B: It includes CNS infections as scrapie, mink encephalopathy, Kuru and Creutzfeldt – Jakob disease. These diseases are collectively called subacute spongiform viral encephalopathy.

Group-C: It consists of two CNS infections of human beings—subacute sclerosing panencephalitis and progressive multifocal encephalopathy.

Visna

- It is slow viral infection of sheep.
- Though it affects all organs of body, pathological changes are more pronounced in brain, lungs and cells of reticuloendothelial system.
- Inflammatory lesions develop in central nervous system but it takes long time (months to years) before clinical manifestations occur.
- The disease has incubation period of 1–2 years.
- There is insidious onset paresis progressing to total paralysis and death.
- Virus can be isolated from CSF, blood and saliva. Culture is done in sheep choroid plexus tissue.

Maedi

- It is caused by lentivirus.
- Virus affects lungs, there is progressive fatal hemorrhagic pneumonia of sheep.
- It has incubation period of 2–3 years.

Group B (Prion Diseases)

Subacute spongiform viral encephalopathies: These are chronic progressive degenerative diseases of CNS.

These diseases are characterized by spongiform degeneration of CNS.

There is progressive vacuolation in dendritic and axonal processes of neurons, extensive astroglial hypertrophy and proliferation.

PRIONS

Prions are unique infectious agents.

There are a many human and animal diseases—the spongiform encephalopathy whose pathology is characterized by development of large vacuoles in CNS. Initially these diseases were thought to be due to slow viral infections. It is now well known that these are caused by prions.

Prions are small proteinaceous infectious particles.

The characteristics of prions include:

1. Small size, less than 100 nm
2. Filterable
3. Lack nucleic acid genome
4. Resistant to heat, disinfectants, irradiations
5. Susceptible to high concentration of phenol, sodium hypochlorite, boiling
6. Slow replication, diseases have long incubation period and late in life
7. Cannot be cultivated
8. Do not cause inflammation or immune reactions

9. Diseases are only restricted to CNS.
10. Basic changes are neurological degeneration and spongiform changes.
11. Diseases are fatal.
12. With the exception of those cases where cases arise by mutation, transmission and spread require exposure to infectious agent. Ways in which these could occur include eating of contaminated food material, use of contaminated medical products (blood, hormones, transplants), the inoculation from contaminated instruments, possible mother to fetus transmission in pregnancy. The disease kuru was transmitted by eating brains of dead humans in funeral rites and now a variant of CJD is probably transmitted by eating contaminated beef products. They are carried in lymphoid cells, eventually being transmitted into neural tissue and CNS.
13. At present, there is no treatment and no vaccine.
14. Prions are host derived glycoproteins.
15. Prions create difficulties in diagnosis as they are not cultured and initially there is no immune reaction or inflammation.

The pathogenic mechanism appears to be proliferation of an abnormal prion protein (PrPsc) which is derived from normal prion protein—PrPee. The accumulation of abnormal protein in CNS causes the pathology.

Prion Diseases

Animals

a. *Scarpie*: Disease of sheep, vertical transmission occurs, or less commonly by contact.
b. *Mink* is scrapie-like disease in mink.
c. *Bovine spongiform encephalopathy* (**mad cow disease**) is present in endemic area and believed to spread by practice of feeding sheep with scrapie infected meat. It is enzootic in UK.

Human Diseases

1. *Creutzfeldt-Jacobs disease*:
   • Presents with dementia, incoordination, ending in death.
   • Iatrogenic infection due to corneal transplant reported.

2. *New variant of CJD 1996*: Age group infected was young persons. (Infection was suspected to be due to ingestion of infected beef.)
3. *Kuru*:
   • It means tremors.
   • It was observed in tribes from New Guinea.
   • Patients presented with progressive cerebellar ataxia, tremors followed by death.
   • Infection was believed to be due to practice of cannibalism and maintained custom of eating dead bodies of relatives after ritual nonsterlilizing cooking.
   • Following abolishing cannibalism, the disease disappeared. Carlton Gajdusek was awarded Nobel Prize (1976) for his contributions in the disease.

Group C: Subacute Sclerosing Panencephalitis

• It is rare sequela of measles virus infection.
• Mental and motor functions are affected, ending fatal in 2–3 years.
• Virus can be demonstrated in CSF, brain tissue. Virus cannot be isolated routinely from CSF or brain.
• Patients show high titer of antibodies. Detection of anti-measles antibody in CSF is pathognomonic of disease.
• Rarely SSPE may occur as rare complication of measles vaccination.

Progressive Multifocal Leukoencephalopathy

• It is subacute demyelinating disease seen in immuno-compromised patients.
• There is deterioration of motor functions, vision, speech and disease ends fatally in 2–3 years.

Laboratory Diagnosis

• Measurement of PrPsc by immunoassay is definitive method of diagnosis.
• Brain MRI shows increased intensity in basal ganglia.
• Stress protein 14-3-3 is raised in CSF.
• Sequencing the PRNP gene to identify mutation is important in familial forms of disease.
• Histopathological examination of brain biopsy shows spongiform degeneration and astrocytic gliosis.

67

Medical Mycology

FUNGI

Characteristics of Fungi

Fungi are **eukaryotic protista.** They possess multi-layered rigid cell wall containing chitin, mannan and other polysaccharides. Cytoplasmic membrane of fungi contains sterols. Cytoplasm possesses true nuclei, nuclear membrane, paired chromosomes, ribosomes, mitochondria and endoplasmic reticulum. They are unicellular (e.g. yeast) or multicellular (e.g. aspergillus). Division takes place by sexual method (e.g. formation of zygospore in mucor), asexual method (e.g. formation of sporangiospores in mucor) or both. They are eukaryotic organisms which exist as saprophytes, parasites or commensals.

Basic Fungal Morphology

- *Yeast cells*: Yeast multiply by budding.
- Bud formed is called blastoconidia.
- *Pseudohyphae*: The chain of elongated yeast cells forms pseudohyphae.
- **True hyphae** are filamentous structures seen in fungi, called molds. **Mycelium** is entangled mass of true hyphae. Hyphae may be aerial which project above the culture medium; vegetative hyphae are within medium. Aerial hyphae bear spores or conidia, help in sexual or asexual method of reproduction. Vegetative hyphae obtain nutrients from medium as they are submerged in the medium.

Fungi are classified by morphological, systematic and clinical classification.

Morphological Classification

A. Yeasts

Fungi in this group show only one morphological from, i.e. yeast. Example of pure yeast is *Cryptococcus neoformans.*

Important characteristics
- Yeast is unicellular.
- It multiplies by budding.
- Yeast cell or bud does not enlarge to form pseudohyphae as seen in *Candida*. Also (filamentous structures) hyphae are absent.
- Colonies are mucoid or pasty.

B. Yeast-like Fungi

It shows yeast cells and pseudohyphae, example is *Candida albicans.*

Important characteristics
- Morphologically, yeast cells and pseudohyphae are present.
- Yeast forms multiply by budding.
- Pasty colonies are produced on culture medium.

C. Molds

Morphologiclly, they show true hyphae, e.g. dermatophytes.
- They are multicellular.
- They have true hyphae (not pseudohyphae).
- Multiplication occurs by sexual method, or asexual method or both (this is covered in systematic classification).
- Colonies have different textures as cottony or velvety, granular.

(**Note.** Even dimorphic fungi form moldy colonies at 22°C).

D. Dimorphic Fungi

These fungi show two morphological forms. The form which is present in soil or **SDA (Sabourad's dextrose agar)** incubated at room temperature is mycelial form and the form seen in tissues as well as on SDA incubated at 37°C shows yeast forms. All the fungi which produce systemic infections are dimorphic fungi. For example, *Histoplasma capsulatum*.

Systematic Classification

It is based on type of sexual spore formation. (Hence there may be overlapping of morphological and systematic classification, e.g. *Aspergillus glacus* which is mold, it shows asexual as well as sexual spore, i.e. ascospore (Fig. 67.1). Zygomycetes of systemic fungi, morphologically fit into molds).

Classes

- *Phycomycetes*: These are lower fungi, they have aseptate hyphae and form endogenous asexual spores in a closed sac-like structure called sporangiospores (within sporangium). They form sexual spore called zygospore (Fig. 67.2) or oospores, e.g. mucor.

  Other three classes are higher fungi;they have septate hyphae and exogenous asexual spores called conidia.

- *Ascomycetes*: These fungi form sexual spores in a sac or ascus. It includes both yeasts and filamentous fungi.
- *Basidiomycetes*: Fungi of this class form sexual spores (basidiospores) on a base or basidium (Fig. 67.3).
- *Fungi imperfecti*: It is a provisional group of fungi whose sexual phases have not been identified.

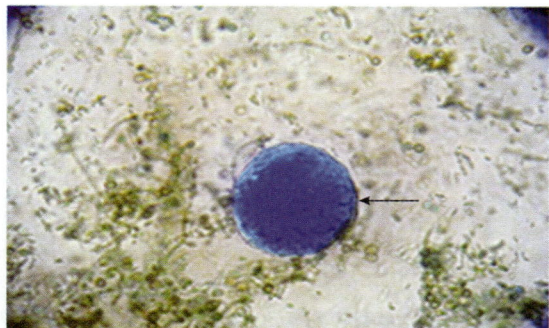

Fig. 67.1: Ascospore

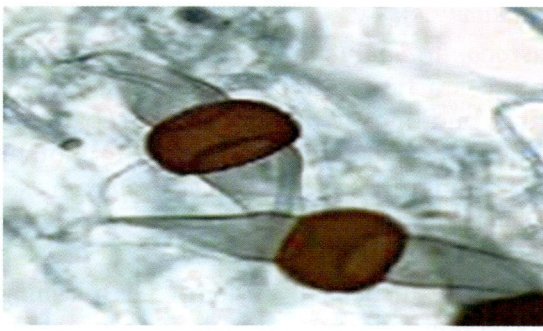

Fig. 67.2: Zygospores

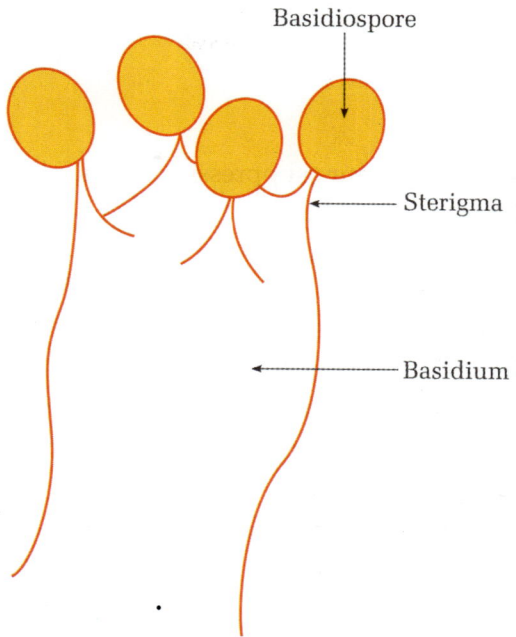

Fig. 67.3: Basidiospore

Pathogenic Classification

Primary pathogenic fungi: They can cause infections in normal healthy individuals. Fungi causing systemic infections (thermally dimorphic fungi) belong to this category.

Opportunistic mycoses (fungi) pathogens: They cause infections in immune suppressed persons, e.g mucormycosis is seen in patients with uncontrolled diabetics.

Clinical Classification

Pathogenic fungi may cause different types of infections:
a. *Superficial mycoses (infections)*: These are of two types:
   i. Surface infection (mycoses)
   ii. Cutaneous (mycoses) infections
b. *Deep mycoses (infection)*: These are of two types:
   i. Subcutaneous (mycoses) infections
   ii. Systemic or deep (mycoses) infection

Apart from this, fungi may cause harm by **allergic reactions** as seen in allergic aspergillosis or fungi produce toxin or they cause poisoning.

Other Classifications of Fungi

a. **Primary pathogenic fungi** which do not require decrease of host defences to produce infections. All systemic or deep mycotic fungi or dimorphic fungi belong to this type.
b. **Opportunistic fungi** cause infection in a patient whose resistance is lowered, e.g. mucor (grows on bread, thus widely present, but causes infection in diabetic patients).

List of (opportunistic) conditions favoring fungal infections are:

1. AIDS
2. Diabetes
3. Patients on immunosuppressive drugs
4. Patients on chemotherapy
5. Transplant recipients
6. Patients on dialysis
7. Premature neonates
8. Patients on antibiotic for longer period

Local decrease in resistance, which is seen in burns patients, patients with dentures (oral candidiasis may occur).

Some Features of Morphological Forms

Types of Budding

It gives idea of fungus involved.

- Broad based budding seen in *Blastomyces dermatitidis*.
- In *Malassezia* percurrent budding is seen.
- Multiple budding is seen in Paracoccidioidomycosis.

HYPHA

It is filamentous structure. It has parallel walls and terminal cell is equal to original cell from which it arises.

PSEUDOHYPHA

The budding yeast cells form chain of elongated yeast cells called pseudohypha.

Hyphae	Pseudohyphae
No constriction at base	Constriction at base
Septa straight and perpendicular	Septa curved
Cell walls are parallel	Cell walls are not parallel
It is formed by apical elongation	Formed by budding

Classification of Hyphae

Hyphae may be septate and aseptate. Aseptate hyphae are characteristics of mucormycosis, i.e. *Mucor, Rhizopus, Rhizomucor, Absidia.*

Septate hyphae are further classified as:

a. *Hyaline (in plain wet mount they have no color)*: These are seen in Aspergillus, dermatophytes, and deep fungi.
b. *Dematiaceous hyphae* have melanin on their wall hence they are dark brown to black. The fungi which cause chromoblastomycosis and phaeohyphomycosis are dematiaceous fungi, e.g. *Phialophora, Cladosporium, Alternaria, Curvularia,* and *Wangiella (exophila) dermatitidis.*

Depending on special shape which is characteristically seen in some fungi (dermatophytes), the hyphae are of different types as:

- *Spiral hyphae*: It is like a spring, seen in *Trichophyton mentagrophytes.*
- *Racket-like hyphae* resemble racket, one end is broad and another is short, (they are present head to head). They are seen in *Trichophyton mentagrophytes.*
- *Favic chandeliers*: Tip of hyphae shows small branches like horns of chandelier. It is seen in *Trichophyton schoenleinii, Trchophyton violaceum* (rarely).
- *Pectinate hyphae*: The end of hypha has branching on one side like comb. It is seen in *Microsporum audouinii.*
- *Nodular hypha*: Nodule-like swelling is seen within hypha. It may be seen in *Trichophyton mentagrophytes.*

Conidia are asexual reproductive structures, while **spores** are sexual reproductive structures. But many times both the terms are interchanged.

Conidia may be produced from the tips of growing hyphae or on specialized hypha called 'conidiophores' or produced directly off the hyphae or within hyphae.

If conidia are small, they are called **microconidia** or larger, called macroconidia. Both microconidia and **macroconodia** may be seen in some dermatophytes in which the morphology of conidia helps to identify the fungus.

SPORES

These are fruiting bodies. They are produced exogenously in contrast to bacterial spores which are endospores.

Types of Asexual Spores

- *Arthrospores*: These are formed by segmentation and fragmentation of hyphae. They are rectangular in shape. Their presence in culture is characteristic, e.g. *Tricosporon, Blastomyces, Sytalidium.*
- *Chlamydoconidia (may also be called as chlamydospores)*: These are thick-walled refractile spores produced on nutritionally deficient media. In Candida species, it's presence is diagnostic of *Candida albicans* (and *C. dublinensis*).
- *Blastoconidia or blastospores*: Budding of yeast cell produces a bud called blastconidia which may further bud, meanwhile it may get separated from mother cell or it remains attached to mother cell. Blastoconidia are seen in *Candida, Cryptococcus*. There are some fungi which form black yeast, e.g. *Wangiella dermatitidis.*

Sexual reproduction is by fusion of cells **(plasmogamy)** and nuclei **(karyogamy)** and meiosis. Asexual production occurs by mitosis.

Sporangiospores: Asexual spores of mucormycosis are present a closed structure called sporangium which after maturity bursts and releases sporangiospores.

Sexual spores: Depending upon class, they are present in a sac (**ascospore**) or **zygospores,** formed by sexual conjugation. They are seen in mucormycosis, hence mucormycosis is also called Zygomycetes.

Laboratory Diagnosis (Figs 67.4 to 67.13)

Specimens to be collected are plucked hairs, nail, skin scraping, blood, tissue, bone marrow, body fluids, respiratory and vaginal secretions, corneal scrapings, and stool.

Microscopy

- *KOH mounts*: 10–20% KOH mount is performed on specimens as nail, skin scraping, and tissue biopsy. KOH is used to dissolve keratin and it makes fungal elements visible.
- *India ink*: It is for demonstration of capsule of *Cryptococcus neoformans* in CSF.
- Gram's smear and special stains used are **PAS, GMS,** and immunofluorescence.
- In Gram's staining, fungal elements, as yeast and hyphae, appear Gram-positive.
- In PAS stain, fungi appear red and in GMS staining, fungi appear black.
- Immunofluorescence is done for *Pneumocystitis*.

Culture

Sabouraud's dextrose agar with chloramphenicol (SDA) is the most common medium used for cultivation of fungi. When growth of fungi appears on SDA, growth characteristics are noted down.

- SDA with chloramphenicol and (actidione) cyclo-heximide inhibts the growth of saprophytic fungi. Its pH is adjusted to neutral (or 4.5 acidic pH).

Following points are observed:

- Colonies on slant, one or few; hyphae slightly projecting form colonies or filling the tube completely (seen in mucor)
- Growth rate
- Color of pigment produced on reverse side of SDA medium.
- Morphology and texture of colony.

Lactophenol Cotton Blue (LPCB) mount: It is prepared from the growth on SDA which stains fungal hyphae, yeast cells, and spore or conidia. Morphology of spores, types of spores, arrangement, hyphal characteristics help in identification of the fungus.

Tease mount: LPCB from colony is done by taking a drop of LPCB on glass slide; colony from medium is taken by bent wire and the colony is teased in LPCB. Coverslip is placed and the preparation is observed under high power. The teasing should be done gently otherwise the arrangement of conidia and other structures is disturbed. If *in situ* morphology needed, slide culture is done.

Slide culture: It is used to observe *in situ* morphology, the procedure is as follows: In a sterile glass petridish, sterile bent glass is placed. At the bottom of petridish sterile filter paper is taken which is moistened with sterile saline. With sterile scalpel, a block of potato dextrose agar is cut from culture plate.With sterile bend wire, fungus growth is taken from SDA slant and four corners of block are inoculated. A sterile coverslip is placed on block and the whole assembly is kept at room temperature (25°C) for 7–8 days. The coverslip is gently lifted and placed on a drop of LPCB. The preparation is observed under high power.When the fungus on block grows, it adheres underside of coverslip, this helps to observe *in situ* morphology.

Newer Methods of Diagnosis

Serology: Antibody or antigen detection, immuno-histochemistry, DNA probes, PCR, detection of fungal metabolites beta-2-glucan.

Antigen detection:
1. Cryptococcal capsular antigen is detected in CSF for diagnosis of meningitis.
2. Enolase antigen is detected for diagnosis of *Candida*.
3. *Pneumocystitis* in respiratory secretion is detected by direct *immunofluorescence* test.

Antibodies detection can be done by following tests but they have the disadvantage that crossreactions occur.
- **CFT**
- **ELISA**
- **LA**
- **Immunodiffusion**

Molecular Methods

- Diagnosis and identification of *Candida* species is possible by **panfungal PCR.**
- DNA probes used for most of the fungal infections.

Fungi of Medical Importance

- **Fungi producing antibiotics:** Penicillin—*Penicillium notatum,* Cephalosporin—*Cephalosporium*. **Simvastatin** is fermentation product of *Aspergillus terreus*.

- **Ergot** is produced from *Claviceps purpura.*
- **Fungi are used as scientific models** to study genetics, biochemical processes and host parasite relationship, e.g. recombinant vaccines for hepatitis B are produced in fungi *Saccharomyces cerevisiae, Hansenula polymorpha* and *Pichia sp.*

Industrial Importance

- In food industry, fungi are used as source of mushrooms (basidiomycetes).
- They are used to alter texture, improve flavor, increase palatability and digestibility of natural and processed food.
- To produce alcohol, *Saccharomyces spp.* are used. Fats are produced from *Endomyces spp,* proteins are produced from *Torulopsis spp.*

Fungi are also used to control pests in farming, e.g. *Beauveria bassiana, Verticillium lecanii,* and *Trichoderma spp.*

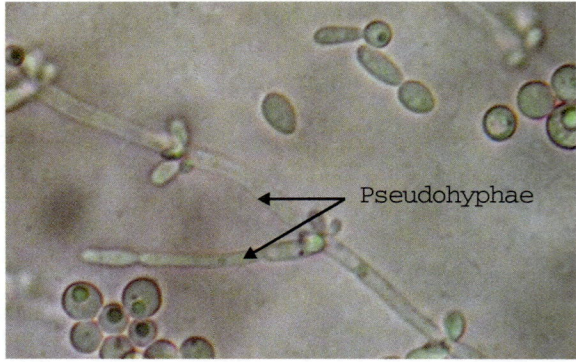

Fig. 67.6: Wet mount showing pseudohyphae

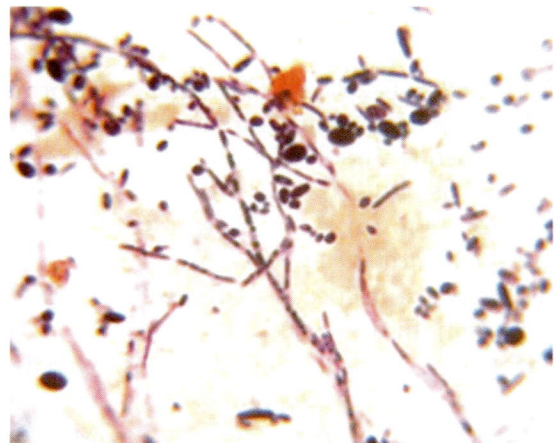

Fig. 67.7: Gram staining showing yeast cell and pseudohyphae

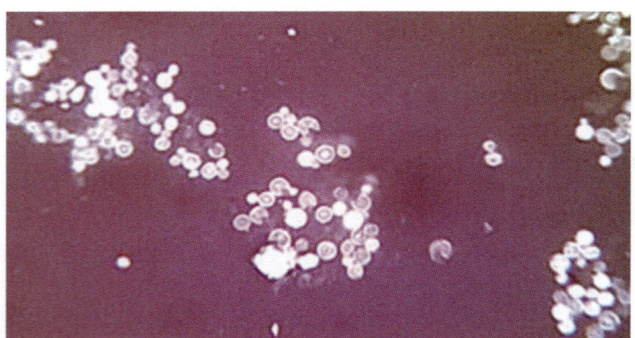

Fig. 67.4: Negative staining showing capsulated yeasts

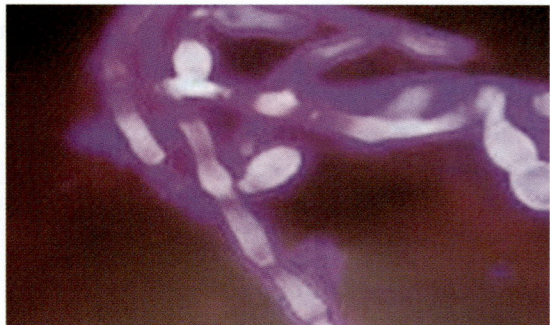

Fig. 67.8: Fluorescent stained smear

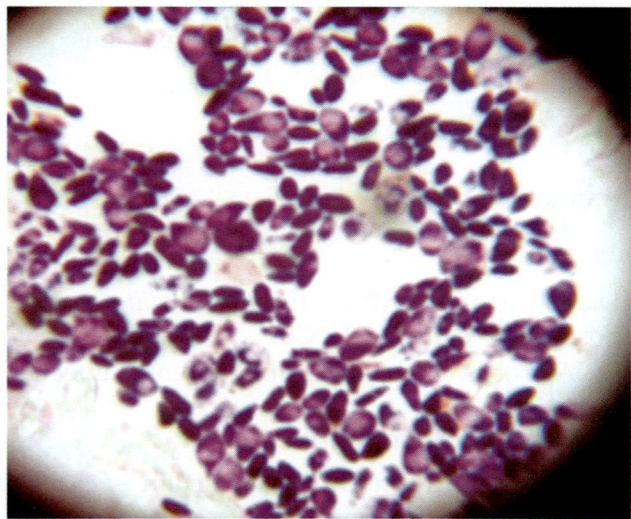

Fig. 67.5: Gram-positive budding yeast cells

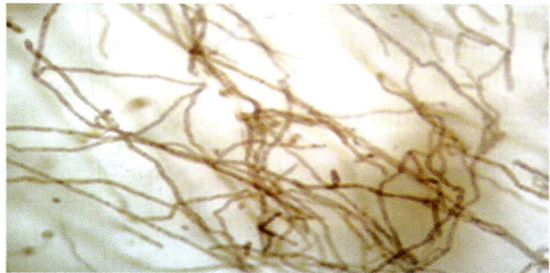

Fig. 67.9: Wet mount showing dematiaceous (brown) hyphae

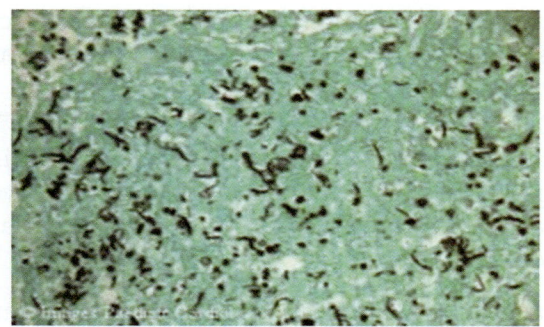

Fig. 67.10: GMS staining showing black fungal elements

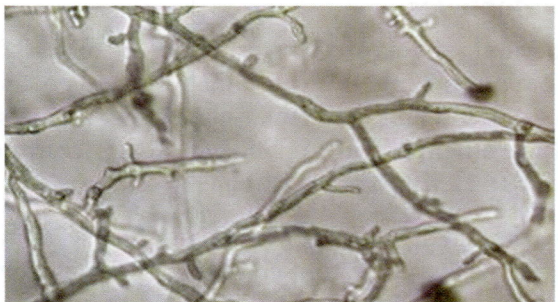

Fig. 67.11: KOH mount showing septate hyphae

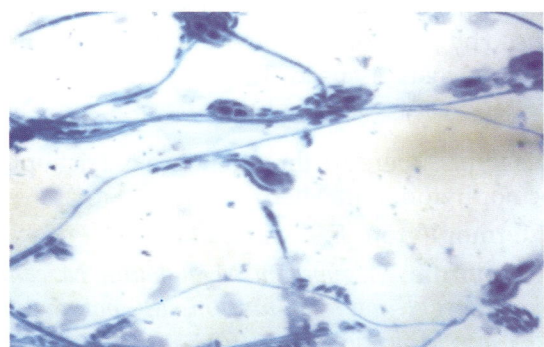

Fig. 67.12. LPCB mount showing fungal elements

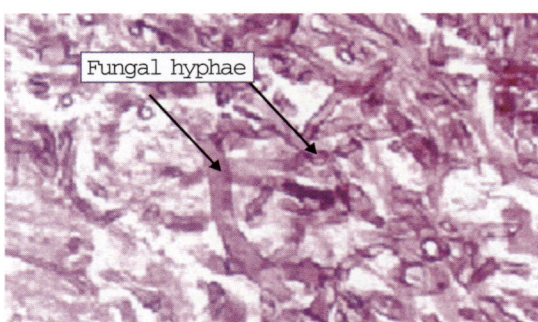

Fig. 67.13: H and E stain

Fungal infections are classified as superficial and deep infections. Superficial infections are further classified as surface infections and cutaneous infection while deep infections are subcutaneous infections and systemic infections.

SUPERFICIAL MYCOSIS

The superficial infections are fungal infections of outer layers of skin, nails and hairs. It is further classified into two types, i.e. surface infections and cutaneous infections.

Surface Infections

These are the infections of dead layers of skin. They do not cause any inflammatory response as there is no contact with living tissue. The examples are tinea versicolor, tinea nigra, and piedra.

Cutaneous infections are infections of cornified layers of skin and its appendages. These infections are caused by a group of fungi of three genera, i.e. trichophyton, microsporum, and epidermophyton and these infections are called **dermatophytes.** If fungi other than dermatophytes cause these infections, they are called **dermatomycosis**.

Tinea Versicolor

It is also called **'pityriasis versicolor'**. It is mild infection of stratum corneum and lesions are in the form of depigmented macules. Occasionally hyperpigmented patches are produced. The fungus causes cosmetic effects only. There is no inflammatory response.

***Causative agent*: Malassezia species (*Malassezia furfur*)**. Formely it was known as *Pityrosporum orbiculare*. It is part of normal flora of body. It is found in areas rich in sebaceous glands. The infections are endogenous. Common sites affected are neck, trunk, shoulder, face, scalp, and arms.

Fungus characteristics: *Malassezia* is lipophilic fungus. It shows round yeast cells. The budding takes place repeatedly at one point. The type of budding shown by this fungus is called percurrent budding.

Medium used for culture is Sabouraud's dextrose agar, and as it is lipophilic fungus, after the material is cultured on SDA, mineral oil is covered over the slant. For identification of fungus, tween hydrolysis tests are used.

Predisposing factor is excessive sweating. The fungus affects melanin production.

- *Malassezia furfur* has also been considered as causative agent responsible for erythematous patchy lesions of dandruff in adults, which may be severe in AIDS patients. Atopic dermatitis and folliculitis are also correlated with this fungus.
- Typical **'fried egg'** like colonies are seen after 5–7 days at 32–35°C.
- Urease test is positive.

- Wood's lamp examination: Scaly lesions show golden yellow fluorescence.

Laboratory diagnosis: The clinical presentation is so classic that usually laboratory diagnosis may not be required. The samples collected are scrapings from the lesions. Tinea versicolor shows fluorescence in Wood lamp examination.

Processing: KOH mount is performed on the collected material. It shows hyphae broken down into pieces and they are plenty round yeast cells. This appearance is described as "**spaghetti meatball"** appearance (Fig. 67.14) or "grapes and banana" appearance. The size of yeast cell varies from 2–7 microns.

Culture is done on SDA with tween 80. Mineral oil is poured over agar slant. The growth occurs in 4–7 days. Smear prepared from colony shows budding cells with pucurrent budding.

Newer tests though not required are **ELISA** and immunofluorescence.

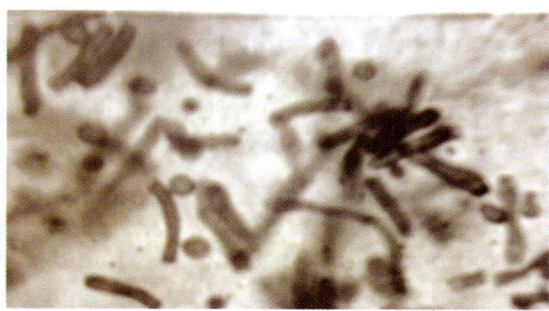

Fig. 67.14: Spaghetii meatball appearance

The fungus responds well to **antifungals like miconazole. Withfield ointment** also can be used.

Tinea Nigra

It is caused by dematiaceous fungus called *Hortaea werneckii.* Thick keratinized sites of body are affected and show dark brown macules. The infection occurs in young group and females have more preponderance for development of this infection. For diagnosis, skin scraping is collected and transported in dry paper fold with clips applied. KOH mount shows short septate brown hyphae and budding cells. Culture is done on SDA which shows black yeasty smooth colony.

Treatment: Topical antifungals, like miconazole, are effective.

Piedra

It is superficial infection of hairs, characterized by formation of **nodules** on hair shaft. It is of two types **black piedra** and **white piedra.** Black piedra is caused by *Piedraia hortae.* White piedra is characterized by greyish white, soft nodules and the condition is caused by *Trichosporon beigelii.*

KOH mount performed on scrapings shows dark hyphae around hair shaft with ascii containing ascospores. In case of white piedra, septate, hyaline hyphae are produced along with blastoconidia and arthoconidia.

Treatment: Local application of antifungal creams, as miconazole, cure the conditon.

Dermatophytes

The dermatophytes are a group of closely related fungi that have the capacity to invade keratinized tissues (skin, hair, and nails) of humans and other animals and produce an infection, dermatophytosis commonly referred to as **ringworm Ortinea.**

Dermatophytosis: It is the infection of skin, hairs and nails caused by fungi grouped as 'dermatophyte' which include three genera—Trichophyton, Microsporum and Epidermophyton.

Dermatomycosis: If infections of skin, hair and nails are caused by fungi other than dermatophytes, the term '**dermatomycosis'** is used. It also includes cutaneous manifestations of systemic fungi.

Etiologic agents: There are three genera, i.e. Trichophyton, Epidermophyton, and Microsporum.

- **Epidermophyton:** *E. flococosum*
- **Microsporum:** *M. gypseum. M. audounii. M. canis, M. cookei, G. gallinae, M. nanum, M. persicolor, M. racemosum M. ferrugineum*
- **Trichophyton:** *T. rubrum, T. mentagrophytes, T. violaceum, T. schoenleinii, T. tonsurans, T. soudanense, T. cocentritum, T. megninii, T. interdigitale, T. equinum, T. erinacei, T. simii.*

Classification of Fungi Based on Ecology and Host Preference

a. **Geophilic:** The source of infection is in soil. The examples of geophilic fungi are *M. cookei, M. gypseum complex, M. nanum, M. persicolor, M. praceox.*

b. **Zoophilic:** These are fungi which cause infection of animals (zoonotic infections). *M. canis, M. mentagrophytes, T. verrucosum, M. gallninae,* and *M. equinum* are the examples of zoophilic fungi.

c. **Anthropophilic:** They are human parasites. *E. floccosum, M. audounii, M. furrugineum, T. cocentricum, T. rubrum, T. megninii, T. schoenleinii, T. soudanense, T. tonsurans,* and *T. violaceum.*

Imortance of Classification Based on Source of Infection (Tables 67.1 to 67.3)

Zoophilic and geophilic dermatophytes in general tend to form lesions that are more inflammatory than those formed by anthropophilic but anthropholic are difficult to treat than others and cause chronic infections.

TABLE 67.1: Endemic geographical distribution of anthrophilic fungi

Species	Major geographic regions
E. floccosum	Cosmopolitan
T. rubrum	Cosmopolitan
T. violaceum	India, West Asia
T. schoenleinii	India, Asia, Africa
T. tonsurans	Cosmopolitan
T. interdigitale	Cosmopolitan
T. cocentritum	Asia, Latin America
M. audouinii	Africa

TABLE 67.2: Endemic geographical distribution of zoophilic fungi

Species	Distribution
M. canis	Cosmopolitan
T. verrucosum	Cosmopolitan
T. mantragrophyte Complex (zoophilic type)	Cosmopolitian
M. gallinae	Cosmopolitan
M. equinum	Cosmopolitan
M. canis var. equinum	Africa, Australia, Europe, New Zealand
M. canis var. distorum	USA, Australia, New Zealand

TABLE 67.3: Endemic geographical distribution of geophilic fungi

Species	Distribution
M. simii	India
M. nanum	Cosmopolitan
M. vanbreuseghemii	India, Russia, Africa, USA
M. persicolor	Cosmopolitan
M. praecox	North America, Western Europe

Clinical Manifestations

Traditionally, infections caused by dermatophytes (ringworm) have been named according to the anatomic location involved, the Latin term designating the body site after the word tinea, e.g., tinea capitis for **ringworm** of the scalp. The clinical manifestations are as follows:

Clinical presentations of dermatophytes

- Tinea capitis is infection of scalp, lesions are favus, kerion and there may be patches of alopecia.
- Tinea corporis (**Tinea glabrosa**) involves smooth non-hairy skin
- Tinea barbae (**barber's itch**) of bearded area on face, neck.
- Tinea cruris—also called (**jock itch**) is infection of groin and perineum.
- Tinea pedis (**Athlete's foot**)—ringworm of foot.
- Tinea mannum—infection of hand
- Tinea ungium involves nails.
- Tinea imbricata—a specific type of Tinea corporis with concentric rings of skin patches.

Laboratory Diagnosis (Figs 67.15 to 67.23)

Collection and transport of specimens: The centers of infected skin patches may consist of the older and poorly viable material, as may portions of older nail plate in onychomycosis. In tinea corporis, where the "rings" of ringworm are well defined, collection is best made by collecting epidermal scales from **near the advancing edges of the rings**.

The lesion is lightly disinfected with alcohol in gauze and then scraped from center to edge, crossing the lesion margin, using a sterile scalpel blade or equivalent. If the lesions have vesicles or bullae, the tops of the vesicles or bullae should be clipped and included in the sample. Suppurating lesions may be sampled with a swab, when it is impractical to obtain scrapings.

Other skin dermatophytoses, such as tinea pedis and tinea manuum, are scraped in such a way that the whole infected area is represented, since an advancing margin is often not evident.

In **tinea** capitis and **tinea barbae,** the basal **root portion of the hair is best sample** for direct microscopy and culture.

Two types of hair infections can be differentiated in wet mount. Ectothrix—arthospores form a sheath around hair while in endothrix the spores are present inside hair shaft. Infected hairs show fluorescence under Wood's lamp (Tables 67.4 to 67.7).

Hairs are best sampled by **plucking,** so that the root is included. If this is not possible due to hair fragility, as in "black dot" tinea capitis, **a scalpel may be used to scrape scales** and excavate small portions of the hair root. **Brushes with stiff bristles,** run firmly across the lesion, have also been used successfully to sample tinea capitis.

The common distal subungual type of tinea unguium is traditionally sampled, after alcohol disinfection, by scraping the debris from beneath the distal end of the nail with a scalpel and collecting scrapings from near the nail bed, where viable inoculum is most likely to be encountered. Close **clipping** of the whole nail end is an alternative to this procedure, as is nail drilling. Superficial white onychomycosis is sampled by scraping material from the white spots on the surface of the nail. Discarding the uppermost layer of material is recommended in order to reduce the presence of contaminants.

Transport of specimens: Sample materials are best transported in dry, strong black paper folded in the manner of a 'herbarium packet'. Moisture of any kind is to be avoided. Black paper allows easy visualization of small skin squames; it should be thin enough to fold tightly at the corners and not "leak" specimen.

Direct Microscopy

KOH mount: It is a highly efficient screening technique in ordinary practice. Scrapings and hairs may be mounted for direct examination in 10–20% KOH or NaOH. The preparation is heated gently. Alkali clears the keratin and debris making the fungal elements visible. If epithelioid cells seen, it means total clearing has not occurred. In skin scraping, the dermatophyte appears as septate hyphae along with arthoconidia. The hyphae should not be confused with **"mosaic fungus"** which is an artifact formed by edges of epidermal cells

(cholesterol crystals deposited around the periphery of epithelioid cells). In endothrix and ectothrix, hyphae and arthoconidia are seen inside and outside along the hair shaft respectively. Hair specimens should be examined without too much delay, otherwise structures may be destroyed.

Modifications: This includes incorporation of Parker blue black ink in (or DMSO) KOH to increase the contrast.

Fluorescent microscope: Two techniques are useful for fluorescence microscopy, the calcofluor white technique and the Congo red technique.

Culture is done on **Sabouraud's dextrose agar** and **dermatophyte test medium** which shows alkalinity generated by dermatophyte growth, as a color change. The red color is due to phenol red indicator. It can, therefore, act as a screening medium.

Identification: Identification characters include colony pigmentation, texture, and growth rate and distinctive morphological structures, such as microconidia, macroconidia, spirals, pectinate hyphae and nodular organs.

A confirmatory test for atypical isolates is the in vitro **'hair perforation test'** of Ajello and Georg. This test relies on the development by certain dermatophytes of specialized perforating organs invading detached hairs and forming conspicuous 'conical pits' at right angles to the long axis. It is positive in *T. mentagrophytes*. *T. mentagrophytes* also gives urease test positive.

TABLE 67.4: Identification of common isolates of dermatophytes			
Trichophyton rubrum	Dark red portwine color pigment	Microconidia plenty, along both sides of hyphae giving "birds on fence" appearance	
Trichophyton mentagrophytes	Dark red pigment	Microconidia in clusters, special hyphae as 'spiral hyphae' seen macroconidia present	Hair perforation test positive
Trichophyton violaceum	Violet pigment	Conidia absent, chlamydospores seen along hyphae	
Epidermophyton floccosum *Microsporum canis*	Khakhi color pigment	Clusters of macroconidia present Numerous macroconidia which are long (10–25 × 35 × 35–110 μ) spindle-shaped, rough, thick walls, the distal end tapers to knob-like ends. Few club-shaped smooth-walled microconidia are seen along the hyphae	
Microsporum gypseum complex	Reverse is yellow or orange or brownish red or purplish red	Macroconidia (8–16 × 22–60 μ) appear in large numbers, symmetric, rough and relative thin walled with no more than 6 cells, ends are rounded not pointed as in *M. canis*	

TABLE 67.5: Fungi causing ectothrix and endothrix

Ectothrix	Endothrix
T. mentagrophytes	T. schoenleinii
M. canis	T. tonsurans
M. gypseum	T. violaceum
M. audouinii	T. soudanense
T. verrucosum	

TABLE 67.6: Fluorescence seen under Wood's lamp

Pathogen	Color of fluorescence
M. canis	Bright green
M. gypseum	Yellow
M. audouinii	Bright green
T. schoenleinii	Dull green
Malassezia furfur	Golden yellow
Corynebacterium minutissumum	Red

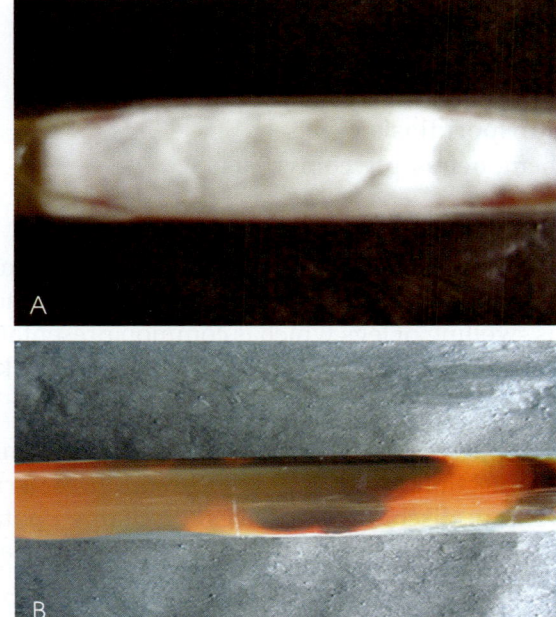

A

B

Fig. 67.15A and B: Colony of *T. rubrum*, on front side (A) 'cottony colony', on reverse side, (B) dark portwine red pigment production

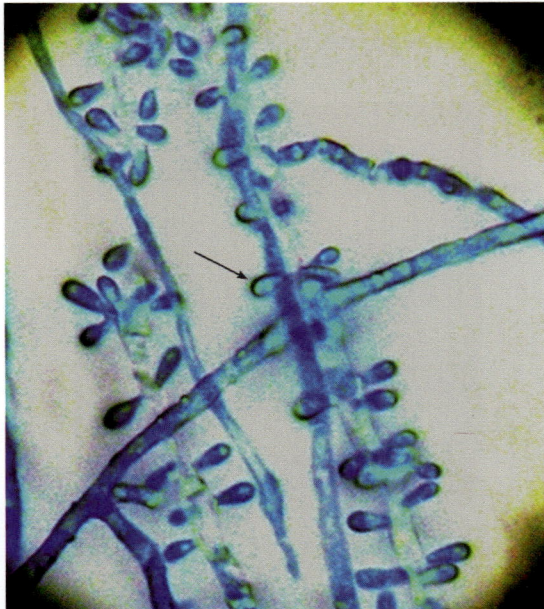

Fig. 67.16: LPCB mount showing microconidia arranged both sides of hyphae (*T. rubrum*)

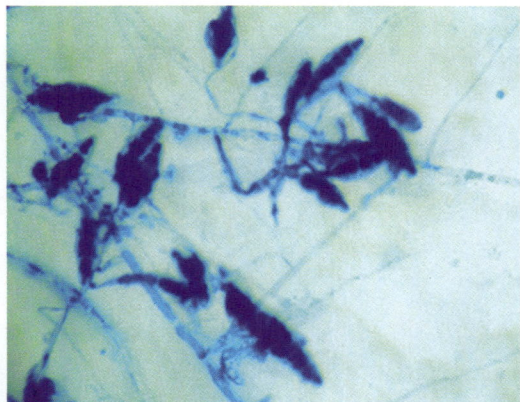

Fig. 67.17: Clusters of macroconidia of *Epidermophyton*

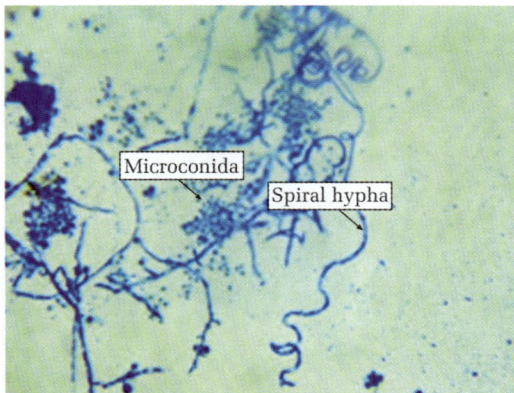

Microconida

Spiral hypha

Fig. 67.18: LPCB mount of *T. mentagrophytes*

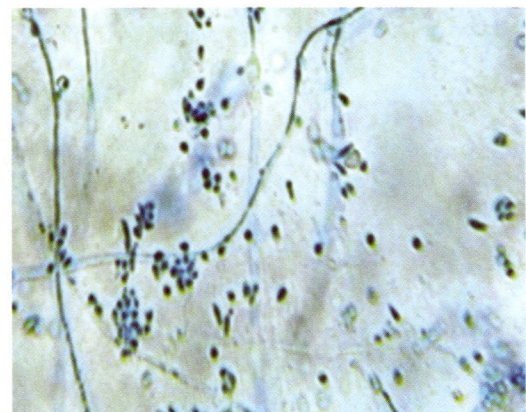

Fig. 67.19: LPCB mount of *T. mentagrophytes* showing microconidia in clusters

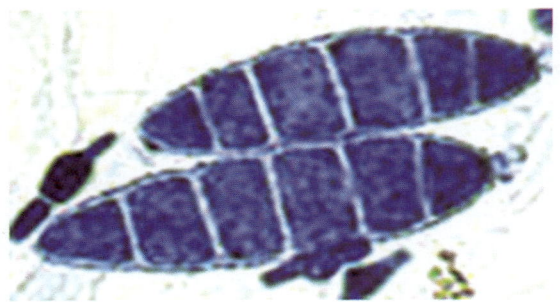

Fig. 67.20: Macroconidia of *Microsporum* spp.

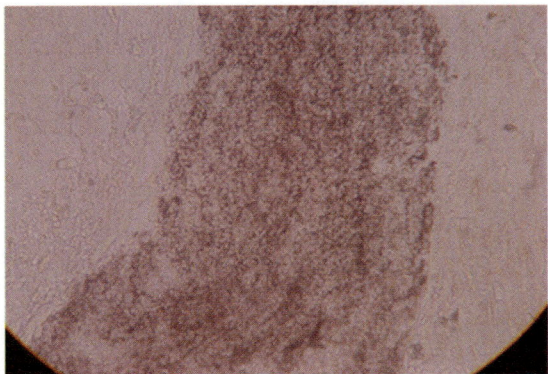

Fig. 67.21: Photograph showing endothrix (hyphae broken into arthroconidia within hair shaft)

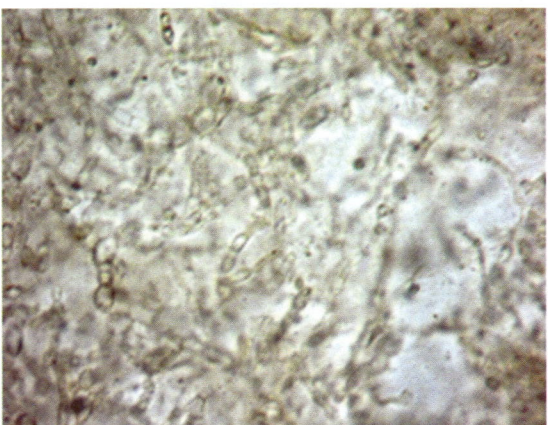

Fig. 67.22: KOH mount of black granule showing hyphae

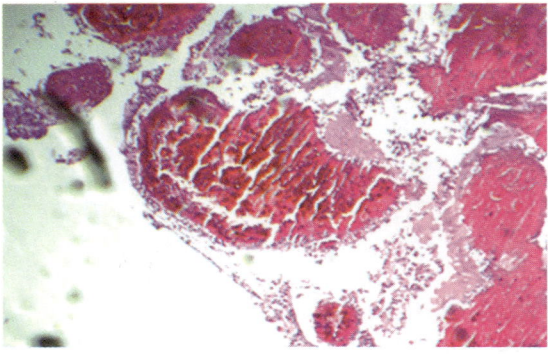

Fig. 67.23: PAS staining of granule

Therapy

- *Local*: Cotrimoxazole, ketoconazole, terbinafine are used for local treatment. The Whitfield ointment (benzoic acid) is outdated.
- *Systemic*: Oral griseofulvin for 4–6 weeks is indicated, for hair infection, prolonged treatment for 3–4 months is given. Other options are oral ketoconazole (200 mg, twice a day), itraconazole (100 mg once in a day).

SUBCUTANEOUS INFECTIONS (MYCOSES)

1. **Mycetoma**
2. **Chromoblastomycosis**
3. **Sporotrichosis**
4. **Rhinosporidiosis**
5. **Subcutaneous phycomycosis**

Mycetoma (Maduromycosis or Pada Valmiki)

It was first reported by Gill from **Madurai,** (South India) hence called **maduromycosis** or Madura foot and as there is swelling of legs which is common presentation, it was called **PadaValmiki =** footwear of Valmiki or **athletes foot.**

Definition: Mycetoma (Fig. 67.24) is chronic granulomatous infection of subcutaneous tissue characterized by swelling, discharging sinuses, discharge contains small granules (these are compact elements of causative agent or micro colonies of organisms).

Predisposing factor is trauma due to vegetative matter, thorn or splinters (carries fungal spores), hence farmers are commonly involved.

Common sites involved are foot, hand, back while uncommon sites are neck, shoulders.

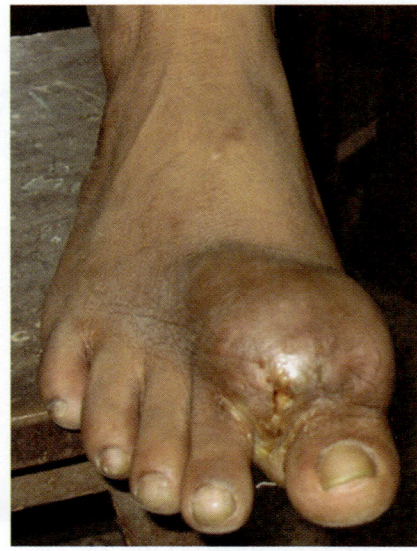

Fig. 67.24: Mycetoma

Types and distribution: When it is caused by Actinomyces it is called actinomycotic mycetoma and when it is caused by fungi it is called eumycotic mycetoma. **Actinomycotic is common in South India while eumycotic is common in North India.** Sometimes similar swelling is caused by pyogenic bacteria like *staphylococci, E. coli,* and *Klebsiella sp* called **botryomycosis.**

Etiological agents of eumycotic mycetoma:

- *Madurella mycetomatis*
- *Madurella grisea*
- *Phialophora (exophilia) jeanselmei*
- *Allescheria boydii*
- *Aspergillus nidulans*
- *Candida spp.*

Of these, first two species cause more than 90% cases of mycetoma in India.

Etiological agents of actinomycotic mycetoma:

- *Nocardia asteroides, Nocardia brasiliensis*
- *Actinomadura maduri*
- *Actinomadura pelliterii*
- *Streptomyces somaliensis*

Laboratory Diagnosis

Samples

- Biopsies
- Directly collect granules from openings of sinuses or apply sterile dressing, call patient after 2–3 days and observe granule on dressing material.

Processing of granule

- *Gross examination*: Note down color, consistency.
- *Gram staining*: Gram-positive filaments may be seen: Actinomycotic filaments are thin while eumycotic filaments are thick. Smears are prepared by crushing the granule in two glass slides.
- In 10% KOH look for hyphae.
- **Modified Z-N** staining with 1% H_2SO_4: **Nocardia** shows acid-fast filaments.
- H and E staining on biosy is helpful.
- **Special stain as PAS, GMS** can be used to stain fungal elements in biopsies.

Culture

- Media inoculated are Sabouraud's dextrose agar for fungi.
- Brain heart infusion agar—supports growth of all pathogens.
- L-J medium used for Nocardia.

Common characteristics of pathogens:

- *Madurella mycetomatis*: Colonies appear in 2 weeks, blackish and lactophenol cotton blue mount from colonies show branching, septate hyphae and chlamydospores along the hyphae.
- *Madurella grisea*: LPCB from colonies show some hyphae wide and some narrow.
- *Nocardia* forms yellow to orange-colored colonies, smear from which shows acid-fast filaments.

Why it is important to differentiate between different groups?

Differentiation is important in treatment point of view, i.e. actinomycotic responds well to antibacterial drugs but eumycotic is difficult to treat with antifungals, even amputation, surgery is required.

Prognosis of actinomycosis is good as compared to eumycotic mycetoma.

How to differentiate the types of mycetoma?

Color of granules: **Eumycotic** mycetoma produce **black-**colored granules (except *Allescheria boydii* which produce yellowish granules) while in case of **actinomycotic mycetoma, the granules are soft** and **white to yellow** except *Actinomadura pelliterii* which produces **red** granules.

KOH mount shows hyphae, if it is eumycetoma.

Treatment

Actinomycotic responds to sulphonamide and for eumycotic, antifungals along with surgery is recommended.

Chromoblastomycosis

Lesions: Warty cutaneous nodules are produced.

Sites: Subcutaneous tissue of the feet and lower legs are commonly involved sites.

Entry: The etiological agents are soil inhabiting fungi of the family Dematiaceae, gain entrance through the skin by traumatic implantation. The disease is mainly tropical and is more common among barefooted agricultural workers and wood cutters.

Fungi Responsible

Fonsecaea (Hormodendrum) species: *F. pedrosoi, F. compactum, F. dermatitidis, Phialophora species—P. verrucosa* and *Cladosporium species—C.carrionii.* Infections caused by *F. pedrosoi* and *P. verrucosa* have been reported to disseminate to other areas, especially brain.

Structures seen in biopsy: **Planate dividing yeast** cells, called **Muriform bodies** or **sclerotic bodies**. This is also called **'Mercedes Benz' sign**. This can be demonstrated by KOH mount or by H and E staining of biopsy.

Biopsy cultured on Sabouraud's dextrose agar shows **black-colored filamentous growth**, for identification LPCB mount from colonies is done.

Treatment: Amphotericin B, 5-fluorocystosine, voriconazole are effective.

Sporotrichosis

- Sporotrichosis is caused by the fungus *Sporothrix (Sporotrichum) schenckii* which is a **dimorphic fungus.**
- *Lesions*: Lesions present on the skin, in subcutaneous tissue and in lymph nodes. Subcutaneous nodules soften and breakdown to form indolent ulcers.
- *Mode of infection*: The fungus is a saprophyte found widely, on plants, thorns and timber. Infection is acquired through thorn pricks or other minor injuries.
- *Geographic distribution*: Worldwide, in India, it is common in **Himachal Pradesh.** Here, the disease is common because of injury by thorn of rose hence called **rose gardener's disease.**
- The fungus spreads from the primary site through lymphatics, but seldom extends beyond the regional lymph nodes. Most cases occur in the upper limb.
- Laboratory diagnosis
- *Biopsy*: KOH mount may show **cigar-shaped yeast cells**, H and E stained slide shows **'asteroid bodies'** which is central fungal mass surrounded by radiating pink-colored material.
- *Culture*: SDA at room temperature shows filamentous growth, LPCB mount from growth shows thin hyphae with 'floret like conidia' while SDA at 37°C shows yeast forms (Fig. 67.25).

- Antigen detection (mannan) is done by LA. (titre >4)
- DNA probe
- Skin test is not used nowadays.

Treatment

- Cutaneous infection: Potassium iodide given locally, orally (250 mg three times a day for 2–4 months).
- For lymphocutaneous infections, fluconazole 400 mg/day, terbinafide 250 mg/day are given.
- Disseminated infections are treated with amphotericin B.

Rhinosporidiosis (Figs 67.26 to 67.29)

- *Infecting agent*: *Rhinosporidium seeberi.*
- *Lesions*: Chronic granulomatous disease, form **friable polyps** in the **nose,** mouth or eye, but rarely seen on the genitalia or other mucous membranes.
- *Geographic distribution*: It is common in India and Sri Lanka. While the disease is generally confined to mucous membranes, hematogenous dissemination has been recorded very rarely.
- *Histologically,* the biopsy shows fungal **spherules** in connective tissue. The spherules are 10–200 µ in diameter and contain thousands of endospores.
- *Mode of infection* not known, infection is probably through stagnant water or aquatic life.

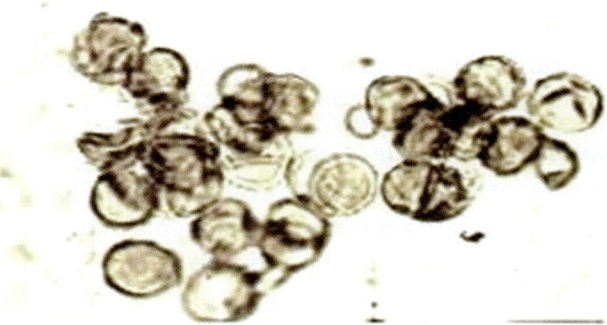

Fig. 67.26: Sclerotic bodies chromoblastomycosis

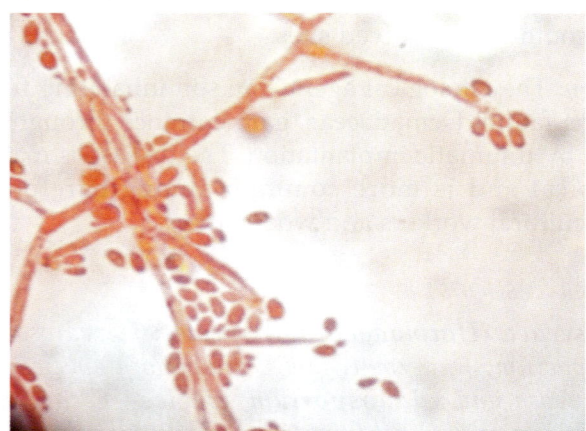

Fig. 67.25: LPCB mount of sporothrix showing floral like arrangement of conidia

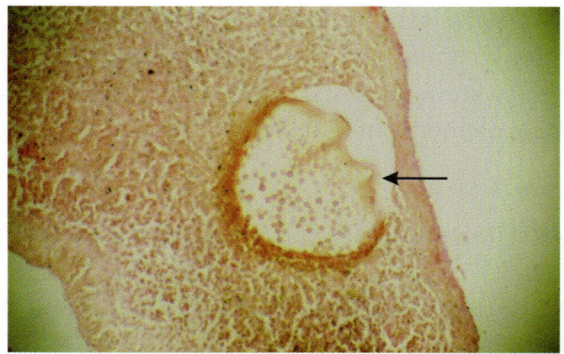

Fig. 67.27: Spherule of *Rhinosporidium seeberi*

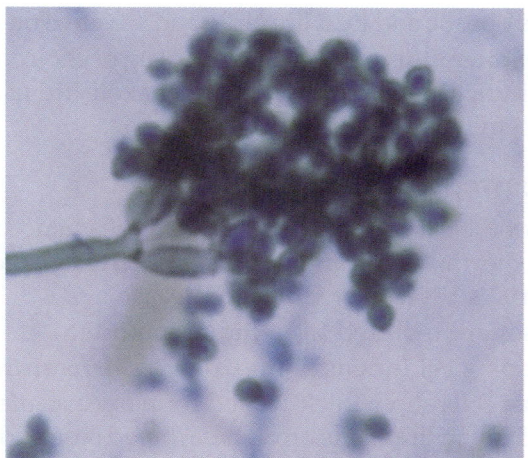

Fig. 67.28: Cladosporium type of sporulation

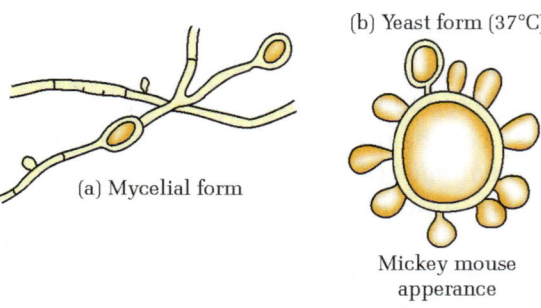

(b) Yeast form (37°C)

(a) Mycelial form

Mickey mouse
apperance

Fig. 67.29: *P. brasiliensis* showing myelial form and yeast form with multiple budding giving Mickey mouse or mariner's ring or pilot's wheel appearance

Laboratory Diagnosis

- Biopsy is stained by H and E, GMS, PAS staining (it has to be differentiated from coccidioidomycosis)
- *Culture*: It is not done, but it has been shown to grow in epithelial carcinoma cell culture.
- *Differential diagnosis*: Rhinoscleroma caused by *Klebsiella rhinoscleromatis*, leprosy, tuberculosis, tumor mass.
- *Treatment*: Radical treatment, dapsone and penta-valent antimony compounds tried.

Subcutaneous Phycomycosis (Zygomycosis) or Entomopthoramycases

- *Lesion*: Painless subcutaneous nodule, may involve whole limb causing swelling.
- *Agent*: *Basidiobolus ranarum*.
- *Mode of infection*: It enters probably by insect bite.
- Biopsy shows aseptate hyphae.
- *Culture*: SDA shows colonies which are wrinkled, LPCB from colony shows broad aseptate hyphae, sexual spores.
- *Treatment*: Surgery and antifungal itraconazole (2–3 months) are the modes of treatment.

SYSTEMIC MYCOSES (DEEP MYCOSIS)

Histoplasmosis (Fig. 67.30)

- Histoplasmosis is an intracellular mycosis of reticulo-endothelial system caused by a dimorphic fungus, *Histoplasma capsulatum*.
- The disease was originally described by Darling hence it was called **Darling disease**, it was related with *Leishmania donovani*.
- *Natural habitat*: Soil enriched with droppings of birds or bats, cats, may be naturally infected.
- *Variants of histoplasma*: **H. capsulatum var. capsulatum** which is ubiquitous, while **H. capsulatum var. dubosii** causes disease in Africa.
- The third variant described '**H. capsulatum var farciminosum** causes epizootic disease in horses and mules.
- The fungus is distributed worldwide, though endemic in USA (states around Ohio river valley).
- Cases of histoplasmosis are reported from all parts of India with increased prevalence in West Bengal. In India, cases have been reported from AIDS patients as well as from patients without HIV.

Pathogenesis

- *H. capsulatum* is transmitted by inhalation of spores (microconidia) present in contaminated air.
- Yeast survives within phagolysosome, travel to lymph nodes and spread to other parts of body.

Clinical Presentation

- Mild as well as disseminated forms are reported from India.
  - It may be mild, self-limiting pulmonary infection.
  - Chronic or acute disseminated disease with poor prognosis. It may occur involving lymph nodes, spleen, liver, adrenals, kidneys, skin, CNS and other organs of the body.

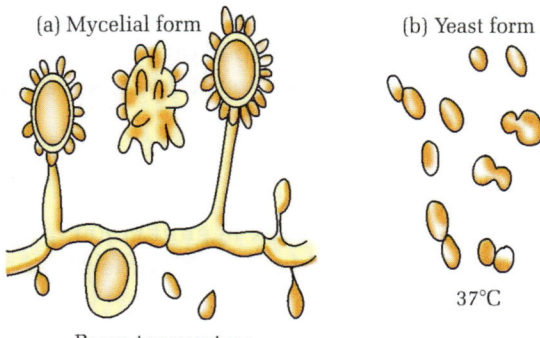

(a) Mycelial form

(b) Yeast form

37°C

Room temperature

Fig. 67.30: (a) Mycelial phase showing tuberculate macro-conidia (cartwheel lke) and a few small microconidia (Histoplasma), (b) yeast form

- Granulomatous and ulcerative lesions may develop on the skin and mucosa.
  - Disseminated infections occur in AIDS patient.
- *Morphological forms*: The fungus is dimorphic (Fig. 67.30).
- **In tissues**, *H. capsulatum* is present inside phagocytic cells in **yeast phase.** They are:
  - Round or oval, yeast-like cells, 2–4 µm in diameter. They fill the cytoplasm of macrophages, mono-cytes and occasionally polymorphonuclear leukocytes.
- On **SDA at 25–30°C (mould phase):**
  - It forms white to tan, fluffy colony with septate branching hyphae with two types of unicellular, asexual spores.
  - Large round, tuberculate macroconidia (8–14 µm) are most prominent and are diagnostic (tuberculous macroconidia called **Cart-wheel**).
  - Small spores or microconidia usually appear first. They are sessile or stalked, smooth-walled, round to pyriform, 2–4 µm in diameter.
- *SDA or brain heart infusion agar at 37°C*: Yeast phase is grown at 37°C. It shows small, round or oval budding yeast cells.
- **Specimens collected** depending upon clinical presentation. These are sputum, bone marrow, peripheral blood, scrapings from dermal or mucosal ulcers and biopsies of lymph nodes and other organs.

Laboratory Diagnosis

- Demonstration of the fungus in tissues is done by GMS stain, H and E, Giemsa stain.
- Culture from these materials is done on SDA and BHIA slants, one set is incubated at 37°C and another at room temperature. Growth appears usually in 2–3 weeks.
- Whitish cottony colonies are produced. Many times yeast forms are not developed on primary isolation. For showing mycelial to yeast form, subculture is done from growth.
- SDA or BHIA or brain heart infusion broths which are incubated for 37°C.
- Serological tests like latex agglutination, precipita-tion and complement fixation become positive two weeks after infection.
- **Kelly's medium is used to demonstrate conversion of mold forms to yeast forms.**
- **Delayed hypersensitivity** to the fungus can be demonstrated by histoplasmin skin test.

- **DNA probe** and **PCR** are rapid and sensitive methods.
- **Treatment:** Amphotericin is the drug of choice. Other antifungals ketoconazole, voriconazole are used for disseminated.

Blastomycosis (Fig. 67.31)

Most of the cases occur in North America hence it was called North American blastomycosis. **It is also called Gilchrist's disease or Chicago disease.**

- Cases are reported from India (imported).
- Aetiological fungus is *Blastomyces dermatitidis*.
- Yeast cells show thick-walled round yeasts of size— 8–15 µm with a single broad base (broad base budding).
- Such budding yeast cells with broad base give **appearance of figure '8'.**
- At 25°C mycelia growth develops which shows hyphae with small pear-shaped conidia.
- Spores enter through air, taken by macrophages, get converted into yeast forms.
- Yeast cell bears a 120 kDa glycoprotein called '*B. dermititidis*' (BAD-1).
- *Lesions*: Suppurative and granulomatous lesions appear in lungs or on skin. It may be asymptomatic or may lead to focal or diffuse consolidation, miliary or abscess formation.
- Cutaneous forms may be papule, nodule or ulcer.
- Soil is considered to be the source of infection, which is acquired by inhalation.
- In tissue and in culture at 37°C, the fungus appears as budding yeast cells, which are large (7–20 µ) and spherical with thick, double contoured walls, the **budding is broad based.**
- SDA or BHIBA at 25°C shows mouldy growth. LPCB from it shows single conidium at the tip of conidio-phore and arthoconidia (Fig. 67.31).

(Samples should be processed in biosafety cabinets only).

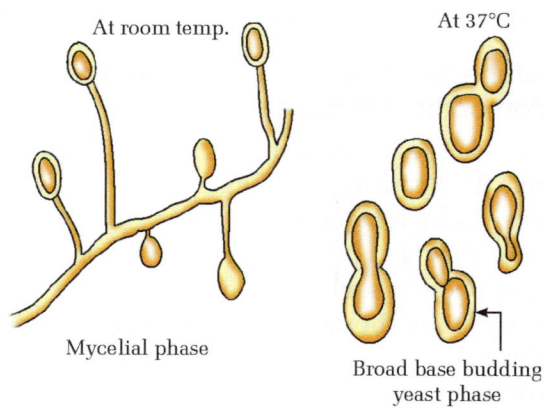

Fig. 67.31: Mycelial and yeast forms (broad based budding) (*Blastomyces dermatitidis*)

Laboratory Diagnosis

- Histopathological section will be stained with H and E or GMS. It shows broad based budding yeasts.
- *Culture*: SDA (two sets, one incubated at room temperature while another at 37°C.
- Brain heart infusion agar is used to demonstrate conversion of yeast form to mycelia form and vice versa.
- Skin test is performed with blastomycin antigen, which is a delayed type of reaction.
- *Detection of antibodies*: Immunodiffusion test has been developed to detect antibodies against antigen of yeast phase (glycoprotein—*B. dermatitidis* adhesion-1 antigen).
- *Antigen detection*: Tests for urine samples are developed.
- *Molecular methods*: These include PCR, DNA probe.
- *Treatment*: Liposomal amphotericin B is the drug of choice. Itraconazole can be tried in immuno-competent patients with mild clinical form.

Coccidioidomycosis

- Agent is *coccidioides immitis*. It is a dimorhic fungus, present in soil (and in rodents Southwest USA)
- Mode of infection is inhalation of arthrospores. After inhalation arthoconidia become round and develop into 'spherules'. Infection may be inapperant or mild infection (influenza-like illness called **Valley** fever or **desert rheumatism or California fever)** or rarely disseminated, forming granulomas.
- Morphological form seen in **tissues** is **spherule,** 15–75 µ, with double wall, and endospores within.
- **Culture at both the temperatures show mycelial forms.** It shows hyphae and **arthroconida.**
- Exoantigen detection can done.
- Molecular method for diagnosis is DNA probe.

Paracoccidioidomycosis

- *Agent*: *Paracoccidioides brasiliensis.* (South American blastomycosis).
- Disease is restricted to South America.
- It causes chronic granulomatous infection of skin, lymph nodes or disseminated disease.
- Yeast phase is found in tissues and culture (SDA) at 37°C while SDA at room temperature shows mycelial growth. Yeast cells show multiple budding giving **"Micky Mouse"** appearance (Fig. 67.29).

OPPORTUNISTIC FUNGAL INFECTIONS

Candidiasis (Figs 67.32 to 67.36)

Candidiasis or candidosis or moniliasis is a primary or secondary mycotic infection caused by members of the genus *Candida* which is yeast-like fungus. The clinical manifestations may be acute, subacute or chronic and it may be localized or become systemic.

Most pathogenic species are *C. albicans*, *C. tropicalis, C. krusei, C. glabrata, C. guilliermondii, C. parapsilosis, and C. viswanathii.*

Loss of normal equilibrium between Candida and host causes pathological disease.

Predisposing factors for candidiasis are: Prolonged antibiotic use, elimination and alteration of bacterial flora, general debility, diabetes mellitus, immunosuppressive agents, chemo-therapy, abnormal leukocyte function, iatrogenic/barrier break, indwelling catheters, hyperalimentation, peritoneal dialysis, and neutropenia, hematological malignances, post-surgical ICU patients, total parenteral nutrition, severe burns, HIV infection.

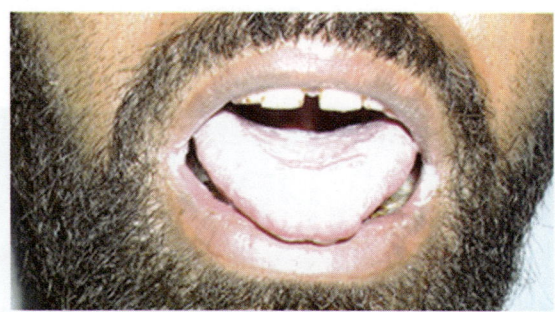

Fig. 67.32: Oral thrush caused by *Candida albicans*

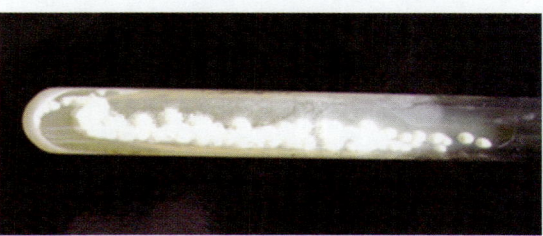

Fig. 67.33: Sabouraud's dextrose agar showing cream pasty colonies of *Candia albicans*

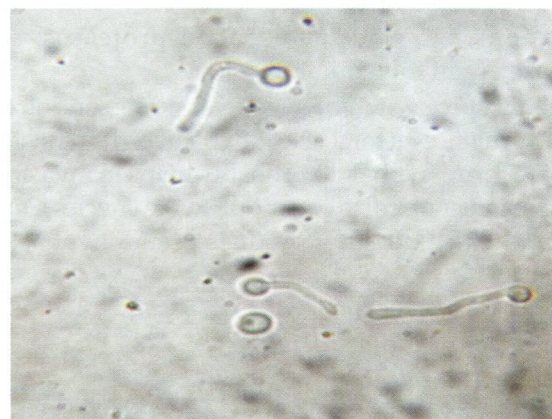

Fig. 67.34: Wet mount showing germ tube

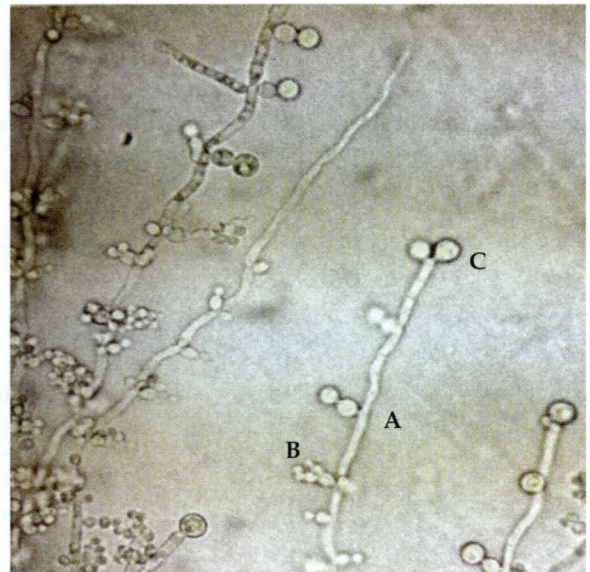

Fig. 67.35: *C.albicans*, A—pseudohypha, B—blastospore, C—chlamydospore

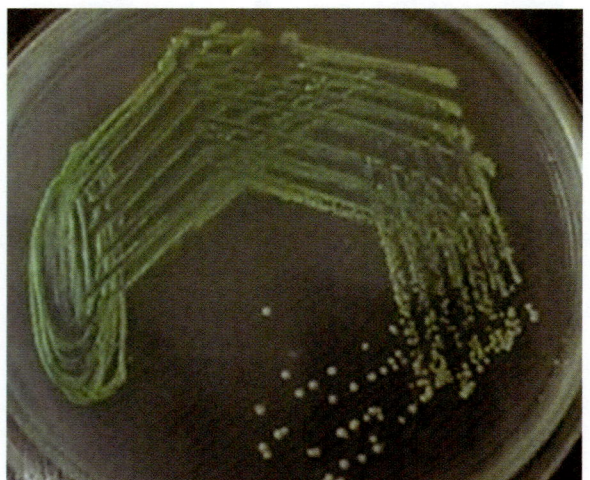

Fig. 67.36: Hichrome agar showing green-colored colonies of *C. albicans*

Virulence Factors

Adhesions, enzymes as aspartyl proteases, serine protease are involved in adhesion.

Phenotypic switch between yeast to pseudohyphae acts as virulence factor. Pseudohyphal form is considered invasive form, hyphal tip probably helps in invasion but invasive infections also occur due to the species *Candida glabrata* which does **not** produce pseudohyphae.

Pathogenesis

A. Cutaneous manifestation
- Intertrigo
- Paronychia and onchomycosis
- Diaper dermatitis

B. Candidal granuloma

C. Mucosal lesions or manifestations
- Oral candidiasis (most common manifestation in HIV patients, it presents mostly as **oral thrush**)
- Esophageal candidiasis (AIDS defining condition)
- Angular cheilitis
- Intestinal
- Vulvovaginitis, balanitis, balanoposthitis
- Chronic mucocutaneous candidiasis (associated primary immunodeficiency of cellular immunity; endocrinopathies are present)
- Ocular candidiasis

D. Systemic manifestations
i. Urinary tract infection (common in diabetics and patients on catheter)
ii. Endocarditis
iii. Pulmonary candidiasis
iv. Meningitis
v. Candidemia (common with children on total parental nutrition in which *C. parapsilosis* is common, (candidemia is also common in premature babies, patients with intravascular catheters)
vi. Dissemination
vii. Arthritis
viii. Osteomyelitis
ix. Endophthalmitis
x. Bronchopulmonary candidiasis

E. Allergic diseases

Laboratory Diagnosis (Flowchart 67.1)

Specimens: Scraping of skin and nails, biopsy specimen of tissue and mucocutaneous lesion, corneal scrapings, vaginal discharge, urine, blood, CSF, pleural fluid, pus, swabs form oral lesions are collected depending on the lesions.

Direct examination
- *Wet mount:* Budding yeast cells, pseudohyphae, pus cells are seen. Presence of pseudohyphae in KOH mount or Grams-stained smear is important as it indicates tissue invasion.
- KOH is done for sputum, skin or nail scrapings, mucus secretions.
- Gram staining shows yeasts and pseudohyphae.
- Calcofluor white highlights fungal elements.
- H and E stain is useful for biopsy to show fungal elements.
- Gomori's methanamine silver stain and PAS are special stains (for histopathology).

Flowchart 67.1 Laboratory diagnosis of *C. albicans*

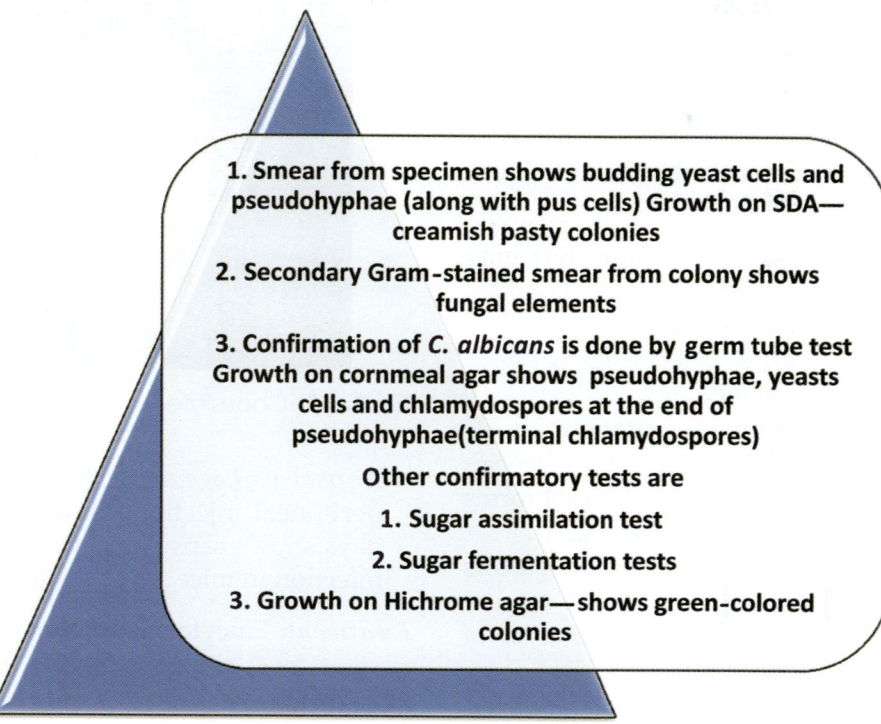

1. Smear from specimen shows budding yeast cells and pseudohyphae (along with pus cells) Growth on SDA—creamish pasty colonies

2. Secondary Gram-stained smear from colony shows fungal elements

3. Confirmation of *C. albicans* is done by germ tube test Growth on cornmeal agar shows pseudohyphae, yeasts cells and chlamydospores at the end of pseudohyphae(terminal chlamydospores)

Other confirmatory tests are

1. Sugar assimilation test

2. Sugar fermentation tests

3. Growth on Hichrome agar—shows green-colored colonies

Culture methods: Sabouraud's dextrose agar within 48 hours produce creamish pasty, smooth colonies. Brain heart infusion broth is used for blood culture.

Tests for identification of *C. albicans* are germ tube test, growth pattern on corn meal agar, sugar fermentation and sugar assimilation tests, green-colored colonies on Hichrome agar.

Germ Tube Test

C. albicans and *C. dublinensis* which is new species (which can be isolated from lesions in AIDS patients) are germ tube test positive. The test is also called **Reynold's Braude phenomenon.**

Definition: Germ tubes are appendages half the width and 3–4 times the length of the yeast cells from which they rise (filamentous outgrowths from blastoconidia). It is differentiated from pseudohyphae by absence of constriction at the base and has parallel wall.

Test procedure:
- Take 0.5 mL normal human or preferably sheep serum in a tube.
- Suspend a very small inoculum of the yeast colony.
- Incubate at 37°C for maximum for 2–3 hours.
- Wet mount prepared from the suspension.
- *Controls*: Known strain of *C. albicans* is used as control.

Microscopic morphology on Cornmeal agar:
- *C. albicans* inoculated on corn meal agar, in 2–3 days. It shows pseudohyphae, clusters of blastoconidia and many terminal chlamydospores which are regularly placed.
- Further identification is done by sugar assimilation tests and sugar fermentation tests.
- *Serological tests*: Detection of antigen—candida enolase antigen testing cell wall mannan and cytoplasmic antigens are detected by ELISA.
- *Detection of antibodies against antigens*: Cell wall components—cell wall mannoprotein (CWMP).
- *Detection of metabolite*: Beta-(1, 3)-D-glucan by 'G' test.
- *Molecular method*: PCR (panfungal PCR).

Treatment

Locally clotrimazole, miconazole oinments are used while for systemic infections, fluconazole is used and for resistant strains of *C. glabrata*, *C. parapsilosis*, *C. krusei*, amphotericin B is used.

Cryptococcosis

It is caused by the yeast *Cryptococcus neoformans*.

Antigenicity, there are 4 types: A, B, C, and D.
1. Infections due to serotypes A and D are common.
2. **Serotypes A and D** are found in excreta of wild and domestic birds (pigeon dropping).

3. **Serotypes B and C** are found in **flowers Eucalyptus camaldulensis.** Infections coincide with distribution of trees.

It is pure yeast. Yeast cells are round or ovoid, 4–20µ in diameter with a prominent polysaccharide capsule.

Source: It is soil saprophyte, particularly abundant in the faces of pigeons and other birds.

Infection: It enters mostly by inhalation, but may sometimes by through skin or mucosa.

Clinical Presentation

Most infections are asymptomatic.

  i. Pulmonary is most common presentation.
 ii. Dissemination of infection leads to visceral, cutaneous and meningeal disease. Visceral forms simulate tuberculosis and cancer clinically.
iii. Cutaneous cryptococcosis varies from small ulcers to large granulomas.

Cryptococcal meningitis is the most serious type of infection seen in AIDS patients.

Diagnosis

CSF

* *India ink* is used for demonstration of capsulated, budding yeast cells. Advantage of the test: Simple, rapid and reporting is done within a few minutes.
* *Antigen detection:* Latex agglutination test is rapid test for diagnosis of cryptococcal meningitis.
* *Culture*: Sabouraud's agar shows smooth, **mucoid,** cream-colored colonies (Fig. 67.37).

Pathogenicity Tests and Tests for Identification

* *Urease test*: Rapid positive.
* Growth on **Bird seed agar brown colonies** are produced.

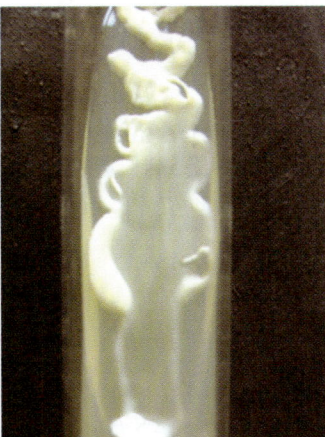

Fig. 67.37: Mucoid growth of cryptococcus neoformans on SDA

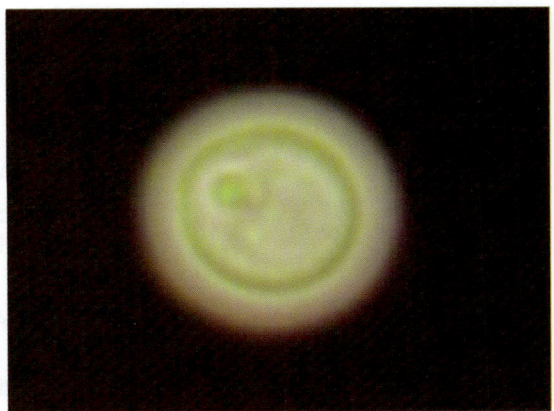

Fig. 67.38: Capsulated yeast suggestive of cryptococcus

* *Animal pathogenicity*: Mice is infected by intra-peritoneal injection. Fluid withdrawn after some days shows capsulated yeast cells (Fig. 67.38). The infection in mice may be fatal.

Treatment: Flucytocin, amphotericin.

ZYGOMYCOSIS

Zygomycetes are characterized by aseptate or sparsely septate hyphae. The fungi are angioinvasive. There are 4 genera, *Mucor, Absidia, Rhizopus and Rhizomucor* associated with human infections. They cause **mucormycosis and entomophthoromycosis.**

Fungi are abundant in soil. Spores are found in air and dust. Organisms usually enter by inhalation or by inoculation.

Predisposing factors: Diabetes mellitus, leukemia or lymphoma, end stage kidney or liver disease are predisposing factors.

Clinical presentation is rhinocerebral zygomycosis, pulmonary, cutaneous, gastrointestinal and disseminated.

Infection of nose causes **sinusitis** which may spread causing orbital involvement. If it spreads further, it can cause cavernous sinus thrombosis which may be fatal. This type of presentation is called **rhino-orbitocerebral mucormycosis.** Fungi may infect GIT in immuno-compromised conditions. If decubitus ulcer is formed, secondary infection by mucorales may occur.

Tissue biopsy shows broad aseptate hyphae demonstrated in KOH mount, Gram's staining, H and E, and GMS.

Culture: As it is saprophytic fungus, **repeated culture** is necessary to prove that the fungus isolated is pathogenic.

Biopsy material is taken on Sabouraud's dextrose agar without cycloheximide, mucorales grow fast, occupy whole tube and cottony growth occurs. (If plate is inoculated, as we open the plate the growth is so heavy that it comes out, hence these fungi are called "**lid lifters**") (Fig. 67.39).

LPCB mount from colonies shows sporangiophore which is a specialized hypha which bearing sporangia. The asexual spores called sporangiospores are produced inside the sporangia. Rhizoids are root-like structures and their position varies (Figs 67.40–67.42).

Treatment consists of surgery and amphotericin B.

Aspergillosis

It is opportunistic fungus. It is angioinvasive (Fig. 67.43).

Important species: *Aspergillus fumigatus* is main opportunistic pathogen followed by *Aspergillus flavus*.

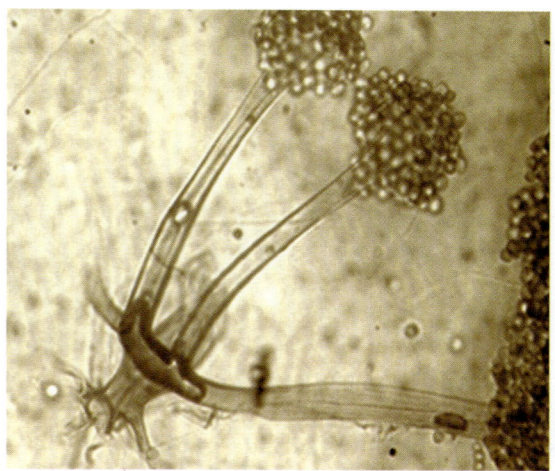

Fig. 67.42: Wet mount of rhizomucor

Fig. 67.39: Growth of mucor on SDA

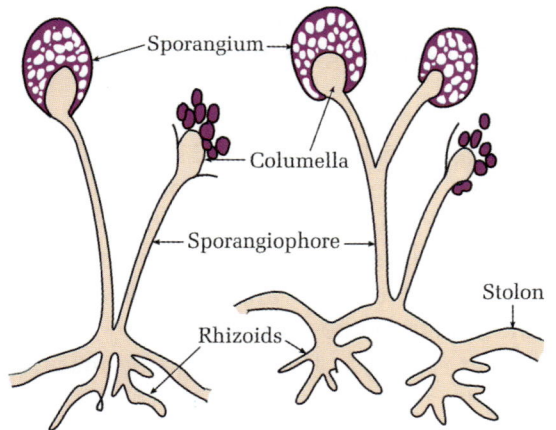

Fig. 67.40: Morphology of mucorales (rhizopus)

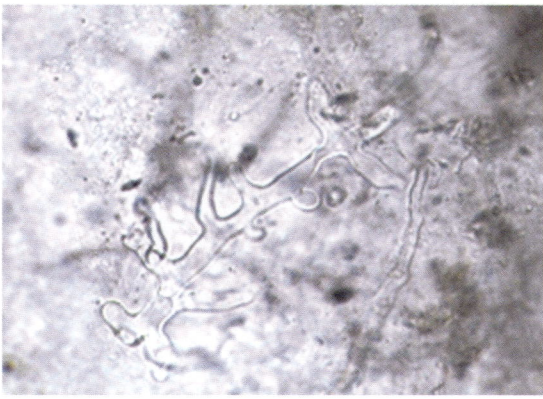

Fig. 67.41: KOH aseptate hyphae

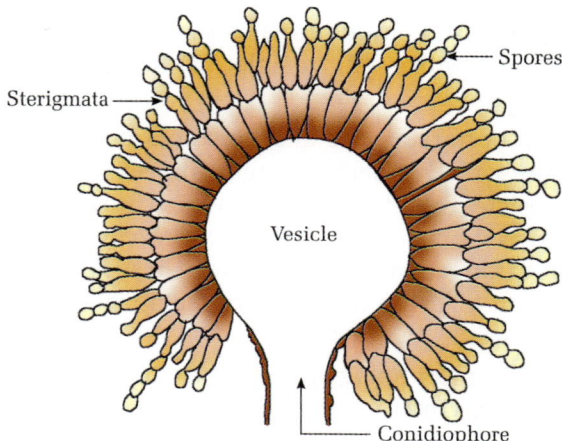

Fig. 67.43: Morphology of Aspergillus spp.

Clinical Features or Lesions or Diseases Produced

- *Pulmonary disease:*
  a. *Allergic bronchopulmonary aspergillosis:* It occurs in atopic persons who are sensitive to fungal spores.
  b. *Bronchopulmonary aspergillosis:* Invasive aspergillosis
  c. *Aspergilloma:* If the fungus grows in a preformed cavity in lungs due to TB or tumor, it causes fungal ball.
- **Aspergillus otomycosis**
- **Aspergillus keratitis**
- *A. flavus* produces **aflatoxin** (Fig. 67.44)
- Aspergillus may cause **sinusitis,** rhinocerebral spread from sinus may occur.

Diagnosis

Note. As it is saprophytic fungus, **repeated culture** is necessary to prove that the fungus isolated is pathogenic.

Sputum: KOH: It shows septate hyphae (with acute angle branching)

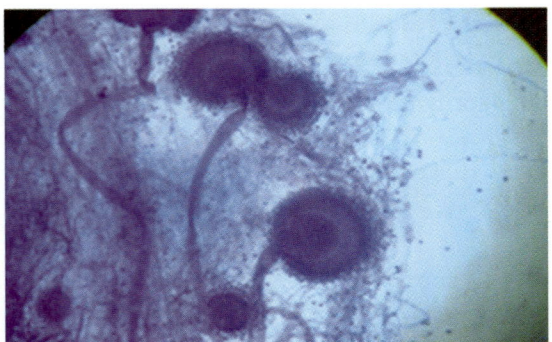

Fig. 67.44: LPCB mount of *A. flavus*

Biopsy: H and E shows septate hyphae.

Culture on SDA shows fast growth. **A. fumigatous produces smoky green colonies while *A. flavus* produces yellow colonies** (Fig. 67.45).

LPCB mount from culture shows following structures: (1) Conidiophore, (2) vesicle, (3) sterigmata, and (4) conidia.

Conidiophore at one end gets enlarged to form a structure called 'vesicle'. Finger-like structures arise from vesicles called 'sterigmata' which are arranged in a single row (uniseriate) as seen in *A. fumigatus* or they may be arranged in two rows as seen in *A. flavus* (called as biseriate). At the tips of sterigmata, round conidia are produced.

In all, the morphology resembles with **'Aspergillum' (used to sprinkle holy water),** hence the name Aspergillus.

Newer Methods of Diagnosis

- Detection of *Aspergillus* specific **galactomannan antigen** in urine or saliva is done by **ELISA.**
- *Antibody detection*: It is useful in chronic invasive aspergillosis and aspergilloma. Titer falls immediately with treatment.
- *Detection of serum IgE* is done for diagnosis of allergic bronchopulmonary aspergillosis.
- *Detection of metabolites*: Detection of 1–3 glucan by **'G' test** or **mannitol** by **gas liquid chromatography.**

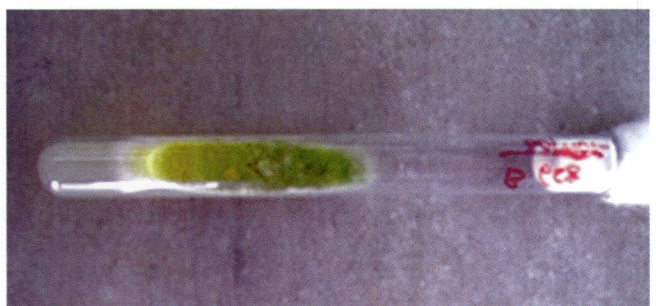

Fig. 67.45: Colony of *A. flavus* on SDA

Treatment

For invasive diseases, caspofungin or amphotericin is given.

Pneumocystis Jirovecii

Pneumocystis is an opportunistic infection of respiratory system leading to atypical pneumonia. It is also called interstitial plasma cell pneumonia.

Causative agent: Initially, pneumocystis was considered to be protozoa, now it has been classified as an ascomycete.

Points in Favor of Protozoa

It does not grow in vitro on fungal culture media but requires tissue cell lines for growth and viability. Absence of ergosterol in cytoplasmic membrane, making it insensitive to antifungals targeting ergosterol synthesis.

Points in Favor of a Fungus

- It takes fungal stains like GMS stain (Fig. 67.46) possesses chitin in cell wall at all stages of life cycle.
- Protein synthesis, elongation factor and thymidylate synthase are homologous to ascomycetes.
- It is r-RNA homology with ascomycetes.

Morphology

Asexual phase of cell division and sexual phase. Three main stages—trophozoite, cyst, sporozoite.

- *Trophozoite*: Pleomorphic, tiny bodies 2–5 µm, appears as clusters, covered with tubular projections.
- *Cyst*: Large—4–6 µm, oval, thick walled, possess up to 8 intracystic bodies or sporozoites.
- *Precyst or sporocyst*: Presumed to be mating stage leading to zygote formation that initiates sporogenesis. It is a transition phase between trophic and cystic phase called precyst.
- *Sporozoite*: Oval, amoeboid or peach shaped, 1–2 µm in length. Extrude out of mature cyst on rupture and subsequently converted to trophozoite.

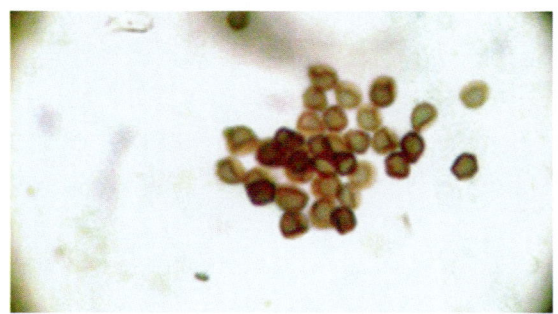

Fig. 67.46: GMS stain: *P. jirovecii* × 1000

Infection is thought to be acquired by **droplet inhalation**. They are deposited in the alveoli of lungs. Alveolar macrophages form the first line defense. Trophic form attaches to the alveolar type 1 epithelial cells. Alveolar type 2 cells undergo hypertrophy, macrophage infiltration, filling of alveolar spaces with eosinophilic foamy material. Necrotic foci and cellular debris in extrapulmonary sites may be seen. It causes **interstitial pneumonia**.

Incubation period is 4 to 8 weeks. Clinical manifestations are classified as pulmonary pneumocystis and extrapulmonary pneumocystitis

Clinical features: Gradually increasing non-productive cough, dyspnea, tachycardia, fever, occasionally sputum production or hemoptysis, chest pain, often chills and night sweats are the common clinical features. Cyanosis appears late, severe.

X-ray: Perihilar haziness, bilateral diffuse interstitial pulmonary infiltrates that gives **ground glass appearance.**

Specimens: Diagnosis is done by detection of trophozoites and cysts in following specimens: (1) BAL—being ideal specimen, (2) induced sputum, (3) lung biopsy.

Various staining methods include GMS, Giemsa, Toluidine blue O. Cysts look like black color 'crushed ping-pong balls' against green background.

Direct immunofluorescence is sensitive and specific method.

Culture: It does not grow on fungal culture media: Cell line tried with limited success is A549 which a cell line derived from human lung adenocarcinoma cells, peripheral blood mononuclear cells from AIDS patients and human embryonic lung fibroblasts.

PCR can be done on BAL fluid and induced sputum.
Treatment: Trimethoprim – sulfamethoxazole, pentamidine, isethionate, atovaquone are used for treatment.

PENICILLOSIS (Fig. 67.47)

Pathogenic species in HIV-infected person is *P. marneffei* which is **dimorphic.** Yeasty growth is seen at 37°C while SDA incubated at room temperature shows moldy growth. The fungus is identified by brush-like arrangement of conidia. *P. marneffei* produces dark red pigment and shows thermal dimorphism.

Oculomycosis

Fungi causing oculomycosis are:
- *Fuserium solani*
- *Aspergillus fumigatus*

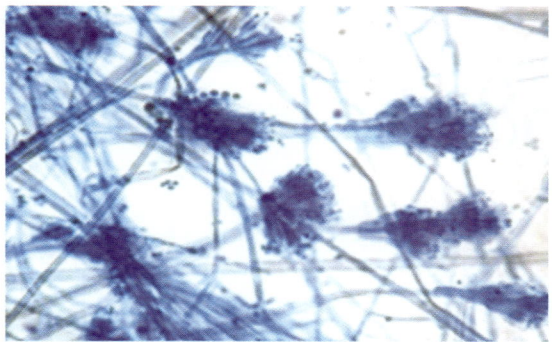

Fig. 67.47: LPCB of penicillium species

- *Aspergillus flavus*
- *Candida albicans*
- *Curvularia*
- *Bipolaris*

Samples collected are corneal scrapings. Diagnosis is based on demonstration of fungal elements in specimens and growth on SDA.

Treatment: Locally nystatin, amphotericin B are applied.

Mycotic Poisoning

Types

Mycetism: Ingestion of fungus itself causes harmfull effects.

Mycotoxicosis: Fungal toxins contaminate the food or grain which is consumed.

Mycetism causes gastrointestinal disease or dermatitis or death—Psilocybin species.

Mycotoxin: **Aflatoxin** is produced by *Aspergillus flavus.* Fungus grows in ground nuts, corn, peas and produce toxin which is toxic to animals and birds. It can cause hematoma; human cases have been reported from India.

Other examples of toxins are:
- Fumonisins are produced by *Fusarium moniliformae* (food—maize).
- Ochratoxins are produced by *Aspergillus ochraceus* (food—cereals).
- *Thrichthecens:* Fusarium graminerium grows on maize, it is used in biological warfare, 'yellow rain in Laos' – necrotic lesions in oral cavity, esophagus, stomach with leucopenia is observed. In 1987, it caused outbreak in **Srinagar.**

Mycetisism
- Claviceps purpurea—ergot poisoning
- Coprine sp—coprine poisoning
- Amantia sp—cyclopeptides poisoning.

68

Normal Flora of Body

INTRODUCTION

Normal flora also called 'indigenous **flora**' includes various types of microorganisms which human body harbours on his skin and mucous membranes.

Resident Flora

Organisms are members of body's normal flora throughout life. This flora temporarily removed with disinfection. They may have benefits in health.

Transient Flora

Organisms visit the mucosa or body surface for a short period. Many of them have capacity to cause disease under certain conditions, meningococci present in throat may spread and cause meningitis, e.g. **MRSA** (in nose, on skin), Gram-negative bacilli as *E. coli, Klebsiella* in upper respiratory tract.

SIGNIFICANCE OF THE NORMAL FLORA

- Normal flora plays an important role in body economy (Flowchart 68.1).
- Normal flora forms may become pathogenic when host defenses become poor, means it acts as pathogen when opportunity occurs.
- Normal flora is natural defence mechanism which prevents or interferes with colonization or invasion by pathogens by competitive inhibition.
- Normal flora raises immune status of host against transient flora.
- Normal flora may cause confusion in diagnosis.
- It is temporary and varies from time to time.
- Commensals from mouth, nasopharynx, and intestine may enter blood and tissues.
- If a person is hospitalized, his flora may change.
- Organisms normally present in intestine produce group B vitamins, also vitamin K and E.

- Shared antigens can confer some immunity to pathogens.

Disadvantages

- They can cause opportunistic infections.
- Abnormal multiplication can cause enteritis and endotoxic shock.
- Production of penicillinase by some flora interferes with antibiotic therapy.
- Normal flora can cause confusion in diagnosis.

Flora depends on area of the body, clothing, occupation, environment. Transient microbial flora occurs more often on skin. Methicillin resistant Staphylococci can colonize hands, groin, and axilla of health care workers. Hair frequently harbours *S. aureus* which acts a reservoir for cross infection.

Normal Flora of Conjunctiva

Diphtheroids (*Corynebacterium xerosis*), *Moraxella, staphylococci,* non-hemolytic streptococci form normal flora of conjunctiva. Conjunctiva is relatively bacteria free due to flushing action of tears.

Normal Flora of Mouth

Aerobic	Anaerobic
Micrococci sp., Bacillus sp.,	Peptostreptococci
Coliforms	Bacteroides sp.
Proteus	Fusobacterium
Candida sp.	Lactobacilli
Corynebacterium sp.	Actinomyces

Nasopharynx: It is sterile at birth. After 2–3 days commensals and pathogens are acquired from mother. Nasopharynx is natural habitat for pathogens of nose, throat, bronchi and lungs.

Flowchart 68.1: Role of normal flora

common source of infection
- Normal flora is source of oppertunistic infections. Staphylococci from skin, nose may cause infection as abscess, stye. *Staphylococcus epidermidis* causes bacteremia in patients with IV catheters as they attach to plastic prosthetic surfaces
- *E. coli* form GIT may act as source of infection to cause UTI.

Immune stimulation
- Antibodies directed against normal flora crossreact with normal tissue components. Bacteria from intestinal flora contain antigens that crossreact with blood group A. This is the source of natural antibodies against blood group antigens.

Keeping out of invaders
- Normal flora inhibits entry of pathogens by competative inhibition.
- They produce inhibitory substances as antibiotics, bacteriocins
- Patients treated with antibiotics that are effective in gut may suffer from overgrowth of *Clostridium difficile* which causes antibiotic-associated diarrhea.

Role in human nutrition and metabolism
- Many intestinal bacteria (*E. coli, Bacteroides*) produce vitamin K, B complex
- Members of intestinal bacteria produce glucouronidases and sulfatases

Source of carcinogen?
- Intestinal flora may produce carcinogens
- Some compounds ingested by person are chemically modified by metabolic activities of normal flora
- Artifical sweetner cyclamate is converted to active bladder carcinogen—cyclohexamine by bacterial sulfatases

Normal flora of throat: *Streptococcus viridans, Pneumococci, Branhamella.*

Normal Flora of Intestinal Tract

Mouth, pharynx and trachea of newborn are not sterile at birth. It contains same organisms as mother's vagina. In first 2–5 days after birth, it is replaced by bacteria from mother and nurse. At 4–24 hours after birth, normal flora starts harboring the GIT. In breastfed babies, it contains *Lactobacillus, staphylococci,* coliform, enterococci while in artificial fed babies it contains, in addition, Grampositive bacilli. Esophagus contains organisms swallowed with saliva and food. Stomach is usually sterile. Duodenum contains 10^3–10^6 bacteria/gm, while jejunum and proximal ileum contain 10^5–10^8 bacteria/gm. Lower ileum and cecum contain 10^8–10^{10} bacteria/gm. In adult, colon and rectum has 10^{11} bacteria/gm (10–20% of fecal mass). In adult feces, 96–99% bacteria are anaerobes, 1–4% aerobes.

Normal intestinal flora: The list include *E. coli, Str. fecalis, Proteus spp., Enterobacter, Pseudomonas aeruginosa, Candida albicans, Bacteroides fragilis, Bifidobacterium, Lactobacilli, Clostridia, Peptostreptococci, Eubacterium sp.*

Normal Flora of the Genitourinary Tract

Males: *Mycobacterium smegmatis, Lactobacillus, Gardnerella vaginalis, Alpha* hemolytic streptococci, *Bacteroides spp, Chlamydia trachomatis, Ureaplasma urealyticum.*

Females: Newborn vagina is sterile. First 24 hours micrococci, enterococci, diphtheroids form the normal flora of vagina. In 2–3 days, glycogen deposition occurs, and vagina has acidic pH similar flora to adult vagina. After 2–3 days up to puberty, glycogen disappears, pH becomes alkaline, micrococci, non-hemolytic streptococci, coliforms, diphtheroids form the normal flora. At puberty, glycogen in vagina reappears. Lactobacillus, *E. coli,* and yeasts produce acid from glycogen lowering of pH which prevents colonization with pathogens. During pregnancy, there is rise in number of *S. epidermidis,* yeasts and *Lactobacillus.* After menopause, it is similar to flora before puberty. Normal adult vaginal flora consists of anaerobic cocci and bacilli, *Listeria,* anaerobic streptococci, *Mycoplasma, Gardenerella vaginalis, Neisseria* and *Spirochetes.*

Normal Flora of Skin

Diphtheroids, staphylococci (aerobic and anaerobic), Gram-negative organism as *E. coli, Proteus* of other intestinal organism, *Candida albicans, Ptyrosporum ovale* from nomral flora of skin. Skin on face, neck, hands buttocks may carry β hemolytic streptococci and staphylococci. Penicillin resistant or methicillin resistant staphylococci may be carried by health professional. Hairs harbour *S. aureus* and may act as source of infection.

Probiotics

Knowledge of normal flora is applied, live organisms given in adequate amount. They are useful to restore normal flora when it lost.
* They are available in the form of capsules or sachet, with bacteria or mixture of bacteria with yeast. For example, *Lactobacillus acidophilus.*
* *Sacchromyces boulardii, Bifidobacterium longum*
* Applications of probiotics:
  – Gastroenteritis pseudomembraneous colitis
  – Necrotising enteritis
  – Lactose intolerance
  – Breakdown bile in gut, helping to reduce cholesterol level by inhibiting reabsorption.
  – Bacterial vaginosis to restore pH by lactic acid producing bacteria.

Prebiotics: These are dietary nondigestible fibers which stimulate growth of commensals.

69

Bacteriology of Water, Milk and Air

Drinking water should be clear, colorless and odorless. It shoud be free from pollution.

Hazards of water pollution:

- Chemical pollutants contain agricultural and industrial wastes, e.g. detergents, solvents, cyanides, minerals, etc.
- Biological hazards come from fecal pollution. It may lead to water-borne diseases.

WATER-BORNE DISEASES

Diseases caused directly by infective agent.

- *Viral*: Hepatitis (A, E), polio, rotavirus
- *Bactrial*: Cholera, typhoid, paratyphoid, shigellosis, E. coli, Yersinia enterocolitica, Campylobacter
- *Protozoa*: Amoebiasis, giardiasis, *Balantidium coli*, cryptosporidiosis
- *Helminths*: Roundworm, whipworm, threadworm.

Diseases due to aquatic hosts:

- *Paragonimus wastermani*, metacercarae, in ingested crustacean
- Clonorchiasis, metacercariae in ingested fish
- *Dracunculus medinensis*: Cyclops
- *Schistosomiasis*: Snail

Other Water-Associated Diseases

If water is not available for bathing, washing clothes following diseases may be transmitted.

- Scabies
- Louse-borne typhus
- Relapsing fever
- Impetigo
- Trachoma
- Schistosomiasis.

Bacterial flora of water: Natural water may contain *Micrococcus, Pseudomonas, Serratia, Flavobacterium, Alcaligenes,* and *Acinetobacter*. Soil bacteria as *B. subtilis, B. megaterium,* and *Klebsiella spp.* may present in water. After fecal contamination, intestinal bacteria as *E. coli, Klebsiella spp., S. faecalis, C. welchii* may contaminate water.

BACTERIOLOGICAL EXAMINATION OF WATER

Collection of Samples

- Water is collected in glass bottles with stoppers.
- **Sampling is done from** tap or pump outlet, reservoir (streams, rivers, lakes and tanks), dug well.
- *Transport*: Samples are to be transported within 1–3 hours.
- Neutralization of chlorine is done with sodium thiosulphate.

Bacteriological testing of water samples includes:

Plate Count

- Water samples are tested for bacterial counts (E. coli) by pour plate method.
- Test is performed in two sets of which one is incubated at 37°C for 1–2 days while another set of media is incubated at 22°C for 3 days.
- If growth is seen in the set of media incubated at 37°C, it is most likely associated with contaminated organic material of human or animal origin. It is an important indicator of dangerous pollution suggesting some defects in filter beds which require quick action.
- Growth plates incubated at 22°C suggest the amount of decomposing organic matter present in water which is contaminated with pathogenic organisms or parasites.

Methods of Analysis

Presumptive coliform test: This test is called presumptive coliform counts, as it is based on the assumption that if coliform counts of water are increased above acceptable levels, it suggests fecal contamination, this indirectly shows the risk of presence of pathogen.

Differential coliform test (Eijkman test)

- After tests for presumptive counts, this test is done to confirm the organism as *E. coli.* (thermotolerant *E. coli*).
- Bottles which showed growth with acid and gas with presumptive counts are subcultured on fresh single strength MacConkey agar which is incubated at 44°C (in water bath) without temperature fluctuations. They are observed after 48 hours.
- Tubes showing gas in Durham's tube are suggestive of *E. coli*. Such tubes showing gases are counted and *E. coli* counts are calculated with using (McCrady's) probability table.
- Further confirmation is done by other biochemical test as indole and citrate.

Membrane filtration method: In this method, 100 mL of water sample or diluted sample is filtered through a membrane filter. The membrane with organisms is placed on a selective broth with indicator. After incubation, number of colonies is counted. This gives presumptive *E. coli* counts in 100 mL of sample.

Multiple tube method or most probable number method (MPN): In this method, 100 mL of water sample is divided into five tubes containing 10 mL and one tube with 50 mL of sterile double strength MacConkey's broth. After overnight incubation, the number of tubes showing growth (color change) is counted. By referring to probability table, the presumptive *E. coli* counts are counted.

Probability table for estimating the MPN of coliform bacilli

Volume of sample in each bottle	50 mL	10 mL
Number of bottles	1	5

The number of tubes giving positive results

50 mL	10 mL	MPN/100 mL
0	0	0
0	1	1
0	2	2
0	3	4
0	4	5
0	5	7
1	0	2
1	1	3
1	2	6
1	3	9
1	4	16
1	5	18+

TABLE 69.1: Standards for drinking water

Mean count	Category	Comments
0	A	Excellent
1–10	B	Acceptable, but make regular checks
10–50	C	Unacceptable. Look for and correct structural faults, disinfect instrument
>50		Grossly polluted. Look for alternative method or carry out necessary repairs and disinfect

Examination for Specific Pathogens

It is done for *Salmonella, Shigella, V. cholerae,* etc.

- *Detection of fecal streptococci:* 5 cc of glucose azide broth is used which is incubated at 45°C, looked for acid production.
- *Detection of C. welchii:* Litmus milk medium is used which is incubated anaerobically at 35°C for 5 days and looked for stormy fermentation.
- *Virological examination: Enterovirus, Echo, Parvo, Reo* and *Adeno viruses* are looked for.

Throughout any year 95% of samples should not contain any coliform organisms in water (Table 69.1).

No samples should contain more than 10 coli form/ 100 mL.

BACTERIOLOGY OF MILK

Sources of infective agents: Milk ducts of udder, milking equipment, the milker and dust in milk, contaminated water, and diseased animals are possible sources of contamination of milk.

Types of Bacteria in Milk of Healthy Cows

Bacteria which may enter milk and possible source is given as follows:

- *Acid forming: S. faecalis,* lactobacilli.
- Staphylococci from utensils and udders
- *Alkali forming: Alcaligenes spp., Achromobacter spp.* from environment.
- *Gas forming:* Coliforms, *C. welchii* and *C. butyricum* from water and hands of milker.

Milk-borne Diseases

Infections primarily of animals which may spread through contaminated milk:

- TB
- Brucellosis
- Salmonellosis

- Q fever
- Cowpox
- Foot and mouth disease
- Anthrax
- Leptospirosis
- *C. fetus*
- *Y. enterocolitica*

Contaminated milk by ticks, rats may spread tick-borne encephalitis, *Streptobacillus moniliformis*

Infections primarily of man which may spread through milk contamination are typhoid, paratyphoid fevers, cholera, TB, shigellosis, ETEC, etc.

Bacteriological Examination of Milk

Viable Count

- Viable counts can be made by serial dilution of milk samples in Ringer's solution incorporating in yeast extract milk agar at 30–37°C for 72 hours.
- *Test for coliforms*: Varying dilutions of milk are inoculated in MacConkey's fluid with Durham's tube at 37°C for 48 hours.

Chemical Tests

Methylene blue tests: It is economical substitute of viable count. Absence of reduction of dye in 30 minutes means, milk is satisfactory.

Resazurin test: The method observes change of color of milk in 10 minutes compared with lovibond comparator.

Phosphatase test: It is checked **for pasteurization**.
- *Principle of the test*: Phosphatase is inactivated during pasteurization.
- 1 mL of milk, 5 mL buffer and disodium phenyl phosphate are incubated at 37°C for 2 hours. Yellow color of P. nitrophenol (milk contains phosphate) will be produced.

Turbidity test: It checks for **sterilization**: Milk (heated at 100°C for 5 minutes) after adding ammonium sulphate, if there is no precipitate formation, means milk sterilized.

Detection of specific pathogens, i.e. TB and *Brucella* may be done. Isolation and identification will be done by culture and inoculation in animals.

BACTERIOLOGY OF AIR

Man respires 500 cu ft air per day.

Sources of Air Pollution

- *Human sources*: Nasal secretions, skin and intestinal organisms from infant napkins.
- Laboratory procedures, dental manipulation, flushing of water closets

Air-borne infections: Hemolytic streptococci, staphylococci, diphtheria, TB, Q fever, psittacosis, etc.

Environmental Sources

- Amount of contamination depends on density of human or animal population, nature of soil, amount of vegetation, atmospheric conditions like humidity, temperature, wind, rainfall, and sunlight.
- Organisms present in air may be *Achromobacter, micrococci, Sarcina,* coliform bacilli, and fragments of molds.

Measurement of Air Contamination

Bacteriological Examination of Air

Sedimentation method or **settle plate method** (Flowchart 69.1). It is used for testing air in surgical theatre, hospital ward.

Method: A sterile dried plate of blood agar is kept open in operation theatre for 30 minutes, after that the plate is closed and incubated at 37°C in incubator. Next day, the type of growth is observed and numbers of colonies are counted.

Slit Sampler

Air is sucked at a rate of one cubic feet (28.3 litre) per 10 minutes. It is directed to culture medium strips present inside the sampler. The culture media are incubated and after overnight incubation, numbers of colonies are counted.

The upper limit of bacterial counts in air in various locations are:
- 50 per cubic feet in office or home
- 10 per cubic feet in general operation theatre
- **1 per cubic feet i**n operation theatre where critical surgeries are performed as **neurosurgery and cardiac surgery.**

Acceptable limits of air pollution

- Factories, offices, homes—50 per cu ft
- Operation theatre—10 per cu ft
- Dressing room, operation theatre for neurosurgery—1 per cu ft
- Single colony of fungus, *Pseudomonas*, or *Staphylococcus aureus* is unacceptable.

Flowchart 69.1: Settle plate method for checking sterility of air in hospital set up

Sterile plate of blood agar is kept

open in operation theatre for 30 minutes

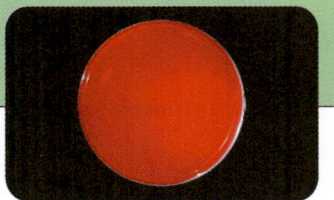

Plate is closed after 30 minutes, brought to laboratory and incubated at 37°C, overnight in a incubater

Next morning observe the number of colonies seen, also note down specifically if there is colony of *Staphylococcus*, fungus, or *Pseudomonas aeruginosa*

If colonies less than 10 and no colony of *Staphylococcus aureus*, or fungus or *Pseudomonas*	If colonies are more than 10 or colony of *Staphylococcus aureus* present/colony of *Pseudomonas* present or colony of fungus present

Conditions in OT are satisfactory

Conditions in OT not good, disinfection (e.g. fumigation required)

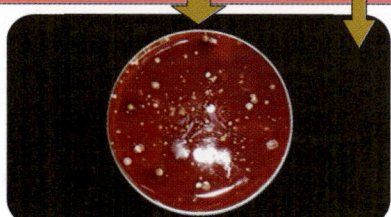

70

Hospital-Acquired Infection

Hospital-acquired infections or nosocomial infections also called healthcare-associated infections are those infections which develop in hospitalized patients; which were not present or in incubation at the time of admission. But those infections which are acquired in hospital stay and manifest after discharge are included in hospital-acquired infections.

Predisposing Factors

- Immune status of the patient, if it is low, that person is susceptible for infection. Patients with burn, diabetes, transplant recipient, malignancy, patients on immunosuppressed drugs, persons suffering from other infections lower the immunity, e.g. AIDS patient.
- Extremes of age, for example, premature babies and infants are susceptible to infections as they have poorly developed immune system.
- Hospital environment: If hospital is unhygienic, chances of infections are more, similarly overcrowding of patients make them susceptible to infection.
- Implanted prosthesis
- Prolonged hospital stay

Sources of Hospital-Acquired Infection
(Flowchart 70.1)

Endogenous

The source of infection is the patient himself; infections arise from organisms present in his own body. For example, nasopharyngeal carriers of *MRSA* which may cause infection to other parts of his body.

Exogenous Source of Infection

The source is other person, or inanimate object. A patient may get cross-infection from another patient or another person like health care worker. Infections

Flowchart 70.1: Sources of hospital-acquired infections

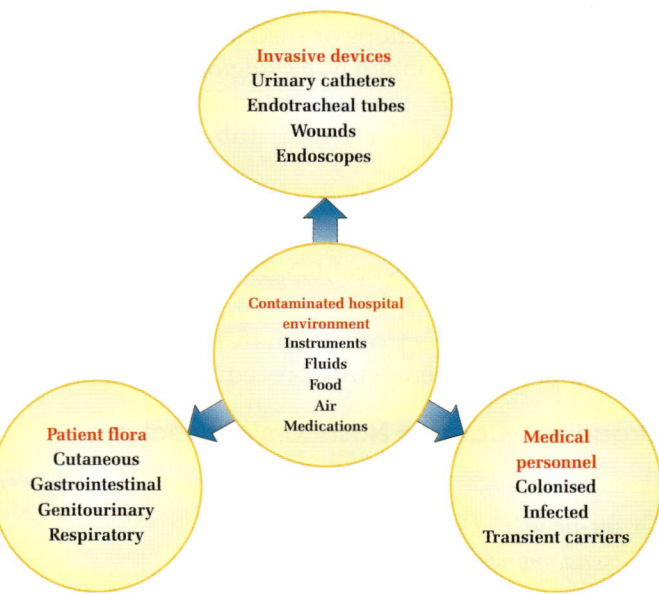

occurring and given by doctors or other staff are called **iatrogenic infections**. For example, meningitis occurring due to lack of asepsis while performing procedure as lumbar puncture, organisms may enter and cause meningitis.

Hospital Environment

- *Quality of air*: It may be contaminated from organisms shed by other patients.
- Dust particles may contain droplet nuclei of respiratory pathogens.
- *Water*: It may be contaminated by bacteria as *Pseudomonas*.
- Wash bowls
- Food
- Disinfectants

- Inanimate objects as bed sheets, clothing, bed pans
- Surface clean or contaminated by other person's secretions and body fluids.

Modes of Transmission of Infection

- *Oral route*: Ingestion of contaminated food or water with pathogens as *Salmonella, Enterobacter, Pseudomonas, E. coli, C. difficile, Rotavirus, Serratia.*
- *Inoculation route or parenteral route*: Infections through contaminated needles, syringes, or other instruments with blood-borne pathogens, as *HBV*, may occur. It may be due to injection of contaminated infusions by bacteria as *Pseudomonas or C. albicans* or through transplant as *Cytomegalovirus.*
- *Air-borne route*: Droplets from other patients suffering from respiratory infections or dust particles containing droplet nuclei from patients shed by body or shed from secretions or shed in beddings. Droplet or aerosol may contain *N. meningitidis, Grp. A streptococci, adenovirus, parainfluenza viruses, B. pertussis, measles, mumps, chickenpox,* tuberculosis, fungal spores.
- *Blood-borne pathogens*: HIV, HBV, HCV.
- *Contact*: Contact of health person may transmit infections (staphylococci, GNB, *C. difficile*, respiratory viruses).
- *Iatrogenic*: Infections transferred during any diagnostic or therapeutic procedure.

Organisms Causing Nosocomial Infections

Bacteria

Gram-negative bacteria

- *Pseudomonas aeruginosa*
- *E. coli*
- *Klebsiella sp.*
- *Proteus sp.*
- *Serratia sp.*
- *Campylobacter*
- *Burkhoderia cepacia*
- *Legionella pneumophila*
- *Salmonella*
- *Shigella*

Gram-positive bacteria

- *Staphylococcus aureus*
- *Streptococcus pyogenes*
- *Enterococci*
- *Streptococcus pneumoniae*
- *Staphylococcus epidermidis*

Other bacteria

- *Nocardia*

- *Clostridium species*
- *Anaerobic cocci*
- *Bacteroides fragilis*

Viruses

- *Hepatitis viruses*
- *Herpes simplex viruses*
- *Influenza and parainfluenza virus*
- *Rhinovirus*
- *Rotavirus*
- *Enteroviruses*
- *HIV*

Fungi

- *Candida albicans, C. parapsilosis and C. glabrata*
- *Aspergillus sp.*
- *Mucor*
- *Pneumocystitis*
- *Histoplasmosis*

Parasites

- *Entamoeba histolytica*
- *Acanthamoeba sp.*
- *Nagleria*

Sequelae of HAI

- Increase in morbidity and mortality
- Residual disability
- Increase in cost of treatment
- Increased length of stay

Factors Influencing Infection

- Age—neonate and elders
- Infected patients
- Immune status of patients
- *Susceptible patients*: Diabetes, immunosuppression, patients in special care units
- Major invasive procedure, diagnostic or therapeutic, may cause lack of sepsis
- Surgical procedure may cause iatrogenic infection
- Relative frequencies of organisms
- Hospital environment heavily laden with pathogens
- Resistance to antibiotics

Wound Infections

Surgical Wound

1–2% overall risk

Organisms causing postoperative wound infections: *Staphylococcus epidermidis, Staphylococcus aureus, Pseudomonas aeruginosa, E. coli, Klebsiella,* and *Candida.*

Types of infections: Infections following intra-abdominal or pelvic surgery, or surgery on urinary tract. Others—stitch abscess, umbilical sepsis, burn infections, injection abscess due to *Clostridium*.

Risk factor

- *Procedure type and length of surgery:* Clean, clean-contaminated (3–9%), contaminated (8.5%)
- Surgical site
- Operator's experience
- Infection at another site
- Shaving a day prior to surgery
- Obesity, diabetes mellitus
- Lack of preoperative antibiotic prophylaxis
- Prolonged stay at hospital (5–24 days)

Organism

- *S. aureus* infects clean wound
- *CONS*
- *Aerobic and anaerobic GNB: E . coli, Klebsiella, Proteus, Pseudomonas,* enterococci may cause infection after abdominal surgery, pelvis surgery.

Prevention

- Maintain strict aseptic measures
- Restrict duration of surgery
- Use chemoprophylaxis, if feseable
- Try to mobilize patient as early as possible.
- Preoperative patient care
- Clipping hair
- Skin disinfection (70% alcoholic solution with povidone iodine or chlorhexidine allow the area to dry)
- Avoid excessive presence and movement of staff
- No staff with a boil or lesion or eczema colonized with *S. aureus* should be allowed in the theatre
- Theatre clothing not to be worn outside theatre

Urinary Tract Infection (UTI)

Risk Factors

- Instrumentation of urinary tract
- *Catheterization:* Poor aseptic precautions while insertion of catheters, disconnection of catheter, contamination during irrigation
- Female sex
- Impaired renal function
- Diabetes mellitus
- Catheter drain, bag colonization
- Catheter >6 days increases risk with resistant organism

Organisms: E. coli, Klebsiella, Proteus, Pseudomonas aeruginosa, Enterobacter, Citrobacter, Acinetobacter, Serratia, Enterococci.

Measures

- Use continuously closed sterile drainage system.
- Reduce unnecessary and prolonged use.
- Proper cleaning of periurethral area to prevent colonization of bacteria.
- Follow standard aseptic techniques.

Bacteremia, Septicemia

Risk Factors

Indwelling intravenous catheter

- Central venous catheter is associated with (hemodialysis) high risk.
- Internal jugular catheter is more risky than subclavian catheter.
- Multilumen catheter is more risky than single lumen catheter.

Organisms which may cause infections are *Staphylococcus epidermidis, Staphylococcus aureus, Enterococcus, Candida sp., Pseudomonas.*

Measures

- Use IV therapy only when indicated.
- Avoid lower extremity for cannulation.
- Use stainless steel needles.
- Disinfect skin properly before cannulation, inspect cannulation site for sepsis.
- Change cannula 48 hourly.

Pneumonia or Lower Respiratory Tract Infections

Predisposing Factors

- Unconsciousness which prevents cough reflexes
- Impaired clearance mechanisms of respiratory tract due to pulmonary disease
- Patients with mechanical ventilation
- Chronic lung disease
- Age >70 years
- Respiratory failure

Measures

- Identify patients at high risk
- Deep breathing and coughing exercises
- Percussion and postural drainage
- Early postoperative mobilization
- Clearing airways at least 6 times a day
- Decontamination of respiratory equipment

- Maintain proper position to prevent aspiration pneumonia.
- Frequent sucking of secretions using sterile methods, especially in tracheostomized individuals.

Management of Outbreaks

WHO defines 'outbreak' as an occurrence of similar illness that are in excess of the normal expectancy for a given location and period of time.

Or

Two or more cases related by time, place and in the same population.

Surveillance is aimed at:
- Identify other infected cases and treating them.
- Tracing of the source of infection and routes of exposure.
- Provide disease or organism fact sheet handouts to all HCWs concerned.
- No new cases and negative cultures for patients and carriers indicate the end of the outbreak.
- On successful control of the outbreak, complete outbreak report prepared to include all the necessary details.

Hospital Infection Control Committee (HICC)

Aim: To lower the risk of infection by:
- Development of an effective surveillance system
- Development of policies and procedures
- Maintenance of continuous education program
- Diagnosis of etiology

Outbreak: Source identified and eliminated.
a. Sampling of possible source is done.
b. Typing of isolate is by various methods as biotype, antibiogram, serotype, bacteriocin, bacteriophage, restriction enzyme analysis.
c. Sterilization systems checked.

Infection Control Team

Members are dean, microbiologist, and medical and nursing staff, medical administrator and statistician.

Functions
- Investigation and controlling outbreaks
- Formulating guidelines for admissions
- Nursing and treatment of infectious patients
- Surveillance on sterilization and disinfectant practices
- Determining antibiotic policies
- Immunization schedules
- Educating personnel on infection control
- Educating hospital staff in waste aggregation and disposal

Infection control nurse (ICN): ICN should be sufficiently senior and experienced, she should full time nurse. There should be one ICN per every 250 beds. ICN everyday reports to infection control officer, direct access to administrative officer on matters of serious breaches of control practices. Activities of infection control nurse include daily visit to wards, checking ward sister's report register, collection and tabulation of daily data of incidence of hospital infection, compilation of ward-wise, discipline-wise or procedure-wise statistics, daily visit to laboratory monitoring and supervision of infection among hospital staff and training of nursing aids and paramedical personnel on correct use of hygiene practices.

Role of Microbiologist

- Diagnosis of infecting agent along with antibiotic susceptibility testing report.
- Maintain record of different pattern of pathogens isolated in different speciality wise and different patient group which will help clinicians for treatment.
- Surveillance of infections, especially drug resistant bacteria as MRSA, ESBL producing Gram-negative bacilli, metallobetalactamase producing bacteria.
- Investigation of outbreak
- Formulate procedures which are designed to control infections like:
  - Catheter care policy
  - Antibiotic policy
  - Disinfectant policy
  - Blood-borne virus infections exposures policies as following needle stick injury, blood splash.

Investigation of Outbreak of Infection

Outbreaks in hospitals are epidemics. They are detected because the incidence of infection seems to be above normal levels for that hospital. Hence **investigations must be made to determine**:
- Extent of infection
- Mode of spread
- Identify persons at risk
- Propose effective methods for control

During investigating outbreak, help of statistician should be taken for analysis of data. The problem with hospital-acquired infections as compared to community-acquired infections is multiple drug resistance among bacteria, which is supported by hospital environment. Epidemiological tests as phage typing and other typing methods are used to find out the common source of infection.

Steps of Investigation of Outbreak

- Formulating the case definitions and exclusion criteria
- Confirmation of the suspected infection
- Reporting of the outbreak

Control the Outbreak

Steps involved in control of outbreak are (Flowchart 70.2):
- Isolation of symptomatic patients
- Frequent and adequate handwashing
- Barrier precautions
- Restrict certain activities depending on the suspected organism
- Confine drainage using appropriate dressing
- All employees not allowed returning to work until asymptomatic, or if required, negative cultures obtained.

Surveillance

- It allows early recognition of problem by noting any change in the number or type of infection.

- Sources of surveillance data are:
  a. *Microbiology laboratory reports*: These can be used for general surveillance, for example monitoring hemodialysis patients regularly, for hepatitis B surface antigen and HCV infection reported in renal units or monitoring of MRSA in hospitals
  b. *Ward rounds*:
     - New cases can be identified by direct inspection; previously identified infections can be followed up.
     - Surveys can also be carried out in wards, e.g. wound infections after different practices or procedures.
  c. Other sources include autopsy reports, staff health records, survey of patients after discharge.

Investigation of an outbreak. (Though there is no universally applicable routine for finding of source of infection but each investigation has epidemiological element and microbiology element.)

Flowchart 70.2: Control measures to prevent or reduce HAI depending upon source of infection

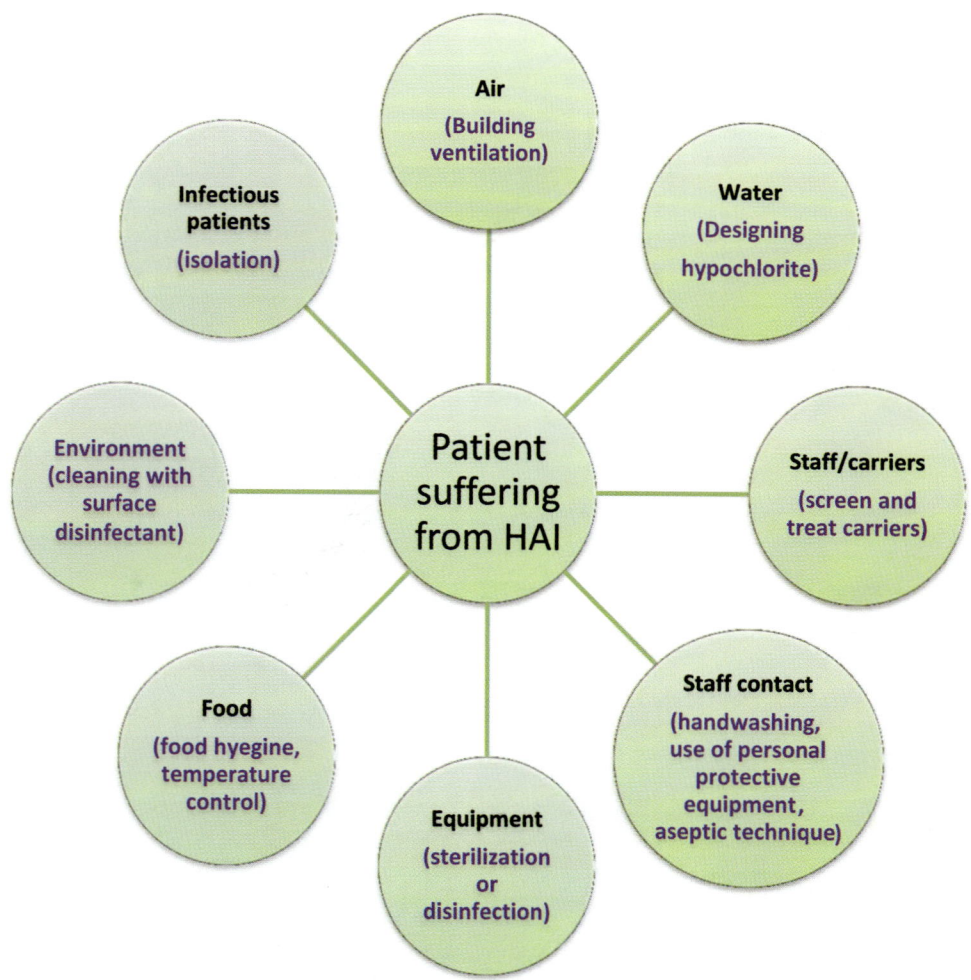

Describe outbreak in epidemic forms: Obtain information of relevant factors:

a. How many people are affected?
b. When they were admitted?
c. When did they develop infection?
d. Are they all from same ward?
e. Are they treated by common doctor; how many of them have been exposed to the same treatments?

The role of microbiology laboratory is to isolate the organisms.

The **identity of infecting organism** can provide some clues as to the source.

- Respiratory and intestinal viruses implicate the source of infection as the patient or the staff.
- Hepatitis indicates spread via contaminated blood products.
- An outbreak of wound infection with *Staph. aureus* is likely to be associated with contact spread from staff.
- Outbreak of *Salmonella* gastroenteritis is more likely to originate from kitchen.
- In addition, the information whether involvement of medical ward or surgical ward or intensive unit is helpful.

71

Gastrointestinal Infections

Gastroenteritis: It is characterized by gastrointestinal symptoms including vomiting, diarrhea and abdominal discomfort.

Diarrhea: It is increased frequency, fluidity or volume of feces and bowl movements relative to routine habit of the individual involving increased fluid and electrolyte loss. Roughly passage of 3 or more motions per day is considered as diarrhea. It is due to infection of small intestine (Table 71.1).

Dysentery: It is an inflammatory disorder of gastrointestinal tract often associated with blood and mucus in feces and accompanied by pain, fever, cramps, usually resulting from a disease of large intestine.

Enterocolitis: It is inflammation involving small and large intestine.

Etiology

Causes of Watery Diarrhea

Bacteria
- *Vibrio cholerae*
- *E. coli (ETEC, EIEC, EAEC, EPEC)*
- *Campylobacter*
- *Yersinia enterocolitica*
- *Aeromonas hydrophila*
- *Plesiomonas shigelloides*
- *Noncholera vibrios*
- *Vibrio parahemolyticus*

Food poisoning agents presenting as watery diarrhea:
- *Staphylococcus aureus*
- *Salmonella typhimurium*

TABLE 71.1: Comparison of different diarrheal diseases

Pathogen	Incubation period	Diarrhea	Vomitings	Abdominal cramps	Fever
Salmonella	6 h–2 d	Watery	+	+	+
Campylobacter	2–11 d	Bloody	–	+	+
Shigella	1–4 d	Bloody	–	+	+/–
Vibrio cholerae	2–3 d	Watery	+	+/–	–
Vibrio parahemolyticus	8h–2 d	Watery	+	+	+
Clostridium perfringens	8h–1 d	Watery	–	+/–	–
Bacillus cereus	–	–	–	–	–
Diarrheal type	8–12 h	Watery	–/+	++	
Emetic type	15 min –4 h				
Yersinia enterocolitca	4–7 d		–	+	–
EPEC	1–2 d	Watery	+	+	+
ETEC	1–7 d	Watery	+	+	–
EHEC	3–4 d	Bloody	+	+	–
EIEC	1–3 d	Bloody	+	+	+

Flowchart 71.1: Definitions of infections of gastrointestinal tract

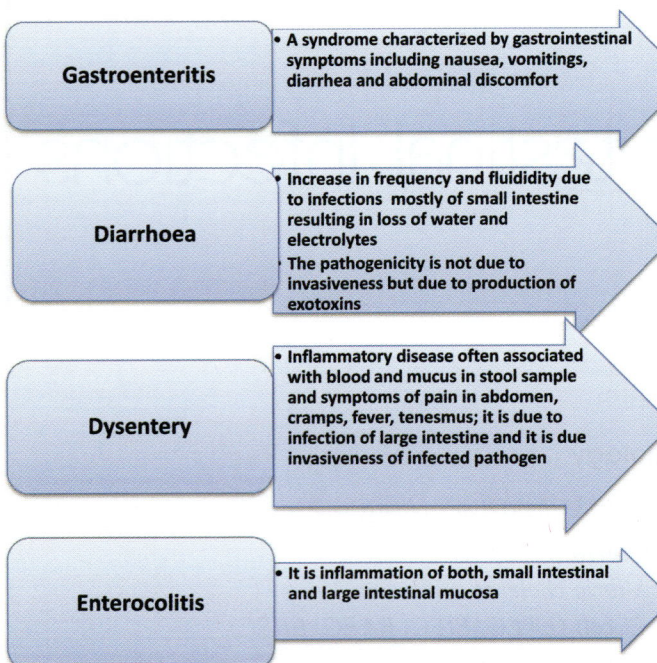

- *Salmonella enteritidis*
- *Clostridium perfringens*
- *Bacillus cereus (diarrhea type)*

Viral agents
- *Rotavirus*
- *Norwalk virus*
- *Astrovirus*
- *Adenovirus*
- *Calcivirus*
- *Coronavirus*

Parasites
- *Cryptosporidium*
- *Isospora*
- *T. solium*
- *T. saginata*
- *Ascaris lumbricoides*
- *Hymenolepsis nana*
- *Ancylostoma duodenale*
- *Necator americans*

Fungal
Candida albicans

Causes of Dysentery
- *Shigella species*
- *Enteroinvasive E. coli*
- *Enterohemorrhagic E. coli*

- *Clostridium difficile*
- *Yersinia enterocolitica*
- *Campylobacter species*
- *Entamoeba histolytica*
- *Balantidium coli*
- *Giardia lamblia*
- *Schistosoma mansoni*
- *Trichuris trichuria*

Pathogenesis
- *Toxic type*: There is preformed toxin in food which is consumed.
- *Infection type*: Pathogenesis is due to invasiveness as in *Shigella*.
- *Toxico-infection*: Organisms enter, multiply and produce toxin.

Collection of Specimens
- Stool sample is collected in sterile wide mouth container.
- In cholera, pass a rubber tube in rectum and allow sample to collect in container.
- Rectal swabs are taken, if stool samples cannot be easily obtained.
- Stool sample can be collected on filter paper.

Transport Media
- V-R medium or autoclaved sea water for *Vibrio*
- Buffered glycerol saline for *Shigella*
- Cary Blair medium is useful for all enteric pathogens including *Campylobacter, Shigella, Vibrio,* and *Salmonella*.

Advantages of Cary Blair Medium
- If clinical diagnosis is not sure, it is used for all enteric bacteria.
- As it is semisolid medium, there is no spillage of material. VTM is used for viruses.

List of bacteria, their incubation period, and clinical presentation is given in Table 71.1.

Gross Examination
- Typical rice watery—*Vibrio cholerae*
- Presence of blood and mucus—dysentery
- Parasitic elements as segments of tapeworms, worms may be seen.

Microscopic Examination
- *Wet mount*: Look for presence of pus cells, parasitic elements (segments of worms, small worms, larvae of *Strongyloides stercoralis*), parasitic eggs, *Trophozoites of Entamoeba* and *Giardia*, Charcot laiden crystals.

- **Iodine mount** is done for parasites (cysts/eggs).
- **Hanging drop preparation**
  - Darting motility should be done if—*Vibrio, Campylobacter, Aeromonas, Plesiomonas* are suspected.
  - **Inhibition of motility** with addition of antisera of *Vibrio* helps in presumptive identification.
  - **Distilled water immobilization test:** *Vibrio* gives test +ve.
- **Gram's staining**
  - It is less important due to normal flora but if predominantly only one organism seen it has importance as cholera—comma-shaped Gram-negative bacilli will be seen.
  - Presence of pus cell: Suspect organisms of dysentery
  - Pus cells and coma-shaped or spiral bacilli: *Campylobacter*
  - It may give clue of food poisoning due to *B. cereus, Clostridium difficile*
- **Modified Z-N stain is done for:** *Cryptosporidium and Isospora.*
- **Electron microscopy** and immune-electron microscopy used for viral cause, e.g. *rotavirus.*
- **Direct IF:** *Cryptosporidium.*

Cultivation

Blood agar for bacteria, specially look for hemo-digestion of *Vibrio cholerae.*

Selective Media

- *TCBS:* It is used for *Vibrio cholerae* (yellow colonies due to sucrose fermentation)
- *XLD:* It is used for *Salmonella* (red colonies with black center) and *Shigella* (pink colonies)
- Special medium used for *Campylobacter* is Campy BAP
- Sorbitol MacConkey's medium used for *E. coli* (VTEC).

Identification is done by biochemical tests and for *Salmonella, Shigella, and Vibrio cholerae,* perform agglutination from colonies with polyvalent and monovalent sera.

Immunological Tests

- **ELISA** is used for detection of **VMA**—virulence marker antigens of *Shigella*
- ELISA is done for *rotavirus* (antigens)
- ELISA is used for detection of toxin of *E. coli.*

Other tests: DNA probes, PCR.

Food Poisoning

Definition: The criteria for diagnosis of food poisoning are:
- There is history of consumption of common food.
- More than one person is involved.
- Same organisms are isolated from feces of patients and food sample. (Identity is proved by typing method.)

Types (Flowchart 71.2)

a. *Toxin type:* Food with preformed toxin is ingested, incubation period short, 1–6 hours. For example, *staphylococcal* food poisoning.

b. *Infection type:* Infective doses of organisms are ingested, which cause infection of GIT, incubation period is 8–24 hours.

c. *Toxic infection type:* Bacteria ingested, cause infection, produce toxin, e.g. *Clostridium perfringens.*

Pathogen	Food responsible for food poisoning
Staphylococcus	Milk, milk products, cream, meat
Bacillus cereus	Chinese fried rice
Salmonella	Poultry, milk, eggs, cream
Clostridium perfringens	Canned food, meat
Clostridium botulism	Honey
Campylobacter	Milk
E. coli	Green salad

Flowchart 71.2: Types of food poisonings

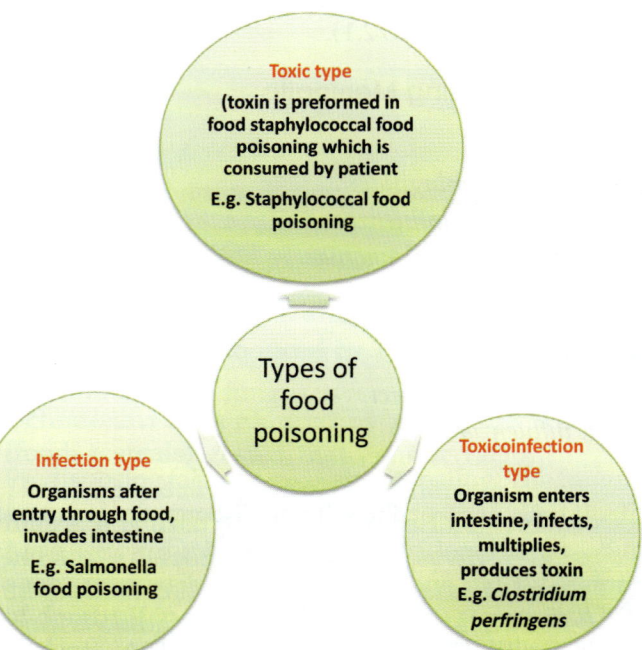

72

Central Nervous System Infections

Invasion of CNS occurs by:
1. Blood vessels and nerves that traverse the wall of skull and vertebral column.
2. Invasion from infected sinuses or ears or from local injury or congenital defects as spina bifida.
3. Rarely, invasion through olfactory nerve may occur.

Microorganisms may cross brain–CSF barriers by:
   i. Growing in the cells of barriers.
   ii. Travelling through intracellular vacuoles or carried by infected WBCs.

Infection of meninges of brain is called **meningitis**. When the organisms cross blood–brain barriers, infection of brain substance takes place which is called **encephalitis** (Table 72.1).

Bacteria Causing Meningitis

Children

- *Neisseria meningitidis*
- *Haemophilus influenzae*
- *Streptococcus pneumoniae*

Neonates and Infants

- *E. coli*
- *Group B streptococci*
- *H. influenzae*

- *Streptococcus pneumoniae*
- *Listeria monocytogenes*
- *Staphylococcus aureus*
- *Staphylococcus epidermidis*
- *Klebsiella species*

Adults

- *Neisseria meningitidis*
- *Haemophilus influenzae*
- *Streptococcus pneumoniae*

Elderly

- *Streptococcus pneumoniae*
- *E. coli*
- *Klebsiella species*

Other causes of bacterial meningitis which may present as **chronic meningitis**
- Tuberculosis
- Syphilis
- Brucellosis
- Leptospirosis
- Lyme disease
- *Nocardia*
- *Actinomyces*
- *Bacteroides fragilis*

TABLE 72.1: CSF findings during CNS infections

	Cells/HPF	Proteins mg/dL microliter	Glucose mg/dL	Causes
Normal	0–5	15–45	45–85	
Septic meningitis	200–20000 mainly neutrophils	High >100	<45	Bacteria, amoebic brain abscess
Aseptic meningitis or encephalitis	100–1000 mainly mononuclear cells	Moderately high (50–100)	Normal	Viruses, TB, leptospira, fungi, brain abscess partially treated

Viral Meningitis (Aseptic Meningitis)

- *Herpes simplex virus*
- *Mumps*
- *Poliovirus*
- *Coxsackie virus*
- *ECHO viruses*
- *Japanese encephalitis virus*
- *Adenovirus*
- *Looping ill*

Viral Encephalitis

- *Herpes simplex virus*
- *Mumps*
- *Varicella-zoster*
- *CMV*
- *Rabies*
- *Polio* and other enteroviruses
- *HIV*
- *Japanese encephalitis viruses*
- *Measles*
- *Rubella*
- *Looping ill*

Symptoms of meningitis are fever, headache, neck rigidity or neck stiffness, altered sensorium.

Fungal Causes of Meningitis

- *Cryptococcus neoformans*
- *Histoplasma capsulatum*
- *Candida albicans*
- *Blastomyces dermatitidis*
- *Coccidioidomycosis*
- *Cladosporium bantianum*
- *Aspergillus species*

Parasitic Infections of CNS

- *Acanthamoeba*
- *Nagleria*
- *Toxoplasma gondii*
- *Cysticercus cellulose*
- *Hydatid disease*
- *Malaria*

Diagnosis of Meningitis

Sample collection: CSF is collected under aseptic precaution by lumbar puncture.

Transportation: It should be immediately transported to the laboratory as delicate bacteria as *Haemophilus influenzae*, pneumococci may lose viability. If there is delay, keep it in **incubator or at room** temperature.

Processing (Flowchart 72.1): CSF is divided into sterile tubes.

First tube: Centrifuge the tube, take the deposit for smear and culture on media. The supernatant is used for antigen detection and for biochemical tests on CSF.

CSF is added to glucose broth or nutrient broth which enriches and acts as a backup.

Microscopy

- *Wet mount*: Note down presence of pus cell and their number under high power field. Increased number >5 cells per mL is suggestive of infection. Predominance of polymorphs indicates bacterial or pyogenic meningitis. Lymphocytic predominance is seen in viral meningitis.
- *India ink or Nigrosin*: It is used to demonstrate capsule of *Streptococcus pneumoniae, Cryptococcus neoformans* and *Haemophilus influenzae.*
- Z-N staining is used for demonstration of acid-fast bacteria suggestive of MTB.

  Tests for detection of antigen of *Cryptococcus neoformans, Streptococcus pneumoniae,* and *Haemophilus influenzae* are based on latex agglutination, countercurrent immune electrophoresis, coagglutination, ELISA.

Culture

- Blood agar with central streak of beta hemolytic *Staphylococcus aureus* (it will provide factor V for *Haemophilus influenzae)* is used for culture.
- Chocolate agar is also used for culture.
- MacConkey's agar is used for Gram-negative bacilli.
- L-J medium is used for MTB.
- Sabouraud's dextrose agar is used for *Cryptococcus neoformans*.

Incubation of Culture Media

- Blood agar and chocolate agar are incubated in candle jar to provide 5–10% CO_2 and guaze piece soaked in saline or water is placed in the incubator to provide 60–70% humidity.
- Bacterial pathogen is identified by colony morphology, Gram's staining smear from colony, biochemical tests.
- L-J medium is checked daily for presence of growth in first week of incubation and then weekly till 8 weeks. Look for rough, buff, tough colonies of MTB. If colonies appear, Z-N stained smear is done from colony and further identification is done by nitrate test, catalase test, arylsulfatase, and niacin test.

Flowchart 72.1: Processing of CSF

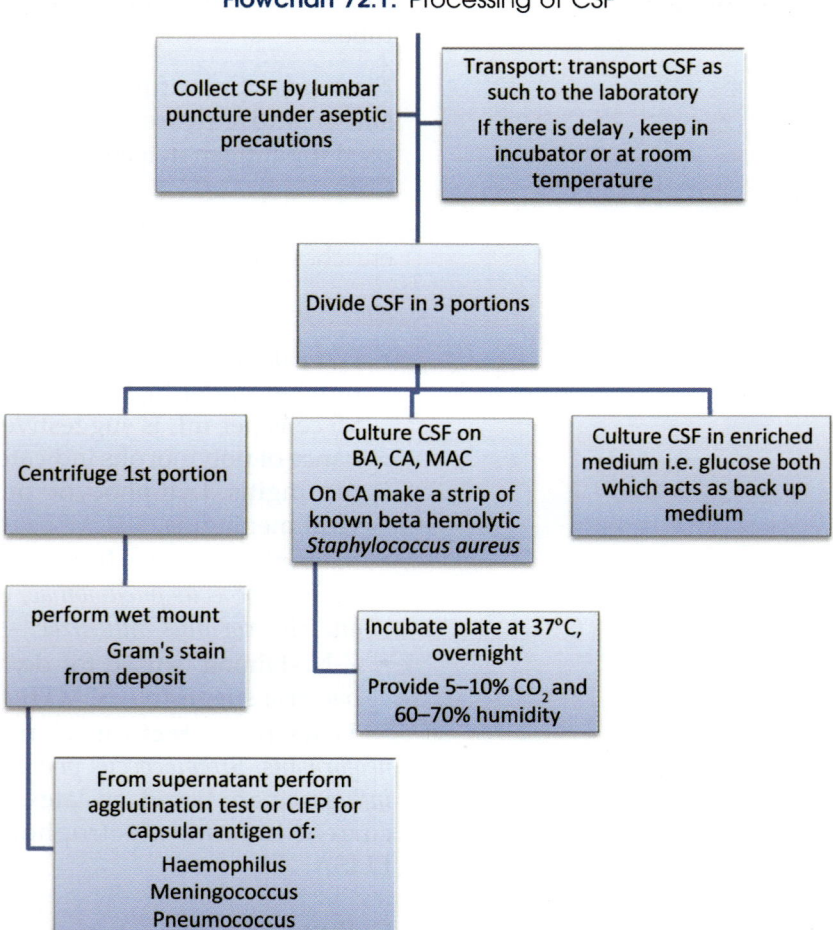

Identification of Cryptococcus Neoformans

Mucoid colonies will be produced on Sabouraud's dextrose agar. Capsulated yeast cells will be seen on India ink preparation. The isolate is further identified by urease test, brown colonies on Niger seed agar. Antigen can be demonstrated by LA, ELISA, CIEP.

73

Respiratory Infections

UPPER RESPIRATORY TRACT INFECTION

Causes of Sore Throat

Viral (2/3 Cases)

- *Adenovirus*
- *E-B virus*
- *Herpes simplex*
- *Coxsackie A virus*
- *Enteroviruses*
- *Rhinovirus*
- *Coronavirus*
- *Parainfluenza virus*
- *Influenza virus*
- *Cytomegalovirus*

Bacterial Causes (1/3 Cases)

- *Streptococcus pyogenes*
- *Corynebacterium diphtheriae*
- *Haemophilus influenzae*
- *Borrelia vincentii along with fusobacteria*
- *Group C and group G streptococci*
- *Staphylococcus aureus*
- *Treponema pallidum* (sore throat in secondary syphilis)
- *Neisseria gonorrhoeae* (sexual contact)

Fungus: *Candia albicans*

Specimens: Nasopharyngeal secretions collected with sterile swabs after local examination.

Findings of Local Examination

- *Yellow pus pocket*: Suspect *Streptococcus pyogenes*, *Staphylococcus aureus*.
- Pseudomembrane on tonsils extending posteriorly is due to *C. diphtheriae*.
- *Dirty patch on tonsils*: Viral agents especially *E-B virus* should be suspected.

- Painful ulcers are seen in *Herpes simplex virus*.
- White curdy patch on tonsils and mouth is due to *C. albicans*.

Transport: Stuart's transport medium; for *Streptococcus pyogenes* use Pike's medium or Amie's medium.

Processing of Samples

Microscopic Examination

1. *Gram staining*: Note down presence of pus cells and Gram-positive cocci in chains, in case of streptococcal infection, yeast cells in case of candidiasis, *Fusobacteria* and *Borrelia* in case of Vincent's angina and Gram-positive bacilli with Chinese letter pattern in case of *C. diphtheriae*.
2. *Negative staining*: It is used to demonstrate capsule of *Streptococcus pneumoniae*.
3. *Z-N staining*: In rare instances, *Mycobacterium tuberculosis* causes primary infection of tonsils. Z-N staining will be helpful.
4. **Direct immunofluorescence** is used for demonstration of *Streptococcus pyogenes*.
5. *Albert staining*: Green bacilli having dark greenish black granules with Chinese letter pattern is characteristic of *C. diphtheriae*.

Culture

- Blood agar with antibiotic disk of **Bacitracin** placed on primary inoculum for rapid identification of *Streptococcus pyogenes*.
- Chocolate agar is inoculated for fastidious bacteria as Pneumococcus and *Haemophilus influenzae*. The plates are incubated at 37°C in candle jar.
- MacConkey's agar is used for Gram-negative bacilli.
- Sabouraud's dextrose agar is used for *Candida*.

Other media used depending on findings of Gram's staining or when the organism is highly suspected.

Quantative Culture

Report the relative number of colonies of *S. pyogenes* on primary culture plate. It has more liked to be pathogenic role when it is numerous (>100 colonies/plate).

Antigen detection: Latex agglutination test is done for capsular organisms as pneumococci and for *Haemophilis influenzae*.

Antibody Detection

- ASO titre for streptococcal infection
- Paul–Bunnel test for glandular fever
- CRP
- For diagnosis of viral infections, CFT, neutralization tests are used.

LOWER RESPIRATORY TRACT INFECTIONS

Pneumonia

It is infection of lungs and production of alveolar exudate.

Bacterial Pneumonia

- *Streptococcus pneumoniae*
- *Haemophilus influenzae*
- *Staphylococcus aureus*
- *Klebsiella pneumoniae*
- *Pseudomonas aeruginosa*
- *Acinetobacter sp.*
- *Bacteroides sp.*
- *Legionella pneumophila*
- *Mycobacterium tuberculosis*

Primary atypical pneumonia

- *Mycoplasma pneumoniae*
- *Legionella pneumophila*
- *Psittacosis*
- *Q fever: Coxiella burnetii*
- *Chlamydia pneumoniae*

Viral Pneumonia

- *Influenza viruses*
- *Respiratory syncytial virus*
- *Parainfluenza virus*
- *Adenovirus*
- *Varicella zoster*

Fungal infections are suspected in AIDS patients:

- *Cryptococcus neoformans*
- *Histoplasma capsulatum*
- *Pneumocystis carinii*
- *Aspergillus sp.*
- *Blastomyces dermatitidis*

(Parasites as *Paragonimus westermani*, amoebiasis, hydatid cyst may be seen as lung infections, they do not present as pneumonia.)

Organisms causing **nosocomial pneumonia** are *Staphylococcus aureus*, *Streptococcus pneumoniae*, *Pseudomonas*, *Acinetobacter*, *Klebsiella sp.*

Clinical Types of Pneumonia

- *Lobar pneumonia*: There is consolidation of one or more lobes or segments of lungs.
- *Bronchopneumonia*: Infection and inflammation of bronchi, terminal bronchioles.
- *Atypical pneumonia*: There is patchy consolidation of lungs.

Laboratory Diagnosis

Laboratory diagnosis of pneumonia caused by *Streptococcus pneumoniae*.

Samples

- Sputum, preferably early morning sample which is concentrated specimen
- Induced sputum
- Bronchoalveolar lavage
- Endotracheal aspirates
- Blood for detection of capsular antigen and CRP
- Blood culture
- Blood for detection of antibodies.

Gross examination: **Rusty sputum** is seen in pneumonia due to *Streptococcus pneumoniae*.

Transport: Samples should be immediately transported to laboratory, in case of viral infection, transport in viral transport medium (VTM).

For Chlamydia, SPS or SPG is used as transport medium.

Microscopy

i. *Gram's staining*: It shows Gram-positive cocci in pairs and pus cells.
ii. *India ink or Nigrosin* is used for demonstration of capsule.
iii. *Fluorescent microscopy*: Phenolic rhodamine for MTB, direct immunofluorescence is used for *Pneumocystis, Chlamydia*.
iv. Z-N staining is used for MTB.
v. Gomori's methenamine silver staining, Giemsa staining for Pneumocystis

Culture

Blood agar and chocolate agar are incubated in candle jar to give 5–10% CO_2. Put **Optochin disc** on blood agar after inoculation of BA plate on primary inoculum.

TABLE 73.1: Serological tests for primary atypical pneumonia

Pathogen	Test	Significant titre
Mycoplasma pneumoniae	CFT IgM, ELISA, latex agglutination	1/16 positive
Legionella	Rapid microagglutination test	1/16
Chlamydia pneumoniae, Psittacosis	Microimmunofluorescence or ELISA	Positive
Coxiella burnetii	CFT using phase I and II antigens	1/200

Blood agar : Look for **alpha hemolysis and optochin sensitivity.**

Chocolate agar: It is good enriched medium, initially colonies are small. With further incubation, they become large with central umbonation giving **draughtsman appearance.**

MacConkey is used, if Gram-negative bacilli are suspected. On blood agar, put a streak of known beta hemolytic *Staphylococcus aureus* for *Haemophilus influenzae.* Use L-J medium for MTB.

Tissue culture media used for Chlamydia and viruses are HeLa and HEp-2.

Chick embryo: Route of inoculation is amniotic cavity for influenza and parainfluenza viruses.

Antigen detection: Capsular antigen of *Pneumococcus, Haemophilus,* and *Cryptococcus* detected by latex agglutination; ELISA and IF are used for detection of antigen of *Chlamydia.*

Antibodies detection:
- Streptococcal MG test, cold agglutination tests are used for atypical pneumonia.

- CFT is used for *Mycoplasma, Coxiella, Chlamydia.*
- ELISA is used for *Chlamydia, Mycoplasma.*

Positive findings

Streptococcus pneumoniae: Alpha hemolysis on blood agar, Gram's staining showing pus cell and Gram-positive cocci in pairs, negative stain showing capsule, perform Optochin test, bile solubility testing, and inulin fermentation.

MTB: Acid-fast bacteria, growth on L-J medium which is rough, buff, tough and confirm MTB by biochemical tests as catalase test, nitrate test, niacin test, growth on medium with PNB.

Molecular test: PCR.

Diagnosis of Primary Atypical Pneumonia (Table 73.1)

- *Microscopy*: Fluorescent microscopy for *Chlamydia.*
- Cultivation on chick embryo yolk sac for Chlamydia, cell cultures for *Chlamydia* are HeLa, HEp-2
- *Antibodies detection*: CFT for Q fever, mycoplasma, indirect immunofluorescence for detection of antibodies for *Legionella.*

74

Zoonotic Diseases

Zoonotic diseases are primarily infections of animals, which can be transmitted to human beings.

Modes of Transmission

- *Arthopods*: Blood-sucking insects infect humans beings. Plague is transmitted by bite of rat flea, rat bite causes rat bite fever, and ticks transmit tick fevers, while mite transmits Scrub typhus. Yellow fever, Japanese encephalitis, KFD, chikungunya are transmitted by mosquitoes, in leishmaniasis the vector is sandfly.

- *Feco-oral route* (contaminated food and water): Unpasteurized milk may cause bovine TB, brucellosis, Q fever. Eggs infected by Salmonella species (trans-ovarian transmission occurs in eggs). Toxoplasmosis occurs through contact with cats. Hydatid disease is due to contact with dogs (eggs contaminate fingers). *Trichinella spiralis* occurs through infected pork while *Tania solium* occurs through infected beef.

- *Bite*: Dog bite in case of rabies

- *Contact with animals or animal products*: Brucellosis, Psittacosis (contact with parrots) anthrax (contact with hides)

- *Through abrasions on skin or mucosa*: Leptospirosis.

Bacterial Infections (Table 74.1)

- Brucellosis
- Plague
- *Yersinia enterocolitica*
- Rat bite fever
- Anthrax
- Salmonellosis
- Leptospirosis
- Scrub typhus
- Tick typhus
- Psittacosis
- *Francisella tularensis*
- *Listeria monocytogenes*
- *Pausteurella multocida*
- Lyme disease
- Q fever
- *Pseudomonas mallei*

Viral Disease (Table 74.2)

- Rabies
- Yellow fever
- *Japanese encephalitis*
- KFD
- *Chikungunya*
- *Marburg*
- *Ebola*

Parasites

- Leishmaniasis
- Toxoplasmosis
- Taeniasis
- *Echinococcus granulosus*
- *Trichinella spiralis*
- Cryptosporidiosis

TABLE 74.1: Bacterial zoonotic diseases

Organism	Mode of infection	Samples collected	Diagnosis by	Serology
Brucellosis	Inhalation, ingestion, contact	Blood for culture Bone marrow culture Send these samples in Castaneda's medium Serum	Blood culture and bone marrow culture	Tube agglutination ELISA
Plague	Bite of rat flea, pulmonary infection is due to inhalation	Bubo aspirate Sputum in pulmonary disease Blood in septicemic disease	Microscopy— bipolar staining Direct immuno-fluorescence	ELISA antibodies detection (anti-F1 antibodies)
Yersinia enterocolitica	Ingestion	Stool sample from case of diarrhea	Stool culture probe	ELISA, DNA
Anthrax	Inhalation, contact with spores	Sample from malignant pustule	Microscopy and culture on BA agar which shows 'medusa head' colony	ELISA
Salmonellosis	Ingestion	Stool	Stool culture	Widal test
Leptospirosis	Entry through mucosa or skin with injury-history of contact with flood, water	Blood culture in EMJH medium Serum	Blood culture	Latex agglutination confirmation by microscopic agglutination
Scrub typhus	Mite	Serum for antibodies detection	Inoculation in mice	Weil- Felix test ELISA test
Psittacosis	Parrots	Culture		ELISA

TABLE 74.2: Viral diseases

Rabies	Bite	Corneal impression smear or skin scrapings from nape of neck	Direct immunofluorescence test	
Japanese encephalitis	Mosquito bite	Serum, CSF	Culture in suckling mice, neutralization, CFT	
Yellow fever	Mosquito bite	Serum, blood	Blood culture in yolk sac of chick embryo, CFT	
Chickungunya	Mosquito (ades)	Blood culture on tissue culture serum	Antibody detection by immuno-chromatography and ELISA, PCR	
KFD		Serum	Immunofluorescence	
Leishmania	Sandfly	Detection of amastigotes in peripheral blood smear inside monocytes Serum	Antibodies detection by aldehyde tests. Specific test: ELISA	
T. solium	Ingestion	Imaging methods Stool sample for detection of eggs	Indirect hemagglutination may be positive	
Hydatid disease	Ingestion	Serum	Serum: Detect antibodies by indirect hemagglutination test Casoni's skin test	
Toxoplasmosis	Ingestion	Serum for antibodies detection Blood for culture in mice by intraperitoneal route	IgM ELISA	

TABLE 74.3: Zoophilic dermatophytes

Disease	Sample	Tests
Microsporum canis	Skin scrapings	KOH—demonstrate fungal hyphae. Culture on SDA
Trichophyton verrucosum	Skin scrapings, nail	KOH—demonstrate hyphae. Culture on SDA
Trichophyton equinum	Nail	KOH—demonstrate hyphae. Culture on SDA

TABLE 74.4: List of vectors and diseases transmitted along with reservoirs

Arthropod vector	Disease transmitted	Causative agent	Reservoirs
Soft ticks	African relapsing fever	*Borrelia duttoni*	Wild rodents, pigs
Hard ticks	Tick-borne typhus Rockey mountain spotted fever	*Rickettsia rickettsii*	Wild rodents, domestic dogs, cats
	Looping ill	*Flavivirus*	Sheep, cattle
	Tularemia	*Fransicella tularensis*	Rabbits, squirrels
	Colorado tick fever	*Arbovrus*	
	Omsk hemorrhagic fever	*Flavivirus*	
Lice	Epidemic typhus	*Rickettsia prowazekii*	Man
	Louse-borne relapsing fever	*Borrelia recurrentis*	Man
Rat flea	Flea-borne typhus	*Rickettsia mooseri*	Rats
	Plague	*Yersinia pestis*	Rats
Mites	Scrub typhus	*Rickettsia tsutsugamushi*	Rodents
	Rickettsial pox	*Rickettsia akari*	House mice
Tsetse fly	African trypanosomiasis	*Trypanosoma brucei rhodesiense*	Wild game
Ruduvid bugs	American trypanosomiasis	*Trypanosoma brucei gambiense*	Man

75

Pyrexia of Unknown Origin

If patient's fever is greater than 38.3°C (101°F) on several occasions and continuously for more than 3 weeks, despite of 1 week intensive ambulatory evaluation or at least three OPD visits or 3 days of hospitalization is called FUO or PUO. This is the definition of **classical PUO or FUO.**

As increasing number of patients with serious diseases are successfully kept alive by improved treatment modalities, FUO in particular risk group can be defined.

- *Nosocomial or hospital-acquired FUO*: Fever on several occasions, in a hospitalized patient receiving acute care, infection not present or incubating at the time of hospitalization and the diagnosis is uncertain after 3 days, despite appropriate investigations including 2 days of incubation of microbiological cultures.

- *Neutropenic FUO*: Fever on several occasions, neutrophil count below 500/mm^3 in peripheral blood or expected to fall below that within 1–2 days and diagnosis is uncertain, after 3 days of appropriate investigations including at least 2 days of incubation of bacterial cultures.

- *HIV associated FUO*: Fever on several occasions, fever of more than 4 weeks duration as an OPD or 3 days duration in hospital, confirmed HIV serology. The diagnosis is uncertain after 3 days of appropriate investigations, including at least 2 days of incubation of microbiological cultures.

Etiology (Flowchart 74.1)

Bacterial Causes

- Enteric fever due to *S. typhi, S, paratyphi A, S. paratyphi B, S. paratyphi C*
- Tuberculosis
- Endocarditis: Oral streptococci, *Staph. aureus,* coagulase negative staphylococci
- Brucellosis

Flowchart 74.1: Mechanisms of fever

Organisms, toxins & other cytokines inducer act as endogenous pyrogenes

Pyrogenic cytokines-IL-1,TNF,IL-6 from mononuclear cells

Anterior Thalamus

PGE2- changes temperature set point

Alteration in autonomic heat loss or preservation mechanisms

Fever

- Abscess: Mixed anaerobic and aerobic flora (*pepto-streptococci, B. fragilis, Prevotella, Porphyromonas*)
- Osteomyelitis: *Staph. aureus, H. influenzae, Salmonella sp.*
- Biliary tract infections: *E. coli, Klebsiella species, Proteus sp,* and other Gram-negative organisms
- Urinary tract infections: Gram-negative facultative anaerobes as *E. coli, Proteus* sp, *Klebsiella* sp., etc.
- Lyme disease: *Borrelia burgdorferi*
- Relapsing fever: *Borrelia recurrentis*
- Q fever
- Tularemia
- Leptospirosis
- Typhus fever
- Psittacosis
- Mycoplasma species

Parasitic Causes

- Malaria
- Amoebic abscess
- Toxoplasmosis
- Leishmaniasis
- Trypanosomiasis

Fungal Causes

- *Candida albicans*
- *Cryptococcus neoformans*
- *Histoplasmosis*
- Coccidioidomycosis
- *Aspergillus species.*

Viral Causes

- AIDS
- Infectious mononucleosis
- Hepatitis viruses

Infective Causes of Fever in Different Groups

Nosocomial

- *Vascular line related*: Staphylococci
- *Other device related*: Staphylococci, *Candida*
- *Transfusion related*: CMV
- *Cholecystitis and pancreatitis*: Gram-negative organisms
- *Pneumonia*: Gram-negative rods including *Pseudomonas*
- *Postoperative abscess*: Gram-negative rods and anaerobes
- Post-gastric surgery: *Candida.*

Neutropenic FUO

- *Vascular line related*: Staphylococci
- *Oral infections*: Candidiasis, *herpes simplex virus*
- *Pneumonia*: Gram-negative rods, *Candida, Aspergillus, CMV*
- Soft tissue infection, e.g. perineal abscess-mixed flora

HIV Associated Fever

- *Respiratory tract infections*: CMV, pneumocystitis, MTB, Mycobacterium avium interacellulare complex
- *CNS infections*: Toxoplasmosis
- *GIT infections*: Salmonella, Campylobacter, Shigella
- Genital tract infection or disseminated: *Neisseria gonorrhoeae, Treponema pallidum.*

Approach to Diagnosis

Stage I in Investigation

Careful history taking, physical examination, and screening test:

- *History:* Take history of travel, occupation, hobbies, exposure to animal, known infectious hazards, antibiotic therapy within last 2 weeks. Some diseases are zoonotic, some are vector-borne, some are endemic in particular area, e.g. leishmaniasis is common in Bihar.
- In physical examination, particularly skin, eyes, lymph nodes, abdomen should be examined. The heart should be auscultated.
- Routine investigations, chest X-ray, blood tests should be performed.

Stage II of Investigations

Stage II involves reviewing the history, repeating the physical examination, specific diagnostic tests and other investigations.

Check up with another physician, if required. As most common causes are infections, proper collections of specimens, examination of specimens is required. The most important investigations include:

- Blood culture
- Serological test for the detection of antibodies, i.e. febrile agglutination tests
- Widal test is done for typhoid fever, tube agglutination test for brucellosis, agglutination test for leptospirosis, Weil-Felix test for rickettsial fever, Paul-Bunnel test for EB virus, streptococcal MG test for primary atypical pneumonia.
- *Other serological tests*
  - ELISA for *CMV, E-BV*
  - CFT for Chlamydia, Rickettsia, Q fever, tularemia,
  - ASO test for rheumatic fever
  - IHA for amoebic abscess
  - ELISA for *HBV, HIV*

Other tests

- Blood test for malaria, filariasis, relapsing fever, and leishmaniasis
- **Urine culture** to rule out urinary tract infection.
- Sputum microscopy and culture for MTB and MOTT
- Look for uncommon or fastidious organisms (nutritionally variant of streptococci)
- Radiological investigations (ultrasound, CT scan, MRI) should be performed.

Stage III of Investigations

It consists of invasive tests: Bone marrow biopsy, liver biopsy and other samples may be collected.

Stage IV of Investigations

Therapeutic trials: Trials of steroids, trial of anti-tuberculosis drugs may be tried and the response is judged.

76

Emerging and Reemerging Infections

Factors Responsible

- Rapid population growth
- Rapid urbanization without planning
- Overcrowding
- Poor sanitation
- Development of resistance to antibiotics by bacteria
- Inadequate health infrastructures
- Increased exposure of humans to vectors and reservoirs of diseases

List of Emerging Infections

From 1973-1991

- *Rotavirus*
- *Parvovirus*
- *Cryptosporidium parvum*
- *Ebola virus*
- *Legionella*
- *Hantaan virus*
- *Campylobacter*
- *Hepatitis E virus*

- *Hepatitis C virus*
- *Shanghi fever*

Since 1993

- Vibrio 139
- *Bartonella henselae—cat-scratch disease*
- *Sin nombre virus*
- *Sabina virus*
- *H5N1*
- *Nipah virus*
- *Coronavirus—SARS*

Reemerging

The term reemerging diseases is used to diseases which were previously controlled by chemotherapy and antibiotics but now they have developed resistance and are often presenting as epidemic forms.

- Multiple drug resistant TB, extensively drug resistant TB
- Drug resistant malaria
- Vancomycin resistant enterococci
- *MRSA*, penicillin resistant pneumococci.

77

Pyogenic Infections

Infections caused by pus producing bacteria are known as pyogenic infections. The infections caused by them include superficial infections, wound infections, abscesses.

Pyogenic Bacteria

Organisms producing pyogenic infection are:
- *Staphylococcus aureus*
- *Streptococcus pyogenes*
- *Staphylococcus epidermidis*
- *Streptococcus pneumoniae*
- *E. coli*
- *Klebsiella pneumoniae*
- *Proteus mirabilis*
- *Pseudomonas aeruginosa*
- *Acinetobacter*
- *Enterobacter*
- *Citrobacter*
- *Provedentia*
- *Haemophilus influenzae*
- *Serratia*
- *Peptostreptococcus*
- *Bacteroides fragilis*
- *Meningococci*
- *C. albicans*

Examples of Pyogenic Infections

Aerobic
- *Skin infections*: Folliculitis, sties, carbuncles, furuncles
- *Wound infections*: Which can be classified as **hospital acquired or surgical wound infections**.
- Burn infections
- *Abscesses*: Lung abscess, liver abscess,
- Cellulitis
- Peritonitis

Anaerobic: Intra-abdominal abscess, injection abscess, brain abscess caused by *B. fragilis*.

> **Importance of gross examination**
> - Pus in *Staphylococcus aureus* infection is creamy and thick in consistency.
> - Pus in streptococcal infection is generally straw color, watery, with lysis of pus cells seen on microscopy.
> - Pus in *Proteus* infection has fishy smell.
> - Pus in *Pseudomonas* infection is sweet, musty or grape-like and often blue pigment will be seen.
> - Pus in case of infection by *Actinomyces* contain small sulfur granule, in fungal mycetoma, black granules are seen.
> - The pus of amoebic liver abscess is ancovy sauce like.
> - Foul smelling pus is seen in anaerobic infections.

78

Bloodstream Infections

Definitions

1. **Bacteremia**: Presence of bacteria in blood is called bacteremia. It may be transient during minor activities as brushing teeth or during dental procedure. Such bacteremia is taken care by phagocytic cells hence it may or may not manifest clinically.

2. **Septicemia**: Presence and multiplication of bacteria in blood and formation of toxic products in blood. For example, septicemia caused by Gram-negative bacteria, in these conditions bacteria are multiplying in blood and toxemia is due to lipopolysaccharides present on cell wall of Gram-negative bacteria.

3. **Toxemia**: Formation of toxic products in blood. Examples of toxemia are infection with bacteria as *Corynebacterium diphtheriae* and gas gangrene in which bacteria have either no invasive power or they are only locally invasive and multiply at the site of infection, produce toxins which enter blood and cause toxemia.

4. **Pyemia**: It means septicemia caused by pyogenic bacteria with multiple abscesses in internal organs as kidney, liver, spleen and brain.

Predisposing Factors

- *Impaired host defenses*: Severe neutropenia, malnutrition, malabsorption, congenital immunodeficiency, diabetes, uremia, hepatic failure, aplastic anemia, immunosuppressive therapy, low birth weight, prematurity, nephrotic syndrome, extreme age, deficiencies of humoral immunity and cell- mediated immunity.
- *Pre-existing localized sepsis*: Urinary tract infection, abdominal sepsis, Gram-negative pneumonia, infection of burns, pelvic inflammatory diseases, peritonitis, osteomyelitis.
- *Instrumentation and surgery*: Surgery of urinary tract, urinary catheterization, cystoscopy, transrectal prostatic biopsy, tracheostomy, intravenous therapy (central venous line), surgery on large intestine.

Etiology

Gram-negative bacilli
- *E. coli*
- *Klebsiella sp.*
- *Proteus sp.*
- *Pseudomonas aeruginosa*
- *Salmonella sp.*
- *Enterobacter*
- *Citrobacter*
- *Providentia*
- *Morganella morganii*
- *Acinetobacter*
- *Bacteroides*
- *Fusobacteria*
- *Brucella sp.*
- *Legionella*
- *Borrelia sp.*
- *Yersinia sp.*
- *Coxiella burnetii*

Gram-positive cocci
- *Staphylococcus aureus*
- *Streptococcus pneumoniae*
- *Streptococcus pyogenes*
- *Enterococci*
- *Group B streptococci*
- *Viridans streptococci*
- *Peptostreptococci*
- *Group C and G streptococci*

Gram-negative cocci
Neisseria meningitidis

Gram-positive bacilli
Bacillus anthracis.

Fungi
- *Candida albicans* and other *Candida species* as *C. tropicalis, C. parapsilosis* and *C. glabrata*
- *Histoplasma capsulatum*
- *Mucor sp.*

- *Aspergillus sp.*
- *Blastomyces dermatitidis*
- *Coccidioides imitis*
- *Cryptococcus neoformans*

Approach to Laboratory Diagnosis

Blood Culture (Fig. 78.1)

Collection of blood: Skin over the vein is disinfected by applying 2% tincture iodine, followed by 80%

Clean the skin with spirit, allow it dry, collect 5–10 ml of blood by venipuncture directly in blood culture media (containing Hartely's broth or tripticase soy broth or brain heart infusion broth or combination of glucose broth and taurocholate broth

Incubate blood cultures for 48 hours

Subculture on solid media (blood agar, MacConkey's medium)

Incubate plates for 18–24 hours at 37°C

After incubation, observe plates, note down colony morphology, prepare smear from colony, note down motility and put up biochemical tests

Also put up antibiotic susceptibility
Report sensitivity pattern along with the pathogen

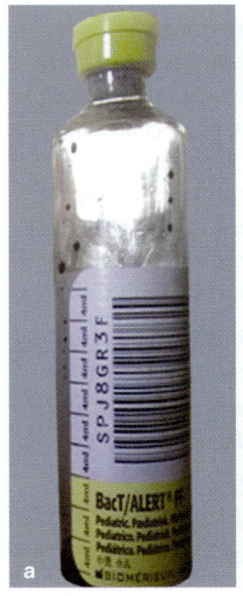 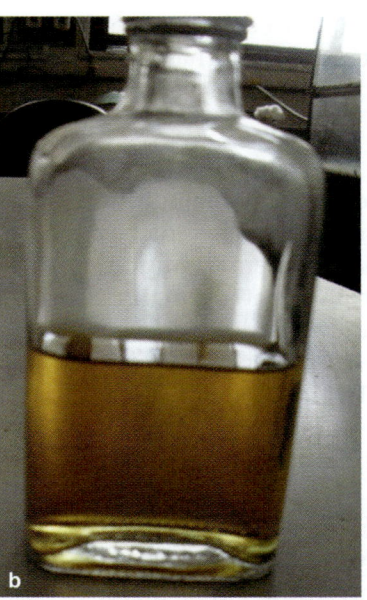

Fig. 78.1: Blood cultue bottles: (a) Automated (for BacT) and (b) conventional

isopropyl alcohol, apply tourniquet. Collect 10 mL of blood in sterile needle and syringe and add it directly to blood culture bottle.

Blood culture media

- Some laboratories use two different bottles; one containing glucose broth which supports the growth of Gram-positive organisms and taurocholate broth which inhibits the growth of cocci
- Trypticase soy broth
- *Brain heart infusion broth*: It has the advantage that it nicely supports the growth of fungi. Other advantage of BHIB is that it also supports growth of anaerobes.
- Thioglycolate broth is used for anaerobes.
- Hartey's broth

Proportion of blood and medium: Blood should be diluted 1:10, to dilute inhibitory substances present in it.

Additives in blood culture bottle

- *SPS*: Sodium polyanethol sulphonate (SPS) has antiphagocytic, anticomplementary activity also it acts as anticoagulant. It also inhibits the action of antibiotic, aminoglycoside. Disadvantage of SPS: It inhibits growth of common *Peptostreptococcus* species.
- If patient has taken antibiotic, it is inhibited by adding enzyme penicillinase.
- Ion exchange resins, which adsorb antibiotic, can be added to blood culture bottle.
- Lysis centrifugation method: It ensures lysis of clot, releases bacteria in the medium.

Castaneda's Blood Culture

Castaneda's blood culture medium is **biphasic medium,** for example, tryptic soy broth and tryptic soy agar. Blood is inoculated in broth and after 48 hours of incubation, it is tilted so that broth runs over the agar slant, thus subculture is not required, as it is required in other media. Manipulations are avoided which will decrease the chances of contamination. This medium minimizes the material. It also reduces the risk of transmission of infection to laboratory workers.

Automated blood culture system: BACTEC system and **Vitek system** are in use.

Processing of blood culture: Blood culture bottles are incubated at 37°C for 48 hours in incubator and after this subculture is done on solid media; Blood agar, MacConkey's medium. The pathogen is identified by colony characteristic, Gram-stained smear from colony and biochemical tests. For identification of *Salmonella typhi*, agglutination is done on slide with polyvalent antiserum (A-G) and then with group D antiserum.

Other methods for diagnosis of bacteremia, septicemia: Limulus amoebocyte assay is used for detection of endotoxin of Gram-negative bacteria.

Automated Blood Culture Systems (Fig. 78.1)

- *BACTEC*: 730: Infrared detection of CO_2 (30 tests)
- *BACTEC*: 660: Infrared detection of CO_2 (600 tests)
- *BACTEC*: 860: Infrared detection of CO_2 (480 tests)
- *BACTEC*: 9240: Fluorescence (240 tests).

BacT/ALERT: Colorimetric CO_2 detection (240/units, 4 units/system (960).

79

Sexually Transmitted Infections

Sexually transmitted diseases or infections are communicable diseases caused by sexual contact.

Etiology

Top 10 Sexually transmitted infections

Organism	Disease
Treponema pallidum	Syphilis—Hard chancre
Haemophilus ducreyi	Soft chancre
Neisseria gonorrhoeae	Gonorrhea
Chlamydia trachomatis	L1, L2, L3-
L1, L2, L3 and D-K	Lymphogranuloma venereum D-K nonspecific urethritis
Herpes simplex virus 1 and 2	Genital herpes
HIV	AIDS
HBV	Hepatitis
HPV	Genital warts
Candida albicans	Vaginitis, balanitis
Trichomonas vaginalis	Vaginitis, vaginal discharge

Other STI or STDs

- *Calmatobacter granulomatis* causes granuloma inguinale.
- *Trichomonas vaginalis* causes vaginitis.
- *Ureaplasma* and *Mycoplasma* cause nonspecific or nongonococcal urethritis.
- *Sarcoptis scabies* causes scabies.
- *Phthirus pubis* causes pediculosis pedis.

Laboratory Diagnosis

Specimens collected are:

- Urethral discharge from cases of gonococcal and nongonococcal urethritis.
- Vaginal discharge from cases of vaginitis.
- Scrapings from ulcers or vesicles.
- *Serum for serological tests*: Antigen detection or antibody detection.
- Swabs from vagina or from ulcers.

Alginate or dacron swabs are recommended over cotton swabs as cotton swab absorbs material and inhibits bacteria, if they are to be used, they are coated with charcoal.

Transport of Specimens

Modified Stuart's transport medium or Amie's medium used, it is recommended to inoculate plates bedside of patient as some of the pathogens are delicate.

Microscopy

Gram's staining

- *Gonococcal discharge*: Observe intracellular Gram-negative diplococci (inside pus cells).
- Observe for Gram-positive budding yeast cell with or without pseudohyphae.
- Observe for **'clue cells'** and other flora in case of bacterial vaginosis. (Clue cells are epithelial cells studded with Gram-negative coccobacilli.) (**Nugent scoring is done**).
- From a suspected case of soft chancre look for bacilli with bipolar staining

Wet mount is done from vaginal discharge, look for budding yeast cells or *Trichomonas vaginalis* and presence of pus cells.

Giemsa staining: Look for inclusion bodies of *Chlamydia*, which are basophilic, surrounding the nucleus like a shield. Look for *Calmatobacterium granulomatis*.

Fluorochrome staining is done for *T. vaginalis*, yeast cells, clue cells.

Direct immunofluorescence is used for:
- *Chlamydia trachomatis*
- *Neisseria gonorrhoeae*
- *Herpes simplex*

Electron microscope is used for viral infections.

H and E staining on biopsy: Look for inclusion bodies of *Molluscum contagiosum*.

Dark ground microscopy is used for *Treponema pallidum*.

Culture
- Modified Thayer-Martin medium for gonococci
- Chocolate agar with isovitalex for *Calmatobacterium*
- For fungus—Sabouraud's dextrose agar for *Candida sp.*

Viral and Chlamydia
- Chick embryo or continuous cell lines used for viruses and *Chlamydia*
- Growth is detected by detection of inclusion bodies or immunofluorescence or genetic probes or PCR.

Detection of Antigen
ELISA: Chlamydia, Cytomegalovirus.

Other tests are LA, immunochromatography tests.

Antibodies Detection
Syphilis: VDRL and specific tests as TPA, TPHA, FTA-ABS.

ELISA for *HIV*

Genetic tests: DNA probes.

PCR is used for most organisms especially for non-cultivable organisms as **HPV, HSV, HCV, HBV, HIV, Chlamydia.**

Syndromic Approach
(This policy is followed by Government of India).

1. Ulcerative Lesions
- *Treponema pallidum* produces hard chancre.
- *Haemophilus ducreyi* produces soft chancre.
- Painful recurrent ulcers are seen in infection with *herpes simplex 2.*
- *Calmatobacterium granulomatis.*
- *Chlamydia trachomatis L-1, L-2, L-3.*

2. Vaginal Discharge
- *Trichomanas vaginalis:* Yellow green purulent discharge, with pH >5.
- *Candidiasis:* White curdy discharge with pH <5.
- *Gardnerella vaginalis:* Grey offensive discharge, pH >5 and **fishy smell** becomes intense after addition of few drops of KOH (**Amide test).**

3. Urethritis
- Gonococccal urethritis
- Nongonococcal urethritis
- *Chlamydia trachomatis*
- *Ureaplasma*
- *Mycoplasma*
- *HSV*
- *Candida albicans*

Laboratory Diagnosis of Gonorrhea

Specimens
- Urethral, cervical smears and swabs.
- Collect discharge after prostatic massage from males in chronic cases or early morning urine or rectal swabs may also be obtained.

Collection of urethral discharge: Patient is asked to hold urine for 3 hours before collection of urethral discharge. In uncircumcised patient, the prepuce is pushed back. One has to milk urethra to ensure discharge of pus from urethra and not from glans penis. The discharge is taken by a sterile platinum loop or swab for preparation of smear and culture.

Direct Gram-Film
Intracellular Gram-negative diplococci in smears is virtually diagnosis of gonorrhea in males (95% cases). It is sometimes difficult to interpret the microscopic findings in the mixed normal flora in females. Asymptomatic carriage in male is much less common about 5% with certain types of gonococci. It is, however, common with females, especially with endocervical lesion.

Culture
Cultures are essential for medicolegal purposes and confirmation. Culture of exudate should preferably be taken directly from the patient using a wire loop and plated beside directly on preheated freshly prepared solid media. The inoculated plates are placed straight into a carbon dioxide incubator. Where there is likely to be any delay, Stuart's transport media may be used.

Media
 i. Chocolate agar
 ii. Thayer-Martin medium
iii. Modified Newyork city medium

Identification

    i. Translucent colonies are formed which are oxidase positive on addition of tetramethyl-p-phenylenediamine dihydrochloride.

    ii. It produces acid from glucose but not lactose, maltose or sucrose.

Other tests

1. Fluorescent antibody test detects gonococcus in smears.

2. Gonococcal complement fixation test (**GCFT**) is of limited value.

Diagnosis of Non-Gonococcal Urethritis or Non-specific Urethritis

Specimens (Smears and swabs from exudate of urethra or cervical discharge). Since the urethral discharge is scanty, patient should be asked to withhold urine for three hours before collection of specimen.

Detection of antigen: Smear made from exudate is examined by immunofluorescence test with a monoclonal antibody or by ELISA for detection of *C. trachomatis*. Smear stained by Giemsa stain shows intracytoplasmic inclusion bodies, suggestive of *C. trachomatis*.

Culture: Specimen should preferably be collected in laboratory or in transport medium and should be quickly transported to laboratory or stored in the refrigerator. Specimen for culture to be collected from urethra, cervix or rectum.

Transport: Specimens are transported in SPS or SPG medium.

    The exudate is inoculated in McCoy or HeLa cell cultures treated with cycloheximide. Tissue cultures are incubated for 3 days.

Identification: Intracytoplasmic glycogen-rich inclusions in tissue culture are detected by Giemsa stain or by immunofluorescence.

Serology: Complement fixing antibody at high level appears in serum and CFT is usually positive. Micro-immunofluorescence or ELISA is useful for detection of species-specific and serovar specific antibody.

Diagnosis of LGV *(C. trachomatis, L1, L2, L3)*

- *Serological tests*: Microimmunofluorescence and complement fixation tests are useful in demonstrating rising titre of antibody.
- *Frei-type skin test* with LGV antigen, once practiced, shows delayed type of hypersensitivity.

- *Isolation*: Chlamydia can be cultivated in a variety of cells from chick embryos and mammals. They also grow in yolk sac of 6–8 day chick embryos. They produce small pock-like lesions on chorioallantoic membrane.
- *Growth is detected in cell cultures by*:
  i. Detection of inclusion bodies by Giemsa staining
  ii. Direct immunofluorescence test
- *Light microscopy*: The chlamydiae are Gram-negative. They stain blue by Castaneda's method. The inclusions in the cell cultures are better stained by Giemsa. Castaneda and Macchiavello methods are more suitable for staining chick embryo yolk sac smears.

Laboratory Diagnosis of Syphilis

Specimens

    i. *Fluid from chancre or scrapings from ulcerated secondary lesions, bubo aspirate*: Dark ground microscope (DGM) examination is done.

    ii. *Blood for serology*: Standard tests for syphilis (VDRL, RPR, VDRL-ELISA), group specific ELISA and specific tests: TPHA, TPPA (*Treponema pallidum* particulate agglutination), FTA-ABS and Western blot are performed.

Diagnosis of Chancroid *(H. ducreyi)*

Smear examination: Gram-film from the exudate shows Gram-negative ovoid bacilli. The bacteria in mass have configuration of "schools of fish".

Culture: Diagnosis is confirmed by isolation of *H. ducreyi* from an ulcer. Exudate is directly cultured on to 20–30% rabbit blood agar or on to chocolate agar with 1% isovitalex and 5% sheep serum, plus 3 mg/L of vancomycin. Plate is incubated at 20–30°C. Colonies are grey surrounded by a zone of faint hemolysis.

Diagnosis of Granuloma Inguinale

Giemsa stain: Tissue smear from the ulcer when stained by Giemsa stain, Donovan bodies may be demonstrated. The Donovan bodies are rounded coccobacilli, 1×2 µm in size, which lie within the cystic spaces in the cytoplasm of large mononuclear cells. Capsule appears as a dense acidophilic zone around the bacterium, resembling a closed safety pin or "**telephone handle**". The pathognomonic mononuclear cell measures 25–90 µm in diameter and contains many cystic areas with Donovan bodies.

Diagnosis of Herpes Genitalis

Specimen: Scrapings from base of the lesions, serum for serology are the specimens collected.

Giemsa or Wright staining or toluidine blue shows characteristic giant cells or intranuclear inclusions.

Cultivation

- Diagnosis is confirmed by tissue culture in human fibroblast cells.
- Growth is rapid, CPE occurs within 24 hours.

Serology: Complement fixation test with patient's serum is still useful in diagnosis of primary infections (antibody titre is usually within 32, especially in genital herpes).

Bacterial Vaginosis

It is a syndrome characterized by increased homogenous white discharge from vagina and malodor often described as rotten fishy smell.

Chemical Examination of Vaginal Fluid

pH: Greater than 4.5, increased pH is partly due to presence of amines and partly due to reduced production of lactate by lactobacilli.

Amide test: When vaginal fluid is mixed with a 10% solution of KOH, fishy (rotten fish smell) odor is immediately liberated. The odor is due to volatile amines present in vaginal fluid.

Saline microscopy: Vaginal discharge contains 'clue cells' (squamous epithelial cells coated with coccobacillary organisms). Leukocytes are virtually absent. Nuegent scoring is performed, look for 'clue cells'.

Gram film shows altered vaginal flora, it is largely replaced by *G. vaginalis* and other anaerobes.

Diagnosis of Trichomoniasis

- *Specimen:* Swab of vaginal discharge to be examined freshly. If delay in transport is inevitable, specimen may be collected in Stuart's transport medium, saline.
- *Microscopy:* Direct wet film shows motile trichmonads and polymorphonuclear leukocytes. Direct microscopy is at least 80% as positive as culture.
- Deposit of early morning first-voided urine or urethral swab is cultured in **Fineberg's** medium and incubated for 5 days and examined for motile protozoa at 2 and 5 days.

Diagnosis of Vulvovaginal Candidiasis

Specimen: Swab from vaginal secretions.

Microscopy

- *KOH mount:* Microscopical examination of vaginal secretions in 10% KOH show yeast cells, pseudohyphae.
- Gram film shows characteristic Gram-positive yeast cells with pseudohyphae.

Culture

Specimen is inoculated in Sabouraud's dextrose agar and incubated for 48 hours at 37°C. The colonies are typically pasty. The fungi are identified by the formation of Germ tubes in serum, formation of chlamydospores in nutritionally poor medium (cornmeal agar), sugar assimilation tests.

Diagnosis of Genital Warts

- Detection of *HPV* is done by polymerase chain reaction.
- Cytological or histological examination of cells in urine is used for detection of inclusion bodies of *HPV*.

80

Universal Safety Precautions (USP)

Components of USP

a. Hand hygiene (washing)
b. Personal protective equipment (PPE)
c. Disinfection and sterilization
d. Management of spills
e. Needle stick injuries management
f. Post-exposure prophylaxis
g. Vaccination against HBV.

Hand hygiene—washing with plain soap and water is very effective.

Personal protective equipment: Gloves, masks, protective glasses or eyeshields, plastic aprons are used.

Precautions for Laboratories

- Mechanical pipetting devices should be used for manipulating all liquids in the laboratory. Mouth pipetting must not be done.
- Use of needles and syringes should be limited and the recommendations for preventing injuries with needles should be followed. Avoid recapping needle.
- Laboratory work surfaces should be decontaminated with an appropriate chemical germicide when work activities are completed.
- Contaminated materials used in laboratory tests should be decontaminated before disposal in accordance with institutional policies for disposal of infective waste.

- Scientific equipment that has been contaminated with blood or other body fluids should be decontaminated and cleaned before being repaired in the laboratory or transported to the manufacturer.
- All persons should wash their hands after completing laboratory activities and should remove protective clothing before leaving the laboratory.

Management of Spills

Immediate measure: Cover spills for 10 min with 1% NaHOCl or bleach and dispose.

Disinfectants effective in inactivating HIV: Chlorine releasing agents, Na-hypochloroide.

Prevent Needle Stick Injuries

- Needles should not be recapped, bent or broken by hand, or removed from disposable syringes, or otherwise manipulated by hand.
- After they are used, disposable syringes and needles, scalpel blades, and other sharp items should be placed in puncture-resistant containers for disposal; the puncture-resistant containers should be located as close as possible to the working area.
- Large bore reusable needles should be placed in a puncture-resistant container for transport to the reprocessing area.

81

Biomedical Waste Disposal

HOSPITAL WASTE

Any waste generated in diagnosis, treatment, immunization or research is called biomedical waste.

Categories of Waste (Table 81.1)

- *Non-hazardous waste*: 80%
- *Biomedical waste (hazardous)*: 15%
- *Hazardous but noninfectious*: 5%
  Hazardous waste is medical or clinical waste.

Biomedical waste management involves

- **Segregation** of waste at the point of generation.
- Disinfection of waste at source, if needed.
- Correct disposal ensuring complete destruction of microorganisms.

Objective of Waste Management Scheme

- Changing the mindset through training.
- Segregating waste so that each type is treated in suitable manner according to the rules.
- Use proper disinfection technology.
- Creating a system where all personnel in the hospital are responsible and accountable for proper waste management.

- Changing use patterns from single usage to multiple usages.
- Minimize health hazards associated with poor hospital waste management.
- Injuries from sharps to all categories of hospital personnel is prevented.
- Nosocomial infection in patient from poor infection control and poor hospital waste management are minimized.
- Risks of infection outside hospital for waste-handlers and eventually the general public are reduced.

The advent of *HBV, HIV* made it necessary that hospital waste disposal systems are improved.

Routes of Transmission of Infection from Infectious Waste

- Through non-intact skin (cuts or raw areas) by cuts and puncture.
- Through mucous membrane, e.g. splashing into eyes.
- Through inhalation of dust particles containing organisms.
- Through ingestion through unwashed hands or contaminated water or food.

TABLE 81.1: Categories of biomedical waste

Category	Biomedical waste	Treatment option
1.	Human anatomical waste	Incineration/deep burial
2.	Animal waste	Incineration/deep burial
3.	Microbiology and biotechnology waste	Autoclaving/microwaving/incineration
4.	Sharps	Disinfection (chemical treatment—mutilation/shredding)
5.	Cytotoxic drugs/discarded	Incineration/destruction and drug's disposal in medicines secured landfills
6.	Solid waste contaminated with blood, body fluids	Incineration/autoclaving/microwving
7.	Solid waste (tubings, catheters, IV sets, etc.)	Autoclaving/microwaving disinfection by chemical treatment and mutilation and shredding
8.	Liquid waste	Disinfection by chemical treatment and discharge into drains
9.	Incineration ash	Disposal in Municipal Landfill
10.	Chemical waste	Chemical treatment and discharge into drains for liquids and secured landfill for solids.

Biomedical waste management protocol contains following things:

- Segregation (Table 81.2), transportation and storage.
- Infectious waste should not be mixed with other wastes.
- Waste should be segregated at the point of generation into appropriate containers or color-coded bags (Table 81.3).
- Containers or bags should have biohazard sign for infectious material.
- If container is to be transported outside, the institution it should have proper information as prescribed.
- Waste should be transported in vehicle authorized for this purpose by competent authority.
- Infectious waste should not be stored beyond 48 hours.

Waste Treatment

- *Chemical disinfection*: It is first step before final disposal of contaminated materials, e.g. sputum, pus.
- *Deep burial*: After disinfection materials are placed in deep trenches. Trenches are filled with soil and covered with lime.
- **Incineration** is safe method for soiled infectious materials, human anatomical waste.
- Laboratories use **autoclave.**
- **Microwaving** is useful for small volume waste which can be disposed at the site of generation.
- **Hydroclave** is equally safe and reliable method.
- Liquid waste is treated with disinfectants or reagents, neutralized and finally flushed in sewer.

TABLE 81.2: Segregation of biomedical waste

Category of waste	Contents	Container
Non-infective household waste	Kitchen, pantry waste, etc.	Black plastic bags to be tied when 3/4th full
Sharps	Needles, scalpel blades, IV line tips, etc.	Puncture-proof sharp containers to be filled only till 3/4th capacity, then close the mouth
Non-sharp infective waste	Soiled linen, cotton, gauze, organs, tissues, used blood bags, catheters, urine bags, Ryle's tube, IV infusion sets, syringes, etc.	Red plastic bags to be tied when 3/4th full
	Human anatomical waste and animal waste, e.g. placenta, organs, etc.	Yellow plastic bags to be tied when 3/4th full

TABLE 81.3: Color coding

Colour coding	Type of container	Waste category	Treatment options
Yellow	Plastic bag	1, 2, and 5	Incineration and deep burial
Red	Plastic bag	3, 6 and 7	Autoclaving/microwaving and chemical treatment
Black	Plastic bag	5, 9, 10 and non-infectious waste	Disposal in secured landfill

82

Urinary Tract Infection

Presence and multiplication of bacteria in urinary system is called urinary tract infection. It is associated with presence of bacteria in significant number, i.e. 1,00,000 per mL in clean catched midstream sample.

Types of UTI

a. *Upper UTI*: Infection of kidney and ureters.
b. *Lower UTI*: Infection of urinary bladder, urethra and prostatic glands.
   i. *Ascending UTI*: Organisms that are present in perineum region cause infection and they travel upward.
   ii. *Descending UTI*: It is due to hematogenous spread.

Clinical Presentation

a. *Frequency and dysuria syndrome*: Dysuria, frequency of micturition sometimes accompanied by suprapubic pain.
b. **Bacterial cystitis** is characterized by significant bacteriuria and often **pyuria** and hematuria.
c. **Abacterial cystitis,** when no bacteria is demonstrated.
d. *Bacterial pyelonephritis*: Characterized by pain in renal area, tenderness, fever accompanied by bacteriuria and **pyuria.**
e. *Covert bacteriuria*: Asymptomatic bacteriuria found during screening of urine.

Predisposing Factors

1. *Age*: Infection increases with age.
2. *Sex*: UTI is common in females due to short urethra, its closeness to anus which has normal flora and urethral trauma during intercourse.
3. *Pregnancy*: Stasis of urine, dilation of ureters and pelvis, incompetence of vesicoureteral valves act as predisposing factors.

4. *Structural or neurological abnormality of urinary tract*: This leads to residual urine and increases chance of infection.
5. Instrumentation and surgery.
6. Diabetes.
7. *Immunosuppression*: Steroids and cytotoxic drugs given to transplant recepient increases infections.
8. Abnormalities of urinary tract predisposing to UTI.

Abnormality	Comments
Vesicoureteral reflux	May cause intrarenal lesions due to back pressure
Urethral stricture	Common causes of obstruction
Ureterocele	
Calculus formation	Common causes of obstruction
Prostatic hypertrophy	
Bladder diverticulum	
Genital prolapse	
Neurogenic bladder	Permanent indwelling catheter

Pathogenicity

Bacteria adhere to epithelial surfaces with the help of pili or colonization factors. Then they spread and cause infection.

Laboratory Diagnosis

Collection and Transport of Specimens

Clean-catched midstream urine collection: Midstream urine sample is best specimen for the diagnosis of **UTI.**

- Cleaning of local parts should be done before sample collection.
- Males should retract prepuce and clean the area with soap and water or mild detergent.
- Females should separate labia with two fingers and should clean the local area.

- Patient should be instructed that during voiding urine, first portion of urine should be discarded and middle portion is taken in sterile wide mouth container.

For diagnosis of renal tuberculosis, whole early morning sample is collected in sterile container for three consecutive days.

- *Stimulation of urination in children*: Urination can be stimulated in children by taping just above pubis with 2 fingers 1 hour after feed: One tap per second is given for 1 minute, an interval of one minute is allowed, then tapping is again done (making noise of water or giving warm bath may stimulate urination).
- *Suprapubic aspiration*: It has the advantage of avoiding contamination of urine from organisms from anterior part of urethra. Disadvantage is that it is an invasive procedure.
- *Note*: If sample is collected by suprapubic aspiration any bacterial count is taken as significant.
- *Catheterization*: A catheter specimen has disadvantage that urethral bacteria may be introduced into bladder.

Transport:
- Urine should be transported and processed as early as possible to avoid multiplication of contaminant bacteria.
- Also biochemical changes occur if there is delay. Pus cells will be disintegrated because of delay. If delay is anticipated, refrigerate the sample.
- Boric acid (1% W/V) may be added to container to prevent multiplication of bacteria. (Urine is processed within one hour of collection.)

Processing of Urine

- *Gross examination*: Look for turbidity when infection occurs. Urine may be reddish, if hematuria is present. (In case of chyluria, urine will be milky white).
- *Wet mount*: It is done to observe pus cells, casts and crystals; the presence of casts and crystals suggests involvement of kidney.
- Presence of more than **5 pus cells per** high power field in **uncentrifuged urine** usually correlates with infection.
- *Gram's staining*: Only one loopful of uncentrifuged urine drop is taken on a slide with standard loop, allowed to air dry and stained with Gram's staining. The one loopful sample should not be spread.
- *Importance of Gram's staining*: Presence of one or more than one bacteria per oil immersion field is used as a simple screening test for significant bacteriuria.

Other Screening Methods

1. *Catalase test*: The enzyme catalase present in pathogens will breakdown H_2O_2 and produce bubbles.
2. *Glucose oxidase test*: It is based upon utilization of small amount of glucose present in urine by bacteria.
3. *Leukocyte esterase test*: This test detects presence of pus cells and thus inflammation. Dipstick is available.
4. *Griess nitrate test*: The Gram-negative bacteria reduce nitrate to nitrites.
5. *Triphenyltetrazolium test (TTC)*: Because of respiratory activity of bacteria, the TTC added to urine shows color change from colorless to pink or red color.

Culture

Semiquantitative Methods

Calibrated loop method
- In this method, a strandard loop which is calibrated and holds 0.001 mL or 0.004 mL of urine is taken. With this loop, urine sample is taken (one loopful) by holding the loop straight in urine container.
- Nichrome wire of SWG 28 is used to make circular loop which holds 0.004 mL of urine, standard loop holding 0.001 mL are also commertially available.
- One loopful is taken on BA and MacConkey's medium. Inoculation is done by "T"streaking method. The plates are then incubated at 37°C in incubator.
- After overnight incubation, the total numbers of colonies are counted on blood agar plate. A single organism present in original sample will multiply overnight and will form one colony forming unit (CFU). The total numbers of organisms in sample are calculated as follows:
  - Total number of bacteria per mL of urine = No. of colonies × 1000. (For loop of 0.001 mL.)

Dip slide technique: In this method, commercially available plastic slides coated with media are used in which MacConkey's medium on one slide and CLED medium on other slide. It is dipped in the urine and incubated. After incubation, colonies are counted.

Quantitative Methods

Pour plate method: Urine sample is diluted tenfold, one mL of urine is added to melted and cooled blood agar (at 45°C), mixed well and then poured in petridish. After overnight incubation, blood agar is observed and total number of colonies produced are counted. Though the method is standard, it is cumbersome.

Other **automated methods** are available based on photometry or Vitek system.

***Interpretation of colonies*: Kass concept of significant bacteriuria** is applied for interpretation of results.

- According to these criteria, 100000 (10^5/mL) or more bacteria per mL of urine collected by clean catched midstream method indicates significant counts and infection of UTI is diagnosed.
- If counts are below 10000 per mL of urine it is considered non-significant and it is due to contamination.
- Colony counts in between 100000/mL and 10000/mL are doubtful significance and a repeat sample is asked for and history especially whether the patient is on diuretic and antibiotic is taken.

Following are the conditions where low counts can be significant:

- Patients partially treated with antibiotics
- Patients on diuretics
- Acute urethral syndrome
- Pure culture of *Staphylococcus aureus* regardless of counts
- Growth of *Candida*—any count significant. This infection is seen in diabetes. Ensure that the sample processed is not collected from bag.

Pyuria is presence of pus cells in urine. **Sterile pyuria** means pus cells are present but routine culture is negative. Consider fastidious organism as *Mycobacterium* (urethritis), *Chlamydia*, *Mycoplasma*, and *Ureaplasma*. **Bacteriuria without pyuria** may be seen in diabetic patients.

Identification

The culture is identified by biochemical tests.

Biochemical reactions of common urinary pathogens are as follows (Table 82.1):

- All members of Enterobacteriaceae are catalase positive and oxidase negative.
- These include *E. coli*, *Klebsiella*, and *Proteus* of which only *Proteus* and *Klebsiella pneumoniae* are urease positive.
- Only *Pseudomonas* is oxidase positive.

Localization of Infection

This is done by direct method as ureteric catheterization.

Indirect tests

- Detection of antibody coated bacteria is done by *Staphylococcus* coagglutination test. If this is positive, it is infection of upper urinary tract.
- Antibodies to infecting organisms in serum: Serum antibodies to 'o' antigen of *E. coli* are found in high titers in patients with pyelonephritis compared to bladder infection.

Antibiotics tested are trimethoprim, cotrimoxazole, ampicillin or augmentin, nalidixic acid, nitrofurantoin (for bladder infections), gentamicin and cefotaxime.

Automated Urine Culture Systems

BAC-T-SCREEN 2000

- *Principle*: Colorimetric filtration—bacteria and leukocytes are trapped in a filter and detected by a residual pink color remaining from saffranin O dye.
- *Detection time*: ≤ 2 minutes.

UTI screen

- *Principle*: Bioluminescence—bacterial ATP is measured by an enzymatic bioluminescence reaction of ATP with luciferin and luciferase.
- Instrument used is Luminometer
- *Detection time*: 10–45 min.

Vitek

- *Photometry*: Detection of growth is based on changes in light transmitted.
- *Detection time*: 1–13 hours, also enumerates and identifies common urinary pathogens.

Etiological Agents

Bacterial Causes

- *E. coli*
- *Proteus mirabilis*
- *Klebsiella sp.*
- *Pseudomonas aeruginosa*

TABLE 82.1: Biochemical tests of common urinary pathogens

Organism	Indole	MR test	VP test	Citrate test	Triple sugar iron agar (TSI)
E. coli	+	+	–	–	A/A with gas
Klebsiella	–	–	+	+	A/A/with gas
Proteus	Variable Positive in *Proteus vulgaris* and negative in *Proteus mirabilis*	+	–	+	K/A, H$_2$S
Pseudomonas	–	–	–	+	No change

- *Enterobacter*
- *Citrobacter*
- *Providentia*
- *Morganella moganii*
- *Acinetobacter sp.*
- *Enterococci*
- *Alkaligenus fecalis*
- *Serratia sp.*
- *Staphylococcus epidermidis*
- *Staphylococcus saprophyticus (infection in young sexually active women)*
- *Staphylococcus aureus*
- *Bacteroides fragilis*

Salmonella may be present in urine but it does not cause UTI.

Hospital-acquired infections are caused by *Pseudomonas, Proteus, Klebsiella sp.,* enterococci, *Enterobacter, Acinetobacter, Serratia.*

Following organisms cause **urethritis**
- *Neisseria gonorrhoeae*
- *Chlamydia trachomatis D-K*
- *Ureaplasma urealyticum*
- *Mycoplasma hominis*

Viral Causes
- *Herpes simplex virus*
- *Adenovirus*
- *CMV*
- *HPV*

Fungal
- *Candida albicans*
- *Cryptococcus neoformans (rarely)*
- *Histoplasma capsulatum (rarely)*

Parasites
- *Schistosoma haematobium*
- *Trichomonas vaginalis.*

83

Antimicrobial Susceptibility Testing

Why test antimicrobial susceptibility?

- To determine whether or not the infecting organism is susceptible to a series of antibiotics that might be used in the treatment of disease.
- To determine susceptibility of the organism to a single concentration of antibiotic, the concentration chosen being related to the concentration found in the infected site.
- These guidelines are usually based on the serum levels attainable by the antibiotic but sometimes related to antibiotic levels in urine, bile, sputum, sinus fluid, etc.
- To produce survey data on the current prevalence of resistant strains in the community or hospital unit.
- Survey data may be used to draw policies for the use of antibiotics.
- In the busy diagnostic laboratory, the most common method of antimicrobial susceptibility testing is disk diffusion method.

ANTIBIOTIC SENSITIVITY TESTS

Procedure

- Solid culture medium is evenly inoculated with the test organism and blotting paper disks containing antibiotics are placed on the surface.
- During incubation, antibiotic diffuses radially from the disk into the medium.
- If the organism is sensitive to the drug in the concentration achieved, its growth is prevented in a circular zone around the disk (zone of inhibition).

Zone is influenced by the sensitivity of the organism. Antibiotic diffuses through the culture medium at the rate that depends on molecular size and chemical nature of antibiotic and the medium. A concentration gradient of antibiotics are formed with higher concentration close to the disk and decreasing, away from it. The critical concentration of antibiotic at which the zone edge is formed depends on sensitivity of organism and is closely related to MIC (minimum inhibitory cocentration). The distance from the disk at which the zone edge is formed is influenced by inoculum size, the growth rate of organism, incubation of the plate before the disk is applied and diffusion from the disk before incubation. The critical density of the organism at which zone edge is formed depends on antibiotic and organism.

Factors Affecting the Results of Diffusion Tests

- *Rate of diffusion of drug*: It depends on molecular weight of the agent. Penicillin has low molecular weight, polymyxin has high molecular weight.
- Chemical interaction of the agent with medium.
- *Culture medium*: An ideal medium would not contain antagonists of antibiotic activity. For example, sulphonamides—action is antagonized by media containing products of folate metabolism. The pH of the medium is 7.3.

Commercial media preferred for antimicrobial susceptibility testing are Mueller-Hinton agar and sensitest agar.

- An ideal medium should support the growth of all pathogens.
- It should not inhibit or enhance growth of any particular organism.
- It should be possible to add serum or BHIA to it for growth of fastidics organisms.

Density of inoculums: Ideal is semiconfluent growth of colonies should be present.

Methods of inoculation: It is done by flooding or swabbing to produce lawn culture of bacteria.

Flooding

1. Prepare suspension of organism of suitable density by diluting young broth cultures or emulsifying colonies in saline or broth. The turbidity of the inoculum is matched with **(0.5%) McFarland's standard.** Semiconfluent growth of colonies will be produced.
2. The suspension is applied to the medium with Pasteur pipette and the plate is tilted from side-to-side to ensure that the surface of medium is completely covered. The plate is then tilted to drain excess inoculum which is removed with Pasteur pipette. It should produce semiconfluent growth.

Swab Inoculation

4 mm loopful of overnight nutrient broth culture or suspension of similar density is placed on the medium. For wet swab method, a sterile swab is dipped into suitably diluted culture; the swab is turned against the side of the tube to remove excess fluid and is streaked across the medium.

Kirby-Bauer Method (Fig. 83.1)

Preparation of Plates

Only Mueller-Hinton medium is used. Defebrinated blood may be necessary for tests on fastidious organisms in which case the medium should be allowed to cool to 50°C before 5% blood is added. The medium should be poured into petridishes kept on a flat horizontal surface to get depth of 4 mm. Poured plates are stored at 4°C, used within one week of preparation.

Before inoculation, plates should be dried. The pH of the medium should be 7.2–7.4.

Preparation of Inoculums

- At least 4 morphologically similar colonies from an agar medium are touched with a wire loop and the growth is transferred to a test tube containing 4 mL of sterile tryptose phosphate broth or tryptic soy broth.
- The tubes are incubated for 2–5 hours at 35–37°C to produce bacterial suspension of moderate cloudiness.
- The density of the suspension is standardized by dilution with sterile saline or broth to a density visually equivalent to barium-sulfate standard. (0.5 McFarland's standard).
- Comparison should be made against a white background with, contrasting black line with the **McFarland's standard.**

Inoculation

- A sterile cotton wool swab is dipped into the suspension and excess is removed by rotation of the swab against the side of the tube above the fluid level.
- The medium is inoculated by even streaking of the swab over the entire surface of the plate in three directions.
- After the inoculum has dried, disks are applied one by one with forceps and pressed gently to ensure even contact with the medium.

Not more than 6 disks are applied on 8.5 cm circular plate and 12 on 13.5 cm circular plate.

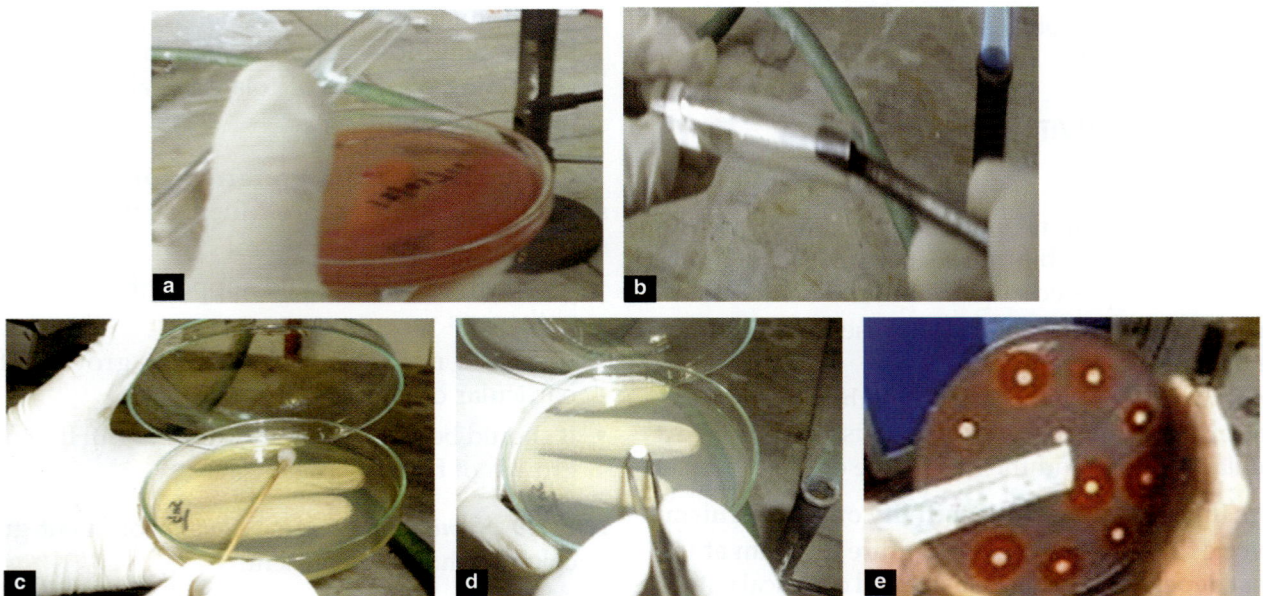

Fig. 83.1: (a) Take colonies from medium, (b) emulsify colonies in broth , (c) swab the MHA plate, (d) put antibiotic disks. Then incubate the plate at 37°C , and (e) Measure the zone of inhibition around the antibiotic disks

(Disks should be stored at 4°C in sealed containers with desiccant and should be allowed to come to room temperature before the containers are opened.)

Incubation: After the disks are placed on MHA, the plate of MHA is incubated for 16–18 hours at 35–37°C.

Reading of Zones of Inhibition

The diameters of zones are measured to the nearest millimeter with calipers, dividers or millimeter rule. The point of abrupt diminution of growth which corresponds with the point of complete inhibition of growth is taken as zero edge.

Interpretation

- *Sensitive*: Infection treatable with normal dosage.
- *Intermediate*: Infection that may respond to therapy with higher dosage.
- *Resistant*: Infection not treatable with this agent.

Control culture: Results of disk diffusion test may vary with number of parameters, hence it is necessary to evaluate results by comparing with the results of control strains of standard organism of known susceptibility. The controls used are:

- *Staphylococcus aureus*: ATCC 25923
- *E. coli*: ATCC 25922
- *Pseudomonas aeruginosa*: ATCC 27853
- *Enterococcus faecalis*: ATCC 29212
- *Haemophilus influenzae*: ATCC 49247
- *Neisseria gonorrhoeae*: ATCC 49226
- **ATCC represents for American type culture collection.**

Stokes Method

It is similar to Kirby-Bauer method, only change is that control and test cultures are grown on the same plate to compare the zones of inhibition produced in the two cultures by the same disks.

The test organism is inoculated on middle third of culture plate and control culture on upper and lower thirds, leaving an uninoculated space of about 5 mm between the test and control areas, which is used for placing disks. After inoculation, disks are placed, three on each side between control and test inocula. The plates are then incubated at 37°C in incubator.

Reading

The results are interpreted by measuring and comparing the zones of inhibition of control and test bacteria.

- *Sensitive*: If zone of inhibition produced by test bacterium is equal to or larger or not less than 3 mm than that of control strain.

- *Intermediate sensitive*: If the zone diameter of test bacterium is at least 2 mm and difference between test and control strain is 3 mm.
- *Resistant*: If the zone of inhibition of test bacterium is less than 2 mm.

Advantages

- Test is simple and reliable
- It can be easily set in routine laboratory.
- As test as well as control bacteria are inoculated on the same plate, the parameter is equal to both and reading is easy to take.

Uses of Minimum Inhibitory Concentration (MIC)

- Indications of MIC for testing antimicrobial susceptibility with *Mycobacterium tuberculosis*.
- For testing antimicrobial susceptibility for the anaerobic organisms.
- For testing antimicrobial susceptibility for fungi.
- For swarming organisms like *Proteus mirabilis*.
- For organisms isolated from the blood of patients with endocarditis, especially that of antibiotics of which the dosage can be varied widely.
- In the investigations of new drugs in comparison with other closely related drugs when their activity can only be compared on a weight basis.

MIC can be obtained by broth dilution or agar dilution method.

Broth Dilution Method (Fig. 83.2)

Twofold dilutions of an antibiotic are prepared and inoculated with the test organism; **the MIC** (minimum inhibitory concentration) is calculated by observing the tube showing no growth.

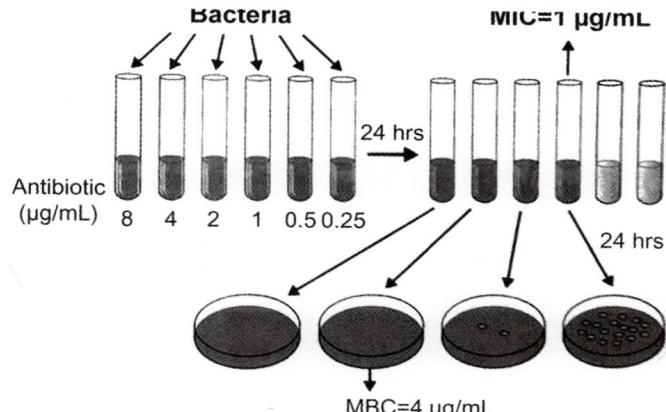

Fig. 83.2: Broth dilution method for determination of MIC and MBC

Minimum bactericidal concentration (MBC) is calculated by subculturing the test tubes showing no visible growth. The minimum dilution which shows no growth is the minimum bactericidal concentration (MBC).

Epsilometer (E) stripes (Fig. 83.3): This E-stripes are commercially available for each antibiotic and organism. The stripe has graded concentration of antibiotic, when it is placed on MHA inoculated with test organism, the point value where the zone of inhibition intersects the stripe is the MIC of the drug. The test is simple to perform. Disadvantage is that E stripes are costly.

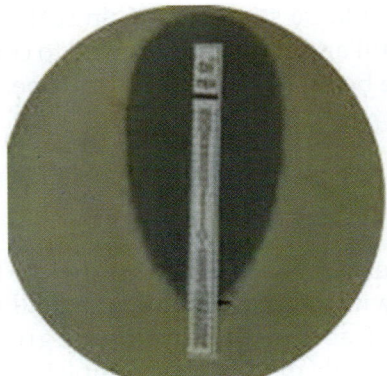

Fig. 83.3: Epsilometer

84

Antimicrobial Chemotherapy

Following are the mechanisms of action of antimicrobials:

1. Inhibition of cell wall synthesis
2. Inhibition of cell membrane synthesis
3. Inhibition of protein synthesis (i.e. inhibiton of transcription and translation of genetic material)
4. Inhibition of nucleic acid synthesis.

Inhibition of Cell Wall Synthesis

All β lactam antibiotics are selective inhibitors of bacterial cell wall synthesis and active against growing bacteria. Attachment of PBP (penicillin binding protein) may result in abnormal elongation of cell, but attachment to another PBP causes defects in cell wall with lysis. When β lactam drug attaches to PBP, transpeptidation reaction is inhibited, peptidoglycan synthesis is blocked. Acitvity of β lactam antibiotics depends upon structural differences in bacteria which is necessary for penetration, binding and activity of the drugs. Penicillins and cephalosporins are major antibiotics in this group.

Inhibition of Cell Membrane Synthesis

Polymyxins consist of cyclic peptides which damage cytoplasmic membrane of bacterial cell. **Nalidixic acids** and novobiocin interfere with biosynthetic functions of cytoplasmic membrane.

Daptomycin binds to cell membrane in Ca ion dependent manner, causing depolarization of bacterial membrane protein. Other drugs acting by inhibition of cell membrane function are amphotericin B, colistin, and imidazoles.

Inhibition of Protein Synthesis

Macrolides, lincosamide, tetracycline, aminogycoside, and chloramphenicol inhibit protein synthesis; the mechanisms of action differ in different groups. Bacteria have 70S ribosomes while humans have 80S ribosomes, hence this group of antibiotics selectively inhibit bacterial protein synthesis.

Macrolides, as erythromycin, clarithromycin, roxithromycin, bind to the 70S subunit of ribosome. They interfere with formation of initiation complexes for peptide chain synthesis.

Lincosamides, as clindamycin and lincomycin, bind to 50S subunit and resemble macrolides in binding sites and mode of action.

Tetracyclines: They bind selectively to 30S subunit of ribosome, inhibit protein synthesis.

Glycyclines: These are synthetic drugs similar to tetracycline. Tigecycline inhibits protein synthesis like tetracycline, but they bind more avidly to ribosomes. This antibiotic is active against large range of Gram-positive and Gram-negative bacteria.

Chloramphenicol: It binds to 50S subunit of ribosomes, interferes with binding of new amino acids to nascent polypeptide chains.

Streptogramins: Quinupristin, dalfopristin, these two drugs act synergistic. They bind irreversibly to different sites on the 50S subunits. They are active against Gram-positive bacteria.

Inhibition of Nucleic Acid Synthesis

Examples of drug acting by inhibition of nucleic acid synthesis are quinolones, pyrimethamine, sulphonamide, trimethoprim and rifampin.

Rifampin inhibits bacterial growth by binding strongly to DNA dependent RNA polymerase of bacteria. Hence, it inhibits bacterial RNA synthesis.

All **quinolones** and fluoroquinolones block DNA gyrases, topoisomerases that play role in DNA replication and repair.

PABA is involved in synthesis of folic acid which is precursor to synthesis of nucleic acids. **Sulphonamides** are structurally similar to PABA and inhibit dihydropteroate synthase.

Trimethoprim inhibits dihydrofolic acid reductase, the enzyme which reduces dihydrofolic acid to tetrahydrofolic acid, leading to synthesis of purines. Sulphonamide and trimethoprim act synergistically and used in treatment of urinary tract infections, systemic *Salmonella* infections, Shigella enteritis, and Pneumocystis pneumonia.

Mechanisms of (Antibiotic) Drug Resistance

Production of enzymes: *Staphylococcus aureus* produces enzyme beta-lactamase that destroys penicillin binding proteins. Gram-negative bacteria are resistant to aminoglycoside due to production of enzymes, adenylating, phosphorylating or acetylating enzymes which destroy the antibiotic.

Production of altered enzymes: Bacteria can produce altered enzyme which can perform its metabolic function.

Types of Drug Resistance

It is of two types, i.e. **intrinsic or inherent drug resistance** and **acquired** resistance.

a. *Intrinsic (inherent) drug resistance:* It is resistance resulting from normal genetic, structural or physiological state of bacteria. It is considered natural and it is consistently inherited characteristic. This type of resistance is predictable, hence once bacterium is isolated, certain aspects of its resistance profile are already known. Following are the examples of intrinsic resistance:

Anaerobic bacteria	Amino glycosides
Klebsiella	Ampicilin
Enterococci	Cephalosporin
Pseudomonas	Sulphonamides, trimethoprim, tetracyclines, chloramphenicol
Aerobic bacteria	Metronidazole
Gram-positive bacteria	Azetreonam
Gram-negative bacteria	Vancomycin

b. *Acquired resistance:* It results from altered physiology, and structure caused by changes in genetic makeup of bacteria.

Resistance may be acquired by:

a. Successful genetic mutations.

b. Acquiring genes of resistance from other bacteria by any of the modes of transfer of genetic resistance.

c. Combination of mutation and genetic transfer events.

Common resistance pathways by which intrinsic resistance or acquired resistance manifests:

1. Bacteria produce enzymes which modify or destroy the drug. For exmple, *Staphylococcus aureus* produces beta-lactamase which destroys penicillin. Other beta-lactamases called **extended spectrum beta-lactamases (ESBL)** are produced by Gram-negative bacilli as *E. coli, Klebsiella*. Due to production of this ESBL, GNB are resistant to all beta-lactam antibiotics as cephalosporins, cephamycins.

   MBLs are metallobeta-lactamases: Lactamases are produced by Gram-negative bacteria as *Pseudomonas, Acinetobacter, E. coli, Klebsiella*, etc.

   Some Gram-negative bacilli are resistant to aminoglycosides (by virtue of plasmid) as they produce phosphorylating or acetylating enzymes that destroy the drug.

2. Decrease uptake or accumulation of antimicrobial agent.

3. Erythromycin resistant bacteria have altered receptor on the 50S subunit of ribosomes produced due to methylation of a 23S ribosomal RNA. Penicillin resistance in *Streptococcus pneumoniae* and *enterococci* is due to altered PBPs.

4. Uncoupling of antibiotic – target interactions have subsequent effect on bacterial metabolism.

5. Any of the above combinations.

85

Postexposure Prophylaxis

Health care workers are at low risk of acquiring HIV during management of patients. Postexposure prophylaxis **(PEP)** is a comprehensive programme in place to deal with anticipated exposure. Most of the exposures do not result in infection. The risk of infection varies with the type of exposure and other factors such as:

1. The amount of blood involved in the exposure.
2. The amount of virus in patients' blood at the time of exposure.

The exposure is defined as a percutaneous injury (e.g. needle stick or cut with a sharp instrument), contact of mucosal membrane or non-intact skin (e.g. when the exposed skin is abraded or chapped or patient has dermatitis), or contact with intact skin when duration of exposure is prolonged with blood or body fluids (semen, vaginal secretions, other body fluids conta-minated with visible blood, CSF, synovial, pleural, peritoneal, pericardial, amniotic fluids).

The PEP program is made on the basis of degree of exposure to *HIV* and *HIV* status of the source from whom the exposure has occurred. The exposure code is categorized as in Flowchart 85.1, *HIV* status code is classified as in Flowchart 85.2, and determination of PEP is given in Table 85.1.

Duration of PEP

It should be started as early as possible, if started after more than 72 hours of exposure, it is of no use, hence not recommended. The health care worker should be tested for *HIV* as per following schedule:

1. Baseline HIV test at the time of exposure
2. Repeat HIV test at 6 weeks following exposure
3. 2nd repeat HIV test at 12 weeks following exposure

Basic regimen	Zidovudine-600 mg in divided doses (300 mg/twice a day or 200 mg/thrice a day for 4 weeks +
	Lamivudine –150 mg twice a day for 4 weeks
Expanded regimen	Basic regimen + Indinavir–800 mg/thrice a day, or any other protease inhibitor

Flowchart 85.1: Exposure code (EC)

Flowchart 85.2: HIV status code

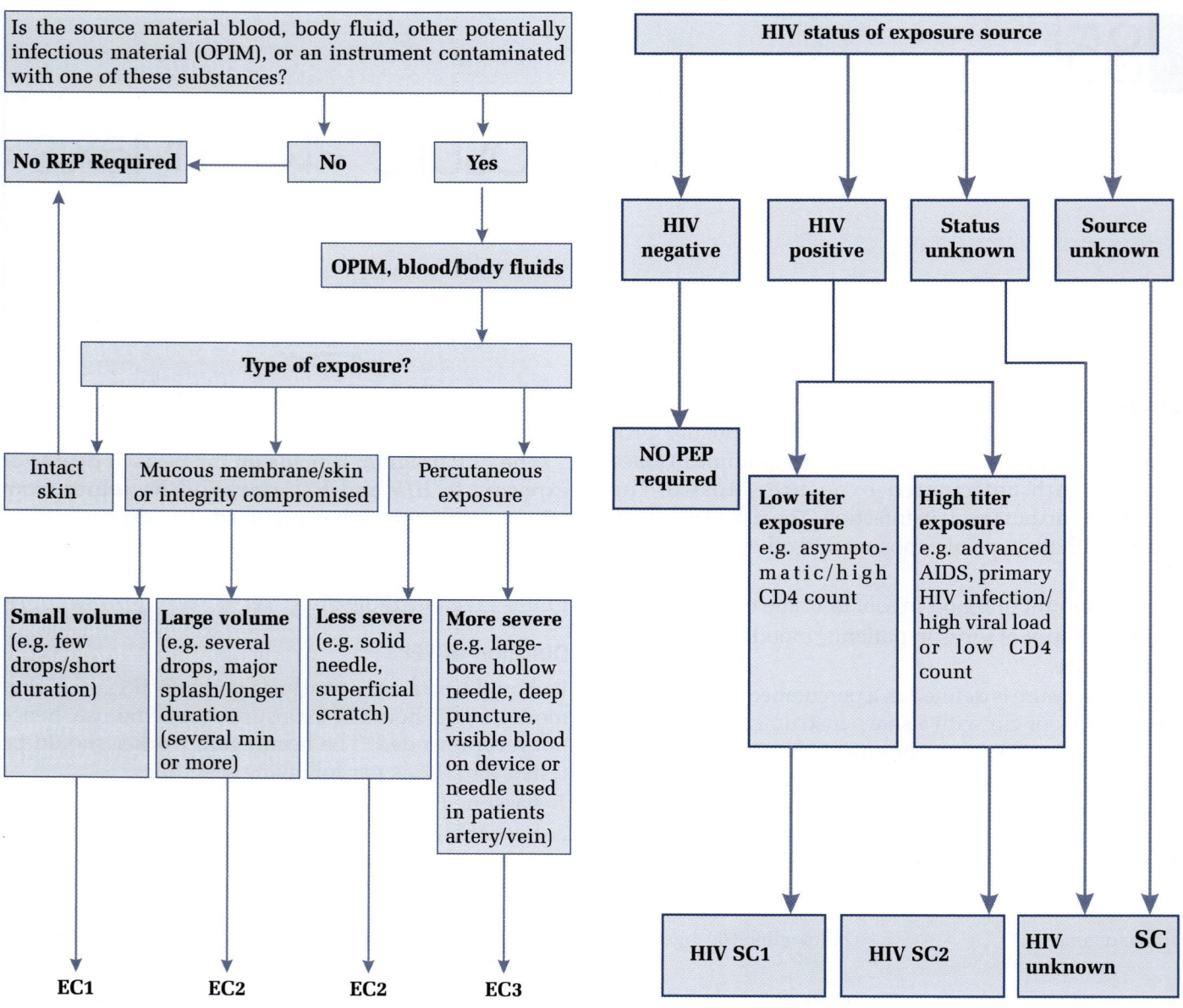

TABLE 85.1: Determination of PEP		
EC	*HIV SC*	*PEP recommendation*
1	1	PEP may not be warranted
1	2	Consider basic regimen (negligible risk)
2	1	Recommend basic regimen (negligible risk)
2	2	Recommend basic regimen
		Most exposure are in this category
2	2	Recommend expanded regimen
3	1 or 2	Recommend expanded regimen
2/3	Unknown	If setting suggests a possible risk (epidemiological risk factors) and EC is 2 or 3, consider basic regimen

86

Immunization

IMMUNOPROPHYLAXIS

Immunization against microorganisms is effective way of controlling infection. Best example is eradication of smallpox which was possible with immunization. The list of 'vaccine preventable diseases' (VMD) includes:

- Diphtheria
- Pertussis
- Tetanus
- Measles
- Mumps
- Rubella
- Poliomyelitis

    Immunoprophylaxis can be classified as **active** immunoprophylaxis (or vaccination) and **passive** immunoprophylaxis (administration of immuno-globulins).

History of vaccination: The terms vaccine and vaccination is obtained from 'Variolae vaccinae' (smallpox of cow); the term used by Edward Jenner for cowpox. Louis Pasteur proposed the term in the honor of Edward Jenner.

Active Immunization (Table 86.1)

Vaccine is an immunological preparation which gives specific protection against infectious diseases. Active immunization gives both humoral or cell-mediated immunity by producing antibodies or by immuno-competent cells (T cell), respectively. Immunological specificity and immunological memory are two important attributes of active immunization. The vaccines used for immunization may be live, killed, acellular or in the form of toxoids, subunit or recombinant vaccines. Vaccines of future prospects are DNA vaccine (gene therapy) and edible vaccines.

Live-Attenuated Vaccines

These are derived from live organisms by attenuation. The **attenuation** is decrease in virulence of the organisms without losing ability to cause infection but retaining their ability to mount immune response (immunogenicity) and generate memory. Attenuation is done by altered growth conditions as passing the organism through foreign host such as live animals, cell cultures or embryonated eggs for prolonged period. **BCG, oral polio, and measles are examples of live-attenuated vaccines.**

Advantages

- They are **more potent** than killed vaccines.
- Vaccinated organisms multiply which result in more antigenic **dose** than what is injected.
- **All major and minor components** of organism which are relevant in protection are present.
- They are capable of giving **local** (mucosal) immunity by producing IgAs as well as **systemic immunity.**

Disadvantages

- Live vaccines are contraindicated in immuno-deficiency diseases or conditions which decrease the immunity as immunosuppressive therapy, cortico-steroids, and some malignant conditions. Pregnancy is also another condition unless the risk of infection is more than the risk of harm caused by vaccine.
- Risk of reversion to virulent strains.
- Risk of remaining virulence (Leuback tragedy).
- Maintenance of cold chain to retain effectiveness specially for oral polio and measles vaccines.

Killed Vaccines or Inactivated Vaccines

- Organisms are inactivated by heat, formaldehyde, betapropionolactone.

TABLE 86.1: Examples of different bacterial and viral vaccines

Bacterial	Viral
Live vaccine	
BCG	Measles vaccine
Typhoral vaccine	Mumps vaccine
Edible typhus vaccine	Rubella vaccine
	Live-attenuated influenza vaccine
	Chickenpox vaccine
	Oral polio vaccine (Sabin)
	Rotavirus vaccine
	Hepatitis A vaccine
	Japanese B encephalitis vaccine (14-14-2 strain)
	Yellow fever 17 D vaccine
Killed or inactive vaccine	
Bacterial	Viral
Typhoid vaccine	Injectable polio vaccine (Salk)
Cholera vaccine	Killed influenza vaccine
Pertussis vaccine	Rabies vaccine
Plague vaccine	Hepatitis A vaccine
	Japanese B encephalitis vaccine (Nakayama strain)
Toxoid vaccine	
DT (Diphtheria toxoid)	
TT (Tetanus toxoid	
Subunit vaccine	
	Hepatitis B vaccine
	HPV vaccine (Human papilloma vaccine)
Cellular fraction vaccine	
Meningococcal vaccine	
Pneumococcal vaccine	
Haemophilus influenzae type b vaccine	
Combined vaccine	
DPT (Diphtheria Pertussis, Tetanus	Measles, mumps, rubella (MMR) vaccine
Pentavalent vaccine (DPT + Hib + Hepatitis B)	
List of commonly used vaccines	

- Killed vaccines are **less efficient,** they produce **weak immune response,** and **systemic immune response** is produced but **does not give local immunity.**
- Killed vaccines require large doses, adjuvant and **multiple doses** are required, may require booster doses.
- They are **stable, safer and cold conditions are not required.**
- They can be given in immunocompromised conditions.
- Killed vaccines are usually given by intramuscular or subcutaneous routes hence **prick** is required for administration.
- The only contraindication is a severe local or general reaction in response to previous dose.
- Examples of killed vaccines are **cholera, influenza, rabies, and pertussis vaccines.**

Toxoids

- Toxoid is a form of toxin which looses its toxicity but ability to mount immune response is retained.

- They are produced from exotoxins inactivated by treatment with formaldehyde, acidic pH.
- Antibody produced against toxoid neutralizes toxic component produced by infection rather than acting on the organism (no anti-infection immunity).
- The commonest toxoids used are tetanus toxoid, diphtheria toxoid.

Cellular Fraction Vaccine or Extracted Vaccines (Bacterial Polysaccharide Vaccines)

These are prepared from extracted cellular fractions of microorganisms. The examples are meningococcal vaccine, pneumococcal vaccine, *haemophilus influenzae* type B vaccine. These are prepared from polysaccharide present in the capsule of bacteria.

Subunit Vaccine

- They are obtained from purified components of pathogenic organisms. Instead of using the whole virus, subviral substance is used for vaccine preparation.

- Hepatitis B vaccine, and human papilloma vaccine are the examples of subunit vaccines.
- For preparation of hepatitis B subunit vaccine, gene producing HBsAg is inserted in chromosome of Baker's yeast (*Saccharomyces cervicae*) and vaccine prepared by **recombinant DNA technology.**

Recombinant Vaccines

The gene coding for antigenic component is cloned in bacteria, yeast. The expressed antigenic protein is used as vaccine after purification. Example is surface antigen of Hepatitis B is used for vaccination.

Newer Vaccines

DNA vaccine: It is in experimental stage. The gene producing protein of interest is injected (by gene gun or liposomal preparation).

Edible vaccine: It is new type of vaccine, the concept is introduced recently. The gene encoding antigenic component is isolated from organism, transferred to suitable plant bacteria which are injected in transgenic plant as banana. The advantages are low cost, production on a large scale, heat stable, induces local immunity.

National Immunization Schedule

Immunization schedule may be different for different countries based on common infections present in that area.

WHO Universal Immunization Programme

It was started (1974) to protect all children from vaccine preventable disease. Later, (2000) it is called **expanded immunization programme (EPI)** and presently the programme **is Universal Immunization Programme (UIP). The national immunization schedule is given in Table 86.2.**

Passive Immunoprophylaxis

Readymade antibodies produced in man or animal are used in conditions in which immediate protection is needed and it is also useful in those conditions in which host cannot mount immune response. For treatment of conditions in which pathogenesis is due to toxin production, passive immunization is useful.

TABLE 86.2: National immunization schedule (India)

Age	Vaccine	Route of administration	Diseases protected
Birth	BCG (0.1 mL)	Intradermal	Tuberculosis
	OPV-0* (2 drops)	Oral	Poliomyelitis
	Hepatitis B	Intramuscular	Hepatitis B
6 weeks	DPT-1 (0.5 mL)	Intramuscular	Diphtheria, Pertussis (Whooping cough, Tetanus
	OPV-1 (2 drops)	Oral	Poliomyelitis
	BCG** (0.05 mL)	Intradermal	Tuberculosis
	Hepatitis B (0.5 mL)	Intramuscular	Hepatitis B
10 weeks	DPT-2 (0.5 mL)	Intramuscular	Diphtheria, Pertussis, Tetanus
	OPV-2 (2 drops)	Oral	Poliomyelitis
	Hepatitis B (0.5 mL)	Intramuscular	Hepatitis B
14 weeks	DPT-3 (0.5 mL)	Intramuscular	Diphtheria, Pertussis, Tetanus
	OPV-3 (2 drops)	Oral	Poliomyelitis
	Hepatitis B (0.5 mL)	Intramuscular	Hepatitis B
9 months	Measles (2 drops)	Subcutaneous	Measles
16–24 months	DPT (0.5 mL)	Intramuscular	Diphtheria, Pertussis, Tetanus
	OPV (2 drops)	Oral	Poliomyelitis
5–6 years	DT#	Intramuscular	Diphtheria, Tetanus
10 years	TTø (0.5 mL)	Intramuscular	Tetanus
16 years	TT (0.5 mL)	Intramuscular	Tetanus
Pregnancy	TTø (0.5 mL)	Intramuscular	Tetanus

Note:
  i. Numbers 1, 2, 3 are number of doses (first, second, third)
 ii. * For institutional births only. OPV-1 is additional and not to be counted for primary course of 3 doses starting at 6 weeks
iii. ** Only for infants not given BCG at birth
 iv. # A second dose of DT to be given to children with no documentary evidence or history of primary DPT immunization
  v. Ø A second dose of TT to be given after one month to those with no record or history or prior DPT, DT or TT immunization
 vi. Ø For prevention of tetanus in the neonate primarily but also for mother
vii. Hepatitis B vaccine is included in immunization schedule in some states of India

TABLE 86.3: Different immunologic preparations with their sources and uses

Immunoglobulin preparation	Source	Indications
Diphtheria antitoxin	Equine	Treatment of diphtheria
Tetanus immunoglobulin (TIG)	Equine, human	Treatment of tetanus
Botulinum antitoxin	Equine, human	Treatment of botulism
Varicella-zoster immunoglobulin (VZIG)	Human	Prophylaxis for immunocompromised contacts of acute cases
Cytomegalovirus immunoglobulin (CMV-IG)	Human	Post-exposure prophylaxis for transplant patients
Rabies immunoglobulin (RIG)	Equine, human	Treatment of rabies and post-exposure prophylaxis in people not previously immunized
Hepatitis B immunoglobulin (HBIG)	Human	Post-exposure prophylaxis for percutaneous, mucosal or sexual exposure
		Post-exposure prophylaxis—newborn of mother with HBsAg positive
Hepatitis A immunoglobulin (HAIG)	Human	Post-exposure prophylaxis for family contacts or travelers
Rubella	Human	Women exposed during pregnancy
Measles	Human	Infants or immunosuppressed contacts of acute cases exposed < 6 days
Rh immunoglobulin (RhIG)	Human	Treatment Rh negative mother after delivery of Rh positive fetus

a. *Human sera*: Normal immunoglobulins can be injected in two forms, i.e. **pooled** or **specific**.
   Pooled immunoglobulins are used for short-term protection against hepatitis A or measles.
b. *Hyperimmune globulins*: These are obtained from **convalescent sera**. Examples are hepatitis B immunoglobulins (HBIG), tetanus immunoglobulin (HTIG), and human rabies immunoglobulin (HRIG).
c. *Animal sera*: Antibodies produced against organisms injected in animals were used previously before human immune globulin. They can produce serum sickness-like immune reactions.

Combined Immunization

In some conditions, immediate protection is required till active immunization produces effective and specific response against particular infection. Immunoglobulins and first dose of vaccine are given at a time (vaccine on one arm limb and immunoglobulin on another arm) followed by full course of immunization.

Newer Vaccines

DNA Vaccine

The most recent development in the vaccine technology is immunization with polynucleotides or genetic immunization or DNA vaccination. DNA vaccines consist of small plasmids obtained from bacterium as *E. coli,* modifying it by removing pathogenic genes (so that pathogenic *E. coli* is not produced) and inserting the gene of interest; **delivery by injection** or by directly into skin by '**gene gun'**.

These are effective but it is not clear whether gene expression will lead to adverse effects as autoimmunity. The DNA vaccines in use (for humans or experiments) are hepatitis B vaccine, HSV, HIV and malaria vaccine. Some of the vaccines are under trials.

Edible Vaccines

- These are also called as **transgenic plant vaccines**.
- It is based on the concept of **expressing viral epitopes and subunits of bacterial toxins in transgenic plants.** The plant will manufacture the vaccine and deliver to the host.
- Some of the foods under trial include banana, potato, and soya bean.
- The advantages of edible vaccines would be:
  - Safe
  - Cheap
  - Ease of administration
- The day is not far off when children will be immunized by munching on foods instead of shots.

Sugar Glass Vaccines

- Saturated solution of sugar, trehalose get converted from liquid to viscous to solid glass-like state called as **sugar glass**. The glass dissolves in contact with water and releases its contents.

- The sugar glass immobilizes, preserves and protects proteins and other molecules from solutions. The vaccine appears to suffer no loss of potency after long periods of exposure to heat or freezing.

Skin Patch Vaccines

Superficial layers of skin are perfect sites of gateways to key area of immune system known as transcutaneous immunizations. Cholera toxin is a good stimulator of immune system. If inactivated cholera toxin mixed with vaccinating agent will produce good antibody response as well as cell-mediated response. This technology is used for vaccination against bacterial and viral infections.

87

Clinical Cases

Case 1

Rohini, 25 years old house wife presented with joints pain affecting elbow followed by wrist. She gave history of fever, cough for which she approached a consultant who gave paracetamol.

On examination, she showed pallor, while cyanosis and clubbing were absent. Her pulse rate was 120/80 mm Hg. The findings of respiratory system, abdomen were normal. On auscultation, cardiac murmur was present suggestive of mitral stenosis.

a. Rohini was suffering from which clinical condition?

b. What is differential diagnosis of the condition?

c. How will you diagnose the condition?

Rohini is presented with history of joint pain, there was fleeting type of arthritis. Probably she had past-episode of sore throat which was missed hence not treated with antibiotics which are recommended for repeated attacks of streptococcal sore throat. Rheumatic fever is diagnosed by ASO test and throat swabs culture for *Streptococcus pyogenes*. The penicillin prophylaxis is advised to prevent recurrence and to prevent further damage.

Case 2

Mr Atul, 35 years laborer developed fever, body ache, malaise. A few days after, he developed dyspnea, right-sided chest pain, productive cough. The sputum sample was collected in a sterile container which showed, rusty sputum (small amount of blood). On examination, his respiratory rate was 40/min, pulse rate 100/min. The total leukocyte count was high (28000 cells/mm^3). Chest X-ray revealed dense infiltration on side.

a. Which is the probable pathogen?

b. Which is this clinical condition?

c. What is the source of infection?

d. What measures can be taken for the prevention of the condition?

Answers

a. The probable pathogen *is Streptococcus pneumoniae.*

b. The condition is community-acquired pneumonia.

c. The source of infection is another patient or carrier shedding the cocci in the environment.

d. Pneumococcal vaccine can be tried for prevention and control.

Case 3

Mr James suffered from profuse watery diarrhea and vomiting since 4 hours. When he was examined, the temperature was normal, also the blood pressure and respiratory rate were also normal. Per abdomen examination showed that there was tenderness; spleen and liver were normal. The tongue was dry, skin showed signs of dehydration. His heart rate was rapid. Patient was also feeling dizziness. Instantly Ringer lactate solution was given intravenously. Ceftriaxone was also given. The patient started showing signs of recovery. Few hours after admission of James, his sister and 2 other members from the same locality presented with watery diarrhea and vomiting.

a. Which is the probable pathogen?

b. Which is the rapid tests for provisional diagnosis of the condition?

c. Which is the gold standard tests for the diagnosis?

d. What is common source of infection?

e. What is the preventable measure?

Mr James presented with classic clinical findings cholera. Other members also had same features within short span of time which suggests a common source, i.e. source of water. This is common water-borne disease, cholera, the pathogen is *VIbrio cholerae.* Distilled water immobilization and immobilization with specific antiserum are rapid tests. The gold standard tests are culture and DNA identification and detection of toxin by DNA probe. The preventive measures include drinking safe water sterilized by boiling for 15 minutes and use of chlorine (bleaching powder) for disinfection of water.

Case 4

Rajesh, 12-year-old boy residing in area with poor sanitation came with fever, abdominal pain and loose motions. Stool sample was collected on admission in hospital which showed mucus and blood. The culture yielded growth of nonlactose fermenter which was identified as *Shigella dysenteriae*.

a. What is likely source of infection?
b. How did pathogen enter his intestinal tract?
c. Which are the virulence factors of the pathogen?
d. What is mode of treatment?

The likely source of infection is contaminated food or water. Modes of infection is feco-oral. The virulence factor of the pathogen is virulence marker antigens (outer membrane proteins).

Case 5

Mr John came to visit India. After seeing Tajmahal, he ate Indian food in a hotel. Next morning he started loose motions. The other Indian friends from his company in which he was working did not suffer from diarrhea. He was brought to hospital with loose motions, muscle cramps, tachycardia. Microscopic examination of stool sample showed no pus cell and sluggishly motile bacilli were seen. On MC agar, lactose fermenting colonies were seen. The results of biochemical tests were as follows: IMViC (++, −, −), TSI (A/A with gas). He recovered with intravenous Ringer's lactate solution and antibiotic, i.e ceftriaxone.

a. What is the cause of diarrhea?
b. Why his other Indian friends did not have loose motions?
c. What is differential diagnosis?

The cause of diarrhea was ETEC. He was classical example of traveler's diarrhea. His friends have probably ETEC as intestinal colonizer because they are living in endemic area. The other organisms which can cause traveler's diarrhea are *Shigella spp., Salmonella, Vibrio*.

Case 6: Typhoid

Mr Anil had high grade fever since 3 days which was increasing progressively. He was admitted in a confused state. His pulse rate was 90/min. Hepato-splenomegaly was present. Peripheral blood smear examination showed slight monocytosis. It was negative for malarial parasite. Serum was tested for antibodies against leptospira and dengue which were negative. His widal test was also negative. Blood culture was done. Nonlactose fermenter was grown, which was urease, oxidase negative and TSI showed K/A with H_2S.

a. What is clinical diagnosis?
b. How diagnosis is justified?
c. Which are the antibiotics used to treat?

Patient had progressively increasing fever, relative bradycardia, and monocytosis. He was suffering from typhoid fever and biochemical parameters were sugges-tive of *S. typhi*. The antibiotics used for treatment are ciprofloxacin, ampicillin, cotrimoxazole, and ceftriaxone.

Case 7: Pseudomembranous colitis

Mr Mangesh, 52 years old male, was hospitalized as he was semiconscious. He was catheterized as he lost bladder control. On 2nd day, he regained consciousness but on 3 day he had fever, chills. He was given ampicillin to which he was responding. On 4th days, he started loose motions, pain in abdomen. His condition improved after withdrawing ampicillin. Microscopic examination revealed presence of RBCs. Gram-stained smear showed Gram-positive bacilli with subterminal spores.

a. What is the clinical condition? Why withdrawal of ampicillin improved diarrhea?
b. Which are the confirmatory tests?
c. How the condition should be managed?

The condition is called "pseudomembranous colitis or antibiotic associated diarrhea". The culprit antibiotic in this case was ampicillin; hence stopping it improved the condition. The patient should be given metro-nidazole. Confirmatory tests are culture on selective medium (CCFA) followed by demonstration of toxin in stool sample. Endoscopic examination is equally helpful.

Case 8: Burn infection

25 years old Sharmila got burns and was hospitalized. Her dehydration and pain was managed successfully. On day 3 of admission, some of the wounds showed discharge. She also developed high grade fever. Her blood culture revealed Gram-negative bacillus, non-fermenter, and oxidase positive. She was given ceftazidime and piperacillin plus tazobactum. Two

other patients in the same burn ward developed septicemia and improved with the same regime.

a. Which is the pathogen?

b. What are the characteristic of the pathogen responsible for causing the clinical condition?

The pathogen is *Pseudomonas aeruginosa*. The characteristics of the pathogen are its simple, minimum growth requirements, its resistance to disinfectants, antibiotics. The pathogen easily survives in environment, e.g. disinfectant solution in which cheatles forceps is kept. That may act as common source of infection.

Case 9: Meningitis due to Meningococci

4-year-old Rajni appeared drowsy since last 3 hours. She had history of fever since 2 days. She also had difficulty in neck movements and vomiting. She was admitted to hospital. Her temperature was 39.5°C, pulse rate 120/minute, blood pressure 110/70 mm Hg. When her neck movements were tested, neck rigidity was present.

Her CSF showed increased opening pressure (300 mm Hg), proteins were raised (90 mg/dL and glucose was 15 mg/dL). The CSF sample was inoculated on chocolate agar with 5–10% CO_2 and humidity. Gram staining showed plenty of pus cells, Gram-negative diplococci; some of which were intracellular and some extracellular.

a. What is the clinical diagnosis and which is the probable pathogen?

b. What is the mode of treatment?

c. How the other children coming in close contact will be prevented?

The patient had fever and neckstiffness. Her CSF findings were suggestive of pyogenic meningitis. Gram-stained smear showed Gram-negative diplococci; it means the pathogen is *Neisseria meningitidis*. The mode of infection is by droplets. The children which were in contact with case can be prevented by rifampicin.

Case 10: UTI due to proteus

A 23 years old female, just married, had 4 days history of mild fever. Since last 2 days, she had chills, discomfort in lower abdomen, increase in frequency and urgency of urine. She never had such experience in life. Wet mount showed pus cells (>5 hpf) and few RBCs. With sterile standard loop, 0.0001 mL of urine sample was inoculated on blood agar and MacConkey's agar. Next day when culture plates were examined there were 100CFU (colonies). On blood agar, thin film

of growth was observed. Urease test was performed which was positive. Trimethoprim sulfamethoxazole was given to her and she got complete relief.

a. What is the clinical diagnosis?

b. Which is the pathogen?

c. What is the colony count?

d. Which antibiotics can be given for treatment of urinary tract infection?

The patient was suffering from urinary tract infection. Mostly she had 'honeymoon cystitis' as infection occurred just after marriage.

The pathogen was *Proteus* as it showed swarming on blood agar and urease test was positive.

The colony count was 10^5/mL which is a significant count according to Kass's concept of significant bacteriuria.

The antibiotics for urine are norfloxacin, nalidixic acid, ciprofloxacin, cotrimoxazole, ceftriaxone, and ceftazidime.

Case 11: Gas gangrene

A 25 years old male had accident and suffered muscle injury of left leg below knee. On admission, the debridement of wound was done. On day 2 of admission, he developed tenderness, fever and swelling. Thin, foul smelling discharge and crepitus were present. X-ray of the leg showed gas shadow. Samples were collected from wound. Muscle pieces were collected; one was transported in RCM medium while other piece was transported as such in a sterile container. Gram-stained smear from 2nd piece showed scanty pus cells, Gram-positive bacilli with truncated ends, Gram-positive bacilli with central spore, Gram-negative bacilli and Gram-positive cocci in clusters. Again debridement was done.

a. What is the clinical diagnosis?

b. How these findings of Gram-stained smear can be explained?

c. What is differential diagnosis?

d. What else is done in treatment of this condition?

The patient was suffering from gas gangrene.

Gram-stained smear showed polymicrobial flora along with gas gangrene group of organisms. The differential diagnosis is anaerobic streptococcal myositis.

Apart from surgical treatment, anti-gas gangrene serum is given to patient and hyperbaric oxygen is given in a special chamber. Metronidazole is the antibiotic given to prevent multiplication of pathogens.

Case 12: Complicated UTI

A 62 years old man was operated for benign enlargement of prostate in private hospital. As needed, catheterization was done postoperatively. The cather was attached to a closed drainage system. On 5th day of catheterization, he developed fever, chills. His temperature was 39°C, pulse rate was 110/min and BP was 100/76 mm Hg. His TLC was 18000/µL of blood. Urine sample was collected from port. The culture showed growth of *Klebsiella pneumoniae* and colony count was 10000/mL.

a. What type of UTI the patient suffered from?

b. Are the counts significant?

The patient was suffering from complicated urinary tract infection.

Though the colony counts are low but in context to clinical presentation, these are suggestive of urinary tract infection.

Case 13: Syphilis

An 18-year-old student came with complain of ulcer on penis. It was painless ulcer. The patient had history of unprotected sex. His serum sample was collected for VDRL test which was reactive with titer 1:4.

a. What is the clinical diagnosis?

b. What is differential diagnosis and how it is differentiated from present illness?

c. Which are the confirmatory tests?

The patient was suffering from syphilis.

The ulcer of syphilis has to be differentiated from ulcer of *Haemophilus ducreyi* (ulcer called as soft chancre). In soft chancre, the ulcer is painful and base is nonindurated.

VDRL test performed early may not give significant titire. A repeat test on paired serum should show 4-fold rise in titer of antibodies.

The confirmatory tests are TPHA, TPI, and FTA-ABS.

Case 14: TB

A 58-year-old man presented with history of cough for 2 weeks. He also gave history of weakness since 6 months and weight loss. Twice he had hemoptysis. His sputum sample was collected in a sterile wide mouth container. The Z-N stained was performed on smear prepared from sputum sample which showed acid-fast bacilli. He was HIV seropositive. His CD4 counts were 300 cells/µL. Tuberculin test was positive which showed induration of 8 mm.

a. What is the clinical condition?

b. Why tuberculin test was weakly reactive?

The patient was suffering from pulmonary TB.

Due to anergy caused by immunocompromised state, tuberculin test shows induration of small size.

Case 15: Chlamydia urethritis

A 20 years old male complained of slight pain during micturation and white-colored urethral discharge since 4 days. The urethral discharge was mucoid and three swabs collected tests. The leukocyte esterase test was positive showing presence of pus cells. Gram's staining was performed which showed pus cells without any organism. One more smear was prepared which was stained with Giemsa stain. It showed presence of intracytoplasmic basophilic inclusion bodies.

a. What is the clinical diagnosis?

b. Which are other sensitive tests for the diagnosis of the disease?

c. How to treat the condition?

The clinical diagnosis is *Chlamydia trachomatis*.

The sensitive methods for the diagnosis include DNA probe, PCR, LCR.

Doxycycline and erythromycin are the antibiotics preferred for treatment of the disease and they are given for 7 days.

Case 16: Haemophilus meningitis

Sangita brought her 2-year-old baby who was suffering from fever since 2 days. The baby was irritable, drowsy and started vomiting. The clinician examined the patient and observed neck stiffness. CSF was collected and sent to culture which was done on blood agar and chocolate agar with filter paper disk containing factor-X and factor-V. Gross examination showed that the sample was turbid. Microscopic examination was done which showed Gram-negative coccobacillary form, Gram-negative bacilli, some of them were short and some of them were long. CRP test on the CSF was positive. Growth was present in between X and V disc. The organism was catalase positive and oxidase positive.

a. What is the provisional diagnosis?

b. Which was the pathogen responsible for the suffering?

c. What is the role of CRP on CSF sample?

d. Which is the simple, cost-effective and rapid method for the diagnosis of the pathogen?

The Gram-stained smear showed pleomorphism and growth of pathogen was present between X and V disks. The pathogen was catalase and oxidase positive; hence it was *Haemophilus influenzae* causing pyogenic meningitis. CRP is positive in pyogenic meningitis which is negative in viral meningitis. The simple, cheap and cost-effective test on CSF is detection of antigen by latex agglutination test.

CASE 17: Cryptococcus meningitis

A 45-year HIV seropositive male with CD4 counts 248 cells/μL was admitted with fever, altered sensorium. CSF was collected under aseptic precautions. Wet mount showed pus cells and budding yeast cells. Mucoid growth was observed on Sabouraud's dextrose agar. The isolate showed urease test positive.

a. Which is the isolate responsible for illness?
b. Which is the sensitive and rapid test for diagnosis of the infection?
c. The patient will be classified into which stage of HIV infection?

The pathogen in this case is *Cryptococcus neoformans* as it is capsulated yeast which produces mucoid colonies on Sabouraud's dextrose agar and urease positive.

The sensitive, rapid test for diagnosis is demonstration of antigen in CSF by latex agglutination test.

The patient is classified in AIDS as *Cryptococcus neoformans* is AIDS defining condition.

Case 18: Ventilator associated pneumonia

A 50-year-old male lost consciousness due to intracranial hemorrhage. He was kept on ventilator. On day 4, tracheotomy was performed. On 7th day of admission, patient had fever, cough. X-ray findings were consolidation suggestive of pneumonia. Sputum sample was collected in a wide mouth container. Gram-stained smear showed pus cells and Gram-positive diplococci in pairs. Alpha hemolytic colonies were produced on blood agar. The inulin fermentative and bile solubility tests were also positive. Patient was started with antibiotics to which it responded.

a. Which was the pathogen responsible for infection?
b. Which is the factor responsible for this condition?

The pathogen was *Streptococcus pneumoniae*.

Due to coma, gag reflexes and cough reflexes get reduced predisposing for infection of lung.

Case 19: Breast abscess

A 30-year-old female, known diabetic, presented with acute pain and swelling of elbow joint. No history of trauma was present. Before this, the patient had fever. There was breast abscess also. Smears prepared from aspirates showed pus cells and Gram-positive cocci in clusters. Patient was given ampicillin and his fever started subsiding.

Which is the serological test which can diagnose the condition?

What is the mode of infection?

Patient had breast abscess earlier from which due to hematogenous spread it has caused osteomyelitis. The pathogen is *Staphylococcus aureus* causing both breast abscess and osteomyelitis. The serological test used for diagnosis of deep seated infections is anti-staphylolysin.

Case 20: Actinomycotic mycetoma

A 35 years old farmer, Ganpat presented with swelling of left foot since 1year, discharging openings since 9 months.

Patient noticed that small sand-like structures coming out of sinuses. When examined local swelling was present with 4 discharging sinuses. Some yellowish granules were present which were collected in a sterile test tube with sterile saline. Granules were washed in saline and processed by standard microbiological process. Gram-stained smear showed Gram-positive thin, branching filaments. Modified Z-N staining was performed by using 1% H_2SO_4 as decolorizing solution. Sabouraud's dextrose agar and L-J medium were inoculated.

a. What is clinical diagnosis?
b. Gram-stained smear and modified Z-N-stained smear findings suggestive of which condition?
c. What is the importance of smear in this case?

The clinical diagnosis is mycetoma as there was swelling, discharging sinuses, and granules.

The findings of Gram-stained smear and modified Z-N-stained smear showed filamentous bacilli suggestive of Nocardia.

The importance of smear is that smear gives the provisional diagnosis of actinomycotic mycetoma or eumycotic mycetoma. Thin filaments are in favor of actinomycotic mycetoma while broad filaments are in favor of eumycotic mycetoma. This is important in treatment point of view as well as prognosis point of view. Actinomycotic mycetoma responds well to antibacterial treatment as sulphonamide, trimethoprim-sulfamethoxazole, while eumycotic mycetoma is difficult to treat.

Appendix

A. Common Pathogens Producing Disease at Different Levels of Respiratory Tract

Conjunctiva	*Streptococcus pneumoniae, Haemophilus influenzae, Neisseria gonorrhoeae, Chlamydia trachomatis, adenovirus, enterovirus, herpes simplex virus*
Middle ear and paranasal sinuses	*S. pneumoniae, H. influenzae, Moraxella catarrhalis, group A streptococci*
Epiglotitis	*H. influenzae*
Larynx–trachea	*Parainfluenza virus, S. aureus*
Bronchi	*S. pneumoniae, H. influenzae, M. pneumoniae, influenza virus, Mycoplasma pneumoniae, measles virus*

B. Classification of Pneumonia Syndromes

Acute	
Person to person transmission	*Streptococcus pneumoniae, Mycoplasma pneumoniae, Haemophilus influenzae, Staphylococcus aureus, Streptococcus pyogenes, Klebsiella pneumoniae, Neisseria menigitidis, Branhamella catarrhalis, Chlamydia pneumoniae, influenza virus*
Animal or environmental exposure	*Legionella pneumophila, Francisella tularensis, Coxiella burnetii, Chlaymidia psittaci, Yersinia pestis, Bacillus anthracis, Pseudomonas pseudomallei (melidiosis), Pasteurella multocida*
Pneumonia in infants and young child	*Chlamydia trachomatis, respiratory syncytial virus, other respiratory viruses, S. aureus, Group B streptococci, Streptococcus pneumoniae, Haemophilus influenzae (type B)*
Nosocomial pneumonia	*Enterobacteriaceae, Pseudomonas aeruginosa, Acinetobacter, S. aureus*
Subacute or chronic	
Pulmonary tuberculosis	*Mycobacterium tuberculosis*
Fungal	*Histoplasma capsulatum, Blastomyces dermatitidis, Paracoccidioidomycosis imitis, Cryptococcus neoformans*
Aspiration pneumonia and lung abscess	Mixed anaerobes and aerobes
Pneumonia in immuno-compromised	*P. carrini, CMV, Nocardia, M. tuberculosis Aspergillus*

C. Some Predisposing Causes and Organisms Causing Osteomyelitis

Predisposing factor	*Etiological agents*
Infancy	*Group B streptococci*
Childhood	*Haemophilus influenzae*
Sickle cell anemia	*Salmonella typhi*
Immunosuppression	*Oppertunistic fungi, Nocardia, Pseudomonas*
Trauma to jaw	*Actinomyces israelii*
Animal exposure	*Brucella*
Pulmonary TB	*Mycobacterium tuberculosis*

D. Most Common Causes of Bacterial Arthritis

- *Staphylococcus aureus*
- *Streptococcus species*
- *Group B streptococci*
- *Haemophilus influenzae type b*
- *Neisseria*
- *Gram-negative bacilli*
- *Anaerobes*

Reactive arthritis

- *Streptococcus pyogenes*
- *Neisseria meningitidis*
- *Neisseria gonorrhoeae*
- *Yersinia enterocolitca*
- *Campylobacter jejuni*
- *Salmonella species*
- *Shigella*
- *Mycoplasma pneumoniae*
- *Chlamydia trachomatis*
- *Hepatitis B virus*
- *Ebstein-Barr virus*

E. Muscle Infections

Pathogenesis	Clinical presentation	Organisms
Localized and spread from a contigious site	Gas gangrene	*Clostridium perfringens, Clostridium novyi, Clostridium sporogenes*
	Synergistic myositis, muscle abscess	*Staphylococcus aureus, Group A Streptococcus*
	Miscellaneous	*Mycobacterium, Nocardia, Actinomyces, fungi*
Hematogenous spread	Bacterial	*Streptococcus pyogenes, group B streptococci, Staphylococcus aureus, Gram-negative bacilli*
	Parasitic, viral	*Trichinella spiralis, ECHO viruses, Coxsackievirus, Epstein-Barr virus*

F. Agents of Lymphadenitis

Bacterial

- *Streptococcus pyogenes*
- *Staphylococcus aureus*
- *Atypical mycobacteria*
- *Corynebacterium diphtheriae*
- *Brucellosis*
- *Franscisella tularensis*
- *Yersinia pestis*
- *Cat scratch agent*
- *Pseudomonas pseudomallei*

Viral

- *Measles*
- *Rubella*
- *EBV*
- *Adenoviruses, types 3, 7*
- *Herpes simplex*
- *CMV*
- *Mumps*
- *HIV*

Fungal

- *Histoplasma capsulatum*
- *Aspergillus*

Parasitic

- *Toxoplasma gondii*
- *Trypanosoma brucei*

G. Skin and Soft Tissue Infections

Vesicles

- *Chickenpox*
- *Varicella zoster*
- Herpetic whitlow
- Hand foot mouth disease—Coxsackie A16
- Orf—parapoxvirus
- Molluscum contagiosum
- Rickettsial pox—Rickettsia tsutsugamushi

Crusted Lesion

- Bullous impetigo—*S. aureus*
- Impetigo contagiosa—*Streptococcus pyogenes*
- Nocardiasis
- Cutaneous leishmaniasis
- Sporotrichosis
- Histoplasmosis
- Ringworm—dermatophytic fungi
- Blastomycosis

Folliculitis

- Furunculosis—*S. aureus*
- Swimmers' itch—*Schistosomiasis*
- Hot-tub folliculitis—*Pseudomonas aeruginosa*

Ucers with or without Eschars

- Anthrax
- Ulcerative tularemia
- Bubonic plague
- Burulis ulcer—*M. ulcerans*
- Cutaneous tuberculosis
- Chancroid (*Haemophilus ducreyi*)
- Leprosy
- Primary syphilis

Bullae

- Staphylococcal scalded skin syndrome
- Necrotizing fasciitis
- *Vibrio vulnificus*

H. Causes of Peritonitis

Primary Bacterial Peritonitis

- *E. coli*
- *S. aureus*
- *Streptococcus pyogenes*
- Enterococci
- Pneumococci

Secondary Peritonitis

E. coli and other Gram-negative bacilli.

Peritonitis in Patients with Continuous Ambulatory Peritoneal Dialysis

- *Staphylococcus aureus*
- *E. coli*
- Enterococci
- *Candida species*

I. Organisms Transmitted by Organ Transplantation

Viruses

- CMV (blood, lung, brain, liver, skin)
- EB virus (blood, lung, brain, liver, skin)
- Herpes simplex virus 1 (blood, lung, liver, skin)
- Herpes simplex 6 (blood, lung, liver, skin)
- Herpes simplex 8 (blood, lung, liver, skin)
- Hepatitis B and C viruses (blood, lung, liver, skin)
- Rabies (blood, lung, brain, liver, skin)
- West Nile virus (blood, lung, brain, liver, skin)
- Bovine spongiform encephalopathy (blood, lung, brain, liver, skin)

Fungi

- *Candida albicans* (blood, lung, liver, skin)
- *Histoplasma capsulatum* (blood, lung, liver, skin)
- *Cryptococcus neoformans* (blood, lung, brain, liver, skin)

Parasites

- *Toxoplasma gondii* (lung, brain)
- *Strongyloides stercoralis* (lung)
- *Plasmodium falciparum* (blood)

J. List of Granulomatous Infections

Bacteria	Fungi	Parasites
Listeria monocytogenes	Cryptococcus neoformans	Toxocara
Rhodococcus equi	Blastomyces dermatitidis	Schistosoma mansonii
Nocardia asteroides	Sporothrix schenckii	Schistosoma japonicum
Treponema pallidum	Coccidioides imitis	
Mycobacterium tuberculosis	Histoplasma capsulatum	
Mycobacterium avium intracellulare complex		
Anaerobic streptococci		
Bacteroides		
Prevotella sp		
Enterobacteriaceae members		
Staphylococcus		
Fusobacteria		
Yersinia enterocolitca		
Yersinia pseudotuberculosis		
Yersinia pestis		
Salmonella typhi/paratyphi		
Francisella tularensis		
Chlamydia trachomatis		
Mycobacterium leprae		
Bartonella henselae/ bacilliformis		
Coxiella burnetii		
Granulomatis		
Burkholderia pseudomallei		
Brucella abortus		

K. Commom Cold Viruses

- *Rhinoviruses*
- *Coronaviruses*
- *Respiratory syncytial virus*
- *Parainfluenza viruses*
- *Coxsackieviruses types A21, B3*
- *Echoviruses types 11, 20*
- *Adenoviruses*

L. Eye Infections

Conjunctivitis, keratitis

Bacteria

- **Neisseria gonorrhoeae**—neonates acquire infection from mother's genital tract, condition is called **ophthalmia neonatorum**. It is preventable by prophylaxis with silver nitrate eye drops (**Crede's solution**).
- *Staphylococcus aureus*—sticky eyes in neonates
- *Haemophilus influenzae*
- *Neisseria meningitidis*
- *Streptococcus pneumoniae*—causes purulent conjunctivitis
- *Pseudomonas aeruginosa*—in presence of foreign body or operation
- *Chlamydia trachomatis* A-D—endemic trachoma (follicular conjunctivitis)
- *Chlamydia trachomatis* D-K—inclusion conjunctivitis

Viruses

- *Adenoviruses*, type-8 causes shipwards eye
- *Herpes simplex virus 1*—dendritic ulcers
- *Varicella zoster*
- *Rubella*—congenital infection—causes cataract

Fungi

- *Fuserium solani*
- *Aspergillus fumigatus*
- *Candida albicans*
- *Curvularia*

Parasite

- *Loa loa*
- *Onchocerca vovulus*

Orbital Cellulitis

- *Staphylococcus aureus*
- *Streptococcus pyogenes*

- *Streptococcus pneumoniae*
- Coliforms
- *Haemophilus influenzae*
- *Bacteroides fragilis*

Choroidoretinitis

- *CMV*—congenital infection
- *Rubella*—congenital
- *Toxoplasma gondii*
- *Toxocara canis*
- *Toxocara cati*

M. Bacteria Responsible for Acute Exacerbation of Chronic Bronchitis

- *Haemophilus influenzae*
- *Streptococcus pneumoniae*
- *Klebsiella pneumoniae*
- *Pseudomonas aeruginosa*
- *E. coli*

N. Organisms Causing Myocarditis and Pericarditis

Viruses

- Coxsackie B1-B6
- Influenza A
- Arboviruses
- Rubella virus

Bacteria

- *Streptococcus pyogenes*
- *Staphylococcus aureus*
- *Streptococcus pneumoniae*
- *Neisseria meningitidis*
- *Neisseria gonorrhoeae*
- *Mycobacterium tuberculosis*
- *Trponema pallidum*
- *Leptospira*
- *Mycoplasma pneumoniae*
- *Chlamydia trachomatis*
- *Coxiella burnetii*
- *Chlamydia psitasii*

Parasites

- *Toxoplasma gondii*
- *Trypanosome cruzi*

Fungus: *Cryptococcus neoformans.*

Organism	Drug of choice	Alternate drugs
Acinetobacter	Imipenem or meropenem	Doxycycline, TMP-SMZ, aminoglycoside, ceftazidime, ciprofloxacin, piperacillin—tazobactum, ticarcillin—clavulanic acid, colistin, tigecycline,
E. coli—sepsis	Cefotaxime, ceftazidime, ceftriaxone, cefepime	Imipenem, meropenem, aminoglycoside, fluoroquinolone, piperacillin-tazobactum
E. coli	Fluoroquinolone	TMP-SMZ, oral cephalosporin
Uncomplicated UTI	Nitrofurantoin	Fosphomycin
Klebsiella pneumoniae	Cefotaxime, ceftriaxone, cefipime, ceftazidime,	TMP-SMZ, aminoglycoside, imipenem, doripenem, fluoro-quinolone, piperacillin tazobactum, ticarcillin—clavulanic acid
Pseudomonas aeruginosa	Aminoglycoside + antipseudomonal penicillin	Ceftazidime, imipenem, meropenem, doripenem+ aminoglycoside, ciprofloxacin, azetreonam + aminoglycoside, cefipime
Proteus mirabilis	Ampicillin	An aminoglycoside, TMP-SMZ, fluroquinolone, cephalosporin, imipenem, meropenem, doripenem, ticarcillin-clavulanic acid, piperacillin – tazobactum, chloramphenicol
Proteus vulgaris *Morganella, Providencia*	Cefotaxime, ceftriaxone, ceftazidime, cefepime	Aminoglycoside, TMP-SMZ, fluoroquinolone, imipenem, meropenem, doripenem, ticarcillin-clavulanic acid, piperacillin –tazobactum , ampicillin, sulbactum, amoxicillin, clavulanic acid
Salmonella—bacteremia	Cefotaxime, ceftriaxone, or fluroquinolone	TMP-SMZ, ampicillin, chloramphenicol
Shigella	Fluoroquinolone	Ampicillin, TMP-SMZ, ceftriaxone, azithromycin
Vibrio cholerae—sepsis *Yersinia enterocolitica*	Tetracycline, TMP-SMX	TMP-SMZ, fluoroquinolone, aminoglycoside, cefotaxime
Enterobacter	Imipenem, meropenem	Aminoglycoside, ciprofloxacin, piperacillin—tazobactum, TMP-SMZ, third generation cephalosporin, azetreonam, tigecycline
Haemophilus—meningitis, other serious infections	Cefotaxime, ceftriaxone	Chloramphenicol, meropenem
Haemophilus—respiratory	TMP-SMZ	Ampicillin, amoxicillin, doxycycline, *infections, otitis* azithromycin, clarithromycin, cefotaxime, ceftriaxone, cefuroxime, fluoro-quinolone, tetracycline, augmentin
Brucella	Tetracycline + rifampin	TMP-SMZ
Campylobacter jejuni	Erythromycin or azithromycin	Fluoroquinolone, tetracycline, gentamicin
Helicobacter pylori	Protein pump inhibitor + clarithromycin + amoxicillin or metronidazole	Bismuth subsalicylate+ metronidazole, tetracycline + proton pump inhibitor or H2 blocker
Burkholderia pseudomallei	Ceftazidime, imipenem	Chloramphenicol + tetracycline, TMP-SMZ, augmentin, meropenem
Burkholderia mallei	Streptomycin+ tetracycline	Chloramphenicol + streptomycin, imipenem
Serratia	Imipenem or meropenem	TMP-SMZ, aminoglycoside, fluoroquinolone, ceftriaxone, cefotaxmine, ceftazidime, cefipime
Yersinia pestis	Streptomycin +/- tetracycline	Chloramphenicol, TMP-SMZ, ciprofloxacin, gentamicin
Streptococcus pneumoniae	Penicillin G or V, amoxycilin	Erythromycin, cephalosporin, vancomycin, TMP-SMZ, clindamycin, azithromycin, clarithromycin, tetracycline, imipenem, meropenem, quinpristin, dalfopristin, llinezolid, tetravancin
Streptococci group A, B, C, G	Penicillin G or V, ampicillin	Erythromycin, cephalosporin, vancomycin, clindamycin, azithromycin, chlarithromycin, linezolid, daptomycin, televancin

(Contd...)

Organism	Drug of choice	Alternate drugs
Viridans streptococci	Penicillin G+ gentamicin	Cephalosporine, vancomycin, televancin
Staphylococcus non penicillinase producing	Penicillin	Cephalosporine, vancomycin, imipenem, meropenem, fluoroquinolone, clindamycin
Staphylococcus penicillinase producing, methicillin susceptible	Penicillinase resistant penicillin	Vancomycin, cephalosporin, clindamycin, augmentin, piperacillin—tazobactum, imipenem, meropenem, fluoroquinolone, TMP-SMZ, linezolid, televancin
MRSA	Vancomicin + gentamicin +/− rifampin	TMP-SMZ, doxycycline, fluoroquinolone, linezolid, quinpristin, dalfopristins, tigecycline, ceftaroline
Enterococcus fecalis	Ampicillin + gentamicin	Vancomycin + gentamicin, or streptomycin, linezolid, quinpristin, dalfopristin, tigecycline
Enterococcus faecium	Vancomycin + gentamicin	Quinprinstin, dalfoprinstin, linezolid, daptomycin
Neisseria gonorrhoeae	Ceftriaxone	Cefixime, cefotaxine, penicillin G
Neisseria meningitidis	Penicillin G	Cefotaxime, ceftriaxone, chloramphenicol, fluoroquinolone
Moraxella catarrhalis	Cefuroxime, fluoroquinolone	TMP-SMZ, cefotaxime, cefodoxime, erythromycin, azithromycin, augmentin, clarithromycin
Actinomyces	Penicillin	Doxycycline, clindamycin, erythromycin
Clostridium, gas gangrene	Penicillin + clindamycin	Metronidazole, chloramphenicol, imipenem, doripenem
Listeria monocytogenes	Ampicillin + aminoglycoside	TMP-SMX
Bacillus	Penicillin, ciprofloxacin or doxycycline for anthrax	Erythromycin, tetracycline, fluoroquinolone
Bacillus cereus	Vancomycin	Imipenem, meropenem, clindamycin
C. diphtheriae	Erythromycin	Penicillin
Chlamydia trachomatis	Tetracycline, azithromycin	Ofloxacin, erythromycin, amoxicillin
Chlamydia pneumoniae	Tetracycline, erythromycin, clarithromycin, azithromycin	Fluoroquinolone
Rickettsia	Doxycycline	Chloramphenicol, fluoroquinolone
Leptospira	Penicillin G	Doxycycline, ceftriaxone
T. pallidum	Penicillin G	Doxycycline, ceftriaxone
Haemophilus—meningitis, other serious infections	Cefotaxime, ceftriaxone	Chloramphenicol, meropenem
Haemophilus—respiratory infections, otitis	TMP-SMZ	Ampicillin, doxycycline, azithromycin, clarithromycin, cefuroxime, cefotaxime, fluoroquinolone, tetracycline, augmentin

LABORATORY ACQUIRED INFECTION

These infections are acquired in laboratory or laboratory associated activities. The severity varies from asymptomatic infection to severe disease, sometimes resulting death. This infection takes place due to occupational exposure or inoculation.

The **most common modes of infections** are:
- Inhalation

- Percutaneous injuries
- Exposure of mucosa with contaminated material or hands
- Ingestion (aspiration during pipette or eating)

Based upon the risk involved to laboratory person, risk of spread in community and availability of effective treatment or prophylaxis, **organisms** are **classified into four groups** as given below.

Group	Definition	Bacteria	Viruses	Fungi	Parasites
Group I	Biological agents that are unlikely to cause human disease	No pathogenic organisms	—	—	—
Group II	Biological agents that can cause human disease and may be hazard to worker; but are unlikely to spread in community; Effective prophylaxis or treatment is available	Clostridium species Corynebacterium diphtheriae Bacillus species (except B. anthracis) Enterobacteriaceae Staphylococcus Streptococcus Calciviruses	Adenoviruses Corona viruses (not SARS) Herpes virus Influenza virus	Cryptococcus neoformans Candida Aspergillus Dermatophytes	All clinically important parasites
Group III	Biological agents that can cause severe human disease and are a serious hazard to worker; they may spread to community; but effective prophylaxis or treatment is available	B. anthracis Brucella species Coxiella burnetii Francisella tularensis M. tuberculosis	Prion Lymphocytic choriomeningitis virus Hantavirus SARS-CoV Encephalitis viruses St.Louis Japanese West Nile Western equine	—	—
Group IV	Same as above except that effective prophylaxis or treatment is NOT available	—	Lassa virus Marburg virus Ebola virus Herpes simiae virus		

BIOTERRORISM—BIOLOGICAL WARFARE

Definition: Bioterrorism is unlawful use of weapon, a type of terrorism where there is intentional and deliberate release of biological agents (bacteria, viruses, fungi, or their products as toxins) which causes mass illness or deaths.

Features of biological agents used as weapons are:

- They can cause high morbidity or mortality in community.
- Potential for easy spread from person to person.
- Should be useful in minimum dose.
- Ease of administration—by aerosols.
- Not easily diagnosed.
- There is no effective vaccine available.
- Easy availability and production.
- Adequate stability in the environment.

History

- Claviceps purpura (rye ergot) was used by Assyrians in the 6th century.
- Anthrax used by Germany to infect mules and horses during 1st world war.
- Japanese forces used Anthrax and Plague bacilli against prisoners.
- *Recent episode*: In the tear 2001, USA World Trade Center attacks during which anthrax spores were used by terrorists. The spores were sent in envelopes to Government agencies and media.

Prevention and preparedness

- Early detection of weapon with efficient diagnostic procedures used recent techniques.
- Quick relief
- Preparing action plan.

  The risk based classification of biological agents causing laboratory-acquired infections is give in table.

Category A: These agents are the highest priority pathogens which can cause great threat to the national security

Such agents can be easily transmitted or disseminated from one person to another Results in high mortality and potential for public threat Might cause public panic Special health prepared awareness is required	• Anthrax (Bacillary antharicis) • Botulism toxin • *Yersinia pestis* (plague) • Tularemia (*Franscisella tularensis*) • Viral hemorrhagic fever agents: Lyssa, Margburg, Ebola, Crimean Congo hemorrhagic fevers.

Category B: These agents are second highest priority pathogens

• Moderately easy to disseminate • Causes moderate morbidity and mortality • Requires special diagnostic capacity	• Meliodiosis (*Burkholderia pseudomallei*) • Glander's disease (*Burkholderia mallei*) • Brucellosis (*Brucella*) • Psittacosis (*Chlamydia psittaci*) • Q fever (*Coxiella burnetii*) • Typhus fever (*Rickettsia prowazekii*) • Toxins: Enterotoxin B of *Staphylococcus aureus*, epsilon toxin of *Clostridium perfringens* • Viral encephalitis • Salmonella, Shigella, *E. coli* O-157 • Water disease—cholera caused for *Vibrio cholerae*

Category C: These agents are the third highest priority pathogens. They are emerging pathogens, to which population lacks immunity

• These agents could be engineered for mass dissemination in the future because of availability, ease of production and ease of dissemination • They have a potential for high morbidity and mortality	• Nipah virus • Hantavirus • SARS coronavirus • Pandemic influenza virus • MDR-TB • Yellow fever virus

Organism	Microscopic characteristic
Acinetobacter	Pairs of Gram-negative coccobacilli (may resist decolorization)
Actinobacillus	Short coccobacilli to short rods
Actinomyces	Gram-positive filament (beaded—irregular staining)
Bacillus species	Gram-positive or Gram variable rods with nonbulging spore
Bacillus anthracis	Gram-positive bacilli arranged end to end, the chain surrounded by capsule-Bamboo stick appearance
Bifidobacterium	Gram-positive rods with bifurcated end (two forks)
Borrelia	Spirochete, do not stain with Gram stain; can be stained with dark ground microscope or phase contrast microscope, show widely opened spirals
Calymmabacterium granulomatis	Giemsa or Wright stained preparations—'Donovan bodies: pleomorphic coccobacilli surrounded by pink capsule, some bacteria give 'safety pin' appearance
Campylobacter	Small, faintly stained, curved Gram-negative rods, 'seagull wings' and 's'shapes
Capnocytophaga	Fusiform Gram-negative rods
Clostridium perfringens	Gram-positive, 'boxcar' shaped' rods
Clostridium tetani	Drumstick or tennis racket because of terminal round bulging spore
Corynebacterium diphtheriae	Gram-positive bacilli, Chinese letter or cuneiform pattern showing 'V'. 'L'shapes, metachromatic granules seen with methylene blue (snapping type of division)
Ehrlichia	Morula (intracytoplasmic inclusion)
Eubacterium	Gram-positive bacilli which may branch
Fusobacterium nucleatum	Thin, fusiform Gram-negative bacilli
Lactobacillus	Long to medium Gram-positive bacilli in chains
Haemophilus influenzae	Pleomorphic, Gram-negative bacilli, few coccobacillary forms

(Contd...)

Organism	Microscopic characteristic (Contd...)
Haemophilus ducreyi	School of fish or rail road tract appearance
Leptospira	Compactly arranged, regular spiral with hooked end resembling umbrella handle
Micrococcus	Gram-positive cocci in tetrads
Mycobacterium kansasii	Long acid-fast bacilli with bands (i.e. cross bars)
Mycobacterium marinum	Acid-fast bacilli with crossbars
Mycobacterium tuberculosis	Thin acid-fast bacilli, straight or slightly curved with beaded appearance; may show branches or serpentine cords
Neisseria species	Gram-negative diplococci with adjacent sides cocave 'kidney bean or coffee bean'
Neisseria elongata	Gram-negative rod
Nocardia	Gram-positive branching filamentous bacilli with tendency to breakdown into coccoid or rods. May show irregular staining
Propionibacterium	Irregular shaped, Gram-positive rods
Spirillium minus	Gram-negative, spiral-shaped bacilli
Stomatococcus mucilaginosus	Gram-positive cocci in tetrads or clusters
Streptobacillus moniliformae	Faintly staining, pleomorphic, Gram-negative rods, filaments may resemble a necklace
Tropheryma whipplei	PAS–positive (red)
Vibrio	Straight or slightly curved Gram-negative rods. Comma-shaped rods arranged in parallel rows giving 'fish in stream appearance'.
Yesinia pestis	Bipolar staining with 'safety pin' appearance
Staphylococcus species	Gram-positive cocci in grape-like clusters
Streptococci	Gram-positive cocci in pairs
Enterococci	Gram-positive oval cocci in pairs, arranged at an angle to each other giving 'spectacle eyed' appearance
Streptococcus pneumoniae	Gram-positive 'lanceolate' shaped cocci in pairs
Diphtheroids	Palisade arrangement of GPB
Clostridium	Gram-positive bacillus with central bulging spore giving 'citron body' appearance
Mycobacterium leprae	Smears prepared from skin lesions stained with modified Z-N stain method (5% H_2SO_4 as decolorizing agent) show bacilli in groups called 'cigar bundles' inside histiocytes or macrophages with 'washout' appearance called 'Virchow's lepra cells'
Vibrio parahaemolyticus	Bipolar staining
Burkholderia pseudomallei	Gram-negative bacilli with 'safety pin' appearance in methylene blue preparation.
Bordetella pertussis	Small Gram-negative coccobacilli. Smear prepared from colony (secondary smear shows bacilli arranged in loose clumps with clear spaces in between giving 'thumb print appraerance'. Bipolar metachromatic granules can be demonstrated by staining with toludine blue
Brucella	Small Gram-negative coccobacilli or bacilli which may be mistaken for Micrococcus, bipolar staining is not uncommon
Treponema pallidum	Thin delicate spirochetes with tapering ends, size about 10 µm × 0.1–.02 µm with ten regular, angular, sharp spirals at about 1 µm
Klebsiella granulomatis	Presence of characteristics intracellular bodies (Donovan bodies). In Giemsa-stained smear, they appear as coccobacilli within cystic spaces in large mononuclear cells. They may show bipolar staining with safety pin appearance
Gardnerella vaginalis	Gram-negative pleomorphic rods with metachromatic granules
Moraxella catarrhalis	Gram-negative cocci in pairs
Capnocytophaga	Gram-negative fusiform bacteria
Kingella	Gram-negative bacilli with tendency to show coccobacillary forms and diplococcal form
Moraxella lacunata	Gram-negative bacilli usually arranged in pairs.
Chlamydia trachomatis	Elementary bodies-spherical bodies, 200–300 nm, reticulate body—500 to 1000 nm (inclusion bodies with elementary bodies within—stain with Giemsa stain, Gimnez stain

DISTINCTIVE COLONIAL CHARACTERISTICS OF SELECTED ORGANISMS

Organism	Colony characteristics
Pseudomonas aeruginosa	• NA: Irregular, flat colonies with metallic sheen and grape-like fruity odor or earthy smell • Mucoid strains isolated from patients with cystic fibrosis • Different colors due to different pigments are produced • Pyocynin-blue pigment, only produced by *Pseudomonas aeruginosa* • Other pigments—pyoverdin-yellow, pyorubrin-red, pyomelanin-brown • 'King' medium: Pigment production is enhanced
Pseudomonas fluorescence and *P. putida*	Produce pyoverdin, a fluorescent pigment
Pseudomonas stutzeri	Dry, wrinkled, adherent colonies, yellow or brown pigment
Burkholderia pseudomallei	NA: Rough, corrugated colonies Ashdown's medium: Wrinkled, purple colonies
Rhodococcus	Salmon pink colonies
Serratia marcescens	Red to pink pigment
Stomatococcus mucilaginosus	Colony strongly adherent to agar surface, 'sticky staph'
Streptobacillus moniliformis	Fried egg colonies, fluff balls or breadcrumb in broth
Streptococcus pneumoniae	Alpha hemolytic, umbilicated(carom coin like or draughtsman shaped or donat like) or mucoid colonies sometimes
Veillonella	Red fluorescence when exposed to U-V light
Vibrio cholerae	• Blood agar: Hemodigestion • TCBS: Yellow colonies due to sucrose fermentation • Mansur's GTTA medium: Translucent colonies with greyish black center (reduction of tellurite to tellurium) surrounded by turbid halo (due to gelatin liquefaction)
Vibrio parahaemolyticus	• Swarm on blood agar • Wagatsuma blood agar (high salt blood agar): β hemolysis (Kanagawa phenomenon)
Yersinia enterocolitica	Bull's eye colonies on CIN medium
Staphylococcus aureus	• NA: Opaque, usually golden yellow pigment (color of pigment may vary from yellow to orange). • Blood agar: β hemolytic, some strains may be nonhemolytic • 'Aluminium paint appearance' on nutrient agar given due to confluent growth. • Mannitol salt agar: Yellow colonies due to mannitol fermentation • Blood potassium tellurite agar-black colonies • DNase agar—halo around colonies, DNase agar with tryphan blue—colonies have pink surrounding • Phenolphthalein phosphate agar—pink colonies
Streptococcus pyogenes	Tiny, pinpoint, beta hemolytic, transparent colonies
Enterococcus	α, β, γ hemolysis Bile esculin agar-black colonies MacConkey agar: Minute magenta pink colonies
Corynebacterium diphtheriae	• Black colonies on blood potassium tellurite agar • Hoyles' potassium tellurite medium—three biotypes give different morphology • Gravis-Daisy head • Intermedius: Frog's egg • Mitis: Poached egg • Tinsdale's medium: Black colonies with brown halo (this property helps to differentiate from colonies of diphtheroids which may produce black colonies without brown halo)
Actinomyces	Thioglycollate broth: *A. israelii* resembles 'fluffy balls' at the bottom BHI-agar: Small, 'spidery' colonies
E. coli	• Blood agar: Moist, low convex • MacConkey agar: Pink flat colonies • Rainbow agar: O-157: black colonies as they are negative for—β glucuronidase • Sorbitol MacConkey agar: *E. coli* produces pink colonies, while EHEC produces pale colonies as it does not ferment sorbitol

(Contd...)

Organism	Colony characteristics
Shigella	MacConkey agar: Nonlactose fermenting colorless colonies DCA: Non-lactose fermenting colorless colonies XLD: Red or pink without black center Hekteonenteric agar: Green color fading towards periphery
Yersinia pestis	• Blood agar: Dark brown colonies due to absorption of heme pigment • MacConkey medium: Pale, non-lactose fermenting colonies • Oil or ghee broth: 'Stalactites growth' hanging from under surface of oil • CIN (cefsulodin, igrasan, novobiocin) agar is a selective medium
Yersinia enterocolitica or pseudotuberculosis	CIN agar: 'Dark red bull eye' appearing colonies in 24 hours
Salmonella typhi	• Wilson-Blair medium: Jet black colonies with metallic sheen due to H_2S production • XLD: Red or pink colonies with black center • SS agar: Colourless colonies with black center • Hektoen enteric agar: Blue green colonies with black center
Haemophilus influenzae	Satellitism around central streak of hemolytic *Staphylococcus aureus* Filde's medium and Levinthal's medium: Iridesence colonies
Campylobacter	Effuse, droplet-like colonies
Legionella pneumophila	Buffered charcoal yeast extract agar: Circular colonies, glistening periphery, granular or speckled opalescence resembling ground glass

IDENTIFICATIONS OF GRAM-POSITIVE BACILLI

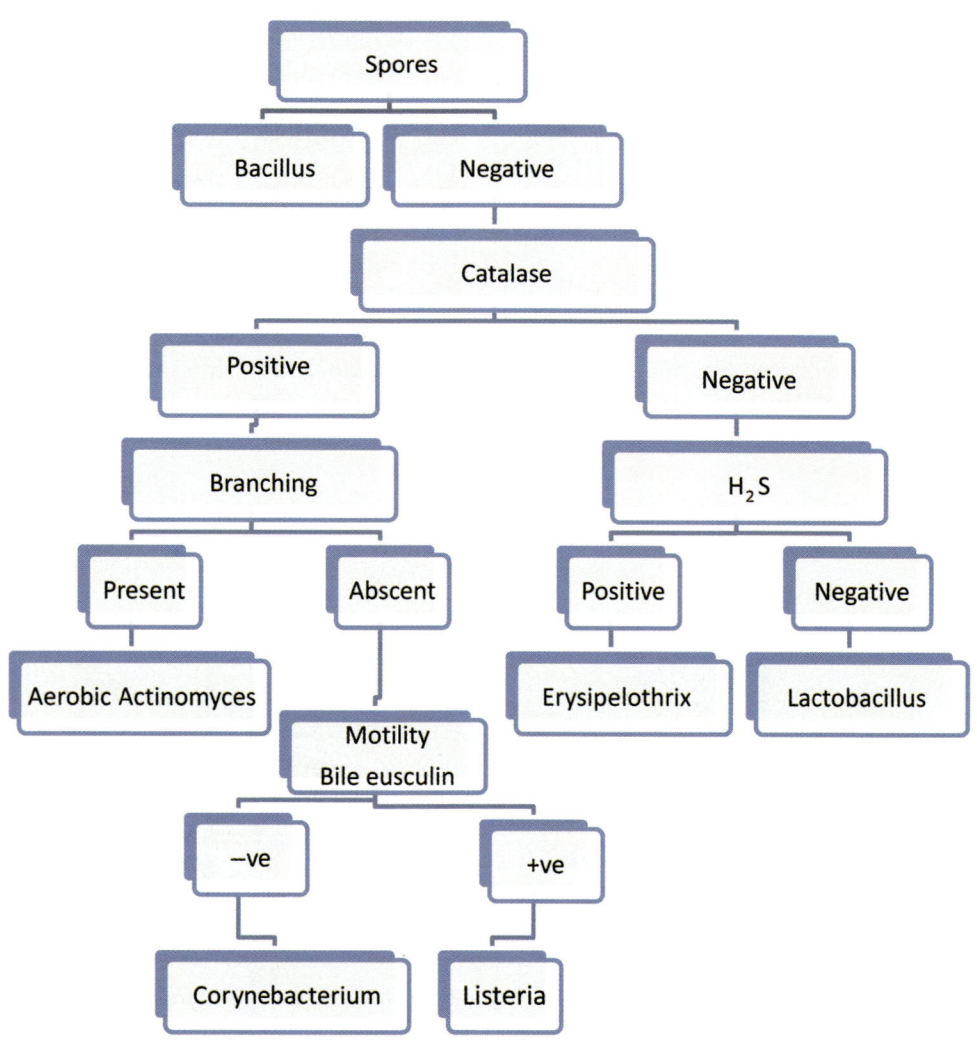

SCHEMATIC WAY TO ORGANIZE BIOCHEMICAL TESTS OF FAMILY ENTEROBACTERIACEAE AND IDENTIFICATION OF ORGANISMS

The family Enterobacteriaceae is divided into three groups based upon reactions of phenylalanine (PPA) and VP test reactions.

1. PPA Positive

- Possibilities are *Proteus* spp., *Providencia* spp. and *Morganella* spp.
- Production of H_2S separates *Proteus* spp. (+VE) from *Providencia* spp. and *Morganella* spp. which are H_2S negative.
- Citrate test separates *Providencia* spp. (positive) from *Morganella* spp. (negative).
- Ornithine decarboxylase also distinguishes *Providencia* spp. (negative) from *Morganella* spp. (positive).
- Indole test differentiates between *Proteus vulgaris* (positive) from *Proteus mirabilis* spp. (negative).

2. Voges-Proskaur Positive (and PPA Negative)

Possibilities

Klebsiella spp., *Enterobacter* spp. and *Serratia* spp.

These organisms can be distinguished as follows:

- **Motility and ornithine decarboxylase:** *Klebsiella* spp. is negative while *Enterobacter* spp. and *Serratia* spp. are positive.
- **Lactose:** *Enterobacter* spp. is lactose positive and *S. marcescens* is lactose negative.
- **DNase test:** *S. marcescens* is positive, *Enterobacter* spp. are negative.
- **Arginine and lysine:** *Enterobacter cloacae* is arginine positive and lysine negative while *Enterobacter*

aerogenes has just opposite reactions (arginine negative, lysine positive).

3. PPA and VP both Negative

Possible organisms are: *E. coli, Edwardsiella tarda, Salmonella* sp., *Shigella* sp. and *Citrobacter* sp.

Citrate test: *Salmonella, Citrobacter* sp. are citrate positive while *E. coli, Edwardesiella tarda, Shigella sp.* are citrate negative.

1. Differentiating *Salmonella sp.* from *Citrobacter sp.* Lysine decarboxylase and ONPG: *Salmonella sp.* is lysine positive and ONPG negative while *Citrobacter sp.* is lysine negative and ONPG positive.
2. Differentiating *Citrobacter koseri* from *Citrobacter frundi*: Indole test: Positive with *Citrobacter koseri* and *Citrobacter frundi* is indole negative.
3. Differentiation between *E. coli, Edwardsiella tarda* and *Shigella sp.*:
   - H_2S production differentiates *E. tarda* (positive) from *E. coli* (negative).
   - Lysine decarboxylase, motility, lactose: *E. coli* is usually lactose positive except few non-motile strains (give reaction like Shigella). Additional biochemical and serogrouping is done for *Shigella sp.* to differentiate from nonmotile strains of *E. coli*.

4. Other Important Reactions

1. Motility: Most members of the family enterobacteriaceae are motile except *Shigella sp.* and *Klebsiella sp.*
2. Urease test: *Proteus sp, Morganella sp.,* and *Klebsiella pneumoniae* and few strains of Citrobacter sp. are urease positive.

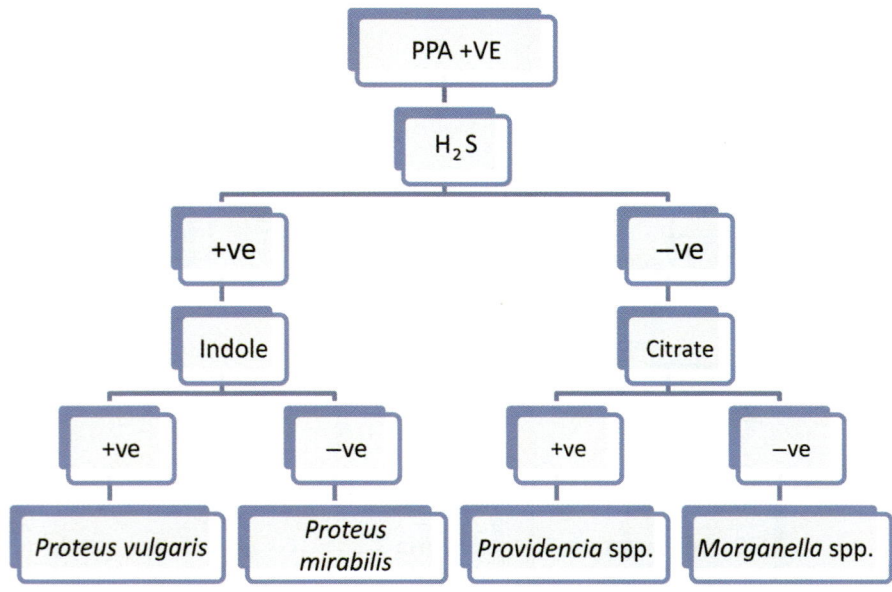

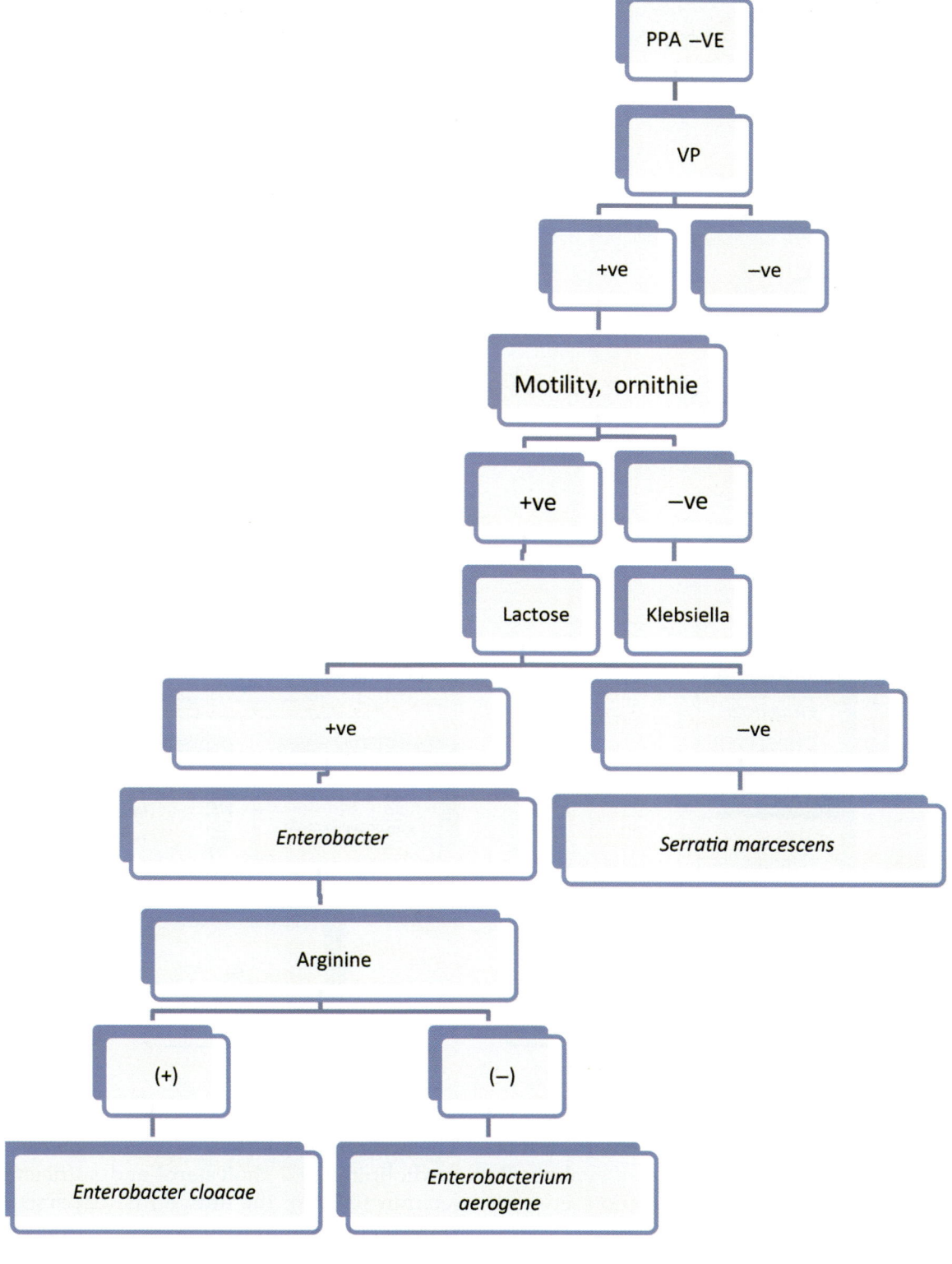

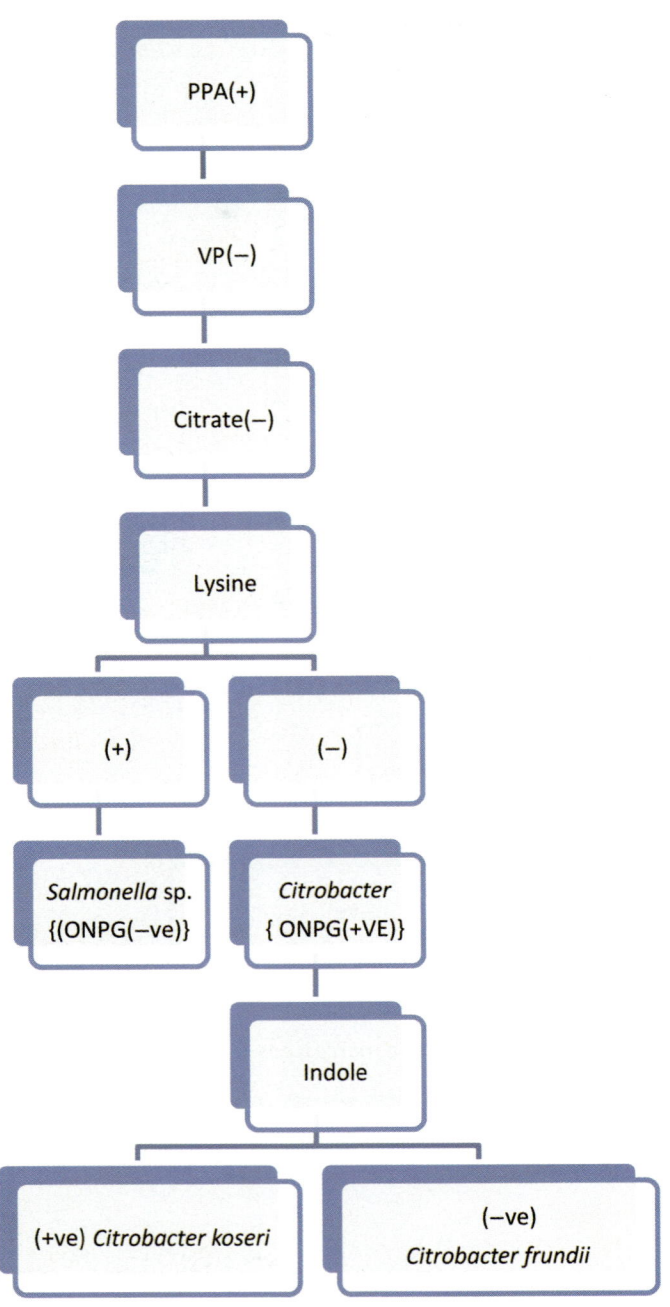

P. VDRL Test

VDRL (Venereal Diseases Research Laboratory) test is used as screening test for the diagnosis of syphilis. It detects syphilitic antibody (reagin) by reaction between patient's serum and standard antigen.

Antigen Used in VDRL

The antigen is composed of cardiolipin and lecithin that have been extracted from beef heart and purified. Cholesterol is added to the alcoholic mixture of cardiolipin and lecithin for the purpose of increasing effective reacting surface.

VDRL Antigen

The antigen is colorless, alcoholic mixture of 0.03% cardiolipin, 0.9% cholesterol and sufficient purified lecithin (0.21%); the antigen is dispersed in screw capped bottles or ampoules.

VDRL buffered saline contains 1% NaCl, pH 6.0 + or –, 0.1.

Requirements for VDRL Test

- Rotating machine adjustable to 180 rpm, circumcising a circle ¾ inch in diameter.
- Ring maker makes paraffin rings approximately 14 mm in diameter.

- Hypodermic needles, without bevels is used for serum tests, (18, 19, 23 gauges) and for spinal fluid (21 or 22 gauge).
- Slides 2 × 3 inches with 12 paraffin or ceramic rings approximately 14 mm diameter for serum tests.
- VDRL slides 2 × 3 cm min., with concavities of 14 mm in diameter and 1.75 mm in depth.
- Syringe, 1 or 2 mL
- Bottles—30 mL, glass stoppered flat bottom for preparing antigenic solution.

Antigen Suspension

Pipette 0.4 mL buffered saline to the bottom of 30 mL round, glass stopered bottle. Add 0.5 mL of antigen directly on to saline while continuously but gently rotating the bottom of surface. Antigen is added drop by drop but rapidly, so that it is added within 6 seconds. Blow the last drop of antigen from pipette without touching to saline. Continue rotation of bottle for 10 sec. Add 4.1 mL of buffered saline with 5 mL pipette. Shake it for 30 times in 10 sec. The antigen solution is ready for use, everyday it should be freshly prepared.

Preparation of serum: Heat clear serum in 56°C in water bath for 30 minutes. Reheat the sera, if they are to be tested 4 hours after original heating period.

VDRL Slide Qualitative Test with Serum

1. Take 0.005 mL of inactivated serum with pipette into ring 1 of paraffin ring or ceramic ring (slide or VDRL tile).
2. Add one drop of antigen solution (1/60 mL) on to each serum with 18-gauge needle and syringe.
3. Rotate slide or tile for 4 minutes (mechanical rotator with diameter ¾ inch, at 180 rpm).
4. Read the test microscopically with 10 × eyepiece and 10 × objectives and look for formation of clumps.

Report the results as follows:

Reading	Report
Large and medium size clumps	Reactive (R)
Small clumps	Weakly reactive (W)
No clumps or slight roughness	Nonreactive (N)

VDRL Quantitative Test

The dilutions of serum tested are undiluted (1:1), 1:2, 1:4, 1:8, 1:16, 1:32, 1:64, 1:128. The dilutions are prepared in tubes by serial dilution method and then taken on slide or tile. Add one drop of antigen to each well, rotate the tile at 180 rpm for 4 minutes, read the results under microscope and find out highest dilution of serum giving the test reactive.

Note:
1. The significant titer of VDRL test is 1:8, but higher titers may be seen depending upon the stage of the disease.
2. If the patient is in secondary syphilis, very high titres will be present in patient's serum, but the test will appear nonreactive if patient's serum is tested without dilution. This (antibody excess) is called prozone phenomenon.
3. VDRL test appears positive in the latent syphilis also.
4. The test becomes positive 7–10 days after appearance of chancre (3–5 weeks after acquiring infection).

Applications of VDRL Test

1. It is a screening test for syphilis.
2. Screening of antenatal females for syphilis is done by VDRL test.
3. It is also used as screening test on donor's blood for donation safety.
4. As VDRL test becomes negative following effective treatment, it has prognostic value also.
5. The frequency of positivity of VDRL test is 70–80% in primary syphilis, 100% in secondary syphilis, and 60–70% in latent or late syphilis.

VDRL Test on CSF for Diagnosis of Neurosyphilis

1. No prior heating is required.
2. Test specimen volume is 0.01 mL; antigen should be diluted with 0.02 mL of saline.
3. Rotation of slide is done for 8 minutes.

Biological False Positive Reactions

Cardiolipin antigen is present on human tissues as well as on *T. pallidum.* Therefore, the test may give false positive reactions in absence of the disease (technical errors ruled out). Conditions in which biological false positive reactions occur are: Pregnancy, acute infections, leprosy, hepatitis, malaria, collegen disorders.

If there is suspicion regarding biological false positive reactions, confirmatory tests for syphilis as TPHA, FTA ABS, and TPI should be performed.

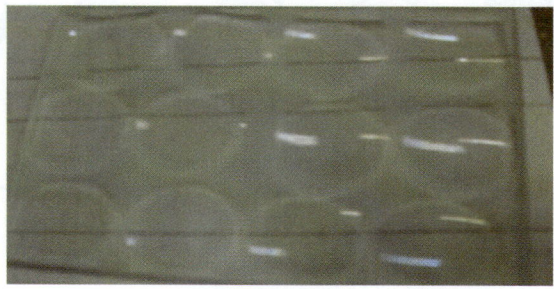

Modifications of VDRL Test

Rapid plasma reagin test (RPR)

1. It contains carbon particles added to VDRL antigen; hence positive reaction is visible with naked eye as clumping of carbon particles is seen.
2. Other advantages of RPR are it can be performed on serum as well as on plasma (hence called plasma test), preheating of serum is not required as choline chloride is added (hence called rapid).

The disadvantage is that it cannot be performed on CSF.

Q. Widal Test

It is performed for the serodiagnosis of typhoid fever. In this test, antibodies against, S. typhi, S. paratyphi 'A' and S. paratyphi 'B' are tested in patient's serum. TH is flagellar antigen of S. typhi, TO is somatic antigen of S. typhi while AH and BH are flagella antigen of S. paratyphi A and B. Somatic antigens of paratyphi A and B are not tested as they crossreact with each other.

Preparation of Antigens of Salmonella for Widal Test

Apart from using commercial kits which use colored antigens, antigens can prepared in the laboratory for Widal test.

S. typhi 901 'O' and 'H' strains laboratory maintained S. paratyphi 'A', S. paratyphi 'B' are used for antigen preparation.

'O' antigen preparation: S. typhi is grown on phenol agar (1:800) to inhibit flagellar H antigen. Growth is scrapped off in saline, mixed with 20 times its volume of absolute alcohol. The preparation is then heated at 40–50°C for 30 minutes and centrifuged. The deposit is resuspended in saline to which chloroform is added as preservative.

H antigen preparation: Salmonella is grown in broth to which 0.1% formalin is added.

Procedure

1. Take 10 test tubes labeled from 1 to 8 in four rows (one row for one antigen).
2. With 1 mL pipette, take 0.9 mL of normal saline in tube no. 1 of each row.
3. To each of the remaining tubes add 0.5 mL of normal saline (tube no. 2 to 8 in each row).
4. To tube no. 1 of each row add 0.1 mL of patients serum to be tested, thus in tube no. 1 of each row has dilution 1:10.
5. Transfer 0.5 mL of diluted sample from tube no.1 to tube no 2. Again transfer 0.5 mL of tube no. 2 to tube no. 3 in each row, mix well.
6. Continue this serial dilution till tube no. 7 of each row.
7. Discard 0.5 mL of diluted serum from tube no. 7 of each row.

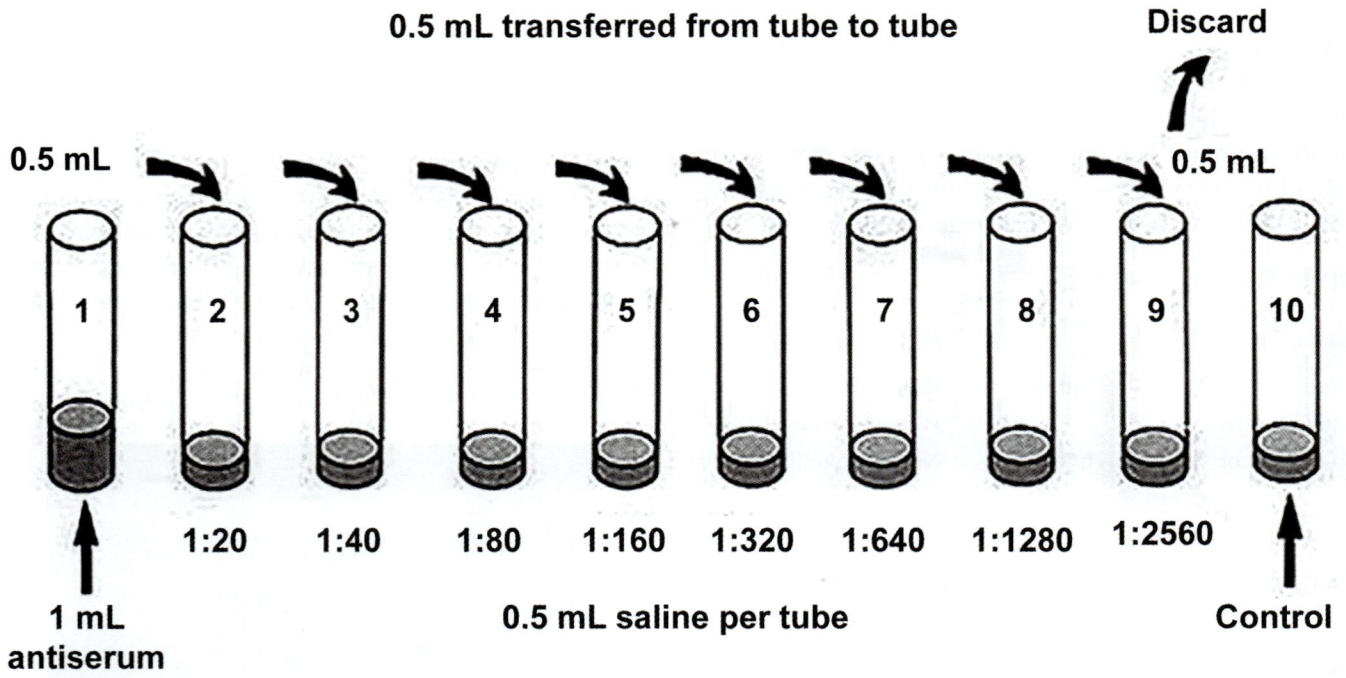

0.5 mL transferred from tube to tube   **Discard**

0.5 mL   0.5 mL

| 1 | 2 | 3 | 4 | 5 | 6 | 7 | 8 | 9 | 10 |

   1:20   1:40   1:80   1:160   1:320   1:640   1:1280   1:2560

1 mL antiserum (1:10)   **0.5 mL saline per tube**   **Control**

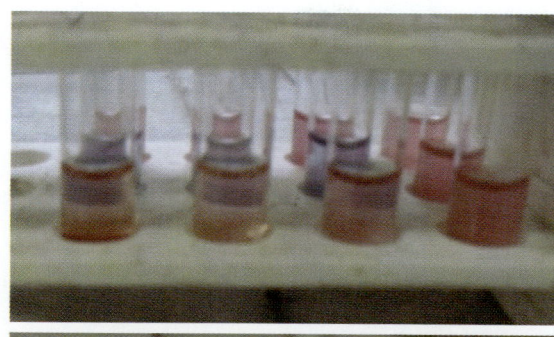

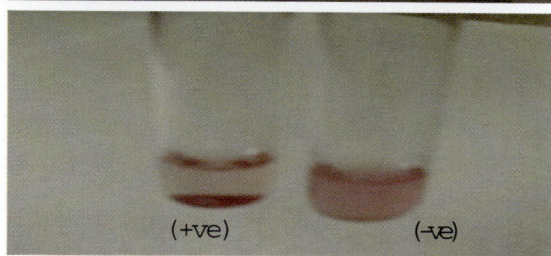

(+ve)   (–ve)

8. Tube no. 10 in each row serves as negative control.

9. To all the tubes of row 1, add 0.5 mL of TH antigen. To all tubes of row 2 add 0.5 mL of TO antigen, to all tubes of row 3; add 0.5 mL AH and to all tubes of row 4, add 0.5 mL of BH.

10. This will give final dilution from tube no. 1 are 1:10 as 1:20, 1:40, 1:80, 1:160, 1:320, 1:640, and 1:2560.

11. Incubate all tubes at 37°C overnight, next day read all the tubes and find out the titers of serum against all four antigens used (TH, TO, AH, BH).

Note. The antigens for Widal test are prepared from *S. typhi* 901 strain.

Interpretation of Widal Test

- 'H' agglutination is seen as cotton woolly clumps. 'O' agglutination is granular disk-like pattern.
- Usually if agglutination is present, clumps are settled down or there is carpet formation with 50% clearing of solution as compared to the negative control.

- If agglutination is not seen, there is no clearing of solution in the tube and the antigen settles down in the form of button. To find out titer, we have to find out highest dilution of patient's serum which shows above finding.

Following points should be kept in mind in interpretation of the test.

- Ideally the results of two tests performed on paired sera are compared, if it shows fourfold rise in titer, it suggests active infection.
- If results of single tests are to interpreted, significant tires of 1:80 or above are considered significant. (Note: The values vary from one manufacturer to another.)
- If endemic titer (overall levels of titers in normal population in that endemic area known as endemic titers) is known, the titers above the endemic titer are taken as significant.
- Patients already on antibiotics may give false negative reaction. Similarly, if serum is collected early in the disease before detectable levels of antibodies are not formed, the test will be negative.

Anamnestic reaction: If the patient had prior infection with the organism or immunization, it will give false positive reaction. If the test is false positive due to prior vaccination, repeat test after 8–10 days doesn't show rise in titer.

Other causes of false positive reactions are patients with autoimmune disorders as rheumatoid arthritis. Even crossreacting antibodies are present in certain infections as *Lepromatous leprosy*, or malaria in which nonspecific polyclonal activation of B cells occurs.

Causes of false negative widal test are patients with protein energy malnutrition and primary immunodeficiency of humoral immunity.

Index